Family Practice
Examination & Board
Review

Family Practice Examination & Board Review

Second Edition

Editors

Mark A. Graber, MD

Professor
Departments of Family Medicine and Emergency Medicine
Roy J. and Lucille A. Carver College of Medicine
University of Iowa
Iowa City, Iowa

Jason K. Wilbur, MD

Assistant Professor (Clinical)
Department of Family Medicine
Roy J. and Lucille A. Carver College of Medicine
University of Iowa
Iowa City, Iowa

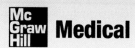

New York Chicago San Francisco Lisbon London Madrid Mexico City Milan
New Delhi San Juan Seoul Singapore Sydney Toronto

Family Practice Examination & Board Review, Second Edition

4 5 6 7 8 9 0   QDB/QDB   12 11

ISBN 978-0-07-149608-7
MHID 0-07-149608-4

This book was set in Janson by International Typesetting and Composition.
The editors were James F. Shanahan and Robert Pancotti.
The production supervisor was Catherine Saggese.
Project management was provided by Preeti Longia Sinha, International Typesetting and Composition.
The cover designer was Aimee Davis.
Front cover photograph: A female patient visiting her general practitioner. (Credit: AJPhoto / Photo Researchers, Inc.)
Quad/Graphics Dubuque was printer and binder.

This book is printed on acid-free paper.

Library of Congress Cataloging-in-Publication Data

Family practice examination & board review / editors, Mark A. Graber,
Jason K. Wilbur.—2nd ed.
p. ; cm.
Includes bibliographical references and index.
ISBN-13: 978-0-07-149608-7 (pbk. : alk. paper)
ISBN-10: 0-07-149608-4 (pbk. : alk. paper)
1. Family medicine—Examinations, questions, etc.   I. Graber, Mark A., MD.
II. Wilbur, Jason K.   III. Title: Family practice examination and board review.
[DNLM: 1. Family Practice—Examination Questions.   WB 18.2 F198   2009]
RC58.F346   2009
616.0076—dc22

2008027736

To Eric Nilles, MD, who is working in Darfur, and to Doctors Without Borders. We can only hope.
— MAG

To my grandfathers, Homer Fritz, who wanted to become a doctor but could not afford medical school, and Kenneth Wilbur, who taught me the value of hard work and a generous spirit.
— JKW

Contents

COLOR PLATES APPEAR BETWEEN PAGES 594 AND 595.

Contributors

Alison C. Abreu, MD
Assistant Professor of Family Medicine and Psychiatry
Roy J. and Lucille A. Carver College of Medicine
University of Iowa
Iowa City, Iowa
Psychiatry

David A. Bedell, MD
Associate Professor of Family Medicine
Roy J. and Lucille A. Carver College of Medicine
University of Iowa
Iowa City, Iowa
Obstetrics and Women's Health

Ottar Bergmann, MD
Fellow, Division of Gastroenterology
Department of Internal Medicine
Roy J. and Lucille A. Carver College of Medicine
University of Iowa
Iowa City, Iowa
Gastroenterology

Christopher J. Berry, MD
Chief Fellow
Division of Cardiovascular Medicine
University of Iowa Hospitals and Clinics
Iowa City, Iowa
Cardiology

Christopher T. Buresh, MD
Assistant Professor of Emergency Medicine
Roy J. and Lucille A. Carver College of Medicine
University of Iowa
Iowa City, Iowa
Emergency Medicine

Katrina Cannon, MD
Veterans Affairs Quality Scholar and Geriatric Fellow
Center for Research in the Implementation of Innovative
    Strategies in Practice (CRIISP)
Iowa City Veterans Affairs Medical Center and
Division of General Internal Medicine
Roy J. and Lucille A. Carver College of Medicine
University of Iowa
Iowa City, Iowa
Care of the Older Patient

Elizabeth C. Clark, MD, MPH
Assistant Professor
Department of Family Medicine
University of Medicine and Dentistry of New Jersey
Robert Wood Johnson Medical School
Somerset, New Jersey
Evidence-Based Medicine

Dana M. Collaguazo, MD
Assistant Professor of Emergency Medicine
Roy J. and Lucille A. Carver College of Medicine
University of Iowa
Iowa City, Iowa
Emergency Medicine

Greg Davis, MD
Pulmonary and Critical Care Medicine Fellow Associate
Department of Internal Medicine
Division of Pulmonary, Critical Care and Occupational
    Medicine
Roy J. and Lucille A. Carver College of Medicine
University of Iowa
Iowa City, Iowa
Pulmonary

Lori J. Day, MD
Fellow, Department of Obstetrics and Gynecology
Roy J. and Lucille A. Carver College of Medicine
University of Iowa
Iowa City, Iowa
Obstetrics and Women's Health

Richard C. Dobyns, MD
Professor of Family Medicine
Roy J. and Lucille A. Carver College of Medicine
University of Iowa
Iowa City, Iowa
End-of-Life Care

Scott A. Frisbie, ATC, PA-C
Steindler Orthopedics
Iowa City, Iowa
Orthopedics and Sports Medicine

Mark A. Graber, MD
Professor
Departments of Family Medicine and Emergency
    Medicine
Roy J. and Lucille A. Carver College of Medicine
University of Iowa
Iowa City, Iowa
Emergency Medicine; Allergy and Immunology; HIV/AIDS;
Endocrinology; Orthopedics and Sports Medicine; Neurology;
Otolaryngology; Care of the Surgical Patient; Substance
Abuse; Patient-Centered Care Final Examination

Emily Greenlee, MD
Clinical Assistant Professor of Ophthalmology
Department of Ophthalmology
Roy J. and Lucille A. Carver College of Medicine
University of Iowa
Iowa City, Iowa
Ophthalmology

Philip Gregory, PharmD
Center for Drug Information & Evidence-Based Practice
Creighton University
Omaha, Nebraska
Editor, Natural Medicines Comprehensive Database
Nutrition and Herbal Medicine

Rajesh Kabra, MD
Fellow, Division of Cardiology
Department of Internal Medicine
Roy J. and Lucille A. Carver College of Medicine
University of Iowa
Iowa City, Iowa
Cardiology

Oladipo A. Kukoyi, MD, MS
Assistant Clinical Professor, UC Davis
Department of Psychiatry and Behavioral Sciences
Medical Director of Inpatient Psychiatry
VA Sacramento Medical Center
Hospital Way, Mather, California
Patient-Centered Care

Colleen M. Kennedy, MD, MS
Assistant Professor of Obstetrics and Gynecology
Roy J. and Lucille A. Carver College of Medicine
University of Iowa
Iowa City, Iowa
Obstetrics and Women's Health

Chirag M. Sandesara, MD
Fellow, Division of Cardiology
Department of Internal Medicine
Roy J. and Lucille A. Carver College of Medicine
University of Iowa
Iowa City, Iowa
Cardiology

Margo Schilling, MD
Associate Professor of Internal Medicine
Division of General Internal Medicine
Roy J. and Lucille A. Carver College of Medicine
University of Iowa
Iowa City, Iowa
Infectious Diseases

Victoria Sharp, MD, MBA
Clinical Associate Professor
Departments of Urology and Family Medicine
Roy J. and Lucille A. Carver College of Medicine
University of Iowa
Iowa City, Iowa
Men's Health

Anne L. S. Sullivan, MD
Associate Professor of Family Medicine
Roy J. and Lucille A. Carver College of Medicine
University of Iowa
Iowa City, Iowa
Adolescent Medicine

Michael E. Takacs, MD
Assistant Professor of Emergency Medicine
Roy J. and Lucille A. Carver College of Medicine
University of Iowa
Iowa City, Iowa
Emergency Medicine

Janeta F. Tansey, MD
Clinical Associate Professor
Department of Psychiatry and
    Program in Biomedical Ethics and Medical Humanities
Roy J. and Lucille A. Carver College of Medicine
University of Iowa
Iowa City, Iowa
Ethics

Rebecca S. Tuetken, MD
Associate Professor of Rheumatology
Department of Internal Medicine
Roy J. and Lucille A. Carver College of Medicine
University of Iowa
Iowa City, Iowa
Rheumatology

Philip N. Velderman, MD
Fellow, Division of Rheumatology
Department of Internal Medicine
Roy J. and Lucille A. Carver College of Medicine
University of Iowa
Iowa City, Iowa
Rheumatology

Michelle Weckmann, MD
Assistant Professor of Psychiatry
Roy J. and Lucille A. Carver College of Medicine
University of Iowa
Iowa City, Iowa
End-of-Life Care

Deborah W. Wilbur, MD
Hematologist/Medical Oncologist
Private Practice
Oncology Associates
Cedar Rapids, Iowa
Hematology and Oncology

Jason K. Wilbur, MD
Assistant Professor (Clinical)
Department of Family Medicine
Roy J. and Lucille A. Carver College of Medicine
University of Iowa
Iowa City, Iowa
*Nephrology; HIV/AIDS; Pediatrics; Men's Health;
Dermatology; Otolaryngology; Care of the Older Patient;
Patient-Centered Care; Final Examination*

Preface

The first edition of this book published four years ago and quickly became established as one of the most relied-upon resources for preparing for family practice board examinations. We are gratified that so many residents, students, and clinicians found the book helpful, and we have appreciated receiving your comments and suggestions over the last few years. Welcome to the second edition of *Family Practice Examination & Board Review*. Our primary goal in writing this book is to help you pass your board exam. **However, there are two crucial differences between this book and other board review books on the market.** First, we have written this book not only to help you pass the boards but also to help you broaden your knowledge of family medicine. Most questions in the book contain a detailed explanation not only of why an answer is right but also why the other answers are wrong. **If the current "state of the art" differs substantially from the answers that will be on the boards (which generally reflect information that is 2 to 3 years out of date), we have made a note of this and have given you the "state of the art" information as well.**

The second difference is that we are not boring. You will find our (sometimes feeble) attempts at humor throughout the book. There is no reason that studying has to be an exercise in tedium and endurance. It should be enjoyable and should provide a surprise every now and again. We have noticed that an occasional reader does not appreciate our sense of humor. Oh well....

We have tried to make this book as broad and as comprehensive as possible. In addition to its use as a board review book for family medicine, it can be used as a general review for primary care physicians, physician assistants, and nurse practitioners. Medical students studying for Step 3 of the licensing exam should find the book helpful as well. However, no board review book can possibly cover the entire scope of family medicine. Ask yourself this question as a guide for using the book: what are the areas in which you are strong and what are the areas in which you need further study? We have provided a "final exam" of 150 questions, with which you can gauge what you have learned. Each answer of the "final exam" is referenced in the book so you can go back and review any topic that you may have missed.

In this book, the use of eponymous medical terms such as Crohn disease, Wegner disease, and Wilson disease reflects the current American Medical Association recommendations for these and similar terms.

We enjoyed writing this book and we hope that you enjoy using it. If you have suggestions or complaints (OK, maybe some of our jokes aren't politically correct), do not hesitate to write us at mark-graber@uiowa.edu or jason-wilbur@uiowa.edu. We take your comments seriously as we endeavor to make studying for the board exam more efficient and more fun.

Mark would like to thank all of the authors for their contributions....sometimes "a bit" over deadline but you know who you are. Thanks also to my family: Hetty, Rachel, and Abe (as always). But not to the dogs...they need to learn to stay either in or out of the house. No more of this back and forth. Finally, thanks to Buckethead, Shawn Lane, Jonas Hellborg, and the soundtrack from "Noir" (the anime) for keeping me awake in the wee hours when text begins to swim across the screen (doing the sidestroke, I think).

Jason thanks his wife, Deb, who has shown great patience during the writing of this book (look...he lives!), and his boys, Ken and Ted, who seem to have changed more than medicine since the first edition. And then there are the growers, producers, and roasters of fine coffee, without whom there would be no fuel for this endeavor. Who would I be without coffee? I get a chill down my spine just thinking about it.

Thank you to David Bedell, who reviewed the chapter on obstetrics and women's health in addition to his other contribution to this book.

Emergency Medicine

Christopher T. Buresh, Dana M. Collaguazo, Mark A. Graber, and Michael E. Takacs

CASE 1

You get a call from a panicked mother because her 4-year-old took some of her theophylline. She thinks it may have been as many as 10 pills but is not clear on the actual number. She is about 35 minutes from the hospital.

Your advice to her is:

A) Give ipecac to promote stomach emptying and reduce theophylline absorption.
B) Do not give ipecac and proceed directly to the hospital.
C) Call poison control and then proceed to the hospital.
D) None of the above.

Discussion

The correct answer is B. Do not give ipecac but proceed to the hospital. Answer A is incorrect for two reasons. First, ipecac is not a particularly effective method of emptying gastric contents. More important, if the patient should start to seize while vomiting as a result of the ipecac, she could aspirate the vomitus causing an aspiration pneumonitis. Answer C is incorrect because you do not want to delay definitive treatment. You can call poison control while the patient is on the way in.

> **HELPFUL TIP:** The FDA has determined that ipecac is ineffective and possibly harmful. It causes myopathy and cardiac problems when used chronically (such as in individuals with anorexia nervosa).

* *

The patient arrives in your ED. She is alert with a tachycardia of 160 beats per minute but with a stable blood pressure. The ingestion occurred about 2.5 hours ago. You decide that the next step is GI decontamination.

Which of the following statements is true about gastric lavage?

A) Except in extraordinary circumstances it should be done only in the first 1.5 hours after an overdose.
B) Patients who have had gastric lavage have higher incidence of pulmonary aspiration than patients who have not.
C) The maximum volume that should be used is 5 liters.
D) It can push pill fragments beyond the pylorus.
E) All of the above are true.

Discussion

The correct answer is E. All of the statements are true. Generally, the efficacy of gastric lavage is limited. The outcome data do not support the use of gastric lavage after the first 1 to 1.5 hours. In a particularly severe overdose or in an overdose that is likely to delay gastric emptying (eg, anticholinergics such as diphenhydramine or tricyclic antidepressants), you might want to try lavage beyond the 1.5 hours, but such circumstances are unusual. Gastric lavage increases the risk of aspiration, can push pill fragments beyond the pylorus, and 5 liters is the maximum volume that should be used.

The next best step to take with this patient is to:

A) Check blood theophylline levels and refer for hemodialysis if markedly elevated.
B) Administer 1 g/kg of charcoal with sorbitol.
C) Prophylactically treat this patient for seizures using lorazepam.
D) Prophylactically treat this patient for seizures using phenytoin.

Discussion

The correct answer is B. Giving charcoal is indicated in almost all overdose situations. Answer A is incorrect because the patient's situation could deteriorate by the time blood levels return. Answers C and D are incorrect because seizure prophylaxis is not indicated in this patient. Although seizures are a major manifestation of theophylline toxicity, they are more likely to occur in patients who take theophylline chronically and have toxic blood levels. Acute ingestions are less worrisome.

> **HELPFUL TIP:** Although standard of care, charcoal has limited or no effect on outcomes. It reduces absorption by about 30% if given within 1 hour of ingestion and likely has no benefit after 1 hour (but it is still the correct answer on the test!).

For which of these overdoses is charcoal NOT indicated?

A) Acetaminophen.
B) Aspirin.
C) Iron.
D) Digoxin.
E) Opiates.

Discussion

The correct answer is C. Charcoal will not bind iron. Some of you may have chosen answer A, acetaminophen. Theoretically, charcoal could interfere with the action of N-acetylcysteine, the antidote for acetaminophen ingestion, by absorbing it. However, this is more of a theoretical concern than an actual one. First, the drugs should be used at different times. Charcoal should be given immediately while N-acetylcysteine is given only after 4-hour levels are available. Second, the doses of N-acetylcysteine recommended are quite

high, and you can give a higher dose if you will be using it with charcoal. Finally, IV N-acetylcysteine is available and is obviously not affected by charcoal. Answers B, D, and E are all incorrect. While we do have antidotes for digoxin and opiates (Digibind, naloxone), charcoal is still indicated to reduce absorption.

Objectives: Did you learn to . . .

- Manage a patient with an acute ingestion?
- Describe the appropriate use of gastric lavage and charcoal administration?
- Identify situations where charcoal may not be indicated?

 QUICK QUIZ: BIOTERRORISM

Oh no! Godzilla is attacking Tokyo with weapons of mass destruction. Which of the following properly describes the isolation requirements of a patient with pulmonary anthrax?

A) No isolation necessary. The patient may be in the same room with an uninfected patient.
B) Respiratory isolation only.
C) Respiratory and contact isolation.
D) Negative pressure room (such as with tuberculosis) plus contact isolation.

Discussion

The correct answer is A. Pulmonary anthrax is not transmitted person-to-person. Contact isolation is indicated in patients with cutaneous anthrax and GI anthrax (where diarrhea may be infectious).

Godzilla is not done yet. Which of the following drugs should be used as prophylaxis against inhaled anthrax should exposure to aerosolized spores be documented?

A) A first-generation cephalosporin.
B) Trimethoprim/sulfamethoxazole.
C) Ciprofloxacin.
D) A third-generation cephalosporin.

Discussion

The correct answer is C. Fluoroquinolones are the drugs of choice when treating individuals exposed to anthrax. Doxycycline may also be used. Cephalosporins and TMP/SMX are not active against anthrax.

Godzilla, frustrated by his failed anthrax attack, is now spreading smallpox. Which of the following is NOT true about smallpox?

A) Isolation is best done at home if possible
B) The patient is infectious until he or she becomes afebrile.
C) All lesions are generally in the same stage of evolution, unlike what is seen in varicella.
D) Smallpox immunization causes an encephalitis in 1:300,000, of which 25% of cases are fatal.

Discussion

The correct answer is B. The patient is infectious until all lesions crust over; the infectious state is not affected by the presence or absence of fever. Answer A is true. Isolation is best done at home since this will limit spread. Answer C is true. All lesions are in a similar state of evolution. Answer D is true, which is why there is not a mass immunization campaign against smallpox.

CASE 2

A 22-year-old female presents to the ED with an overdose. She has a history of depression, and there were empty bottles found at her bedside. The bottles had contained clonazepam (a benzodiazepine) and nortriptyline (a tricyclic). The patient is unconscious with diminished breathing and is unable to protect her own airway.

The BEST next step is to:

A) Intubate the patient.
B) Begin gastric lavage and administer charcoal.
C) Administer flumazenil, a benzodiazepine antagonist, to awaken her and improve her respirations.
D) Administer bicarbonate.
E) None of the above.

Discussion

The correct answer is A. This patient should be intubated. Remember that in any emergency situation that the ABCs (**a**irway, **b**reathing, and **c**irculation) are the priority. Answer B is incorrect because, as noted above, patients who are lavaged have a higher incidence of pulmonary aspiration—an even greater concern in the obtunded patient. In fact, airway protection is **mandatory** before undertaking lavage. Answer C is incorrect. Flumazenil **will** reverse the benzodiazepine. However, we know from experience that seizures in patients who have had flumazenil are particularly difficult to control. This would be particularly problematic in a patient

with a mixed overdose, such as with a tricyclic, where seizures are common. Thus, it is recommended that flumazenil be used only as a reversal agent after procedural sedation in patients who are not on chronic benzodiazepines.

* *

You notice that the patient begins to have an abnormal ECG tracing.

Which of the following findings would you expect to find in a tricyclic overdose?

A) Normal QRS complex.
B) 2nd- and 3rd-degree heart block.
C) Widened QRS complex.
D) Sinus tachycardia.
E) All of the above.

Discussion

The correct answer is E. All of the above findings can be seen with a tricyclic overdose. In fact, the most common presenting rhythm is a narrow-complex sinus tachycardia. As toxicity progresses, you can get a prolonged PR interval, a widened QRS complex and a prolonged QT interval. Heart blocks (2nd- and 3rd-degree) herald a poor outcome and may be seen late in the course. Asystole is not a primary rhythm in tricyclic overdose and tends to reflect the end-stage of another arrhythmia.

* *

YIKES! The patient becomes unresponsive and you look at the monitor. You obtain the ECG as shown in Figure 1–1.

What is the patient's rhythm?

A) Monomorphic ventricular tachycardia.
B) Sinus tachycardia with a bundle branch block.
C) Paroxysmal supraventricular tachycardia.
D) Torsade de pointes.
E) None of the above.

Discussion

The correct answer is D. This is torsade de pointes (literally "twisting of the points"), which is a subtype of polymorphic ventricular tachycardia. It can be recognized by the varying amplitude of the complex in a somewhat regular pattern. Answer A is incorrect because the complexes are not monomorphic. Answer B is incorrect for two reasons. First, there are no P waves visible. Second, sinus tachycardia should not have varied amplitude. Answer C is incorrect because, again, there are no P waves and the complexes are polymorphic.

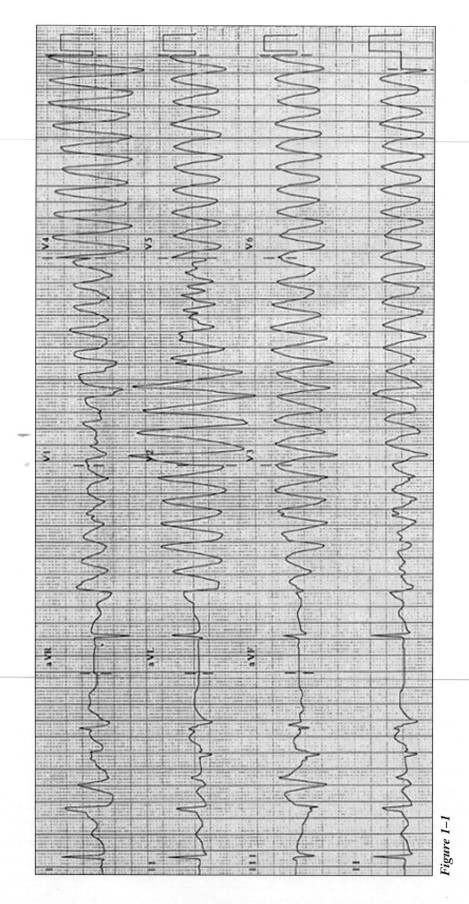

Figure 1–1

This patient needs treatment posthaste. After taking care of the ABCs, what is the one BEST drug for the treatment of this arrhythmia in a patient with a tricyclic overdose?

A) Beta-blockers.
B) Lidocaine.
C) Sodium bicarbonate.
D) Procainamide.
E) Amiodarone.

Discussion

The correct answer is C. The treatment of choice for arrhythmias in patients with a tricyclic overdose is sodium bicarbonate. Raising the pH and administering sodium seems to "prime" the sodium channels in the heart reversing the toxicity of the tricyclic. Procainamide and quinidine should not be used because they act in similar fashion to tricyclics and may worsen the problem. Lidocaine can be used as can amiodarone, but they are not the best choices. Beta-blockers can worsen hypotension and should be avoided.

* *

This is not your patient's lucky day. She begins to seize after the administration of the bicarbonate.

The treatment of choice for this seizing patient is:

A) Lorazepam.
B) Repeating the bolus of sodium bicarbonate and increasing the bicarbonate drip.
C) Phenytoin (Dilantin).
D) Fosphenytoin (Cerebryx).
E) None of the above.

Discussion

The correct answer is A. Benzodiazepines are the treatments of choice in tricyclic-induced seizures. While most seizures are self-limited, it is important to control seizures because the resultant acidosis can worsen tricyclic toxicity. Answer B is incorrect. This patient is already alkalinized, and sodium bicarbonate is not particularly effective in tricyclic induced seizures. Answer C is incorrect because phenytoin can be used, but benzodiazepines and phenobarbital should be administered first if possible. Phenytoin is not a particularly good antiepileptic drug in tricyclic overdose. Answer D is incorrect for two reasons. First, since fosphenytoin is metabolized to phenytoin, the caveats above also apply

for it. Second, it requires adequate circulation and renal and hepatic function for adequate metabolism and blood levels. If your patient becomes hypotensive with poor liver and renal perfusion, adequate drug levels might not be achieved. Finally, both phenytoin and fosphenytoin can cause hypotension—not what you need in this unstable patient.

* *

The patient's seizures stop and she is admitted to the intensive care unit.

 HELPFUL TIP: A patient who is asymptomatic 6 hours after a tricyclic overdose is unlikely to have any serious consequences from the ingestion. The patient can be "medically cleared" at that point for admission to the psychiatric unit. Note that "symptomatic" includes tachycardia or mild confusion. We are talking about the entirely asymptomatic patient here.

Objectives: Did you learn to . . .

- Describe the role of flumazenil in toxicologic emergencies?
- Manage a tricyclic overdose?
- Recognize ECG findings in a tricyclic overdose?
- Recognize torsade de pointes and its treatment?

QUICK QUIZ: DESIGNER AND CLUB DRUGS

An 18-year-old male presents after a party. He is having alternating episodes of combative behavior interspersed with episodes of coma. He becomes almost apneic during the episodes of coma. He has alternating bradycardia (while in coma) and tachycardia (when awake). The patient is also having myoclonic seizures. His serum alcohol level is zero.

The most likely drug causing this is:

A) Ecstasy (MDMA).
B) GHB (gamma hydroxybutyrate, aka liquid ecstasy).
C) Methamphetamines.
D) LSD (lysergic acid diethylamine, aka "acid").
E) Opiate overdose.

Discussion

The correct answer is B. The episodic coma and bradycardia interspersed with episodes of extreme agitation are almost pathognomonic of GHB overdose. Answer A is incorrect because MDMA causes an amphetamine-like reaction with agitation, hypertension, hyperthermia, tachycardia, etc. Answer C is incorrect for the same reason. Answer D is incorrect because LSD rarely (if ever) causes coma. Answer E is incorrect because patients with opiate overdoses are generally somnolent or comatose without interspersed episodes of agitation.

The main point of this case is to be aware of the increased use of GHB (aka "Georgia home boy," "grievous bodily harm," and other names) and of the toxicity associated with it. It is odorless and has slight salty taste. It has become a drug of choice for date rape. The toxicity tends to be self-limited and can be treated with intubation if needed along with tincture of time. The half-life is only 27 minutes.

QUICK QUIZ: TOXIDROMES

A patient presents to the hospital with a diphenhydramine overdose.

Which of the following signs and symptoms are you likely to find in this patient?

A) Bradycardia, dilated pupils, flushing.
B) Bradycardia, pinpoint pupils, flushing.
C) Tachycardia, dilated pupils, diaphoresis.
D) Tachycardia, dilated pupils, flushing.
E) Tachycardia, pinpoint pupils, flushing.

Discussion

The correct answer is D. This patient has an anticholinergic toxidrome. Toxidromes are symptom complexes associated with a particular overdose that should be recognized immediately by the clinician. Common toxidromes are listed in Table 1–1.

CASE 3

A patient presents to your office with neck pain after a motor vehicle accident. He was restrained and the airbag deployed. He notes that he had some lateral neck pain at the scene. He continues to have lateral neck pain.

Which of the following IS NOT a criterion for clearing the cervical spine clinically?

A) Absence of all neck pain.
B) Normal mental status including no drugs or alcohol.
C) Absence of a distracting injury (such as an ankle fracture).

Table 1–1 TOXIDROMES

Drug Class	Examples	Signs and Symptoms
Anticholinergic	Tricyclics, diphenhydramine, scopolamine, loco weed (jimson weed), some mushrooms, etc	Tachycardia, flushing, dilated pupils, low-grade temperature, and confusion. *Mnemonic:* Dry as a bone, red as a beet, mad as a hatter, blind as a bat
Opiates	Morphine, heroin, codeine, oxycodone, etc	Pinpoint pupils, hypotension, hypopnea, coma, hypothermia
Cholinergic	Organophosphate or carbamate pesticides, some mushrooms	Lacrimation, salivation, muscle weakness, diarrhea, vomiting, miosis. *Mnemonic:* Moist as a slug, eyes like a mole, weak as a kitten
Sympathomimetic	Cocaine, ecstasy, methamphetamine	Tachycardia, hypertension, elevated temperature, dilated pupils (mydriasis)
Gamma hydroxybutyrate	GHB, liquid ecstasy, etc	Alternating coma with agitation, hypopnea while comatose, bradycardia while comatose, and myoclonus

D) Absence of paralysis or another "hard" sign that could be caused by a neck injury.

E) All of the above are needed to clear the cervical spine clinically.

Discussion

The correct answer is A. Patients can have lateral neck pain and still have their cervical spines cleared clinically. However, no one will fault you for obtaining radiographs in patients with lateral muscular (eg, trapezius) neck pain. Patients with central neck pain (eg, over the spinous processes) **do need** radiographs to clear their cervical spine. All of the other criteria are required in order to clinically clear the cervical spine (Table 1–2).

 HELPFUL TIP: The most common cause of missed fractures is an inadequate series of radiographs. An adequate series of radiographs for the cervical spine includes an AP film, a lateral film including the top of T-1, and an odontoid film. CT should be done if radiographs are negative and there is still clinical suspicion of a fracture. Flexion-extension views add little and should be avoided.

* *

The patient's daughter, aged 4 years, was in the same motor vehicle accident and also had her cervical spines cleared by radiograph. However, you get a call from the ED 48 hours after the initial accident that the child is paralyzed from just above the nipple line down (never a good thing; the lawyers are probably close behind). You review the initial radiographs with the radiologist, they are negative as is a CT of the cervical spine bones done after the onset of the paralysis.

Table 1–2   CLEARING THE CERVICAL SPINE CLINICALLY

No central neck pain on questioning or palpation

No distracting, painful injury (eg, bone fracture, etc)

No symptoms or signs referable to the neck (paralysis, stinger-type injury, etc)

Normal mental status including no drugs or alcohol; including any retrograde amnesia, etc

The most likely cause of this patient's paralysis is:

A) Missed transection of the thoracic cord.

B) Conversion reaction from the psychological trauma of the accident.

C) Subarachnoid hemorrhage.

D) SCIWORA syndrome.

Discussion

The correct answer is D. This likely represents SCIWORA syndrome (**s**pinal **c**ord **i**njury **w**ithout **r**adiologic **a**bnormality). This occurs from stretching of the cord secondary to flexion/extension-type of movement in an accident. Patients with SCIWORA syndrome may be paralyzed at the time of initial presentation (in the event of cord transection) or may have a delayed presentation up to 72 hours after the injury. Answer A is incorrect because a cord transection would present with paralysis immediately at the time of injury. Answer B is incorrect because this child is 4 years old, and conversion reaction is unlikely in children. Additionally, conversion reaction **is always** a diagnosis of exclusion. Answer C is incorrect because this is not the presentation of a subarachnoid hemorrhage (headache, stiff neck, perhaps focal neurologic symptoms).

The next step in the management of this patient is:

A) IV methylprednisolone to reduce cord edema.

B) Fluid restriction and diuretics to reduce cord edema.

C) Mannitol to reduce cord edema.

D) Neurosurgical intervention to decompress the cord.

E) None of the above.

Discussion

The correct answer is A. Patients with a cord injury should be treated with IV methylprednisolone 30mg/kg bolus (3 g in an adult) followed by a 5.4mg/kg drip for 24 hours. The efficacy of this therapy in spinal cord injury is limited, and its efficacy in SCIWORA is unknown. However, it is currently considered the standard of care. Neither diuretics nor mannitol will be useful in this situation. Answer D is incorrect because the process of SCIWORA involves stretching of the cord (and subsequent dysfunction) rather than cord compression such as would be seen with a bony injury.

The father is, understandably, irate that his child is now paralyzed. You can tell him that the natural history of SCIWORA syndrome in THIS CHILD is likely to be which of the following?

A) Continued paralysis with the necessity of long-term, permanent adaptation to the injury.
B) Progression of the injury over the next week to include further paralysis in an ascending fashion.
C) Resolution of paralysis and sensory symptoms over the next several months.
D) Resolution of all symptoms except sensory symptoms of the next several months.
E) Large lawsuit payout on the way. Do not pass go, do not collect $200 (adjusted for inflation).

Discussion

The correct answer is C. Generally, patients with SCIWORA syndrome regain their strength and sensory abilities over time. **However, this depends on when they present with symptoms!** Patients who present with paralysis right after the accident may have complete cord transection and thus will not regain function. For this reason, it is important to obtain an MRI on all patients with SCIWORA syndrome (and any trauma-induced paralysis for that matter).

Objectives: Did you learn to . . .

- Clinically "clear" the cervical spine and decide when to order cervical spine radiographs?
- Describe causes of missed cervical spine fractures?
- Understand the physiology, natural history, and management of SCIWORA syndrome?

CASE 4

A hard-core alcoholic presents to the ED after drinking a bottle of automobile winter gas treatment (Rothschild Vintage, 1954). He is intoxicated, has a headache, and describes a "misty" vision, such as might be seen during a snowstorm. He is tachycardic and tachypneic. You start an IV and administer IV saline. You obtain a blood gas, which shows a mild metabolic acidosis.

A metabolic acidosis is consistent with all of the following ingestions EXCEPT:

A) Ethylene glycol.
B) Methanol.
C) Ethanol (eg, vodka, gin, etc).
D) Petroleum distillates (eg, non–alcohol-containing gasoline products).

Discussion

The correct answer is D. Ethylene glycol, methanol, and ethanol can all cause a metabolic acidosis. Hydrocarbons (eg, gasoline products) do not cause a metabolic acidosis. The main manifestation of hydrocarbon toxicity is secondary to the inhalation of the hydrocarbon and the resulting pneumonitis.

* *

This patient's electrolytes are as follows: sodium 135 mEq/L, potassium 4.0 mEq/L, bicarbonate 12 mEq/L, chloride 108 mEq/L, BUN 12 mg/dL, Cr. 1.0 mg/dL.

This patient's anion gap is:

A) 13
B) 15
C) 23
D) Unable to calculate the anion gap with the information provided.

Discussion

The correct answer is B. By convention, the anion gap is calculated without using a major cation, potassium. Thus, the anion gap is calculated as follows:

$$sodium - (chloride + bicarbonate).$$

In this patient the anion gap is

$$135 - (108 + 12) = 15$$

The normal gap is 12 or less.

 HELPFUL TIP: In methanol ingestions, the severity of acid-base disturbance is generally a better predictor of outcome than serum methanol levels.

All of the following are causes of an anion gap acidosis EXCEPT:

A) Lactic acidosis.
B) Diabetic ketoacidosis.
C) Renal tubular acidosis.
D) Uremia.
E) Ingestions such as methanol.

Discussion

The correct answer is C. See Table 1–3 for more on causes of anion gap acidosis.

Table 1–3 CAUSES OF ACIDOSIS

Causes of an **elevated** anion gap acidosis	Lactic acidosis Diabetic ketoacidosis Ingestions such as ethanol, methanol, etc Uremia Alcoholic ketoacidosis
Causes of a **normal** anion gap acidosis	GI bicarbonate loss (eg, chronic diarrhea) Renal tubular acidosis (types I, II, and IV) Interstitial renal disease Ureterosigmoid loop Acetazolamide and other ingestions Small bowel drainage

Which of the following findings IS NOT frequently seen in patients with methanol ingestion?

A) Hypopnea.
B) Optic disk abnormalities.
C) Abdominal pain and vomiting.
D) Basal ganglia hemorrhage.
E) Meningeal signs, such as nuchal rigidity.

Discussion

The correct answer is A. Hypopnea is not commonly seen in methanol poisoning until the patient is close to death. In fact, the reverse is true. Tachypnea is a frequent finding in methanol overdose. This makes sense. The patient is trying to compensate for a metabolic acidosis by blowing off CO_2. Optic disk abnormalities, abdominal pain and vomiting, basal ganglia hemorrhage, and meningeal signs are all seen as part of methanol toxicity. It is thought that many of these signs and symptoms are secondary to CNS hemorrhage.

* *

You can test for ethanol at your hospital but do not have a test for methanol on a stat basis and want to be sure that this patient is not just saying he has a methanol ingestion in order to obtain alcohol (a treatment for methanol ingestion—break out the single malt scotch!).

What test is most likely to help you determine if the patient has methanol ingestion?

A) CBC.
B) BUN/creatinine.
C) Liver enzymes.
D) Serum osmolality.
E) Amylase and lipase.

Discussion

The correct answer is D. With a measured serum osmolality, you can calculate the osmolar gap. Subtract the total **measured** serum osmoles from the osmoles known to be due to ethanol (each 100 mg/dL of ethanol accounts for approximately 22 osmoles). If there is an elevated osmolar gap, it is evidence of a circulating, unmeasured osmole. In this case, it would be methanol. So, for example:

Measured serum osmolality = 368
Blood alcohol = 200 mg/dl or about 44 osmoles
Calculated osmolality = 2(Na) + BUN/2.8
+ glucose/18 = 280 + 6 + 8 = 294
So, osmolar gap = 368 – (294 + 44) = 30

This means that there are 30 unmeasured osmoles which could, in this case, represent methanol. Thus, we know that the patient is not simply drunk.

* *

You decide that there is sufficient evidence that this patient has ingested methanol in order to institute treatment.

Appropriate treatment(s) for this patient include:

A) Fomepizole (4-MP).
B) Cimetidine.
C) Ethanol.
D) A and C.
E) All of the above.

Discussion

The correct answer is D. Both fomepizole (4-MP) and ethanol are used for methanol ingestion. The idea is to slow down the metabolism of the methanol. The toxicity of methanol is caused by formic acid, which is a byproduct of methanol metabolism. Ethanol is metabolized by alcohol dehydrogenase, the same enzyme that breaks down methanol. Thus, methanol metabolism is competitively inhibited by ethanol. The same holds true for fomepizole which is a competitive inhibitor of alcohol dehydrogenase. Fomepizole and ethanol can both be used for ethylene glycol ingestion as well. Answer B is incorrect. While cimetidine does reduce alcohol metabolism, the effect size is so small as to be negligible.

Objectives: Did you learn to . . .

- Recognize manifestations of alcohol ingestion?
- Identify causes of metabolic acidosis with elevated and normal anion gaps?
- Use the osmolar gap to narrow the differential diagnosis of metabolic acidosis?

QUICK QUIZ: BETA-BLOCKER OVERDOSE

Which of the following has been shown to be useful in β-blocker overdose when conventional, adrenergic pressors are ineffective?

A) Calcium chloride.
B) Glucagon.
C) Milrinone.
D) All of the above.

Discussion

The correct answer is D. In β-blocker overdoses, the following findings may be observed: bradycardia, AV block, hypotension, hypoglycemia, bronchospasm, nausea, and emesis. When an overdose has been identified, the usual treatments are employed (eg, pressure support, airway protection, charcoal, etc). If conventional pressors have failed, glucagon in a dose of 3–5 mg IV bolus and a drip at 1–5 mg/hr may be effective in treating β-blocker overdose. It is generally preferred over atropine in this situation. Milrinone and other phosphodiesterase inhibitors may also be used but are considered third-line. Likewise, calcium is considered a third-line agent in β-blocker overdose. Calcium chloride may potentiate the action of glucagon.

QUICK QUIZ: TOXICOLOGY

The best therapy for seizures secondary to isoniazid ingestion is:

A) Lorazepam.
B) Phenytoin.
C) Pyridoxine.
D) Thiamine.
E) Phenobarbital.

Discussion

The correct answer is C. Isoniazid is a B_6 antagonist. Thus, pyridoxine is the drug of choice in isoniazid-induced seizures. These seizures are often resistant to conventional therapy. Look for this type of overdose in patients who are being treated for tuberculosis (either active or latent disease).

QUICK QUIZ: TOXICOLOGY

Whole-bowel irrigation is most appropriate for which of these overdoses?

A) Aspirin.
B) Sustained-release verapamil.
C) Ethanol.
D) Acetaminophen.
E) Sertraline.

Discussion

The correct answer is B. Whole-bowel irrigation is best used in patients who have taken sustained-release tablets and in patients with a pill bezoar.

QUICK QUIZ: TOXICOLOGY

Which of the following can be used to increase the metabolism of alcohol in an intoxicated patient?

A) IV fluids.
B) Charcoal.
C) Forced diuresis.
D) GABA antagonists such as flumazenil.
E) None of the above.

Discussion

The correct answer is E. The rate of alcohol metabolism is fixed with zero-order kinetics at lower doses (fixed metabolic rate) and first-order kinetics at higher doses (rate proportional to levels). Generally, this rate is in the range of 9–36 mg/dL/hr with 20 mg/dL/hr being the accepted norm. At this point, there are no available agents to increase the metabolism of ethanol. Answer B is incorrect because ethanol is absorbed too rapidly for charcoal to be of any benefit.

CASE 5

A family of four come into your ED after being exposed to carbon monoxide (CO). They were in an idling car and were running the engine and heater to stay warm. You want to get a carboxyhemoglobin level on the whole family but cannot get a blood gas from the youngest child.

What is your response?

A) Check an oxygen saturation, and if the oxygen saturation is normal, be reassured.
B) Check a venous carboxyhemoglobin level.
C) Check a venous carboxyhemoglobin and correct for the difference between venous and arterial samples.
D) None of the above.

Discussion

The correct answer is B. A venous carboxyhemoglobin is just as accurate as an arterial carboxyhemoglobin, and it is much less painful to draw. Answer A is incorrect because the pulse oximeter does not reflect hypoxia in carbon monoxide poisoning. Thus, pulse oximetry is useless in determining the carboxyhemoglobin level. Answer C is incorrect because there is no correction needed.

When determining which patients need hyperbaric oxygen on the basis of a carboxyhemoglobin level, the level to rely upon is:

A) The carboxyhemoglobin level on arrival to the ED.
B) The carboxyhemoglobin level at 4 hours after exposure.
C) The carboxyhemoglobin level projected to "time zero" (eg, at the time of exposure).
D) None of the above.

Discussion

The correct answer is C. A major consideration regarding the initiation of hyperbaric oxygen therapy is the patient's clinical situation. More severely ill patients with CO poisoning (eg, severe acidosis, unconscious,

unresponsive, etc) should be considered candidates for hyperbaric oxygen. Also, treatment should be based on the carboxyhemoglobin level projected to time zero. This is the level that gives the most accurate information about the degree of exposure. The rest of the answers are incorrect.

* *

The father has a headache and a time zero carboxyhemoglobin level of 12%. The mother, who is pregnant, is asymptomatic and has a carboxyhemoglobin level of 16%, and one of the children, aged 6 years, has a level of 18% while another has a carboxyhemoglobin level of 23% and was asymptomatic at the scene.

The first step in the treatment of these patients is:

A) Start an IV and administer saline.
B) Start n-acetylcysteine which is a free radical scavenger.
C) Start CPAP to maximize air flow by keeping the airways from collapsing.
D) Administer 100% oxygen.
E) Intubate the most severe patient, 100% oxygen for the others.

Discussion

The correct answer is D. Because CO competitively binds to hemoglobin in place of oxygen and in fact has greater affinity for hemoglobin than oxygen, high-flow 100% oxygen is the cornerstone of treating CO poisoning. Thus, **the first step in CO poisoning is to administer 100% oxygen.** The rest of the answers are incorrect. If the patient is not ventilating well, intubation would be appropriate. However, because your patients are breathing well, there will be no advantage (and a substantial downside) to intubation.

Which of the following can be seen with carbon monoxide poisoning?

A) Rhabdomyolysis.
B) Cardiac ischemia.
C) Long-term neurologic sequelae, including dementia.
D) Pulmonary edema.
E) All of the above.

Discussion

The correct answer is E. All of the above can be seen with carbon monoxide poisoning. Additional findings include acidosis, seizures, syncope, and headache.

Answer C deserves a bit more discussion. Long-term neurologic sequelae can develop days to months after the exposure and can include cognitive deficits, focal neurologic deficits, movement disorders, and personality changes. Such neurologic sequelae do not appear to be related to the level of carboxyhemoglobin but are more likely to occur when a patient has lost consciousness during his or her CO exposure. It appears that using hyperbaric oxygen in the appropriate patient will reduce long-term neurologic sequelae.

* *

Your closest diving chamber is about 90 minutes away and will hold only one patient at a time. You need to make a decision about whom to send for hyperbaric oxygen.

Which patient will benefit most from hyperbaric oxygen therapy?

A) Asymptomatic pregnant mother, time zero carboxyhemoglobin of 16%.

B) Asymptomatic 6-year-old, time zero carboxyhemoglobin of 18%.

C) Asymptomatic 8-year-old, time zero carboxyhemoglobin of 23%.

D) Adult male with mild headache only, time zero carboxyhemoglobin level of 12%.

Discussion

The correct answer is A. Criteria for hyperbaric oxygen include mental status changes, carboxyhemoglobin level >25%, acidosis, cardiovascular disease, and age >60 years. Obviously, these are relative criteria. An otherwise normal 61-year-old with a mild exposure need not have HBO. **Pregnancy is an indication for HBO therapy** because fetal hemoglobin has a high affinity for carbon monoxide and the fetus is highly susceptible to carbon monoxide.

All of the following are well-established consequences of hyperbaric oxygen EXCEPT:

A) Seizures.
B) Psychosis.
C) Myopia.
D) Ear and pulmonary barotraumas.
E) Direct pulmonary oxygen toxicity.

Discussion

The correct answer is B. All of the rest are found as a result of hyperbaric oxygen. Answer C, myopia, is actually found in up to 20% of patients being treated with hyperbaric oxygen. It is due to direct toxicity of oxygen on the lens and usually recovers within weeks to months.

Objectives: Did you learn to . . .

● Diagnose and manage patients with carbon monoxide poisoning?
● Describe complications of carbon monoxide poisoning?
● Identify patients who may benefit from hyperbaric oxygen therapy?
● Describe the complications of hyperbaric oxygen therapy?

CASE 6

A 50-year-old immigrant from a country in the developing world is brought to your ED after being bitten by a stray dog. The bite was unprovoked and is on the patient's abdomen. The patient has no other health history of note and has not taken antibiotics for over a year. You irrigate the wound and are deciding about closure. There is a 3-cm laceration on the abdomen.

All of the following are true about dog bites EXCEPT:

A) They tend to be primarily crush type injuries.
B) In general, the infection rate is similar to a laceration from any other mechanism (eg, knife cut), except on the hands and feet.
C) The primary organism in infected dog bites is *Staphylococcus aureus*.
D) Primary closure of dog bite wounds is an acceptable option (except perhaps on the hands and feet).
E) They always require antibiotics.

Discussion

The correct answer is E. All of the rest are true statements. Dog bites (except for those from little poodles named Fifi) tend to be crush injuries (as contrasted with cat bites, which are primarily puncture wounds). The infection rate is about the same as other lacerations. Bites on the hands and feet tend to have a higher rate of infection. Most dog bite infections are polymicrobial with *S. aureus* playing a large role and *Pasteurella* playing a smaller, but still significant, role. Other organisms include *Streptococcus* species and Gram-negative species. Dog bites do not generally require antibiotic prophylaxis, except under certain circumstances (eg, immunocompromised, large or complicated wound, etc).

You are concerned about rabies prophylaxis. Which of the following is (are) viable options?

A) Isolating the suspect animal for 3 days.
B) Euthanizing the suspect animal and examining its liver.
C) Administering rabies immune globulin IM.
D) Administering rabies immune globulin IV followed by rabies vaccination series.
E) Administering rabies immune globulin by infiltrating it around the wound followed by rabies vaccination series.

Discussion

The correct answer is E. You should infiltrate rabies immune globulin around the wound and then begin the rabies vaccination series. As much of the immune globulin as possible should be infiltrated around the wound and the rest should be given IM at a different site. Answer A is incorrect because animals need to be isolated for **10 days,** not 3. Answer B is incorrect. The animal can be euthanized but the brain should be examined—not the liver. Answers C and D are both incorrect methods of administering the vaccine/immune globulin.

Which of the following require rabies prophylaxis in all cases?

A) Stray rabbit bites.
B) Stray rat bites.
C) Stray bat bites.
D) Stray squirrel bites.
E) Stray snake bites.

Discussion

The correct answer is C. All bats should be considered rabid unless available for observation and testing. See Table 1–4 for detailed recommendations. Go to the CDC Web site for information about rates of infection in wild animals in your area.

In patients who have completed the primary tetanus vaccine series, the current CDC recommendations for administering a tetanus booster (Td) are:

A) Every 10 years unless the patient has sustained a contaminated wound, in which case the booster should be within 5 years.

Table 1–4   GUIDELINES FOR RABIES PROPHYLAXIS

Always assume rabid unless animal available for testing	Foxes, bats, raccoons, skunks, dogs, cats, ferrets, other carnivores
Judge on an individual basis	Rodents (squirrels, rats, mice, etc), lagomorphs (rabbits, etc)
Never require rabies prophylaxis	Non-mammals (snakes, lizards, etc)

B) Every 10 years regardless.
C) Every 10 years to the age of 70.
D) The primary series of 3 shots and then with each potentially contaminated wound.
E) None of the above.

Discussion

The correct answer is A. Patients should receive a tetanus booster (Td) every 10 years. For a contaminated wound, the Td booster should be documented within the last 5 years. Answer B is incorrect because patients should have a booster when they have a contaminated wound if they have not had one within the last 5 years. Answer C is incorrect because patients should have boosters for life according to the CDC, although Medicare does not cover routine Td boosters and many patients older than 65 years choose to forego it for cost reasons. Answer D is incorrect because patients do not need boosters with every contaminated wound. This offers no additional protection but does increase the risk of side effects.

 HELPFUL TIP: Individuals should receive at least one dose of Tdap (tetanus, diphtheria, and acellular pertussis) between 11 and 18 years and a single dose between 18 and 64 years. Additionally, health-care workers should receive a single dose of Tdap.

 HELPFUL TIP: If the patient has not had a primary series of tetanus immunizations, administer tetanus immune globulin **and** start the primary tetanus series.

You have irrigated this patient's wound. Which of the following statements is true about irrigating a wound and wound infections?

A) Povidone-iodine as a 50% irrigation solution (eg, Betadine) in the wound will decrease the infection rate.

B) Irrigation with normal saline is the only recommended method of cleaning a wound.

C) Irrigation with normal saline and irrigation with tap water are equally effective in reducing wound infection rates.

D) Use of epinephrine with lidocaine in a wound increases the rate of infection.

E) Irrigation of a wound with either alcohol or hydrogen peroxide will reduce the rate of wound infection.

Discussion

The correct answer is C. Infection rates are the same whether the wound is irrigated with normal saline or tap water. **We are not recommending that you start using tap water as an irrigation solution!** This is **not** standard of care although it is just as effective. Answer A is incorrect. Povidone-iodine is toxic to tissue and polymorphonuclear leukocytes and actually may **increase** infection rates unless a solution of 1% or less is used. Full-strength povidone-iodine **can** be used on intact skin as a cleanser but should not be used in a wound. Answer B is incorrect because other solutions (poloxamer 188, balanced salt solutions, etc) can be used but are more expensive and do not offer any benefit in reduction of infection rates. Answers D and E are incorrect. As with povidone-iodine, alcohol may be used for cleaning skin but should be kept out of the wound. It is toxic to tissue and acts a fixative. Hydrogen peroxide is also toxic to tissue and should not be used in open wounds.

How long after a laceration occurs can the wound be closed primarily?

A) 6 hours.

B) 12 hours.

C) 18 hours.

D) 24 hours.

E) Any of the above can be correct depending on the wound.

Discussion

The correct answer is E. There is no arbitrary time limit to when a wound can be closed. Facial wounds may be closed up to 24 hours after injury for cosmetic reasons, while you may not want to close other, contaminated wounds more than 12 hours after injury. Some wounds you may not want to close at all (eg, bites to the hand, wounds contaminated with grease, etc), rather allowing them to close by secondary intention.

Objectives: Did you learn to . . .

• Describe the indications for rabies prophylaxis?

• Recognize the issues that arise with animal bites and indications for closure and/or prophylactic antibiotics?

• Describe a method for tetanus prophylaxis in a patient who has not had primary tetanus vaccination?

• Understand current recommendations for Td booster administration?

• Use various wound irrigation solutions for cleansing wounds?

• Decide upon the time frame for wound closure?

 QUICK QUIZ: EMERGENCY MEDICINE

A patient presents to your office after sustaining a wound to his index finger which was caused by an industrial, high-pressure paint sprayer. There is evidence of a puncture wound on the index finger but no other evidence of injury although the finger is stiff.

Appropriate management of this patient would be:

A) Tetanus prophylaxis and soaking the finger.

B) Tetanus prophylaxis, antibiotics, and reassurance.

C) Open exploration in the operating room by an orthopedic surgeon.

D) Tetanus prophylaxis, radiograph, and reassurance if the radiograph is normal.

E) None of the above.

Discussion

The correct answer is C. This patient needs to go to the OR to have the wound explored. While underwhelming on initial presentation, injuries from high pressure paint sprayers and grease guns can be quite severe with paint or grease tracking up the tendons into the hand or forearm. For this reason, all patients with a high pressure injury require surgical exploration.

CASE 7

A 52-year-old male presents to your ED via ambulance complaining of a headache after a fall. He was working and fell approximately 10 feet. He notes no injury except for head and neck pain. A quick survey reveals that he has a blood pressure of 128/86, pulse 100, and respirations 12. There was no loss of consciousness at the scene. He "saw stars" and was clumsy, dazed, and slow at the scene without any focal neurologic deficit. He is now back to his baseline.

A concussion is defined as:

A) Any neurologic symptoms (eg, clumsy, dazed, or slow) after head injury.
B) Loss of consciousness followed by return to baseline.
C) Loss of consciousness with continued neurologic symptoms.
D) Requires confusion after head trauma regardless of whether the patient lost consciousness or not.

Discussion

The correct answer is A. A concussion is defined as **any** neurologic symptom after head trauma. Note that a concussion does not require a loss of consciousness. For this reason, Answers B and C are incorrect. Answer D is incorrect because manifestations of concussion are not limited to confusion but also include protracted vomiting, transient amnesia, slowed mentation, dizziness, and other neurologic symptoms.

* *

Your patient opens his eyes on his own, follows commands, answers all orientation questions correctly, but appears unsteady when ambulating.

His Glasgow Coma Scale (GCS) is:

A) 5
B) 10
C) 14
D) 15
E) 20

Discussion

The correct answer is D. The GCS is a scale used to indicate the severity of neurologic dysfunction and is often applied to victims of head trauma. Only the maximum score of 15 is considered a normal GCS. There are three components to the GCS, as listed in Table 1–5.

 HELPFUL TIP: My chair and refrigerator each have a GCS of 3. Remember that **nothing** can have a GCS less than 3.

Table 1–5 GLASGOW COMA SCALE

Eye opening *Mnemonic:* "4 eyes"	Spontaneous = 4 To speech = 3 To pain = 2 No response = 1
Verbal response *Mnemonic:* "Jackson 5"	Alert and oriented = 5 Disoriented conversation = 4 Nonsensical speech = 3 Moaning = 2 No response = 1
Motor response *Mnemonic:* "6 cylinders"	Follows commands = 6 Localizes pain = 5 Withdraws from pain = 4 Decorticate flexion = 3 Decerebrate extension = 2 No response = 1

Independent of other factors, an entirely normal Glasgow Coma Scale score of 15 indicates that:

A) The patient does not require a head CT scan.
B) There is essentially no possibility that this patient has an intracranial injury requiring surgical intervention.
C) There is little or no possibility that this patient has any focal intracranial bleed.
D) There is up to a 4% chance this patient will need neurosurgical intervention.
E) None of the above.

Discussion

The correct answer is D. In appropriately selected patients (eg, those with a significant mechanism of injury), about 18% with a GCS of 15 will have some intracranial lesion, and up to 4% will eventually require neurosurgical intervention. These are generally patients who have a depressed skull fracture but a normal GCS. Answers A, B, and C are incorrect because a normal GCS in and of itself does not allow one to forego head CT in patients with a significant mechanism of injury Remember that the GCS is **not** linear; a GCS of 14 is bad. Patients with a GCS of 14 **must** have a CT scan—unless another factor in the clinical decisionmaking dictates otherwise (eg, patient/family wishes, dementia).

In an adult patient with a significant head injury, which of the following is NOT an indication for a head CT scan?

A) Intoxication with drugs or alcohol.
B) Vomiting once or more.
C) Amnesia or memory deficit.
D) Age greater than 40 years.
E) Seizure.

Discussion

The correct answer is D. Older patients are at greater risk of developing serious intracranial injuries, but ≥60 years is usually used as an indication. While there is no "upper limit of normal" for vomiting after head trauma, the best data available suggests that any vomiting after head trauma in an adult indicates the need for a head CT scan. The currently recommended criteria for a CT of the head in various age groups are listed in Table 1–6.

The patient is noted to have a subdural hematoma on CT scan. Which of the following is true regarding the use of prophylactic phenytoin in head trauma?

A) It reduces the incidence of seizures but does not affect overall outcome.

Table 1–6 INDICATIONS FOR HEAD CT SCAN BY AGE

Age	Indications for Head CT Scan after Trauma with a Significant Mechanism
Adult	• Intoxication • Age >60 • Any memory deficit • Vomiting (number of times undefined) • Seizure • Headache
Child >2 yrs	• Loss of consciousness • Amnesia • Seizure • Headache • Persistent vomiting • Irritability • Behavioral changes
Child <2 yrs, >3 mos	Any of the above as well as: • Any unusual behavior • Large scalp hematoma
Infant <3 mos	Any of the above as well as: • A significant mechanism • Any scalp hematoma

B) It reduces the incidence of seizures and reduces adverse outcomes.
C) It is ineffective at reducing the occurrence of seizures.
D) It is best given as an IV push bolus with cardiac monitoring.

Discussion

The correct answer is A. Phenytoin reduces the incidence of seizures after head trauma (NNT 10 for 1 week to prevent 1 seizure) but has no effect on overall outcome. Answer B is incorrect because phenytoin does not change outcomes. Answer C is incorrect because phenytoin can reduce posttraumatic seizure. Answer D is incorrect because phenytoin must be given as a loading dose of 18 mg/kg IV at a maximal rate of no more than 50 mg/minute.

* *

You are going to have to transfer this patient for neurosurgical intervention to drain the subdural hematoma. It is about a 4-hour drive by ambulance to the nearest facility that has a neurosurgeon.

Which of the following is indicated as prophylaxis against increased intracranial pressure in this patient?

A) Hyperventilation after intubation.
B) IV mannitol.
C) Keeping the head of the bed elevated at 30 degrees.
D) IV dexamethasone.
E) None of the above.

Discussion

The correct answer is E. None of the above is indicated as prophylaxis for increased intracranial pressure. Answer A is incorrect for two reasons. First, this patient does not need to be intubated. Second, routine hyperventilation as prophylaxis for increased intracranial pressure is of no benefit. This has been well studied. What happens is that hyperventilation **does** cause vasoconstriction reducing intracranial blood flow and therefore intracranial pressure. However, hyperventilation also causes ischemia around the area of the injury and may worsen outcomes. Answer B is incorrect because prophylactic mannitol, like prophylactic hyperventilation, confers no benefit. Answer C is incorrect. Elevating the head of the bed does reduce intracranial pressure but also reduces perfusion pressure and is therefore a wash; there is no discernible benefit.

Answer D is incorrect because steroids are not useful acutely in **head trauma** (versus spinal cord trauma). However, steroids are useful in cerebral edema secondary to tumor.

Objectives: Did you learn to . . .

- Use the Glasgow Coma Scale?
- Recognize which patients with head trauma are appropriate for head CT scan?
- Describe indications for seizure prophylaxis in head trauma?
- Manage patients presenting with potential intracranial injuries?

CASE 8

A 23-year-old male is in a bar fight. He said he had only two beers and was just standing there minding his own business when he was jumped by three other guys (yeah, right!). He presents to you about 1 hour after the event with facial trauma. His vitals are normal and he is mentating well (with the exception of some impaired judgment secondary to the alcohol). His blood alcohol level is 150 mg/dL, showing that he is legally intoxicated. On exam you notice that the patient has some epistaxis and a quite swollen nose. Additionally, there is one avulsed tooth and one tooth that is displaced.

The best way to transport an avulsed tooth is:

A) In sterile water.
B) In the buccal mucosa after thorough washing with soap.
C) In a glass of milk.
D) Wrapped in saline-soaked gauze.
E) Under a pillow.

Discussion

The correct answer is C. The best way to transport an avulsed tooth is either: 1) in a glass of milk or 2) in the buccal mucosa or under the tongue in a patient in whom risk of aspiration is not a concern. Answer A is incorrect because sterile water is hypotonic and may damage the tooth root decreasing the success rate of reimplantation. Answer B is incorrect because **washing the tooth with soap** is not appropriate. Again, you want to maintain the viability of the root if possible. Answer D is incorrect as well. If this is the only option available to you, it is better than

nothing, but a glass of milk or under the buccal mucosa is preferred. Answer E is correct only if you are hoping for the tooth fairy to leave you a dollar.

* *

You call the dentist, who is out of town. A dentist will not be available for at least 12 hours.

Your best course of action at this point is:

A) Continue to keep the tooth viable in a glass of milk.
B) Continue to keep the tooth viable in the buccal mucosa.
C) Clean the tooth and keep it sterile and dry for reimplantation in 12 hours realizing that a bridge will probably be needed to hold the tooth in position.
D) Reinsert the tooth into the socket yourself.

Discussion

The correct answer is D. If there is going to be any delay in reimplantation by a dentist, the best course of action is to reinsert the tooth into the socket yourself. Answers A, B, and C are all incorrect because they will reduce the rate of successful reimplantation.

 HELPFUL TIP: **Primary teeth should not be reinserted into the socket!** They ankylose to the bone preventing the eruption of the permanent tooth and cause a cosmetic deformity.

 HELPFUL TIP: Any patient who is in the ED and says he had only two beers and was minding his own business is probably not telling the truth on either account.

* *

You now turn your attention to this patient's nose. You are trying to decide whether or not to do a radiograph of the patient's nose.

The BEST timing for a radiograph of the nose is:

A) As soon as possible after the trauma, once other injuries are stabilized and more important problems are addressed.
B) As soon as possible to assure that there are no bone fragments threatening the brain.

C) There is no need for a radiograph acutely. You can wait for 3 or 4 days.

D) There is never any indication for nasal radiographs.

Discussion

The correct answer is C. There is no need for radiographs acutely except in extraordinary circumstances. The reason to do a radiograph is to document a fracture **and** to assist in reduction. Because of swelling, it is difficult to get a good cosmetic result reducing a nasal fracture acutely. Thus, a radiograph is indicated in 3–4 days **only** if there is evidence of nasal deformity once swelling has resolved. If there is good cosmesis, a radiograph is unnecessary just to document a fracture. Answers A, B, and D are incorrect because, as noted above, there is no reason to do a radiograph at all unless there is evidence of deformity once the swelling as resolved.

You get the epistaxis stopped and examine the nasal mucosa. Which one of these is considered an emergency?

A) Closed nasal fracture.

B) Septal hematoma.

C) Trauma to Kiesselbach plexus.

D) All of the above.

Discussion

The correct answer is B. A septal hematoma is considered an emergency. The problem is that the perichondrium, which supplies nutrition to the septum, is no longer in contact with the septum because of the intervening hematoma. Thus, the septal cartilage can necrose, leading to a perforated septum. Septal hematomas should be drained acutely and the nose packed to keep the perichondrium in contact with the septal cartilage. Answer A is incorrect (see previous question). Answer C is incorrect. Kiesselbach plexus is in the anterior nose and is a venous plexus. Bleeding is easily controlled and generally is self-limited.

* *

You continue to evaluate this patient and note that he has the loss of upward gaze in the right eye, the side on which he was hit. All of the other extraocular motions are intact.

The most likely diagnosis in this patient is:

A) Blowout fracture with entrapment of the inferior rectus.

B) Blowout fracture with dysfunction of the superior rectus.

C) Injury to cranial nerve III which controls the superior AND inferior rectus muscles.

D) Volitional refusal to perform upward gaze on the right side in this intoxicated patient.

Discussion

The correct answer is A. The most likely diagnosis is blowout fracture with entrapment of the inferior rectus. The force of a blow to the globe is transmitted to the inferior orbital wall, which is the weakest point in the orbit. This can cause entrapment of the contents of the inferior orbit, including the inferior rectus, causing an inability to perform upward gaze. Due to disconjugate gaze, patients with entrapment of the inferior rectus muscle from a blowout fracture may complain of diplopia.

Answer B is incorrect because a blowout fracture generally refers to the inferior orbital wall, which would not entrap the superior rectus. Additionally, patients with an entrapped superior rectus would have difficulty with downward gaze. Answer C is incorrect because it is unlikely that being hit in the face would cause an injury to CN III. Additionally, a CN III lesion would also affect other extraocular muscles except for the lateral rectus (CN VI) and the superior oblique (CN IV). Answer D is incorrect because it is impossible to move the eyes independently of one another unless you are a chameleon or particularly talented.

 HELPFUL TIP: Fluid in the maxillary sinus on radiograph is considered presumptive evidence of a blowout fracture given the proper clinical situation. You may also see fat, etc, herniated into the sinus in the area of the fracture even if the fracture itself is not visible. If there is any question, CT scan should resolve the issue.

* *

The patient has had a long night of partying and it is 3:00 AM Saturday when you call your consultant about the blowout fracture. The consultant is not happy about being called for an intoxicated patient at 3:00 AM. He refuses to see the patient acutely and wants you to send him to the office in 3 days (Tuesday morning).

Your response is:

A) To call another consultant; a blowout fracture should be attended to immediately.

B) Do nothing; evaluation in 2–3 days for a blowout fracture, even with inferior rectus entrapment, is appropriate.
C) Start steroids to reduce muscle edema to facilitate the spontaneous release of the entrapped muscle.
D) Start antibiotics and hospitalize the patient so that he can be seen in the morning when the consultant makes rounds.
E) Stick pins in a voodoo doll of your consultant.

Discussion

The correct answer is B. While blowout fractures with muscle entrapment require close follow-up, there is no need to intervene acutely. In fact, a decision to operate may be delayed for up to 14 days. If the entrapment spontaneously resolves (not uncommon) and there is no diplopia or other complicating symptoms, surgery is not needed. The other answers are all incorrect because acute intervention is not required in this patient. Answer E, however, may be of some benefit.

 HELPFUL TIP: In the pediatric population, however, immediate surgical repair should be undertaken in trapdoor fractures. A trapdoor fracture is one in which there is significant entrapment of the inferior rectus muscle. If the muscle is left entrapped in the pediatric population, restriction and fibrosis may occur, so immediate surgery is warranted. **Oral steroids** at a dose of 1 mg/kg may also facilitate decreased edema in the first 7 days limiting ultimate fibrosis. In patients with significant sinus disease, antibiotics may be considered, usually a penicillin or cephalosporin.

* *

The patient above has a friend who was also in the altercation. He, too, was just minding his business as was everyone in the bar—that is why the fight started! He has a simple laceration of the chin, which you repair. This patient has a blood alcohol level of 150 mg/dL (the legal limit in most states is 80 mg/dL). Since he is intoxicated, the nurses are reluctant to allow the patient to leave because of liability issues. He seems initially very cooperative and competent. However, the nurse manager reminds you of the legal issues. The patient is getting more agitated; he wants to go home.

Your response is:
A) Sedate the patient with haloperidol and observe him until sober.
B) Sedate the patient with a benzodiazepine and observe him until sober.
C) Call the police to remove the patient from your ED.
D) Use restraints on the patient and observe him until sober, as sedative drugs may prolong time in the ED.
E) Let the patient leave the ED with a competent adult.

Discussion

The correct answer is E. The patient was initially cooperative and competent. Competence **is not** based on a blood alcohol level but rather on your judgment of the patient's ability to make rational decisions. We allow patients on narcotics to make decisions about their care all of the time, despite having narcotics on board. There are patients who will be competent and safe at a blood alcohol of 200 mg/dL and others who may be impaired at 80 mg/dL. So, judge competence individually.

Objectives: Did you learn to . . .
- Treat acute dental trauma?
- Diagnose and manage nasal and periorbital trauma?
- Care for the intoxicated patient with minor trauma?

CASE 9

A 17-year-old female fell asleep with her contact lenses in her eyes last evening. This morning she notes quite a bit of eye pain and photophobia. You evert the eyelids and find no evidence of a foreign body. When you stain her eye, you find a corneal ulcer. The treatment for this patient is:

A) Debridement with a burr and systemic antibiotics.
B) Debridement with a cotton swab and systemic antibiotics.
C) Topical antibiotics, cycloplegia, and referral to ophthalmology.
D) Copious irrigation, systemic antibiotics, and cycloplegia.

Discussion

The correct answer is C. This is an ophthalmologic emergency that requires topical antibiotics, cycloplegia (for pain control), and referral to an ophthalmologist.

These ulcers can become quite deep and result in a ruptured globe.

* *

You consult with your ophthalmologist who would like you to start a cycloplegic agent in this patient prior to referral.

The drug you would choose for a cycloplegic agent is:

A) Pilocarpine eye drops.
B) Timolol eye drops (eg, Timoptic).
C) Tetracaine eye drops.
D) Cyclopentolate eye drops.

Discussion

The correct answer is D. Cyclopentolate is the only cycloplegic agent listed above. Pilocarpine is a miotic agent. Timolol is a β-blocker used in the treatment of glaucoma. Tetracaine eye drops are a topical anesthetic.

If your patient just had a simple corneal abrasion, you would not have had to think so hard! Regarding corneal abrasions, you realize that:

A) Patching an eye after a corneal abrasion reduces pain and promotes healing.
B) If a topical antibiotic is needed after a large corneal abrasion, gentamicin ophthalmic ointment is the drug of choice.
C) Tetracaine is a good topical anesthetic and should be considered for home use in patients with a painful corneal abrasion.
D) Patients should avoid wearing contact lenses until the eye has been healed for at least a week.

Discussion

The correct answer is D. Answer A is incorrect because patching an eye may actually increase pain and decrease healing. Whether or not to use a patch should be a matter of patient comfort only. Answer B is incorrect because gentamicin ophthalmic ointment (as well as other topical aminoglycosides) actually reduce healing of the cornea, and antibiotics are not necessary unless there are signs of infection. Answer C is incorrect because patients should never be sent home with a topical anesthetic. It reduces healing and can lead to further injury if the patient, whose eyes are now insensate, continues a harmful activity, rubs his/her eyes, etc.

HELPFUL TIP: To differentiate a topical ophthalmologic problem from iritis, put in some tetracaine. If the pain resolves it is likely **but does not prove** that the problem is superficial (eg, corneal abrasion, etc). Posttraumatic iritis is manifest by ciliary flare, anterior chamber cells, and marked photophobia.

Objectives: Did you learn to . . .

● Recognize a corneal ulceration and treat it appropriately?
● Treat corneal abrasions?
● Understand the proper use of cycloplegic agents?

QUICK QUIZ: EYE TRAUMA

You are on call for your group and a welder who was welding and grinding presents at 2:00 AM with severe bilateral eye pain. When he left work at 5:00 PM the day before, he did not notice any problem. He notes that he was wearing his dark goggles some of the time while he was welding but did quite a bit of work without goggles as well.

The most likely diagnosis in this patient is:

A) Foreign body.
B) Ultraviolet (UV) keratitis.
C) Globe penetration secondary to the welding and a foreign body.
D) Iritis.

Discussion

The correct answer is B. This patient likely has ultraviolet (UV) keratitis. UV keratitis is found in patients who are welders or have been out in the sun for an extended period of time (at the beach, skiing, tanning bed, etc). UV keratitis generally presents as severe, bilateral eye pain about 6–10 hours following the activity. It is treated with cycloplegic agents and pain medication, often requiring narcotics. Answers A, C, and D are incorrect because they generally present unilaterally. Additionally, in the cases of Answers A and C, they should present directly after the event rather than 9 hours later, as in this patient. However, always consider globe penetration and rule it out clinically.

HELPFUL TIP: Patients who have a foreign body in the eye following a high-speed injury (eg, grinding wheel) should be assumed to have a globe perforation until proven otherwise.

 QUICK QUIZ: ORTHOPEDIC EMERGENCIES

Which of the following is most commonly associated with significant vascular injury?

A) Pubic ramus fracture.
B) Knee dislocation.
C) Shoulder dislocation.
D) Elbow dislocation.
E) Ankle dislocation.

Discussion
The correct answer is B. Knee dislocations (**not patellar dislocations**) are highly associated with injury to the popliteal artery. **All** patients who have had a dislocated knee should have an angiogram to document vascular integrity since vascular injury is a major cause of limb loss and morbidity. Answer A is incorrect because pubic ramus fractures are relatively minor injuries without vascular involvement, requiring only pain control. Shoulder dislocations are commonly associated with injury to the axillary nerve. Elbow dislocations can be associated with injury to the median nerve and brachial artery. However, arterial injuries are much less common than with knee dislocations. Ankle dislocations are rarely associated with vascular injury.

CASE 10

A 55-year-old male farmer is injured by a cow that pins him against a fence. His leg was trapped against the fence for a several minutes. Being a typical midwestern farmer, he ignores the injury until later that afternoon when he presents to your office complaining of severe pain in the calf area. A radiograph is normal, and the patient has normal distal pulses. The calf (his leg, not the cow) is tender with increased pain on passive stretch. His pain seems to be out of proportion to his injury.

Which of the following is true?

A) Since the patient has excellent pulses, a compartment syndrome is not likely.

B) Compartment syndrome is defined as compartment pressure >30 mm Hg.
C) Compartment syndrome is associated only with significant crush injuries or fractures.
D) Pain out of proportion to the injury is a red flag for compartment syndrome.
E) His calf (the leg, not the cow) likely has mad cow disease.

Discussion
The correct answer is D. Pain out of proportion to the injury is a red flag for compartment syndrome. Answer A is incorrect because pulses can be maintained until there is significant increase in compartment pressures and significant injury to muscle and nerves. Answer B is incorrect because it is difficult to define a specific cut off for compartment syndrome. Some patients tolerate higher pressures and others cannot tolerate 30 mm Hg (normal compartment pressure is zero). However, when the pressure gets above 20–30 mg Hg, strong consideration should be given to the presence of compartment syndrome. Answer C is incorrect. Compartment syndrome can be due to a number of factors including electrical injury, excessive muscle use, tetany, reperfusion after ischemia, etc.

 HELPFUL TIP: Traditionally, we are taught the "5 Ps" of compartment syndrome: **p**ulselessness, **p**aresthesia, **p**allor, **p**ain, and **p**aralysis. But this is misleading. Pain may be the only symptom. By the time the others are present, there may be significant disruption of vascular supply and extensive injury.

* *

You decide that it is likely that this patient has compartment syndrome.

Which of the following labs will be the most helpful in guiding treatment for this patient?

A) CBC.
B) Urinalysis.
C) Glucose.
D) Sodium.
E) PT/PTT.

Discussion
The correct answer is B. One of the major complications of compartment syndrome is rhabdomyolysis.

This will manifest itself as a urine which is dipstick-positive for blood but with a negative microscopic exam for red blood cells. The positive dipstick is picking up myoglobin in the urine. This can be confirmed by a serum CPK. CBC, glucose, sodium, and coagulation studies may be appropriate depending on the clinical situation but are not useful in establishing the presence of myoglobinuria.

> **HELPFUL TIP:** Myoglobin can be measured in the urine. However, many laboratories have stopped doing this test, favoring the positive dipstick/negative microscopic exam approach. **There can be false-negative dipstick findings.** Thus, check a CPK as well if rhabdomyolysis is a consideration.

* *

The patient has a positive dipstick for blood with no red blood cells on microscopic exam (presumptive myoglobinuria). His serum CPK is 32,000, which is >5 times the upper limit of normal, so you make the diagnosis of rhabdomyolysis.

The most common adverse consequence and greatest danger of rhabdomyolysis is:

A) DIC.
B) Acute renal failure.
C) Seizure from hypocalcemia.
D) Acute gout from hyperuricemia.
E) Cardiac arrhythmia from hyperkalemia.

Discussion

The correct answer is B. Myoglobin precipitates in the renal tubules causing acute renal failure. Answer A, DIC, can occur but is rare. Answer C, seizures from hypocalcemia, have not been reported in this condition, nor has Answer D, gout. The potassium elevation from rhabdomyolysis generally does not reach a level sufficient to cause arrhythmias.

The primary treatment for rhabdomyolysis is:

A) Mannitol infusion.
B) Saline infusion.
C) Furosemide.
D) Dialysis.

Discussion

The correct answer is B. The most important treatment for rhabdomyolysis is saline infusion with alkalinization of the urine. Mannitol (answer A) can be used to increase urine flow, but this is really a treatment that is secondary to good hydration and urine alkalinization. Furosemide (answer C) is not used in rhabdomyolysis. Loop diuretics will actually acidify the urine and are contraindicated. Dialysis (answer D) is what we are trying to avoid using saline.

> **HELPFUL TIP:** In patients with rhabdomyolysis, try to maintain urine output of 200–300 cc/hr for an adult. Alkalinize the urine using sodium bicarbonate. Remember that in order to alkalinize the urine you have to maintain an adequate serum potassium level, otherwise the body will reabsorb potassium in exchange for hydrogen ions causing urine acidification.

* *

The patient is able to maintain urine output after you institute saline.

What treatment are you going to suggest for the underlying compartment syndrome?

A) Fasciotomy.
B) Immobilization and traction.
C) Hot packs and elevation of the affected limb.
D) Ice and elevation of the affected limb.

Discussion

The correct answer is A. The treatment of compartment syndrome is fasciotomy. A rapid surgical or orthopedic consultation is critical in the treatment of compartment syndrome.

The patient does well and everyone is happy except the cow who is still fated to his lot in life as a cow.

Objectives: Did you learn to . . .

• Recognize manifestations of compartment syndrome and understand that compartment syndrome can be present with pain alone?
• Identify patients at risk for compartment syndrome and rhabdomyolysis?
• Manage compartment syndrome?
• Diagnose and treat rhabdomyolysis?

CASE 11

A 24-year-old black male presents to the ED complaining of fever, chills, and dyspnea. He has chest pain that is respirophasic (pleuritic) in nature. He is noted to be tachypneic with a respiratory rate of 36 and an oxygen saturation of 90%. He has a history of sickle-cell anemia and has had a number of sickle-cell crises in the past. He is up to date on immunizations, including *S. pneumonia* and *Haemophilus influenzae* vaccines.

The patient's current symptoms are MOST suggestive of:

A) Pneumothorax.
B) Pulmonary embolism.
C) Acute chest syndrome.
D) Sickle cell-related pericarditis.

Discussion

The correct answer is C. This patient likely has acute chest syndrome, which is associated with sickle-cell anemia and may be indistinguishable from pneumonia. Acute chest syndrome is characterized by pleuritic chest pain, fever, cough, chills, dyspnea, rales, and rhonchi. The etiology is unknown but it may be secondary to infarction of the lung and/or fat emboli.

All of the following are recommended in the initial treatment of acute chest syndrome EXCEPT:

A) Hydroxyurea.
B) Oxygen.
C) IV normal saline.
D) Morphine.

Discussion

The correct answer is A. Hydroxyurea, while useful for the chronic treatment of sickle-cell anemia, is not indicated for the treatment of acute chest syndrome. It can reduce the incidence of acute chest syndrome by 50% when used chronically, however. Other treatments include IV antibiotics to cover for community-acquired pneumonia (although acute chest syndrome is **not bacterial**). It is prudent to cover these patients with antibiotics because they are de facto splenectomized and the initial presentation of acute chest syndrome can be easily confused with pneumonia.

* *

The patient continues to be hypoxic despite your therapy. His CBC shows a slight elevation in the WBC count and a hemoglobin of 11 g/dL. A chest radiograph indicates progression of infiltrates.

The next step in treating this patient is:

A) Fresh frozen plasma.
B) Pentoxifylline.
C) Packed red blood cells.
D) Exchange transfusion.

Discussion

The correct answer is D. Patients who have acute chest syndrome and remain hypoxic with progressing infiltrates are candidates for exchange transfusion to bring the level of HbS to <30% of the total. Simply administering blood (answer C) will not resolve the problem because HbS will still be present in significant amounts. If this patient had a more significant anemia, packed red cell transfusion would be a more viable option. Answers A and B are also incorrect. Fresh frozen plasma has no role in the treatment of acute chest syndrome, nor does pentoxifylline.

* *

Your patient recovers from this episode. He has had numerous painful crises in the past, as well as hospitalizations for other reasons. You have an opportunity to provide some patient education. You answer your patient's questions and then review potential manifestations of sickle cell anemia.

Which of the following may be a manifestation of sickle-cell disease?

A) Joint and bone pain.
B) Acute abdominal pain.
C) Acute sequestration syndrome.
D) Aplastic crisis.
E) All of the above.

Discussion

The correct answer is E. All of the above can be associated with sickle-cell anemia (keep reading for additional information).

Which of the following infections is a common cause of aplastic crisis in sickle-cell anemia?

A) Parvovirus B-19.
B) Influenza virus.
C) CMV virus.
D) Parainfluenza virus.
E) None of the above.

Discussion

The correct answer is A. Patients with sickle-cell anemia can develop aplastic anemia in response to a parvovirus B-19 infection. Also, Epstein-Barr virus and some bacteria have also been reported to cause aplastic crisis in patients with sickle-cell anemia.

Acute sequestration syndrome is a manifestation of sickle cell anemia.

In which age group does acute sequestration syndrome occur?

A) Less than 5 years.
B) 5–12 years.
C) 12–25 years.
D) Greater than 25 years.

Discussion

The correct answer is A. Acute sequestration syndrome occurs when the spleen sequesters red blood cells, leading to a drop in hemoglobin. The presentation can be quite dramatic with severe left upper quadrant pain and profound anemia, sometimes resulting in hypovolemic shock and death. Because it requires a functional spleen, it is most common in children <5 years. Patients with sickle-cell anemia who are >5 years generally do not have a functioning spleen; most often it has infarcted so that acute sequestration syndrome no longer occurs. The mortality is 15% per episode, and 50% recur.

Objectives: Did you learn to . . .

- Recognize acute chest syndrome?
- Manage a patient with acute chest syndrome?
- Use exchange transfusion in a patient with sickle-cell anemia?
- Recognize various other manifestations of sickle-cell anemia?

CASE 12

A 52-year-old truck driver presents to your ED after being out in subzero (Fahrenheit) temperatures for several hours trying to repair his truck. He is hypothermic when you use a rectal thermometer with appropriate calibration. His initial core temperature is noted to be 28°C. He has a pulse of 24, a blood pressure of 70/30, and slow mentation. He is awake, however.

The appropriate first-line treatment for this patient is:

A) Atropine.
B) Epinephrine.
C) Dopamine.
D) Lidocaine.
E) None of the above.

Discussion

The correct answer is E. The hypothermic heart is generally resistant to drugs. Thus, the best treatment for this patient is rewarming. If the patient has poor perfusion, rapid rewarming with CPR if indicated is the treatment of choice.

 HELPFUL TIP: The typical progression of hypothermia-related cardiac findings is: sinus bradycardia, atrial fibrillation with a slow ventricular response, ventricular fibrillation, and finally asystole. The classic ECG finding in hypothermia is the Osborn (J) wave, a slow positive deflection at the end of the QRS.

All of the following are acceptable methods of rewarming this patient EXCEPT:

A) Active external rewarming (eg, hot packs, etc).
B) Immersion in 40°C water.
C) Passive external rewarming (eg, blankets).
D) Heated, humidified oxygen.
E) Thoracic lavage with warm fluids.

Discussion

The correct answer is C. Patients with a temperature of below 30°C generally do not have enough endogenous heat production to rewarm themselves effectively. Thus, external or internal **active** rewarming is indicated. All of the other options are correct methods of rewarming this patient. Extracorporeal blood warming is also effective. Heated lavage fluids (eg, gastric and rectal) are generally not very effective because of the limited surface area involved. Additionally, this type of lavage can potentially cause electrolyte abnormalities.

Rapid rewarming of the extremities is associated with:

A) Alkalosis, hypokalemia.
B) Acidosis, hypokalemia.
C) Acidosis, hyperkalemia.
D) Alkalosis, hyperkalemia.
E) None of the above.

Discussion

The correct answer is C. Rewarming of the extremities can lead to return of cold blood to the core leading to a paradoxical drop in body temperature. Additionally, hypothermia causes lactic acidosis with hyperkalemia in the extremities; as the peripheral blood is rewarmed and mobilized, systemic metabolic acidosis with hyperkalemia may result.

Which of the following is NOT associated with an increased risk of hypothermia?

A) Diabetes mellitus.
B) Obesity.
C) Alcohol use.
D) Old age.
E) Chronic illness.

Discussion

The correct answer is B. Obese patients have a smaller body mass to surface area ratio and do not have an increased risk of hypothermia. Answer C, alcohol use, causes patients to be relatively insensate to cold (thus the term "liquid jacket") and also causes a peripheral vasodilatation, increasing heat loss. Thermoregulation is impaired as individuals age. Thus, old age (answer D) is associated with a greater propensity towards hypothermia. Diabetes (answer A) and any chronic illness (answer E) can also predispose to hypothermia.

* *

The patient's mental status clears and he complains that his fingers and toes, which were numb and cold, are now quite painful. You note that there is probably freezing of tissue (frostbite).

The BEST method of rewarming the areas with frostbite is:

A) Slowly in tepid water.
B) Rapidly in the hottest water he can stand (tested by you to assure that there will be no burns).
C) Using a hot air source such as a hair dryer.
D) Using moist heat via a heating pad.

Discussion

The correct answer is B. Frostbitten parts should be rewarmed as quickly as possible in hot water between 37° and 40°C. Water cooler or hotter than this can lead to incomplete thawing and increased tissue loss. The other methods (answers A, C, and D) are not recommended. **Do not rewarm parts that may become**

frozen again (for example if you are in the field). Refreezing will cause additional damage.

* *

The patient has a lot of pain after thawing and reperfusion. You control the pain with morphine.

Which of the following is the most appropriate dose of morphine in this 100-kg male?

A) 2 mg IV.
B) 4 mg IV.
C) 6 mg IV.
D) 8 mg IV.
E) 10 mg IV.

Discussion

The correct answer is E. The correct dose of IV morphine is 0.1 mg/kg or 10 mg in this 100-kg male. Similarly, the correct dose of meperidine (Demerol) is 100 mg (1 mg/kg) and the dose of hydromorphone is 0.015 mg/kg. However, there really is no "fixed" dose of narcotic pain medication in the ED. Titrate the dose until the patient obtains pain relief.

* *

It is 2 days later. The patient is noted to have black eschar on the multiple fingers and toes. There is no obvious perfusion to these areas.

The best course at this point is:

A) Debridement of the nonviable tissue.
B) Skin grafting over open areas after debridement.
C) Observation for a number of weeks despite the black eschar.
D) Amputation of the nonviable distal digits.

Discussion

The correct answer is C. It can take weeks for the proper demarcation line for debridement and grafting to become apparent. Thus, aggressive intervention at this point is counterproductive and may lead to additional tissue loss. For this reason, answers A and D are incorrect. Skin grafting is also not appropriate at this time because debridement of the eschar is not appropriate.

Objectives: Did you learn to . . .

- Identify severe bradycardia in hypothermia and treat it appropriately?
- Manage a patient with hypothermia?
- Use methods of rewarming and identify complications of rewarming?

- Recognize risk factors for hypothermia?
- Diagnose and manage frostbite?

 QUICK QUIZ: TOXICOLOGY

Which of the following is true about the ingestion of household bleach?

A) Patients who drink household bleach are at a high risk of esophageal and gastric burns.

B) Oral burns are a good predictor of esophageal burns.

C) All patients who ingest household bleach should be referred for gastroscopy to rule out burns.

D) Household bleach ingestions are generally benign and require no treatment if the patient is not symptomatic.

Discussion

The correct answer is D. Most **household** bleach ingestions are benign and need no therapy if the patient is asymptomatic. However, **this does not extend to industrial bleach or drain cleaner.** There is a high risk of esophageal and gastric burns with industrial bleach. Answer B is incorrect. The oral mucosa may be normal in **industrial bleach or drain cleaner** ingestion and there may still be significant esophageal and gastric burns. For this reason all patients with **drain cleaner or industrial bleach ingestion** should have gastroscopy. Answer C is incorrect. Patients with household bleach ingestions do not require gastroscopy.

CASE 13

A 26-year-old male was working outside in the heat and humidity. The outside temperature reached 105°F with 90% humidity. He usually lives in northern Canada and works as a penguin herder; he is in Iowa on a job detasseling corn. (Don't believe it? Look at www.teamcorn.com.) His friends noticed that he became confused, complained of headache and muscle cramps, and became lightheaded. On arrival to your ED, he is not sweating and is lethargic. His rectal temperature is 41.5°C.

All of the following are indicated in the treatment of this patient EXCEPT:

A) Pack the patient in ice to reduce core temperature.

B) IV fluids.

C) Use a fan on the patient to promote evaporative cooling.

D) Administer glucose if the patient is hypoglycemic.

Discussion

The correct answer is A. Packing patients in ice is contraindicated. Total body immersion in ice water is useful but packing the person in ice actually reduces cooling for two reasons. First, it causes cutaneous vasoconstriction reducing cooling. Second, it does not allow conductive cooling such as would be seen in ice water submersion. The appropriate treatment of heat exhaustion/heat stroke (heat stroke being defined as CNS dysfunction with a change in the level of consciousness) is cool water-soaked blankets and towels with fans aimed at the patient. This allows evaporative cooling and also conductive heat loss (to the water in the towels). Antipyretics are generally not effective because by this point the patient's endogenous thermoregulation is kaput.

Which of the following is NOT a contributing factor to heat exhaustion/heat stroke?

A) Use of stimulants such as ephedra or amphetamines.

B) Dehydration.

C) Anticholinergic drugs.

D) Thin body habitus.

E) Extremes of age.

Discussion

The correct answer is D. A thin body habitus is not a risk factor for heat stroke/exhaustion; the opposite is true. Obesity predisposes to heat stroke/exhaustion because there is less evaporative surface area per kg of weight. All of the others predispose to heat-related illness. Answers A and C reduce sweating and, in the case of answer A, increase metabolic rate. Both of these predispose to heat-related disease. Of particular note is answer E. Small children, while thin, sweat less readily than do adults. This predisposes them to heat-related disease.

 HELPFUL TIP: Up to 80% of patients with heat stroke will not have a prodrome of nausea, lightheadedness, confusion, headache, etc which is seen in heat exhaustion. Make sure you check hepatic enzymes in patients in whom you suspect heat stroke. They are almost uniformly elevated and normal liver enzymes should cause you to question your diagnosis.

Objectives: Did you learn to . . .

- Recognize and manage heat exhaustion/heat stroke?
- Recognize risk factors for heat exhaustion/heat stroke?
- Locate penguin habitats? Penguins do not live at the North Pole, so the patient could not have been working as a penguin herder.

CASE 14

A 19-year-old female presents to the ED with complaints of wheezing. She has a history of asthma and you have been following her since her eighth birthday. Generally, she has mild asthma not requiring an inhaled steroid. However, over the past several months things have accelerated so that she now uses her rescue inhaler daily. On exam she is tachypneic, using accessory muscles of respiration, with a respiratory rate of 30 and wheezing in all fields. Her oxygen saturation is 95% and pulse is 110 with a normal blood pressure. Her blood gas is as follows: pH 7.40, CO_2 40 mm Hg, O_2 92 mm Hg, and HCO_3 24 mEq/L.

A normal blood gas in this patient suggests that:

A) This is a mild exacerbation and should respond well to therapy.
B) She has a respiratory acidosis.
C) She has a respiratory alkalosis.
D) This is a severe exacerbation that will require aggressive therapy.
E) None of the above.

Discussion

The correct answer is D. A pH of 7.4 with a CO_2 of 40 mm Hg in a patient who is asthmatic and tachypneic is a bad sign. The CO_2 **should** be low in a tachypneic patient because the patient will be blowing off CO_2. Thus, a normal CO_2 and normal pH indicate that the patient is retaining CO_2. This is another case where looking at the patient is more important than looking at the labs. Answers B and C are both incorrect because the blood gas indicates neither acidosis nor alkalosis.

Which of the following tests are indicated in routine evaluation of a patient with an asthma exacerbation?

A) Chest x-ray.
B) CBC.
C) Arterial blood gas.
D) All of the above.
E) None of the above.

Discussion

The correct answer is E. None of the above tests is indicated in the routine evaluation of an asthma exacerbation. A chest x-ray should be reserved for those patients in whom pneumonia or other pulmonary process is suspected. A CBC is not going to change your therapy in the routine asthma exacerbation and is not indicated. Likewise, an ABG is unnecessary in most asthma exacerbations. It can be used to assist in your clinical evaluation to determine whether or not the patient is retaining CO_2; however, even in the "crashing patient" an ABG is not necessary because **intubation is a clinical decision and should not be based on the blood gas.**

You decide to initiate therapy for this patient. Of the following options, the initial treatment of this patient is:

A) Subcutaneous epinephrine.
B) Albuterol MDI (metered-dose inhaler) with spacer.
C) Nebulized ipratropium.
D) Oral steroids.
E) IV steroids.

Discussion

The correct answer is B. The initial treatment for this patient—and any patient presenting with an asthma exacerbation—is a bronchodilator, in this case albuterol. It makes little difference whether this is via nebulizer or MDI, as long as one uses adequate doses. One albuterol nebulization is equal to about 8–10 puffs of an albuterol MDI with a spacer. Answer A is incorrect because subcutaneous epinephrine is second- or third-line treatment of asthma. Answer C is incorrect. While ipratropium is effective in asthma, it is secondary to albuterol in the treatment of asthma. Answers D and E are incorrect. Steroids are indicated, but bronchodilator therapy is the primary treatment in acute asthma exacerbations.

* *

There is no albuterol MDI available to you in your ED, so the patient receives nebulized albuterol. However, she continues to wheeze.

How many albuterol treatments can this patient safely receive?

A) 1 every other hour.
B) 1 per hour.
C) 2 per hour.

D) 3 per hour.

E) Continuous nebulization of albuterol is safe.

Discussion

The correct answer is E. Albuterol can be administered via nebulizer continuously if needed, even in the pediatric age group. Tachycardia, one of the main side affects of albuterol treatment, will often **improve** with continuous albuterol. This occurs because the patient's tachycardia is often driven by hypoxia. Once the asthma is adequately treated, oxygenation improves, and the pulse comes down.

* *

The patient does not respond well to albuterol alone, so you request the addition of ipratropium. At this point you want to order steroids.

Which of the following statements about steroids is true?

A) IV steroids are superior to PO steroids in the treatment of asthma.

B) All patients who are steroid-dependent should have additional steroids even if they have already taken their dose for the day.

C) The effective dose range for steroids in asthma is well established.

D) Only patients requiring admission should have oral or parenteral steroids.

Discussion

The correct answer is B. All patients who are steroid-dependent should get steroids if they present to the ED with an acute exacerbation of asthma. Answer A is incorrect. Intravenous steroids and oral steroids have the same efficacy in acute asthma exacerbations. Thus, the choice of route depends mostly on convenience, cost, and physician preference. Answer C is incorrect. Multiple steroid dosing regimens and ranges of doses have been used in asthma with success. Answer D is incorrect. Discharged patients who have anything more than a minor asthma exacerbation should receive steroids.

Which of the following is true about the role of theophylline in the treatment of acute asthma?

A) Theophylline/aminophylline should be used in cases unresponsive to 2–3 doses of nebulized albuterol since it has added benefits when used with an inhaled beta-agonist.

B) Patients who get theophylline/aminophylline have more side effects than do patients who get continuously nebulized albuterol and get no benefit from the drug.

C) If you choose to use theophylline/aminophylline the therapeutic goal is a serum level of 20 micrograms/dL.

D) None of the above is correct.

Discussion

The correct answer is B. Patients who are treated with theophylline have more side effects, including tachycardia, nausea, and arrhythmias, than do patients who get continuously nebulized albuterol. Theophylline/aminophylline have essentially no role in the treatment of acute asthma exacerbations. There is no benefit to theophylline or aminophylline over **optimal** beta-agonist therapy (eg, continuous nebulized albuterol if required). Answer C is incorrect because if used at all, the therapeutic goal for theophylline is a serum level of 15 micrograms/dL.

 HELPFUL TIP: Magnesium sulfate (2 g over 10 minutes in adults, 25 mg/kg in children) can be used in patients with status asthmaticus. Magnesium is a direct smooth muscle relaxant. Not all patients will respond, and in patients who will respond you can expect a 60- to 90-minute effect. Avoid using magnesium in patients with renal failure since they may become toxic.

* *

The patient responds to nebulizers and steroids. You decide to send her home.

Which of the following is true?

A) You should discharge the patient on 2 puffs of an albuterol MDI via spacer to be used PRN.

B) You should place the patient on a steroid taper.

C) You should discharge the patient on 8–10 puffs of an albuterol MDI via spacer to be used every 6 hours around the clock.

D) You should start the patient on a steroid inhaler.

E) None of the above.

Discussion

The correct answer is D. The patient should be started on a steroid inhaler to prevent recurrent exacerbations.

She has been using her albuterol daily, indicating poor control. Overlapping this with oral steroids will give the inhaled steroid a chance to work while the patient is being covered with the oral steroids. Answer A is incorrect. The proper dose of albuterol via MDI is 6–10 puffs PRN. Answer B is incorrect because patients **do not need a steroid taper** if they are not on chronic steroids and will be taking steroids for no more than 10 days. You can simply treat the patient (eg, with prednisone 40 mg PO QD for 5–10 days) and then stop. No taper is needed. **Note that this is not true for patients on chronic steroids who clearly do need a taper.** Answer C is incorrect because scheduled albuterol is not as effective as PRN use. Additionally, albuterol can certainly be used more than every 6 hours.

Objectives: Did you learn to . . .

- Recognize clinical and blood gas manifestations of a severe asthma exacerbation?
- Evaluate a patient presenting with an asthma exacerbation?
- Initiate treatment for asthma in the ED?
- Recognize the pitfalls in using theophylline/aminophylline for asthma?
- Formulate a plan for discharging an asthma patient from the ED?

CASE 15

A 7-year-old presents to the ED with wheezing and hives after being stung by a bee. He was evidently throwing rocks at a yellow jacket nest when he was stung. On exam the patient has hives and wheezing with a normal blood pressure for his age. He is mildly tachycardic.

Potentially useful treatments for this patient includes all of the following EXCEPT:

A) IV Diphenhydramine.
B) Subcutaneous epinephrine.
C) Subcutaneous diphenhydramine.
D) Intravenous cimetidine.

Discussion
The correct answer is C. Subcutaneous diphenhydramine can cause skin necrosis and is contraindicated. Either IV or IM diphenhydramine can be used. Of the others, subcutaneous epinephrine should be used in the patient with anaphylaxis who fails to respond to diphenhydramine and cimetidine or who has respiratory distress, hypotension, etc. Intravenous H_2 blockers (eg, cimetidine, ranitidine) are particularly effective in the treatment of anaphylaxis and should be used routinely in these patients.

The family is concerned that the stinger may still be in the patient's skin. The proper response is to:

A) Remove the stinger with forceps.
B) Remove the stinger using a double-edged razor or credit card.
C) Leave the stinger embedded in the skin.
D) Not worry about looking for a stinger in this patient.

Discussion
The correct answer is D. The one Hymenoptera (bees, wasps, etc) that leaves the stinger in the skin is the honeybee. Because this patient was stung by a yellow jacket, there will be no stinger to find in this child. As for the other answers, either A or B would be appropriate treatment if a stinger was present. The only thing that seems to make a difference in the amount of venom injected is the length of time the stinger is in the skin and not the mechanism by which is removed. So, remove the stinger as quickly as possible by whatever means available.

* *

The patient responds well to the therapy as noted above. You are going to discharge him and want to write his prescriptions.

The patient should be discharged with which of the following?

A) Diphenhydramine Q 6 hours for the next 48 hours.
B) Cimetidine for Q 12 hours for the next 48 hours.
C) An anaphylaxis ("bee sting") kit.
D) All of the above medications.

Discussion
The correct answer is D. Patients can have biphasic reaction mediated by "slow reacting substance of anaphylaxis" which is now believed to be a neutrophil chemotactic factor. This recurrence may occur up to 48 hours after the initial event. Thus, prescribing medications to prevent the recurrence is prudent. Also, the patient should have a "bee sting" kit available.

* *

The parents are concerned about this child who likes to play outside. They worry that he will get stung again.

You let them know that:

A) Any sting should be treated as an emergency.
B) He will continue to be allergic to "bee stings" in the future.
C) He should take prophylactic medication before going out to play in the woods or other areas where he might get stung.
D) None of the above.

Discussion

The correct answer is D. Individuals who are allergic to one species of Hymenoptera are not necessarily allergic to others. Generally, the allergy is species specific. Thus, most stings will be benign in an allergic patient **unless** it is a sting from the offending species. Answer B is incorrect. Many children tend to outgrow "bee sting" allergies. This is in contrast to adults in whom reactions tend to get worse over time. Answer C is incorrect. Obviously the child should be careful not to irritate yellow jackets, but prophylactic treatment is not routinely indicated.

 HELPFUL TIP: Adults with a systemic allergic reaction to an insect sting have a 30% to 60% risk of experiencing another systemic reaction upon re-sting; therefore, adults are more likely to benefit from venom testing and prophylaxis. All patients with a history of anaphylaxis should be provided with an anaphylaxis kit.

Objectives: Did you learn to . . .

- Describe the physiology and natural course of bee sting reactions?
- Treat a patient with an anaphylactic reaction to a bee sting?

CASE 16

A 14-year-old white male presents to the ED with acute onset left testicular pain when running, 1 hour prior to presentation. His past medical history is negative, he is on no medications, and he has no allergies. He denies any trauma to the region. He states that his pain is severe and only on the left. The pain is increased with ambulation and movement. He denies nausea, vomiting, diarrhea, fever, chills, dysuria, hematuria, or penile discharge.

His vital signs and physical exam are as follows: temperature 37.0°C, pulse 110, respirations 18, blood pressure 120/85. He is a well-nourished, well-developed male in distress secondary to pain. Abdomen: Normal bowel sounds, nontender, soft, no masses. Genitourinary: Circumcised male, no penile lesions, no discharge; left testicle tender to palpation but has a normal lay in the scrotum. The cremasteric reflex is normal bilaterally.

What is the significance of the normal lay and cremasteric reflex?

A) The cremasteric reflex should be abnormal in epididymitis.
B) The presence of a cremasteric reflex effectively rules out testicular torsion.
C) The normal lay of the testicle in the scrotum effectively rules out testicular torsion.
D) The presence or absence of a cremasteric reflex is not helpful in ruling out testicular torsion.

Discussion

The correct answer is D. The presence or absence of a cremasteric reflex is neither sensitive nor specific enough to confirm or rule out the presence of testicular torsion. Likewise, the lay of the testicle can be normal in patients with testicular torsion. An abnormal testicular lay and absence of the cremasteric reflex may point towards testicular torsion. However, you cannot rely on these findings to rule out testicular torsion.

The LEAST likely diagnosis in this patient is:

A) Torsion of testis.
B) Epididymitis.
C) Torsion of appendix testis.
D) Torsion of appendix epididymis.
E) Testicular tumor.

Discussion

The correct answer is E. Testicular tumors are generally painless. Testicular torsion (answer A) is characterized by acute onset of unilateral testicular pain, often during activity such as running. It has a bimodal age distribution, during the first year of life and again during puberty. The differential diagnosis is dependent on the patient's age. If the patient is <15 years, the differential consists of testicular torsion, epididymitis, torsion of appendix testis/appendix epididymis, orchitis, hydrocele, and varicocele. In patients >15 years, the differential includes all of these diagnoses plus testicular tumor.

What is the most reliable method for diagnosing testicular torsion?

A) Doppler (Duplex color).
B) Radionuclide scan.
C) Surgical exploration.
D) Checking the cremasteric reflex.
E) MRI.

Discussion

The correct answer is C. **Every patient with suspected testicular torsion should have surgical exploration of the scrotum.** All of the other studies are adjunctive. For example, radionuclide scan has a false negative rate of about 20%. Surgical exploration is the only definitive diagnostic tool. The window of opportunity for surgery is about 6 hours, after which the testicle may not be salvaged. Orchiopexy should be performed on the involved and uninvolved sides to prevent torsion.

Objectives: Did you learn to . . .

- Examine a patient presenting with acute scrotal pain?
- Generate a differential diagnosis for scrotal pain based on the patient's age?
- Evaluate a patient with suspected testicular torsion?

QUICK QUIZ: UROLOGY

What is the most common agent causing epididymitis in a 21-year-old male?

A) *E. coli.*
B) *Neisseria gonorrhoeae.*
C) *Chlamydia trachomatis.*
D) *Pseudomonas* species.
E) *Ureaplasma urealyticum.*

Discussion

The correct answer is C. In young males, epididymitis is usually the result of sexually transmitted diseases. Of these, *Chlamydia trachomatis* is currently the most common etiologic agent. *Neisseria gonorrhoeae* is the second

most common in this age group. It is therefore essential to treat for both agents when the diagnosis of epididymitis is suspected.

QUICK QUIZ: UROLOGY

What is the most common agent causing epididymitis in a 55-year-old male?

A) *E. coli.*
B) *Neisseria gonorrhoeae.*
C) *Chlamydia trachomatis.*
D) *Pseudomonas* species.
E) *Ureaplasma urealyticum.*

Discussion

The correct answer is A. Gram-negative rods are the most common cause of epididymitis in older men. Of these, *E. coli* is the most common etiologic agent, followed by *Klebsiella* and *Pseudomonas* species.

CASE 17

A 22-year-old white female college student presents to the ED with dysuria and urinary frequency of 2-days duration. She denies any abdominal/pelvic pain, flank pain, hematuria, fever, chills, vaginal discharge, nausea, vomiting, or diarrhea. Her LMP was 2 weeks ago and she is not sexually active. She is on oral contraceptives to treat menstrual cramps and denies any allergies. Her past medical history is negative. She states she has never been sexually active.

A urine beta-HCG is NOT indicated for which of the following patients who presents with abdominal pain?

A) A 32-year-old female who has had a tubal ligation.
B) A 16-year-old female who by history has never been sexually active.
C) A 25-year-old female who has had a normal period 1 week ago and states she couldn't possibly be pregnant.
D) A 24-year-old, married, professional female who is taking oral contraceptives and had a normal last menses.
E) A 25-year-old male.

Discussion

The correct answer is E. Of course males do not need a pregnancy test (although the HCG may be elevated in testicular cancer). All female patients of reproductive age, except for those who have had a hysterectomy, must have a pregnancy test as part of the evaluation of abdominal pain. There are several reasons for this position. First, many patients may not be candid about their sexual activity. In fact, in one study, almost 33% of patients who said they could not possibly be pregnant, including one who denied ever having intercourse, were pregnant. Second, the failure rate of tubal ligation is up to 3% over 10 years depending on the technique used (laparoscopic tubal ligation is the least reliable). And, almost all of the pregnancies in patients who have had a tubal ligation are ectopic.

 HELPFUL TIP: When examining a patient whose history is consistent with vulvovaginitis, remember that a KOH preparation is only 65% to 80% sensitive for *Candida* and treatment based on symptoms and physical findings is certainly reasonable.

* *

You get a urinalysis on this patient, mostly out of habit. The UA shows 5–10 WBCs/HPF, 2 + bacteria, 2 + leukocyte esterase, and 1 + nitrite.

Which of the following antibiotic regimens IS NOT indicated for the treatment of simple cystitis?

A) 3-day course of trimethoprim-sulfamethoxazole (TMP-SMX).
B) 3-day course of a fluoroquinolone.
C) 7-day course of nitrofurantoin.
D) Single dose of fosfomycin.
E) Single dose of cephalexin.

Discussion

The correct answer is E. The usual causative agents for uncomplicated cystitis are Gram-negative organisms such as *E. coli*. In areas that have high rates of resistance to TMP-SMX (≥30% of isolated *E. coli* bacteria resistant), it is wise to use a quinolone as the first line agent; however, quinolones are more costly. All of the above regimens are usually effective for treating cystitis except a single dose of cephalexin. Cephalexin is effectively used in pregnant females, although a 7-day course is recommended. Fosfomycin has a lower cure rate than the other regimens and is more expensive; therefore, it is not generally recommended.

All of the following patients with pyelonephritis should be admitted EXCEPT:

A) 22-year-old G1 P0 female <24 weeks pregnant, but hemodynamically stable.
B) 22-year-old female unable to tolerate PO fluids or medications.
C) 22-year-old female with unreliable social situation and/or compliance.
D) 22-year-old female with an unclear diagnosis or extreme pain.

Discussion

The correct answer is A. The old adage that all pregnant patients with pyelonephritis must be admitted has gone out of favor. It is safe to send patients home who are <24 weeks' gestation, compliant, have stable vital signs, and are accessible by telephone. Patients should be given clear instructions to return for any complications. All of the other situations require in-hospital care.

Objectives: Did you learn to . . .

- Decide which patients should have a urine beta-HCG in the ED?
- Provide appropriate antibiotic treatment to a patient with an uncomplicated UTI?
- Identify patients with pyelonephritis who require hospital admission?

CASE 18

A 63-year-old male presents to the ED with a 2-day history of fever, urinary frequency, dysuria, and difficulty initiating the urinary stream. He also relates having some perineal pain. On exam, his vitals are stable except for a temperature of 102°F. His rectal exam is remarkable for a tender, warm, edematous prostate. There are no perirectal masses and the stool is heme-negative. He has no penile lesions, discharge, scrotal masses, or tenderness. He does not exhibit any costovertebral angle tenderness. His UA is positive for 10 WBCs/HPF, 1 + nitrite, 1 + leukocyte esterase.

What is the most likely diagnosis in this patient?

A) Pyelonephritis.
B) Perirectal abscess.
C) Epididymitis.
D) Acute prostatitis.
E) Cystitis.

Discussion

The correct answer is D. This patient's symptoms most closely fit those of someone with acute prostatitis. Although his urinalysis is also consistent with pyelonephritis or cystitis, his exam findings are more suggestive of acute prostatitis; he lacks costovertebral angle tenderness (pyelonephritis) and he has a significant temperature, which argues against a simple cystitis. In the past, prostatic massage was recommended when obtaining a urine specimen; this practice is to be avoided since it is quite painful and bacterial seeding into the bloodstream may occur. In the absence of scrotal tenderness, epididymitis is also quite unlikely.

What should be included in the treatment regimen for this patient?

A) Oral fluoroquinolone or TMP-SMX for 21–30 days.
B) Instructions for hydration, sitz baths, stool softeners, NSAIDs.
C) Admission for IV antibiotics if patient appears toxic or hemodynamically unstable.
D) Foley or suprapubic catheter if urinary retention is a problem.
E) All of the above.

Discussion

The correct answer is E. Patients with acute prostatitis should be treated for 21–30 days with PO antibiotics to prevent chronic prostatitis. Treatment should be initiated with a quinolone while urine cultures are pending, since sulfa resistance is high in some areas of the country.

* *

While this patient is still in the ED, he develops acute urinary retention. A Foley catheter is placed without difficulty and 300 cc of slightly cloudy urine is obtained. Your patient feels much better and thanks you for alleviating his pain. You decide to discharge him home with the Foley catheter and a leg bag after discussion with a urologist and scheduling follow-up.

Which of the following IS NOT a cause of urinary retention?

A) Phimosis, urethral stricture, BPH, calculi.
B) Anticholinergics, sympathomimetics, narcotics, antipsychotics.
C) Psychogenic.
D) Cauda equina syndrome, diabetes, spinal cord injuries, herpes.
E) All of the above can cause urinary retention.

Discussion

The correct answer is E. All of the above can cause urinary retention in men. The most common cause of acute urinary retention by far is BPH. The categories of acute urinary retention may be divided into neurogenic (spinal cord injuries, cauda equina syndrome, diabetes, syringomyelia, herpes, etc), obstructive (BPH, phimosis, paraphimosis, calculi, urethral stricture, etc), pharmacologic (anticholinergics, antihistamines, narcotics, antipsychotics, tricyclics, etc), and psychogenic, which is a diagnosis of exclusion.

 HELPFUL TIP: Sending patients home on an α-blocker (eg, doxazosin) may reduce the need for recatheterization after the catheter is removed.

Objectives: Did you learn to . . .

- Recognize the clinical presentation of prostatitis?
- Treat a patient with prostatitis?
- Identify causes of urinary retention in a male?

 QUICK QUIZ: UROLOGY

Which of the following is characterized by a swollen, painful foreskin which cannot be reduced back to its normal position?

A) Phimosis.
B) Paraphimosis.
C) Balanoposthitis.
D) Meatal stenosis.

Discussion

The correct answer is B. Paraphimosis is a condition in which the foreskin is retracted, swollen, and unable to reduce into its normal position. Ice and steady manual compression often permit reduction. Surgery is indicated if manual reduction fails. Phimosis (answer A) is a condition in which the distal foreskin is too tight to be retracted to allow exposure of the glans. It is often confused with penile adhesions in males <2 years. Balanoposthitis (answer C) is a form of cellulitis involving the foreskin and glans in the uncircumcised male, associated with poor hygiene. Treatment is with warm soaks, antibiotics, and possible circumcision. Meatal stenosis (answer D) is common in circumcised males, associated with an inflammatory reaction involving the meatus. Symptoms that indicate the need for surgical treatment include spraying of the urine stream or dorsal deflection of the stream.

 QUICK QUIZ: UROLOGY

Until what age is it normal to have adhesions between the glans and foreskin in uncircumcised males?

A) Adhesions are always abnormal.
B) 6 months.
C) 1 year.
D) 2 years.
E) 3 years.

Discussion

The correct answer is E. Some adhesions are normal in males <3 years. However, the foreskin should be fully retractable in uncircumcised males aged 3–5 years. Before this, no action need be taken.

CASE 19

A 20-year-old female presents to your ED complaining of lower quadrant abdominal pain. She is on "the patch" for contraception and has been faithfully using it. She has had regular menses and has not noticed any change in her pattern of menses. Her pain had a sudden onset but is not associated with any vaginal bleeding. On vaginal exam, you find marked cervical motion tenderness but no palpable adnexal mass.

Based on this information you decide that:

A) The absence of an adnexal mass effectively rules out ectopic pregnancy.
B) If a patient becomes pregnant, all forms of contraception reduce the risk of ectopic pregnancy.
C) The fact the patient has had normal periods effectively rules out an ectopic pregnancy.
D) Cervical motion tenderness effectively clinches the diagnosis of pelvic inflammatory disease.
E) None of the above is true.

Discussion

The answer is E. None of the above is true. Answer A is incorrect because only 10% of patients with an ectopic pregnancy will have a palpable mass in the adnexa. Answer B is incorrect because both IUD and tubal ligation **increase** the risk of ectopic pregnancy if the patient becomes pregnant. Answer C is incorrect because 15% to 20% of patients with ectopic pregnancy have no history of missed menses. Answer D is incorrect because cervical motion tenderness can be present not only in PID but also in other illnesses such as ovarian torsion, ectopic pregnancy, etc.

Risk factors for ectopic pregnancy include all of the following EXCEPT:

A) Prior ectopic pregnancy.
B) History of pelvic inflammatory disease.
C) Treatment for infertility.
D) Older age.
E) Oral contraceptive use.

Discussion

The correct answer is E. All of the others increase the risk of an ectopic pregnancy. Other risk factors include cigarette smoking, recent elective abortion, IUD, and tubal ligation.

* *

You decide that this patient may have an ectopic pregnancy. A urine HCG test is positive for pregnancy.

The significance of a positive pregnancy test is that:

A) An ultrasound will be able to detect an ectopic pregnancy if one is present.
B) The serum level of HCG is at least 1,000 IU/L.
C) Combined with the patient's abdominal pain and cervical motion tenderness, it effectively rules in an ectopic pregnancy.
D) The urine HCG is 98% sensitive for pregnancy 7 days after implantation.

Discussion

The correct answer is D. Answer A is incorrect. The pregnancy test is positive very early and ultrasound may not be positive by an experienced operator until 6 weeks' gestation. Answer B is incorrect. The urine may be positive at serum HCG levels of 25–50 IU/L. Patients do not have an HCG level of 1,000 IU/L until 6 weeks of pregnancy. Answer C is incorrect because patients with a normal pregnancy may also have abdominal pain and cervical motion tenderness.

* *

The patient's serum HCG is 440 IU/L. You order an ultrasound and find no evidence of an intrauterine **or** ectopic pregnancy.

Your next step is to:

A) Reassure the patient that she does not have an ectopic pregnancy.
B) Recheck the HCG in 48 hours.
C) Refer for a laparoscopy to rule out ectopic pregnancy.
D) Recheck an HCG in 1–2 weeks.
E) Follow the patient clinically.

Discussion

The correct answer is B. The HCG should double in a normal pregnancy every 1.8–3 days. If the HCG **is not** doubling in this time frame, it is likely an ectopic pregnancy. Remember, the fact that you did not see an ectopic pregnancy on ultrasound is irrelevant. The HCG is generally **at least** 1,000 IU/L before anything is seen on ultrasound. By an HCG of 6,000 IU/L, you should certainly be able to see a pregnancy on ultrasound. Answer A is incorrect for the above reasons. Answer C is incorrect. This is invasive and not needed. Answer D is incorrect because of the time frame; the HCG should be rechecked in 24–48 hours. An ectopic may well rupture within 1–2 weeks. Answer E is incorrect. If you follow the patient clinically, you are basically saying that you will wait until the ectopic ruptures before addressing the problem.

You recheck the HCG in 48 hours and it is now 1,000 IU/L (prior level 440 IU/L). Your interpretation is that:

A) This patient does not likely have an ectopic pregnancy.
B) This patient has a molar pregnancy.
C) This patient has a blighted ovum.
D) The patient has fetal demise of an IUP.
E) All of the above are possible.

Discussion

The correct answer is A. Since the HCG doubled normally, it is **not** likely that this is an ectopic pregnancy, a blighted ovum (answer C), or intrauterine fetal demise (answer D). In all of these conditions, the HCG

would not double. Answer B is incorrect because in a molar pregnancy, the HCG would rise precipitously.

Objectives: Did you learn to ...

- Evaluate a fertile female who has pelvic pain?
- Diagnose and manage an ectopic pregnancy?

QUICK QUIZ: EMERGENCY MEDICINES: OVARIAN TORSION

Which of the following is typical of ovarian torsion?

A) Periumbilical pain gradually migrating to both the right and left quadrants.
B) Sudden onset of colicky abdominal pain in one of the lower quadrants.
C) Sudden onset of colicky abdominal pain with vaginal bleeding.
D) All of the above can be presentations of ovarian torsion.

Discussion

The correct answer is B. Patients with ovarian torsion present with sudden onset of severe lower abdominal pain. The pain is frequently colicky. Since only one ovary is involved, the pain is located in one side or the other. Spontaneous torsion/detorsion may also occur so that the pain may remit spontaneously. Ovarian torsion can be diagnosed by Doppler ultrasound, which examines flow to the ovaries.

CASE 20

A middle-aged unresponsive, disheveled patient is brought by EMS to your ED. The EMS had been called by the patient's girlfriend, who had seen him lying in the grass outside his home this morning. He has spontaneous respirations and has a pulse.

What should be your first steps in assessment and treatment?

A) Oxygen by non-rebreather mask, stat serum glucose, naloxone.
B) Oxygen by non-rebreather mask, ECG, Head CT.
C) Oxygen by non-rebreather mask, intubate, ECG, head CT.
D) Intubate, ECG, head CT.

Discussion

The correct answer is A. There are several causes of unresponsiveness that can be immediately corrected. A helpful algorithm to recall in the initial treatment for an unresponsive patient is "DON'T": **D**extrose, **O**xygen, **N**aloxone, **T**hiamine. Answer A is correct because naloxone and oxygen are administered and a glucose is checked. If rapid blood sugar is unavailable, empirical administration of dextrose would be appropriate. Rapid treatment of hypoxia, hypoglycemia, and narcotic overdose can improve mental status and thus avoid intubation. ECG and head CT may be indicated later in the evaluation.

* *

The patient is found to be hypothermic, hypoglycemic, and hypoxic. He is placed on oxygen and given warm normal saline, an amp of D50W, and naloxone. The patient now is saturating at 98% on non-rebreather mask (NRB). He is responding to painful stimuli by moaning and withdrawing his extremities but is not opening his eyes; he still has no gag reflex.

What is your next step?

A) Intubate.
B) Obtain head CT.
C) Obtain ECG.
D) Obtain blood cultures.
E) Admit to the ICU.

Discussion

The correct answer is A. Although the patient has improved and has a normal oxygen saturation, his level of consciousness is still too low to protect his airway. Thus, he should be intubated before further diagnostic studies are performed. A simple method to determine need for intubation is the Glasgow Coma Scale (see Table 1–5). Patients with a GCS of 8 or less should be intubated as they cannot protect their airway from aspiration of oral secretions and/or emesis. The rhyme "GCS of 8, intubate" assists in recollection of this rule. This patient has a GCS of 7 (eyes 1, verbal 2, movement 4) and therefore should be intubated before other studies or admission.

* *

The patient's girlfriend arrives and gives further history that he is an alcoholic and had told her he had quit drinking 2 days prior. She states he has had a seizure in the past when he stops drinking. He starts to seize before your eyes.

What should you do now?

A) Give lorazepam and admit for probable delirium tremens (DTs).
B) Give lorazepam, obtain a head CT, blood cultures, and ECG.
C) Give lorazepam, extubate, and admit for probable DTs.
D) Give phenytoin and admit for probable DTs.
E) Give lorazepam, obtain head CT and ECG.

Discussion

The correct answer is B. Even though it is easy to assume the patient had a seizure from DTs which may have resulted in hypoxia, hypothermia, and hypoglycemia, this kind of thinking can lead to errors. It is still possible that the patient has a spontaneous or traumatic brain hemorrhage. It is also possible that the patient is septic; remember that hypothermia can be seen with sepsis. Thus, blood cultures should be obtained and possibly an LP performed. Finally, an ECG can show a myocardial infarction or arrhythmia that may also result in seizure. Answer D is incorrect because phenytoin is not the drug of choice for an actively seizing patient; a benzodiazepine such as lorazepam should be administered. Answer C is incorrect. The patient still has a GCS of less than 8 and is unable to protect his airway so he should not be extubated.

Objectives: Did you learn to . . .

- Rapidly assess and treat an unresponsive patient?
- Use the GCS to determine need for intubation?
- Assess and treat a seizing patient?

CASE 21

You are working in a rural ED and get a call that the volunteer fire service is bringing an unresponsive, adult male patient status post MVC. They bring the patient on a backboard with a c-collar.

The primary survey of a trauma patient includes all of the following EXCEPT:

A) Check for pulses.
B) Immobilize the c-spine.
C) Glasgow Coma Scale.
D) Abdominal exam.
E) Unclothe the patient.

Discussion

The correct answer is D—what you do **not** want to do in the primary survey. The primary survey is the initial evaluation performed on each trauma patient as specified by the algorithm ABCDE: **A**irway assessment includes c-spine immobilization, opening the airway by jaw thrust/chin lift, and when indicated, intubation, bag-valve mask or cricothyrotomy. **B**reathing includes listening for breath sounds, administering oxygen, and treating pneumothoraces. **C**irculation requires assessment of blood pressure by checking pulses and treatment of hypotension and tachycardia with crystalloids and blood. **D**isability is the rapid neurologic exam for potential cord injury and GCS. **E**xposure involves disrobing the patient and rolling him or her to assess any injury to the back.

* *

On the primary survey, the patient was not protecting his airway and was intubated with an 8 Fr endotracheal tube (ETT) with rapid sequence intubation. The patient is noted to have breath sounds on the right but no breath sounds on the left.

What is the next best step in evaluation and treatment of this patient?

A) Remove the ETT; you must be in the esophagus
B) Get a chest x-ray to confirm tube placement
C) Do needle decompression of left chest
D) Insert a left chest tube
E) Check ETT for depth at the teeth and position.

Discussion

The correct answer is E. This patient has breath sounds on the right; therefore, esophageal intubation is unlikely, making answer A incorrect. The most likely and easily recognizable source of absent breath sounds on the left is a right main stem intubation. Thus, looking at the depth of placement of the ETT at the teeth (answer E) is the initial evaluation indicated. The ETT should be placed at about 3 times the size of the ETT ($3 \times 8 = 24$ cm) assuming that the size of ETT was correctly chosen. This is an important calculation to remember as it also applies to pediatric patients. A chest x-ray can also evaluate for right main stem intubation but should not be the first step. A pneumothorax may be the cause of unilateral breath sounds, but right main stem intubation should be considered first.

* *

You now note that there is an open chest wound to the left lateral rib cage that you didn't notice before. What is the initial treatment of this new finding?

A) Needle thoracostomy.
B) Chest tube placement.
C) Occlusive dressing.
D) Chest x-ray.

Discussion

The correct answer is C. This patient has an open "sucking" chest wound. Each time the patient inspires, air can be sucked into the chest cavity acting as a one-way valve. This can result in a tension pneumothorax. Thus, apply an occlusive dressing to the wound (eg, petrolatum gauze).

* *

The patient continues to have absence of breath sounds on the left, is hypotensive, and has distended neck veins. The presumed diagnosis is a tension pneumothorax.

What should you do now?

A) Chest x-ray.
B) Chest tube placement through wound.
C) Chest tube placement through separate site.
D) Remove occlusive dressing.

Discussion

The correct answer is D. The occlusive dressing itself may cause a tension pneumothorax, so its placement should be followed immediately by chest tube placement. If a tension pneumothorax develops before the tube is placed, removing the dressing can usually alleviate the tension component. EMS will often place a dressing that is closed only on three sides to serve as a release valve and avoid this possibility. The diagnosis of tension pneumothorax is clinical. The time required to obtain a chest x-ray may result in the death of the patient. When placing a chest tube in a patient with an open wound, never pass the tube through the wound as it is likely to follow the path of the initial penetration into lung parenchyma.

 HELPFUL TIP: Needle thoracostomy is also useful in a tension pneumothorax and is the treatment in most cases.

* *

The patient now has a chest tube in place but remains hypotensive. Two large-bore (18-gauge or larger) IVs were established. No external source of bleeding is identified.

When should blood be administered?

A) Immediately.
B) If persistent hypotension after 1 L of normal saline.
C) If persistent hypotension after 2 L of normal saline.
D) If persistent hypotension after 4 L of normal saline.
E) If FAST exam shows intraabdominal free fluid.

Discussion

The correct answer is C. If a patient arrives hypotensive with no signs of external bleeding, 2 L of crystalloid (normal saline) should be given immediately. If the patient continues to be hypotensive, packed red blood cells should be started along with additional normal saline. The FAST exam is a rapid bedside ultrasound to identify free fluid in the trauma patient's abdomen and pericardial sac. Persistent hypotension with positive FAST exam is an indication for emergent exploratory laparotomy.

Which of the following findings is a contraindication to placing a Foley catheter in this male trauma victim?

A) Rectal blood.
B) Blood at the urethral meatus.
C) Penile erection.
D) All of the above are contraindications.

Discussion

The correct answer is B. Contraindications to Foley placement in the trauma patient include: high riding, soft boggy prostate; blood at the urethral meatus; perineal hematoma. A retrograde urethrogram should be performed prior to Foley placement to assess urethral injury. Penile erection is not a contraindication and is suggestive of a spinal cord injury. Rectal blood and vaginal bleeding do not indicate urethral injury but should be noted in the secondary survey.

Objectives: Did you learn to . . .

- Employ the primary assessment of a trauma patient?
- Treat an open chest wound?
- Resuscitate an unstable trauma patient?
- Describe the contraindications to Foley placement in a trauma patient?

 QUICK QUIZ: CHEST PAIN

A 54-year-old female presents to your ED with a chief complaint of chest pain. She states it came on suddenly while she was working in her garden. She describes it as "sharp" and it radiates through to her back. She reports difficulty breathing. Her past medical history is pertinent for hypertension, breast cancer, and obesity. She is a smoker.

Based on this history, what diagnosis can be excluded from your differential?

A) Acute myocardial infarction.
B) Aortic dissection.
C) Pulmonary embolism.
D) Pneumothorax.
E) None of the above.

Discussion

The correct answer is E. The patient's history is most suggestive of pulmonary embolism with her complaint of sharp chest pain, trouble breathing, cancer history, and smoking. However, at this point in time, all of the etiologies listed—and more—must be considered. Women often have atypical presentations of cardiac chest pain. In addition, patients often use the term "sharp" to describe intense or strong pain.

 QUICK QUIZ: AORTIC DISSECTION

In aortic dissection, the blood pressure is different between the extremities in 15%.

What limb should you use to guide blood pressure management?

A) Right arm.
B) Left arm.
C) Either lower extremity.
D) The limb with the highest BP.
E) The limb with the lowest BP.

Discussion

The correct answer is D. An aortic dissection may impair the blood flow to certain extremities due to the false lumen. The blood pressure should be maintained at or below normal (SBP 120) in the extremity with the highest BP. This will decrease the forces propagating the dissection.

HELPFUL TIP: Patients with an aortic dissection should be started on a β-blocker and vasodilator drip (nitroglycerin, nitroprusside) to control blood pressure and minimize stress to the aortic wall.

CASE 22

A mother brings her 3-year-old child to the ED. She states that the child has been vomiting and complaining of abdominal pain all afternoon. He has had between 15 and 20 episodes of emesis; the last 2 have contained small amounts of bright red blood. He has had a little nonbloody diarrhea. He has not been tolerating fluids and is beginning to look a little listless. On exam you find the child to be ill appearing with normal color, but he seems less alert and interactive than you would expect. His vitals reveal a temperature of 36.5°C, a pulse of 170, a respiratory rate of 28, and a blood pressure of 98/58.

His abdomen is slightly and diffusely tender. He has dry mucous membranes.

In general (not specifically in this patient) what is the initial treatment of a moderately dehydrated child?

A) 20 cc/kg bolus of D5 1/2NS.
B) 10 cc/kg bolus of isotonic crystalloid fluid.
C) Oral challenge of a small amount of electrolyte solution.
D) 12.5 mg promethazine suppository.

Discussion

The correct answer is C. Many children who are vomiting and have diarrhea will be able to tolerate small (5 cc) sips of fluid administered every few minutes. Oral fluids should be attempted prior to IV therapy. In children who are severely dehydrated, as evidenced by altered mental status or change in skin turgor, IV fluid resuscitation should begin immediately. If IV rehydration is considered appropriate, use normal saline in 20 cc/kg aliquots. Therefore, answers A and B are not correct. Promethazine (answer D) is an antiemetic that has been used in children in the past. However, promethazine has received a "black box" warning from the FDA for children <2 years, as there is a risk of respiratory depression.

* *

You obtain some lab work and notice that the child has normal renal function but low serum bicarbonate, indicating a possible metabolic acidosis. In speaking with his mother, you discover that earlier in the day he was playing unsupervised in the bathroom, where she keeps her prenatal vitamins. Upon questioning the child, he states that he ate a bunch of "candy" in the bathroom (about 3 hours ago).

What component of prenatal vitamins is most concerning for toxicity?

A) Folic acid.
B) Iron.
C) Calcium.
D) Vitamin D.

Discussion

The correct answer is B. Iron can continue to be absorbed while it remains in the GI tract. Iron is a direct irritant to the gastrointestinal mucosa and interferes with the electron transport chain and aerobic metabolism. Folic acid, calcium, and vitamin D are all well tolerated in high doses, as their absorption from the gastrointestinal tract is limited.

The nurse asks if you should add on an iron level to the blood that was drawn 3 hours after the ingestion. You respond:

A) "No. Iron levels are not helpful."
B) "No. It's too early. We need to wait until at least 12 hours have elapsed."
C) "Yes. If it's normal, we don't need any further treatment."
D) "Yes. It may help us determine the severity of toxicity."

Discussion

The correct answer is D. The iron level between 2–4 hours after ingestion is the most accurate; beyond this period the majority of the iron is moving intracellularly and cannot be measured. For slow-release iron, serum concentrations should be measured at 6–8 hours after ingestion. These measures will give you a peak serum iron concentration that correlates well with the severity of toxicity. **However, a low serum level of iron does not mean the symptomatic patient is OK. Treatment is based on clinical findings and *not* serum iron levels.**

How do patients with iron toxicity present?

A) Abdominal pain, vomiting, and diarrhea.
B) Hematemesis, shock, and coma.
C) Relatively asymptomatic.
D) All of the above.

Discussion

The correct answer is D. Patients who have had an iron overdose classically pass through five phases. The first phase is characterized by nausea, vomiting, diarrhea, and abdominal pain. There may be hematemesis and hematochezia as the gastrointestinal mucosa becomes irritated. The second phase is a relatively asymptomatic period as the GI symptoms resolve. During this quiet phase iron is absorbed and transported to the periphery where it causes the interruption of aerobic metabolism. In the third phase, patients become hypotensive, acidotic, and can develop multisystem organ failure and coma. It is this shock that is the usual cause of death in iron toxicity. The fourth phase is heralded by hepatic necrosis. Liver failure, which does not occur in all patients, is the second most frequent cause of death in cases of iron toxicity. Finally, patients may develop bowel obstructions 2–4 weeks or longer after the ingestion due to stricture at the site of mucosal irritation (Table 1–7).

Assume the patient took iron tablets and not prenatal vitamins. What is the best next step in treatment for this patient?

A) Whole bowel irrigation with polyethylene glycol solution.
B) Gastric lavage.
C) Activated charcoal.
D) Syrup of Ipecac.

Discussion

The correct answer is A. Treatment for iron toxicity involves whole bowel irrigation with polyethylene glycol solution to flush the iron out of the GI tract. There are various doses and rates of administration published, but 10–15 mL/kg/hr, up to 2,000 cc/hr, seems to be a reasonable place to start. This requires the placement of a nasogastric tube. If a patient does not tolerate the volume of the infusion, the rate should be decreased by 50%. The irrigation should continue until the rectal effluent is clear and there are no visible pill fragments. If follow-up radiographs demonstrate persistent iron tablets in the stomach, consider the possibility of a bezoar having formed, which may require endoscopic or surgical intervention for removal. Gastric lavage and vomiting induced by syrup of Ipecac (answers B and D) are both treatments that entail a fair amount of risk. They are usually effective only if the ingestion has happened within the last hour. In addition, there is the risk of aspiration and subsequent pneumonitis. Iron, lithium, and lead will not adsorb to activated charcoal (answer C); therefore it is of no benefit in such cases.

Table 1–7   MANIFESTATIONS OF IRON TOXICITY

First phase	Hours 0–6 (rarely >6 hours)	Vomiting and diarrhea, often bloody Metabolic acidosis Shock
Second phase (silent or quiescent phase)	3–48 hours (time variable)	Resolving acidosis Resolving hypovolemia Frequently, asymptomatic
Third phase	12–48 hours (time variable)	GI hemorrhage Lethargy, coma, shock Cardiovascular collapse Metabolic acidosis Renal failure (variable)
Fourth phase	2 days or more	Hepatotoxicity Hepatic necrosis Coma
Fifth phase	2–4 weeks	GI obstruction due to strictures and scarring

HELPFUL TIP: Patients who are entirely asymptomatic from the time of supposed iron ingestion to 6 hours afterwards **and** do not have any radiographic evidence of iron in the GI tract are not at risk for toxicity. They can be safely discharged with close follow-up. The caveat is that chewable multivitamins are not radioopaque and will not show up on x-ray.

 HELPFUL TIP: The much touted "deferoxamine challenge" to see if there is free iron in the blood, it is not an accurate predictor of toxicity. The test is done by giving an individual a single challenge dose of deferoxamine and seeing if the urine changes to a "vin rosé" color reflecting circulating free iron. However, this again does not predict who needs therapy since the iron may already be working its evil in the periphery.

The patient is symptomatic (vomiting and diarrhea) and also has an iron level is 650 micrograms/dL, which puts him at significant risk for toxicity. What is your next step?

A) Correction of acid-base disturbance and aggressive fluid resuscitation.
B) EDTA.
C) Deferoxamine.
D) A and B.
E) A and C.

Discussion

The correct answer is E. In addition to symptoms and acidosis, an iron level >500 micrograms/dL or ingestion of more than 60 mg/kg of elemental iron are considered high-risk situations, and chelation with deferoxamine is warranted. Deferoxamine is used to chelate iron, while EDTA is a chelation treatment for lead poisoning. Fastidious supportive care, with correction of the patient's volume and acid-base disturbances, is imperative. Ensuring that the patient is euvolemic is especially important when using chelation therapy, given that the major side effect of deferoxamine is hypotension. The dose of deferoxamine is 15 mg/kg/hr for 24 hours, but may be slowed down if the patient becomes hypotensive.

 HELPFUL TIP: Dialysis does not remove iron from the blood stream nor the intracellular space, where the majority of it will be found. Dialysis may be indicated to treat renal failure or persistent profound acidosis.

Objectives: Did you learn to . . .

- Rehydrate a child with GI symptoms?
- Recognize the manifestations of iron poisoning?
- Manage a child with an iron ingestion?

CASE 23

A 25-day-old female newborn is brought to the ED by her parents. They state that she has not been eating well this morning and has felt warm. They got a temperature of 100.2°F with an axillary digital thermometer at home. They have not noticed any rhinorrhea, cough, or rashes. The newborn is having 5–6 wet diapers per day and 5–6 yellow seedy stools per day. She has not had any sick contacts. She slept normally last night, but was a little hard to wake up from her morning nap today. She was the 7.5-lb product of an uncomplicated term gestation, born via normal spontaneous vaginal delivery to a GBS negative mother. There were no complications in the early neonatal period and she was discharged with the mother at 2 days of life after receiving routine neonatal care. At her 2-week weight check she seemed to be gaining weight well and her doctor had no concerns.

Which of these is not a common cause of serious infections in newborns <1 month?

A) *Listeria monocytogenes.*
B) *Neisseria meningitides.*
C) Group B *streptococcus.*
D) *Pseudomonas aeruginosa.*

Discussion

The correct answer is D. *Pseudomonas* infections are not commonly seen in the neonatal period. *Listeria monocytogenes* (answer A) is an obligate intracellular anaerobe that is transmitted transplacentally from mother to newborn. *Neisseria meningitides* (answer B) is a Gram-negative diplococcus that colonizes the respiratory tract of up to 15% of healthy individuals. It is usually spread through close contact. Group B *streptococcus* (GBS) (answer C) is a Gram-positive organism that colonizes the genital tract of normal healthy women. GBS may be the most common cause of bacterial infection in the newborn. The peak incidence of GBS disease is in the first 7 days of life, but there may be a delayed presentation out to 30 days.

HELPFUL TIP: Look carefully for cold sores or other vesicular lesions on newborns with rashes. Also try to get a history of any close contacts between the patient and people with cold sores. Herpesvirus infection can be devastating to newborns, and they may require treatment with acyclovir.

* *

The newborn is seen in her father's arms. She appears to have normal color and tone. She is sleeping, but arouses after some stimulation. She seems fussy, but can be consoled by her parents. She appears to be well-hydrated, and has a completely normal physical exam. Vitals: temperature 38.1°C rectally, pulse 165, respiratory rate 32.

What further evaluation is indicated now?

A) Complete blood count, blood cultures, catheterized urine for analysis and culture.
B) Complete blood count, blood cultures, bag urine for analysis and culture.
C) Complete blood count, blood cultures, chest radiograph, catheterized urine for analysis and culture.
D) Complete blood count, blood cultures, catheterized urine for analysis and culture, lumbar puncture.

Discussion

The correct answer is D. It is important that a complete evaluation and septic workup be performed on all infants <2 months without a definite source of infection. This includes complete blood count, blood cultures, catheterized urine specimens for analysis and culture, and a lumbar puncture. A chest x-ray need not be done in the patient without respiratory symptoms. LP is mandatory. Even if you suspect a pneumonia or urinary tract infection, a lumbar puncture should still be considered, as it is impossible to tell if the bacteria have spread hematogenously to the meningeal space.

HELPFUL TIP: Do not delay antibiotic therapy to obtain a lumbar puncture. Lumbar punctures performed within 2–4 hours of receiving antibiotics should still yield valid results.

HELPFUL TIP: Some would argue that a bag urine should be done as the initial urine exam. While not as specific as a cath urine, bag urine is more sensitive for UTI. If the bag UA comes back positive, a cath specimen should be sent for culture.

You are awaiting lab results. Should you play World of Warcraft or start antibiotics? You decide to start antibiotics. Which antibiotics are most appropriate for empiric therapy in this patient?

A) Ampicillin and gentamicin.
B) Ceftriaxone.
C) Valacyclovir.
D) Amoxicillin with or without clavulanate.
E) Any of the above are equally valid choices.

Discussion

The correct answer is A. Ampicillin and gentamicin cover all of the common causes of serious bacterial infection in the newborn, and both antibiotics penetrate into the cerebrospinal fluid (CSF) well. Ceftriaxone also penetrates the CSF well, but is highly bound to albumin and may displace bilirubin that has already bound. There have been case reports of kernicterus following the administration of ceftriaxone in newborns, so its use is not recommended in children <1 month. If there is concern for a herpesvirus infection, acyclovir IV would be preferred over valacyclovir, but neither of these is used on an empiric basis routinely. Amoxicillin, with or without clavulanate, does not provide adequate CSF penetration.

What is the appropriate disposition for this patient?

A) Admission to the general pediatrics floor.
B) Admission to the pediatric intensive care unit.
C) Monitor for 3 hours in the ED, and decide based on laboratory results.
D) Discharge with 24-hour follow-up.

Discussion

The correct answer is A. This patient does not look toxic and can probably be managed appropriately on a general pediatrics floor instead of in an intensive care unit. This patient should be admitted, regardless of what the laboratory results demonstrate. Some experienced practitioners will discharge a nontoxic febrile patient from the ED if he/she is >3 months and has follow-up within 24 hours. However, there is some risk inherent in this practice—namely that deterioration in the patient's condition may go unrecognized at home and that the family will fail to follow up. The standard of care is to admit all patients who have a fever when they are ≤1 month.

 HELPFUL TIP: With the advent of the polyvalent pneumococcal vaccine and the implementation of universal screening for group B streptococcus, the incidence of occult serious bacterial infection is falling. It may be that in the near future, the way in which febrile infants <3 months are evaluated and treated will change. However, the practice outlined in Table 1–8 represents the current standard of care.

Table 1–8 CURRENT RECOMMENDATIONS FOR EVALUATING THE FEBRILE CHILD

Age	Evaluation Procedures
<28 days	• These neonates are assumed to have bacteremia and potential seeding of the CSF, even if a source is discovered. • Workup should include cultures of blood, urine, CSF, and stool (if GI symptoms present), and CXR (if respiratory symptoms present). • CBC and/or CRP can be obtained, but the decision about whether or not to proceed with evaluation should not be based on these results. • Neonates should be admitted for IV antibiotics until cultures are negative.

1–3 months	• It is safest to assume that infants are still unable to contain bacterial infections at this age.
	• Infants at low-risk of having a serious bacterial infection have the following labs:
	  • WBC <15,000/mm^3 with band count <1,500/mm^3
	  • Normal urinalysis
	  • Normal CSF
	  • Stool microscopy <5 WBC/HPF if diarrhea present
	• If no source is found on exam, it is reasonable for infants who meet these low-risk criteria to be managed with intramuscular ceftriaxone in the ED/clinic—if follow-up can be arranged to receive a second dose in 24 hours.
	• It should be emphasized that these infants are still vulnerable to dissemination of bacterial infections. Therefore, those with an obvious source, those who appear clinically ill, or those who do not meet the low risk criteria should be cultured and admitted for IV antibiotics until cultures are negative.

3–36 months	• Management of fever in this age group is somewhat controversial, as the advent of Prevnar (pneumococcal vaccine) and continued use of HIB vaccine will presumably reduce the risk of invasive bacterial disease. • It is generally accepted that well-appearing infants who have temperature <39°C do not require further evaluation or antibiotics. • Up to 5% of infants who have temperature >39°C and who appear clinically well will have positive blood cultures (occult bacteremia), putting them at risk for serious infections. One approach is to obtain screening WBC on those who have temperature >39°C. If WBC >15,000/mm^3 or bands >1,500/mm^3, then further evaluation of blood, urine, and CSF should be considered.

HELPFUL TIP: Even when present, otitis media **is not** considered a source of fever when evaluating the neonate. You should continue with your clinical and laboratory evaluation as if you did not even see the ears!

Objectives: Did you learn to . . .

- Describe common infections in the early neonatal period?
- Evaluate the febrile newborn?
- Manage the febrile newborn?

CASE 24

A 6-month-old male is brought to the ED by his father. His father states that he was doing well earlier this morning, but that a few hours ago he began coughing and seemed to be having some difficulty breathing. He has had a little bit of rhinorrhea for the last 36 hours but no fevers. He has been taking his bottle and rice cereal well. His father states that there have been no changes in his stools. He is fully vaccinated, has no significant past medical history, and has had no known sick contacts.

What is the most common cause of respiratory distress in a 6-month-old?

A) Pneumonia.
B) Foreign body aspiration.
C) Bronchiolitis.
D) Second-hand smoke exposure.

Discussion

The correct answer is C. Bronchiolitis is very common, especially in the winter months. It is usually caused by the respiratory syncytial virus, but can also be caused by parainfluenza, influenza, and human metapneumovirus. Bronchiolitis is usually associated with profuse rhinorrhea, bronchospasm, and mucus plugging of the bronchiole tree. Although pneumonia is a serious cause of respiratory problems, it is not terribly common in infants. Foreign body aspiration is something that always must be considered in an infant, especially a 6-month-old who is becoming more mobile. Second-hand smoke exposure can cause chronic irritation to the respiratory tract and can exacerbate bronchospasm, but it is infrequently the sole cause of respiratory distress.

What is the most serious complication of bronchiolitis?

A) Subconjunctival hemorrhage from severe cough.
B) Decreased oral intake as a result of nasal congestion.
C) Increased risk of developing asthma later in childhood.
D) Apnea.

Discussion

The correct answer is D. All of the possible answers are complications of bronchiolitis. But, in our opinion, apnea is the worst.

* *

Because you are a physician who always likes to be prepared, you calculate the size of endotracheal tube you would need in the event that you would have to intubate this infant if he was to get worse suddenly.

What size endotracheal tube would you want to have ready?

A) 3.0 and 3.5 uncuffed.
B) 3.0 and 3.5 cuffed.
C) 4.0 and 4.5 uncuffed.
D) B or C.

Discussion

The correct answer is D. Luckily, most EDs now employ a length-based guide to estimating children's weight, such as the Broselow-Luten tape. This guide usually lists the appropriate doses for emergency drugs, Foley catheter sizes, chest tube sizes, nasogastric tube sizes, appropriate laryngoscope blade sizes, and endotracheal tube sizes. However, it is good to have a backup system in case such a guide is unavailable.

A good formula to remember is the child's age in years added to 16, with the sum divided by 4 ([Age + 16]/4). In this case, with a 6-month-old infant, the result would be between 4 and 4.5, meaning that you should be ready with 4.0 and 4.5 uncuffed endotracheal tubes. It is also a good practice to have the next size smaller available. In the past, the dogma has been that only uncuffed endotracheal tubes should be used in children <8 years. However, it is now acceptable to use cuffed endotracheal tubes in small children if you subtract 1 from the size of the uncuffed endotracheal tubes.

* *

As you examine the infant, you note that he is mildly tachypneic with some suprasternal, subcostal, and intercostal retractions. He makes a wheezing whistling sound on inspiration that seems to get worse the harder he breathes. He also has a brassy-sounding cough that does not seem to be productive.

What is the most likely diagnosis at this point?

A) Pneumonia.
B) Croup.
C) Laryngomalacia.
D) Asthma.

Discussion

The correct answer is B. Croup, or laryngotracheo-bronchitis, is a common infection of the upper and lower respiratory tract. It is most commonly caused by parainfluenza virus, but may also be caused by influenza and respiratory syncytial virus. Classically, this affects children <5 years, although it is occasionally seen in older children. As the glottis swells, children develop a wheeze/whistle on inspiration and a characteristic brassy "seal-like" barking cough. The vast majority of cases are mild. Occasionally, however, children may require control of the airway due to hypoxia. Answer A, pneumonia, is an infection of the lower airways that can be either bacterial or viral in nature. These children generally have a fever and productive cough. They may be tachypneic and have an increased work of breathing, but they usually do not have inspiratory stridor. Answer C, laryngomalacia, is a congenital disorder where the epiglottis is unusually large and more flimsy than normal. These children usually develop symptoms at a few weeks of age and present with inspiratory stridor that gets worse with crying. It tends to be a little better when the child is calm and in the supine position. Laryngo-malacia resolves spontaneously in the majority of children as the epiglottis becomes more firm and the airway diameter increases, but some children will require surgical intervention to facilitate feeding and growth. The child in this vignette is presenting with a new problem, as opposed to a chronic one, so this is not laryngomalacia. Answer D, asthma, is another disease of the lower airways, and wheezing is expiratory in nature.

* *

You decide to do a radiograph of this child's neck to aid in the diagnosis (although this is certainly not necessary or advocated in most cases—but this is a board review book, not real life).

You are most likely to see which of the following on cervical radiograph?

A) Thumb sign.
B) Sign of Lesser-Trélat.
C) Spine sign.
D) Retropharyngeal space swelling.
E) Steeple sign.

Discussion

The correct answer is E. Radiographs in croup show the "steeple sign," which is a subglottic narrowing of the trachea from edema, giving it a steeple-like appearance. Answer A, the thumb sign, is seen in epiglottitis. Answer B, the sign of Lesser-Trélat, is the sudden development of numerous seborrheic keratoses in a patient with internal malignancy—it is rare, not seen in children. Answer C, the spine sign, is loss of progressive radiolucency of the spine on lateral chest radiograph. This is seen when something—classically an infiltrate indicative of pneumonia—is overlaying the lower thoracic spine making the vertebral bodies appear denser. Answer D, retropharyngeal space swelling, is seen in retropharyngeal abscess.

What is the most appropriate definitive therapy for this patient at this time?

A) Epinephrine 0.01 mg **SQ**.
B) Nebulized albuterol.
C) Dexamethasone 0.6 mg/kg PO/IM/IV.
D) High-flow oxygen and prepare to intubate.

Discussion

The correct answer is C. Corticosteroids help decrease the glottic edema. One dose of dexamethasone 0.3–0.6 mg/kg (maximum of 10 mg) can be given via multiple routes (PO/IM/IV) and is usually sufficient to improve the airway swelling enough to allow the child to breathe comfortably. The advantage of dexamethasone over prednisone or another corticosteroid is that its long half-life obviates the need for further dosing at home. While waiting for the dexamethasone to work, racemic epinephrine is **commonly administered via nebulizer**. This usually leads to significant clinical improvement and gives time for the steroid to begin to take effect. Subcutaneous epinephrine is usually unnecessary. Albuterol, while helpful for bronchospasm, does not do anything to treat the glottic edema that is causing the majority of the respiratory distress. Intubation is not indicated at this point if the child is not in impending respiratory failure, hypoxic, or minimally responsive.

HELPFUL TIP: While classically we have used racemic epinephrine, the "d" isomer is inactive. Additionally, racemic epinephrine is more expensive and must be kept refrigerated if a multidose vial is used. L-epinephrine, 5 cc of 1:1000, delivered by nebulizer is as—if not more—effective, than racemic epinephrine, is cheaper, and is the same dose for everyone—a benefit if you are mathematically challenged.

* *

You administer the appropriate dose of dexamethasone to the child along with a treatment of nebulized epinephrine. He improves markedly. You watch him for 2 hours. He is able to tolerate oral fluids well, and is active and playful. He still has a brassy cough, but no inspiratory stridor.

What should his disposition be?

A) Admit for 23 hours of observation.
B) Administer second dose of racemic epinephrine and reevaluate.
C) Discharge to home with close outpatient follow-up.
D) Administer albuterol and reevaluate.

Discussion

The correct answer is C. If the child is free of stridor while at rest, he can be safely discharged with close outpatient follow-up (within 24 hours) as long as the parents are reliable, able to monitor the child, comfortable with the plan, and able to return if the child's condition should deteriorate. After administering dexamethasone and epinephrine, it is imperative to observe children for at least 2 hours. If children redevelop stridor at rest, they should receive a second dose of epinephrine. Any child who needs a second treatment has more severe croup, is at higher risk of having complications, and should be considered for hospital admission.

 HELPFUL TIP: Contrary to what many of us were taught, patients who get nebulized epinephrine do not necessarily need to be admitted if they are doing well 2 hours after epinephrine administration.

Objectives: Did you learn to . . .

- Describe common causes of respiratory distress in children?

- Manage pediatric airway problems?
- Treat children with croup?

QUICK QUIZ: CROUP

You treat a child who has croup with epinephrine and dexamethasone. Two hours later his oxygen saturation on room air improves to 92%.

Your next step is to:

A) Admit the patient to the hospital for further treatment.
B) Discharge the patient for follow-up in your office the next day.
C) Discharge the patient with instructions to use a cool mist humidifier.
D) Discharge the patient with a course of azithromycin just in case it is bacterial.
E) None of the above.

Discussion

The correct answer is A. An oxygen saturation of 92% is distinctly abnormal in a child of this age. He or she should be running 95% or better. Sending this child home would not be a great idea.

BIBLIOGRAPHY

ACEP Clinical Policies Committee; Clinical Policies Subcommittee on Seizures. Clinical policy: Critical issues in the evaluation and management of adult patients presenting to the emergency department with seizures. *Ann Emerg Med.* 2004;43(5):605-25.

American College of Emergency Physicians Clinical Policies Subcommittee (Writing Committee) on Critical Issues in the Management of Patients Presenting to the Emergency Department with Acetaminophen Overdose, Wolf SJ, Heard K, Sloan EP, Jagoda AS. Clinical policy: critical issues in the management of patients presenting to the emergency department with acetaminophen overdose. *Ann Emerg Med.* 2007;50(3):292-313.

Baren JM, Brennan J, Brown L, Rothrock SG. *Pediatric Emergency Medicine.* Philadelphia, Pa: Saunders Health Sciences;2007.

Ford MD, Delaney KA, Ling LJ, Erickson T. *Clinical Toxicology.* Philadelphia, Pa: WB Saunders; 2001.

Herz AM, Greenhow TL, Alcantara J, et al. Changing epidemiology of outpatient bacteremia in 3- to 36-month-old children after the introduction of the heptavalent-conjugated pneumococcal vaccine. *Pediatr Infect Dis J.* 2006;25(4):293-300.

Leung AKC, Sigalet DL. Acute abdominal pain in children. *Am Fam Physician.* 2003;67:2321-26.

Ma OJ, Tintinalli JE, Kelen GD, et al. *Emergency Medicine Manual.* 6th ed. New York, NY: McGraw-Hill;2003.

Marx JA, Adams J, Rosen P, el al. *Rosen's Emergency Medicine: Concepts and Clinical Practice.* 6th ed. Elsevier Health Sciences; 2005.

Mokhlesi B, Leikin JB, Murray P. Adult toxicology in critical care: Part II: Specific poisonings. *Chest.* 2003; 123(3):897-922.

Pang D, et al. Spinal cord injury without radiographic abnormality in children—the SCIWORA syndrome. *J Trauma.* 1989;29(5):654.

Panju AA, et al. Is this patient having a myocardial infarction? *JAMA.* 1998;280(14):1256.

Rogers RL, McCormack R. Aortic disasters. *Emerg Med Clin North Am.* 2004;22(4):887-908.

Steiner RW. Treating acute bronchiolitis associated with RSV. *Am Fam Physician.* 2004;69(2):325-30.

Tenebein M, Shannon M. The poisoned patient: is gastrointestinal decontamination all washed up? Two responses. *Pediatr Emerg Care.* 1998;14:380-381.

Touger M, Gallagher EJ, Tyrell J. Relationship between venous and arterial carboxyhemoglobin levels in patients with suspected carbon monoxide poisoning. *Ann Emerg Med.* 1995;25(4):481-483.

Rajesh Kabra, Chirag M. Sandesara, and Christopher J. Berry

CASE 1

A 35-year-old female presents to the ED with a 1-hour history of chest pain that resolved spontaneously. The pain is described as a pressure radiating to both arms. The patient is a smoker but has no family history of cardiac disease. She has no history of hypertension, diabetes, or other significant risk factor for cardiac disease. The patient is diaphoretic and has a normal blood pressure. She blames the diaphoresis on the fact that it is hot outside with high humidity and she has just walked in from the parking lot. She looks relatively calm and comfortable. You push on her chest wall, and this reproduces the pain. She is now otherwise chest-pain-free.

Which of the following is true about this patient's physical findings and history?

A) Pain radiating to both arms makes it unlikely that this patient's pain is cardiac.
B) The physical findings that are most highly associated with cardiac disease include hypotension, diaphoresis, and a new S_3 gallop.
C) The absence of risk factors makes it unlikely that this patient has cardiac disease.
D) That the pain is reproducible on palpation of the chest wall effectively rules out cardiac disease.
E) None of the above.

Discussion

The correct answer is B. The findings that are most likely to be associated with cardiac disease are hypotension, diaphoresis, and a new S_3 gallop. Answer A is incorrect because pain radiating to both arms can still be associated

with cardiac disease. Right arm radiation or bilateral arm radiation increases the likelihood of the pain's being cardiac, as compared to left arm radiation. Women with acute myocardial infarctions (AMIs) experience more chest pain radiating to the right arm/shoulder and the front neck area compared to men. Answer C is incorrect. The absence of risk factors has little bearing on whether or not this patient has heart disease. The only risk factors that change the prior probability enough to be useful in decision-making are male gender and diabetes. Smoking, hypertension, family history, etc do not change the prior probability of cardiac disease enough to allow them to be used to rule out or rule in cardiac disease. Answer D is incorrect. Approximately 15% of patients with cardiac disease will have their pain reproduced by chest wall pressure. This is probably because of the patient's inability to discriminate between the types of pain (cardiac vs. chest wall). Therefore, although one can reproduce the pain on chest wall pressure it does not 100% reliably rule out cardiac disease.

**

You decide that further testing is warranted, including an ECG and cardiac enzymes.

Which of the following statements is true?

A) A normal ECG in the ED effectively rules out cardiac disease.
B) The serum troponin is more sensitive than the CPK-MB in the first 6 hours after a myocardial infarction (MI).
C) Serum troponin is an unreliable marker of cardiac ischemia in patients with renal failure.

D) The serum troponin is 100% specific for MI.
E) Troponin and CPK cannot be used to make decisions about who to admit in the ED.

Discussion

The correct answer is E. Except in cases where the chest pain has been continuous for over 12 hours, a normal troponin and/or CPK-MB do not rule out cardiac disease. If they did, we would not admit patients for a "rule out" but would rather rely on the single level drawn in the ED. Answer A is incorrect because 9% of patients with an MI will have a normal ECG in the ED. Only 50% of those with an MI have a diagnostic ECG in the ED. Additionally, those with angina may have a normal ECG. Thus, a normal ECG does not rule out cardiac disease. Answer B is incorrect since the CPK-MB is more sensitive in the first 6 hours than is the troponin (about 84% versus 74%). Answer C is incorrect. Patients with renal disease may have a mildly elevated troponin at baseline due to poor clearance, but troponin can still be useful in these patients if it is elevated. Also, an increased troponin is associated with increased short-term and in-hospital mortality. Answer D is incorrect because we now know that other processes, such as pulmonary emboli, can elevate the serum troponin.

All of the following statements are true EXCEPT:

A) All MI present with chest pain.
B) Dyspnea may be the only presenting symptom of MI.
C) Patients with MI can present with syncope.
D) The elderly and diabetics are more likely to present with atypical symptoms.
E) Neither A nor C is a true statement.

Discussion

The correct answer is A. This statement is not true. Many elderly and diabetic patients will present with painless MIs. As high as 30% of MIs are pain free. Answer B is a true statement because, especially in the elderly, dyspnea may be the only presenting symptom due to left ventricular failure secondary to ischemia. Answer C is a true statement because syncope (as well as light-headedness and fatigue) can be presenting symptoms of an MI. Answer D is a true statement because the elderly and diabetics may present with atypical symptoms. Answer E is incorrect because answer C is a true statement.

* *

Her ECG shows nonspecific ST-T changes.

Which of the following drug(s) is/are indicated in the initial management of this patient?

A) Aspirin.
B) Thrombolytic such as TPA or streptokinase.
C) Heparin.
D) A and B.
E) A and C.

Discussion

The correct answer is A. Because you are not sure that this patient has an MI or unstable angina, there is no indication for thrombolytic therapy or heparin. Additionally, since she is currently pain free, heparin carries more of a risk than a benefit at this juncture. However, all patients with possible angina or an MI should have aspirin unless they are truly allergic (hives, anaphylaxis). Answer B is incorrect because thrombolytics are indicated for an MI, which has not been proven in this patient.

 HELPFUL TIP: Current use of warfarin or aspirin should **not** preclude the administration of aspirin in the ED for a patient with chest pain that may be cardiac in origin. Unless there is a real allergy to aspirin, it must be given to chest pain patients in the ED.

* *

The patient tells you that she is allergic to aspirin, which causes hives and bronchospasm. She can, however, take other NSAIDs without difficulty.

Which of the following is an acceptable substitute for aspirin now?

A) Dipyridamole.
B) Clopidogrel (Plavix).
C) Ibuprofen or naproxen.
D) Celecoxib (Celebrex).
E) Salsalate.

Discussion

The correct answer is B. Clopidogrel in a loading dose of 300 mg can be used as a substitute for aspirin in the setting of unstable angina or MI. Answer A is incorrect because dipyridamole (in combination with aspirin) is indicated only for TIAs. It is a relatively weak platelet inhibitor. Answer C is incorrect because neither ibuprofen nor naproxen has been shown to be of benefit in angina/MI, and they are reversible platelet inhibitors that do not give adequate platelet inhibition. Additionally, both can block the effect of aspirin by making binding sites on platelets unavailable. Answers D and E are incorrect because neither drug inhibits platelets to a significant degree and thus would be of no use in this situation.

* *

The patient has a minor recurrence of her pain. You order sublingual nitroglycerin which gives her complete relief of her pain.

What can you deduce from her response to sublingual nitroglycerin?

A) The patient's pain is related to her heart.
B) Since she did not get hypotensive, it is unlikely that she had an anterior wall MI.
C) Since her pain is relieved, it meets the standard of care to discharge the patient on aspirin with PRN nitroglycerin and to schedule her for outpatient follow-up.
D) You believe that this patient has unstable angina. To prove it, an immediate exercise stress test is an acceptable alternative to admission.
E) None of the above.

Discussion

The correct answer is E, none of the above. Answer A is incorrect because relief with nitroglycerin is not specific for cardiac disease. Although cardiac pain may respond to nitroglycerin, esophageal spasm may also respond to nitrates. Answer B is incorrect since hypotension in response to nitroglycerin is not usually due to an anterior wall MI (keep going for more on this one, fearless reader). Answer C is incorrect because if you believe that this patient has unstable angina, she should be admitted to the hospital regardless or whether or not her pain has resolved with sublingual nitroglycerin. Alternatively, if you believe that this patient does not have cardiac disease, she can be discharged regardless of the response to nitroglycerin. Answer D is incorrect because unstable angina is a contraindication to exercise stress testing. If you do not believe that this patient has angina and have decided that she is very low risk, stress testing acutely may be

appropriate. If you believe that the patient has cardiac pain, she should be ruled out and stabilized before undergoing exercise testing. The fact that the patient's pain has been relieved with nitroglycerin does not mean that this patient did not have myocardial damage.

* *

The patient's pain recurs again in the ED. You suspect that she is having an MI but do not yet have unequivocal proof, such as ECG changes or elevated enzymes. The patient becomes markedly hypotensive in response to another dose of sublingual nitroglycerin.

Which of the following is true?

A) Further nitroglycerin is contraindicated in this patient.
B) Hypotension caused by nitroglycerin is usually unresponsive to IV saline.
C) Hypotension caused by nitroglycerin may be indicative of a right ventricular infarction, which is most commonly associated with an inferior wall MI.
D) Hypotension caused by nitroglycerin is diagnostic of cardiogenic shock, suggesting that this patient will have a poor outcome.
E) Since this patient is hypotensive, her interests are best served by a cardiology consult and immediate intervention in the cath lab.

Discussion

The correct answer is C. Hypotension in response to nitroglycerin may be indicative of a right ventricular infarct, which is most commonly associated with an inferior wall MI. Since the right ventricle is dependent on filling pressure, NTG, which drops the preload, will frequently result in hypotension in those with a right ventricular infarct. Answer A is incorrect because hypotension from sublingual nitroglycerin is not a contraindication to additional nitrates once the patient's blood pressure is stable. A typical sublingual dose is 400 micrograms (0.4 mg). A typical IV dose starts at 20 micrograms per minute. Thus, the sublingual dose is quite a bit larger than the IV dose. In such a situation, you could consider starting IV nitroglycerin at 10–20 micrograms per minute and titrating up as the blood pressure allows. Answer B is incorrect because hypotension from NTG is usually responsive to a saline bolus. Answer D is incorrect because hypotension from NTG does not indicate cardiogenic shock. Certainly patients with cardiogenic shock will be hypotensive, but hypotension from NTG does not

...ie cardiogenic shock. Answer E is incorrect. Patients with an MI may need to go to the cath lab quickly especially if they are hypotensive. However, this patient may or may not have an MI and the blood pressure will likely recover.

* *

You tell the patient that she may have a right ventricular infarction. Understandably, she is quite worried about this.

You let the patient know that:

A) She will likely continue to have problems with right ventricular functioning in the future.
B) She will need to increase her salt intake in order to increase preload and right ventricular filling pressure.
C) Her right ventricular function should return to normal or close to normal following her infarction.
D) A and B.
E) None of the above.

Discussion

The correct answer is C. Most patients will have return of right ventricular functioning following an MI. Answer A is incorrect because answer C is correct. Answer B is incorrect because there will be no need to increase right ventricular filling pressure (which is what IV saline does acutely) once right ventricular function returns to normal.

* *

You consider other options in this patient, including the possibility that this does not represent cardiac disease.

Which of the following is true?

A) Giving a GI cocktail (eg, Maalox and lidocaine) can reliably differentiate cardiac from esophageal/GI causes of chest pain.
B) A normal chest radiograph and symmetrical pulses in the upper extremities reliably rule out a thoracic aortic dissection.
C) Most patients with a spontaneous pneumothorax should be treated with a chest tube.
D) The absence of risk factors for cardiac disease (eg, smoking, elevated LDL, etc) can be used to decide whom to admit for chest pain.
E) Pain is a consistent finding in approximately only 60% of patients with a pulmonary embolism.

Discussion

The correct answer is E. Only a small majority (59%) of pulmonary emboli have pain as a feature. Answer A is incorrect because approximately 20% of patients with cardiac pain will have their pain relieved by a GI cocktail. Answer B is incorrect because only 50% of patients with an aortic dissection will have unequal pulses and blood pressures, and only 75% will have an abnormal CXR. The consideration of an aortic dissection mandates a chest CT scan or angiogram. Remember that approximately 20% of the population will have unequal blood pressures in the upper extremities at baseline. Answer C is incorrect because most patients with spontaneous pneumothorax can be treated with a pigtail catheter with a Heimlich valve placed in the second anterior intercostal space. This type of treatment reduces the morbidity associated with a chest tube. Answer D is incorrect because the presence or absence of risk factors is good at predicting trends in populations but should not be used to determine whom to admit. For example, in one study 77% of patients with an MI did not have elevated cholesterol. Ignore risk factors when making admission decisions (although risk factor modification is ultimately very important).

 HELPFUL TIP: CXR findings in patients with thoracic aortic dissection may include widened mediastinum, obliterated aortic knob, pleural capping, tracheal deviation, depression of left main stem bronchus, esophageal deviation, and loss of the paratracheal stripe.

* *

The patient's pain continues despite treatment with nitroglycerin, and you obtain another ECG (Figure 2–1).

Which of the following is true regarding this ECG?

A) This injury pattern on ECG is most consistent with an anterior wall MI.
B) In this situation, intervention in the cath lab with percutaneous transluminal coronary angioplasty (PTCA) and stent placement is superior to TPA or streptokinase.
C) In this situation, TPA is always preferred over streptokinase and has been shown to be superior in every comparison.

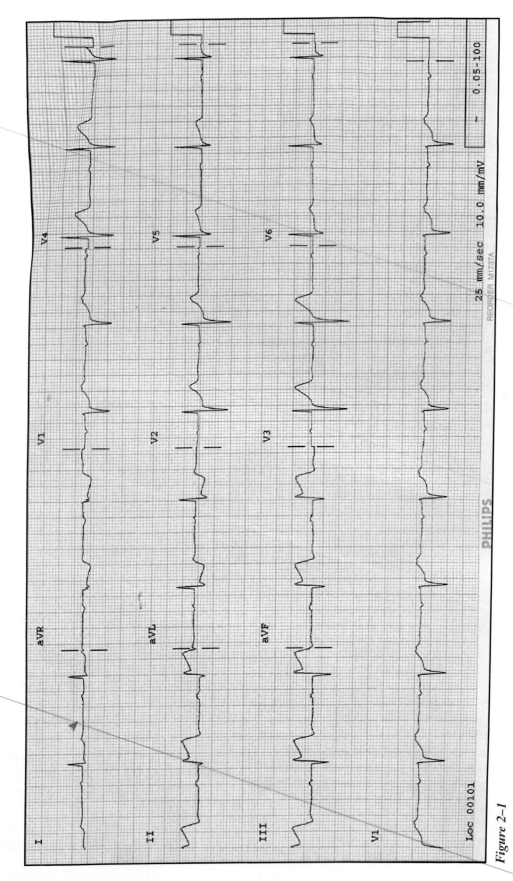

Figure 2–1

D) This injury pattern is classic for pericarditis.

E) The presence of these ECG changes proves that this patient's pain is not from an aortic dissection.

Discussion

The correct answer is B. Intervention in the cath lab with PTCA and/or stent placement is superior to thrombolytic therapy in the treatment of MI. Answer A is incorrect because this pattern is indicative of an inferior wall, not an anterior wall, MI. You will note that this ECG shows ST elevations in leads II, III, and aVF (inferior leads) along with reciprocal ST-segment depression in the anterior leads. An anterior wall MI is defined by ST elevations in leads V_3, V_4, and V_5, and an anteroseptal MI shows ST elevations in leads V_1, V_2, and V_3. Answer C is incorrect because not all trials show that t-PA is superior to streptokinase. More recent trials suggest a 1% absolute benefit to t-PA. However, this was mostly in subgroup analysis. Answer D is incorrect because patients with pericarditis should have ST elevations in all leads (although an ECG is only 80% sensitive for pericarditis). Answer E is incorrect because patients with an aortic dissection can present with an abnormal ECG that looks similar to an infarct pattern. Therefore, ECG changes do not prove that the patient does not have an aortic dissection.

**

You are considering other drugs that might be useful in this patient.

Which of the following drugs has been shown unequivocally to limit infarct size?

A) Nitroglycerin.
B) Metoprolol.
C) Heparin.
D) Oxygen.
E) Morphine.

Discussion

The correct answer is B. The drugs that have been shown to limit infarct size in patients with an MI include metoprolol (and other β-blockers), thrombolytics, and aspirin. Nitroglycerin, heparin, oxygen and morphine are all useful in treating the chest pain of an MI, but there is no evidence that they limit infarct size.

**

You now have all the evidence that you need to show that this patient is indeed having an ongoing MI. Since your rural hospital is just around the corner from nowhere, you decide to initiate thrombolytic therapy.

All of the following are valid indications, contraindications, or cautions for the use of thrombolytic therapy EXCEPT:

A) At least 1 mm of ST-segment elevation in at least two adjacent limb leads or at least 1–2 mm of ST-segment elevation in at least two adjacent precordial leads.
B) Absence of prior history of hemorrhagic stroke or any history of CVA within the last year.
C) No active bleeding including menstrual bleeding.
D) No history of recent head trauma.
E) No pregnancy.

Discussion

The correct answer is C. It is not a true statement. Although active internal bleeding is a contraindication to the use of thrombolytics, menstrual bleeding is not. Although there are no controlled trials, anecdotal evidence suggests that thrombolytics are safe with menstrual bleeding. Answer A is incorrect because it is a true statement. In addition to these ECG criteria, the presence of a new complete bundle branch block in addition to characteristic pain also indicates the patient will benefit from thrombolysis. Patients with only ST-segment depression or a normal ECG, even with symptoms, do not benefit. Answers B, D, and E are incorrect because they are true statements. Additional criteria for and contraindications to the use of thrombolytics are listed in Tables 2–1 and 2–2.

**

The patient is given a thrombolytic, which is indicated in this case. However, the patient develops a new left bundle branch block. Additionally, the ECG shows evidence of a first-degree heart block (a prolonged PR interval) although the heart rate remains adequate at 80 beats per minute.

The proper response to this is to:

A) Insert a Swan-Ganz catheter to monitor central pressures.
B) Insert a temporary pacemaker regardless of the heart rate.
C) Administer atropine to this patient.
D) Administer isoproterenol to this patient.
E) Do nothing, other than observe this patient.

Table 2–1   ACC/AHA GUIDELINES FOR THE MANAGEMENT OF PATIENTS WITH ST-ELEVATION MYOCARDIAL INFARCTION

Class 1 recommendations for the use of thrombolytics in myocardial infarction

At least 1 mm of ST-segment elevation in at least two adjacent limb leads or at least 1 to 2 mm of ST-segment elevation in at least two adjacent precordial leads. Or the presence of a new complete bundle branch block that obscures the ST segment analysis plus a history suggestive of myocardial infarction, less than 12 hours since the onset of pain, age <75 years (although treating those >75 years is still a class 2)

Class 2 recommendations for the use of thrombolytics in myocardial infarction

At least 1 mm of ST-segment elevation in at least two adjacent limb leads or at least 1 to 2 mm of ST-segment elevation in at least two adjacent precordial leads and age >75 years

At least 1 mm of ST-segment elevation in at least two adjacent limb leads or at least 1 to 2 mm of ST-segment elevation in at least two adjacent precordial leads and presenting 12–24 hours after onset of infarction

Blood pressure of >180 systolic and >100 diastolic in a patient with a "high risk" myocardial infarction (eg, the high risk of the MI mitigates the warning about thrombolytic use in uncontrolled hypertension)

J Am Coll Cardiol 2004;44:671–719.

Table 2–2   ACC/AHA GUIDELINES FOR THE MANAGEMENT OF PATIENTS WITH ST-ELEVATION MYOCARDIAL INFARCTION

Class 3 Absolute contraindications to the use of thrombolytic therapy in MI

Previous hemorrhagic stroke at any time or stroke within the last 12 months

Known intracranial neoplasm

Active internal bleeding (but not menstrual bleeding)

Suspected aortic dissection

Relative contraindications to the use of thrombolytic therapy in MI

Uncontrolled hypertension (>180/110) at time of presentation

History of bleeding diathesis, ongoing anticoagulation (INR >2-3)

Trauma, including traumatic CPR within 2–4 weeks, major surgery within 3 weeks

Noncompressible vascular punctures (eg, subclavian line)

Internal bleeding within the last 2–4 weeks

Pregnancy

Peptic ulcer disease (bleeding or not)

Severe, chronic hypertension

J Am Coll Cardiol 2004;44:671.

Discussion

The correct answer is B. For patients presenting with an MI, a transvenous pacemaker should be inserted, and in the interim a transcutaneous pacemaker should be placed in case complete heart block or advanced degree AV block develops. Answer A is incorrect because a Swan-Ganz catheter will be of no help in arrhythmias. Answer C is incorrect because atropine is indicated for symptomatic bradycardia and not for just a bundle branch block. Answer D is incorrect for the same reason as C. Additionally, isoproterenol is arrhythmogenic and is no longer recommended in general. Answer E is incorrect because B is correct. See Tables 2–3 and 2–4 for more on arrhythmia and pacemakers in the setting of AMI.

The patient requires heparin with the thrombolytic that you choose. Which of the following dosing regimens is the best accepted for use with thrombolytics?

A)   Enoxaparin 30 mg SQ every 12 hours.
B)   Enoxaparin 1 mg/kg SQ every 12 hours.
C)   Heparin 5,000 unit bolus and a drip at 1,000 U/hr.
D)   Heparin 100 units/kg bolus with a drip at 25 U/kg/hr.
E)   None of the above represents the best dosing option in this situation.

Table 2–3   TYPE OF HEART BLOCK ASSOCIATED WITH INFARCTION

Anterior myocardial infarction	Bundle branch blocks Mobitz type II second-degree heart block
Inferior myocardial infarction	Bradycardia from: Mobitz type I second-degree heart block, third-degree heart block

Table 2–4   CLASS I INDICATIONS FOR PACEMAKER IN PATIENTS WITH AN ACUTE MYOCARDIAL INFARCTION

New left bundle branch block + first degree AV block
New right bundle branch block + left anterior fascicular block + first degree AV block
Mobitz type II heart block (class 1)
Third-degree heart block (class 1)
Symptomatic bradycardia unresponsive to atropine

Discussion

The correct answer is B. For anticoagulation, the dose of enoxaparin is 1 mg/kg SQ every 12 hours. Answer A is incorrect because 30 mg SQ every 12 hours is the dose for DVT prophylaxis and not for anticoagulation. Answer C is incorrect. This is the classic way that heparin has been dosed but it is **not** the best choice listed. Answer D is incorrect. The **correct** dose for heparin **when given with a thrombolytic** is 60 U/kg bolus (maximum of 4,000 U) with a drip of 15 U/kg/hr (maximum dose of 1,000 U/hr). The bottom line here is that either enoxaparin or heparin can be used in this setting, and they are more or less equivalent (maybe some slight advantage to enoxaparin). If you choose to use heparin, do not use fixed-dose heparin but rather weight-based dosing.

* *

The patient receives her thrombolytic and enoxaparin, and she is admitted to the hospital to a monitored bed. You get a call from the nursing staff 5 hours later. Evidently the rhythm strip shows 3 PVCs per minute. However, the patient remains pain free and is hemodynamically stable. The nurse on the floor has discussed this with another physician who was on the floor, and he suggested prophylactic lidocaine for this patient.

The nurse is calling you for an order for lidocaine. Your response is:

A) Give lidocaine.
B) Give amiodarone which works better than lidocaine.
C) Give no antiarrhythmic at this point in time.
D) Check labs including potassium and magnesium.
E) C and D.

Discussion

The correct answer is E. In the setting of an MI, the general indication for antiarrhythmics is complex arrhythmias (PVC couplets, triplets, nonsustained ventricular tachycardia [<30 seconds], or >10 PVCs per minute). Over 90% of patients will have isolated PVCs in the peri-infarct period, and there is no association with increased mortality. Correcting hypokalemia and hypomagnesemia can help reduce arrhythmias, and checking these labs is certainly appropriate. The use of prophylactic lidocaine (answer A) has fallen out of favor and is proarrhythmic. The same is true for prophylactic amiodarone (answer B), which can cause torsade de pointes.

* *

The patient remains pain free while in the hospital. She is ready to be discharged 4 days later.

Which of the following tests is the MOST appropriate for this patient prior to discharge?

A) Coronary angiography.
B) Submaximal stress test.
C) Full Bruce protocol, symptom-limited stress test.
D) Spiral CT to assess for coronary artery calcification.

Discussion

The correct answer is B. Submaximal stress testing is considered the standard of care. Patients with a positive submaximal stress test can be referred for catheterization. Patients with a borderline stress test can be sent for a radionuclide study. Coronary angiography is **not** routinely recommended for all patients who have had an MI unless they are considered to be at high risk (eg, continued symptoms, positive screening test [such as submaximal stress test], CHF, etc). Answer C is incorrect because a symptom-limited, full protocol stress test should be done only 14–21 days after an infarction. Answer D is incorrect because spiral CT to assess for coronary artery calcification has no role in risk stratification after an MI.

The patient passes her stress test with flying colors. Patients after an MI should be routinely discharged on all of the following medications EXCEPT:

A) Aspirin.
B) β-Blocker.
C) Continuous nitroglycerin (eg, patch or isosorbide).
D) Lipid lowering agent, if appropriate.
E) Sublingual nitroglycerin for PRN use.

Discussion

The correct answer is C. There is no benefit to scheduled nitrates unless needed for a specific indication (eg, recurrent angina). All post-MI patients should be discharged on aspirin, β-blocker, statin (in most cases), nitroglycerin PRN, and an ACE inhibitor.

* *

This patient had an ST elevation MI (STEMI or Q-wave MI).

Which of the following statements is true?

A) Patients with a non-STEMI (non-Q-wave MI) have the same or a bit worse long-term outcomes than do patients with a STEMI (Q-wave MI).
B) Patients with a non-STEMI (non-Q-wave MI) have worse in-hospital outcomes when compared to patients with a STEMI (Q-wave MI).
C) Unstable angina and non-STEMI (non-Q-wave MI) can be readily differentiated from each other on presentation.
D) None of the above is true.

Discussion

The correct answer is A. Although it is contrary to what many of us were taught, patients with a non-Q-wave MI (now called non-ST elevation MI) actually have the same or perhaps even slightly worse long-term outcomes than do patients with a STEMI (Q-wave MI). This makes sense; there is still myocardium left to infarct after a non-STEMI. As to the other answers, patients with a STEMI do have worse in-hospital outcomes; and unstable angina and non-STEMI look similar on ECG with T-wave inversion, etc, but without the ST elevations that are classically seen in a transmural infarction.

* *

It is 2 months later. The patient has read about coronary artery disease (CAD) and has some questions about cholesterol. She wants to know what risk factors you consider when determining what her cholesterol goal should be.

The following are all considered cardiac risk factors when calculating target cholesterol EXCEPT:

A) Male >45 years.
B) First-degree female relative with CAD >65 years.
C) Smoking.

D) Hypertension.
E) HDL cholesterol of <40 mg/dL.

Discussion

The correct answer is B. Female relative with CAD <65 years, not >65 years, is a risk factor. If the patient has an HDL >60mg/dL, this counts as a protective factor and cancels out one of the risk factors. See Table 2–5 for a complete list of cardiac risk factors.

* *

The patient read about risk factors that are considered equivalent to having CAD as she was deciding whether or not to start lipid-lowering therapy.

All of the following are considered CAD equivalents when determining whether or not to start a statin EXCEPT:

A) Diabetes mellitus.
B) Symptomatic carotid disease.
C) Peripheral vascular disease.
D) Severe, sustained hypertension (>180/110).
E) All of the above are considered CAD equivalents.

Discussion

The correct answer is D. Severe hypertension is **not** considered a CAD equivalent risk factor when deciding whether a patient should be started on lipid-lowering therapy. In addition to diabetes, symptomatic carotid disease, and peripheral vascular disease, other CAD equivalent risk factors include abdominal aortic aneurysm and multiple risk factors that elevate the risk of CAD to >20% in the next 10 years (Table 2–6).

* *

Table 2–5   RISK FACTORS FOR CORONARY ARTERY DISEASE

First-degree male relative with CAD <55 years or first-degree female relative with CAD <65 years
Smoking
HDL <40mg/dL
Hypertension
Age: males >45 years, females >55 years
Elevated LDL

Table 2–6 CALCULATING 10-YEAR CORONARY ARTERY DISEASE RISK IN MEN AND WOMEN

Estimate of 10-Year Risk for Men	Estimate of 10-Year Risk for Women

(Framingham Point Scores)

Age	Points (Men)		Age	Points (Women)
20–34	–9		20–34	–7
35–39	–4		35–39	–3
40–44	0		40–44	0
45–49	3		45–49	3
50–54	6		50–54	6
55–59	8		55–59	8
60–64	10		60–64	10
65–69	11		65–69	12
70–74	12		70–74	14
75–79	13		75–79	16

Men — Points

Total Cholesterol	Age 20–39	Age 40–49	Age 50–59	Age 60–69	Age 70–79
<160	0	0	0	0	0
160–199	4	3	2	1	0
200–239	7	5	3	1	0
240–279	9	6	4	2	1
≥280	11	8	5	3	1

Women — Points

Total Cholesterol	Age 20–39	Age 40–49	Age 50–59	Age 60–69	Age 70–79
<160	0	0	0	0	0
160–199	4	3	2	1	1
200–239	8	6	4	2	1
240–279	11	8	5	3	2
≥280	13	10	7	4	2

Men — Points

	Age 20–39	Age 40–49	Age 50–59	Age 60–69	Age 70–79
Nonsmoker	0	0	0	0	0
Smoker	8	5	3	1	1

Women — Points

	Age 20–39	Age 40–49	Age 50–59	Age 60–69	Age 70–79
Nonsmoker	0	0	0	0	0
Smoker	9	7	4	2	1

HDL (mg/dL)	Points (Men)		HDL (mg/dL)	Points (Women)
≥60	–1		≥60	–1
50–59	0		50–59	0
40–49	1		40–49	1
<40	2		<40	2

Men

Systolic BP (mmHg)	If Untreated	If Treated
<120	0	0
120–129	0	1
130–139	1	2
140–159	1	2
≥160	2	3

Women

Systolic BP (mmHg)	If Untreated	If Treated
<120	0	0
120–129	1	3
130–139	2	4
140–159	3	5
≥160	4	6

Men

Point Total	10-Year Risk %
<0	<1
0	1
1	1
2	1
3	1
4	1
5	2
6	2
7	3
8	4
9	5
10	6
11	8
12	10
13	12
14	16
15	20
16	25
≥17	≥30

10-Year Risk _____ %

Women

Point Total	10-Year Risk %
<9	<1
9	1
10	1
11	1
12	1
13	2
14	2
15	3
16	4
17	5
18	6
19	8
20	11
21	14
22	17
23	22
24	27
≥25	≥30

10-Year Risk _____ %

The patient wants to know about something she read about "crap" and cardiac disease. A light bulb goes off and you realize she wants to know about CRP (C-reactive protein).

Which of the following best represents the role of CRP in cardiac disease in 2008?

A) CRP should be measured in all patients in whom cardiac disease is suspected.

B) CRP should be measured only in patients with cardiac risk factors but in whom it is not clear whether treatment is indicated (eg, those with a 10-year-risk of CAD of 10%–20%).

C) CRP should be measured in patients with known heart disease in order to monitor inflammation and risk.

D) CRP should be measured in patients who are not being treated for cardiac disease and who are considered low risk (<10% risk of CAD in next 10 years) based on cholesterol, etc. An elevated CRP suggests that these patients should be treated.

E) None of the above.

Discussion

The correct answer is B. We are talking about the highly sensitive CRP here, which is indicated only in those in whom the 10-year CAD risk is 10% to 20%. **This is a Class IIa recommendation. There is still conflicting evidence about the use of CRP in this situation.** Answer C is incorrect because the CRP is not something that is monitored to dictate therapy. Answer D is incorrect. Those individuals at very low risk do not benefit from CRP measurements. In those with cardiac disease, intensive treatment should be undertaken regardless of the CRP.

The best available evidence suggests:

A) An elevated CRP is **not** an independent risk factor for cardiac events when risks such as homocysteine and cholesterol are taken into account.

B) Treatment with steroids to reduce inflammation will reduce the risk of coronary events in those with an elevated CRP.

C) CRP must be measured on at least two occasions before taking any action.

D) Statins have been shown in several randomized trials to reduce the risk of death in those with an elevated CRP.

E) None of the above.

Discussion

The correct answer is C. The CRP can be elevated as a result of multiple factors including infectious causes. Thus, a single measurement may not reflect a patient's true baseline level. Answer A is incorrect because an elevated CRP seems to be an independent risk factor even when cholesterol is taken into account. We do not know about homocysteine, however. Answer B is incorrect. There is no evidence about the use of steroids in patients at risk for CAD because of elevated CRP, but steroids are unlikely to be useful. Answer D is incorrect because it is not known if statins reduce mortality in patients with elevated CRP and no previous history of coronary artery disease (CAD). The PRINCE trial randomized patients without any history of coronary artery disease to statin or placebo and it demonstrated a statistically significant decrease in CRP levels in patients with statin therapy and no change in CRP levels in patients taking a matched placebo. The trial was not designed to address mortality outcomes. Answer E is incorrect because answer C is correct.

* *

The next day, you obtain fasting labs. The patient has normal electrolytes and the following cholesterol panel: LDL 110 mg/dL, HDL 35 mg/dL, TRG 150 mg/dL. You review the ATP III (Adult Treatment Panel III, National Cholesterol Education Panel) guidelines to determine your next step in the treatment of this patient based on these labs.

Given the lipid profile above, you:

A) Consider the LDL to be too high and start an HMG CoA reductase inhibitor (statin). According to ATP III, this action is mandated in patients with cardiac disease and this level of LDL.

B) Consider the lipid profile to be in the normal range, so that no further intervention should occur. According to ATP III, no action is mandated in patients with cardiac disease and this level of LDL.

C) Consider the LDL to be too high and recommend diet and other lifestyle modifications. According to ATP III, this action is mandated in patients with cardiac disease and this level of LDL.

D) Repeat the lipid profile because this patient clearly was not fasting and the LDL cannot be relied upon since her triglycerides are so high.

Discussion

The correct answer is C. The first step is to change the patient's lifestyle and diet. This includes exercise, weight loss if indicated, and a low-fat diet. Even in patients who have cardiac disease, statins are not mandatory for those with an LDL between 100 mg/dL and 130 mg/dL unless 6 months of dietary modifications have failed to reduce the LDL to <100 mg/dL. Even though there is not a firm recommendation to start statins with a normal LDL in those who have had a recent MI, there are some data that suggests a benefit to the use of statins even in those with a normal LDL. Answer A is incorrect because lifestyle modification for 6 months is indicated before starting a drug. Answer B is incorrect because for a patient who has cardiac disease, this LDL is **not** considered optimal. Answer D is incorrect. There is no reason to suspect that the patient was not fasting, and the triglyceride level is not too high to calculate LDL (generally with a TRG >400 LDL cannot be reliably calculated).

If you choose to start a statin on this patient, what will your goal be?

A) LDL <130 mg/dL.
B) LDL <100 mg/dL.
C) LDL <110 mg/dL.
D) LDL need not be a goal if you can reduce the triglycerides.
E) None of the above.

Discussion

The correct answer is B. The LDL goal is <100 mg/dL in those with a history of CAD or those with >20% risk of a cardiac event in the in the next 10 years. Other goals set forth by ATP III include LDL <130 mg/dL in patients with two or more risk factors for cardiac disease and LDL <160 mg/dL in patients with 0 or 1 risk factor (Table 2–7).

The patient tries diet and exercise, but her lipids do not change. You are not surprised; you are a realist. You start a statin on this patient, and her liver enzymes (AST and ALT) rise to two times the upper limit of normal. You recheck them in 2 weeks but they remain the same.

The proper response at this point is to:

A) Stop the statin because of the elevated liver enzymes.
B) Start a different statin since this is not a "class effect."
C) Do nothing. These elevated liver enzymes are not a problem.
D) Add cholestyramine to help ease the burden on the liver.
E) Consider a liver biopsy to rule out other causes of elevated liver enzymes.

Discussion

The correct answer is C. Statins can be continued as long as the elevation of liver enzymes is less than three

Table 2–7 LDL CHOLESTEROL GOALS AND CUTPOINTS FOR THERAPEUTIC LIFESTYLE CHANGES (TLC) AND DRUG THERAPY IN DIFFERENT RISK CATEGORIES

Risk Category	LDL Goal	LDL Level at Which to Initiate Therapeutic Lifestyle Changes (TLC)	LDL Level at Which to Consider Drug Therapy
CHD or CHD Risk Equivalents (10-year risk >20%)	<100 mg/dL	≥100 mg/dL	≥130 mg/dL (100–129 mg/dL: drug optional)*
2+ Risk Factors (10-year risk ≤20%)	<130 mg/dL	≥130 mg/dL	10-year risk 10–20%: ≥130 mg/dL 10-year risk <10%: ≥160 mg/dL
0–1 Risk Factor†	<160 mg/dL	≥160 mg/dL	≥190 mg/dL (160–189 mg/dL: LDL-lowering drug optional)

*Some authorities recommend use of LDL-lowering drugs in this category if an LDL cholesterol <100 mg/dL cannot be achieved by therapeutic lifestyle changes. Others prefer use of drugs that primarily modify triglycerides and HDL eg, nicotinic acid or fibrate. Clinical judgment also may call for deferring drug therapy in this subcategory.

†Almost all people with 0-1 risk factor have a 10-year risk <10%, thus 10-year risk assessment in people with 0-1 risk factor is not necessary.

times the upper limit of normal. However, the liver enzymes should be monitored. Generally, the elevation in liver enzymes will resolve with discontinuation of the medication if this is what you choose to do. However, never assume that this is a drug effect if there is a reason to believe that the patient could have another disease, such as hepatitis C. Answer A is incorrect since the levels are only two times normal. Answer B is incorrect for two reasons. First, there is no need to act to change the drug at this point. Second, elevated liver enzymes are a class effect. Answer D is incorrect because you do not need to add another drug at this time, and cholestyramine will do nothing to ease the burden on the liver. Answer E is incorrect. If you want to check for other causes of elevated LFTs, biopsy certainly is not the next step!

* *

In patients on statin therapy who are NOT having problems with liver enzymes, how often should you check liver enzymes?

A) Initially, then every 12 weeks.
B) Initially, at 12 weeks, then every 3 months.
C) Initially, at 12 weeks, then annually.
D) Initially, at 8 weeks, then every 6 months.
E) Initially, at 12 weeks, then every 6 months.

Discussion

The correct answer is C. This is currently the recommendation. The other answers are incorrect.

* *

The patient returns to your office in 2 weeks for a recheck. This patient did not meet her LDL goal with just one drug. In fact, her LDL went up a bit. You decide that the patient needs a second drug.

Which of the following is the *safest* drug to add to a statin in order to control this patient's LDL?

A) Niacin.
B) Gemfibrozil.
C) Cholestyramine.
D) Probucol.
E) Fluvastatin.

Discussion

The correct answer is C. Cholestyramine is the safest of the drugs listed above. It is not systemically absorbed and has very few side effects (constipation primarily).

Answer A is incorrect because niacin can elevate liver enzymes, can cause rhabdomyolysis, and has other side effects. Thus, while it is a good choice for many patients, it is not the safest drug listed here. Gemfibrozil and probucol can reduce triglycerides and LDL. However, probucol is no longer available because it may increase mortality, and the combination of gemfibrozil and a statin can cause rhabdomyolysis (as can the use of a statin alone). Again, gemfibrozil is often used with a statin but is not the safest choice. Fluvastatin is another statin, and so it has the same potential problems.

Which of the following is not classified as a bile acid sequestrant?

A) Ezetimibe.
B) Colestipol.
C) Colesevelam.
D) All of the above are bile acid sequestrants.

Discussion

The correct answer is A. Ezetimibe (Zetia) is not a bile acid sequestrant but rather reduces cholesterol absorption by blocking at the brush border of the small intestine. This is a mechanism that is different from any of the other lipid-lowering agents. It is relatively safe but expensive and less potent than the statins. Even in combination with statins the additional lowering of LDL is 15% to 18%. Answers B and C bind bile acids to reduce serum cholesterol.

Side effects of ezetimibe include which of the following?

A) Diarrhea.
B) Arthralgia.
C) Angioedema.
D) Liver enzyme elevation.
E) All of the above.

Discussion

The correct answer is E. Answer C, angioedema, deserves special mention. As with ACE inhibitors, angioedema has been reported with the use of ezetimibe during postmarketing research. The rate of occurrence is not known. However, it can be life-threatening although no deaths have been reported to date. All of the other side effects are known to occur at a rate greater than with placebo.

* *

Due to GI side effects, the patient is unable to tolerate bile acid sequestrants. You feel that the potential benefits of further lipid-lowering therapy outweigh the risks, and you decide to start this patient on niacin to lower her LDL and elevate her HDL. She returns to your office in 2 weeks complaining of muscle aching and weakness. She also has some depressive symptoms such as anhedonia and sleep disturbance. You want to evaluate the patient to make sure that she does not have myopathy secondary to the medications she is taking. Her CPK and aldolase are normal.

From this you can conclude that:

A) She does not have myopathy since her muscle enzymes (CPK and aldolase) are within normal limits.
B) Her fatigue and aches are a manifestation of her depression and sleep disturbance.
C) You can continue her statin and niacin since the CPK is normal.
D) She still may have statin-related myopathy despite a normal CPK and aldolase.

Discussion

The correct answer is D. The patient still may have statin-induced myopathy despite a normal CPK and aldolase. Answer A is incorrect because Answer D is correct. There are several crossover trials that demonstrate myopathy in patients with normal muscle enzymes. The mechanism is thought to be a mitochondrial dysfunction. Answer B is incorrect, and the reverse may be true (myopathy causing poor sleep and anhedonia). Answer C is incorrect because she may indeed have a myopathy, and a trial of one or both drugs is warranted.

* *

You stop her medications and her symptoms improve over the course of several weeks. Everybody is happy—except the manufacturers of atorvastatin and ezetimibe, who would have liked this case to end with the patient taking their drugs, preferably twice a day.

 HELPFUL TIP: Metamucil or other psyllium products are useful in reducing serum cholesterol and provide a nondrug alternative. At least 7 grams of soluble fiber daily are required.

Objectives: Did you learn to . . .

- Define the accuracy of the initial history, ECG, and labs in the diagnosis of cardiac disease in the ED or office?
- Recognize the role and significance (or lack thereof) of risk factors, such as diabetes, family history, smoking, and hypertension, in the decision of whether or not to admit a patient to the hospital for chest pain?
- Generate a differential diagnosis of chest pain?
- Identify the roles of various diagnostic tests in the evaluation of chest pain?
- Treat a patient with an AMI?
- Describe the role of lipid-lowering therapy in the treatment of cardiac disease and as prophylaxis?
- Identify some of the potential side effects of lipid-lowering medications?

 QUICK QUIZ: HYPERTENSION

According to JNC 7, a blood pressure of 120/80 is classified as:

A) Normal.
B) Prehypertension.
C) Hypertension.
D) None of the above.

Discussion

The correct answer is B. The other answers are incorrect. See Table 2–8 for the JNC 7 classification scheme for hypertension.

CASE 2

You are seeing a patient in the ED with chest pain. The ECG shows elevated ST segments in leads V_1, V_2, and V_3 with reciprocal changes inferiorly. You have run

Table 2–8   JNC 7 CLASSIFICATION OF HYPERTENSION

<120/80: Normal
120/80–139/89: Prehypertension
140/90–159/99: Stage 1 hypertension
>160/100: Stage II hypertension

through the standard medications, but the patient continues to have pain. You consult a cardiologist who suggests the use of a glycoprotein IIB/IIIA inhibitor.

Which of the following is true about the glycoprotein IIB/IIIA inhibitors?

A) They are best used in patients who are not candidates for PTCA and stenting.

B) They cause no increase the rate of intracranial bleeding.

C) They are useful in all groups of patients with acute coronary syndrome.

D) They are most effective in patients going to PTCA and/or stenting.

Discussion

The correct answer is D. The glycoprotein IIB/IIIA inhibitors are most effective in patients who are undergoing PTCA or stenting. The GUSTO V trial showed **no** difference in 30-day mortality in patients **who were not** scheduled for catheterization. Answer A is incorrect because the glycoprotein IIB/IIIA inhibitors are best in those patients going for PTCA/stenting. Answer B is incorrect because glycoprotein IIB/IIIA inhibitors do increase rates of intracranial and other bleeding. Answer C is incorrect because patients who have an acute coronary syndrome that is well controlled with other drugs (eg, heparin, metoprolol, ASA, etc.) are not likely to benefit from glycoprotein IIB/IIIA inhibitors.

Bosch and Marragut conclude the following for the Cochrane collaboration:

> Intravenous glycoprotein IIA/IIIB blockers reduce the risk of death at 30 days and markedly that of death or MI at 30 days and at 6 months in patients submitted to percutaneous coronary revascularization at a price of a moderate increased risk of severe bleeding. In contrast, in patients with unstable angina/non-ST-segment elevation MI, these agents do not reduce mortality, only slightly reduce the risk of (the combined endpoints) of death or MI, and slightly increase the risk for severe bleeding.

CASE 3

A 53-year-old male with a history of hypertension and smoking, but no family history of cardiac disease, presents to your office complaining of a typical angina-type chest pain. The pain is substernal, radiates to his left arm, and is associated with exertion. The patient notes that this same pain has been going on for the last 6 months

and has not changed at all in duration, intensity, or characteristic. It generally lasts 5 minutes or so and resolves with rest.

You tell the patient that:

A) Without doing any test, the probability that this pain is cardiac is >85%.

B) If his ECG in the office is normal, his pain is unlikely to represent cardiac disease.

C) Even with risk factors, his probability of having CAD with typical angina is still only 50% or so.

D) The only intervention indicated at this point are lifestyle modifications (eg, stop smoking) and addressing his cholesterol and hypertension.

E) It is likely that he has unstable angina.

Discussion

The correct answer is A. A 50-year-old male with classic angina symptoms has a >85% probability of having coronary artery disease. Answer B is incorrect because patients with angina who are pain free may have a normal electrocardiogram (as will many patients with active angina or even an MI). Therefore, his pain could still be cardiac in origin. Answer C is incorrect because, based on demographic data, his risk of CAD is much greater than 50%. Answer D is incorrect because he needs a further evaluation and treatment for his chest pain. Answer E is incorrect since this pain represents stable angina. There has been no change in quality, duration, amount of exertion required to bring on symptoms, etc., thus eliminating unstable angina as a diagnosis.

* *

You send the patient home on aspirin and with a prescription for sublingual nitroglycerin for PRN use. You schedule the patient for a stress test.

All of the following are considered absolute contraindications to exercise stress testing EXCEPT:

A) Left bundle branch block.

B) Presence of severe CHF.

C) Significant aortic stenosis.

D) Myocarditis.

E) Unstable angina.

Discussion

The correct answer is A. A left bundle branch block is a **relative—not absolute—**contraindication to stress testing and limits the usefulness of the test. One should add an imaging modality, such as myocardial perfusion scanning or echocardiography, in cases of left bundle branch block. The remaining answers are absolute contraindications to exercise stress testing. Other contraindications include: acute MI (within 2 days), dissecting aneurysm (but not asymptomatic abdominal aneurysm), recent pulmonary embolism, thrombophlebitis, blood pressure of >200/120, and hemodynamically significant arrhythmias. There are also a number of relative contraindications including significant systemic disease (uncontrolled thyroid disease, diabetes mellitus), inability to complete the test, etc. See Table 2–9 for a list of relative and absolute contraindications.

Exercise stress testing is *best* suited to which group of individuals?

A) Men with an intermediate probability of cardiac disease.
B) Women with a high risk of cardiac disease.
C) Men at a high risk of cardiac disease.
D) Men at a low risk of cardiac disease.
E) Women with a low risk of cardiac disease.

Discussion

The correct answer is A. Stress testing is best suited to patients with an intermediate pretest probability of

cardiac disease (between 25%–75%). Answers B and C are incorrect since patients with a high risk of cardiac disease should go directly to another study, such as thallium testing, stress echocardiography, etc. Answers D and E are incorrect because these are not the best groups in which to use exercise stress testing. There will be a greater proportion of false-positive results in these low-risk patients. Exercise stress testing in these groups is best used to allay patient fears that they do not have cardiac disease, not to prove they do have cardiac disease. **However, a false-positive stress test may lead to other unnecessary invasive testing!**

This patient has a negative stress test. Your next step is to:

A) Reassure the patient that he does not have cardiac disease.
B) Suggest a chest CT scan to rule out possible aortic aneurysm.
C) Schedule the patient for another cardiac test such as stress echocardiogram, exercise thallium test, or angiography.
D) Schedule the patient for endoscopy to rule out gastroesophageal disease as a cause of these symptoms.
E) None of the above.

Table 2–9   CONTRAINDICATIONS TO EXERCISE STRESS TESTING

Absolute contraindications	• Acute myocardial infarction within 2 days
	• Dissecting aneurysm
	• Recent pulmonary embolism
	• Active thrombophlebitis
	• BP >200/120
	• Hemodynamically significant arrhythmias
	• Severe CHF
	• Severe aortic stenosis
	• Active myocarditis, pericarditis, or endocarditis
	• Inability to complete test
Relative contraindications	• Left bundle branch block
	• Moderate aortic stenosis
	• Hypertrophic cardiomyopathy
	• Electrolyte disturbance
	• High grade AV block
	• Tachyarrhythmias or bradyarrhythmias including uncontrolled atrial fibrillation

Discussion

The correct answer is C. This patient who is in his fifties and who has a classic history for angina has >90% pretest probability of cardiac disease. Thus, it is likely that the negative stress test is a false-negative. Men >40 years and women >60 years who have classic angina have a pretest probability of cardiac disease of 87% and 91%, respectively. **A stress test probably should not have been done in this patient in the first place** since a negative test just leads to further testing (as would have a positive test, probably resulting in angiography). For this reason, answer A is incorrect. Answers B and D are incorrect. Initiating a workup for another cause of chest pain is premature because we still have not proven that this patient does not have cardiac disease.

* *

You are considering whether to do a thallium stress test or a stress echocardiogram.

Which of the following is true?

A) Stress echocardiography is more sensitive for cardiac disease than is a thallium test.
B) Stress echocardiography is more specific than is stress thallium.
C) Thallium testing is more specific for cardiac disease than is stress echocardiography.
D) None of the above is true.

Discussion

The correct answer is B. Stress echocardiography is more specific for cardiac disease than is thallium testing. Alternatively, thallium testing is more sensitive. Remember that positive and negative predictive values of these tests will vary depending on the pretest probability of disease in the patient **and** severity of disease. Table 2–10 summarizes these data.

Table 2–10 OVERALL SENSITIVITY AND SPECIFICITY OF NONINVASIVE CARDIAC TESTING

	Sensitivity	Specificity
Exercise stress testing	45%–68%	77%
Thallium stress testing (SPECT)	88%	77%
Stress echocardiography	76%	88%

You decide to send the patient for a thallium stress test. However, because his exercise capacity is limited, you choose to stress him chemically. The patient is taking theophylline for COPD.

The LEAST desirable method of stressing this patient is:

A) Adenosine.
B) Dobutamine.
C) Dipyridamole.
D) All of the above are equally acceptable methods of chemically stressing this patient.

Discussion

The correct answer is A. Theophylline (and caffeine) interact with adenosine, attenuating the affect of the adenosine. Thus, adenosine would not be a good choice for stressing this patient. Likewise, caffeine is verboten in those undergoing an adenosine test. All of the other answers are acceptable methods of chemically stressing this patient.

The patient's thallium stress test shows a nonreversible defect. The best interpretation of this is that it indicates:

A) Attenuation artifact from breast tissue.
B) Prior MI.
C) Angina.
D) Anomalous cardiac circulation.
E) It is not significant and therefore adds no value to this test.

Discussion

The correct answer is B. A nonreversible defect suggests prior MI. A reversible defect suggests inducible ischemia. Answer A is incorrect because breast attenuation occurs mostly in women. Answer C is incorrect because angina is manifested by a reversible deficit.

* *

Since there was no reversible defect on the thallium stress test, you conclude that there is no myocardium currently at risk. However, the patient continues to have chest pain and now at an increasing frequency with less exertion. He is asymptomatic when he presents to your office. He was noted at the last visit to have an elevated glucose at 350 mg/dL.

What is the next step in the evaluation or treatment for this patient?

A) Stress echocardiogram to document what segments are involved.
B) Start the patient on insulin to control his blood sugars.
C) Proceed directly to cardiac catheterization.
D) Since there were no reversible deficits on thallium stress, schedule the patient to see a gastroenterologist.
E) Give a trial of NSAIDs to help differentiate chest wall pain from other causes.

Discussion

The correct answer is C. Answer A is incorrect because we already have done a noninvasive test. We already know what segment has previously been infracted, as noted on the thallium stress test. Answer B is incorrect for two reasons. First, addressing his diabetes will not address the immediate problem of what you must presume is unstable angina. Second, insulin is not necessarily the first drug to use in this patient who presumably has type 2 diabetes. Certainly the blood glucose needs to be addressed but so does the chest pain. Answer D is incorrect. The sensitivity of thallium testing is in the 88% range (see Table 2–10), so it will miss 12% of disease. Thus, we still have not proven in this high-risk patient that he does not have treatable cardiac disease causing his chest pain. Answer E is incorrect for the same reason.

 HELPFUL TIP: NSAIDs may block the benefit of aspirin by reversibly binding to platelets, competing against aspirin as it irreversibly binds to the same sites on platelets. Always stop NSAIDS in the patient admitted for possible CAD.

* *

The patient has a catheterization done that shows 3-vessel disease including left main coronary artery disease. The cardiologist calls you with the report the next day and suggests PTCA with stenting since, in his opinion, this is the best modality for diabetics and diabetics are high-risk candidates when it comes to surgery.

Your opinion is that:

A) Patients generally have better outcomes in terms of control of angina with stenting when compared to coronary artery bypass grafting (CABG).
B) Diabetic patients do particularly well with stenting when compared to CABG.
C) Medical control of symptoms is indicated as the best management in this diabetic patient with 3-vessel disease.
D) You would like to send this patient for CABG.
E) None of the above.

Discussion

The correct answer is D. This patient should probably have surgery for his 3-vessel disease because diabetics generally have **worse** outcomes with stenting than do nondiabetics based on results from the BARI trial (see below). Answer A is incorrect because a percentage of patients with stents go on to have an open CABG. Answer B is incorrect. Diabetic patients do particularly poorly with stents when compared to other patients. Diabetics have a much higher rate of secondary occlusion. Answer C is incorrect. The indications for CABG are significant left main coronary artery disease (>50%) or 3-vessel disease with evidence of LV dysfunction (ejection fraction <50%). This patient has left main vessel disease and thus medical control is **not** the best option for this patient.

 HELPFUL TIP: Drug-eluting stents decrease reocclusion rates in diabetics and others compared to bare metal stents. Women who have multiple stents and multivessel disease are also at a higher risk of restenosis, as are patients with a small poststenting lumen size. **Early reocclusion secondary to thrombosis is higher with drug-eluting stents. This is because it takes the body longer to cover these stents with fibroblasts. Thus, clopidogrel should be used for a full year in patients who have a drug-eluting stent inserted.**

* *

Your patient has a CABG and comes into your office complaining of chest pain and fever 3 weeks after the surgery. He has had the pain and fever for 4 days and does not seem to be getting any better. He has no cough, no sputum production, and the pain seems to be worse when he lies down. He reports no dyspnea and has 97% oxygen saturation on room air. The wound from the surgery is well healed, and a chest radiograph shows no evidence of abnormalities.

Which of these studies is LEAST likely to be abnormal in this patient?

A) ECG.
B) V/Q scan.
C) Echocardiogram.
D) Sedimentation rate.
E) CBC.

Discussion

The correct answer is B. A V/Q scan is not likely to be positive in this patient. This patient is unlikely to have a pulmonary embolism given the duration of symptoms because the pain is worse when he lays down, and because he is febrile, reports no dyspnea, and has a normal oxygen saturation. This **could** still be a pulmonary embolism, but it would be less likely than other, more plausible explanations. The most likely diagnosis in this patient, given the lack of other symptoms, is postpericardotomy syndrome. This is similar to Dressler syndrome, which occurs after an MI and presents with fever and chest pain several days to weeks after the inciting event. The white blood count is often elevated, as is the sedimentation rate. The ECG can also be helpful as can an echocardiogram.

You obtain an ECG on this patient which shows a pattern consistent with pericarditis. Which of the following patterns can be seen in a patient with pericarditis?

A) Diffuse ST segment elevation.
B) Normal ECG.
C) Left bundle branch block.
D) ST elevations in anterior leads with reciprocal ST depressions in inferior leads.
E) A and B.

Discussion

The correct answer is E. Both diffuse ST segment elevations and a normal ECG can be seen with pericarditis. The initial ECG is only 80% sensitive for pericarditis. Small (low voltage) QRS complexes or electrical alternans can also be seen with pericarditis. Answer C is incorrect because bundle branch blocks have nothing to do with pericarditis. Answer D is incorrect because ST elevations with reciprocal depressions are likely due to MI and **not** to pericarditis.

✳ ✳

You decide to treat this patient for pericarditis based on echocardiogram and ECG findings consistent with this diagnosis.

Which of the following drugs might be helpful in this patient?

A) Heparin.
B) Warfarin.
C) Furosemide.
D) Indomethacin.
E) None of the above.

Discussion

Answer D is correct. You must prescribe an antiinflammatory in this patient. You can use aspirin, an NSAID, or steroids. Generally, indomethacin or aspirin are considered first-line drugs with steroids being reserved for those who fail NSAID therapy. Answers A and B are incorrect. **Do not** use anticoagulation, either heparin or warfarin, in patients with pericarditis. This can cause bleeding into the pericardial sac and tamponade. Answer C is incorrect because furosemide will likely make this patient worse. Patients with increased pericardial pressures are dependent on circulating preload volume in order to fill the right heart. Decreasing the preload may worsen this patient's dyspnea.

✳ ✳

The patient returns the next day and is feeling more short of breath. On exam you notice JVD and peripheral edema.

The best initial treatment for this patient is:

A) Furosemide.
B) Nitroglycerin.
C) IV saline.
D) Morphine.
E) Ethacrynic acid.

Discussion

The correct answer is C. This patient is in pure right heart failure secondary to cardiac tamponade. He is preload dependent. The treatment is to increase his preload by using IV saline. All the other options reduce the preload and will worsen this patient's symptoms.

✳ ✳

You give a bolus of IV saline, but the patient remains dyspneic with elevated neck veins and has a pulsus paradoxus of 14 mm Hg.

The NEXT step for this patient is:

A) Change the patient to steroids from indomethacin.
B) Perform a pericardiocentesis.
C) Start a positive inotrope (eg, dopamine) to improve right heart function.
D) Start an afterload reducer to reduce cardiac demand.
E) None of the above.

Discussion

The correct answer is B. The patient is clearly not doing well if he is getting more short of breath and not responding to your treatment. The pulsus paradoxus is 14 mm Hg; a positive test is an inspiratory reduction in systolic pressure >10 mm Hg. This is indicative of cardiac tamponade, but may be seen in constrictive pericarditis or severe asthma. This patient's clinical picture is consistent with decompensated cardiac tamponade, and drastic action is indicated to relieve the symptoms of right-heart failure. The definitive treatment is pericardiocentesis. Answer A is incorrect because more drastic action is required. You would be correct to change the patient to prednisone if he were failing an NSAID but was not decompensated. Answer C is incorrect because an inotrope will do little to help this problem. Answer D is incorrect for two reasons: first, this is a right-sided heart problem and reducing afterload (systemic vascular resistance) will not help the right heart, which pumps against pulmonary resistance; second, most drugs that reduce systemic vascular resistance will also decrease preload to some degree, worsening the symptoms of tamponade.

You perform a pericardiocentesis and the patient gets better. The case has a happy ending and nobody gets sued. Of course a good outcome never protected anyone from a lawsuit.....

Objectives: Did you learn to . . .

- Evaluate a patient with typical anginal chest pain?
- Describe the test characteristics of various types of noninvasive cardiac testing?
- Become familiar with the interpretation of noninvasive cardiac testing?
- Recognize various indications for PTCA with stent placement versus coronary artery bypass grafting (CABG)?
- Understand the physiology, presentation, and treatment of postpericardotomy syndrome?
- Treat pericarditis and cardiac tamponade?

 QUICK QUIZ: HYPERTENSION

According to JNC 7, the blood pressure goal in a patient with diabetes is:

A) 100/50.
B) 110/70.
C) 130/80.
D) 140/90.
E) None of the above.

Discussion

The correct answer is C. The goal for a diabetic patient (or any patient with underlying renal disease) is 130/80 or lower.

CASE 4

A 24-year-old male presents to your clinic with a 10-hour history of an irregular heart rate. He is generally well but has a history of hypertension (too many super-jumbo burgers....with bacon and salt...), which he has been trying to control with exercise and diet. He has been successful and blood pressures have been normal. There is no prior history of cardiac disease or palpitations. He did "have a bit to drink" celebrating....well, he doesn't quite remember *what* he was celebrating but he is sure it was important. There is no family history of heart disease and the patient does not smoke. You have known the patient and his family for 20 years and know that he has never had a heart murmur. Vital signs reveal an irregular pulse of 130 beats per minute and a blood pressure of 160/100 mm Hg (likely from anxiety since this patient is generally normotensive). The patient is afebrile and has normal respirations. He has no heart murmur. The ECG is shown in Figure 2–2.

The most appropriate diagnosis is:

A) Multifocal atrial tachycardia.
B) Wandering atrial pacemaker.
C) Atrial fibrillation.
D) Ventricular tachycardia.
E) Accelerated junctional rhythm.

Discussion

The correct answer is C, atrial fibrillation. This is characterized by the lack of P waves and an irregularly irregular rhythm. At some points on this ECG, one could argue for the presence of atrial flutter P waves;

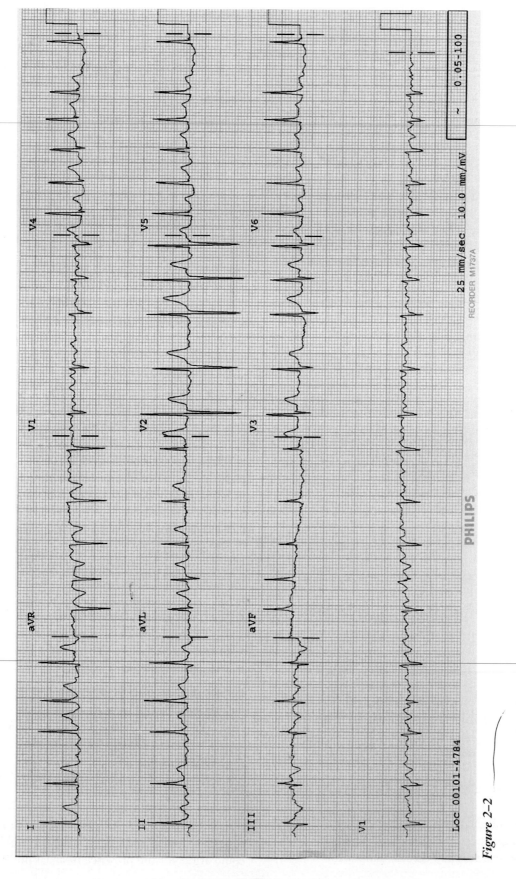

Figure 2–2

but we do not see the regular QRS complexes that should occur with atrial flutter, so atrial fibrillation is the more appropriate diagnosis. Answers A and B are incorrect. Although both multifocal atrial tachycardia and a wandering atrial pacemaker are irregularly irregular, both have P waves. Answer D is incorrect. Ventricular tachycardia is a wide complex tachycardia and is regular. Answer E is incorrect. Although there are no P waves in an accelerated junctional rhythm, it should be a regular, organized rhythm.

What is the most likely cause of this patient's dysrhythmia?

A) Congenital prolonged QT syndrome.
B) Hypertrophic cardiomyopathy.
C) Alcohol.
D) Marijuana use.
E) Ischemic cardiac disease.

Discussion

The correct answer is C. The most likely cause of atrial fibrillation in this 24-year-old is alcohol (aka "holiday heart"). It occurs after episodes of significant alcohol intake. The underlying mechanism is not known. Answer A is incorrect because prolonged QT typically causes polymorphic ventricular tachycardia (especially torsade de pointes). Answer B, hypertrophic cardiomyopathy, is unlikely since the patient has never had a murmur, and hypertrophic cardiomyopathy generally presents with signs of aortic outlet obstruction (syncope or angina with exercise). Answer D is incorrect because marijuana is not implicated in causing atrial fibrillation. Answer E is incorrect because a patient who is 24 is unlikely to have ischemic cardiac disease.

Other states that can cause atrial fibrillation include all of the following EXCEPT:

A) Valvular disease, especially mitral disease.
B) Hyperthyroidism.
C) Stroke.
D) CHF.
E) Acute pulmonary embolism.

Discussion

The correct answer is C. Stroke does not generally cause atrial fibrillation. Certainly stroke and other intracranial injuries can be associated with arrhythmias. However, these are generally isolated PVCs. Stroke may also be associated with CHF and ischemic changes on the ECG, but it is rarely an isolated cause of atrial fibrillation. However, the reverse is true: stroke may be the result of thromboembolic phenomena caused by atrial fibrillation. Valvular heart disease, hyperthyroidism, CHF, and pulmonary emboli (PE) are all causes of atrial fibrillation. Valvular heart disease, CHF, and PE all have a similar mechanism: stretching of the atrium leading to atrial irritability. Atrial fibrillation is found in 10%–20% of those with hyperthyroidism, especially in the elderly. The majority of patients will spontaneously convert once their hyperthyroidism is controlled, but they should be anticoagulated until they are in normal sinus rhythm and for 4–6 weeks thereafter.

* *

The patient confides that he was indeed at a bachelor party yesterday and had a bit too much to drink. This is quite unusual for the patient. He generally drinks 2 to 3 beers per week. The patient's pulse increases to 160 but he remains asymptomatic.

The INITIAL goal for this patient is:

A) Anticoagulation.
B) Immediate cardioversion.
C) Transesophageal echocardiogram to rule out vegetations.
D) Rate control.
E) Administer thiamine.

Discussion

The correct answer is D, rate control. The patient does not need **immediate** anticoagulation. Thus, answer A is incorrect. Answer B is incorrect because this patient is not hypotensive and is asymptomatic aside from palpitations. If the patient were hypotensive or had evidence of end-organ hypoperfusion (ie, cardiac ischemia), urgent cardioversion would be appropriate. Answer C is incorrect because the purpose of an echocardiogram is to assess for vegetations. This may be important to do at some point (although it can be argued that for atrial fibrillation of 10 hours or less, it is superfluous) but it is not the immediate goal. Answer E is incorrect for two reasons: first, thiamine will not help with rate control or his arrhythmia; second, the patient is not a chronic alcoholic or malnourished and thus would not need thiamine in any event.

* *

The patient's heart rate remains elevated at 160 bpm with occasional forays into the 170 bpm range.

Which of the following is the best drug to administer to this patient?

A) Digoxin.
B) Lidocaine.
C) Amiodarone.
D) Adenosine.
E) Verapamil.

Discussion

The correct answer is E, verapamil. Answer A is incorrect. Digoxin will be of limited use since it takes at least 30 minutes to have an effect. It can be used in those with atrial fibrillation secondary to CHF but will still not help with rate control acutely. Answer B is incorrect because lidocaine is indicated for a wide complex tachycardia. Answer C is incorrect. Amiodarone will work as a treatment for atrial fibrillation but is a second-line drug because it can cause torsade de pointes. It can be used in patients with atrial fibrillation and congestive failure, whereas verapamil or another calcium channel blocker might be contraindicated. Answer D is incorrect. Adenosine is ultrashort-acting, blocks the AV node, and can be used to convert a paroxysmal supraventricular tachycardia or slow the rate of the arrhythmia temporarily if you are not sure what the diagnosis is (eg, rapid atrial flutter vs. PSVT). However, adenosine will not reduce the ventricular rate in atrial fibrillation since it does not require the AV node to propagate. Thus, verapamil is the best choice. Diltiazem can also be used in this situation, as could a β-blocker.

* *

You realize that 50% of atrial fibrillation will spontaneously convert to normal sinus rhythm. A transthoracic echocardiogram was performed and did not demonstrate any structural heart disease. Thus, you choose to watch the patient. At 24 hours he still is in atrial fibrillation, although the rate is controlled well with verapamil.

The next step in the management of this patient is (remember, he is generally normotensive):

A) Start warfarin.
B) Start heparin and warfarin at the same time.
C) Use low-molecular-weight heparin so the patient does not need to be hospitalized and start warfarin at the same time.

D) Start heparin and wait until the patient's PT/PTT/INR are stabilized before starting warfarin.
E) Start aspirin.

Discussion

The correct answer is E. In this patient, there is no indication to anticoagulate as he meets criteria for lone atrial fibrillation—atrial fibrillation occurring in a patient <65 years and without structural heart disease, hypertension, diabetes, or prior thromboembolic event. For this patient, therapy with aspirin is sufficient. Answer A is incorrect as this patient meets criteria for lone atrial fibrillation and will not have any benefit from warfarin. Answers B, C, and D are incorrect because this patient does not need warfarin and heparin.

 HELPFUL TIP: In patients with atrial fibrillation and current thrombosis, you would want to start heparin and warfarin at the same time. This could be done either as an outpatient (with low-molecular-weight heparin) or as an inpatient, as the situation dictates.

* *

Since the patient remains in atrial fibrillation and does not want to take drugs for years, you decide to cardiovert him.

How long must you wait after the patient has been anticoagulated before cardioverting the patient?

A) 1 week.
B) 3 weeks.
C) 3 months.
D) Only until therapeutic on warfarin.
E) There is no need to wait before cardioversion in this patient.

Discussion

The correct answer is B. If the patient has been in atrial fibrillation for >48 hours, one should wait until the patient has been anticoagulated (target INR 2–3) for 3 weeks before attempting cardioversion. This is based on recommendations from expert consensus. If atrial fibrillation has been present for <48 hours, you can proceed directly to cardioversion. Some physicians may order a transesophageal echocardiogram to assess for thrombus formation before cardioversion; this approach is acceptable, but not necessary, as long as the patient has been in atrial fibrillation for <48 hours.

All of the following can be used to cardiovert atrial fibrillation EXCEPT:

A) Ibutilide.
B) Electrical cardioversion.
C) Quinidine.
D) Digoxin.
E) Procainamide.

Discussion

The correct answer is D. Digoxin does not work to cardiovert atrial fibrillation. Digoxin may facilitate cardioversion in patients by reducing CHF and atrial stretching. However, it does not directly convert atrial fibrillation. All of the other drugs convert atrial fibrillation. Because of potential induction of arrhythmias with the other agents, electrical cardioversion (answer B) is becoming the preferred method of restoring normal sinus rhythm.

Objectives: Did you learn to . . .

- Recognize the clinical and ECG presentation of atrial fibrillation?
- Use rate-controlling drugs to treat a patient with atrial fibrillation?
- Appropriately employ anticoagulation in atrial fibrillation?
- Identify appropriate situations for cardioversion of atrial fibrillation?

QUICK QUIZ: ANTIHYPERTENSIVE AGENTS

A 70-year-old male complains of impotence and requests sildenafil (Viagra) for erectile dysfunction, which you believe is secondary to vascular disease. Which of the following antihypertensive drugs can cause prolonged hypotension when used with sildenafil?

A) Peripheral α-blockers.
B) Calcium channel blockers.
C) An ACE inhibitor.
D) Diuretics.
E) β-Blockers.

Discussion

The correct answer is A. The peripheral α-blockers (doxazosin, prazosin, tamsulosin) can cause symptomatic hypotension when combined with sildenafil or other drugs of this class (tadalafil [Cialis], vardenafil [Levitra]). This hypotensive effect is more severe when these drugs are combined with a nitrate, such as sublingual nitroglycerin. Therefore, nitrates should not be administered within 24 hours (or longer in patients with renal or hepatic dysfunction) of these drugs. None of the other drugs (answers B–E) causes this hypotensive effect when combined with sildenafil.

CASE 5

A 65-year-old male with a history of newly identified atrial fibrillation is referred to you for medical clearance for surgery. He has a history of hypertension and hypercholesterolemia. He has normal cardiac function otherwise with a normal ejection fraction and no valvular disease on echocardiogram. His atrial fibrillation has not been addressed since it was picked up by the surgeon at a preop visit. His heart rate is 80 beats per minute when you see him, his rhythm is irregularly irregular, and he has no signs of heart failure.

Which of the following options would be appropriate for this patient?

A) Anticoagulate the patient with warfarin and allow him to stay in atrial fibrillation.
B) Place the patient on aspirin and allow him to stay in atrial fibrillation.
C) Give digoxin to cardiovert the patient.
D) Strongly suggest cardioversion to this patient since sustained normal sinus rhythm yields the best long-term outcomes.
E) Add furosemide to prevent the development of CHF and edema.

Discussion

The correct answer is A. Outcomes of patients in atrial fibrillation who are rate controlled and anticoagulated are actually **better** than are the outcomes in those in whom normal sinus rhythm is maintained using antiarrhythmics. **A rhythm-control strategy, even if apparently successful, is not considered a reason to discontinue anticoagulation.** Answer B is incorrect because aspirin should be used only in patients with lone or low-risk atrial fibrillation (see below) and in patients who have contraindications to anticoagulation with warfarin. Answer C is incorrect; digoxin may help with rate control in atrial fibrillation but does not convert atrial fibrillation and is proarrhythmic. It works best for rate control in those who are sedentary. Answer D is incorrect because trying to maintain normal sinus rhythm with antiarrhythmics has not been shown to be advantageous. Answer E is incorrect because the patient exhibits no features of CHF and fluid retention.

* *

In discussing this patient's care with the surgeon, she asks if this patient really needs anticoagulation because of his "lone atrial fibrillation." You believe that her assumption is incorrect.

The criteria for lone atrial fibrillation, which allows one to use *aspirin rather than warfarin* as an antithrombotic drug, include all of the following EXCEPT:

A) No history of hypertension.
B) Age <50 years.
C) Absence of heart failure.
D) No prior history of stroke or transient ischemic attack.
E) No history of diabetes mellitus.

Discussion
The correct answer is B. The term "lone atrial fibrillation" has been used to identify patients with atrial fibrillation with a very low risk of thromboembolism. The clinical criteria include the following: no history of hypertension, diabetes mellitus, transient ischemic attack or stroke, heart failure, coronary artery disease or significant valvular disease. In addition to these clinical criteria, there should be no echocardiographic evidence of structural heart disease. Although 60 years has been a cut-off in the past, recent data suggest that patients >65 years can be considered for aspirin therapy if they meet all of the other criteria for "lone A-fib."

* *

The reason this 65-year-old male initially came to see you is because of right upper quadrant pain that you have diagnosed as cholelithiasis. He needs surgery to remove his gallbladder.

Which of the following approaches is the best for controlling his anticoagulation given that he needs surgery?

A) Stop the warfarin several days before surgery to allow his INR to normalize. Restart the warfarin after surgery.
B) Hospitalize the patient a couple of days ahead of time and start heparin. Then stop his warfarin. Restart the warfarin after surgery.
C) Use low-molecular-weight heparin at home and stop the warfarin once this is started. Restart the warfarin after surgery.
D) Stop the warfarin several days before surgery to allow his INR to normalize. Start heparin after surgery and simultaneously restart warfarin.

Discussion
The correct answer is A. For patients with atrial fibrillation who are undergoing surgery or invasive diagnostic procedures, it is reasonable to interrupt anticoagulation for up to 1 week without substituting heparin. The risk of perioperative bleeding with heparin is actually greater than the risk of thromboembolism from atrial fibrillation. Answers B, C, and D are incorrect because the patient does not need heparin.

* *

The patient has his surgery and returns to your clinic for a postoperative checkup 1 month after his surgery. You check his INR and it is noted to be 5.2. There is no active bleeding.

The most appropriate action now is to:

A) Hospitalize the patient for observation since he is at a high risk of bleeding.
B) Give the patient 5 mg of vitamin K orally.
C) Give the patient 2 units of fresh frozen plasma to reverse his anticoagulation.
D) Hold the next warfarin dose and reduce the maintenance dose.
E) A, B, and C.

Discussion
The correct answer is D. The risk of bleeding in a relatively healthy patient with an INR of 5.2 is very low. Thus, simply holding next one to two doses of warfarin and reducing the maintenance dose of warfarin is appropriate. Answer A is incorrect because the patient does not need hospitalization. Answer B is incorrect because it will be difficult to reanticoagulate the patient after vitamin K is administered. Answer C is incorrect because there is no active bleeding.

* *

The patient misunderstands your instructions and takes an **extra** dose of warfarin that evening and for the next 2 days. He returns to your clinic and his INR is now 13.

What is the most effective form of therapy indicated for this patient now?

A) 5 mg vitamin K IV.
B) Fresh frozen plasma.
C) 1 mg vitamin K PO.
D) 5 mg vitamin K PO.
E) 20 mg vitamin K IV.

Discussion

The correct answer is D. Giving this patient 5 mg of PO vitamin K is the best solution. This has been found to lower the INR while still allowing the patient to be anticoagulated relatively easily after treatment. Answer B is incorrect because there is no call for FFP in this asymptomatic patient. The other answers are incorrect because there is no advantage to higher doses of vitamin K in this patient, and the higher doses will make continued anticoagulation more difficult.

 HELPFUL TIP: If the INR is ≤5, simply hold the next dose of warfarin. If it is 5–9, hold one or two doses or administer PO vitamin K (1 mg is generally recommended but up to 5 mg can be used). If the INR is 10–20, administer 5–10 mg of vitamin K PO. If the INR is >20 rapid reversal of INR is indicated with FFP and vitamin K. Hospitalization, vitamin K, and FFP are appropriate regardless of the INR if there is **active bleeding** (intracranial hemorrhage) or if the patient will need an invasive procedure in the near future (eg, a few hours).

Objectives: Did you learn to . . .

- Weigh the advantages and disadvantages of rate control versus rhythm control strategies for atrial fibrillation?
- Define lone atrial fibrillation?
- Manage anticoagulation and atrial fibrillation vis-à-vis surgery?
- Manage the overanticoagulated patient?

CASE 6

A 62-year-old female presents to your office with a history of occasional palpitations, which are of great concern to her. She notes that she feels a racing heart that lasts for a matter of seconds and occurs every 7 days or so. However, when she has the symptoms, she generally will get 4 to 5 episodes during that day. She notes no associated cardiac symptoms such as chest pain, dyspnea, lightheadedness, etc.

Which of the following modalities would be the best way to diagnose this patient's condition?

A) ECG.
B) Holter monitor.
C) Stress echocardiography.
D) Event monitor.
E) Electrophysiologic (EP) study.

Discussion

The correct answer is D. The patient can wear an event monitor for up to 1 month and can push a button when she notices the symptoms. This rhythm is then stored and sent to the reader of the event monitor to examine. Answer A is incorrect because she is having only intermittent symptoms that will probably not show up on an ECG. Clearly, an ECG is indicated in this patient, but it is not the way to diagnose the presenting complaint. Answer B is incorrect because a Holter monitor will record only for a short period of time (24–48 hrs). This patient's symptoms occur only episodically and may not be found on a time-limited recording. Answer C is incorrect because a stress echocardiogram is not primarily used to detect arrhythmias but rather ischemia. Answer E is incorrect because we do not know if this patient is even having a significant arrhythmia at this point. Once we know that there is a significant arrhythmia, an EP study might be indicated.

* *

The event monitor shows that the patient is having nonsustained episodes of monomorphic ventricular tachycardia lasting less than 4 beats each. She is otherwise asymptomatic.

The best approach at this point is to:

A) Start an antiarrhythmic such as quinidine or mexiletine to control the heart rhythm.
B) Refer the patient to a cardiologist for an EP study to determine the best drug to control this rhythm.

C) Implant an automatic defibrillator to prevent sudden death.
D) Implant a pacemaker.
E) Check serum potassium, magnesium, TSH.

Discussion

The correct answer is E. The first step in determining the treatment of this patient is to make sure that there is not an underlying metabolic abnormality that could predispose to this rhythm abnormality.

* *

You check a panel of laboratory studies including thyroid function tests, electrolytes, magnesium, glucose, CBC. They are all within normal limits. You suggest that the patient avoid potential triggers such as caffeine and sympathomimetics.

The next step for this patient is to:

A) Start an antiarrhythmic such as quinidine or mexiletine to control the heart rhythm.
B) Refer the patient to a cardiologist for an EP study to determine the best drug to control this rhythm.
C) Implant an automatic defibrillator to prevent sudden death.
D) Start a β-blocker.
E) Order transthoracic echocardiogram to rule out structural heart disease.

Discussion

The correct answer is E. Nonsustained ventricular tachycardia may have an adverse prognosis in the presence of structural heart disease like hypertrophic cardiomyopathy or ischemic heart disease. An echocardiogram as well as a stress test may be helpful in ruling them out. There is no evidence that nonsustained, asymptomatic ventricular tachycardia worsens outcomes **as long as the patient has no underlying cardiac disease**. In an otherwise healthy, asymptomatic, patient, the risk of trying to use drugs to suppress ventricular ectopy leads to worse outcomes than doing nothing. Quinidine, mexiletine, amiodarone, and other antiarrhythmics all have proarrhythmic effects. Generally, there is more sudden death in these patients if they are treated with drugs than if they are watched. Therefore, answer A is incorrect because these drugs will increase mortality. Answer B is incorrect since the patient has asymptomatic, self-limited episodes. The reason to do an EP study is to see if there is an inducible arrhythmia and to determine treatment. This

patient does not need treatment. Answer C is incorrect because this patient has asymptomatic ventricular tachycardia. Thus, an implantable defibrillator is not indicated. A β-blocker may be used after initial evaluation for symptomatic relief.

* *

The echocardiogram is normal, and the patient does well for the next 3 months but then becomes symptomatic with prolonged episodes of ventricular tachycardia. Although all of the episodes are self-limited, the patient has had two episodes of syncope.

Which of the following is the next best step in treating this patient?

A) Sotalol.
B) Implantable defibrillators.
C) Amiodarone.
D) Electrophysiologic study.
E) Tocainide (an oral lidocaine equivalent).

Discussion

The correct answer is D. An electrophysiologic study is indicated to induce and characterize the ventricular tachycardia. Certain types of ventricular tachycardia respond very well to radiofrequency ablation. Answer B is incorrect. Implantable defibrillator would be the correct choice for patients with ischemic heart disease and left ventricular dysfunction and symptomatic ventricular tachycardia. However, this patient does not have any underlying CHF.

Objectives: Did you learn to . . .

- Evaluate a patient with palpitations?
- Manage nonsustained, asymptomatic, ventricular tachycardia?

CASE 7

A 22-year-old female presents to your office with a history of palpitations. You are able to capture the arrhythmia on the monitor in your office: the rhythm strip shows evidence of isolated premature atrial contractions (PACs). You take a history from this patient. She is taking no other medications and there is no family history of any similar problems.

All of the following are salient points of the history with regards to PACs EXCEPT:

A) Aged cheese consumption.
B) Caffeine use.
C) Tobacco use.
D) Alcohol use.
E) COPD.

Discussion

The correct answer is A. Aged cheese **can** cause problems in combination with monoamine oxidase inhibitors (MAOIs). In combination with an MAOI, aged cheese and other sources of tyramine can cause a hypertensive emergency. However this patient is not taking any medications. All of the other conditions and drugs listed can cause PACs. Although there are conflicting data about the strength of the association, caffeine, COPD, tobacco, and alcohol can all cause an increase in sympathetic tone, leading to PACs. Neurologic abnormalities (eg, stroke) can also be associated with PACs, as can some drugs (eg, theophylline).

Which of the following statements about PACs is true?

A) Mitral valve prolapse is associated with PACs.
B) Mitral valve stenosis is associated with PACs.
C) Bicuspid aortic valve is associated with PACs.
D) None of the above is true.

Discussion

The correct answer is B. Anything that can cause an increase in left atrial pressures (and therefore atrial wall stretching) is associated with an increase in the number of PACs. Mitral stenosis causes increased pressures in the left atrium, wall stretching and enlargement and thus predisposes to PACs. Answer A is incorrect. Although multiple problems have been blamed on mitral valve prolapse, a study done as part of the Framingham study showed that the symptoms blamed on mitral valve prolapse (anxiety, PACs, tachycardia, etc) are no more prevalent in those with mitral valve prolapse than in those without it. Answer C is incorrect. A bicuspid aortic valve **may** cause PACs as a result of CHF when the patient decompensates and has increased left-sided heart pressures. However, a bicuspid aortic valve itself is not a source of PACs. Similarly, hypertrophic cardiomyopathy, other causes of CHF, drugs (eg, theophylline and digoxin), and neurologic diseases can be associated with PACs.

* *

The patient is bothered by her PACs. She is rather aware of them and finds them disconcerting.

What is the best pharmacologic therapy to consider now?

A) Sotalol.
B) Metoprolol.
C) Traysolol.
D) Amiodarone.

Discussion

The correct answer is B. A β-blocker may help to reduce this patient's PACs. Answer A is incorrect because, while sotalol can be used for both atrial and ventricular arrhythmias, it is proarrhythmic and can cause torsade de pointes. Thus it should be reserved for those with severe arrhythmias. Answer C is incorrect because Traysolol (trade name for aprotinin) is an enzyme that is used to reduce bleeding during surgical procedures. Answer D is incorrect because, like sotalol, amiodarone is proarrhythmic, and its use should be limited to those with significant arrhythmias.

Objectives: Did you learn to . . .

- Recognize causes of PACs?
- Treat a patient with bothersome PACs?

 QUICK QUIZ: VALVULAR DISEASE

Surgery is indicated in which of these patients with valvular disease?

A) An asymptomatic patient with severe mitral regurgitation and a left ventricular ejection fraction of <60%.
B) An asymptomatic patient with a bicuspid aortic valve.
C) Asymptomatic aortic regurgitation with a left ventricular ejection fraction of <50% on echocardiogram.
D) Only symptomatic valvular lesions should be approached surgically.
E) A and C.

Discussion

The correct answer is E. Once patients with mitral regurgitation and aortic regurgitation become symptomatic, the morbidity and mortality increase significantly. Thus, these patients should be operated on **before** they become symptomatic. Patients should have routine echocardiography yearly if they have severe disease. In addition to evaluating the valve, echocardiography allows you to evaluate ventricular function.

CASE 8

A 74-year-old male presents to your office with a chief complaint of a "long cold" with a cough for 5 months. He has also noticed that he gets up to urinate twice a night although he has no trouble with his urine stream, starting urination, or dribbling afterwards. He has been a bit more tired lately and notices that his exercise tolerance has decreased to several blocks, limited mainly by shortness of breath. He has had no episodes of chest pain. He has no history of asthma or COPD and has not had any new exposures to drugs or chemicals. He has a history of hypertension and noncompliance with medical recommendations. He is taking no medications except for 1 aspirin per day. His pulse is 100 with a blood pressure of 160/95. He looks pretty well. On exam you find only trace pitting edema of the lower extremities.

Which of the following is NOT a possible cause of cough in this patient?

A) CHF.
B) Asthma.
C) Deconditioning.
D) COPD.
E) GERD.

Discussion

The correct answer is C. Deconditioning may cause dyspnea on exertion but should not cause a cough. The purpose of this question is to point out that a chronic cold or chronic cough in an elderly person can be due to myriad causes, including occult CHF. Do not make the assumption that the patient's diagnosis (eg, a chronic cold), disguised as the chief complaint, is necessarily the correct diagnosis.

Given the symptom complex above (dyspnea on exertion, nocturia, cough, and trace edema) what is the MOST likely cause of this patient's symptoms?

A) Sarcoidosis.
B) Diabetes with polyuria.
C) Pneumonia.
D) Wegner granulomatosis.
E) CHF.

Discussion

The correct answer is E, CHF (this is the cardiology review section, after all). There are several clues that point to CHF. First, the patient notes nocturia. Although this can be due to prostate troubles in a male, it was stipulated that the patient had no other problems with urination that might indicate prostatism. Nocturia can reflect volume overload, such as with early CHF or early renal failure. Patients cannot mobilize excess fluid during the day (eg, they develop edema while upright) but are able to do so at night, as the recumbent position facilitates fluid mobilization from the lower extremities. Thus, they develop nocturia. Second, the patient has pitting edema. Answer A, sarcoidosis, is incorrect because it is unlikely to have initial onset in a 75-year-old. Answer B, diabetes, is incorrect because because the patient has only nocturia and not true polyuria. If the patient was having polyuria during the day, diabetes might be a more serious consideration. Answer C is incorrect because these symptoms have been continuing for 6 months. Answer D is incorrect because Wegner is generally a disease of young adults (age of onset usually in the forties) and generally has other systemic symptoms associated, including fever, weight loss, arthralgias, etc.

* *

You decide that this patient may have CHF and decide to do an ECG in your office. The ECG shows no evidence of prior or ongoing ischemia. There are no signs of atrial enlargement or ventricular hypertrophy.

The proper conclusion is:

A) The patient does not have cardiac chamber enlargement or hypertrophy and therefore it is unlikely to be CHF.
B) The absence of evidence for an infarct makes CHF unlikely.
C) Regardless of the ECG results, clinical judgment alone is sufficient to make the diagnosis of CHF, being correct 85% of the time.
D) The patient's edema is likely from venous insufficiency.
E) Despite a normal ECG, further testing is needed in this patient to evaluate for CHF.

Discussion

The correct answer is E. Further testing is needed to determine if this patient has CHF. Answer A is incorrect because only 30% to 60% of moderate-to-severe left ventricular hypertrophy (LVH) is detectible on ECG. Answer B is incorrect because patients with diastolic dysfunction (discussed below) may not have any evidence of prior ischemia or MI. Answer C is incorrect. The clinical diagnosis of CHF is incorrect up to 50% of the time. For this reason, confirmation is required before embarking upon a therapeutic adventure for CHF. Answer D is incorrect because the patient has other symptoms of CHF (exertional dyspnea, etc) that make simple venous insufficiency unlikely.

* *

You decide on further testing. Assuming every test is easily available to you (which might not be the case depending on the setting in which you work), what is the ONE BEST test that you would use to determine if this patient has CHF?

A) Echocardiography.
B) Brain natriuretic peptide (BNP) level.
C) Chest radiograph looking for evidence of pulmonary edema (Kerley B lines, etc.).
D) SPECT thallium test.
E) Adenosine thallium testing.

Discussion

The correct answer is A. Echocardiography is the procedure of choice for the diagnosis of CHF for two reasons. First, you can assess left ventricular systolic function as well as look for diastolic dysfunction to determine if this is systolic or diastolic heart failure. Second, you can evaluate the potential causes of heart failure including valvular heart disease, ischemic heart disease and pericardial disease. Answer B is incorrect because the BNP will give you less information about the patient than will echocardiography. Among patients with dyspnea, BNP is highly sensitive for the detection of acute CHF. In addition, a low BNP effectively rules out acute CHF with 99% negative predictive value. However, the positive predictive value of BNP is limited; conditions other than heart failure like chronic renal failure, cor pulmonale, and pulmonary embolism can also elevate BNP. Specifically, a BNP of <100 pg/mL effectively rules out CHF. A BNP of 100 pg/mL–500 pg/mL is indeterminate and may not be related to cardiac disease. A BNP >500 pg/mL is specific for CHF. In this patient with a high pretest probability of CHF, BNP will most likely be elevated and helpful if over 500 pg/mL. Answers D and E are incorrect

because SPECT thallium and adenosine thallium testing are better used to diagnose ischemic cardiac disease.

* *

The patient has an echocardiogram which shows an ejection fraction of 40% and regional wall motion abnormalities.

This is most consistent with a diagnosis of:

A) CHF secondary to myocarditis.
B) CHF from systolic dysfunction secondary to ischemic disease.
C) Diastolic dysfunction.
D) CHF secondary to constrictive pericarditis.
E) CHF from valvular disease.

Discussion

The correct answer is B. Regional wall motion abnormalities suggest that this patient has infarcted or poorly perfused myocardium at the present time ("hibernating myocardium"). Answer A is incorrect because those with myocarditis should have a more global hypokinesis. Answer C is incorrect given low ejection fraction. Diastolic dysfunction is associated with a hypertrophied left ventricle and a **preserved** ejection fraction. Echocardiogram in constrictive pericarditis generally shows normal left ventricular systolic function. It may reveal pericardial thickening, dilated inferior vena cava or hepatic veins, abnormal septal motion and abnormal mitral and tricuspid flow dopplers. Therefore answer D is incorrect. Answer E is incorrect. Absence of significant valvular stenosis or regurgitation make valvular disease unlikely etiology of CHF.

 HELPFUL TIP: Methamphetamine and cocaine can lead to left-sided heart failure and should be considered as a possible etiology in the appropriate patient.

Which of the following is the most appropriate next strategy to work up this patient's CHF?

A) Cardiac MRI to assess myocardial viability.
B) Coronary angiogram.
C) Measure serial troponins to rule out acute coronary syndrome.

D) Electrophysiologic study to assess for inducible ventricular arrhythmia.

E) CT to assess calcium scores.

Discussion

The correct answer is B. Ischemic heart disease is the most common etiology for heart failure associated with systolic dysfunction. Coronary angiogram remains the gold standard to evaluate for coronary artery disease. Answer A is incorrect because it does not help in the initial workup of heart failure. Assessment of myocardial viability is important in the evaluation of patients with chronic CAD and resting left ventricular dysfunction eligible for revascularization. Coronary angiograms provide information about anatomy and feasibility of revascularization but do not predict recovery of function. Answer C is incorrect because this patient does not have chest pain or ECG changes to suggest acute cardiac ischemia. Answer D is incorrect as there is no indication for an electrophysiologic study in the absence of any arrhythmia.

* *

The coronary angiogram shows diffuse coronary artery disease; no coronary lesions are considered to be amenable to angioplasty or bypass surgery. You decide to initiate medical therapy in this patient. In addition, you advise the patient regarding the nonpharmacologic therapies for heart failure treatment.

These include all of the following EXCEPT:

A) Fluid restriction of <2 liters per day.

B) Sodium restriction of <2 g sodium per day.

C) Dietary consultation.

D) Cardiac risk factor modification.

E) Weekly weight monitoring.

Discussion

The correct answer is E. The keystone of an effective heart failure treatment regimen is sodium as well as fluid restriction. Frequently overlooked, these are the most common causes of heart failure exacerbation. It is imperative to get dietary consultation for every patient with newly diagnosed heart failure. Cardiac risk factors including hypertension, diabetes and hyperlipidemia need to be treated with the same aggressiveness as in a patient with an acute coronary syndrome. The patient should be advised about **daily** weight monitoring rather than weekly monitoring. A weight gain of more than 3–5 lbs may necessitate additional doses of furosemide.

* *

You wish to start an appropriate drug regimen for this patient's heart failure.

All of the drugs below have been shown to decrease mortality in patients with CHF secondary to systolic dysfunction EXCEPT:

A) Digoxin.

B) Metoprolol.

C) Angiotensin converting enzyme inhibitors (ACE inhibitors).

D) Hydralazine and long-acting nitrates used in combination.

E) Spironolactone.

Discussion

The correct answer is A. **Digoxin has not been shown to increase survival and may worsen outcomes, especially in women.** Thus, if using digoxin in CHF, a lower dose than has been used in the past is currently recommended. Digoxin does reduce hospitalizations and improves symptoms in those with systolic dysfunction and can be appropriately used for symptom control if other treatments are not working. All of the other drugs (answers B–E), including the combination of isosorbide dinitrate and hydralazine, have been shown to decrease mortality. However, hydralazine and isosorbide dinitrate are generally reserved for those patients who are unable to tolerate ACE inhibitors or angiotensin receptor blockers (ARBs). None of the traditional loop diuretics such as furosemide, bumetanide, etc, has been shown to positively affect mortality.

* *

You start this patient on furosemide for diuresis and lisinopril for systolic dysfunction. You also decide to initiate metoprolol for its survival benefits. However, the patient's symptoms worsen.

Which of these is true about the use of metoprolol in CHF?

A) It is the only β-blocker indicated for use in CHF.

B) The best use is in those patients who are still symptomatic since it will help control symptoms.

C) It should only be initiated in patients with well-controlled CHF who are not currently having significant symptoms.

D) β-Blockers can lead to significant hypokalemia when combined with diuretics, so potassium levels should be monitored closely.

E) β-Blockers are contraindicated in patients who have a combination of COPD and CHF.

Discussion

The correct answer is C. β-Blockers are **not** indicated for patients who are significantly symptomatic. While they do decrease mortality, they can increase symptoms. Therefore, they are best initiated in the stable patient who is relatively well controlled. Even then some patients cannot tolerate the introduction of β-blockers without a worsening of symptoms which may require additional diuresis, discontinuation of the β-blocker or a reduction in dose. Answer A is incorrect. Other β-blockers have been used in CHF, including carvedilol (now available as a generic). Answer B is incorrect because β-blockers may worsen heart failure symptoms and thus should not be initiated in a patient who is symptomatic. Answer D is incorrect because β-blockers do not cause hypokalemia. Answer E is incorrect. β-Blockers can be used in patients with COPD with the same caveats that apply to any other patient: if the patient is becoming more symptomatic on the β-blocker, reduce the dose or discontinue the drug.

* *

You reduce the dose of metoprolol and consider starting this patient on another medication.

Which of the following patients is (are) good candidate(s) for spironolactone therapy?

A) A patient with NYHA class I and II CHF.

B) A patient with NYHA class III and IV CHF.

C) Both A and B.

D) Neither A nor B.

Discussion

The correct answer is B. Spironolactone has been shown to decrease mortality in patients with New York Heart Association (NYHA) class III and IV CHF. It has not been studied in class I and II heart failure. Serum potassium needs to be monitored closely after initiation of spironolactone, especially since it will generally be used with an ACE inhibitor or ARB, both of which can increase the serum potassium. This drug should be avoided in patients with renal insufficiency or patients with serum potassium >5 mEq/L.

* *

You treat this patient with metoprolol, lisinopril, furosemide, and aspirin. This regimen seems to help, and the patient's symptoms improve. However, a few weeks later he presents to the ED with increased dyspnea. There have been no changes in his medications, and he assures you that he is taking his medications as directed. His exam reveals that he has elevated JVP, rales over the lower half of his lung fields bilaterally, and pedal edema.

Common causes of decompensation in patients with otherwise stable CHF include all of the following EXCEPT:

A) Inactivity.

B) Fever.

C) Arrhythmia.

D) Dietary indiscretion.

E) Ischemia.

Discussion

The correct answer is A. Inactivity will not generally cause an exacerbation of CHF. The major causes of increased CHF include dietary indiscretion (increased salt intake "Say, can you pass the potato chips?"and increased fluid consumption), increased metabolic demand (from infection), anemia, medication noncompliance, arrhythmia, and ischemia. The inappropriate use of medications, such as some calcium channel blockers, and the institution of β-blockers are also common causes of exacerbations of CHF.

* *

This patient notes that he did have some chest pain earlier in the day. You want to initiate therapy. You take his vitals, and his pulse is 100, blood pressure 140/95 mm Hg, oxygen saturation 89% on room air, and respiratory rate 32.

Besides oxygen, the ONE BEST drug to initiate first in ED to treat this patient with CHF is:

A) Furosemide.

B) Digoxin.

C) A positive inotrope, such as dobutamine.

D) Nitroglycerin.

E) An ACE inhibitor.

Discussion

The correct answer is D. Nitroglycerin is the one best drug to initiate. This patient will benefit from nitroglycerin for two reasons. First, the patient has told you that he had chest pain earlier today. Thus, it is likely that this patient's CHF exacerbation is due to ischemic disease. Nitroglycerin will help this. Second, the goal here is to restore normal cardiac function by causing vasodilation and decreasing preload and afterload. Nitroglycerin will do both of these. Answer A, furosemide, is a good drug but not the one best drug. By inducing diuresis, furosemide will also significantly decrease preload and provide symptomatic relief. Remember not all CHF patients are fluid overloaded. Answer B is incorrect because it will take some time for digoxin to have a significant impact on this patient's symptoms. Answer C is incorrect because dobutamine is a second-line drug reserved for those not responding to more conservative therapy. Answer E is technically not incorrect, but it is not the best answer. There is ample evidence that ACE inhibitors can be used in acute CHF exacerbations either IV (eg, enalapril) or sublingual (eg, captopril). However, these drugs should be reserved as second-line therapy for patients who do not respond to more conservative measures.

* *

You treat the patient with nitroglycerin. He improves, and you admit him to the floor. While in the hospital, the patient develops some additional chest pain that lasts for 10 minutes and responds to additional sublingual nitroglycerin. His BNP is noted to be elevated. His hemoglobin (Hb) is 9.5 g/dL and hematocrit (HCT) is 32%. You have records from the office, and this is not a lot different from his baseline Hb and HCT. He is still in congestive failure (although, as noted above, better than when he was admitted). The pathologist tells you that there is blood available in the laboratory to transfuse this patient if you so choose. There is a problem, of course: he is in CHF and now is somewhat tachycardic at 110.

You tell the pathologist that:

A) Hb of 9.5 g/dL is not an indication for transfusion.
B) Transfusing this patient is inappropriate since he is already in CHF and may become more fluid overloaded with a blood transfusion.
C) You would like to go ahead with transfusing this patient.
D) Making this patient's blood more viscous with a transfusion will increase the stress on his heart.
E) A and B.

Discussion

The correct answer is C. This patient should be transfused. One of the indications for transfusion is symptomatic CHF and/or ischemia in a patient who is anemic. Transfusion will increase blood oxygen carrying capacity and oxygen delivery. There is evidence that keeping a patient's Hb above 13 g/dL if he has had an MI will decrease mortality and complications. Even though it sounds counterintuitive since you are adding fluid to a potentially fluid-overloaded patient, this is the thing to do. Obviously you will need to do it with some care, giving the blood slowly and using diuretics to prevent fluid overload as you go. Answer A, not transfusing this patient, would be the correct choice in a hemodynamically stable patient without CHF or angina. However, both angina and CHF are indications for transfusion in the anemic patient. Answer B is incorrect because this patient should be transfused carefully as noted above. Answer D is incorrect because transfusing this patient to a normal hemoglobin and hematocrit will not cause excess blood viscosity.

 HELPFUL TIP: Nesiritide (Natrecor), a BNP analogue, can be used for CHF but is expensive, contributes to renal failure, and likely increases mortality. Nesiritide can produce prolonged hypotension, which limits the dose that can be used. **This is a therapy of last resort.**

Objectives: Did you learn to . . .

• Recognize atypical presentations of CHF in the elderly?
• Describe the sensitivity and specificity of an ECG for left ventricular hypertrophy?
• Evaluate a patient with CHF?
• Manage a patient with CHF and understand the role of β-blockers, ACE inhibitors, ARBs, digoxin, and spironolactone in the treatment of CHF?
• Describe the role of BNP measurement in the evaluation of CHF and of nesiritide in the treatment of heart failure?

CASE 9

Your patient with CHF does well and is discharged from the hospital after 2 days. You are just beginning to think that the authors are tired of writing questions about CHF....but you are wrong. The patient's 70-year-old wife shows up with shortness of breath. Her physical examination is consistent with heart failure. Since you have learned so much from this case already, you send her to get an echocardiogram. You also get the recommended office tests of CBC, electrolytes, ECG, thyroid functions, etc. The results of the echocardiogram show a concentric thickening of the left ventricle with an ejection fraction of 75%.

This is most consistent with:

A) Ischemic cardiomyopathy.
B) Diastolic dysfunction.
C) Viral cardiomyopathy.
D) Hypertrophic cardiomyopathy.
E) None of the above.

Discussion

The correct answer is B, diastolic dysfunction. Answer A is incorrect because there would be evidence of regional wall motion abnormality if there had been an old MI. Also, this patient has a preserved ejection fraction which is consistent with diastolic dysfunction rather than the decreased ejection fraction associated with ischemic cardiomyopathy. Answer C is incorrect. Viral cardiomyopathy is associated with a dilated ventricle rather than a hypertrophic one, and there is a global dyskinesia with decreased ejection fraction. Answer D is incorrect. Hypertrophic cardiomyopathy is usually associated with asymmetric septal hypertrophy rather than concentric hypertrophy of the left ventricle. Hypertrophic cardiomyopathy may lead to diastolic dysfunction in addition to left ventricular outflow tract obstruction.

Diastolic dysfunction is associated with which of the following?

A) A prolonged history of untreated hypertension.
B) Poor relaxation of the ventricular wall.
C) Hemochromatosis.
D) A and B.
E) B and C.

Discussion

The correct answer is D. Diastolic dysfunction is associated with long-standing hypertension as well as a stiff ventricular wall that does not relax to allow good filling during diastole (therefore diastolic dysfunction).

Answer C is incorrect because hemochromatosis produces a dilated cardiomyopathy rather than diastolic dysfunction.

Diastolic dysfunction represents APPROXIMATELY what percentage of CHF?

A) <5%.
B) 10%.
C) 25%.
D) 50%.
E) >75%.

Discussion

The correct answer is D. Diastolic dysfunction represents between 40% and 60% of patients with CHF when looking at the population as a whole. The other answers are incorrect. As discussed above, patients with CHF need an echocardiogram to determine what type of CHF they have.

 HELPFUL TIP: Diastolic dysfunction occurs more commonly in elderly individuals with the prevalence increasing with age.

Diastolic dysfunction can be the mechanism of heart failure in which of the following settings?

A) Chronic hypertension.
B) Hereditary hypertrophic cardiomyopathy.
C) Aortic stenosis with a normal left ventricular ejection fraction.
D) Amyloid disease of the heart.
E) All of the above primarily manifest as CHF occurring by diastolic dysfunction.

Discussion

The correct answer is E. All the listed conditions can cause diastolic heart failure with normal or near-normal left ventricular systolic function, and evidence of diastolic dysfunction (eg, abnormal left ventricular filling and elevated filling pressures). Amyloidosis can also cause conduction system abnormalities.

Which of the following drugs is the LEAST desirable in patients with diastolic dysfunction?

A) Diuretics.
B) ACE inhibitors.

C) Nitrates.

D) Digoxin.

E) Negative inotropes such as β-blockers and calcium channel blockers.

Discussion

The correct answer is D. Of the medications used to treat systolic heart failure, the least desirable drug in diastolic dysfunction is digoxin (and other positive inotropes, such as milrinone). This makes sense. The problem here is not a lack of contractility but the opposite—a lack of muscle relaxation. The goals of therapy are blood pressure control, the use of diuretics to relieve congestion and edema, treatment of ischemia, and control of the heart rate and elimination of tachycardia (Table 2–11).

Which of the following drugs is theoretically the BEST choice for the treatment of diastolic dysfunction?

A) ACE inhibitors.

B) β-Blockers.

C) Diuretics.

D) Hydralazine.

E) ARBs.

Discussion

The correct answer is B. β-Blockers, especially metoprolol, are useful as initial therapy in diastolic dysfunction. Two problems with diastolic dysfunction are that the left ventricle does not relax, and there is decreased filling of the left ventricle with tachycardia. β-blockers address both of these problems by slowing the heart to permit better filling during diastole, and helping to relax the myocardium to promote a less restrictive filling pattern. If a patient fails β-blockers, calcium channel blockers, such as verapamil and diltiazem, should be considered the next best options (although verapamil is better studied). Unlike systolic dysfunction, the treatments for diastolic dysfunction are not well established, and there is no convincing evidence that β-blockers or ACEI's reduce mortality.

Objectives: Did you learn to . . .

● Understand the pathophysiology of diastolic dysfunction?

● Treat a patient with diastolic dysfunction?

QUICK QUIZ: CHF

Which of the following statements is true?

A) ACE inhibitors are more effective in CHF than are ARBs (angiotensin receptor blockers).

B) ARBs are more effective in CHF than are ACE inhibitors.

C) ARBs and ACE inhibitors have the same efficacy in the treatment of CHF.

D) Combination of ACE inhibitors and ARBs is the most effective treatment of CHF.

Discussion

The correct answer is A. Angiotensin converting enzyme inhibitors remain the first choice for inhibition of the renin-angiotensin system in chronic HF, but ARBs can now be considered a reasonable alternative. Experience with ARBs in controlled clinical trials of patients with HF is considerably less than that with ACE inhibitors. Therefore, unless there is a contraindication (angioedema, cough, etc) ACE inhibitors should be used in CHF. The combination of ACE inhibitors and ARBs increases the risk of side effects like hyperkalemia with no significant improvement in mortality.

 HELPFUL TIP: CHF is a terminal illness with a 5-year survival of only 50%. This is worse than many cancers.

CASE 10

The "congestive heart failure couple," as they now call themselves, are doing so well that the wife refers her cousin to you. Her cousin, a 65-year-old male, arrives at your office and you immediately notice the smell of tobacco leaching from his clothing. The small burns in his clothing confirm to you that he smokes, and he informs you that he has smoked three packs per day "since I was born." He recently has noticed some swelling in his feet and increased shortness of breath. He denies a history of cardiac disease. An ECG performed in the office shows right axis deviation and a right bundle branch block. An echocardiogram shows that he has normal left ventricular function but a

Table 2–11   TREATMENTS FOR HEART FAILURE DUE TO DIASTOLIC DYSFUNCTION

Goal	Treatment*	Daily Dose of Medication†
Reduce the congestive state	Salt restriction	<2 g of sodium per day
	Diuretics	Furosemide, 10–120 mg
		Hydrochlorothiazide, 12.5–25 mg
	ACE inhibitors	Enalapril, 2.5–40 mg
		Lisinopril, 10–40 mg
	Angiotensin II–receptor blockers	Candesartan, 4–32 mg
		Losartan, 25–100 mg
Maintain atrial contraction and prevent tachycardia	Cardioversion of atrial fibrillation	
	Sequential atrioventricular pacing	
	β-Blockers	Atenolol, 12.5–100 mg
		Metoprolol, 25–100 mg
		Verapamil, 120–360 mg
	Calcium-channel blockers	Diltiazem, 120–540 mg
	Radiofrequency ablation modification of atrioventricular node and pacing	
Treat and prevent myocardial ischemia	Nitrates	Isosorbide dinitrate, 30–180 mg
		Isosorbide mononitrate, 30–90 mg
	β-Blockers	Atenolol, 12.5–100 mg
		Metoprolol, 25–200 mg
	Calcium-channel blockers	Diltiazem, 120–540 mg
		Verapamil, 120–360 mg
	Coronary-artery bypass surgery, percutaneous coronary intervention	
Control hypertension	Antihypertensive agents	Chlorthalidone, 12.5–25 mg
		Hydrochlorothiazide, 12.5–50 mg
		Atenolol, 12.5–100 mg
		Metoprolol, 12.5–200 mg
		Amlodipine, 2.5–10 mg
		Felodipine, 2.5–20 mg
		Enalapril, 2.5–40 mg
		Lisinopril, 10–40 mg
		Candesartan, 4–32 mg
		Losartan, 50–100 mg
Measures with Theoretical Benefit in Diastolic Heart Failure		
Promote regression of hypertrophy and prevent myocardial fibrosis	ACE inhibitors	Enalapril, 2.5–40 mg
		Lisinopril, 10–40 mg
		Ramipril, 5–20 mg
		Captopril, 25–150 mg
	Angiotensin-receptor blockers	Candesartan, 4–32 mg
		Losartan, 50–100 mg
		Spironolactone 25–75 mg

*Treatments listed for the first four goals are those generally used in clinical practice. Angiotensin-converting–enzyme (ACE) inhibitors, angiotensin-receptor blockers, and spironolactone inhibit the renin–angiotensin–aldosterone system and thus have a theoretical benefit, but more data are required to show that they reduce the risk of heart failure.

†The list of medications is not comprehensive but rather includes examples that are in common clinical use or have been included in studies of pathophysiologic mechanisms in diastolic dysfunction or heart failure or were included in larger trials that generally were not designed to assess outcomes in diastolic heart failure. Candesartan is the only agent studied in a randomized, controlled trial involving patients with diastolic heart failure. A more exhaustive list of antihypertensive agents can be found in the guidelines of the Seventh Report of the Joint National Committee on Prevention, Detection, Evaluation, and Treatment of High Blood Pressure.

Aurigemma, GP, Gaasch, WH. Clinical Practice, Diastolic heart failure. *N Engl J Med* 2004;351:1097.

hypertrophied right heart with paradoxical bulging of the ventricular septum into the left ventricle.

This clinical picture is most consistent with which of the following?

A) Constrictive pericarditis.
B) Chronic mitral valve prolapse.
C) Cor pulmonale.
D) Old right ventricular infarction with subsequent dysfunction.
E) Atrial myxoma.

Discussion

The correct answer is C, cor pulmonale. A typical picture of cor pulmonale is right ventricular hypertrophy with paradoxical bulging of the septum into the left ventricle, right axis deviation on ECG, and partial or complete right bundle branch block. Answer A is incorrect. Constrictive pericarditis is associated with pericardial thickening, dilated inferior vena cava or hepatic veins, abnormal septal motion, and abnormal mitral and tricuspid flow dopplers. Answer B is incorrect because mitral valve prolapse, in the absence of mitral regurgitation is not likely to be hemodynamically significant. Answer D is incorrect because with a right ventricular infarct, you would expect to see a poorly functioning right ventricle. Answer E is incorrect because an atrial myxoma is in the atrium and would not cause right ventricular hypertrophy.

Cor pulmonale may result from all of these disease processes EXCEPT?

A) Sickle cell anemia.
B) Left ventricular failure.
C) Pulmonary embolism.
D) Chronic obstructive lung disease.
E) Interstitial lung disease.

Discussion

The correct answer is B. Cor pulmonale is the term used for right-sided heart failure caused by diseases primarily affecting the lungs and pulmonary vasculature. This excludes pulmonary hypertension due to primary disease of the left side of the heart or congenital heart disease.

Besides stopping smoking, the best treatment for this patient's cor pulmonale and pulmonary hypertension is:

A) Continuous prostacyclin infusion.
B) Continuous, low-flow oxygen.
C) Calcium channel blockers.
D) Nitroglycerin.
E) Antibiotics to reduce pulmonary inflammation secondary to infection.

Discussion

The correct answer is B. In this patient who is a smoker with cor pulmonale, the best drug is continuous, low-flow oxygen. This will help to reverse the pulmonary vasoconstriction caused by chronic hypoxia. You must do everything you can to get him to stop smoking. His disease process will progress much faster if he continues to smoke. Answer A is incorrect because prostacyclin infusion is useful in primary pulmonary hypertension, not this type of cor pulmonale. Answer C is incorrect. In some cases of primary pulmonary hypertension, calcium channel blockers, which serve as direct vasodilators to dilate the pulmonary vascular bed, can be useful. However, this is not the best choice for this patient and he needs to be started under controlled conditions. Answer D is incorrect because patients with cor pulmonale are dependent on high right-sided heart filling pressures to get blood through the pulmonary vasculature. Nitroglycerin will reduce preload, worsening this patient's symptoms. Answer E is incorrect. Antibiotics might be needed in this patient for pneumonia, bronchiectasis, etc., but they are not going to help with the treatment of cor pulmonale.

Objectives: Did you learn to . . .

- Diagnose cor pulmonale?
- Describe causes of cor pulmonale?
- Treat a patient with cor pulmonale?

CASE 11

A 65-year-old male presents to your clinic for a complete history and physical. You notice that his abdominal exam reveals a pulsatile mass which you suspect may represent an aortic aneurysm. This finding is confirmed by ultrasound. The radiologist reports that the patient has a 3.5-cm abdominal aortic aneurysm without evidence of leak or thrombus formation.

The best advice to this patient is:

A) Have the aortic aneurysm fixed now while he is still healthy.

B) Have a follow-up ultrasound every 3 months.
C) Have a stent placed to prevent further aortic dilatation.
D) Have an angiogram in the next several days to rule out vascular disease below the aorta (femoral arteries, iliac arteries, etc.).
E) Have a repeat ultrasound at 1 year.

Discussion

The correct answer is E. Patients with an abdominal aortic aneurysm <4 cm in diameter should have an ultrasound yearly to check progression. Those with an aneurysm 4–5 cm in diameter should have an ultrasound every 6 months for follow-up. Answer A is incorrect (see next question for an explanation). Answer B is incorrect because E is correct. Answer C is incorrect. A stent is not indicated now. Answer D is incorrect. The only reason to do an angiogram now is if the patient is symptomatic or you are planning surgical intervention.

* *

The patient is really worried that this aneurysm will rupture and kill him.

You tell him that the benefit of having the aneurysm repaired is greater than the risk of the surgery when the aneurysm reaches:

A) 4.5 cm.
B) 5.0–5.5 cm.
C) 5.5–6.0 cm.
D) >6.0 cm.
E) No repair is indicated until the patient becomes symptomatic.

Discussion

The correct answer is B. The risk of the surgery outweighs the benefits until the aneurysm reaches somewhere between 5.0–5.5 cm. The other answers are incorrect. It would be an especially bad idea to wait until an aneurysm is symptomatic, as a ruptured aortic aneurysm can be lethal in a matter of minutes.

* *

The patient goes to Texas (or Arizona or Florida....somewhere warmer than Iowa) for the winter as part of the re-establishment of human annual migration. When he returns, he calls you complaining of back pain that is somewhat sharp and radiating into his legs. You meet him in the ED and suspect that he is having a dissection of his aneurysm.

All of the following are true EXCEPT:

A) A substantial number of patients with an aortic dissection will have palpable pulses below the level of the dissection.
B) Patients may have an elevated LDH and microangiopathic findings on RBC examination.
C) Blood pressure should be kept on the high side to ensure perfusion below the area of the aneurysm.
D) The pain may migrate down from the chest to the lower abdominal area over time.
E) The pain may be episodic.

Discussion

The correct answer is C. One does **not** want to keep the blood pressure on the high side. Reducing the blood pressure is the initial treatment of choice for a dissecting aneurysm. Answers A, B, D, and E are all true statements. Patients may have an elevated LDH and microangiopathic findings on RBC smear as a result of trauma and cell lysis. Although the classic teaching is that pain of a dissection migrates from the chest area to the lower abdomen, most patients **do not** have this pattern of pain. So, answer D is a true statement although patients may not have this migrating pattern of pain. Answer E is often true of pain in aortic dissection—it may be episodic.

* *

The patient has a blood pressure of 160/105. Clearly this is too high in a patient who has an ongoing dissection. You decide to treat this patient before transferring him to a tertiary care center where he can be surgically managed. The best medication(s) to use in this patient to control his blood pressure is (are):

A) Sublingual nifedipine plus metoprolol.
B) Amlodipine.
C) Intravenous hydralazine.
D) Intravenous labetalol plus nitroprusside.
E) Intravenous nitroglycerin.

Discussion

The correct answer is D. The goal of therapy here is not only blood pressure reduction but also control of shear forces on the aorta, which requires the prevention of tachycardia. Intravenous β-blockers such as labetalol, propranolol, metoprolol or esmolol are the first-line agents. Nitroprusside can be added if the blood pressure control remains suboptimal even after β-blockade. In this scenario, nitroprusside should never be given without β-blockade, as it may cause tachycardia induced by vasodilation and thus further aortic shear stress. The same rationale is true for not using intravenous hydralazine (answer C) in this scenario. Answer A is incorrect for two reasons. First, nifedipine should **never** be used sublingually. Syncope, heart block, MI, stroke, and other serious adverse consequences have been reported. Second, nifedipine increases heart rate causing an increase in shear forces on the aorta. Answer B is incorrect because amlodipine does nothing to reduce heart rate and is not titratable to any useful degree. Answer E is incorrect because nitroglycerin alone causes reflex tachycardia, increasing shear forces on the aorta.

 HELPFUL TIP: Short-acting dihydropyridine calcium channel blockers (eg, immediate-release nifedipine) should generally be avoided when treating angina, hypertension, and other cardiovascular disease. The effects on blood pressure are unpredictable, and mortality is greater. Use long-acting preparations, such as amlodipine and extended-release nifedipine.

Objectives: Did you learn to . . .

- Identify the treatment options and timing of treatment of an abdominal aortic aneurysm?
- Manage a patient with a dissecting aneurysm?

CASE 12

A 60-year-old male presents with dizziness and palpitations. The patient has a blood pressure of 100/60 mm Hg and a pulse of 160. His ECG is shown in Figure 2–3.

Which of the following are appropriate options in the treatment of this patient?

A) Amiodarone, lidocaine, defibrillation, metoprolol.
B) Amiodarone, lidocaine, defibrillation, diltiazem.
C) Amiodarone, lidocaine, cardioversion, diltiazem.
D) Procainamide, lidocaine, adenosine, defibrillation.
E) Procainamide, lidocaine, cardioversion, amiodarone.

Discussion
The correct answer is E. The rhythm is stable ventricular tachycardia. Procainamide, lidocaine, amiodarone, and cardioversion can all be used for ventricular tachycardia. Answer A is incorrect for two reasons: the rhythm is ventricular tachycardia and is stable, and neither metoprolol nor defibrillation is appropriate. Defibrillation could be appropriate if the patient was unstable or pulseless. Answer B is incorrect because of the inclusion of diltiazem, a calcium channel blocker, and defibrillation. Answer C is incorrect because of the inclusion of diltiazem. Answer D is incorrect because adenosine, which is used for atrial arrhythmias, is included and because defibrillation is inappropriate.

 HELPFUL TIP: Procainamide is no longer in the ACLS protocols. It takes too long to load and is not as effective as other drugs.

* *

The patient does not respond to IV amiodarone and you choose to cardiovert him.

Which of the following is the recommended energy (in joules) for an initial attempt at cardioversion?

A) 100 joules, monophasic.
B) 360 joules, monophasic.
C) 200 joules, biphasic.
D) 360 joules, biphasic.
E) None of the above.

Discussion
For purposes of the test, the correct answer is A. For cardioversion of ventricular tachycardia, start with 100–200 joules for monophasic waveforms and 50–100 joules for biphasic waveforms. The rest of the answers are incorrect. The ACC/AHA guidelines, revised in 2005, reflect a more simplified approach to cardioversion and defibrillation.

HELPFUL TIP: No more "shock, shock, shock, everybody shock." For defibrillation, escalating doses of electricity are out of the new protocols. Start with a single shock at 360 joules with a monophasic defibrillator **or** 200 joules if using a biphasic defibrillator.

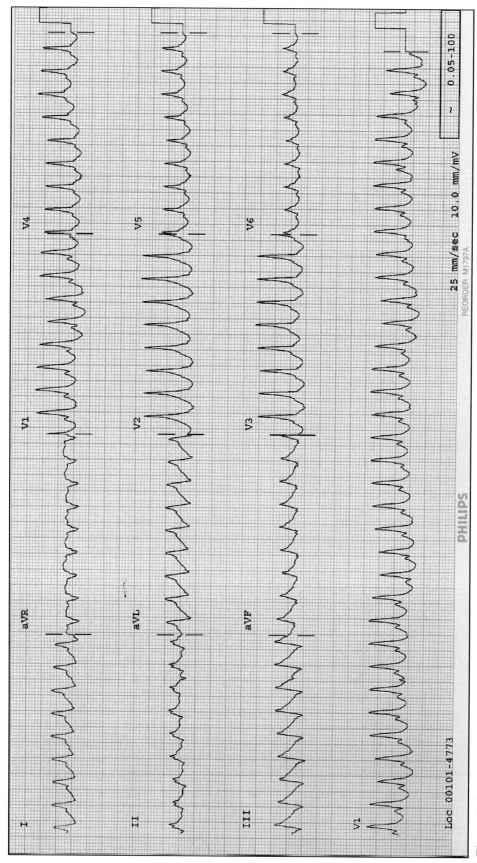

Figure 2–3

* *

You cardiovert the patient, and the rhythm is on the monitor (Figure 2–4).

Of the following, what is the FIRST step you will take?

A) Reshock the patient at the same energy level.
B) Check another lead to assure the readout is accurate.
C) Give epinephrine, 1mg IV.
D) Begin CPR to restore circulation.
E) Give atropine, 1mg.

Discussion

The correct answer is B. This rhythm is asystole. It is important to check another lead and make sure that all of the leads are connected properly. Answer A is incorrect because cardioversion/defibrillation are not routinely indicated in the treatment of asystole. Answers C, D, and E are incorrect because it is important to ensure that the patient actually is in asystole.

* *

You check additional leads and the patient is in asystole. You decide to try epinephrine and atropine.

What is the appropriate intravenous dose of atropine in this situation?

A) 0.5–1.0 mg with a total maximum of 2 mg.
B) 0.5–1.0 mg every 5 minutes.
C) A single dose of 1–2 mg.
D) 0.5–1.0 mg with a maximum of 0.04 mg/kg.
E) 0.05–1.0 mg with a maximum of 0.02 mg/kg (2 mg in a 100-kg patient).

Discussion

The correct answer for the board examination is D. The rest of the answers are incorrect.

* *

This does not work and you place the patient on an external pacemaker. The pacer captures and the patient is saved!

Note: The new guidelines suggest using 0.5–1.0 mg aliquots of atropine to a maximum of 3 mg. The dose is no longer a maximum of 0.04 mg/kg. However, this dose change will not likely be on the board examination for several years.

Objectives: Did you learn to . . .

● Recognize and manage ventricular tachycardia and asystole?

CASE 13

A 75-year-old female presents to your office with complaints of episodic palpitations with episodes of light-headedness that are **not** concurrent with the palpitations. You perform an electrocardiogram in your office, and the rhythm is shown in Figure 2–5.

What rhythm does this represent?

A) First-degree heart block.
B) Second-degree heart block type I (Wenckebach).
C) Second-degree heart block type II.
D) Third-degree heart block.
E) Atrial flutter with variable block.

Discussion

The correct answer is C. This is a second-degree heart block, Mobitz type II. Answer A is incorrect. First-degree heart block is characterized by a prolonged PR interval without any blocked beats. The upper limit of normal of the PR interval is 0.2 seconds. A fixed PR interval >0.2 seconds without dropped beats is considered first-degree heart block. A second-degree heart block, Mobitz type I (Wenckebach), is defined by a progressively prolonged PR interval ending with a nonconducted P wave and a dropped beat. Your patient's ECG shows a second-degree heart block, type II. This is characterized by a **fixed PR interval** with an intermittently nonconducting P wave and resultant

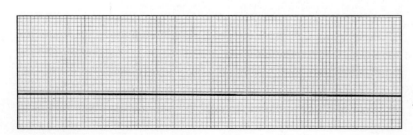

Figure 2–4

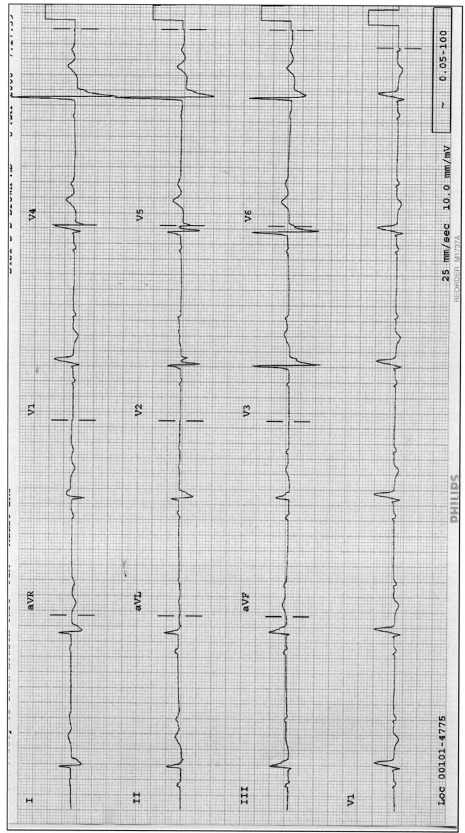

Figure 2–5

dropped beats. A third-degree heart block is characterized by no consistent pattern between the P waves and the QRS complex. Answer E is incorrect because, by definition, atrial flutter is represented by a rapid atrial rate. In this patient, the rate is slow.

* *

By the time the patient arrives at the hospital, she is having a rapid, chaotic rhythm, which appears to be atrial fibrillation on the monitor. It seems as though there are also episodes of atrial flutter with 2:1 block.

The most likely diagnosis in this patient is:

A) Sick sinus syndrome (bradycardia-tachycardia syndrome).
B) Hypothyroidism.
C) Hyperthyroidism.
D) Hyperkalemia.

Discussion
The correct answer is A. The most likely diagnosis in this patient is sick sinus syndrome, (aka "tachy-brady" syndrome and "bradycardia-tachycardia" syndrome). This syndrome is most common in elderly individuals and reflects the replacement of the SA node with fibrous tissue. Answer B is incorrect because hypothyroidism should cause bradycardia without intermittent tachycardia. Answer C is incorrect because hyperthyroidism should cause tachycardia without bradycardia. Answer D is incorrect because hyperkalemia generally causes a widened QRS complex on ECG and eventually ventricular tachycardia.

Treatment for this syndrome generally includes which of the following?

A) Mexiletine.
B) Hydralazine.
C) Quinidine.
D) Pacemaker.
E) Implantable defibrillator.

Discussion
The correct answer is D. Generally, patients with sick sinus syndrome become symptomatic because of the bradycardia episodes. Thus, pacing is necessary. Answers A and C are incorrect because mexiletine and quinidine are aimed primarily at ventricular arrhythmias; sick sinus syndrome is a problem with the SA node. Answer B is incorrect because hydralazine is an

afterload reducer with no direct effect on cardiac rhythm. Answer E is incorrect because patients with sick sinus syndrome do not have ventricular fibrillation, and thus there is no need for a defibrillator.

 HELPFUL TIP: In addition to the pacemaker, it is often necessary to add a β-blocker, digoxin, or a calcium channel blocker to address the supraventricular tachycardia (eg, PSVT or atrial fibrillation).

Objectives: Did you learn to . . .

• Identify and differentiate second-degree heart blocks?
• Diagnose and treat sick sinus syndrome?

CASE 14

A 58-year-old male smoker with a history of type 2 diabetes mellitus presents with complaints of easy fatigability and pain in his thighs when exerting himself. The pain is no worse going downhill than uphill. The thigh pain resolves after resting. He has some nighttime pain as well. He works as a carpenter, and the leg pain is now limiting his ability to work. He will not quit smoking; you have gone down that road with him many times, and again he refuses to do so today. The patient states that his symptoms are better when he hangs his leg over the side of the bed at night.

The etiology of this patient's leg pain is most likely:

A) Peripheral venous disease (eg, venous insufficiency, varicose veins).
B) Spinal stenosis.
C) Diabetic neuropathy.
D) Peripheral arterial disease (eg, arterial occlusion).
E) None of the above.

Discussion
The correct answer is D. Most patients with lower extremity peripheral arterial disease (PAD) are asymptomatic. Intermittent claudication is the classic presenting symptom. When rest pain is present, relief of symptoms occurs by making the affected area dependent (eg, hanging legs over the side of the bed letting

gravity help increase blood flow). The pain associated with diabetic neuropathy begins distally, has a burning quality to it, and is not typically relieved with rest. Patients often notice it more at rest (eg, during the night). Patients with PAD will often have worsening of their symptoms when the leg is dependent. Spinal stenosis is often made worse by walking downhill and better when walking uphill (a kyphotic position opens up the foramen).

* *

The patient's exam shows decreased pulses in the lower extremities bilaterally. You would like to confirm your suspicion that he has peripheral vascular disease.

What is the first study you would order in this patient?

A) Spiral CT to confirm vascular calcification.
B) Ankle-brachial index.
C) Color Doppler to assess flow.
D) Arteriography.
E) None of the above is the recommended first test.

Discussion

The correct answer is B. The ankle-brachial index (ABI) is sensitive and specific for PAD in the lower extremity. The pressure in the ankle should be higher than that in the brachial artery in a normal person. Highest sensitivity is achieved by measuring pressures in both brachial arteries and both dorsalis pedis and posterior tibial arteries. Neither spiral CT nor color Doppler is the recommended test for the diagnosis of peripheral vascular disease. Arteriography is an option but should be reserved for patients in whom surgery is a consideration and who have the diagnosis of peripheral vascular disease.

 HELPFUL TIP: Duplex ultrasonography which combines Doppler waveform analysis and velocities can also be used to diagnose PAD and is helpful in determining the location of disease. Also, segmental pressures can be used to help localize the blockage.

* *

The ABI results for this patient are normal. However, you strongly suspect claudication.

The next step should be:

A) Arteriography.
B) Repeat ABI after an exercise stress test.
C) Magnetic resonance arteriography (MRA).
D) CT arteriography.
E) None of the above.

Discussion

The correct answer is B. In patients in whom you strongly suspect peripheral vascular disease, ABIs after exercise can be positive when a resting test is negative. This would be the least invasive and most cost-effective test of the options given.

* *

The postexercise ABIs are as follows: 0.9 in the right leg, 0.4 in the left leg.

The proper interpretation of this information is:

A) 95% probability of some degree of occlusive disease in the right leg, advanced occlusive disease in the left.
B) No occlusive disease in the right leg, mild disease in the left.
C) Moderate occlusive disease on both sides.
D) None of the above.

Discussion

The correct answer is A. A normal ABI should be ≥1.0. An ABI of 0.9 is 95% sensitive for finding some degree of occlusive disease on arteriography. An ABI of 0.41–0.9 represents disease that is usually associated with claudication, while an ABI of 0.4 represents advanced disease. Paradoxically, an ABI >1.30 represents noncompressible arteries and may be a marker for artery calcification. In these cases, a toe-brachial index (TBI) should be measured.

* *

You decide to start the patient on a medication to help control his claudication.

Which of the following statements is correct?

A) Pentoxifylline is relatively contraindicated in heart failure.
B) Cilostazol is the best choice for claudication in patients with heart failure.
C) β-Blockers are good arterial dilators and are thus useful in claudication.

D) The main mechanism of action of pentoxifylline and cilostazol is selective vasodilation.

E) None of the above is correct.

Discussion

The correct answer is A. Cilostazol (Pletal) and pentoxifylline (Trental) are phosphodiesterase inhibitors. Their mechanism of action in improving walking distance is poorly understood. Other phosphodiesterase inhibitors (such as milrinone) increase mortality in patients with heart failure. Thus, pentoxifylline and cilostazol should be used with extreme caution, if at all, in patients with heart failure. Selective β-blockers cause arterial constriction, not arterial dilation. Answer D is incorrect. The purported benefit of pentoxifylline is to increase RBC malleability and thus reduce the viscosity of blood in the microcirculation. It has no vasodilating effects. However, cilostazol does have some vasodilating effects. Therapeutic benefit with these drugs may take several weeks. A dedicated and supervised exercise program is of paramount importance and underutilized. Pharmacologic therapy of PAD should include antiplatelet therapy and cardiovascular risk factor modification.

 HELPFUL TIP: PAD is a CAD equivalent. Address all risk factors aggressively.

* *

The patient fails a trial of pentoxifylline and a trial of cilostazol. You decide that the next step for this patient is to send him for an arteriogram in order to assess for bypass, stenting, etc. As noted, the patient has a history of diabetes mellitus type 2. He is taking metformin.

The correct management strategy when sending this patient for a dye study (eg, arteriography) is to:

A) Ensure that the patient is well hydrated and start the patient on N-acetylcysteine the day of the procedure in order to protect his kidneys.

B) Ensure that the patient is well hydrated and hold his metformin the day of the procedure and restart it the next day.

C) Ensure that the patient is well hydrated and stop the metformin for 48 hours prior to the procedure and restart 48 hours after the procedure.

D) Ensure that the patient is well hydrated and hold the metformin the day of the procedure and restart it 48 hours later.

E) None of the above.

Discussion

The correct answer is D. You should hold the metformin the day of the procedure and ensure that the patient is well hydrated. You can then restart the metformin 48 hours after the procedure. Answers A, B, and C are incorrect.

Indications for further intervention for peripheral artery disease (eg, bypass, stenting, or PTA) include all of the following EXCEPT:

A) Rest pain.

B) Persistent pain that interferes with day-to-day functioning.

C) Tissue loss.

D) 80% occlusion of the femoral artery.

Discussion

The correct answer is D. Classic indications for invasive treatment of lower extremity PAD are: (1) salvage of a threatened limb (rest pain, nonhealing ulceration, or gangrene) or (2) improvement in functional capacity. An 80% occlusion of the femoral artery in and of itself is not an indication for percutaneous or surgical revascularization in a patient who is asymptomatic.

* *

The patient sees the light, but does not go into it, and quits smoking. The case ends happily.

 HELPFUL TIP: No anticoagulation regimen seems to prevent reocclusion of lower extremity arteries after stenting. Patients should, however, continue on their current antithrombotic regimen as indicated for cardiovascular disease (ASA, warfarin, etc).

Objectives: Did you learn to . . .

- Recognize symptoms and signs of peripheral vascular disease?
- Order appropriate diagnostic tests for a patient suspected of having peripheral vascular disease?
- Develop an understanding of the agents used to treat peripheral vascular disease?
- Modify metformin dosing to prevent problems with contrast studies?

CASE 15

A 75-year-old male presents to your office for a complete physical before prostate surgery. On exam, you notice a 3/6 midsystolic murmur radiating to the neck. S_1 and S_2 are normal. An echocardiogram notes mild aortic stenosis. Currently he is asymptomatic.

The indications for valve replacement surgery include:

A) Grade 4/6 murmur.
B) Requirement for major, semielective surgery such as prostatectomy.
C) Moderate aortic stenosis without symptoms.
D) Severe aortic stenosis with evidence of left ventricular dysfunction.
E) All of the above.

Discussion

The correct answer is D. Answer A is incorrect because the loudness of the murmur does not always correlate with its functional significance. Answer B is incorrect. As long as the lesion is not hemodynamically significant (eg, left ventricular dysfunction), this patient should tolerate surgery. Answer C is incorrect because surgery is not usually necessary in patients without symptoms. Severe aortic stenosis with symptoms is also an indication for valve replacement surgery.

The patient would like to know how often he should have a repeat echocardiogram since he has mild disease. Your answer is:

A) Every 3–5 years.
B) Every year.
C) Every 6 months.

D) When he develops symptoms.
E) None of the above.

Discussion

The correct answer is A. Patients with mild aortic stenosis who are asymptomatic can be followed by echocardiogram every 3–5 years. Although the valve area in population-based studies of aortic stenosis decreases an average of 0.1 cm² per year, individual variation is quite marked. Patients with severe disease should have yearly echocardiography to evaluate for left ventricular dysfunction (Table 2–12).

* *

Two years later, the patient returns for a checkup and states that he believes he has been having symptoms from his aortic stenosis.

All of the following can occur with symptomatic aortic stenosis EXCEPT:

A) Left-to-right intracardiac shunt.
B) Exertional dyspnea.
C) Syncope.
D) Angina.

Discussion

The correct answer is A. Intracardiac shunts do not occur with aortic stenosis. If you got this one wrong, back to anatomy for you! An isolated, fixed valvular lesion as an adult cannot cause intracardiac shunting.

Which of the following statements about aortic valve disease is NOT true?

A) Aortic stenosis can be treated quite effectively with valvulotomy.

Table 2–12   **RECOMMENDED INTERVALS FOR ECHOCARDIOGRAPHIC EVALUATION**

Lesion	Mild Disease	Significant Disease
Aortic stenosis	Every 2 years (moderate disease)	Every year
	Every 3–5 years (mild disease)	
Aortic regurgitation	Any change in symptoms	Every year
Mitral stenosis	No need for regular echocardiography	
	Therapy based on symptoms	
Mitral regurgitation*	Periodically	Every 6–12 months

*Recommendations vary.

B) There are no known medical treatments that reduce the need for aortic valve replacement.

C) Risk factors for the development of aortic stenosis are similar to coronary artery disease.

D) Valve replacement surgery is the preferred treatment for symptomatic aortic stenosis.

Discussion

The correct answer is A. Valvulotomy is not effective in the treatment of aortic stenosis and carries a high risk for cerebral embolism. Valve replacement surgery is preferred. The epidemiological risk factors for aortic stenosis and coronary artery disease are similar (as is their pathophysiology).

Objectives: Did you learn to . . .

- Recognize symptoms of aortic stenosis?
- Manage a patient with aortic stenosis?
- Evaluate aortic valve disease and determine long-term follow-up vis-à-vis periodic echocardiograms?

 QUICK QUIZ: VALVULAR DISEASE

Which of the following symptom complexes are associated with mitral valve prolapse?

A) Chest pain, palpitations, dyspnea.
B) Chest pain, syncope, dyspnea.
C) Anxiety, chest pain, palpitations.
D) Increased risk of death.
E) None of the above.

Discussion

The correct answer is E. Although mitral valve prolapse has been implicated as a cause of many bad symptoms (chest pain, palpitations, dyspnea, anxiety, syncope, and an increased risk of death), recent evidence suggests no increase in these symptoms beyond that in the general population. Thus, patients with mitral valve prolapse can be reassured that the incidental finding on echocardiography is of no long-term significance.

CASE 16

A 35-year-old male presents to the office with upper respiratory symptoms. He is taking no medications except for some pseudoephedrine for his cold. You notice when looking at his vital signs that his blood pressure is 180/106. Repeat measurement confirms that the blood pressure is elevated at 175/103.

What is your initial approach to this patient?

A) Start a chronic antihypertensive since he is at a risk for a stroke within the next couple of days with a blood pressure at this level.

B) Administer clonidine in the office to reduce the blood pressure to a safe level of about of 150/100.

C) Watch the patient over the next 2 weeks and get additional blood pressure readings before deciding what to do.

D) Schedule the patient for outpatient labs and electrocardiogram.

Discussion

The correct answer is C. The diagnosis of hypertension requires two elevated blood pressures on two different occasions. This patient's elevated blood pressure could be situational, related to decongestant, etc. Answers A and B are incorrect because a blood pressure of 175/103 does not pose a risk of acute stroke, and the pressure need not be lowered acutely unless there is evidence of end-organ injury (eg, angina, CHF, hypertensive encephalopathy, etc). Answer D is incorrect because you cannot establish that this patient has hypertension based on just one office blood pressure measurement.

* *

The patient returns to your office with six blood pressures taken over a period of 2 weeks at a local pharmacy. The majority of the blood pressure readings are in the 120/80 range with only two of the six readings suggesting that the patient is hypertensive. The patient states that the elevated blood pressures were while he was under stress at work.

Your best response at this point is to:

A) Start an antihypertensive.
B) Send the patient for a 24-hour ambulatory blood pressure measurement.
C) Don't worry about the blood pressure since the majority of the readings were within a normal range.
D) Get a nephrology consult to help in decision making.

Discussion

The correct answer is B. One way to determine if a patient with contradictory readings is hypertensive is to perform 24-hour ambulatory blood pressure monitoring. This can be useful in patients who have elevated blood pressures in the office but not at home or vice versa. It can also be used if you do not trust the blood pressure readings taken outside of your office. Answer A is incorrect since you have not yet established that this patient is hypertensive. Answer C is incorrect since you have not yet established that this patient is not hypertensive. Answer D is incorrect because you are smarter than that and should be able to work through this kind of case yourself!

The following are all well-accepted indications for 24-hour ambulatory blood pressure monitoring EXCEPT:

A) Suspected white-coat hypertension.
B) Patients in whom it is difficult to control the blood pressure.
C) Patients having hypotensive symptoms on antihypertensive treatment.
D) Routine follow-up after initiating antihypertensive treatment.
E) Evaluation of patient for autonomic dysfunction.

Discussion

The correct answer is D. One need not do 24-hour ambulatory blood pressure monitoring to document response to antihypertensive therapy in patients in whom most or all measurements post-treatment are normal. All of the other answer choices are considered reasonable indications for 24-hour ambulatory blood pressure monitoring.

* *

Elevated blood pressure in response to stress (especially in the physician's office) is called "white-coat hypertension."

Which of the following statements is true about white-coat hypertension?

A) As long as the majority of blood pressure readings are normal the patient does not require treatment because there is no increased risk of adverse cardiac outcomes.
B) Patients with white-coat hypertension have an intermediate risk for adverse outcomes when compared to patients with normal blood pressure and those with chronically elevated blood pressure.
C) White-coat hypertension is more common in young patients.

D) Patients with white-coat hypertension have an elevated left ventricular mass when compared to patients with normal blood pressures.
E) B and D.

Discussion

The correct answer is E. Patients with white-coat hypertension have outcomes that are intermediate between normotensive and hypertensive patients. Additionally, they have an elevated left ventricular mass. Surprisingly, white-coat hypertension is more common in the elderly.

According to the JNC 7 guidelines, hypertension is defined as an ambulatory 24-hour monitor average blood pressure of:

A) 135/85 during the day and 125/75 at night.
B) 140/90 during the day and 130/85 at night.
C) 130/85 during the day and 125/85 at night.
D) 140/90 over 24 hours.

Discussion

The correct answer is A. Patients with an average blood pressure of >135/85 during the day and >125/75 at night are defined by JNC 7 as being hypertensive. Another published criterion is a blood pressure of >140/90 >40% of the time.

* *

The ambulatory blood pressure monitor reveals that the patient is hypertensive (>140/90 >40% of the time).

The initial evaluation of hypertension includes the following:

A) History, physical, CBC, urinalysis, glucose, BUN, creatinine, electrolytes, ECG, lipids.
B) History, physical, CBC, urinalysis, glucose, BUN, creatinine, electrolytes, lipids.
C) History, physical, CBC, urinalysis, glucose, BUN, creatinine, electrolytes, ECG, lipids, echocardiography.
D) History, physical, and labs only as indicated by history and physical.

Discussion

The correct answer is A. History, physical, CBC, urinalysis, glucose, BUN, creatinine, electrolytes, ECG, and lipids are the generally agreed-upon initial workup of the hypertensive patient. Answer C includes echocardiography, which is not recommended as part of the routine evaluation but may be indicated if signs of cardiac disease are present.

* *

The patient's ECG comes back showing evidence of left ventricular hypertrophy (LVH).

This finding suggests that:

A) You should initiate this patient's therapy with an ACE inhibitor because ACE inhibitors promote cardiac remodeling.
B) The patient has diastolic dysfunction.
C) You should recommend an echocardiogram for this patient.
D) You should order a B-natriuretic peptide (BNP) level to screen for LVH and early CHF.

Discussion

The correct answer is C. The sensitivity of ECG for LVH is only in the 30% to 60% range with a specificity of 80%. Thus, a positive ECG is not enough to embark on a therapeutic adventure for LVH. For this reason, an echocardiogram should be done to confirm the diagnosis of LVH. Answer B is incorrect. Long-standing hypertension and significant LVH can cause diastolic dysfunction. However, you cannot conclude that this patient has diastolic dysfunction on the basis of an ECG, especially in the absence of symptoms. Answer D is incorrect because the sensitivity of the BNP as a screening tool in an asymptomatic population is poor.

* *

The echocardiogram is normal. You have decided to start this patient on treatment for his hypertension.

Based on outcome data, the BEST drug to start this patient on is:

A) An ACE inhibitor, such as lisinopril.
B) An α-blocker, such as doxazosin.
C) A β-blocker, such as metoprolol.
D) A thiazide diuretic, such as hydrochlorothiazide.
E) A calcium channel blocker, such as amlodipine.

Discussion

The correct answer is D. The ALLHAT study suggests that the one best drug to start for hypertension is a thiazide diuretic (specifically, chlorthalidone was used in ALLHAT). This recommendation can be modified if there is a compelling reason for starting another agent. The next two questions are examples.

Which of the following drugs is the BEST choice as the initial agent for the treatment of hypertension

in a patient with diabetes and known microalbuminuria?

A) Lisinopril.
B) Metoprolol.
C) Doxazosin.
D) Verapamil.
E) Amlodipine.

Discussion

The correct answer is A. In a diabetic patient who has proteinuria, an ACE inhibitor is indicated to slow the progression of renal disease. An ARB or nondihydropyridine calcium channel blocker (verapamil, diltiazem) is a viable alternative for those who cannot tolerate an ACE inhibitor. However, ACE inhibitors are still first line.

Which of the following drugs might you want to use as the initial agent for the treatment of hypertension in a 72-year-old male with a history of symptomatic benign prostatic hypertrophy?

A) Amlodipine.
B) Doxazosin.
C) Captopril.
D) Losartan.
E) Verapamil.

Discussion

The correct answer is B. Doxazosin is an α-blocker that is useful in the treatment of symptomatic BPH. None of the other choices can be used for this indication. The α-blockers are also antihypertensives, and thus serve a useful purpose by treating two diseases with one drug. Note: There is some evidence that α-blockers do not confer as much benefit for the hypertensive patient as other classes of drugs (see ALLHAT trial results). Thus, α-blockers are not the best choice in general.

These two examples emphasize that thiazides are recommended as initial therapy in most cases of hypertension unless there is a compelling reason to use another agent. Another example would be a patient with CAD and angina starting on a β-blocker as initial treatment rather than a thiazide (since the β-blocker may improve angina symptoms and is indicated for CAD).

* *

Remember the 35-year-old patient? You start him on hydrochlorothiazide, but his blood pressure does not respond at a dose of 25 mg per day.

The best approach for such a patient is to:

A) Push his hydrochlorothiazide to its maximum (50 mg).
B) Stop the hydrochlorothiazide and start another medication.
C) Rely on exercise and diet to normalize the blood pressure.
D) Start a second drug before you have maximized the dose of the first drug.
E) Start a workup for secondary causes of hypertension.

Discussion

The correct answer is D. The thinking on this has changed in the past several years. Most experts, and the JNC 7 guidelines, now recommend a low dose of two drugs rather than pushing one drug to its maximum. This is for two reasons. First, most patients will eventually require two drugs. Second, you can get good blood pressure control while minimizing the side effects seen at a higher dose of a single drug. Answer A is incorrect because you get little if any additional blood pressure benefit with hydrochlorothiazide doses above 25 mg per day. Low-dose hydrochlorothiazide (12.5 mg) provides the greatest blood pressure reduction per mg of drug, compared to higher doses. Answer B is incorrect because a patient with this level of blood pressure elevation will generally require more than one drug to achieve a normalized blood pressure. Answer C is incorrect because the majority of patients are unable to maintain an adequate diet or exercise regimen to effectively treat blood pressure. Exercise and dietary change are laudable goals and should be encouraged in all patients. However, exercise and diet are not likely to normalize blood pressure in most hypertensive patients. Answer E is incorrect because this patient has not yet proven to be resistant to treatment.

* *

You decide to start this patient on diltiazem as a second agent.

Which of the following side effects is most characteristic of diltiazem and other calcium channel blockers?

A) Dehydration.
B) Cough.
C) Dependent edema.
D) Hypokalemia.
E) Elevated cholesterol.

Discussion

The correct answer is C. As a class, calcium channel blockers tend to cause peripheral edema. Dehydration and hypokalemia can be caused by diuretics. Cough and hyperkalemia are characteristic of ACE inhibitors. Diuretics can also increase cholesterol, while β-blockers can increase triglycerides.

* *

Although the patient is on two medications, he remains hypertensive. The blood pressure has barely moved. With your thorough history taking, you have ruled out excess alcohol intake (often an occult cause of hypertension). The patient is compliant with his medications.

Further investigations that might be helpful in determining the cause of hypertension in this patient include all of the following EXCEPT:

A) Checking the potassium level while the patient is taking his drugs to rule out hyperaldosteronism.
B) Assessing for renal artery stenosis.
C) Checking a 24-hour urine for glucocorticoids.
D) Checking a 24-hour urine for catecholamines.

Discussion

The correct answer is A. This is **not** what you would want to do because when checking the serum potassium level for hyperaldosteronism, the patient must be off all diuretic medications and have an unrestricted salt intake. Hypertension is secondary to another cause in about 1% of patients with mild hypertension, but up to 10% to 45% of those with severe, difficult-to-control hypertension. Secondary causes of hypertension include hyperaldosteronism, renal artery stenosis, pheochromocytoma, Cushing disease, sleep apnea, primary hyperparathyroidism, and others. All of the other answer choices can be a part of a workup for secondary hypertension caused by renal artery stenosis (answer B), Cushing disease (answer C), and pheochromocytoma (answer D). See Table 2–13.

You decide to check this patient for renal artery stenosis. The most sensitive test for renal artery stenosis is:

A) Doppler ultrasound.
B) Captopril renal scan.
C) Serum renin level.
D) MR angiography.

Table 2–13 CAUSES OF SECONDARY HYPERTENSION

Drugs, including over-the-counter medications

Sleep apnea

Endocrine:

- Hyperaldosteronism
- Pheochromocytoma
- Thyroid disease
- Cushing syndrome (innate or iatrogenic)

Vascular:

- Renal artery stenosis
- Coarctation of the aorta

Renal disease

Discussion

The correct answer is D. When angiography is used as the gold standard, MR angiography is the most sensitive test for renal artery stenosis, followed by captopril-enhanced Doppler ultrasound, followed by captopril renal scan (90%, 63%, and 33%, respectively). Frequently, renal artery stenosis is an incidental finding when the patient has angiography for another indication. In these cases, intervention is usually not needed so long as blood pressure control is adequate.

 HELPFUL TIP: Consider an evaluation for renal artery stenosis in a patient who has a positive clinical captopril challenge. If you start an ACE inhibitor and see a dramatic decline in renal function in a few days, renal artery stenosis is the likely culprit.

* *

Your patient does not have any identifiable cause for secondary hypertension. You add a third agent, and his blood pressure comes under control.

 HELPFUL TIP: Adding spironolactone to the regimen of a patient with difficult-to-control blood pressure can often be helpful even in the presence of another diuretic. Watch for hyperkalemia with ACE inhibitors, however.

Objectives: Did you learn to . . .

- Evaluate a patient with initial high blood pressure readings?
- Select initial antihypertensive therapy?
- Appropriately tailor the treatment of hypertension, based on patient-specific characteristics?
- Use and interpret 24-hour ambulatory blood pressure monitoring?
- Understand the concept of white-coat hypertension?
- Generate a differential diagnosis and an appropriate evaluation of secondary hypertension?

 QUICK QUIZ: HYPERTENSION

Black patients tend to have LESS of a response to which of the following antihypertensives?

A) Calcium channel blockers and ACE inhibitors.
B) ACE inhibitors and diuretics.
C) β-Blockers and ACE inhibitors.
D) Calcium channel blockers and diuretics.

Discussion

The correct answer is C. In comparison with white patients, black patients tend to be more resistant to ACE inhibitors, β-blockers, and ARBs. They tend to respond better to diuretics. Of course, this is a generalization and therapy should be individualized to the patient.

CASE 17

A 31-year-old woman presents for prepregnancy counseling. She has a history of stage I hypertension and a heart murmur; she was told several years prior to see a physician before becoming pregnant. She has dyspnea when climbing stairs but performs normal activities of daily living with minimal difficulty. She takes lisinopril 10 mg daily for her blood pressure. On physical examination, heart rate is 82 bpm and blood pressure is 138/90 mm Hg. Height is 5′6″ and weight is 160 lbs. She appears well. Lungs are clear to auscultation. Neck veins are not visible with the exam table at 30 degrees and carotid upstrokes are normal.

Regarding the management of her chronic hypertension during pregnancy, which is the most appropriate next step?

A) Discontinue lisinopril; begin methyldopa and recheck blood pressure in 2 weeks.

B) Increase lisinopril to 20 mg daily and recheck blood pressure in 2 weeks.

C) Make no changes at this time.

D) Discontinue lisinopril; recheck blood pressure in 2 weeks.

E) Either A or D is correct.

Discussion

The correct answer is E. ACE inhibitors are contraindicated in pregnancy; therefore, a woman contemplating pregnancy should discontinue the medication or replace it with a safer alternative. For a woman capable of conceiving, ACE inhibitor use is discouraged unless no better alternative exists. Women with chronic hypertension which is mild (systolic blood pressure 140–160 mm Hg) have a low risk for cardiovascular complications during pregnancy and can be managed with nondrug therapy. An equally acceptable strategy is to select a medication regarded as safe during pregnancy; methyldopa, nifedipine, or labetalol would be preferred.

Which of the following statements about cardiovascular physiology in pregnancy is NOT true?

A) Blood volume and cardiac output increase by approximately 50% during pregnancy.

B) Heart rate increases by 10 to 20 beats per minute, peaking in the third trimester.

C) Systemic arterial pressure increases during the first trimester, reaches a peak in midpregnancy, and remains at that level until labor and delivery.

D) Left ventricular ejection fraction remains constant or increases slightly throughout pregnancy.

E) A temporary rise in venous return immediately following delivery may lead to a substantial rise in left ventricular filling pressure and cardiac decompensation in women with certain types of heart disease.

Discussion

The correct answer is C. Systemic arterial pressure decreases during the first trimester, reaches a nadir during the second trimester and returns to prepregnancy levels in the third trimester. The rest of the statements are true. Answer E receives special note. Immediately following delivery, relief of caval compression may cause a rise in venous return, despite blood loss, leading to clinical deterioration in some women with heart disease.

**

An echocardiogram is obtained. The report documents moderate left atrial enlargement and normal left ventricular size and function. There is thickening and restriction of the anterior mitral leaflet consistent with mitral stenosis. The mitral valve is amenable to treatment. Moderate to severe pulmonary hypertension is reported.

The following lesions and/or disorders are considered high risk (and contraindications to) pregnancy EXCEPT:

A) Repaired tetralogy of Fallot (TOF).

B) Severe aortic stenosis.

C) Left ventricular ejection fraction <40%.

D) Symptomatic mitral stenosis.

E) Marfan syndrome with an increased aortic root diameter.

Discussion

The correct answer is A. A repaired TOF does not increase the risk during pregnancy beyond that of the general population. All of the other answer choices are associated with a high risk of maternal complications in pregnancy. Women with Marfan syndrome and no cardiac complications (including normal root diameter) have a reasonably low risk of complications but a favorable outcome is not guaranteed.

The next most appropriate management strategy in this woman who still desires pregnancy is:

A) Counsel her on the risk of pregnancy and inform her that you will treat her to the best of your ability.

B) Refer her for balloon valvuloplasty of her mitral valve.

C) Refer her for mitral valve replacement.

D) Refer her for tubal ligation.

E) None of the above.

Discussion

The correct answer is B. In an anatomically favorable mitral valve, balloon valvuloplasty (or valvotomy) is the procedure of choice due to its lower complication rate (compared to surgical mitral valve replacement) and obviates the need for chronic anticoagulation. Most patients will benefit substantially from the procedure and the improvement in the amount of the stenosis will allow a woman to tolerate a pregnancy.

Objectives: Did you learn to . . .

- Manage stage I hypertension during pregnancy?
- Recognize normal cardiac physiological changes associated with pregnancy?
- Identify cardiac lesions with high complication rates in pregnancy?
- Analyze the treatment options in mitral stenosis?

CASE 18

You have a patient who is mildly hypertensive and you decide to check baseline labs. The patient's potassium is low at 3.0 mEq/L. Being the good physician that you are, you recheck the potassium before getting too excited, and it is 2.9 mEq/L.

Of the following, the MOST LIKELY cause of low potassium in this patient is:

A) Hyperaldosteronism.
B) Hypoaldosteronism.
C) Spuriously low potassium because of an elevated glucose.
D) Metabolic acidosis.

Discussion

The correct answer is A. Hyperaldosteronism can cause hypokalemia and hypertension. Aldosterone increases the secretion of potassium, which leads to hypokalemia. Answer B is incorrect because hypoaldosteronism, such as that seen with adrenal failure secondary to adrenal destruction, causes hyperkalemia and hypotension. Answer C is incorrect because elevated glucose does not result in a spuriously low potassium; if you chose answer C, maybe you were thinking of sodium. Answer D is incorrect because a metabolic acidosis should cause an elevated potassium rather than a low one.

 HELPFUL TIP: The serum potassium goes up by approximately 1 mg/dL for every 0.1 decrease in the pH from 7.4. Thus, the potassium would go from 4 mg/dL to 6 mg/dL if the pH changes from 7.4 to 7.2.

**

You suspect that the patient has hyperaldosteronism.

Which of the following is true?

A) Many patients with hyperaldosteronism have normal serum potassium.
B) In hyperaldosteronism, the plasma aldosterone-to-renin ratio is usually high.
C) All antihypertensives should be stopped before checking a plasma renin level.
D) If a confirmatory 24-hour urine is done, the urine potassium should be low to confirm the diagnosis of hyperaldosteronism.
E) A and B.

Discussion

The correct answer is E. Many patients with hyperaldosteronism will have normal serum potassium levels. Additionally, the plasma aldosterone-to-renin level is usually high. Answer C is incorrect because, although ACE inhibitors and spironolactone (and perhaps all diuretics) should be stopped before renin and aldosterone levels are drawn, other antihypertensives (eg, calcium channel blockers) will have little effect on plasma renin levels. Answer D is incorrect because hyperaldosteronism causes potassium wasting, so the urine potassium should be elevated.

You diagnose this patient with hyperaldosteronism. The MOST COMMON cause of hyperaldosteronism is:

A) Adrenal adenoma.
B) Idiopathic.
C) Pituitary adenoma.
D) Aldosterone-secreting tumor such as small-cell carcinoma.
E) Renal artery stenosis.

Discussion

The correct answer is A. Adrenal adenoma is the most common cause of hyperaldosteronism. The second most common cause is idiopathic.

Accepted approaches to the treatment of hypertension caused by hyperaldosteronism include all of the following EXCEPT:

A) Unilateral adrenalectomy in the case of adrenal adenoma.
B) Liberalized sodium intake.
C) Use of a potassium-sparing diuretic.
D) Use of a combination of amiloride and hydrochlorothiazide.

Discussion

The correct answer is B. Liberalizing sodium intake will actually cause volume expansion, which is counterproductive and can lead to further hypokalemia. Once the patient is hypervolemic, there will be a spontaneous diuresis (aka "aldosterone escape") leading to increased hypokalemia. The exact mechanism of aldosterone escape is not known, but it occurs after a weight gain of approximately 3 kg from fluid retention. It is probably related to the release of atrial natriuretic peptide, among other mechanisms.

Objectives: Did you learn to . . .

- Identify laboratory abnormalities that occur in hyperaldosteronism?
- Evaluate a patient suspected of having hyperaldosteronism?
- Initiate treatment for hyperaldosteronism?

 QUICK QUIZ: HYPERTENSION

A 28-year-old female you have known for a year returns for routine follow-up of hypertension. Because she is a single mother with no insurance, you treat her with the "flavor of the month" ARB available in your sample closet. Lately, she "really feels it" when her blood pressure is high. She reports good compliance with her medication, but she occasionally has systolic blood pressures around 250 mm Hg. When her pressures are this high, she has blurry vision, headaches, diaphoresis, and palpitations (but no chest pain or dyspnea). Her pressure today is 148/92 mm Hg. You want to order a test to evaluate for secondary hypertension in this patient. She can afford only one.

Which test do you choose?

A) Renal ultrasound and Doppler study of the renal arteries.
B) 24-hour urine for catecholamines.
C) Plasma metanephrines.
D) Serum creatinine.
E) Echocardiogram.

Discussion

The correct answer is C. This patient is experiencing symptomatic paroxysmal hypertension with underlying essential hypertension. Although she is unlikely to actually have a pheochromocytoma, it is important that you perform some sort of diagnostic test. Answer B is not strictly incorrect, but urine catecholamines are less sensitive than plasma metanephrines and are more difficult to obtain. Plasma metanephrines have been shown in various studies to have a sensitivity for pheochromocytoma of 85% to 100%. On the downside, the specificity of plasma metanephrines is not agreed upon, with some studies showing a specificity less than that seen with urine catecholamines and metanephrines. To get an accurate sample for plasma metanephrine measurement, the patient should have blood drawn in the morning while fasting and should avoid caffeine, tobacco, stimulants, and acetaminophen prior to the test. If the test is negative, no further investigation into pheochromocytoma is necessary. If the test is positive, tumor should be confirmed by other means (eg, MRI, etc.). Answers A, D, and E are incorrect because these tests will not address a primary cause of paroxysmal hypertension.

 HELPFUL TIP: The use of drug samples actually increases overall drug costs. Samples are a form of advertising designed to increase drug sales otherwise they wouldn't be in your sample closet....

CASE 19

A 40-year-old female presents to your office with blood pressures in the range of 140–159 mm Hg systolic and 90–99 mm Hg diastolic taken over a number of weeks. You have verified these numbers and have decided that she does indeed have hypertension. She has no other risk factors for cardiac disease but tends to be sedentary and have a relatively poor diet.

How long are you willing to try lifestyle modifications before starting medications?

A) Start medications now.
B) 1–3 months.
C) 3–6 months.
D) 6–12 months.

Discussion

The correct answer is D. In patients without any other risk factors for cardiovascular disease and stage 1 hypertension (defined as systolic 140–159 and diastolic 90–99), you can prescribe a trial of lifestyle modification for up to 1 year. Patients with stage 1 hypertension and another risk factor can be tried on lifestyle modification for up to 6 months.

Lifestyle changes recommended by JNC 7 include which of the following?

A) Low-sodium diet.
B) Alcohol intake of 2 drinks or less per day.
C) Exercise.
D) Weight loss.
E) All of the above.

Discussion

The correct answer is E. All of the other answer choices, including moderate alcohol intake, are recommended lifestyle modifications per JNC 7. You should not encourage people to start drinking, but limit them to two drinks a day if they do drink. This will lead to a reduction in blood pressure of 2–4 mm Hg. A final lifestyle modification is the adoption of a DASH diet. The acronym stands for "**d**ietary **a**pproach to **s**top **h**ypertension." The DASH diet includes fruits, vegetables, and low-fat dairy products.

* *

A year later your patient is not meeting with much success. Initially, she lost weight, but then she found it, then found some more. She has a number of drug allergies, including a rash with hydrochlorothiazide and wheezing with atenolol. You want to start her on an ACE inhibitor, but she is concerned about potential side effects.

Which of the following side effects is (are) associated with the use of ACE inhibitors?

A) Cough.
B) Dependent edema.
C) Hypokalemia.
D) Angioedema.
E) A and D.

Discussion

The correct answer is E. Both chronic dry cough and angioedema (more common in blacks) are side effects of ACE inhibitors. Hyperkalemia is another potential concern. These side effects may not occur immediately.

Objectives: Did you learn to . . .

- Identify hypertensive patients appropriate for lifestyle modification?
- Recommend lifestyle modifications to a hypertensive patient?
- Recognize common side effects of ACE inhibitors?

What is the rhythm on the rhythm strip shown in Figure 2–6?

A) Second-degree heart block, type I.
B) Second-degree heart block, type II.
C) Third-degree heart block with junctional escape rhythm.
D) Sinus rhythm with nonconducted PACs.

Discussion

The correct answer is B. This is a Wenckebach block, also known as second-degree heart block type I or Mobitz type I AV block. Note the progressive prolongation of the PR interval before a nonconducted P wave on the rhythm strip in Figure 2–7 (arrows indicate P waves).

The proper treatment for an asymptomatic patient with this rhythm is:

A) Treat any underlying causes identified and observe.
B) Place temporary pacemaker followed by permanent pacemaker.
C) Give atropine followed by permanent pacemaker.
D) None of the above.

Discussion

The correct answer is A. Wenckebach/second-degree heart block type I can be treated with observation as long as any underlying cardiac disease is treated. You should also stop any medications that might be contributing to this rhythm disturbance, such as digoxin and other AV node blocking agents. Pacemaker is appropriate for selected patients, usually those with symptoms. Atropine is used in the emergent setting.

What is the proper diagnosis of the ECG shown in Figure 2–8?

A) Anterior wall MI.
B) Posterior wall MI.
C) Pericarditis.
D) Hyperkalemia.
E) Inferior wall MI.

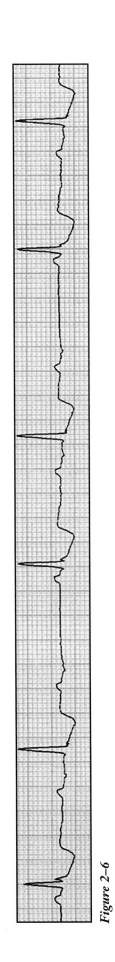

Figure 2–6

Figure 2–7

103

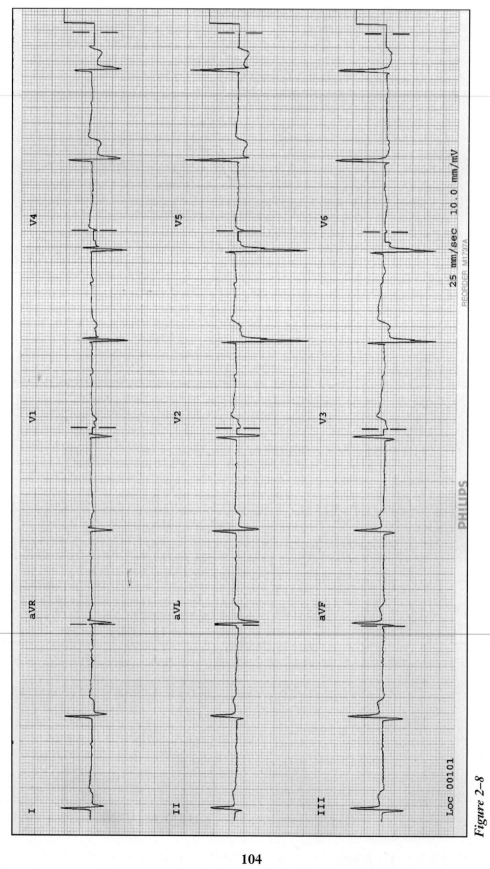

aVR V1 V4

aVL V2 V5

aVF V3 V6

I

II

III

Loc 00101

25 mm/sec 10.0 mm/mV

REORDER M1737A

PHILIPS

Figure 2–8

Discussion

The correct answer is E. See Figure 2–9. This is an inferior wall MI. Note the ST elevations in leads II and III, and aVF with reciprocal changes in leads V_2–V_5 (indicator arrows).

CASE 20

A patient presents with a history of light-headedness when he stands. He has the ECG shown in Figure 2–10.

What is the rhythm?

A) Atrial flutter with 4:1 block.
B) Atrial fibrillation with slow ventricular response.
C) Atrial tachycardia with third-degree heart block.
D) Mobitz type I (Wenckebach).

Discussion

The correct answer is C. This is an atrial tachycardia with a third-degree heart block. The P wave preceding each QRS complex is indicated with an arrow on the ECG shown in Figure 2–11. While the atrial rate (approximately 190 bpm) could still be sinus, the P wave axis (nonsinus) suggests an atrial tachycardia. Note that there is no consistent relationship between the P waves and the QRS complexes, giving the diagnosis third-degree heart block.

The appropriate treatment for this patient with atrial tachycardia and third-degree block is:

A) Pacemaker.
B) Isoproterenol.
C) Lidocaine.
D) Atropine.

Discussion

The correct answer is A. The treatment for a third-degree heart block is a pacemaker. Atropine will increase the atrial rate, but that is not the problem here. The problem is conduction from the atrium to the ventricle. Isoproterenol will increase the ventricular rate but is arrhythmogenic and may cause hypotension. Lidocaine is not indicated in this patient.

 HELPFUL TIP: Atrial tachycardia with block is classic for digitalis intoxication. If this patient were on digoxin, you would treat with Digibind.

The drug of choice for the rhythm on the rhythm strip in Figure 2–12 is:

A) Atropine.
B) Procainamide.
C) Quinidine.
D) Metoprolol
E) Lidocaine.

Discussion

The correct answer is D. This is an accelerated junctional rhythm which generally occurs only in the setting of cardiac ischemia. Slowing down this rhythm with metoprolol is acceptable. Note the absence of P waves. Using a Class I antiarrhythmic can extinguish this rhythm, causing asystole (usually considered a bad outcome).

The patient also has inferior wall ischemia (Figure 2–13). The indicator arrows point to depressed ST segments in the inferior leads.

The rhythm shown in Figure 2–14 is best described as:

A) Atrial flutter with 2:1 block.
B) 2:1 second-degree heart block, Mobitz type II.
C) Sinus bradycardia.
D) Third-degree heart block.

Discussion

The correct answer is B. This rhythm strip represents second-degree heart block, Mobitz type II. Notice that the PR interval is constant and there are dropped beats See Figure 2–15, with indicator arrows showing P waves with no associated QRS complexes.

The electrocardiogram shown in Figure 2–16 is consistent with which of the following?

A) Pericardial effusion.
B) Pneumothorax.
C) Pulmonary embolism.
D) Cardiac contusion.
E) None of the above.

Discussion

The correct answer is A. This is an example of electrical alternans. Note the low QRS voltages which alternate in height from beat-to-beat. This type of pattern is seen with pericardial effusion.

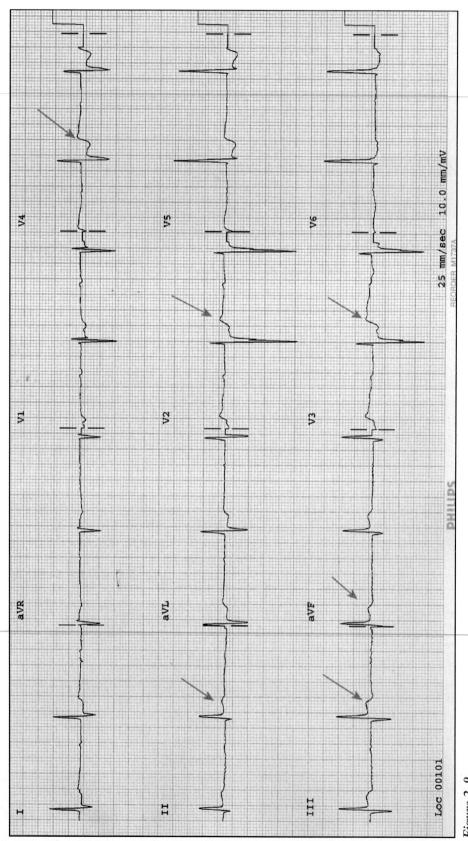

Figure 2–9

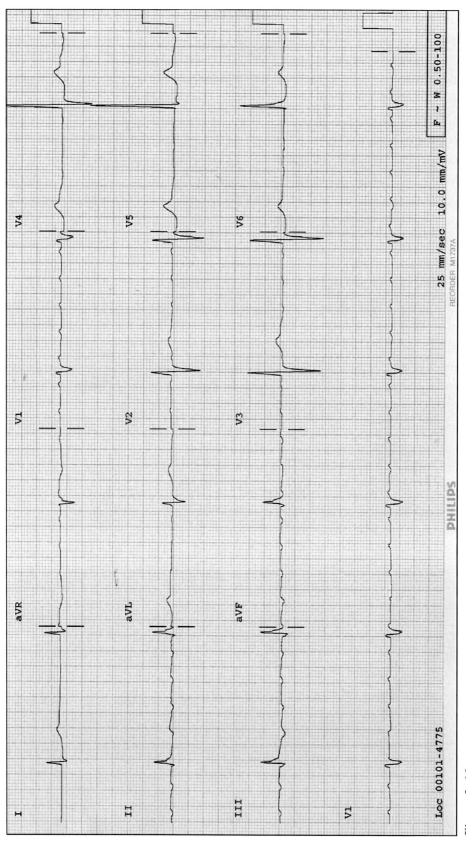

Figure 2–10

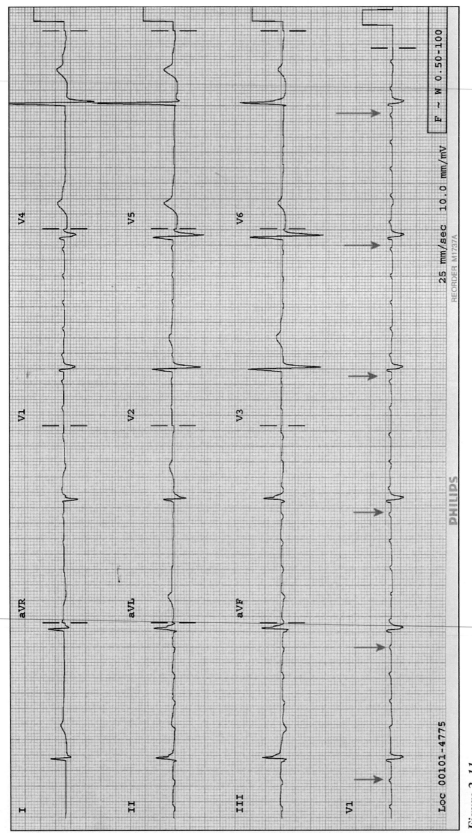

Figure 2-11

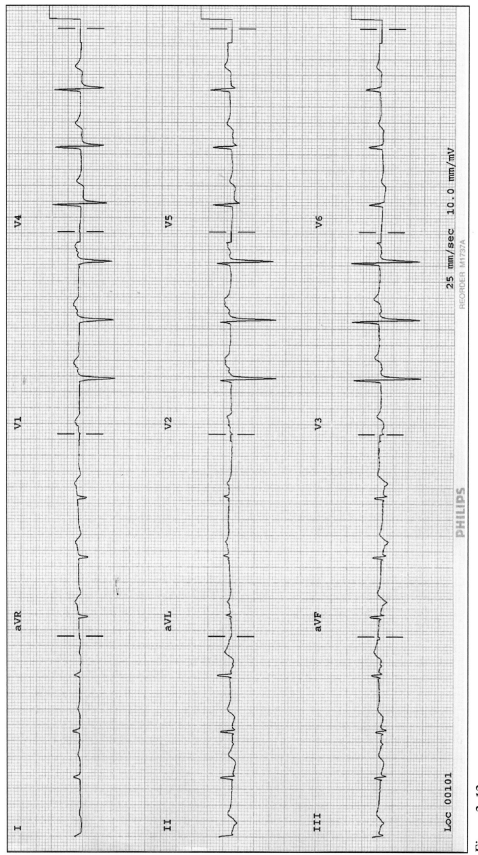

Figure 2–12

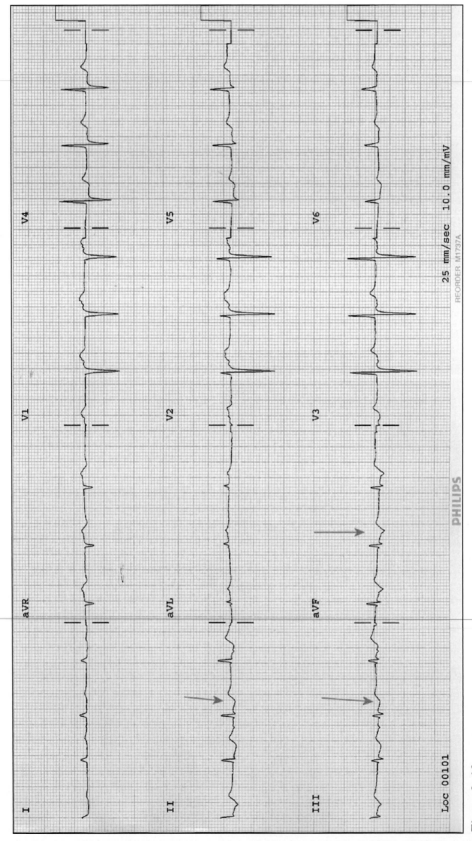

Figure 2–13

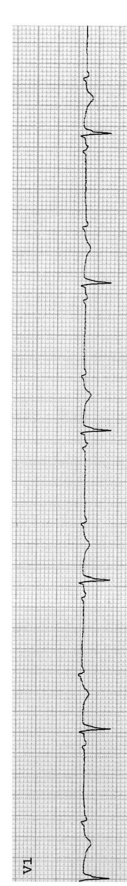

Figure 2–14

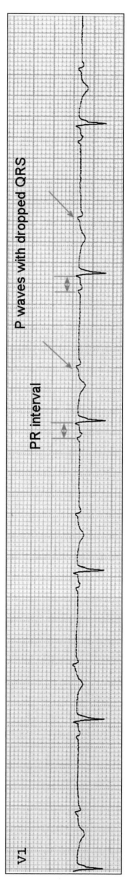

P waves with dropped QRS

PR interval

Figure 2–15

111

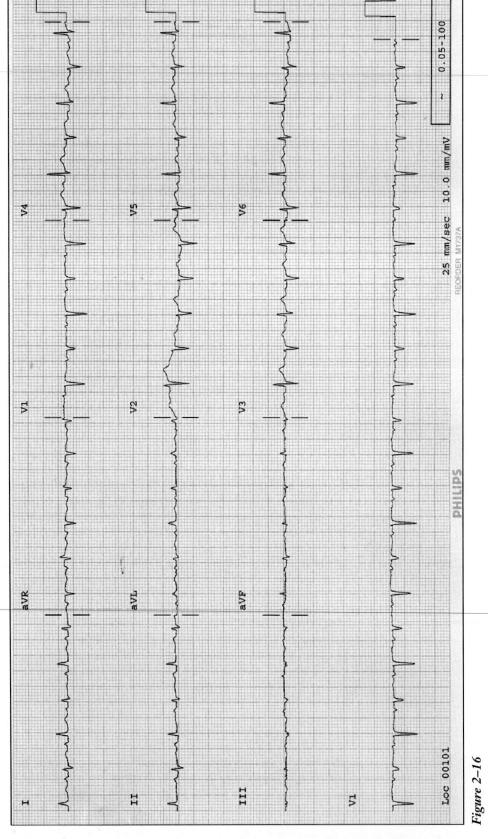

I   aVR   V1   V4

II   aVL   V2   V5

III   aVF   V3   V6

V1

Loc 00101   PHILIPS   REORDER M1737A   25 mm/sec   10.0 mm/mV   ~ 0.05-100

Figure 2–16

The ECG in Figure 2–17 is consistent with which of the following?

A) Anterior MI.
B) Anterolateral myocardial infarction.
C) Pericarditis.
D) Early repolarization.
E) Left ventricular hypertrophy.

Discussion

The correct answer is C. This ECG is consistent with pericarditis. This ECG demonstrates several findings that indicate pericarditis, including sinus tachycardia, diffuse ST elevations, and PR depression shown in Figure 2–18.

CASE 21

A 24-year-old female presents to the ED with a history of tachycardia and the rhythm strip shown in Figure 2–19. Her blood pressure is stable at 115/70 with an oxygen saturation of 98% on room air. There are no associated symptoms of chest pain, dyspnea, etc.

The appropriate treatment for this patient is:

A) Adenosine 6 mg IV followed by 12 mg IV.
B) Diltiazem 5 mg/kg IV.
C) Verapamil 25 mg IV.
D) Digoxin 0.5 mg IV.
E) Defibrillation.

Discussion

The correct answer is A. There are several treatment options for paroxysmal supraventricular tachycardia (PSVT). These include adenosine, diltiazem, and verapamil. Many physicians prefer using the calcium channel blockers over adenosine. Answer B is incorrect because the dose for diltiazem is 0.25 mg/kg IV, not 5 mg/kg. Answer C is incorrect because the dose for verapamil is 2.5–5.0 mg IV, not 25 mg IV. Answer D is incorrect because digoxin is the least preferred agent due to slow onset of action. The initial dose of digoxin is 0.5-1 mg IV. Although cardioversion is also an option, in a hemodynamically stable patient, medication should be tried first. Answer E is incorrect because defibrillation is never recommended for a perfusing rhythm.

**

You treat the patient with adenosine but there is no response. Thus, you choose to try a calcium channel blocker. Unfortunately, the patient rapidly deteriorates with the calcium channel blocker and the heart rate actually increases, so you successfully cardiovert the patient. The ECG done after cardioversion is shown in Figure 2–20.

The ECG represents:

A) Normal ECG.
B) Wolf-Parkinson-White syndrome.
C) Right bundle branch block.
D) Right axis deviation.
E) Left ventricular hypertrophy.

Discussion

The correct answer is B. This is an ECG demonstrating Wolf-Parkinson-White (WPW) pattern. When combined with documented tachyarrhythmia, it is referred to as WPW syndrome. Note the short PR interval as well as the delta wave (Figure 2–21).

The ECG shown in Figure 2–22 represents which of the following?

A) Left bundle branch block.
B) Right bundle branch block.
C) Left anterior fascicular block.
D) Left posterior fascicular block.
E) None of the above.

Discussion

The correct answer is C. For those of us who can't remember these things, any patient with a net negative force in lead II has a left anterior fascicular block. For those of you who can remember these things, left anterior fascicular block (LAFB) is present when the QRS axis is –45° to –90°, there is a rS pattern (with small r waves) in leads II, III, and aVF and a qR pattern (with small q waves) in I and aVL. Because the QRS is narrow, neither LBBB nor RBBB can be correct. Left posterior block is quite uncommon due to the size of the posterior fascicle.

The ECG shown in Figure 2–23 represents which of the following?

A) Left bundle branch block.
B) Right bundle branch block.
C) Left anterior fascicular block.
D) Left posterior fascicular block.
E) None of the above.

Discussion

The correct answer is A. This ECG represents a left bundle branch block (LBBB). Criteria include QRS

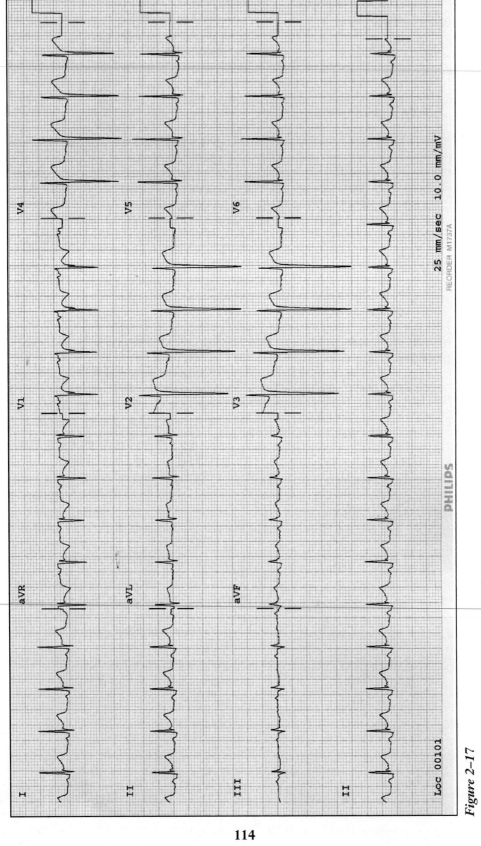

Figure 2–17

114

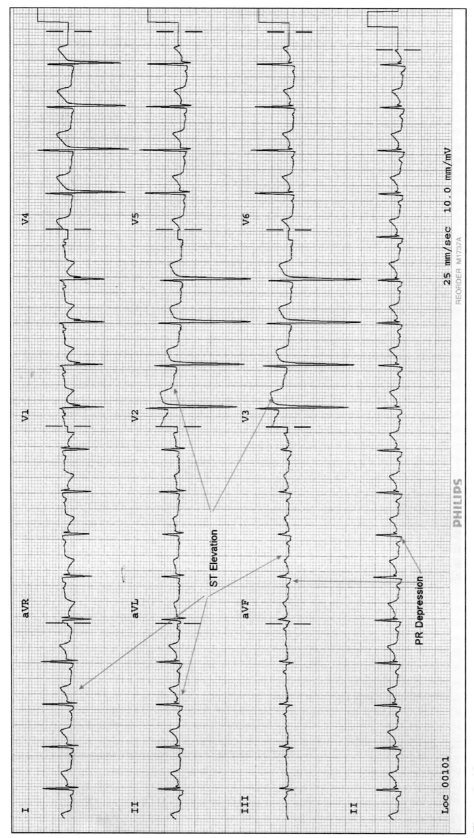

Figure 2–18

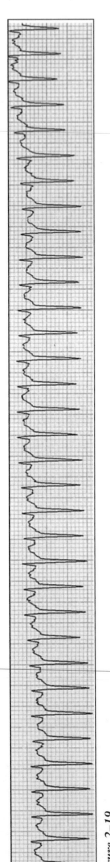

Figure 2-19

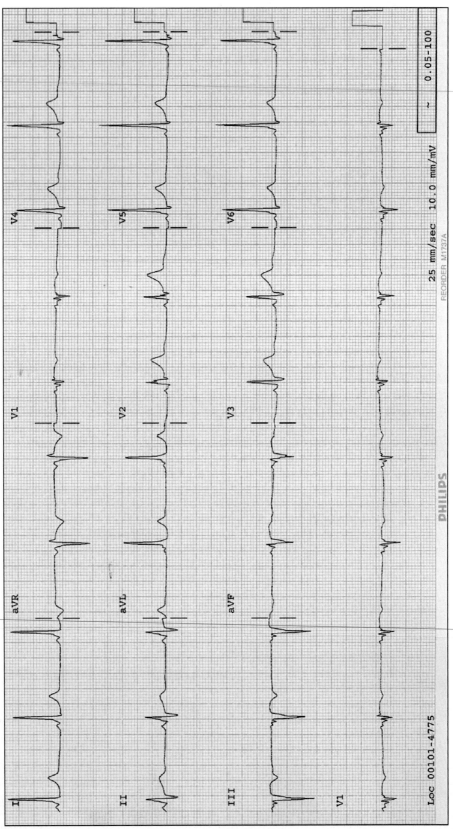

Figure 2-20

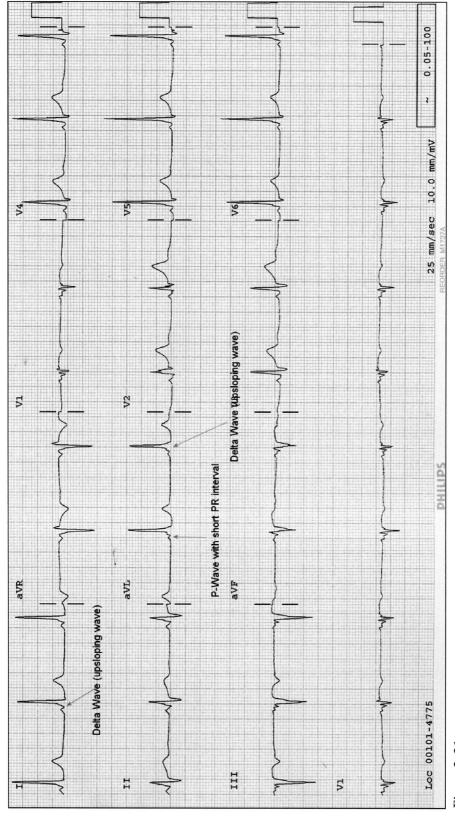

Figure 2–21

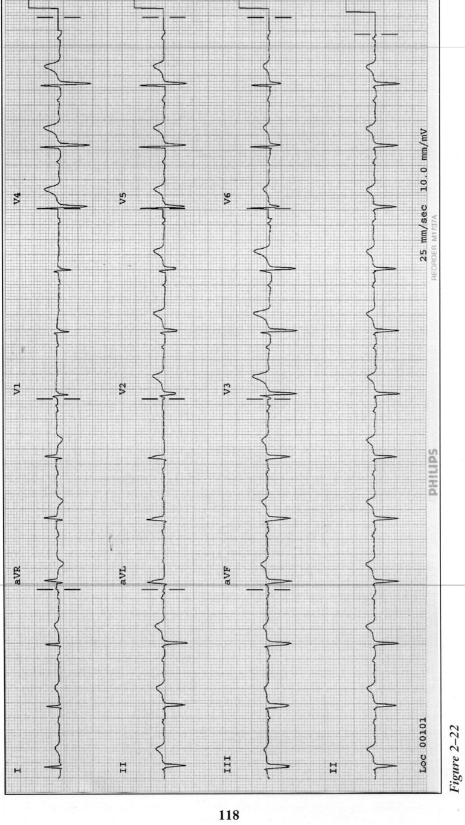

Figure 2-22

118

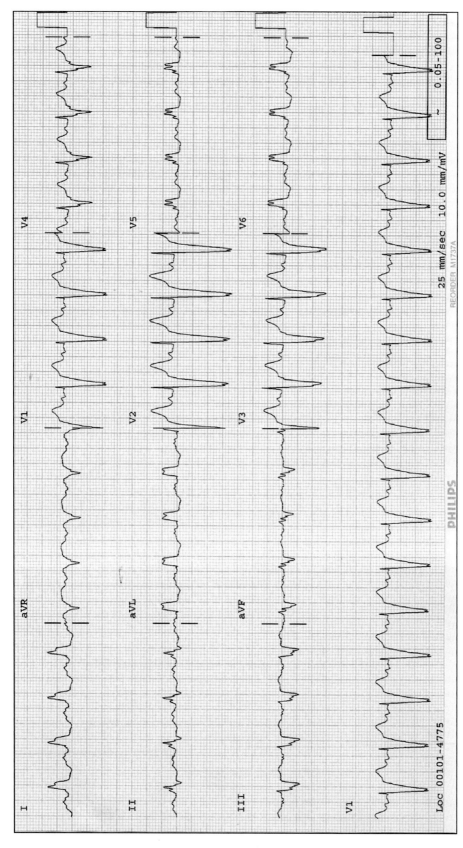

Figure 2–23

width ≥0.12 ms, upright (monophasic) QRS in leads I and V₆, and a mostly negative QRS in V₁.

The ECG shown in Figure 2–24 represents which of the following?

A) First-degree block.
B) Right bundle branch block.
C) Left anterior fascicular block.
D) All of the above.
E) None of the above.

Discussion

The correct answer is D. This ECG represents a first-degree AV block, a right bundle branch block, and a left anterior fascicular block. The right bundle branch block is defined by a QRS width of ≥0.12 ms (>3 small blocks) and a rsR′ ("rabbit ears") in chest leads V₁–V₃. This patient also has an LAFB (see the ECG in Figure 2–22 for criteria).

CASE 21

A 75-year-old patient presents to your ED with the ECG shown in Figure 2–25.

What is the most likely electrolyte abnormality in this patient?

A) Hypokalemia.
B) Hyperkalemia.
C) Hyponatremia.
D) Hypermagnesemia.
E) Hypercalcemia.

Discussion

The correct answer is B, hyperkalemia. Note the peaked T waves across the precordium. Note also that the patient has early repolarization.

All of the following are potential causes of this patient's hyperkalemia EXCEPT:

A) Metabolic acidosis.
B) ACE inhibitors.
C) Angiotensin receptor blockers.
D) Renal failure.
E) Furosemide.

Discussion

The correct answer is E. Furosemide will cause hypokalemia rather than hyperkalemia. All the other answer choices are potential causes of hyperkalemia. Other causes of hyperkalemia include a potassium load from muscle breakdown (eg, rhabdomyolysis, burns, transfusion of old blood) and other exogenous sources of potassium such as penicillin, potassium supplements, and water softeners. Consider also Addison disease and hypoaldosteronism. Digoxin toxicity is also a possibility.

* *

You confirm the diagnosis of hyperkalemia by sending a potassium and then a confirmatory sample (never get fooled by hemolysis!!). The patient's potassium is 8.0 mEq/L, presumably due to acute renal failure. His pH is normal and he is not taking digoxin.

Appropriate therapies for this patient at this time include which of the following?

A) Kayexalate (sodium polystyrene sulfonate).
B) Insulin and glucose.
C) IV bicarbonate.
D) Calcium gluconate.
E) All of the above.

Discussion

The correct answer is E. Kayexalate (answer A) will bind potassium in the GI tract and help remove it from the body. Remember that nothing is free: the potassium is exchanged for sodium, so Kayexalate can worsen CHF. Insulin and glucose (answer B) will drive potassium intracellularly and decrease the serum potassium but will not remove potassium from the body. The same is true of sodium bicarbonate (answer C). Note that sodium bicarbonate is useful even when the pH is normal. Calcium gluconate (answer D) (and calcium chloride) will stabilize the myocardium and make it less prone to arrhythmias. Again, this does not help remove potassium from the body. Diuretics such as furosemide can be used to remove potassium from the body in patients with good renal function. β-Agonists will drive potassium into the cell and cause modest (transient) decreases in serum potassium. Dialysis may be necessary, especially when renal failure is present.

 HELPFUL TIP: Do not use calcium gluconate in hyperkalemia caused by digoxin. It will worsen the problem by increasing binding of digoxin to cardiac muscle.

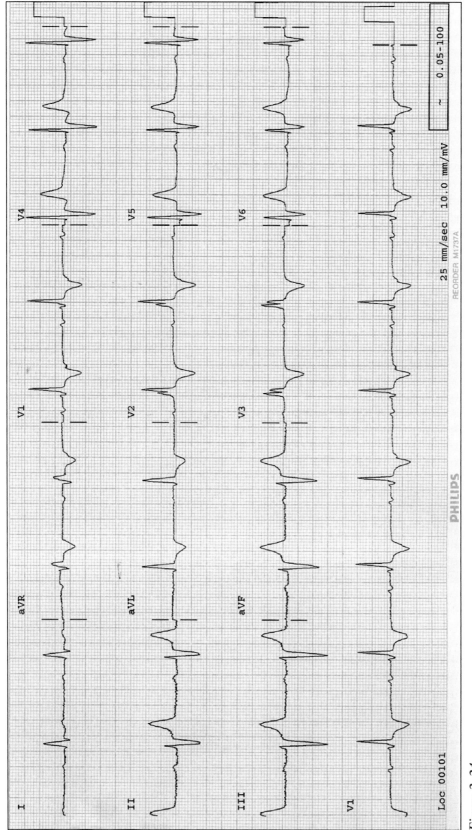

Figure 2–24

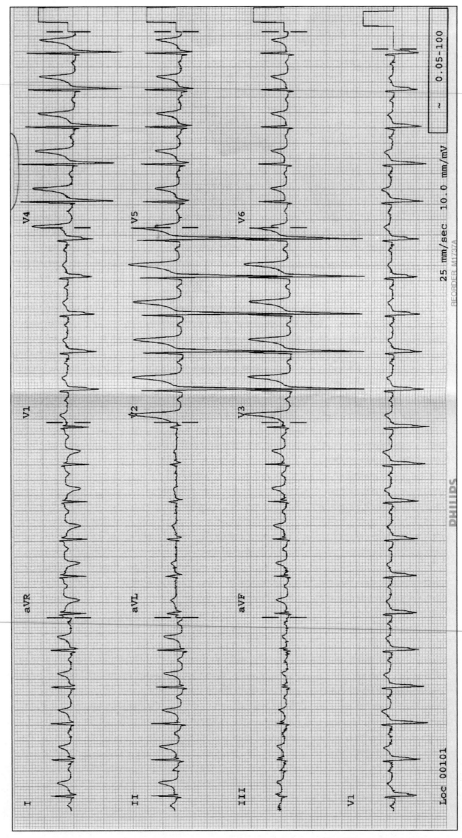

Figure 2-25

What is the rhythm shown in Figure 2–26?

A) Atrial fibrillation.
B) Normal sinus rhythm with multiple PACs.
C) Third-degree heart block with rapid rate.
D) Multifocal atrial tachycardia.

Discussion

The correct answer is D. This is a multifocal atrial tachycardia.

Note the multiple morphologies of the P waves indicated by arrows in Figure 2–27. This is generally associated with severe pulmonary disease and theophylline use.

All of the following are treatments for multifocal atrial tachycardia EXCEPT:

A) Calcium channel blocker.
B) β-Blocker.
C) Magnesium.
D) Improving pulmonary function and reducing hypoxia.
E) Adenosine.

Discussion

The correct answer is E. All of the others are indicated in the treatment of multifocal atrial tachycardia. Adenosine may slow the rhythm temporarily but is not considered a treatment for this rhythm.

CASE 22

A 28-year-old woman with no significant past medical history presents to clinic with complaints of shortness of breath. The patient first noted dyspnea over 1 year ago which she attributed to lack of physical conditioning. She began a walking program but has been unable to improve her stamina. She becomes dyspneic with less activity than 1 year ago. If she exerts herself beyond a brisk walk, she becomes lightheaded, presyncopal, and feels a tightness in her chest. She also notes generalized fatigue. Your examination discloses a heart rate of 105 bpm and normal blood pressure. Resting transcutaneous oximetry is 92% at rest. BMI is 24 kg/m². She has JVD but clear lungs. A grade 2/6 midsystolic murmur is heard over the left upper sternal border. Electrocardiogram is shown in Figure 2–28.

What is the most likely diagnosis?

A) Coronary artery disease.
B) Pulmonary hypertension (PHTN).
C) Asthma.

D) Congenital aortic stenosis.
E) Mitral valve prolapse.

Discussion

The correct answer is B. The physical examination is consistent with right ventricular pressure overload. This is supported by the electrocardiogram demonstrating right atrial enlargement, right axis deviation, and right ventricular hypertrophy. Coronary artery disease is almost unheard of in a woman <30 years with no risk factors. Asthma may cause her symptom complex but is not supported by her examination. Aortic stenosis should not cause resting hypoxemia nor evidence of right ventricular hypertrophy.

Note: Findings that suggest right ventricular hypertrophy on the ECG: Right axis deviation, right atrial abnormality (p wave >2.5 boxes tall in lead II), right ventricular hypertrophy (tall R in V_1), strain pattern in leads II, III. The arrows in Figure 2–29 point to some of these findings. Often patients with pulmonary hypertension will have an intraventricular conduction delay with R-R′ in V_1 (not shown on this ECG).

The following tests may be helpful in elucidating the cause of pulmonary hypertension EXCEPT:

A) Chest x-ray and pulmonary function studies.
B) V/Q scan.
C) ANA, HIV-1, 2 and liver function studies.
D) Nasopharyngoscopy.
E) Polysomnogram.

Discussion

The correct answer is D. An important part of the workup for pulmonary hypertension is defining the etiology and potentially reversible causes. There is no cookbook approach, and diagnostic workup should be tailored by the history and physical examination. Chest radiography and PFTs can identify chronic lung disease causing (or contributing) to pulmonary hypertension. A V/Q scan, or possibly chest CT, is done to exclude chronic thromboembolic pulmonary disease. Connective tissue disease, HIV and cirrhosis are known to cause pulmonary hypertension. Sleep apnea is an important, treatable cause of PHTN. Nasopharyngoscopy has no role in this workup.

* *

An echocardiogram confirms severe pulmonary hypertension and changes consistent with right ventricular pressure overload. No intracardiac shunt is identified. The remainder of her diagnostic workup fails to

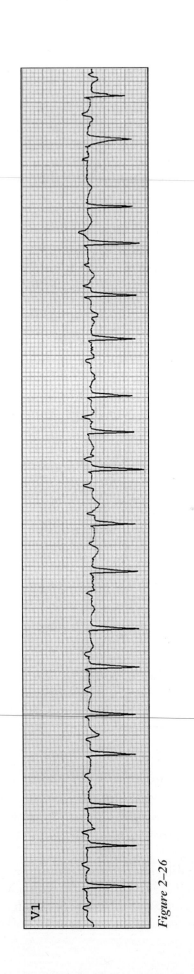

Figure 2–26

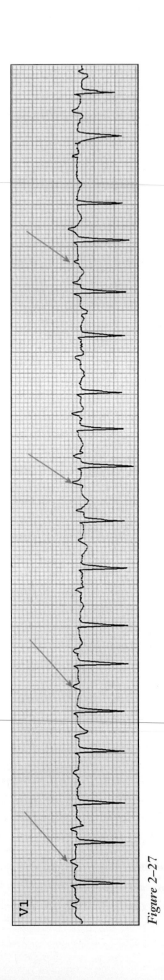

Figure 2–27

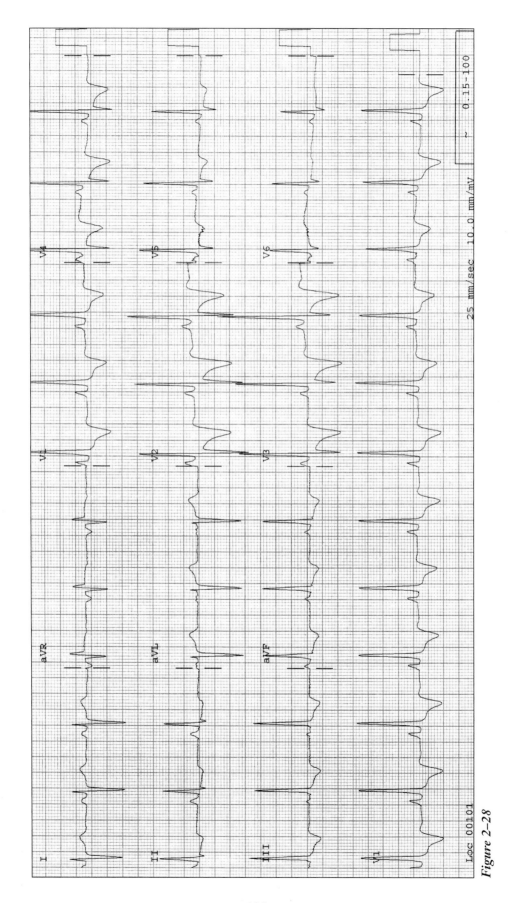

Loc 00101

25 mm/sec 10.0 mm/mV ~ 0.15-100

Figure 2–28

125

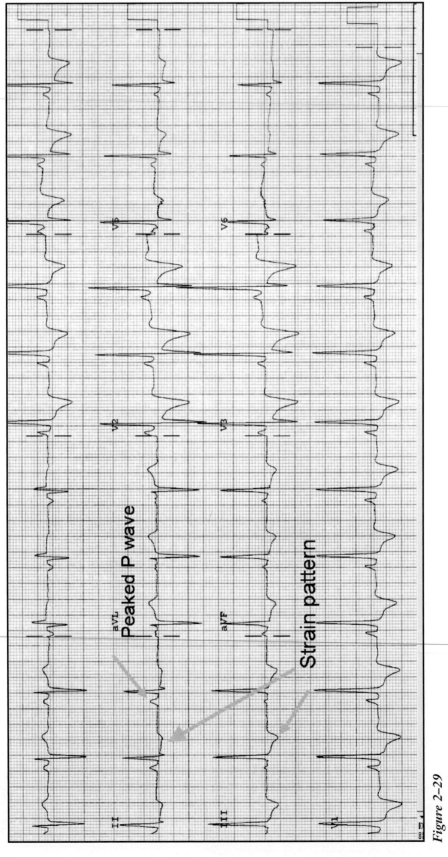

Figure 2–29

identify a secondary cause of pulmonary hypertension. A right heart catheterization confirms severe pulmonary hypertension but fails to identify a shunt. A vasodilator challenge (with adenosine) is performed and no change in pulmonary pressure is elicited. She is given a diagnosis of idiopathic pulmonary arterial hypertension (PAH). The treatment of pulmonary hypertension is, in general, very specialized and a cardiologist should be involved. Exceptions include pulmonary hypertension from chronic hypoxia (smoking, sleep apnea) which is amenable to primary care management. Chronic pulmonary emboli can also be managed by the primary care practitioner.

 HELPFUL TIP: Additional therapy for pulmonary hypertension may include prostacyclin, phosphodiesterase inhibitors (sildenafil or other drugs of this class tadalafil [Cialis], vardenafil [Levitra]). Some patients require anticoagulation. Management is best done in conjunction with a cardiologist.

Objectives: Did you learn to . . .

- Suspect pulmonary hypertension on the basis of history and physical?
- Order baseline studies for the evaluation of new onset pulmonary hypertension?
- Identify patients with PHTN appropriate for anticoagulation?

BIBLIOGRAPHY

Adan V. Diagnosis and treatment of sick sinus syndrome. *Am Fam Physician*. 2003;67(8):1725.

Bosch X, Loma-Osorio P, Marrugat J. Platelet glycoprotein IIB/IIIA blockers for percutaneous coronary intervention and the initial treatment of non-ST segment elevation acute coronary syndromes. Cochrane Database of Systematic Reviews. *Cochrane Review*. 2006:4.

Bouknight DP. Current management of mitral valve prolapse. *Am Fam Physician*. 2000;61(11):3343.

Braunwald E, et al. Management of patients with unstable angina and non-ST-segment elevation myocardial infarction. *J Am Coll Cardiol*. 2002;40:1366.

Carabello BA, Crawford F. Valvular heart disease. *N Engl J Med*. 1997;337(1):32.

Eagle KA, et al. Perioperative cardiac evaluation for noncardiac surgery update. 2002. Available at http://www.acc.org/clinical/guidelines/perio/update/periupdate_index.htm.

Elkayam U. Pregnancy and Cardiovascular Disease. *Braunwald's Heart Disease: A Textbook of Cardiovascular Medicine*. Saunders, Philadelphia. 2005.

Gibbons RJ, et al. Management of patients with chronic stable angina update. Available at http://www.acc.org/clinical/guidelines/stable/update_index.htm.

Goyle KK. Diagnosing pericarditis. *Am Fam Physician*. 2002;66(9):1695.

Gregoratos G, et al. ACC/AHA/NASPE 2002 Guideline update for implantation of cardiac pacemakers and antiarrhythmia devices. Available at www.acc.org/clinical/guidelines/pacemaker/incorporated/index.htm.

Harris GD. Heart disease in children. *Prim Care*. 2000;27(3):767.

Hazinski MF, Cummins RO, Field JM. *Handbook of Emergency Ccardiovascular Care for Healthcare Providers*. Dallas: American Heart Association; 2000.

Hebbar AK. Management of common arrhythmias: Part I. Supraventricular arrhythmias. *Am Fam Physician*. 2002;65(12):2479.

Hebbar AK. Management of common arrhythmias: Part II. Ventricular arrhythmias in special populations. *Am Fam Physician*. 2002;65(12):2491.

Hirsh J, et al. American Heart Association/American College of Cardiology Foundation guide to warfarin therapy. *J Am Coll Cardiol*. 2003;41:1633.

Hunt SA, et al. Evaluation and management of heart failure. Available at www.acc.org/clinical/guidelines/failure/hf_index.htm.

Laussen PC. Neonates with congenital heart disease. *Curr Opin Pediatr*. 2001;13(3):220.

McLaughlin VV, McGoon MD. Pulmonary arterial hypertension. *Circulation*. 2006;114:417.

Moodie DS. Diagnosis and management of congenital heart disesase in the adult. *Cardiol Rev*. 2001;9(5):276.

National Heart, Lung and Blood Institute. The Seventh Report of the Joint National Committee on Prevention, Detection, Evaluation, and Treatment of High Blood Pressure (JNC 7). Available at www.nhlbi.nih.gov/guidelines/hypertension.

National Heart, Lung and Blood Institute. Third Report of the Expert Panel on Detection, Evaluation, and Treatment of High Blood Cholesterol in Adults (Adult Treatment Panel III). Available at www.nhlbi.nih.gov/guidelines/cholesterol.

Roden DM. Risks and benefits of antiarrhythmic therapy. *N Engl J Med*. 1994;331:785.

Ryan TJ, et al. ACC/AHA Guidelines for the management of patients with acute myocardial infarction. *Circulation*. 1999;100(9):1016.

Shammash JB. Perioperative assessment and perioperative management of the patient with nonischemic heart disease. *Med Clin North Am*. 2003;87(1):137.

Shipton B. Valvular heart disease: review and update. *Am Fam Physician*. 2001;63(11):2201.

3
Pulmonary

Greg Davis

CASE 1

A 42-year-old male who works in a hog confinement area presents to your office complaining of cough, fever, wheeze, and dyspnea. He and some other workers were moving moldy hay, and they all came down with the same symptoms which started between 4 and 8 hours after work. On examination, he is febrile with a respiratory rate of 28. He is able to talk in complete sentences. There are slight crackles when you auscultate the lungs.

The most likely diagnosis is:

A) "Farmer Lung" (hypersensitivity pneumonitis).
B) Toxic organic dust syndrome.
C) Reactive airway disease.
D) Hydrogen sulfide poisoning.
E) Bronchiolitis obliterans.

Discussion

The correct answer is B. Toxic organic dust syndrome occurs when moldy or decomposed hay and other organic material is moved. Endotoxins are aerosolized and inhaled, leading to the symptoms. The tip off here is that everyone on the job site was affected. Answer A is incorrect. Because hypersensitivity pneumonitis is specific to the individual, generally the patient who presents will be the only worker at the site to have problems. Answer C is incorrect because everyone is involved and febrile which is not consistent with reactive airway disease. Answer D is incorrect. Hydrogen sulfide poisoning presents as a toxic pneumonitis with

pulmonary edema, dyspnea, hypoxia, and loss of consciousness. Hydrogen sulfide also acts as a direct cellular toxin which binds to cytochrome oxidase system, similar to cyanide. Additionally, hydrogen sulfide exposure comes when cleaning manure pits, not when moving hay (as anyone in Iowa would know). Answer E is incorrect. Bronchiolitis obliterans is a chronic illness rather than an acute one.

Appropriate treatment for this patient includes:

A) Antibiotics.
B) Intubation and mechanical ventilation.
C) Supportive care.
D) A and B.
E) A and C.

Discussion

The correct answer is C. Supportive care is the usual treatment for toxic organic dust syndrome. Answer A is incorrect. Antibiotics are not needed because the syndrome is mediated by endotoxins rather than direct infection. Answer B is incorrect because this patient is not in significant respiratory distress.

 HELPFUL TIP: Remember that other work exposures can cause fever, including "metal fume fever" caused by zinc, Teflon byproducts, contaminated humidifier water, etc.

CASE 2

This patient's brother, who also works on a farm, notes that every time he unloads hay he has fever, cough, dyspnea, and sputum production. It tends to resolve in 2–5 days but reoccurs when he is reexposed to hay. None of the other workers on the farm is affected, and they are beginning to wonder if he is malingering. His exam reveals tachypnea and fine rales. There is no wheezing present. A chest radiograph is normal.

The most likely cause of this patient's symptoms is:

A) *Thermoactinomyces candidus.*
B) *T. sacchari.*
C) *Botrytis cinerea.*
D) *Cryptostroma corticale.*
E) None of the above.

Discussion

The correct answer is A. This patient presents with classic symptoms of hypersensitivity pneumonitis or, in this case, Farmer Lung. This is caused by exposure to the *Actinomyces* species. Acute findings include fever, chills, cough, dyspnea, chest tightness, etc. Frequently, the radiograph is normal, but a high-resolution CT may show evidence of pneumonitis in about 50% of cases. Answer B, *T. sacchari*, is involved in hypersensitivity pneumonitis from sugar cane (aka "Bagassosis"). Answer C, *Botrytis cinerea*, is involved in hypersensitivity pneumonitis from grapes (aka "Spaetlese lung"). Answer D, *Cryptostroma*, is involved in "Maple Bark Stripper Lung."

The correct treatment for this patient with Farmer Lung includes:

A) Antibiotics.
B) Inhaled steroids.
C) Oral steroids.
D) Leukotriene inhibitors.
E) Bronchioalveolar lavage (BAL).

Discussion

The correct answer is C. Oral steroids are effective in the treatment of hypersensitivity pneumonitis. Neither antibiotics (answer A) nor inhaled steroids (answer B) is of any benefit. Answer E, bronchioalveolar lavage, can be used as a diagnostic tool. One would expect to see lymphocytes on BAL.

You would advise this patient to:

A) Get a new job.
B) Apply for disability.
C) Use a respirator at work and avoid exposure to this toxin if possible.
D) Sue the employer.
E) Take up worm farming or monoculture in rhubarb.

Discussion

The correct answer is C. Wearing an appropriate respirator at work can be beneficial. Avoiding exposure is even better.

* *

The patient is unable to change jobs or wear a respirator (because it itches and he "keeps forgetting it"). He returns to see you 3 years later. He now has a chronic cough, weight loss, dyspnea, fatigue, and clubbing of the fingers.

Further evaluation will most likely reveal:

A) Bronchogenic carcinoma.
B) Air space disease (eg, a pneumonia-like picture).
C) Decreased carbon monoxide diffusing capacity (decreased DLCO).
D) Markedly abnormal BAL with lymphocytosis.
E) Obstructive changes on pulmonary function testing.

Discussion

The correct answer is C. Hypersensitivity pneumonitis can become chronic if exposure is not limited. In these cases, patients will generally have systemic complaints such as fatigue and possibly weight loss; fever will be absent. Dyspnea and clubbing of the fingers is also generally noted, reflecting chronic pulmonary disease. Along with this finding, pulmonary fibrosis can occur and the DLCO may be decreased. Answer A is incorrect. Hypersensitivity pneumonitis does not lead to lung cancer. Answer B is incorrect. Although acute hypersensitivity pneumonitis causes alveolitis, chronic hypersensitivity pneumonitis causes pulmonary fibrosis with an occasional micronodular pattern. Answer D is incorrect. BAL in chronic hypersensitivity pneumonitis does not contain the markedly elevated lymphocyte count that is seen with acute hypersensitivity pneumonitis. Answer E is incorrect. One would see a restrictive pattern on pulmonary function testing, not an obstructive pattern.

> **HELPFUL TIP:** If you have a patient with recurrent "pneumonia," consider hypersensitivity pneumonitis.

Objectives: Did you learn to . . .

- Recognize the clinical presentations of toxic organic dust syndrome and hypersensitivity pneumonitis?
- Manage patients with lung disease related to agricultural exposures?

QUICK QUIZ: ASTHMA

All of the following populations are at increased risk for developing asthma EXCEPT:

A) Obese children.
B) Female children.
C) Children exposed to tobacco.
D) Children with atopy.

Discussion

The correct answer is B. Male children have a greater prevalence of asthma. Adult females catch up so that there is gender equity in young adulthood, and >40 years the prevalence is higher in females. Obesity is a risk factor. A meta-analysis in 2007 concluded that overweight and obese persons have increased incidence of asthma, with the incidence increasing with increasing BMI. Childhood exposure to tobacco, including secondhand smoke in the home, increases the likelihood of developing asthma by a factor of 2. Adolescent smoking has an even stronger association with asthma. Atopy (as measured by eosinophilia or IgE levels) has been strongly associated with airway hyperresponsiveness and asthma. Another important risk for developing asthma is exposure to a variety of indoor and outdoor allergens and pollutants. Of note, frequent respiratory infections seem to be protective.

CASE 3

A 20-year-old woman with no significant past medical history presents with a 2-month history of episodic shortness of breath. These symptoms began with an upper respiratory tract infection. She has fits of coughing and trouble catching her breath with exertion. She states that her breath "sounds like whistles" at times. She tried a friend's albuterol inhaler with some

improvement and wonders if she has asthma. On exam she is breathing comfortably at 16 times per minute and her arterial oxygen saturation is 96% on room air. Her lungs are clear to auscultation, and the remainder of her exam is unremarkable. You want to better categorize this patient's disease.

Which of the following tests is most appropriate to order now?

A) Spirometry.
B) Chest x-ray.
C) Arterial blood gas.
D) Methacholine challenge.

Discussion

The correct answer is A. Because this patient has symptoms of bronchospasm, spirometry will be essential in determining if there is objective evidence of obstructive lung disease. However, spirometry results are often normal in mild cases of asthma, especially when the patient is asymptomatic. Bronchoprovocation testing, with methacholine or histamine (answer D), may be useful in such cases, but should follow basic spirometry. Although a chest x-ray (answer B) may reveal an unsuspected process, it is not indicated in otherwise healthy patients with symptoms of bronchospasm. Bacterial pneumonia is a potential precipitant of bronchospasm that may be diagnosed on chest x-ray, but this patient has no constitutional symptoms (such as fever) associated with serious bacterial infection. Arterial blood gas levels (answer C) may be helpful when a patient presents with respiratory distress but certainly not in this office setting.

> **HELPFUL TIP:** A normal blood gas in a patient with an asthma exacerbation and tachypnea is an ominous sign that signals impending respiratory failure. The carbon dioxide ($PaCO_2$) should be low in a patient who is tachypneic. Thus, a normal-appearing arterial blood gas with a normal carbon dioxide level is an indication of respiratory muscle fatigue and early respiratory failure.

If this patient has mild asthma, which of the following pulmonary function test results would you expect to find?

A) Forced vital capacity (FVC) 50% of predicted.
B) Forced expiratory volume in 1 second (FEV₁) 100% of predicted.
C) FEV₁/FVC ratio <0.7.
D) Total lung capacity (TLC) 50% of predicted.
E) FEV₁/TLC <0.7.

Discussion

The correct answer is C. Patients with asthma will have a decreased FEV_1. The FVC may fall as well, but FEV_1 falls first and to a greater degree as the lung becomes obstructed. The ratio of FEV_1/FVC is very sensitive to airflow limitations, and FEV_1/FVC <0.7 (not predicted, just the ratio of the 2 numbers) is virtually diagnostic of obstructive airway disease. A decreased FEV_1/FVC ratio is often the first sign of airway obstruction, even with technically "normal" values of FVC and FEV_1. Answer A is incorrect because FVC should not be so low in mild asthma. Answer B is incorrect because FEV_1 should be low, not normal. Answer D is incorrect because the TLC is normal or elevated in asthma, and it is not measured by spirometry.

Office spirometry shows the following:

Normal FVC

FEV_1 82% predicted

FEV_1/FVC 0.68

These findings are most consistent with which of the following?

A) Normal spirometry.
B) Obstructive lung disease.

C) End-stage emphysema.
D) Interstitial fibrosis.

Discussion

The correct answer is B. Always go first to the FEV_1/FVC ratio. In this case, it is <0.70, which is suggestive of airway obstruction. The information provided here lacks data regarding reversibility, so you could not differentiate between chronic obstructive pulmonary disease (COPD) and asthma. But this is clearly not severe emphysema, so answer C is incorrect. Interstitial fibrosis (answer D) is generally marked by a restrictive pattern on spirometry, but it cannot be diagnosed by spirometry alone. Answer A is incorrect. Flow rates (eg, FEV_1) are decreased in interstitial lung diseases but usually in proportion to lung volumes, and FEV_1/FVC is often normal or elevated (Table 3–1).

* *

Six months after you discuss her findings and prescribe inhaled β-agonist therapy, the patient returns with complaints of continued wheezing and difficulty breathing. Her symptoms are brought on by cold weather and exercise and she uses her inhaler two times per week. She woke up 2 nights over the last 6 months with shortness of breath and coughing. Her albuterol still works for these symptoms, but she finds them bothersome and asks, "Why haven't I gotten over this?"

How would you categorize this patient's respiratory state?

A) Mild intermittent asthma.
B) Mild persistent asthma.

Table 3–1 PFT RESULTS COMPARING OBSTRUCTIVE AND RESTRICTIVE DISEASE (may not be applicable for all forms of lung disease)

PFT Result	Obstructive Pattern	Restrictive Pattern
FEV_1	<80% predicted	Decreased in proportion to loss of lung volume
FVC	Decreased	<80% predicted
FEV_1/FVC	<0.7	>0.7
FEF_{25-75}	<50% predicted	Decreased in proportion to loss of lung volume
TLC	Normal or elevated	Decreased
DLCO	Normal or elevated in asthma; normal or decreased in COPD	Decreased in intrinsic restrictive lung disease; normal in neuromuscular or musculoskeletal restrictive disease

KEY: FEV_1 = forced expiratory volume in one second; FVC = forced vital capacity; FEF_{25-75} = forced expiratory flow at 25%–75% vital capacity; TLC = total lung capacity; DLCO = diffusing capacity of the lung for carbon monoxide.

C) Moderate persistent asthma.

D) Severe persistent asthma.

E) This patient does not have asthma.

Discussion

The correct answer is A. According to the National Asthma Education and Prevention Program (NAEPP, Table 3–2), your patient meets the criteria for mild intermittent asthma. In such patients, mild symptoms correspond to an FEV_1 (not an FEV_1/FVC ratio) that is >80% predicted.

Which of the following is most appropriate for this patient since she has mild intermittent asthma?

A) Add theophylline.

B) Add montelukast.

C) Continue albuterol as needed.

D) Schedule albuterol every 4 hours.

E) Prednisone 5 mg daily.

Discussion

The correct answer is C. As discussed, this patient appears to have mild intermittent asthma. She is in no respiratory distress, is oxygenating normally, and is still responding well to albuterol by her report. Although there is some debate about the role of inhaled steroids in mild intermittent asthma, the NAEPP and most experts do not recommend their use. Oral prednisone is certainly not indicated in this case. She should be

Table 3–2   CATEGORIZATION OF SEVERITY OF ASTHMA

Category of Severity	Frequency of Symptoms
Mild intermittent asthma	Daytime symptoms ≤2 days/week
	Nighttime symptoms ≤2 nights/month
Mild persistent asthma	Daytime symptoms >2 days/week (but not daily)
	Nighttime symptoms >2 nights/month
Moderate persistent asthma	Daily symptoms
	Nighttime symptoms >1 night/week
Severe persistent asthma	Continual daytime symptoms
	Frequent nighttime symptoms

continued on a short-acting inhaled β_2-agonist, such as albuterol, without the addition of another medication. Answer D is incorrect. Scheduled albuterol demonstrates less effective symptom control than does PRN use.

 HELPFUL TIP: One nebulized treatment of albuterol is equal to 8–10 puffs of an albuterol MDI via a spacer. The traditional "2 puffs QID" is almost homeopathic. Using an MDI via a spacer works as well as a nebulizer in essentially all situations as long as an adequate dose is prescribed. So, when sending patients home from the ED or writing a prescription for albuterol, make sure you write for appropriate doses.

* *

Your patient goes on to develop more frequent recurrent symptoms, such that she is using her albuterol inhaler more than 3 times per week, although her nighttime symptoms are rare.

Which medication is the most appropriate next step in treating this patient's asthma?

A) Inhaled triamcinolone.

B) Inhaled salmeterol.

C) Inhaled cromolyn sodium.

D) Inhaled ipratropium.

E) Oral montelukast.

Discussion

The correct answer is A. Your patient now has mild persistent asthma and should be started on an inhaled steroid. When asthma symptoms become more persistent (ie, when they occur >2 days per week or the patient awakens from sleep >2 times per month), the inflammatory component of the disease should be addressed while simultaneously treating the bronchospastic component with β_2-agonists. Antiinflammatory drugs are the mainstay of chronic asthma therapy, and inhaled corticosteroids are the most efficacious with the fewest side effects.

Although ipratropium, cromolyn sodium, and montelukast have a place in asthma treatment, none of these medications is a first-line agent. Ipratropium works through its bronchodilatory effects, while cromolyn sodium is a mast cell stabilizer. Montelukast is a leukotriene inhibitor. The long-acting inhaled β_2-agonists, such as salmeterol, are useful primarily in patients with nocturnal symptoms or as supplemental therapy after inhaled steroids are employed.

 HELPFUL TIP: Remember the "Rule of Twos": any patient who has >2 asthma exacerbations per week requiring rescue medication or who wakes with nocturnal symptoms >2 times per month should be on an antiinflammatory drug, preferably an inhaled corticosteroid.

 HELPFUL TIP: The leukotriene inhibitors (eg, montelukast, zafirlukast) add little or nothing to maximized inhaled steroid therapy in most patients. They are clearly not as effective as inhaled steroids. They should be used only when a patient has failed inhaled steroids and should be added to the regimen; they are not a substitute for an inhaled steroid.

* *

Your patient does quite well over the next year, having very few exacerbations. She continues to use her corticosteroid inhaler as prescribed. Over the winter, she visits you twice because of increasing difficulties with rhinorrhea. On examination, you note slightly edematous nasal mucosa and nasal polyps. You prescribe intranasal steroids.

One night when you are on call, she comes in severely dyspneic with audible wheezing. She talks in two- or three-word phrases and reports a headache today, which she treated with aspirin. Her asthma attack started about an hour after the aspirin dose. She denies fever, rhinorrhea, nasal congestion, and sore throat. Her respiratory rate is 40, heart rate 120, and oxygen saturation 88% on room air. She has poor air movement on auscultation of her lung fields.

Which of the following is the most likely reason for this patient's acute exacerbation of asthma?

A) Viral upper respiratory infection.
B) Sinusitis.
C) Noncompliance with inhaled albuterol.
D) Sensitivity to aspirin.
E) Noncompliance with nasal steroids.

Discussion
The correct answer is D. It is likely that this patient has aspirin sensitivity. Up to 10% of adults with asthma have the clinical triad of asthma, aspirin sensitivity, and nasal polyposis. Patients with asthma should be warned about the potential for exacerbations resulting from consumption of aspirin and NSAIDs. The drug-induced bronchial constriction caused by these medications can have an abrupt onset with severe symptoms. Patients with aspirin sensitivity can be desensitized with daily administration of small amounts of aspirin, but this should be done carefully with close supervision.

Although viral upper respiratory infections frequently cause exacerbations of asthma, your patient did not report antecedent symptoms of such an infection. Likewise, there is no reason to believe she has sinusitis (answer B) or has become noncompliant with her medications (answer D), although reaffirming medication compliance is always warranted. Answer C is incorrect because noncompliance with a rescue inhaler would not cause an asthma exacerbation.

* *

Initial treatment with nebulized inhaled albuterol 2.5 mg fails to result in significant clinical improvement in oxygen saturation, respiratory rate, or apparent work of breathing. However, with nasal cannula oxygen, her saturation improves to 92%.

Which of the following interventions do you apply next?

A) High-dose nebulized albuterol (5–7.5 mg).
B) Aminophylline IV.
C) Epinephrine IV.
D) Nebulized ipratropium.
E) A and D.

Discussion
The correct answer is E. The initial treatment of acute asthma exacerbations focuses on bronchodilation with the use of inhaled β_2-agonists and inhaled anticholinergics (eg, ipratropium). Albuterol can be administered by continuous nebulization. The addition of ipratropium

increases bronchodilation and can be beneficial when albuterol alone is not working. Treatment for the inflammatory component is also important in this situation and oral or IV corticosteroids are appropriate. Aminophylline (answer B) adds nothing to maximized β-agonist therapy in acute asthma. Additionally, it has serious arrhythmogenic potential and has fallen out of favor. Epinephrine (answer C) is not appropriate unless the patient's respiratory status is decompensating.

 HELPFUL TIP: All patients with an asthma exacerbation should be discharged on an oral steroid for short-term use. Steroids are effective within 1–2 hours and, in addition to their antiinflammatory action, act by upregulating β receptors in the lungs.

 HELPFUL TIP: Magnesium sulfate, 2 g IV over 10 minutes, can be of use in asthmatics with an acute exacerbation who are not responding well to albuterol, ipratropium, and steroids. It has minimal side effects (transient flushing and mild hypotension), but should not be used in patients with a history of renal failure because they can become hypermagnesemic. Another potentially helpful—although more controversial—modality is heliox (helium and oxygen mixture) which increases laminar flow and may improve ventilation. Both modalities have somewhat mixed results in clinical trials.

* *

After a brief hospitalization, your patient recovers nicely. Prior to this incident involving aspirin, she had been free of exacerbations for about a month.

In addition to a short course of oral steroids, which of the following medication regimens do you prescribe for this patient with aspirin-sensitive asthma at discharge?

A) Inhaled triamcinolone and inhaled albuterol as a "rescue."
B) Inhaled triamcinolone, oral montelukast, and inhaled albuterol as a "rescue."

C) Oral montelukast and inhaled albuterol as a "rescue."
D) Inhaled albuterol as a "rescue."
E) Inhaled salmeterol and inhaled triamcinolone.

Discussion
The correct answer is B. Leukotriene inhibitors (eg, montelukast, zafirlukast) do not have a well-defined role in asthma management. However, these medications have demonstrated effectiveness in reducing symptoms and improving peak flow in patients with aspirin-sensitive asthma. Answer C is incorrect. Leukotriene inhibitors should be used only in asthma patients who are already using a corticosteroid inhaler—or those who cannot tolerate inhaled corticosteroid therapy. Answer D is incorrect. This patient has had frequent exacerbations in the past and one recently resulting in admission to a hospital; as such, she must be treated with antiinflammatory medications. Although answer E offers an antiinflammatory agent, there is no rescue inhaler, and patients with asthma must always have access to a short-acting inhaled bronchodilator. See Table 3–3 for an approach to chronic asthma management.

 HELPFUL TIP: For an acute asthma exacerbation, there is no need to do a steroid taper if the patient is not on chronic steroids (eg, has not been on steroids within the month). You can administer up to 10 days of prednisone (eg, 40 mg a day) and safely stop without a taper. This does not increase the rate of bounce-backs over a taper, nor does it result in significant adrenal suppression. But this rule does not apply to steroid-dependent patients.

* *

Which of the following medications, when used alone as maintenance therapy in persistent asthma, is associated with an increased risk of asthma-related mortality?

A) Inhaled fluticasone.
B) Inhaled salmeterol.
C) Oral zafirlukast.
D) Oral prednisone.

Table 3–3 STEPWISE APPROACH TO CHRONIC ASTHMA THERAPY

Step 1: Inhaled short-acting β₂-agonist as "rescue" therapy.
Step 2: Add a low- or moderate-dose inhaled corticosteroid.
Step 3: Increase to a high-dose inhaled corticosteroid or add an inhaled long-acting β₂-agonist.
Step 4: Increase to a high-dose inhaled corticosteroid or add an inhaled long-acting β₂-agonist (whichever was not done in Step 3).
Step 5: Consider adding other antiinflammatory drugs: leukotriene inhibitors and mast cell stabilizers (cromolyn sodium and nedocromil).
Step 6: Consider adding oral theophylline.
Step 7: Consider adding oral steroids (to be used **chronically** as a last resort due to the morbidity associated with long-term steroid therapy; oral steroids are one of the drugs of choice for an **acute** asthma exacerbation.)

Discussion

The correct answer is B. Inhaled salmeterol, when used alone as a controller agent for asthma, has been associated with a 2- to 4-fold increase in the risk of death related to asthma or other respiratory conditions. Thus, the FDA has mandated a "black box" warning be applied to salmeterol-containing products. It is not known whether inhaled steroid therapy is protective, but NAEPP guidelines recommend adding long-acting inhaled β-agonists only after inhaled steroids are already in use. Inhaled salmeterol and the alternative agent formoterol have a place in asthma management because they improve symptoms, improve spirometry, and reduce exacerbations, but they should be used cautiously and only with an inhaled steroid.

 HELPFUL TIP: The importance of patient education in asthma cannot be overstated. Patients diagnosed with asthma should receive a written plan of action, detailing when to increase β₂ agonist use and when to start an oral steroid. Although there is no proven major benefit to home peak flow monitoring, this may serve to get patients more involved in management of their illness. A home peak flow meter can be used as a part of the educational process and to enhance communication between the healthcare practitioner and the patient.

Objectives: Did you learn to . . .

- Identify triggers of bronchospasm?
- Evaluate symptoms of wheezing and dyspnea?
- Diagnose mild intermittent and mild persistent asthma?
- Prescribe appropriate medications for mild intermittent and mild persistent asthma?
- Describe the triad of asthma, aspirin sensitivity, and nasal polyposis?
- Manage an acute exacerbation of asthma in the emergency department?

 QUICK QUIZ: SPIROMETRY

A 60-year-old female who smokes two packs of cigarettes per day complains of shortness of breath and fullness in her throat. You obtain spirometry in the office and the results are given here along with the flow/volume loop.

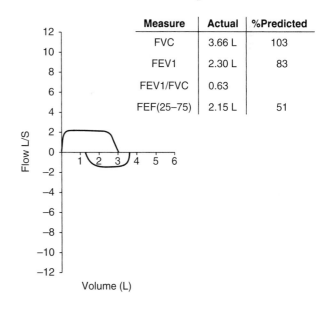

Measure	Actual	%Predicted
FVC	3.66 L	103
FEV1	2.30 L	83
FEV1/FVC	0.63	
FEF(25–75)	2.15 L	51

How do you interpret these findings?

A) Chronic obstructive lung disease.
B) Restrictive lung disease.

C) Fixed upper airway obstruction.

D) Poor patient effort.

Discussion

The correct answer is C. The flattened flow/volume loop is consistent with a fixed upper airway obstruction. In this patient, the FEV_1 may look like obstructive disease, so you have to attend to the flow/volume loop. Some examples of flow/volume loops are shown here:

rales. The cardiac exam is normal except for tachycardia. There is no edema.

What is the BEST first step in caring for this patient?

A) Administer nebulized albuterol.

B) Administer IV corticosteroids.

C) Administer oxygen by nasal cannula.

D) Obtain arterial blood gas.

E) Secure the airway with intubation.

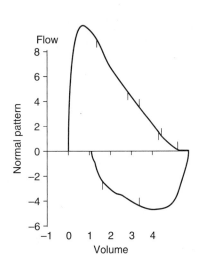

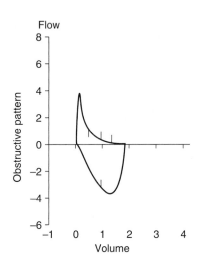

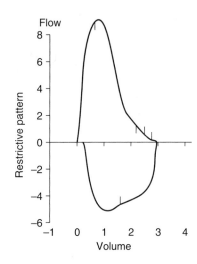

CASE 4

A 67-year-old male presents to the ED where you are working. He is unable to give much history due to shortness of breath. His wife tells you he has been having increasing shortness of breath over the past week, and was trying to make it until tomorrow, when he has an appointment with his primary doctor. He has not had fever, chest pain, or hemoptysis. He has been using nebulized albuterol and ipratropium every 3 hours, instead of his usual twice-a-day. He quit smoking—but that was only 2 days ago—and he was smoking one pack of cigarettes per day for 50 years. His medical history includes coronary artery bypass grafting 3 years ago and emphysema with an FEV_1 of 0.9 L. He is on aspirin, atenolol, and isosorbide dinitrate in addition to his nebulizers.

On examination, he is alert but using accessory muscles of respiration. His respiratory rate is 28, blood pressure 160/70, pulse 110, and temperature 37.4°C. On room air, his oxygen saturation is 81%. On lung auscultation, there are diffuse bilateral wheezes but no

Discussion

The correct answer is C. The administration of oxygen to a hypoxemic patient should not be delayed in order to perform a diagnostic workup or to administer other, less urgent therapies. Start with a low flow via nasal cannula and increase it as needed. High-flow O_2 may cause worsening hypercapnia in COPD. The classic teaching has been that this is due to a change in respiratory drive. The theory is that COPD causes a switch from carbon dioxide levels driving respiration to oxygen levels driving respiration. Although this may be partly true, further study has suggested that the main reason COPD patients are at risk of worsening hypercapnia is due to loss of hypoxic pulmonary vasoconstriction and worsening ventilation-perfusion mismatch that occurs with excess oxygen delivery. Regardless of cause, the most important point remains—give as much oxygen as needed to oxygenate the patient. Do not withhold oxygen because of these theoretical concerns. You are in an ED and can intubate the patient if needed. The onset of action of corticosteroids, whether given intravenously or orally, is on the order of hours rather than minutes; it is not the first priority in this patient. Answer E is incorrect. The patient does not need emergent endotracheal intubation now; he has mild hypoxemia and bronchospasm, and should be given a trial of bronchodilators and oxygen prior to such an intervention.

When initiating supplemental oxygen by nasal cannula, you instruct the nurse to keep the patient's oxygen saturation:

A) Between 95% and 100%.
B) Between 90% and 95%.
C) Below 90%.
D) At whatever saturation he looks most comfortable.

Discussion

The correct answer is B. The primary goal of supplemental oxygen is to reduce the risk of tissue hypoxia. Maintaining oxygen saturations above 90% (or PaO_2 60–65 mm) will ensure tissue oxygenation. Higher oxygen saturations may result in CO_2 retention and hypercapnia, as noted above. Answer D is of special note. Patients with COPD who look comfortable may be hypercapnic and have CO_2 narcosis. Thus, while comfort is a goal, it may not be the best judge of clinical status in patients with COPD exacerbations.

* *

The patient receives albuterol and ipratropium via nebulizer and reports some relief of dyspnea. His respiratory rate is now 26, and his oxygen saturation is 85% with 4 L/min of nasal cannula oxygen. Arterial blood gas reveals a pH of 7.25, PCO_2 70, and PO_2 53.

What would be the next step in management?

A) Obtain a chest x-ray.
B) Start aminophylline.
C) Begin noninvasive positive pressure support (CPAP or BIPAP).
D) Administer IV antibiotics.
E) Perform endotracheal intubation and mechanical ventilation.

Discussion

The correct answer is C. This patient is retaining CO_2 despite tachypnea and is in impending respiratory failure. He is also not oxygenating well despite low-flow oxygen. Noninvasive positive pressure support (CPAP, BIPAP) can relieve hypercapnia and improve oxygenation without requiring intubation and its associated morbidity.

A chest x-ray may be helpful in the diagnostic evaluation, but should not delay efforts to improve his respiratory status. Often IV antibiotics are used for empiric therapy in severe exacerbations of COPD, but again, improving the respiratory status comes first. You saw in the asthma case (Case 3) that aminophylline adds nothing to the treatment of asthma or COPD in the ED and has a significant downside. Although this patient's respiratory status is tenuous, he is not in imminent respiratory failure, and intubation is not warranted now.

* *

After several hours of noninvasive positive pressure ventilation, your patient is doing well and he is transferred out of the intensive care unit. When you see him the next day, his medications include inhaled bronchodilators, ceftriaxone, azithromycin, and prednisone. A chest x-ray shows no evidence of infiltrate. He is weaned from the positive pressure support and is now on 2 L/min of oxygen by nasal cannula. He appears comfortable, with a respiratory rate of 14 and an oxygen saturation of 95%.

You decide to discharge the patient on which of the following medication regimens?

A) Prednisone 40 mg daily for 10 days and inhaled albuterol as needed.
B) Prednisone tapering over 30 days and inhaled ipratropium and albuterol as needed.
C) Prednisone 40 mg daily for 10 days; inhaled ipratropium and albuterol QID; and inhaled albuterol as needed.
D) Prednisone tapering over 30 days; inhaled ipratropium and albuterol QID; and inhaled albuterol as needed.

Discussion

The correct answer is C. Current recommendations for the treatment of exacerbations of COPD focus on a combination of anti-inflammatories and bronchodilators. A 10-day course of prednisone, which does not need to be tapered, is recommended for its potent anti-inflammatory effect. Longer courses of acute treatment do not offer any further benefit but are associated with more adverse effects (although patients on chronic steroids do need a taper lest you induce adrenal insufficiency). Some patients will fail when you attempt to withdraw steroids and may be steroid dependent. Although pulmonary function does not improve to a greater degree, **COPD** patients have greater symptomatic control if inhaled bronchodilators are scheduled rather than used as needed during an **acute** exacerbation. The combination of albuterol and ipratropium is superior to either drug used alone. The patient should also have a "rescue" inhaler available, typically a β₂-agonist like albuterol.

* *

The chest x-ray shows no infiltrates; therefore, antibiotic therapy for **pneumonia** is not warranted. The use of antibiotics in exacerbations of COPD without obvious bacterial infection is controversial (more on this later . . .).

Which of the following decreases stable COPD?

A) Inhaled tiotropium.
B) Inhaled salmeterol.
C) Inhaled ipratropium.
D) Inhaled corticosteroid.
E) None of the above.

Discussion

The correct answer is E. Aside from oxygen, no medical therapy has clearly demonstrated a mortality benefit for stable COPD. Inhaled tiotropium has the advantage of once-daily dosing. Tiotropium is an inhaled anticholinergic that improves COPD symptoms and spirometry results.

HELPFUL TIP: Contrast asthma and COPD management. Both start with a short-acting bronchodilator (albuterol and ipratropium respectively). For treating mild persistent asthma (or worse) the next step is the addition of an inhaled steroid—then a long-acting bronchodilator. For treating moderate COPD (or worse) the next step is the addition of a long-acting bronchodilator (eg, salmetarol, famoterol)—then a second long-acting bronchodilator (tiotropium) and only then does one add an inhaled steroid. **Inhaled steroids should be used in those with moderately severe to severe COPD who have failed bronchodilators. There is no benefit in patients with mild or moderate COPD who respond to bronchodilators and there is a downside (an increase in pneumonia).**

* *

Prior to discharge, your patient asks if he should also be taking antibiotics. Based on clinical findings and a negative chest x-ray, you do not think that he has pneumonia, but you decide to finish a 5-day course of azithromycin (a fortune cookie said that you should).

You explain to your patient that antibiotics may be useful in COPD:

A) When given daily to chronically suppress infection.
B) When sputum volume and purulence are increased.
C) When given the first 10 days of each month.
D) When a fortune cookie says so.
E) Only when broad-spectrum agents (eg, respiratory fluoroquinolone) are used.

Discussion

The correct answer is B. Antibiotics are indicated for significant acute exacerbations of COPD and for increased sputum volume and purulence. These recommendations are somewhat soft, and numerous guidelines exist in the literature. What is clear is that one-third of exacerbations are caused by environmental change (eg, increased air pollution, heat, and humidity), one-third are viral, and about one-third are bacterial. Answer E is incorrect because there is no agent of choice for COPD exacerbations, and more narrow-spectrum antibiotics (doxycycline, amoxicillin, etc.) are recommended for outpatient treatment.

* *

The patient is discharged from the hospital in good condition and no longer requires supplemental oxygen. At follow-up 1 month later, he feels that he is back to his baseline level of dyspnea on exertion after walking one mile. Did he quit smoking? No. But you persist in your belief in disease prevention.

In order to reduce his risk of mortality and serious morbidity, you recommend smoking cessation and which of the following?

A) Polyvalent pneumococcal vaccine.
B) Annual chest CT.
C) Annual chest x-ray.
D) Supplemental oxygen used PRN.

Discussion

The correct answer is A. The pneumococcal vaccine currently available for adults has been shown to reduce the risk of invasive pneumococcal disease and related morbidity and mortality. It may also reduce the risk of pulmonary infections in patients with COPD. The vaccine does not reduce the risk of pneumonia in patients with no underlying lung disease but does decrease the risk of severe pneumonia in this population. Annual radiographic screening exams, such as chest CT (answer B) and x-ray (answer C) have not yielded a survival benefit and are not currently recommended. Supplemental oxygen (answer D) may be useful in patients with exertional or rest hypoxemia but will not reduce morbidity or mortality when used PRN.

 HELPFUL TIP: The polyvalent pneumococcal vaccine is recommended in patients of all ages with COPD and in all persons >65 years. Additionally, the influenza vaccine should be given to all patients with COPD annually and can reduce serious illness and death in patients with COPD by 50%.

Criteria for the use of continuous low-flow oxygen in those with COPD include all of the following EXCEPT:

A) PO_2 <55 mm Hg.
B) Oxygen saturation <88%.
C) PO_2 of <59 mm Hg with evidence of cor pulmonale.
D) Episodic sleep-apnea-related desaturations at night.

Discussion

The correct answer is D. Episodic sleep-apnea-related oxygen desaturations, although a cause for concern and amenable to treatment (eg, CPAP), are **not** one of the criteria for the use of continuous low-flow oxygen. Why would such a patient need oxygen during the day? Answer C deserves special note. Evidence of cor pulmonale can include "p-pulmonale" on ECG, peripheral edema, or a hematocrit >55%. This does not mean that you should not treat nocturnal desaturations, only that they are not an indication for **continuous** low-flow oxygen.

Concerning hypoxemic patients with COPD, which of the following is true?

A) Patients on continuous, low-flow O_2 become oxygen-dependent and cannot function without it.
B) Continuous low-flow O_2 used for at least 8 hours a day helps to reverse pulmonary hypertension.

C) Continued smoking is a contraindication to the use of continuous low-flow home O_2 because patients are spontaneously combusting right and left.
D) Low-flow O_2 used 24 hours a day significantly enhances survival.
E) None of the above.

Discussion

The correct answer is D. Patients who use low-flow O_2 at home for 24 hours a day have an improved rate of survival. Patients should be encouraged to use O_2 at least 15 hours a day if possible. Answer B is incorrect because patients need at least 12–15 hours of O_2 per day to have any significant benefit with regard to pulmonary hypertension. Answer C is incorrect. Smoking while on O_2 is not a good idea, but patients can go outside to smoke. When was the last time you heard about a patient catching on fire because of home O_2 (not that they shouldn't be careful)?

* *

Over the next year, you see this patient on several occasions. He continues to smoke cigarettes. He complains of increasing dyspnea with exertion. Exam reveals a thin, elderly male with a normal respiratory rate. His lung fields are clear. His oxygen saturation on room air is 91% at rest and drops to 87% with ambulation. On office spirometry, he has an FEV_1 of 0.7 L with no improvement after inhaled albuterol.

Which of the following interventions is most likely to reduce this patient's risk of mortality from COPD?

A) Inhaled corticosteroids.
B) Intermittent antibiotics.
C) Smoking cessation.
D) Theophylline.
E) Oral corticosteroids.

Discussion

The correct answer is C. It's still not too late. Smoking cessation is the most important step for this patient (and any patient with COPD). Unfortunately, most COPD treatments except for continuous low-flow oxygen have had disappointingly little effect on disease progression and mortality.

In addition to supplemental oxygen, all of the following interventions/treatments are indicated for this patient EXCEPT:

A) Inhaled bronchodilators.
B) Pulmonary rehabilitation.
C) Antitussives.
D) Inhaled corticosteroids.
E) Smoking cessation.

Discussion

The correct answer is C. Although many patients with COPD are bothered by cough and would like to treat it, antitussives are contraindicated in COPD. Mucociliary clearance is disrupted in COPD, and coughing is thought to serve a protective role against pulmonary infection. All patients with COPD benefit from symptomatic therapy with inhaled bronchodilators, specifically β_2-agonists and anticholinergics, even if they do not have a spirometric response to bronchodilator therapy. Likewise, pulmonary rehabilitation and smoking cessation will benefit patients at different stages in the disease process. Answer D is of special note. As noted above, there is little benefit and some downside to inhaled corticosteroids in COPD (those with fixed disease that have <12% reversibility with β-agonists). **If the patient has disease that is reversible with albuterol, steroids will probably be useful.** Approximately 15% of COPD patients will respond to inhaled corticosteroids and albuterol. These are the patients who have a bronchospastic component to their disease.

* *

Your patient has a nephew who is in veterinary school and swears lung volume reduction surgery works for hamsters with COPD. Your patient is wondering if lung reduction surgery works in humans.

Your response is:

A) Lung reduction surgery increases the survival of patients with COPD. Go for it!
B) Perioperative mortality is as high as 25% and there is no proven survival benefit. You do not recommend the surgery.
C) There is no evidence that lung reduction surgery improves symptoms. Flip a coin.
D) Patients with the most severe disease fare the best. Wait until the disease progresses.

Discussion

The correct answer is B. The perioperative mortality for lung reduction surgery is up to 25%. There is no evidence that lung reduction surgery (answer A) can improve survival in patients with COPD. Lung reduction surgery makes intuitive sense: remove some of the dead space and nonfunctioning lung and the rest of the lung will have a larger thoracic cavity to expand. It may turn out to be beneficial in certain subgroups (eg, those with upper-lobe emphysema), but a validation study has not been done to confirm these results. Answer C deserves special note. Improvement in symptoms and quality of life has been seen in several subgroups, but dedicated studies in these populations have yet to be done. Answer D is incorrect. The more severe the disease, the worse the patients fare with surgery.

* *

While you are on call, your patient presents in the early morning hours with severe dyspnea unresponsive to nebulized albuterol and ipratropium at home. He was feeling fine earlier in the day but had sudden onset of dyspnea. His respiratory rate is 36, pulse 120, blood pressure 150/86, temperature 36.9°C, and oxygen saturation 79% on 5 L/min oxygen by nasal cannula. His neck veins are flat; he has unilateral left leg swelling. The patient shows no signs of improvement after nebulized albuterol and ipratropium in the ED. You start noninvasive positive pressure ventilation (BIPAP) with 50% inspired oxygen. Within a few minutes, he appears less distressed, but his blood gas shows pH 7.45, $PaCO_2$ 33 mm Hg, and PaO_2 45 mm Hg. His oxygen saturation is 84%.

In addition to hypoxemia, what does this blood gas suggest?

A) Metabolic acidosis.
B) Metabolic alkalosis.
C) Respiratory acidosis.
D) Respiratory alkalosis.

Discussion

The correct answer is D. Based on the pH, this patient is slightly alkalotic. Since his baseline gases are not available, you cannot tell if he retains CO_2 when in his usual state of health. Assuming he does not retain CO_2, his normal $PaCO_2$ should be 40 mm Hg. In an acute respiratory alkalosis, the $PaCO_2$ should fall 1 mm Hg for every 0.008 increase in pH above 7.4. In this patient:

$$\text{Change in } PaCO_2 = (7.45 - 7.40)/0.008 = 6.25$$

If your patient normally has a $PaCO_2$ of 40 mm Hg and the alkalosis is entirely due to increased respiratory rate, his $PaCO_2$ should be 33.75, which is very close to the measured $PaCO_2$ of 33 mm Hg. This formula can be used to determine the contribution of the CO_2 to the pH. If his pH was 7.53, you would know that he had a mixed respiratory and metabolic alkalosis. If the pH was 7.4, you would know that he had a mixed respiratory alkalosis and metabolic acidosis.

**

A chest x-ray shows hyperinflation, and an ECG shows sinus tachycardia. Blood tests are pending. Because the patient has failed to respond to the usual therapy for a COPD exacerbation, you begin to consider alternate explanations for his current condition.

Which of the following is the most likely diagnosis given his current history and symptoms?

A) Pneumonia.
B) Acute bronchitis.
C) Pulmonary embolism.
D) Cor pulmonale.

Discussion

The correct answer is C. This patient had sudden onset of dyspnea, unilateral leg edema, and respiratory distress unresponsive to usual COPD treatments. All of these are more consistent with a pulmonary embolism (PE) than with an exacerbation of COPD, which should have progressed more gradually. PEs can present with signs and symptoms very similar to COPD—dyspnea, pleuritic chest pain, cough, respiratory distress, and hypoxemia. His alveolar-arterial oxygen (A-a) gradient is high, as calculated by the following equation:

$$\text{A-a gradient} = [(FiO_2 \times 713) - PaCO_2/0.8] - PaO_2$$
$$= [(0.5 \times 713) - (33/0.8)] - 45 = 270.25$$

An approximation of a patient's normal A-a gradient can be determined by the following formula:

$$\text{Normal A-a gradient} = 2.5 + (0.21 \times \text{age in years}).$$

A high A-a gradient represents ventilation/perfusion mismatch and should raise concern for PE. A diagnosis of pneumonia should be considered if the patient has fever, worsening cough, and/or an infiltrate on chest x-ray. Acute bronchitis does not present with such severe symptoms. Cor pulmonale presents with typical signs and symptoms of right heart failure—edema, increased jugular venous pressure manifested as JVD, and, possibly ascites.

 HELPFUL TIP: An elevated A-a gradient suggests a ventilation/perfusion mismatch and occurs in a number of conditions, including atelectasis, a right-to-left shunt, ARDS, air embolism, and bronchiectasis with impaired gas exchange. Thus, an elevated A-a gradient is not specific for PE. Likewise, a normal A-a gradient and normal oxygen saturation do not rule out PE! In patients without underlying lung disease, the PIOPED study found no difference in the oxygen saturation and A-a gradient among patients with and without PE.

**

Heparin is initiated, and the patient requires intubation and ventilation. A saddle PE is found on chest CT. Despite aggressive therapy, your patient lacks pulmonary reserve and ultimately succumbs to this disease process. You list PE as the immediate cause of death, with COPD as a secondary cause.

Objectives: Did you learn to . . .

- Recognize a patient who has COPD?
- Develop a plan to manage hypoxemia and hypercapnia?
- Manage medications for acute exacerbations of COPD?
- Direct therapy for chronic COPD?
- Identify causes of dyspnea other than COPD presenting in a patient with known COPD?

CASE 5

A 50-year-old male who is a heavy drinker with a history of squamous cell carcinoma of the neck presents to your office complaining of abdominal pain. He has not had any nausea or vomiting. He has been coughing and expectorating bloody sputum and notes a low-grade fever, chills, and mild dyspnea starting about 1 week ago. He does not have chest pain. His squamous cell carcinoma was treated with external beam radiation several years ago. Examination reveals an afebrile male

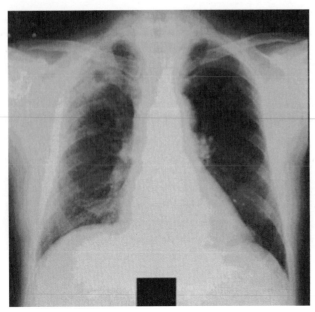

Figure 3–1

in mild distress. His vital signs are normal, and his lungs sound clear. The abdominal exam reveals only mild epigastric tenderness. The chest x-ray is available for your review (Figure 3–1). Your colleague, who is on call today, walks by and asks if you have any admissions for her.

You consider this 50-year-old man with a cough and reply:

A) "Yes. This man will need the ICU."
B) "Yes. This man will need a respiratory isolation room."
C) "No. I'm sending this man home with metronidazole."
D) "No. I'll work up this man as an outpatient."

Discussion

The correct answer is B. Because he is expectorating bloody sputum and has a cavitary lesion on chest x-ray (right upper lobe), this man should be admitted to a respiratory isolation room until tuberculosis can be ruled out. He will need further evaluation and possibly intravenous antibiotic therapy, both of which may be accomplished during his hospitalization. Answer A is incorrect. There is no need to send this man to the ICU based on his current picture. Answer C is incorrect for two reasons. First, metronidazole alone is not an appropriate therapy for this man. Second, this might not represent an infectious process and requires further investigation.

What is the best next step in the diagnosis of this process?

A) Bronchoscopy.
B) Sputum cultures.
C) Blood cultures.
D) Chest CT.
E) Open lung biopsy.

Discussion

The correct answer is D. The chest x-ray demonstrates a cavitary lesion in the right upper lobe. Chest CT is warranted for further characterization of the lesion. From history, exam, and chest x-ray, it is not possible to determine whether the lesion is an abscess or a malignant process. An indolent course with low-grade fever is characteristic of lung abscess. However, the preexisting squamous cell carcinoma has potential to have spread to the lungs, and squamous cell carcinoma is known to cause cavitations. Culture of sputum and blood (answers B and C), including evaluation of first morning sputum for AFB, will be an essential part of the assessment. These tests, however, may not yield as much information as chest CT, and sputum culture should be done in conjunction with cytology and Gram stain. Bronchoscopy (answer A) should be postponed until CT results are available. Bronchoscopic biopsy (answer E) is potentially detrimental if the lesion is an abscess since the airway could flood with pus if the entire cavity wall is penetrated.

* *

Chest CT further confirms a parenchymal abscess in the right upper lobe with cavitation and air within the cavity. Bronchoscopy reveals pus in the airway and extrinsic compression of the bronchi. A lavage sample is obtained, but biopsies are not taken because of the clinical impression that this is a lung abscess.

What organisms are most commonly isolated in lung abscesses?

A) Anaerobic bacteria.
B) Aerobic bacteria.
C) Tuberculosis.
D) Mixed aerobic/anaerobic bacteria.

Discussion

The correct answer is A. Anaerobes are isolated most often, followed by mixed anaerobic/aerobic bacteria, followed by aerobic bacteria alone.

* *

Gram stain of sputum demonstrates gram positive cocci and gram negative rods. Cultures are pending. Tuberculin skin test is negative.

What is the most appropriate therapy for this patient?

A) Refer for surgical drainage.
B) Oral levofloxacin.
C) Intravenous clindamycin.
D) Intravenous metronidazole.
E) Intravenous ceftriaxone.

Discussion

The correct answer is C. The most important aspect in treatment appears to be the use of an antibiotic active against anaerobes. Intravenous clindamycin is the usual choice for lung abscess due to its coverage of anaerobes and *S. pneumoniae*. Metronidazole is less effective, failing in up to 50% of cases of putrid lung abscess. A β-lactam with β-lactamase inhibitor (eg, piperacillin/tazobactam) is another good choice. Ceftriaxone and levofloxacin offer poor coverage of anaerobes. Surgical drainage of lung abscesses is needed in only 5% to10% of cases.

Objectives: Did you learn to . . .

- Recognize the presence of a cavitary lesion on chest x-ray?
- Identify the common causes of cavitary lesions?
- Decide when to place a patient in respiratory isolation?
- Manage a patient with a lung abscess?

CASE 6

A 53-year-old male is accompanied by his wife to your office and complains of a cough for 6 weeks. It is more bothersome at night. He denies sputum production, shortness of breath, chest pain, and wheezing. He takes an antacid once or twice per day to settle his stomach. He smoked three packs of cigarettes per day until 1 year ago, when he quit cold turkey. He takes hydrochlorothiazide for hypertension and a daily aspirin and states that he is healthy otherwise. He has no cardiac disorders. His wife reports that he snores at night, and she adds, "He's always hacking and clearing his throat." The review of systems is negative. In order to sleep better, he has recently started to have a shot of whiskey before going to bed.

What is the most likely cause for the cough?

A) Gastroesophageal reflux.
B) Lung cancer.
C) Antihypertensive medication.
D) Alcohol abuse.
E) Congestive heart failure.

Discussion

The correct answer is A. This patient appears to have a chronic cough that is most likely due to gastroesophageal reflux disease (GERD). He takes antacids and exhibits throat clearing, which can be a subtle sign and is not typically identified by patients as reflux. Additionally, he drinks alcohol at bedtime, further predisposing to reflux. He has a history of smoking, which places him at increased risk for developing a bronchogenic carcinoma, but a lung mass would not be a common cause for cough. Aspirin is associated with bronchospasm in some people, but it would not usually present as cough in a patient with no history of asthma. Hydrochlorothiazide is not known to cause cough. Also, it is unlikely that symptoms would be isolated to the nighttime if his cough was medication related.

 HELPFUL TIP: Remember that ACE inhibitors may cause cough in 5% to 20% of patients taking them. For patients who develop a cough and are on an ACE inhibitor, a brief trial off the medication may save a costly workup for chronic cough. Usually symptoms resolve within 1 week but may persist for 1 month. Cough caused by an ACE inhibitor may first occur up to 6 months after initiation of treatment.

* *

On physical examination, you note a mildly overweight male in no distress. His vital signs are normal. His lungs are clear to auscultation. The nasal and oropharyngeal mucosae are intact, moist, and not inflamed. The remainder of the exam is unremarkable. Chest x-ray is remarkable for flattened diaphragms but is otherwise negative. You suspect GERD, but also entertain other diagnoses.

Which of the following is your next step in managing this patient's cough?

A) Start a proton pump inhibitor.
B) Start an inhaled steroid.
C) Order 24-hour esophageal pH monitoring.
D) Obtain spirometry.
E) Obtain a chest CT.

Discussion

The correct answer is A. An empiric trial of an effective gastric acid-suppressing medication is likely to relieve the cough if the diagnosis is accurate. The American College of Chest Physicians (ACCP) recommends starting therapy with a proton pump inhibitor rather than an H_2-blocker (answer B). The usual antireflux measures, such as avoiding fatty foods, alcohol, and food before bedtime, should be instituted as well. Prescribers must be aware that sometimes a complete resolution of cough takes months. A 24-hour pH monitor (answer C) is invasive and often not necessary if an empiric trial of gastric acid suppression resolves the problem. Answer E is incorrect. Starting the evaluation of chronic cough with a chest x-ray is part of the ACCP recommendations, but CT scan is not indicated with a negative chest x-ray. If the cough does not resolve with empiric therapy, spirometry (answer D) should be considered.

* *

The patient does not respond after 2 months of empiric treatment, and he is becoming more concerned. The examination is unchanged. Spirometry is normal with a normal flow volume loop.

Which of the following management options is LEAST likely to benefit this patient?

A) Combination antihistamine and decongestant.
B) Inhaled corticosteroid.
C) Inhaled β_2-agonist.
D) Antibiotics.

Discussion

The correct answer is D. This patient has no signs or symptoms of sinusitis or bacterial pulmonary infection, so treating with an antibiotic is inappropriate and unlikely to help. However, some form of empiric therapy might be tried. He could have postnasal drainage without signs on physical exam, and empiric therapy with combination antihistamine and decongestant may improve the cough. Inhaled corticosteroids and β_2-agonists are the mainstay of chronic asthma therapy, and may help relieve this patient's chronic cough. This patient could yet have "cough variant asthma" despite normal spirometry results.

 HELPFUL TIP: The evaluation of chronic cough should proceed in a logical manner. Usually, history and physical will find the cause. If this is unrevealing, consider a stepwise evaluation including addressing each of the etiologies in a serial fashion (Table 3–4). If this still does not give you an answer, consider a methacholine challenge test to see if you can reproduce the symptoms that would lead you to a presumptive diagnosis of asthma with normal spirometry.

Cough receptors are located where?

A) Upper respiratory tract.
B) Epicardium.
C) Esophagus.
D) Stomach.
E) All of the above.

Discussion

The correct answer is E. A cough can originate from sources other than the lungs.

The three most common causes of chronic cough (cough lasting >8 weeks) are:

A) Postnasal drip, asthma, GERD.
B) GERD, COPD, congenital lung disease.
C) Lung cancer, postnasal drip, COPD.
D) Obstructive sleep apnea, respiratory infections, asthma.

Table 3–4 CAUSES OF ACUTE AND CHRONIC COUGH

Acute	URI, pertussis, allergic rhinitis, COPD, exacerbation, asthma, acute sinusitis
Chronic	GERD, postnasal drip, asthma, chronic sinusitis, allergic/vasomotor rhinitis, ACE inhibitors, eosinophilic bronchitis, chronic bronchitis, postinfectious asthma

Discussion

The correct answer is A. Epidemiologic studies have demonstrated that most cases of chronic cough are due to postnasal drainage, asthma, or GERD. Most cases of chronic cough seem to have only a single cause, although some will have more than one cause. Empiric therapy should be aimed at these top three causes. Of course, infection (pertussis in particular), malignancy, and other causes of cough are important to consider—and potentially rule out—as well.

 HELPFUL TIP: Look in the ears—cerumen impaction can cause a chronic cough and is often overlooked. Remember medications, especially ACE inhibitors (as above). Other drugs that can cause cough include amiodarone, olanzapine, and some asthma medications (eg, albuterol, montelukast).

Objectives: Did you learn to . . .

- Recognize the most common causes of chronic cough?
- Evaluate a patient with chronic cough?
- Develop a management plan for chronic cough?

CASE 7

You see a 38-year-old female in follow-up for a recent episode of sinusitis. The illness has been present for about 6 weeks and has not responded to 2 weeks of appropriate antibiotics. She continues to have intermittent nosebleeds, fatigue, arthralgias, low-grade fevers, and night sweats. Two new complaints have surfaced: she has a cough productive of white sputum and she occasionally expectorates quarter-sized clots of blood. She has pleuritic chest pain, but denies dyspnea, tobacco use, or any history of cardiac or pulmonary disease.

She is afebrile with a respiratory rate of 16, blood pressure 120/74, and pulse 92. Her oxygen saturation is 98% on room air. There is dried blood in the nares, but the oropharynx is clear. Cardiac and pulmonary exams are unremarkable.

Which initial test is most appropriate?

A) Chest x-ray.
B) Sputum cytologic analysis.
C) Bronchoscopy.
D) Chest CT.
E) CBC.

Discussion

The correct answer is A. Hemoptysis is alarming to the patient and the physician. A stepwise approach is warranted. Chest x-ray is the first step. Sputum for cytology might help if the suspicion for lung cancer was substantial, but the yield is likely to be low here. She may eventually require bronchoscopy if initial studies are unrevealing. However, this is premature. Chest CT is likely to be part of the evaluation, but a chest x-ray should be performed first. Obtaining blood for a CBC is also important, although likely to be normal in the setting of minor hemoptysis. See Table 3–5 for a list of causes of hemoptysis.

You obtain the chest x-ray shown in Figure 3–2. You get the following laboratory results back:

CBC: Leukocytosis, thrombocytosis and normochromic, normocytic anemia

ESR: 70 mm/hr

Urine dipstick: Positive for protein, heme, and white cells

Which of the following tests will best assist you in the diagnosis of this patient?

A) Antineutrophil cytoplasmic antibody (ANCA).
B) Antiglomerular basement membrane antibody.
C) Antinuclear antibody (ANA).
D) A and B.
E) A and C.

Table 3–5 CAUSES OF HEMOPTYSIS

Vascular	PE, vasculitides (Goodpasture, Wegener), arteriovenous malformation
Neoplastic	Bronchogenic carcinoma, metastatic disease
Connective tissue	Lupus, rheumatoid arthritis
Cardiac	CHF, mitral stenosis
Infectious	TB, bronchitis, pneumonia, abscess
Drugs	Anticoagulants, cocaine, solvents
Miscellaneous	Trauma, foreign body, epistaxis, hematemesis

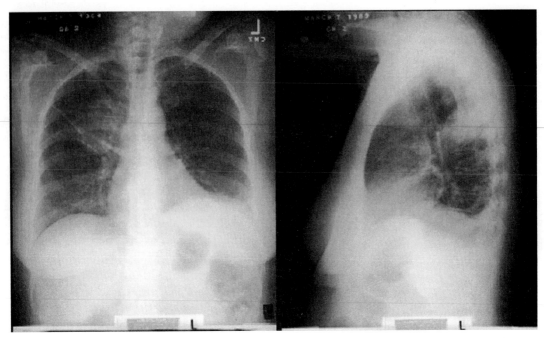

Figure 3–2

Discussion

The correct answer is D. This patient is presenting with the classic triad of Wegener granulomatosis: disease of the upper respiratory tract, lower respiratory tract, and kidneys. She has some of the additional signs and symptoms associated with Wegener granulomatosis as well. Common findings include pleuritic chest pain, myalgias, arthralgias, ptosis, fever, weight loss, and purpuric skin lesions, among others.

The antineutrophil cytoplasmic antibody (ANCA), and especially c-ANCA, which is more specific for Wegener, is present in up to 90% of patients with Wegener. An ANA is not helpful in diagnosing Wegener: An antiglomerular basement membrane antibody may be helpful in diagnosing Goodpasture syndrome, which can be clinically easily confused with Wegener: they both present with respiratory and renal involvement. Thus, anti-GBM antibody will be helpful in differentiating these two (but about 10% of patients with Goodpasture will also have Wegener).

Which of the following is NOT a radiographic finding of Wegener granulomatosis?

A) Nodules that may be cavitary.
B) Alveolar opacification.
C) Pleural opacities.
D) Widened mediastinum.

Discussion

The correct answer is D. A widened mediastinum is not one of the classic findings in Wegener granulomatosis. However, one may on occasion see hilar adenopathy. All of the other choices can be found in Wegener. In the patient's x-ray (see Figure 3–2), a right upper-lobe mass is easily distinguished. In a young, nonsmoking female presenting with these symptoms, such a lung mass should lead to the consideration of Wegener or possibly an infectious process. She is less likely to have a malignant process.

 HELPFUL TIP: A major and more common cause of hemoptysis is bronchitis—more likely in smokers and older patients.

＊＊

The diagnostic evaluation is in progress. Laboratory tests are pending, and a chest CT is scheduled. You have arranged for a pulmonologist to see her. When you are next on call, the physician covering the ED calls you to admit her for "massive hemoptysis." When you arrive, the patient looks comfortable and has normal vital signs. She begins a fit of coughing, expectorating several ounces of bright red blood. Her systolic blood pressure falls to 80 mm Hg. Her respiratory rate is 40. Her work of breathing has increased considerably. The situation does not improve after 5 minutes of observation, and her O_2 saturation is now 83%.

What is your first action in this situation?

A) Arrange emergent bronchoscopy.
B) Transfuse 2 units of blood.
C) Perform endotracheal intubation.
D) Provide bolus IV normal saline.
E) Call for emergent surgical evaluation.

Discussion

The correct answer is C. Massive hemoptysis is variably defined as 100–600 mL of blood expectorated per day, and it can result in hemodynamic compromise and asphyxiation. The main cause of mortality with hemoptysis is not hypovolemia, but rather asphyxiation from blood in the lungs. As with any patient in acute respiratory distress, the airway must be controlled first. The best choice here is to perform intubation. Since this patient is known to have a potential source for bleeding in the right lung, intubation of the left mainstem bronchus may protect the left lung from the blood. Also, placing this patient on her right side (so that the bleeding source is dependent) may protect the left lung. If available, emergent bronchoscopy may allow identification and tamponade of the bleeding site. Emergent surgery is indicated if the bleeding remains brisk and not responsive to other interventions. Blood products should be available and transfused as appropriate. Fluid resuscitation is important. However, before any of these other measures is undertaken, the airway must be protected.

The patient stabilizes in the ICU. You plan to start treatment for her Wegener.

 HELPFUL TIP: The 5-year mortality of untreated Wegener granulomatosis is 90%. These patients need aggressive treatment! Cyclophosphamide + steroids seem to be the best combination.

Objectives: Did you learn to . . .

● Perform an appropriate evaluation on a patient with hemoptysis?

● Recognize the major causes of hemoptysis?
● Diagnose Wegener granulomatosis?
● Identify massive hemoptysis?

CASE 8

A 35-year-old African American female presents with dyspnea, worsening over the last 2 months. She also complains of cough, generalized fatigue, and intermittent low-grade fevers. She does not smoke. Chest x-ray shows hilar adenopathy and small bilateral pleural effusions. Spirometry is consistent with a restrictive pattern.

Of the following, which is the most likely diagnosis?

A) Wegener granulomatosis.
B) Sarcoidosis.
C) Bronchogenic carcinoma.
D) Pneumonia.

Discussion

The correct answer is B. The findings of hilar lymphadenopathy and a restrictive pattern on spirometry are most consistent with sarcoidosis. The chest x-ray findings do not support the diagnosis of Wegener granulomatosis (see Case 6). Bronchogenic carcinoma is unlikely in this relatively young nonsmoker. The clinical history is not typical of pneumonia, and chest x-ray shows no infiltrate. Tuberculosis, although not a choice, should also be considered, and the appropriate history and testing should be completed. TB and sarcoidosis often present in a similar fashion.

Which of the following is NOT commonly associated with sarcoidosis?

A) Hypercalcemia.
B) Elevated angiotensin-converting enzyme levels.
C) Reduced diffusion capacity.
D) Hypothyroidism.
E) Facial or peripheral nerve palsy.

Discussion

The correct answer is D. Sarcoidosis is marked by the presence of non-caseating granulomas. While sarcoid can infiltrate the thyroid, it rarely if ever causes hypothyroidism. Pulmonary sarcoidosis includes a decreased diffusion capacity and decreased vital capacity. Other laboratory findings include hypercalcemia, hypercalciuria, elevated liver and pancreatic enzymes, and elevated angiotensin-converting enzyme levels. Neurologic involvement occurs in up to 5% of patients and frequently presents as facial paralysis but may present as any CNS lesion. Peripheral nerves may also be involved.

Which of the following is NOT found as a part of sarcoidosis?

A) Erythema nodosum.
B) Myocardial infarction.
C) Cardiac arrhythmias.
D) Elevated liver enzymes.
E) Vision loss.

Discussion

The correct answer is B. Although there is cardiac involvement with sarcoidosis, the manifestations are bundle branch block, cardiac arrhythmias, and sudden death. Many organs can be affected by sarcoidosis, including the skin, eye, heart, lung, liver, nervous system—anywhere granulomas form.

Which of the following is true about angiotensin-converting enzyme (ACE) levels in sarcoidosis?

A) An elevated ACE level is specific for sarcoidosis.
B) ACE often correlates with disease severity in sarcoidosis.
C) ACE inhibitors are effective in the treatment of sarcoid.
D) All of the above.

Discussion

The correct answer is B. One can follow ACE levels to track the progress of the disease. However, since treatment is based on symptoms, following ACE levels is not recommended. Answer A is incorrect. ACE levels may be elevated in silicosis, miliary TB, and asbestosis, among others. Answer C is incorrect. ACE inhibitors are not used to treat sarcoid.

**

This patient is found to have only pulmonary sarcoidosis with some mild systemic symptoms.

Which of the following is the best initial choice for management?

A) Observation.
B) Oral corticosteroids.
C) Oral antibiotics.
D) Inhaled corticosteroids.
E) Methotrexate.

Discussion

The correct answer is A. This patient has apparent pulmonary-limited disease and has minimal systemic symptoms. Nearly 50% of patients with sarcoidosis may have spontaneous resolution of their symptoms without treatment. **Treatment may prolong the disease process.** If her pulmonary or systemic symptoms worsen or are causing major life problems, she should be started on oral steroids. Systemic corticosteroid therapy is the mainstay of treatment for sarcoidosis. Methotrexate and other immune-modulating drugs may be employed as well and offer a steroid-sparing effect, but these are not first-line agents. Evidence for the use of inhaled corticosteroids is lacking. Antibiotics are not effective.

Objectives: Did you learn to . . .

- Recognize the clinical manifestations of sarcoid?
- Manage a patient with mild sarcoidosis?

CASE 9

A 57-year-old male with no prior medical history presents with a 1-week history of right rib pain and low back pain. The rib pain is worse with deep breaths and especially bothers him at night. There has been no trauma. He has lost 20 pounds in the last 3 months. He has a cough productive of white sputum. He denies any other symptoms. He smokes one to two packs of cigarettes per day but does not drink alcohol.

Vital signs show temperature 36.5°C, pulse 95, blood pressure 110/70, and respiratory rate 16. On room air, his oxygen saturation is 96%. There is no adenopathy. His lung sounds are clear on the left and decreased on the right. There is dullness to percussion and decreased tactile fremitus over the right lower lung field.

Based on this patient's history and physical exam, what do you expect to find on chest x-ray?

A) Normal chest x-ray.
B) Cavitary lung lesion.
C) Pleural effusion.
D) Expanded lung fields.
E) Pneumothorax.

Discussion

The correct answer is C. A physical exam can be misleading. But in general, this patient's findings suggest pleural effusion. Everything is diminished in pleural effusion: there is dullness to percussion, decreased breath sounds, decreased tactile fremitus, and decreased voice transmission. A cavitary lung lesion presents with either a normal exam or findings similar to an infiltrate (eg, crackles, increased fremitus, and dullness to percussion). Expanded lung fields on chest x-ray are often seen in patients with COPD or asthma, and exam findings include prolonged expiratory phase, wheezing, and resonance to percussion. Pneumothorax presents with hyperresonance to percussion, decreased breath sounds, and decreased fremitus.

 HELPFUL TIP: Chest radiographs have a low sensitivity for rib fractures. However, this is not a problem. The presence or absence of a rib fracture is generally irrelevant. What we are interested in is whether or not there is anything underlying the rib fracture, such as a pulmonary contusion or hemothorax.

* *

The chest x-ray shows obliteration of the right hemidiaphragm, and the posterior costophrenic angle is obscured on the lateral view, consistent with pleural effusion. There is also a right upper-lobe lung mass.

Which of the following is the minimum testing required in all patients before performing a thoracentesis for diagnostic purposes?

A) Supine chest x-ray.
B) Chest CT.
C) Lateral decubitus chest x-ray.
D) Chest ultrasound.
E) Apical view chest radiograph.

Discussion

The correct answer is C. Prior to performing a thoracentesis, you must know whether the effusion is loculated

or freely flowing. A decubitus film, with the affected side down, will allow you see the effusion "layer out" unless it is loculated. A supine chest x-ray may allow the effusion to layer out too, but you will not be able to see it as well. Chest CT and ultrasound are excellent modalities for quantifying effusions, but are generally more expensive.

Relative and absolute contraindications to thoracentesis include all of the following EXCEPT:

A) Herpes zoster in the area of needle placement.
B) Coagulopathy.
C) Diaphragmatic rupture.
D) Positive pressure ventilation.
E) History of recurrent laryngeal nerve injury or compromise.

Discussion

The correct answer is E. Absolute contraindications include chest wall compromise (eg, burn, cellulitis, herpes zoster, ruptured diaphragm) and cases where chest tube thoracostomy would be more appropriate. Relative contraindications are poor patient cooperation, coagulopathy, anticoagulation therapy, very small effusions (<10 mm on decubitus film view), positive pressure ventilation, and pleural adhesions.

* *

On right lateral decubitus view, the effusion does not layer freely. It appears loculated.

What is the next most appropriate step?

A) Referral for surgical drainage.
B) Place a chest tube to drain the effusion.
C) Perform diagnostic thoracentesis at the bedside.
D) Perform ultrasound-guided thoracentesis.

Discussion

The correct answer is D. The patient has a loculated pleural effusion based on decubitus x-ray. Loculated pleural effusions are difficult to successfully drain blindly with the usual bedside technique. Ultrasound-guided thoracentesis is a good first step in evaluating this effusion, although it may not be successful in accessing all loculations. Referral to a thoracic surgeon may eventually be necessary, but this would not be the first step. Placing a chest tube into a loculated effusion blindly is not recommended, and the diagnostic study should be obtained first unless the patient is in urgent need of a therapeutic thoracentesis.

* *

Ultrasound-guided thoracentesis is successful in obtaining fluid. The fluid is amber and cloudy, with a pH 7.3, LDH 800 IU/L, glucose 65 mg/dL, total protein 5.5 g/dL, WBC 1,300/mm³, RBC 50,000/mm³. Serum studies done the same day include LDH 155 IU/L, glucose 99 mg/dL, and total protein 7.0 g/dL. Cytology, Gram stain, and culture of the pleural fluid are pending.

Which of the following is the most accurate statement regarding the pleural fluid analysis?

A) The fluid is due to infection.
B) The fluid is due to cancer.
C) The fluid is a transudate.
D) The fluid is an exudate.

Discussion

The correct answer is D. Pleural effusions are broadly categorized as exudates and transudates (Tables 3–6 and 3–7). Such a categorization helps to narrow the differential diagnosis. In this case, several elements of the pleural fluid are consistent with an exudate.

LDH and protein can be used to determine whether the pleural fluid is transudative or exudative. A pleural fluid LDH >2/3 the upper limit of normal serum LDH, a pleural LDH:serum LDH ratio >0.6, and a pleural protein:serum protein ratio >0.5 are all suggestive of an exudate. All three of these indicators point to an exudate in this case. Also, exudative effusions tend to have a higher degree of cellularity than transudative effusions. With the information given, it is difficult to determine if the effusion is related to infection, cancer, or some other process.

Table 3–6 CATEGORIZATION OF PLEURAL FLUID AS AN EXUDATE OR TRANSUDATE

Exudate characterized by

- Pleural fluid to serum protein ratio >0.5
- Pleural fluid to serum LDH ratio >0.6
- Pleural fluid LDH >150 mg/dL (two-thirds the upper limit of normal serum LDH)

Table 3–7 CATEGORIZATION OF PLEURAL EFFUSIONS BY CLASS (TRANSUDATIVE VS. EXUDATIVE)

Type of Effusion	Potential Causes
Transudative effusions	Heart failure, cirrhosis, nephritic syndrome, atelectasis, myxedema, pulmonary embolism, urinothorax
Exudative effusions	Bronchogenic carcinoma, metastatic neoplasm, mesothelioma, pneumonia, TB, chylothorax, pancreatitis, esophageal rupture, collagen vascular diseases (rheumatoid arthritis, Sjögren), trauma, drugs (nitrofurantoin, amiodarone, methotrexate), heart failure with diuretic therapy, pulmonary embolism

Note: CHF and PE can cause both exudative and transudative effusions.

* *

The pleural fluid cytology comes back negative. The patient's symptoms and exam have not changed. Repeat radiograph still shows an upper lobe mass.

What is the most appropriate next step in approaching this pleural effusion?

A) Await pleural fluid culture results.
B) Perform bedside chest tube drainage of the effusion.
C) Refer for surgical evacuation of the effusion.
D) Refer for bronchoscopy.
E) Place a chest tube for chemical pleurodesis.

Discussion

The correct answer is D. The effusion is clearly exudative, and the patient appears to have a lung mass. Biopsy of the lung mass via bronchoscopy is indicated. A negative pleural fluid cytology does not rule out lung cancer. Positive cytology indicates advanced stage lung cancer. Chest tube drainage of a loculated pleural effusion is not recommended. Surgical evacuation of the fluid would be indicated if the patient were symptomatic. If the effusion grows, or is drained and recurs, it may respond to pleurodesis. Otherwise, pleurodesis is not indicated at this time.

HELPFUL TIP: Patients with malignant pleural effusions are not likely to benefit from surgery since the tumor is not localized and resectable. Long-term outcomes with a malignant pleural effusion are bleak.

Objectives: Did you learn to . . .

- Recognize the historical and physical exam findings of pleural effusion?
- List potential etiologies of pleural effusion?
- Narrow the differential diagnosis based on pleural fluid findings?
- Decide when to perform diagnostic and therapeutic thoracentesis?
- Decide when to perform chest tube drainage?

CASE 10

A 60-year-old male presents to the ED for a cough. His symptoms began with a cold 2 weeks ago, and the other symptoms have improved, but the cough has persisted. He has mild production of white sputum with no hemoptysis. The patient denies fevers, night sweats, chills, and weight loss. He has had no chest pain or dyspnea. He smokes one pack of cigarettes per day, works in construction, and does not have a regular doctor. With some pride, he says, "I haven't seen a doctor in over 30 years." On physical examination, you find a fit-appearing male in no acute distress. His vital signs are normal. His lung sounds are diminished bilaterally, but the remainder of the exam is unremarkable. While breathing ambient air, the patient's oxygen saturation is 94%. You obtain a chest x-ray as shown in Figure 3–3.

Your next step is to:

A) Prescribe a 5-day course of azithromycin.
B) Refer the patient to a pulmonologist.
C) Order a high resolution CT scan of the chest.
D) Have the patient return to you in 3 months to repeat a chest x-ray.
E) Reassure the patient and have him return as needed.

Discussion

The correct answer is C. The chest x-ray in Figure 3–3 shows a single nodule in the right lower lobe. The nodule is round, less dense than bone, and appears to be

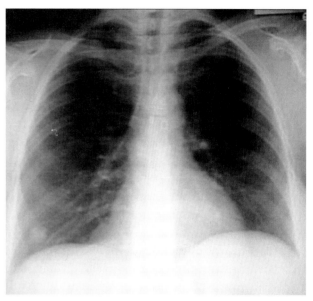

Figure 3–3

>1 cm in diameter. These are sometimes called coin lesions. There are no other abnormalities. The most appropriate next step in the evaluation is to order a high resolution CT scan of the chest. Treatment with azithromycin is inappropriate in this setting, as this patient has no signs of pulmonary infection on exam or chest x-ray. Referral to a pulmonologist is premature without first investigating the nodule by CT scan. Delaying further imaging and evaluation is also inappropriate since 15% to 75% of solitary pulmonary nodules ≥8 mm are ultimately diagnosed as cancer (depending on multiple factors including size).

Which of the following is NOT considered a benign pattern of calcification on CT scan?

A) Diffuse, homogeneous calcification.
B) Central calcification.
C) Laminar calcification.
D) Spiculated, irregular calcification.
E) "Popcorn" calcification.

Discussion

The correct answer is D. We are accustomed to thinking of calcified nodules as benign, but that is not always the case. Irregular, spiculated calcification is not reassuring. The other answer choices are considered indicative of a benign lesion. Two patterns on CT are relatively specific for cancer: a scalloped border and the corona radiata sign, which is composed of fine linear strands extending out from the nodule.

All of the following are useful to help assess the risk of cancer in a patient with a solitary pulmonary nodule EXCEPT:

A) Smoking status.
B) Age.
C) Diameter of the nodule.
D) Gender.

Discussion

The correct answer is D. Determining the probability of cancer in patients with a solitary pulmonary nodule (SPN) is an inexact science. Although men are slightly overrepresented in lung cancer, this is generally thought to be due to greater smoking rates in men and to occupational hazards. Gender itself does not help to risk-stratify patients with a SPN. The diameter of the nodule is also important. If the diameter is <8 mm, the risk of cancer is low. When the diameter is ≥3 cm, the SPN is now referred to as a "pulmonary mass" and is highly likely to be cancerous. SPN >3 cm in diameter should be considered cancer until proven otherwise.

 HELPFUL TIP: Female smokers are equally or more likely to be diagnosed with lung cancer compared with male smokers. However, female smokers are less likely to *die* of lung cancer.

* *

Later that week, your patient returns with his CT scan in hand. His cough is somewhat better (therapeutic CT scan?). You review the CT with him. It shows a round, smooth nodule measuring 2 cm in diameter and located in the periphery of the right lower lobe. There are no calcifications in the nodule and no other abnormalities.

Which of the following is the most appropriate next step?

A) Referral for bronchoscopy.
B) High-resolution CT scan every 3 months.

C) Chest x-ray every 3 months.
D) Bone scan.
E) Referral to a thoracic surgeon.

Discussion

The correct answer is E. This patient needs a biopsy. There are several factors that put your patient at higher risk of having a malignant cause for the SPN, including his age and tobacco use. Although the nodule is smooth on CT, its size is >8 mm and there are no calcifications. This patient should be referred for transthoracic fine-needle biopsy or open biopsy.

Answer A is tempting but incorrect. Bronchoscopy is insensitive in the peripheral lung, especially when the lesion is relatively small. Answers B and C are incorrect. Repeat imaging over time may delay a diagnosis of malignancy. Without symptoms of bone pain or confirmation that the SPN is a cancer that might metastasize to bone, a bone scan (D) will have a very low yield.

* *

Your patient returns from the surgeon much relieved. Fine-needle biopsy proved the SPN to be a hamartoma. Now your patient wants to quit smoking for good, and he thinks that he will need some assistance. You recommend nicotine replacement products and bupropion, but your patient claims to have had an allergic reaction to bupropion. Fortunately, you know of an effective alternative.

To assist with tobacco cessation, you prescribe which of the following?

A) Varenicline.
B) Fluoxetine.
C) Olanzapine.
D) Metoprolol.
E) Clonidine.

Discussion

The correct answer is A. Recent randomized trials have demonstrated the effectiveness of the nicotine partial agonist, varenicline (Chantix). This FDA-approved medication appears to be at least as effective as bupropion as an aid to smoking cessation. Fluoxetine and other SSRIs have not demonstrated a benefit. In schizophrenic patients, the use of atypical antipsychotic medications may aid in smoking cessation when compared to typical antipsychotics. Clonidine is sometimes used to help patients who are withdrawing from narcotics, and it may have some limited role in smoking cessation but is not very effective.

 HELPFUL TIP: The most common side effects of varenicline include insomnia, abnormal dreams, and nausea. Some patients have become depressed and suicidal. Use this—and all—medication with care.

Objectives: Did you learn to . . .

● Weigh risk factors when evaluating a solitary pulmonary nodule?
● Evaluate a solitary pulmonary nodule?
● Assist a patient with smoking cessation?

CASE 11

A 74-year-old male is seen in the ED for weakness, cough, and fatigue. His wife relates an incomplete recovery since his myocardial infarction last year. He continues to have poor appetite and she thinks that he may be depressed.

The patient is short of breath and confused. His wife speaks for him. Over the past week, he has become weaker and developed vomiting and diarrhea. Yesterday he developed a fever, chills, and a new cough productive of white sputum. His past medical history is otherwise remarkable for a cholecystectomy. He is taking aspirin, metoprolol, and simvastatin.

On examination, his temperature is 39°C, respiratory rate 30, pulse 90, and blood pressure 140/80. Oxygen saturation on room air is 90%. He is thin, pale, and oriented to person only. The lung examination is remarkable for rales in the left lower field, with dullness to percussion and increased tactile fremitus. The remainder of the exam is normal.

The chest x-ray shows a left lower lobe infiltrate. Other laboratory data currently available: hemoglobin 12.4 g/dL, WBC 14,100/mm³, platelets 340,000/mm³, creatinine 1.9 mg/dL, BUN 50 mg/dL, and normal electrolytes, troponin, and CK. An ECG shows normal sinus rhythm.

What is your next step in managing this patient's medical condition?

A) Place a chest tube on the left.
B) Perform chest CT.
C) Administer inhaled bronchodilators.
D) Administer parenteral antibiotics.
E) Perform intubation and mechanical ventilation.

Discussion

The correct answer is D. Given the clinical picture and chest x-ray findings, the patient most likely has community-acquired pneumonia. Therefore, the administration of parenteral antibiotics is the best choice. Answer A is incorrect. Since there is no effusion, a chest tube would be useless. Answer B is incorrect. CT is not required in this straightforward case of pneumonia. Answer C is incorrect. The patient is not wheezing and there is no indication for bronchodilators at this time. Answer E is incorrect. Since your patient's respiratory status is stable, he does not require intubation.

 HELPFUL TIP: Time counts—the goal is to get the patient antibiotics ASAP, and absolutely within 6 hours of his presentation. This means making sure he gets appropriate antibiotics in the ED. Remember: it is impossible to tell a **typical** versus an **atypical** pneumonia by radiograph. Do not base your therapy for community-acquired pneumonia on the appearance of the radiograph. Atypical organisms can cause lobar consolidation and typical pneumonias can appear diffuse. Treatment guidelines make no mention of radiographic appearance.

* *

The Pneumonia Severity Index (PSI) is a popular guideline used for deciding whether or not to admit a patient with pneumonia.

If you employ this guideline, which factor will carry the most weight in deciding to admit your patient to the hospital?

A) Presence of pleural effusion.
B) Respiratory rate.
C) Presence of infiltrate on chest x-ray.

D) Oxygen saturation.

E) Heart rate.

Discussion

The correct answer is B. Although somewhat cumbersome, the PSI is a useful tool to stratify patients based on risk and to decide whether to hospitalize. However, it should be used only as a tool: the final decision on admission rests on the clinician's judgment in a particular case. In a common sense manner, the PSI accounts for age, comorbidities, physical exam findings, and laboratory and radiologic data. The PSI assigns certain points to each indicator, and a score is calculated to determine the overall risk (Table 3–8). A score of ≤90 points indicates that a patient is at low risk of death caused by pneumonia.

 HELPFUL TIP: A simpler but less well-validated tool exists for determining disposition in a patient with pneumonia is the acronym **CURB-65.**

Confusion (based upon a specific mental test or disorientation to person, place, or time)

Urea (BUN) >20 mg/dL

Respiratory rate >30 breaths/minute

Blood pressure <90/60

Age >65 years

Patients with one or two positive criteria should be admitted.

Based on patient-specific characteristics and your knowledge of causative factors involved in pneumonia, which of the following is LEAST likely to be the agent causing this patient's infection?

A) *Mycoplasma pneumoniae.*

B) *Streptococcus pneumoniae.*

C) *Haemophilus influenzae.*

D) *Pseudomonas aeruginosa.*

Discussion

The correct answer is D. When a pathogen is identified in adult community acquired pneumonia, it is usually *S. pneumoniae*. *S. pneumoniae* makes up 40% to 60% of all cases of community-acquired pneumonia in

Table 3–8   PNEUMONIA SEVERITY INDEX

Characteristic	Points Assigned*
Demographic factor	
Age	
Men	Age (yr)
Women	Age (yr) –10
Nursing home resident	+10
Coexisting illnesses†	
Neoplastic disease	+30
Liver disease	+20
Congestive heart failure	+10
Cerebrovascular disease	+10
Renal disease	+10
Physical-examination findings	
Altered mental status‡	+20
Respiratory rate ≥30/min	+20
Systolic blood pressure <90 mm Hg	+20
Temperature <35°C or ≥40°C	+15
Pulse ≥ 125/min	+10
Laboratory and radiographic findings	
Arterial pH <7.35	+30
Blood urea nitrogen ≥30 mg/dl (11 mmol/liter)	+20
Sodium <130 mmol/liter	+20
Glucose ≥250 mg/dl (14 mmol/liter)	+10
Hematocrit <30%	+10
Partial pressure of arterial oxygen <60 mm Hg§	+10
Pleural effusion	+10

*A total point score for a given patient is obtained by summing the patient's age in years (age minus 10 for women) and the points for each applicable characteristic. The points assigned to each predictor variable were based on coefficients obtained from the logistic-regression model used in step 2 of the prediction rule.

†Neoplastic disease is defined as any cancer except basal- or squamous-cell cancer of the skin that was active at the time of presentation or diagnosed within one year of presentation. Liver disease is defined as a clinical or histologic diagnosis of cirrhosis or another form of chronic liver disease, such as chronic active hepatitis. Congestive heart failure is defined as systolic or diastolic ventricular dysfunction documented by history, physical examination, and chest radiograph, echocardiogram, multiple gated acquisition scan, or left ventriculogram. Cerebrovascular disease is defined as a clinical diagnosis of stroke or transient ischemic attack or stroke documented by magnetic resonance imaging or computed tomography. Renal disease is defined as a history of chronic renal disease or abnormal blood urea nitrogen and creatinine concentrations documented in the medical record.

‡Altered mental status is defined as disorientation with respect to person, place, or time that is not known to be chronic, stupor, or coma.

§In the Pneumonia PORT cohort study, an oxygen saturation of less than 90% on pulse oximetry or intubation before admission was also considered abnormal.

the elderly. Nontypeable *H. influenzae* composes about 5% to 10% of cases. *Mycoplasma* is implicated in 5% of all cases of pneumonia in adults, and it is more common in young adults. *P. aeruginosa* pneumonia is uncommon in healthy elders and more likely to occur in patients with serious underlying lung disease or immunodeficiency. Approximately 5% of patients or more are infected with multiple agents.

* *

Based on your assessment of his risk, you decide to admit this patient to the hospital. An IV is in place.

Which of the following IV antibiotic regimens do you choose?

A) Penicillin.
B) Azithromycin.
C) Penicillin and gentamicin.
D) Azithromycin and ceftriaxone.
E) Piperacillin/tazobactam and ciprofloxacin.

Discussion

The correct answer is D. For community-acquired pneumonia treated in the hospital setting, the optimal antibiotic regimen must offer good coverage of *S. pneumoniae*, *H. influenzae*, and atypical organisms like *Mycoplasma* and *Chlamydia* species. Most *S. pneumoniae* bacteria are resistant to penicillin and approximately 20% to 30% are resistant to macrolides as well. Therefore, these agents should not be used alone in the treatment of pneumonia in hospitalized patients. Gentamicin has no activity against *S. pneumoniae* but has a role in *P. aeruginosa* infections. Ceftriaxone offers good Gram-negative coverage and activity against *S. pneumoniae*. Azithromycin covers atypical organisms. An alternative yet effective regimen would be monotherapy with a respiratory fluoroquinolone such as moxiflocacin or levofloxacin. The combination of piperacillin/tazobactam with ciprofloxacin is reserved for patients with more severe pneumonia, requiring ventilation and ICU care.

* *

Initial blood cultures grow *S. pneumoniae*. Sputum Gram stain and culture are negative. The patient initially does well and does defervesce after 2 days of IV antibiotics. However, on day 3 he again spikes a fever. He looks moderately ill. Your exam reveals increased dullness to percussion on the left. There is no JVD or peripheral edema. The radiograph is shown in Figure 3–4.

The most likely diagnosis now is:

A) Anaerobic abscess.
B) Development of resistant *Streptococcus pneumonia*.
C) Parapneumonic effusion.

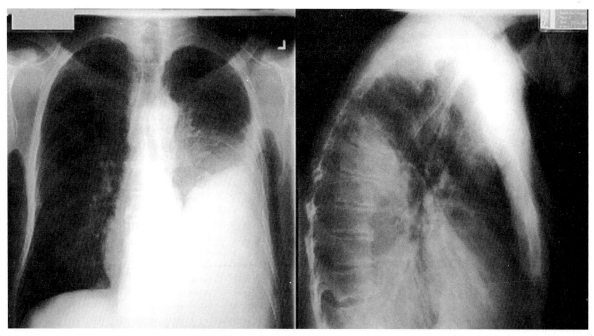

Figure 3–4

D) Transudate secondary to heart failure.
E) Drug-induced transudate.

Discussion

The correct answer is C. The most likely problem in this patient is a parapneumonic effusion. An anaerobic abscess is unlikely given that there are no air/fluid levels and the fact that the fluid appears to be in the pleura. Answer B is incorrect. Development of resistance should take more than 3 days, especially since this patient is on two drugs. Answer D is incorrect because this patient does not have a history of CHF, is febrile, and has no JVD, etc. Answer E is incorrect. None of the drugs that he is on is known to cause pleural effusions.

You place a chest tube to drain the pleural effusion and continue the current antibiotic regimen. The patient does well and is discharged 1 week later on clarithromycin after sensitivities conclude that his organism is sensitive.

* *

Six weeks after the onset of illness, the patient returns for follow-up to ensure clearing of the chest x-ray. He is feeling well. He is alert and oriented, and has clear lungs to auscultation. Percussion and tactile fremitus are normal. There is no lymphadenopathy in the neck or supraclavicular areas. The x-ray still shows left lower lobe infiltrate, unchanged in size from the initial x-ray. The pleural effusion has resolved.

Which of the following is the most appropriate next step in the evaluation and management of this patient?

A) Chest CT.
B) Chest x-ray in 2 weeks.
C) Chest x-ray in 6 weeks.
D) Prescribe amoxicillin/clavulanate.

Discussion

The correct answer is C. Bacterial pneumonia can rarely late 3-5 months to clear on x-ray. Thus, repeating the chest x-ray in 2 weeks (answer B) is unlikely to show resolution. In elderly patients, the chest x-ray takes longer to normalize than in younger patients. The patient is clinically doing well, and does not require treatment for a persistent pulmonary infection (answer D). Chest CT (answer A) would give more

information, but in the absence of systemic symptoms, such as weight loss, persistent cough, hemoptysis, or fever, it is unlikely to change the management at this point. It is important to consider that this infiltrate may represent a neoplastic process if it does not resolve within several months.

 HELPFUL TIP: Even with extensive evaluation (blood culture, sputum culture, etc.) an infectious agent is identified in only 50% of cases of pneumonia. Thus, treatment is usually empiric. Sputum cultures do not alter antibiotic therapy or disease outcome in most patients with pneumonia, and 30% of patients with pneumonia are not able to produce sputum. Blood cultures are of little or no value in pneumonia but are still recommended in most guidelines for hospitalized patients. If possible, do blood cultures before initiating therapy.

 HELPFUL TIP: Although infrequently a cause of routine community-acquired pneumonia, *Staphylococcus aureus* is a common cause of bacterial pneumonia during influenza epidemics.

* *

In one of life's coincidences, the next day you diagnose this patient's 36-year-old, healthy son with a community-acquired pneumonia. Besides a fever, cough, and left lower lobe infiltrate on chest x-ray, he feels fine.

Which of the following drug regimens is appropriate for the treatment of this patient in the outpatient setting?

A) Cephalexin (Keflex) 250–500 mg PO QID and penicillin V 250 mg TID for 10 days.
B) Clarithromycin 500 mg BID for 10 days.
C) Doxycycline 100 mg BID for 10 days.
D) B or C.
E) C or D.

Discussion

The correct answer is D. The treatment of community-acquired pneumonia requires that one cover both typical and atypical organisms. Answer A does not cover atypical organisms. Guideline recommended choices for the outpatient treatment of community-acquired pneumonia include doxycycline (answer C) and macrolides such as clarithromycin (answer B). Additional options include the respiratory fluoroquinolones such as moxifloxacin, gemifloxacin, or levofloxacin. Of the appropriate regimens, doxycycline and erythromycin are the least expensive, but erythromycin is associated with a high rate of gastrointestinal intolerance.

A respiratory fluoroquinolone is the recommended choice for the outpatient treatment of community-acquired pneumonia in patients with serious underlying disease such as diabetes, COPD, etc. These medications have a high degree of oral bioavailability and are active against penicillin-resistant *Streptococcus pneumoniae*. However, respiratory fluoroquinolones should be not be used in all cases. The IDSA/ATS consensus guidelines recommend that respiratory fluoroquinolones be reserved for patients with serious underlying disease.

 HELPFUL TIP: The usual duration for antibiotic therapy in pneumonia is 10–14 days. Although this duration is the standard of care, there is no evidence to prove that this length of time is any more or less effective than any other.

Objectives: Did you learn to . . .

- Recognize the clinical presentation of community-acquired pneumonia in different patient populations?
- Differentiate community-acquired from nosocomial pneumonia?
- Determine the appropriate disposition for a patient with community-acquired pneumonia?
- Initiate outpatient and inpatient treatment for community-acquired pneumonia?

CASE 12

A 21-year-old female college student presents to the ED in the middle of the night. She complains of sudden onset of chest pain a few hours earlier while she was studying. The pain is sharp in nature, located under her left breast, and is nonradiating. Breathing deeply and pressing on her left chest make the pain worse. She denies any history of cardiac or pulmonary disease. Her only medication is an oral contraceptive. She smokes about 10 cigarettes per day, binges on alcohol on the weekends, and smokes marijuana about once a month. Other than a nonproductive cough and mild shortness of breath, her review of systems is negative.

On physical examination, you find an obese female in mild distress. She is holding her arm against her left chest, splinting. Her temperature is 38°C, pulse 110, respiratory rate 24, and blood pressure 130/82. Her oxygen saturation on room air is 95%. She is able to answer questions in full sentences. Her cardiovascular exam is remarkable only for tachycardia. The lung fields are clear to auscultation and percussion. Her ECG shows sinus tachycardia. The chest x-ray is shown in Figure 3–5. The results of CBC, troponin, CK, D-dimer, and a complete metabolic panel are pending.

Your interpretation of this chest x-ray is:

A) Pneumonia.
B) Pneumothorax.
C) Cardiomegaly.
D) Blunted costophrenic angle on the left.
E) Hampton hump and Westermark sign.

Discussion

The correct answer is D. Your patient's chest x-ray findings are not specific for any disease process. There is blunting of the left costophrenic angle, which may be the result of a small pleural effusion. There is no infiltrate, pneumothorax, or enlargement of the heart. Answer E is incorrect. Hampton hump and Westermark sign are chest x-ray findings associated with pulmonary embolus. Hampton hump is a pleural-based, wedge-shaped defect representing a site of pulmonary infarct. Westermark sign is a paucity of pulmonary vascular markings downstream from the embolus.

* *

An ABG on room air shows: pH 7.42, $PaCO_2$ 40 mm Hg, and PaO_2 100 mm Hg.

Because of the results of her ABG, you are able to say:

A) This is clearly not a pulmonary process.
B) Her oxygenation is normal.
C) She is at high risk for PE.
D) She has no risk for PE.

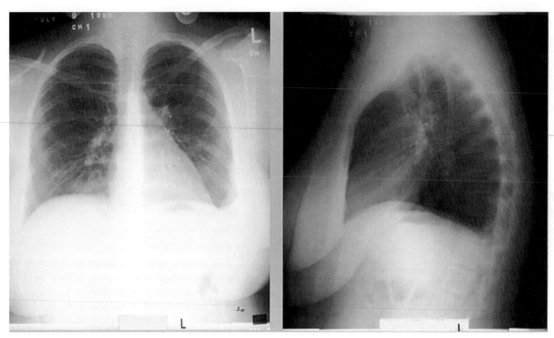

Figure 3–5

Discussion

The correct answer is B. The patient is breathing ambient air with a FiO$_2$ of 21%, and the A-a gradient is about 10 (see calculation of A-a gradient earlier in the chapter), which is normal. With a normal A-a gradient and oxygen saturation, you have good evidence that this patient's overall oxygenation is normal. Answer C is incorrect. Her normal oxygenation reduces her risk of having a PE. However, she is still at some risk for PE; therefore answers A and D are incorrect. Note that normal oxygenation does not rule out PE.

> **HELPFUL TIP:** Only 88% of patients with a PE are hypoxic, 70% have dyspnea or tachypnea, 65% have pleuritic pain, and as low as 30% are tachycardic. You need to have a high clinical suspicion in the right situation despite the lack of the classic triad. To make things worse, the troponin and BNP can be elevated in patients with a PE.

* *

You order nebulized albuterol, and the patient reports slight improvement in her symptoms. As comfort measures, you place her on nasal cannula oxygen and give a dose of acetaminophen. Her blood tests are unremarkable. You go in to reevaluate the patient, and she is now complaining of pain and swelling in the left leg. You confirm that the left calf is tender and edematous, measuring 2 cm more in circumference than the right calf.

Which of the following tests do you order now?

A) Lower extremity Doppler ultrasound.
B) D-dimer.
C) Ventilation/perfusion scan.
D) Chest CT.

Discussion

The correct answer is A. Given the findings consistent with left leg deep venous thrombosis (DVT), your patient is now at a higher risk of having a PE. Your objective is to diagnose a thromboembolic phenomenon—not to confirm PE. In this patient, lower extremity Doppler exam will have the highest yield for diagnosing thrombotic disease. If you find a clot in the leg, you are done. She will require anticoagulation and there is no need to try to prove that she has a PE.

Answer B is incorrect. D-dimer, a degradation product of cross-linked fibrin, is only useful when the clinical suspicion for thromboembolism is low. Remember that it is critical that you know the method being used by your hospital. D-dimer assessed by latex agglutination performs less well than D-dimer by ELISA. Latex agglutination D-dimers have a negative likelihood ratio for DVT of 0.20–0.32 (the range is given because there are several latex agglutination assays). When evaluated for diagnosing PE, the negative likelihood ratio ranges from 0.13–0.36. The ELISA D-dimer tests are more helpful, having DVT negative likelihood ratio ranging from 0.10–0.25 and for PE from 0.07–0.13. Answers C and D are incorrect at this stage of the workup for two reasons. First, you are likely to diagnose DVT with lower extremity Doppler—a less expensive test. Second, a Doppler avoids radiation.

 HELPFUL TIP: The likelihood ratio (LR) is one of the most clinically helpful tools related to diagnostic tests. Simply stated, it is the ratio of likelihoods of a given test result in those with the problem and those without. A LR is a characteristic of a test result that has the power to move you from the pretest probability to the posttest probability. A test result with a LR of 1 means you are no better off after the test than before. On the other had, a LR >10 or <0.1 can move you significantly toward or away from a diagnosis. On the nomogram in Figure 3–6, you can find the posttest probability by placing a straight edge on the pretest probability and the LR, and see where you cross the posttest probability line. Give it a shot with the LRs and your best bet of pretest probability in this case. The LRs above are related to negative test results. With D-dimer testing, a positive test is almost useless clinically, as the positive likelihood ratios range from 1.5 to 2.6.

* *

According to the Doppler, your patient has a clot in the left popliteal, posterior tibialis, and superficial femoral veins with complete occlusion. Because of her abnormal vitals and her status as a dorm-dwelling college student, you decide to admit her.

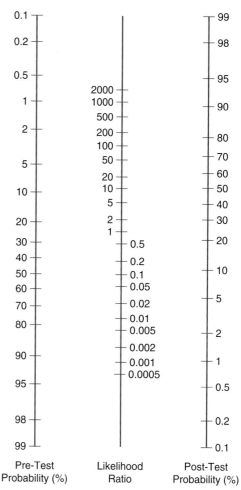

Figure 3–6 **Reproduced from the Centre for Evidence-Based Medicine. Available at http://www.cebm.net**

Which of the following is the most appropriate therapy to initiate?

A) Aspirin.
B) Ibuprofen and cephazolin.
C) Aspirin and warfarin.
D) Low-molecular-weight heparin and warfarin.
E) Unfractionated heparin until therapeutic INR achieved then start warfarin.

Discussion

The correct answer is D. Despite its name, the superficial femoral vein is considered to be in the deep venous system; thus, your patient has a DVT and probably a PE. She must be started on anticoagulant therapy immediately. Subcutaneous low-molecular-weight heparin and intravenous unfractionated heparin are acceptable choices. Answer E is incorrect because heparin does not affect the INR directly. In order to transition to oral medication quickly, your patient should also receive a first dose of warfarin as soon as possible. Treatment with warfarin alone is inappropriate because it will not reach its therapeutic goal for at least 5 days. Aspirin and warfarin are not used in combination to treat DVT or PE.

If she had venous thrombus formation in the superficial veins, she could be treated with aspirin or NSAIDs alone. Superficial thrombophlebitis with cellulitis is treated with NSAIDs and antibiotics. When superficial thrombus is identified and extends above the knee, repeat Doppler examination of the involved extremity in 1 week is recommended due to a high frequency of propagation of the thrombus into the deep venous system.

* *

In your discussion of risk factors, you convince the patient to stop smoking and discontinue her oral contraceptive pill.

All of the following are risk factors for developing DVT and PE, EXCEPT:

A) Hyperlipidemia.
B) Obesity.
C) Heart failure.
D) COPD.
E) Pregnancy.

Discussion

The correct answer is A. Hyperlipidemia is not associated with an increased risk of DVT and PE. The other answer choices are risk factors. In addition to these, all of the following are associated with an increased risk of venous thromboembolism: cancer, stroke, major trauma, surgery (especially orthopedic surgery), tobacco use, bed rest, oral contraceptives and female hormone replacement therapy, hereditary or acquired hypercoagulable states, and a history of previous venous thromboembolism.

* *

At hospital discharge, you review anticoagulation with your patient. Her goal INR will be 2–3.

For your patient, the optimal length of treatment with anticoagulation is:

A) 6 weeks.
B) 6 months.
C) 12 months.

D) Indefinite.
E) Unknown.

Discussion

The correct answer is E. The decision about length of anticoagulation therapy should involve at least three considerations: risk of bleeding, risk of recurrent DVT or PE, and personal and social factors that may contribute to the patient's ability to comply with medical therapy and frequent blood tests. Randomized trials comparing different lengths of therapy have yielded conflicting results, and the optimal duration of therapy is unknown.

Most patients with a first-time diagnosis of DVT or PE should receive warfarin therapy for at least 3 months and more often 6 to 9 months. Patients without an identifiable risk factor (see previous question) may benefit from longer durations of therapy—6 to 12 months. Patients with recurrent venous thromboembolism should be anticoagulated indefinitely. For patients with a modifiable risk factor (eg, smoking, oral contraceptives) who can have this addressed (as in this patient who quits smoking and quits oral contraceptives), 3 to 6 months is probably adequate.

HELPFUL TIP: Warfarin is in no way "protective." Once it is stopped, the patient goes back to his or her pretreatment risk of recurrent thromboembolic event; thus, the need for lifelong therapy in patients with more than one thromboembolic event.

HELPFUL TIP: Provide graduated compression stockings for patients after a DVT to help prevent postphlebitic syndrome. The preponderance of evidence suggests that stocking use after a symptomatic DVT reduces the risk of postphlebitic syndrome—but not the risk of recurrent DVT.

* *

Your patient does well, completes her course of warfarin, and has no further episodes over the next 2 years. She develops gallstones and plans to have an elective laparoscopic cholecystectomy. A surgeon colleague sends her back to see you for a preoperative evaluation. You find no evidence of cardiac, pulmonary, or hematologic disease. She is no longer on warfarin and is doing well.

Which of the following postoperative management strategies do you recommend?

A) Aspirin 81 mg PO daily.
B) Warfarin 5 mg PO daily.
C) Unfractionated heparin 5,000 units subcutaneously daily.
D) Enoxaparin 40 mg subcutaneously daily.
E) No antiplatelet or anticoagulant drugs.

Discussion

The correct answer is D. Even for a relatively minor surgical procedure, where anesthesia is used for 30 minutes or less and the postoperative recovery is usually quick, your patient is at moderate risk for venous thromboembolism. Her history of DVT and presumed PE put her in a higher risk category, and she requires prophylaxis. Of the choices available, enoxaparin would be the most appropriate. Low-molecular-weight and unfractionated heparin are both acceptable for prevention of DVT and PE in the postoperative period. Studies have shown that low-molecular-weight heparin has efficacy equal to or greater than unfractionated heparin. Additionally, unfractionated heparin must be dosed every 8–12 hours, rather than once a day. Thus, answer C is incorrect. Answer A is incorrect. Aspirin is sometimes used postoperatively, but the dose should be 160 mg per day or greater. Also, in comparison with heparin and its derivatives, aspirin is less efficacious in the prevention of thrombus. Answer B is incorrect. Warfarin alone is not appropriate in this setting due to its extended onset of action.

The optimal length of time that patients require prophylaxis for venous thromboembolism after surgery is not known. Arguments can be made for prophylaxis until the patient is ambulating several hundred feet per day.

Objectives: Did you learn to . . .

- Evaluate a patient with pleuritic chest pain?
- Interpret a normal ABG in the setting of chest pain?
- Identify patients in the emergency department at risk for PE?

- Diagnose and treat DVT/PE?
- Interpret test results using likelihood ratios to move you from the pretest probability to posttest probability?
- Identify patients at risk for developing DVT/PE in the perioperative setting?
- Prevent DVT/PE in the perioperative setting?

 QUICK QUIZ: PULMONARY EMBOLISM

In a patient with a low clinical probability of PE and normal or low-probability V/Q scan, what is the probability that the patient actually has a PE?

A) 0%.
B) 2% to 4%.
C) 9% to 13%.
D) 20% to 24%.
E) >50%.

Discussion

The correct answer is B. You might consider using your own estimates in the likelihood ratio chart in Figure 3–6. A patient with a low clinical probability of PE and a normal or low-risk V/Q scan has about a 2% to 4% risk of having a PE. A patient with a **high** clinical probability and a **high**-probability V/Q scan has a 96% to 98% chance of having a PE (eg, 2% to 4% of patients we treat will not have had a PE).

 QUICK QUIZ: PULMONARY EMBOLISM

The best initial step to take in a patient who is hypotensive from a PE is to:

A) Begin pressors such as dopamine.
B) Begin a thrombolytic.
C) Increase fluids.
D) Decrease fluids because of the risk of CHF after a PE.
E) A and D.

Discussion

The correct answer is C. The best thing to do for a hypotensive patient with a PE is to increase IV fluids (ie, give a bolus). This is because hypotension in the setting of a PE is likely due to right heart failure. The pulmonary vascular pressure is increased and the right heart needs additional preload to compensate. Answer A is incorrect because pressors are not the best choice in this circumstance. They will increase blood pressure a bit but do nothing to correct the hemodynamic problem. Answer B is incorrect. Providing thrombolytics is not the first thing you would do. Thrombolytics have a very spotty record in treating massive PE, with some studies showing an increase in mortality.

QUICK QUIZ: PULMONARY EMBOLISM

Which of the following is true about the diagnosis of PE?

A) While not sensitive, findings on ECG are specific for PE if they are present.
B) The majority of patients with PE will have a "Hampton hump" on the chest radiograph.
C) V/Q scan is most useful for patients who have a completely normal chest radiograph.
D) It is rare to misdiagnose a PE.
E) The mortality rate of PE in all comers is approximately 30%.

Discussion
The correct answer is C. V/Q scan is the most useful in patients who have a normal or near normal chest radiograph. A V/Q scan is less likely to be diagnostic in a patient with metastatic cancer, multiple infiltrates, severe COPD, etc. This does not make it useless, just less helpful. Answer A is incorrect. The most common findings on ECG are nonspecific ST-T changes. The reason to do an ECG on patients in whom PE is suspected is to rule out other causes of chest pain. The ECG is neither sensitive nor specific enough to rule in or rule out PE. Answer B is incorrect. The chest radiograph may be normal with a PE and is generally nondiagnostic. Additionally, if PE is suspected, your workup should proceed regardless of the chest x-ray results. Answer D is incorrect because it is thought that most PEs are undetected. Are they clinically significant? Probably not. But the next piece that breaks off might be. Answer E is incorrect because the overall mortality from a PE is about 15%, not 30%.

HELPFUL TIP: Pulmonary angiography is the traditional gold standard for diagnosing PE. However, emerging evidence suggests that clinically significant PEs will be diagnosed with proper utilization of clinical, laboratory, and CT diagnostic strategies.

HELPFUL TIP: In patients with recurrent venous thromboembolism or an idiopathic (no identifiable risk factors) initial venous thromboembolism, you may consider an evaluation for a hypercoagulable state. Minimal initial evaluation includes CBC, activated partial thromboplastin time, and prothrombin time. Additional tests for hypercoagulable state: factor V Leiden mutation, prothrombin gene mutation, protein C and S deficiency, antiphospholipid antibodies, antithrombin III deficiency, and hyperhomocystinemia. **The greatest risk for having a second PE/DVT is having a first PE/DVT.** Finding a hypercoagulable state does not change the risk of a second event beyond the risk posed by an idiopathic first event.

CASE 13

While you are covering the ED, a 60-year-old female comes in by ambulance. She is unresponsive, and her husband states that he found her 30 minutes ago surrounded by bottles of pills and an empty bottle of vodka. She has a history of COPD, hypertension, osteoarthritis, and depression. The EMTs brought in her pill bottles, which include lorazepam, acetaminophen/hydrocodone, hydrochlorothiazide, aspirin, and nortriptyline. Only a few tablets are left in the bottle of hydrochlorothiazide. She is wearing a nonrebreather face mask with 50% oxygen. Her respirations are shallow with a rate of 8. The remainder of her vitals: temperature 36°C, blood pressure 90/50, and pulse 90. Oxygen saturation is 88% and increases to 94% with some assisted breaths. One nurse is obtaining a blood gas while another gives naloxone. You decide that this patient cannot protect her airway and choose to intubate her. You estimate her weight at 70 kg.

The respiratory technician asks for initial ventilator settings. You decide on the following:

A) Rate 20/min, FiO$_2$ 30%, tidal volume 500 mL.
B) Rate 14/min, FiO$_2$ 100%, tidal volume 700 mL.
C) Rate 10/min, FiO$_2$ 100%, tidal volume 200 mL.
D) Rate 14/min, FiO$_2$ 40%, tidal volume 1000 mL.

Discussion
The correct answer is B. You know very little about this patient, including her blood gases. A safe strategy is to

start with routine initial ventilator settings and observe her response. You can obtain a blood gas now and another after she has been on the ventilator for 5–10 minutes. Generally, O_2 saturation and CO_2 equilibrate in 3–5 minutes in patients with appropriate lung function (witness how quickly patients in the ED increase their oxygen saturations when you put on a couple of liters of oxygen by nasal cannula). A rate of 14 is close to the physiologic normal. FiO_2 of 100% is used to ensure adequate oxygenation, but it should be reduced quickly to avoid oxygen toxicity while still maintaining the patient's arterial oxygenation. Initial tidal volume is estimated based on the patient's weight: 8–10 mL/kg, which would be 560–700 mL in this 70-kg woman (keep in mind that if patients have acute lung injury, lung protective ventilation strategies use tidal volume of 6 mL/kg to improve outcomes).

> **HELPFUL TIP:** Ventilated patients with obstructive disease generally need more time for exhalation.

**

The blood gas drawn just before intubation shows pH 7.16, $PaCO_2$ 60 mm Hg, PaO_2 40 mm Hg.

These findings imply which of the following processes?

A) Metabolic acidosis.
B) Metabolic alkalosis.
C) Respiratory alkalosis.
D) Mixed metabolic/respiratory acidosis.
E) Mixed metabolic/respiratory alkalosis.

Discussion
The correct answer is D. The pH is acidotic. In a patient whose baseline $PaCO_2$ is not known to you, you might assume her $PaCO_2$ is usually 40 mm Hg, which is the accepted normal for most patients. If this is true and the acidosis is purely due to acute respiratory changes, a rise in $PaCO_2$ should be accompanied by a fall in pH equal to 0.008 × (change in $PaCO_2$ from baseline) = 0.008 × 20 = 0.16, resulting in a pH of 7.24. However, this patient's pH is measured at 7.16, lower than expected for a pure respiratory acidosis presenting acutely. Thus, you can determine that the acidosis is both metabolic and respiratory in nature. Indeed, one of the medications she may have taken in her overdose

includes aspirin, a salicylate that can cause a metabolic acidosis.

**

Your patient is on assist-control mode of ventilation. A nasogastric tube, 2 IVs, and a bladder catheter are in place. Gastric lavage yielded no pill fragments, and she has received activated charcoal. She was given IV N-acetylcysteine. Her blood pressure has improved to 112/67, and her oxygen saturation is 99%. Her chest x-ray shows an endotracheal tube terminating 3 cm above the carina and no infiltrates. Thirty minutes after you intubated her, with the ventilator rate at 14 breaths/min, FiO_2 100%, and tidal volume at 700 mL, you obtain another ABG: pH 7.35, $PaCO_2$ 45, PaO_2 130. She takes 6–8 spontaneous, assisted breaths, while the ventilator provides the remaining breaths. She appears to be perfusing her periphery well.

It turns out that the patient did not take a tricyclic overdose. Her main problems are the alcohol, acetaminophen, and narcotics.

Your next action is to:

A) Decrease the tidal volume to allow for permissive hypercapnia.
B) Increase the tidal volume to achieve a pH of 7.45–7.50.
C) Reduce FiO_2 while maintaining oxygen saturations >90%.
D) Change to pressure support ventilation.

Discussion
The correct answer is C. Your patient is perfusing well, and her PaO_2 and measured oxygen saturation are much improved. You should now decrease the FiO_2, with the goal being to achieve a FiO_2 of less than 60% while maintaining adequate perfusion and oxygen saturation. Answer A is incorrect. However, permissive hypercapnia (the CO_2 may be allowed to rise to >80 mm Hg as long as the patient tolerates it) may be useful in ventilated patients with ARDS or asthma. Allowing the CO_2 to rise allows you to reduce the ventilator's volume and pressure settings. This reduces the risk of barotrauma. But remember that you still need to maintain oxygenation. Contraindications to the use of permissive hypercapnia include cerebrovascular disease, hemodynamic instability, seizures, and cardiac arrhythmias. Answer B is incorrect. Your patient is doing reasonably well with her slightly acidotic pH, which has corrected very quickly. It may be inadvisable to attempt

to increase her pH beyond 7.40, as she may develop respiratory alkalosis that can then lead to cardiac arrhythmias. Because of her low respiratory rate, she should remain on some type of assisted volume-cycled ventilation. Pressure support ventilation, as its name implies, only augments patient-triggered breaths with increased airway pressure.

In this patient, which of the following ventilator management techniques will unequivocally decrease her FiO$_2$ requirement?

A) Increase the respiratory rate.
B) Increase the positive end expiratory pressure (PEEP).
C) Decrease the tidal volume.
D) Addition of inhaled nitric oxide (NO).

Discussion

The correct answer is B. Two standard techniques are usually employed to improve a patient's oxygenation: increasing FiO$_2$ and increasing PEEP. PEEP maintains positive pressure in the airways at the end of expiration. Its use increases lung compliance and decreases ventilation/perfusion mismatching, resulting in better oxygenation. Since FiO$_2$ >60% over periods longer than 48 hours may result in oxygen toxicity, PEEP may be employed to reduce the need for high levels of FiO$_2$. Low levels of PEEP are useful in patients with COPD to prevent airway collapse. High levels of PEEP can cause barotrauma, and patients on large amounts of PEEP must be weaned carefully. Answers A and C are incorrect. Increasing respiratory rate or tidal volume will cause increases in minute ventilation, which reduces PaCO$_2$, but has little affect on PaO$_2$. Decreasing minute ventilation, through decreased respiratory rate or tidal volume, causes CO$_2$ retention and increased PaCO$_2$. Answer D is incorrect. Nitric oxide has been shown to improve oxygenation in select patients with severe pulmonary hypertension and ARDS, but its use is not appropriate in this patient.

* *

You follow the patient during her hospitalization. The next day she is more alert and is able to follow commands. Her ventilator requirements have decreased. You consider extubation.

All of the following parameters predict a poor outcome for attempted weaning from ventilation EXCEPT:

A) Minute ventilation supplied by ventilator is <10 L/min.
B) PaO$_2$ <55 mm Hg with FiO$_2$ >35%.
C) Frequency of breaths to tidal volume ratio >100 breaths/min/L.
D) Physical exam findings of increased respiratory effort.

Discussion

The correct answer is A. Preparing to withdraw a patient from mechanical ventilation—typically called weaning or liberation—relies considerably on physician judgment, but a few objective parameters can be helpful. In general, the patient to be liberated must be awake, alert, and cooperative. She should have reasonably good oxygenation on a lower FiO$_2$, have PEEP <8 cm H$_2$O, and be able to generate adequate inspiratory pressures. Minute ventilation from the ventilator of <10 L/min is associated with greater success with weaning.

Poor prognostic indicators include a minute ventilation from the ventilator >10 L/min, PaO$_2$ <55 with FiO$_2$ >35%, breath frequency/tidal volume (in liters) >100 breaths/min/L, and signs of increased respiratory effort (eg, nasal flaring, accessory muscle use). Patients with poor cardiopulmonary reserve or who have significant underlying disease may also have difficulty weaning. Allow patients a period of breathing on their own (eg, a T-piece) before extubating. This way, if the patient fails, you can simply hook her back up to the ventilator.

 HELPFUL TIP: Minute ventilation (for the patient) is calculated by multiplying respiratory rate by tidal volume. Thus, a person getting 12 breaths/minute from the ventilator at 700 mL/breath generates a minute ventilation = 12 × 700 = 8.4 L/min.

Objectives: Did you learn to . . .

- Identify patients in need of intubation and mechanical ventilation?
- Recognize a mixed respiratory/metabolic acidosis?
- Calculate expected pH changes in acute respiratory acidosis?
- Institute ventilation with appropriate initial ventilator settings?

- Identify potential complications of ventilation?
- Wean a patient from the ventilator?

CASE 14

A 52-year-old male smoker presents for a 3-month history of productive cough. He reports multiple episodes of pneumonia and continues to produce copious amounts of purulent sputum. Chest x-ray is unremarkable. Chest CT shows enlarged peripheral airways with thickened airway walls in the lower lobes bilaterally. Sputum culture grows several types of bacteria, including *Pseudomonas aeruginosa*.

Which of the following do you recommend as initial therapy?

A) Prolonged oral corticosteroids.
B) Prolonged antibiotics.
C) Chemotherapy.
D) Supplemental oxygen.
E) Wedge resection of the affected lung tissue.

Discussion

The correct answer is B. This patient's findings are consistent with the diagnosis of bronchiectasis, a chronic inflammatory disease of the medium-sized bronchi. Appropriate initial therapy consists of prolonged courses of antibiotics, up to 6 months at a time. Doxycycline, amoxicillin/clavulanate, and trimethoprim/sulfamethoxazole are often used. Respiratory quinolones demonstrate some limited use in patients with *Pseudomonas*. Patients should be directed to discontinue tobacco use and take inhaled bronchodilators. Resection of the affected lung tissue may be necessary, but should not be the initial therapy. Supplemental oxygen therapy is used if oxygenation is poor. Chemotherapy and prolonged oral corticosteroids are not used to treat bronchiectasis.

 HELPFUL TIP: Patients with bronchiectasis are often treated with intermittent or daily antibiotics to prevent acute exacerbations. One regimen is to alternate between trimethoprim/sulfamethoxazole and doxycycline, taking one of these antibiotics for the first 10–14 days of the month.

In most adults who have bronchiectasis, its cause is:

A) Genetic.
B) *Pseudomonas* infection.
C) Tobacco smoking.
D) Allergic bronchopulmonary aspergillosis (ABPA).
E) Unknown.

Discussion

The correct answer is E. There are limited data regarding the etiology of bronchiectasis, but many conditions and environmental exposures seem to have an association. In most patients, no cause is identified. Children are more likely than adults to have an identified etiology of their bronchiectasis, and the most common causes in children are foreign-body aspiration, cystic fibrosis, and gastroesophageal reflux. Identified etiologies in adults include those mentioned for children and pulmonary infections, ABPA, COPD, rheumatic diseases, and cigarette smoking.

Objectives: Did you learn to . . .

- Identify findings consistent with bronchiectasis?
- Treat a patient with bronchiectasis?

 QUICK QUIZ: DYSPNEA

A 75-year-old male presents to your office with emphysema diagnosed elsewhere. He reports dyspnea on exertion after 1–2 blocks. He smokes 10 cigarettes per day and does not have underlying cardiac disease. Physical examination is remarkable for fine crackles in both lung bases. You review his chest x-ray (Figure 3–7). He has no pulmonary function testing on record.

Of the following tests, which is the most likely to confirm or alter the diagnosis?

A) Spirometry, diffusing capacity, lung volumes.
B) Spirometry, arterial blood gas, diffusing capacity.
C) Arterial blood gas, diffusing capacity, lung volumes.
D) Arterial blood gas, lung volumes, chest CT.

Discussion

The correct answer is A. This case demonstrates a commonly seen phenomenon: patients who smoke and have dyspnea are assumed to have obstructive lung disease, particularly emphysema. However, pulmonary function tests are required to make the diagnosis of

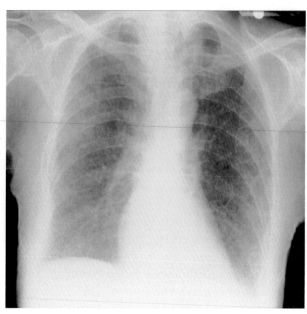

Figure 3–7

Which of the following assessment of this patient's lung disease is most accurate?

A) Severe obstructive disease, with hyperinflation and air trapping, and a compensated respiratory acidosis.

B) Moderate obstructive disease, hyperinflation and air trapping, and a compensated respiratory acidosis.

C) Restrictive pattern, decreased diffusing capacity, and compensated respiratory acidosis.

D) Severe obstructive disease, with hyperinflation and air trapping, and respiratory acidosis without metabolic compensation.

Discussion

The correct answer is A. This patient has an obstructive pattern on spirometry—FEV_1 is severely diminished. Obstructive lung disease is graded on a mild-moderate-severe scale. FEV_1 65%–80% is mild, FEV_1 50%–65% is moderate, and FEV_1 <50% is severe obstruction. Hyperinflation and air trapping are typical of obstructive lung disease and are manifested by an elevated residual volume on pulmonary function testing. A residual volume (RV) of >135% is considered abnormal and represents air trapping. An elevated TLC of >120% defines hyperinflation. The diffusing capacity, as measured by DLCO, is low in the following disease states: emphysema (as in this patient), interstitial lung disease (eg, sarcoid, alveolitis, pulmonary radiation, pulmonary toxicity from drugs such as amiodarone, pulmonary fibrosis), Pneumocystis pneumonia, and pulmonary vascular disease. Anemia will also cause a low DLCO—so a hemoglobin or hematocrit should always be ordered with DLCO.

obstructive disease. Furthermore, this patient's chest x-ray shows increased interstitial markings in the lower lung fields, which point to another disease process. Based on the chest x-ray, interstitial lung disease seems likely. This disease process is associated with a restrictive pattern on pulmonary spirometry. Lung volumes and diffusing capacity will provide a more complete picture. In interstitial lung disease, spirometry shows a FEV_1/FVC ratio >0.7, a decreased diffusing capacity, and decreased total lung capacity (the hallmark of restrictive lung disease). Answers B through D are incorrect because arterial blood gas is unlikely to help diagnose restrictive lung disease.

QUICK QUIZ: SPIROMETRY

A 63-year-old female smoker is scheduled to see you in clinic tomorrow. You are reviewing her chart and find a report of pulmonary function tests from last year when she was in her usual (but poor) state of health. Results show an FEV_1 of 0.57 L (29% predicted), FVC 2.64 L (88%), FEV_1/FVC =0.21, DLCO 33%, total lung capacity 140% predicted, residual volume 180% predicted. Arterial blood gas on room air reveals pH 7.35, PCO_2 55 mm Hg, PO_2 59 mm Hg, and HCO_3 30.

> **HELPFUL TIP:** DLCO can be increased by pulmonary hemorrhage, polycythemia, massive obesity, left-to-right intracardiac shunting, asthma, left heart failure (increase capillary volume in the lungs).

QUICK QUIZ: PULMONARY INFECTIONS

A 72-year-old woman you admitted to the hospital for pneumonia is having worsening dyspnea and hypoxia. She is decompensating despite 3 days of antibiotic therapy with intravenous levofloxacin (since levofloxacin achieves the same blood levels orally as IV, the Medicare police will soon be after you). According to her husband, the couple had been working on their Iowa farm, and made a trip to an old barn to collect manure a week before the patient developed a cough and fever. The barn was noted to be the home of numerous birds. Her respiratory rate is 32, and her oxygen saturation is 89% on 5 L/min of oxygen by nasal cannula. Chest x-ray reveals a diffuse interstitial infiltrate, enlarged mediastinal nodes, and normal heart size.

Which of the following is the most likely culprit for the cause of her current illness?

A) *Streptococcus pneumoniae.*
B) *Haemophilus influenzae.*
C) *Coxiella burnetii.*
D) *Histoplasma capsulatum.*
E) *Blastomyces dermatiditis.*

Discussion

The correct answer is D. The case described here is classic for an environmental exposure to a large dose of *Histoplasma* organisms. *Histoplasma* occurs most commonly in the Mississippi and Ohio River valleys, causing a self-limited disease in most individuals. Patients who have *Histoplasma* infection frequently develop calcified mediastinal lymph nodes after resolution of the infection. Diagnosis can be made by urinary antigen or bronchoscopic biopsy. The bacterial causes are unlikely to be important factors here, as she was on a broad-spectrum antibiotic for 3 days with no improvement. *Coxiella burnetii*, the agent causing Q fever, is rare and tends to affect workers exposed to fresh animal material, such as placentas. *Blastomyces* is found in the same regions as *Histoplasma*, but the site of exposure tends to be more moist, unlike the dry environment inside a barn.

CASE 15

A 42-year-old female comes to your office with a history of asthma that has been difficult to control. She relates symptoms that have been worsening over the last 4–6 weeks. She received two courses of oral corticosteroids during that time. Her symptoms improved with this therapy but quickly returned after completing the steroids. She denies fever, chills and night sweats, but complains of a **chronic cough productive of brownish-colored sputum**. Her review of systems is otherwise negative. She is a homemaker in a suburban area and has no pets. Physical examination reveals wheezing throughout all lung fields, but is otherwise within normal limits. Spirometry values are decreased from her baseline. Laboratory evaluation includes normal CBC (aside from a very few eosinophils), normal C-reactive protein, and an elevated IgE level of 1,250 ng/mL. A high-resolution CT scan of the chest reveals central bronchiectasis.

What is the most likely diagnosis?

A) Hypersensitivity pneumonitis.
B) Acute eosinophilic pneumonia.
C) Allergic bronchopulmonary aspergillosis.
D) Bacterial pneumonia.
E) Churg-Strauss vasculitis.

Discussion

The correct answer is C. This patient's history points to the diagnosis of allergic bronchopulmonary aspergillosis (ABPA), which is characterized by the presence of severe asthma, brownish mucus plugs, peripheral eosinophilia, elevated serum IgE, and central bronchiectasis. Answer A is incorrect but a bit tricky. First, there is no history of exposure to a causative agent. Second, let's focus on symptoms. Constitutional symptoms are present in the acute form of hypersensitivity pneumonitis (eg, fever). However, they need not be present in the subacute and chronic forms of the disease. So, based on symptoms, this could be hypersensitivity pneumonitis. However, the radiologic findings of hypersensitivity pneumonitis would include interstitial lung disease, rather than central bronchiectasis. Therefore, this is not likely hypersensitivity pneumonitis. Answers B and D are incorrect. Note that she has no significant constitutional symptoms that might be more typical of acute eosinophilic pneumonia or bacterial infection. You would also expect an infiltrate on the chest CT. Answer E is incorrect. Churg-Strauss vasculitis is characterized by transient patchy interstitial infiltrates, fever, weight loss, elevated sedimentation rate, abnormal liver enzymes, and a peripheral blood eosinophilia >1,000/micrograms/L. Remember that this patient has a normal CBC. Extrapulmonary manifestations distinguish this entity from other eosinophilic conditions.

Which of the following would be the next best step in confirming the diagnosis?

A) Sputum cultures.
B) Transbronchial biopsy.
C) Methacholine challenge.
D) Allergy skin testing for *Aspergillus* species.
E) p-ANCA.

Discussion

The correct answer is D. Most, but not all of the following criteria need to be present in order to make the diagnosis of ABPA (Table 3–9). Transbronchial biopsy is unnecessarily invasive, and the other tests will not help to confirm the diagnosis.

The most appropriate treatment would include which of the following?

A) Antibiotics.
B) Oral corticosteroids.
C) Leukotriene receptor antagonist.
D) Levalbuterol.
E) Inhaled ipratropium bromide.

Discussion

The correct answer is B. Oral corticosteroids are the treatment of choice for ABPA. Patients are typically treated for several months with tapering doses rather than short courses of steroids. Serum IgE levels and chest x-rays are used to monitor response to treatment.

QUICK QUIZ: ASTHMA

A 24-year-old women with asthma notes shortness of breath and daily wheezing. She requires the use of an inhaled β$_2$-agonist 1–2 times per day. On physical exam she appears comfortable and in no acute distress. **This patient has no production of chronic, brown sputum (in contrast to the case above).** On skin testing, this patient had positive results to several mold species.

Which of the following would be most likely associated with a severe asthma exacerbation in this patient?

A) *Alternaria.*
B) *Helminthosporium.*
C) *Aspergillus.*
D) *Epicoccum.*
E) *Cladosporium.*

Discussion

The correct answer is A. Airborne fungal spores have been implicated in causing asthma exacerbations, especially during the summer and fall seasons. Several studies have shown a relationship between severe asthma attacks and sensitivity to the mold species, *Alternaria alternata*. Although *Aspergillus fumigatus* is a key factor in the pathogenesis of allergic bronchopulmonary aspergillosis, it has not been commonly implicated in causing severe asthma exacerbations. Appropriate treatment is inhaled steroids.

Objectives: Did you learn to . . .

- Identify the clinical presentation of allergic bronchopulmonary aspergillosis?
- Diagnose and treat a patient with allergic bronchopulmonary aspergillosis?

CASE 16

A 16-year-old female comes to your office with complaints of sneezing spells, itchy watery eyes, and nasal congestion for the past 2 years. These symptoms are worse during the spring and fall and when she plays with her cat. She denies any other constitutional symptoms and has no other past medical history. She has tried over-the-counter loratadine without relief. She has lived in the same residence for the past 6 years and denies any other environmental exposures.

Her examination reveals pale nasal mucosa and swollen nasal turbinates bilaterally. Her lungs and skin are clear. You are not certain if this is allergic or vasomotor rhinitis.

The most effective way to determine if this is allergic is to:

Table 3–9   CRITERIA FOR THE DIAGNOSIS OF ALLERGIC BRONCHOPULMONARY ASPERGILLOSIS (ABPA)

- Asthma
- Central bronchiectasis
- Elevated total serum IgE
- Immediate skin test reactivity to *Aspergillus*
- Elevated serum specific IgE and/or IgG to *Aspergillus fumigatus*
- Peripheral blood eosinophilia
- Pulmonary infiltrates

A) Do a methacholine challenge test.
B) Do a Hansel stain of nasal mucus.
C) Check overall IgG levels.
D) Perform a nasal mucus electrophoresis to visualize allergic bands.

Discussion

The correct answer is B. The best way to determine if this is allergic is to do a Hansel stain of the nasal mucous. This will show eosinophils if it is allergic. If this is vasomotor rhinitis, eosinophils will be absent. Answer A is incorrect. A methacholine challenge test is helpful in diagnosing asthma, not allergic rhinitis. Answers C, IgG levels, and D, nasal mucus electrophoresis, are incorrect because they have no use here.

Which of the following would be the MOST APPROPRIATE next step in managing her symptoms?

A) Recommend allergen-impermeable encasements for mattress and pillow.
B) Use topical decongestant sprays.
C) Change classes of antihistamines.
D) Refer for allergy evaluation, including percutaneous aeroallergen skin testing.
E) Recommend a HEPA air filter for the home.

Discussion

The correct answer is C. Although all of the above answer choices may provide relief for allergic symptoms, the most appropriate would be to change the class of antihistamines. Antihistamines (and NSAIDs) are grouped into classes based on chemical structure. One class may be helpful for a patient when another class does not work.

The other answer choices are suboptimal. Without skin testing, avoidance measures may be needless, costly, and ineffective. Allergen-impermeable encasements are currently recommended for patients with dust mite allergy. Although filters are often recommended for pet allergies, there has been controversial data regarding their effectiveness in reducing allergic symptoms. Topical decongestant sprays are an inappropriate choice secondary to the addictive nature of these medications and the risk of causing rebound symptoms. Removing a pet from the bedroom may reduce—but not eliminate—allergen exposure. Further evaluation should be performed prior to recommending any such lifestyle modifications.

BIBLIOGRAPHY

Cahill K, Stead L, Lancaster T. Nicotine receptor partial agonists for smoking cessation. *Cochrane Database Syst Rev.* 2007;24(1):CD006103.

Centers for Disease Control and Prevention. Antiviral Agents for Seasonal Influenza: Information for Health Professionals. Accessed October 31, 2007, at http://www.cdc.gov/flu/professionals/antivirals/index.htm.

Centre for Evidence-Based Medicine. http://www.cebm.net

Gravenstein S, Davidson HE. Current strategies for management of influenza in the elderly population. *Clin Infect Dis.* 2002;35:729.

Irwin RS, Madison MJ. The diagnosis and treatment of cough. *N Engl J Med.* 2000;343(23):1715.

Laszlo G. Standardisation of lung function testing: helpful guidance from the ATS/ERS Task Force. *Thorax.* 2006;61:744.

Mandell LA, et al. Infectious Diseases Society of America/American Thoracic Society consensus guidelines on the management of community-acquired pneumonia in adults. *Clin Infect Dis.* 2007;1(44)suppl2:S27.

Marik PE. Aspiration pneumonitis and aspiration pneumonia. *N Engl J Med.* 2001;344(9):665.

National Asthma Education and Prevention Program, Expert Panel Report 3. Guidelines for the diagnosis and management of asthma. 2007. Accessed October 31, 2007, at http://www.nhlbi.nih.gov/guidelines/asthma/asthsumm.pdf.

Naureckas ET, Solway J. Mild asthma. *N Eng J Med.* 2001;345(17):1257.

Ost D, Fein AM, Feinsilver SH. The solitary pulmonary nodule. *N Eng J Med.* 2003;348(25):2535.

Rabe KF, Hurd S, Anzueto A, et al. Global strategies for the diagnosis, management, and prevention of chronic obstructive pulmonary disease: GOLD executive summary. *Am J Respir Crit Care Med.* 2007;176(6):532.

Shanthi P, Jones P. Corticosteroid therapy in pulmonary sarcoidosis: a systematic review. *JAMA.* 2002;287(10):1301.

Swenson SJ, et al. CT screening for lung cancer: five-year prospective experience. *Radiology.* 2005;235:259.

Van Belle, et al (for the Christopher Study Investigators). Effectiveness of managing suspected pulmonary embolism using an algorithm combining clinical probability, D-dimer testing, and computed tomotraphy. *JAMA.* 2006;295(2):172.

4
Allergy and Immunology

Mark A. Graber

CASE 1

A 15-year-old girl has a history of acute difficulty breathing when playing basketball. Her symptoms include **inspiratory** wheezing, increased respiratory rate, throat tightness, and chest discomfort. Premedication with adequate doses of albuterol has minimal effect.

What is the most likely diagnosis?

A) Exercise-induced asthma.
B) Gastroesophageal reflux disease.
C) Musculoskeletal chest pain.
D) Hyperventilation.
E) Vocal cord dysfunction.

Discussion

The correct answer is E. Vocal cord dysfunction (VCD) is one of the most common asthma mimics. Patients with VCD present with hoarseness, coughing, dyspnea, and loud **inspiratory wheezing**, along with other symptoms mentioned above. Pulmonary function testing indicates airway obstruction due to an extrathoracic component. Paradoxical inspiratory vocal cord adduction causes airflow restriction at the level of the larynx, thereby resulting in a flattened inspiratory loop on flow-volume diagram. VCD presents a diagnostic challenge, and often leads to unnecessary treatment for asthma. In this patient, a β_2-agonist was ineffective, even though she displays symptoms with exertion. Answer A is incorrect. The distinction between VCD and asthma may be less clear in other patients because the two disorders sometimes coexist. Answers B, C, and D are incorrect. The clinical history does not support

the diagnoses of gastroesophageal reflux disease, musculoskeletal chest pain, or hyperventilation.

* *

You make the diagnosis of VCD. However, the patient also complains of rhinorrhea, itchy eyes, sneezing, and itchy nose. Because you realize that we need to discuss this in this book, you refer her for allergy testing.

With regards to RAST (radioallergosorbent testing) for allergic rhinitis, which of the following is true?

A) RAST is less expensive than traditional skin testing.
B) RAST is more sensitive than traditional skin testing.
C) RAST has a limited role in testing those with allergic rhinitis
D) Antihistamine use is a contraindication to the use of RAST.

Discussion

The correct answer is C. RAST will be negative in up to 25% of those with a positive skin test, has poorly reproducible results, and is more expensive. Thus, skin testing remains the procedure of choice for identifying allergens. RAST can be used if skin testing is unavailable.

Which of the following medications does NOT need to be discontinued prior to aeroallergen skin testing?

A) Intranasal steroid spray.
B) Atenolol.
C) Amitriptyline.

D) Cyproheptadine.

E) Azelastine nasal spray.

Discussion

The correct answer is A. Intranasal steroid sprays do not need to be discontinued prior to skin testing as they do not interfere with immediate-type hypersensitivity reactions. They are not antihistaminic in nature, as opposed to amitriptyline, cyproheptadine, and azelastine, which may all blunt dermal reactivity. Although azelastine is administered as a nasal spray, its administration may interfere with skin test reactivity within 2 days of usage. β-Blockers, such as atenolol, have been shown to affect skin test reactivity and should be avoided in patients undergoing skin testing.

* *

Aeroallergen skin prick and intradermal testing reveals positive reactions to dust mites, cats, ragweed pollen, and tree pollens. The patient relates that she gets considerable nasal congestion and has tried over-the-counter decongestants with no relief.

Which of the following interventions would provide the most relief for her nasal symptoms?

A) Diphenhydramine 25 mg PO BID.

B) Nasal saline irrigations BID.

C) Montelukast 10 mg PO QHS.

D) Intranasal steroid spray daily.

E) Ipratropium bromide nasal spray BID.

Discussion

The correct answer is D. Intranasal corticosteroids would provide the most relief in this patient by addressing nasal congestion in addition to the other nasal symptoms mentioned. Although antihistamines (answer A) are very helpful in relieving nasal symptoms such as rhinorrhea, nasal itching, and sneezing, they are generally not as effective for nasal congestion. Likewise, montelukast (answer C) is a leukotriene modifier which is approved for treatment of allergic rhinitis, but studies suggest that intranasal steroids are superior. Additionally, nasal steroids are nonsystemic (although a bit may be absorbed). Ipratropium (answer E) is mainly effective for rhinorrhea only, while nasal saline irrigations (answer B) promote thinning of nasal secretions and drainage, but neither predictably improves nasal congestion.

 HELPFUL (AND REALLY COOL) TIP: Nasal steroids also seem to improve ocular symptoms. Whether some of the drug gets up the nasolacrimal ducts or is otherwise aerosolized into the eye is unclear. But it works equally for all nasal steroids. Obviously, do not put nasal steroids directly in the eye.

* *

The patient returns to you 1 year later, having tried intranasal steroid sprays and high-dose antihistamines, without gaining significant relief. She has instituted appropriate avoidance measures during the interim, also without improvement in symptoms. You recommend allergen immunotherapy.

All of the following statements are true regarding allergen immunotherapy EXCEPT:

A) Patients should carry emergency epinephrine to all immunotherapy shot appointments.

B) It is unnecessary to stop β-blocker therapy prior to starting immunotherapy.

C) Patients should be observed in the office for at least 30 minutes after immunotherapy injections.

D) At least 3 years of immunotherapy should be given to avoid recurrence of symptoms.

Discussion

The correct answer is B. It has been shown that patients taking β-blockers may be at increased risk of having more severe systemic reactions to immunotherapy, because these medications attenuate the response to epinephrine. Patients should be treated with an alternative antihypertensive during immunotherapy. The rest of the answer choices are true. The current practice parameters for allergen immunotherapy recommend that emergency epinephrine should be readily available for treatment of systemic allergic reactions associated with immunotherapy (answer A). To monitor for these immediate reactions, patients should be observed in the office setting for at least 30 minutes after immunotherapy shots are administered (answer C). Based on studies of seasonal symptom scores, it is generally recommended that allergen immunotherapy be continued for 3 to 5 years (answer D).

HELPFUL TIP: β-Blockers should be stopped in patients with a history of anaphylaxis if possible. β-Blockers amplify anaphylaxis and make it more difficult to treat.

Objectives: Did you learn to . . .

- Recognize symptoms of vocal cord disfunction?
- Recognize symptoms of allergic rhinitis?
- Provide appropriate management for allergic rhinitis?
- Describe the role of immunotherapy in treating allergic rhinitis.

QUICK QUIZ: ALLERGIC REACTIONS

A 52-year-old male with common variable immunodeficiency receives his first infusion of intravenous immunoglobulin (IVIG) therapy. Ten minutes into the infusion, he complains of difficulty breathing and generalized pruritus. Based on the traditional classification of hypersensitivity reactions, which of the following best categorizes this patient's reaction?

A) Type I–immediate hypersensitivity reaction.
B) Type II–cytotoxic reaction.
C) Type III–immune complex reaction.
D) Type IV–delayed-type reaction.

Discussion

The correct answer is A. Based on the clinical history and timing of the above event, you should suspect an immediate hypersensitivity reaction (type I). Type I reactions typically occur within seconds to minutes after exposure to the offending agent and are due to cross-linkage of IgE antibodies that are bound to surfaces of mast cells or basophils, with subsequent release of mediators such as histamine. Pruritus, urticaria, angioedema, laryngeal edema, and possible generalized anaphylaxis can occur. Type II reactions occur when IgG or IgM antibodies are directed against antigens on the individual's own tissues. Consequent complement activation leads to cell destruction. Examples of type II reactions include hemolytic anemia and acute graft rejection. Type III reactions are characterized by formation of IgG or IgM antigen-antibody complexes which cause tissue damage by forming deposits within blood vessel walls and basement membranes. Examples of type III reactions include localized Arthus reactions

(severe local reaction plus fever such as can be seen with too frequent use of tetanus toxoid) and serum sickness, which may occur 1–4 weeks after drug use. Type IV reactions are mediated by sensitized T lymphocytes and usually occur 24–72 hours after exposure. An example is contact dermatitis, such as poison ivy.

QUICK QUIZ: CAN I HAVE THAT BANANA OR NOT?

All of the following may be associated with cross-reactivity in latex-allergic patients EXCEPT:

A) Celery.
B) Banana.
C) Avocado.
D) Kiwi.
E) Chestnut.

Discussion

The correct answer is A. Latex-fruit cross-reactivity may occur with banana, avocado, passion fruit, kiwi, and chestnut, but not celery. Symptoms of oral allergy syndrome can include oral pruritus with or without angioedema of the lips, tongue, palate, and posterior oropharynx. Cross-reactivity has been reported between ragweed antigens and the gourd family and banana. Birch pollen allergy may result in sensitivity to apple, carrot, parsnip, celery, hazelnut, and potato.

QUICK QUIZ: PENICILLIN ALLERGY

A 34-year-old pregnant female receives her prenatal care from you. She has positive laboratory testing for syphilis. She has a history of possible penicillin allergy as a child. The patient is unable to recall the specifics regarding her reaction.

What is the best treatment option for this patient?

A) Give a test dose of penicillin.
B) Give an alternative antibiotic.
C) Proceed with penicillin desensitization.
D) Skin test for penicillin; if positive, perform penicillin desensitization procedure.
E) Skin test for penicillin; if negative, give penicillin at full treatment dose.

Discussion

The correct answer is D. This patient requires treatment for syphilis for which penicillin is the drug of choice. The best treatment option would include skin testing for penicillin followed by desensitization if skin testing is positive. If skin testing is positive, there is approximately a 60% risk of an immediate reaction to penicillin. If skin testing is negative, there is still a 2% risk of an immediate reaction. Therefore, prior to full treatment doses, a test dose of penicillin (answer E) should be given to ensure that the patient can tolerate the medication. Penicillin desensitization should not be performed without skin testing since a costly desensitization procedure may be avoided if skin testing is negative. Test-dosing with penicillin would not be safe without negative skin testing, as very little drug would be necessary to bring about a severe IgE-mediated reaction if true penicillin allergy does exist.

 HELPFUL TIP: The large majority of patients who report penicillin (and other) allergies are not truly allergic. In the case of penicillin, 0.5% of those with reported penicillin allergy had skin reactions and <10% had **any** reaction to a full dose of penicillin. Many patients misinterpret an adverse reaction (such as nausea) as an allergy.

 HELPFUL TIP: There is essentially no cross reactivity between penicillin and third-generation cephalosporins. As long as the patient did not have true anaphylaxis, feel comfortable using these drugs in penicillin-allergic patients.

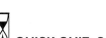 **QUICK QUIZ: CONTRAST ALLERGY**

A 57-year-old male with chest pain is scheduled for an elective cardiac catheterization. You remember that the patient has a history of generalized urticaria with lip and tongue angioedema shortly after receiving contrast dye for a CT scan several years back.

Which of the following interventions should be recommended for this patient prior to undergoing the planned procedure?

A) Use of higher-osmolality radiocontrast media if possible.
B) Administration of prednisone, diphenhydramine, and ephedrine as premedications.
C) Administration of prednisone and diphenhydramine as premedications.
D) Percutaneous and intradermal skin testing with radiocontrast media.
E) Desensitization procedure for radiocontrast media.

Discussion

The correct answer is C. This patient will require the premedication for this elective procedure. The appropriate premedication regimen for contrast dye allergy includes: (1) diphenhydramine 50 mg IM/PO 1 hour before procedure, and (2) prednisone 50 mg PO 13 hours, 7 hours, and 1 hour before procedure. Answer A is incorrect. Anaphylactoid reactions to radiocontrast material are typically non-IgE-mediated; however, they can be severe and life threatening. Use of **lower-osmolality** radiocontrast media is associated with fewer adverse reactions and is appropriate for contrast-allergic patients. Skin testing (answer D) **can** be done, but it is of very limited predictive value and **should not** be done. Answer E is incorrect. There is no desensitization procedure available.

 HELPFUL TIP: There is no cross-reaction between shellfish and iodine-based contrast material. The allergy to seafood is an allergy to the protein (tropomyosins) in the seafood not to the iodine. Think about it for a second. How many people have you seen have an anaphylactic reaction to iodized salt?

CASE 2

An 18-month-old boy comes to clinic with a history of eczematous rash covering his extremities and face. His parents state that it worsens after the ingestion of certain foods. He has had increased fussiness during the last several months, as well as some difficulty gaining weight. Food allergy is suspected.

Which of the following foods is NOT commonly implicated in food allergy?

A) Milk.
B) Corn.
C) Wheat.
D) Soy.
E) Egg.

Discussion

The correct answer is B. Corn is not often implicated in food allergies (a good thing too since we live in Iowa). Although many foods are potentially antigenic, the great majority of food allergies involve only a few foods. Studies have shown that eight foods account for 93% of reactions, and these foods are, in order of frequency: egg, peanuts, milk, soy, tree nuts, fish, crustacean, and wheat. Although food allergies may be outgrown, sensitivity to peanut, tree nuts, fish, and crustacean tend to be life-long.

* *

Two months later, this infant required an ED visit after developing increased work of breathing, wheezing, and an urticarial rash after eating. He is tested by both percutaneous skin testing and RAST and is found to have egg allergy.

Which of the following vaccinations should NOT be given to this patient in light of his egg allergy?

A) MMR vaccine.
B) Inactivated polio vaccine.
C) *Hemophilus influenzae* B vaccine.
D) Conjugated pneumococcal vaccine (Prevnar).
E) Influenza vaccine.

Discussion

The correct answer is E. Influenza vaccine should not be given to individuals with egg allergy. Of particular note is answer A. It had been common practice to withhold measles vaccination (MMR) from children with a history of anaphylactic reaction to egg; the measles vaccine is prepared in chick-embryo fibroblast cultures. However, the MMR is safe to use in these children. Answers B, C, and D are incorrect. These vaccines do not contain egg-related products and can be given safely to this patient.

Objectives: Did you learn to . . .

- Identify common food allergens?
- Recognize important associations between food allergy and selected vaccines?

CASE 3

A 34-year-old female establishes care in your clinic. Her medical history consists of intermittent abdominal pain and two anaphylactoid episodes in the past with unclear etiology. She has received multiple laparoscopic procedures which were unrevealing. During the initial interview, she relates several past episodes of lip and tongue swelling, for which she has not sought medical assistance. She has tried diphenhydramine without significant improvement. The swelling episodes resolve without intervention after 3–4 days.

Which of the following laboratory tests would be most helpful in establishing the diagnosis in this patient?

A) ANA.
B) C3 complement level.
C) C4 complement level.
D) CBC.
E) SS-A and SS-B.

Discussion

The correct answer is C. This patient's presentation should raise concern for hereditary angioedema (HAE), or C1-esterase inhibitor deficiency. This entity is clinically characterized by recurrent episodes of angioedema involving any part of the body. It can present with laryngeal angioedema (the major cause of death) and recurrent abdominal pain (generally with a normal white count and **always** without peritoneal signs). Most attacks are precipitated by trauma, medical procedures, emotional stress, menstruation, oral contraceptive use, infections, or the use of medications. HAE is caused by a C1-esterase inhibitor deficiency which allows an over-exuberant activation of the complement cascade. For this reason, patients with C1-esterase inhibitor deficiency have chronically low levels of C2 and C4. They may have normal levels of C1 esterase inhibitor but have a nonfunctional allele. Thus, answer C is the correct answer and C4 levels should be low if the patient has C1-esterase inhibitor deficiency and is having angioedema. You can also check a C1-esterase inhibitor level keeping in mind that the nonfunctional allel may give a false negative test (eg, the presence of a nonfunctional C1 esterase inhibitor).

In this patient, which medication would be most helpful in preventing further episodes?

A) Emergency epinephrine.
B) Oral diphenhydramine.
C) Fresh frozen plasma.
D) Androgens (eg, danazol).
E) No prophylactic treatment is available.

Discussion

The correct answer is D. Prophylactic treatment in the form of attenuated androgens (danazol) is available. Attenuated androgens appear to work by up-regulating the synthetic capability of hepatic cells that make C1-esterase inhibitor, thus raising the C4 level and reducing the number and severity of acute exacerbations. Since purified C1-esterase inhibitor concentrate is not available in this country (but is available in Europe, the UK, etc), the only available treatment for acute episodes of HAE is fresh frozen plasma (FFP) which contains C1 esterase inhibitor. Answer C is incorrect because FFP is not for prophylactic use in HAE except perhaps in preparation for surgery. Answers A and B are incorrect. Emergency epinephrine and antihistamines have not generally been effective as HAE is not allergic in nature.

 HELPFUL TIP: Make sure patients with HAE receive the hepatitis B vaccination series as they may require blood products for acute treatment of angioedema.

Objectives: Did you learn to . . .

- Recognize a patient with hereditary angioedema?
- Provide appropriate acute and chronic treatment for hereditary angioedema?

This section is about immunodeficiency syndromes. As Dante put it "Abandon hope all ye who enter here." The main points and the most important cases follow. Table 4.1 at the end of this chapter reviews the findings in a number of other immunodeficiency syndromes. Main points:

- Rule out the obvious: Does the patient have HIV, cancer, lupus, or other chronic disease or is he/she on immunosuppressing drugs that predispose to recurrent infections?
- 1% to 3% of patients are heterozygous for an IgG subtype deficiency, the most common type of immunoglobulin deficiency. These patients may be asymptomatic or may present with recurrent sinusitis,

otitis, skin infections, etc. IgG deficiency can be diagnosed by immunoglobulin electrophoresis. These patients often do not have an appropriate response to vaccinations.

- 1 in 700 patients is IgA deficient. It may be hereditary but it can also be caused by several drugs (including captopril and thyroxin). Usually this resolves upon stopping the drug. Most patients with IgA deficiency are asymptomatic although some have recurrent sinus and GI infections. These patients frequently develop autoimmune disease and may have anaphylaxis to blood products.
- Symptomatic immunoglobulin deficiencies can be treated with IVIG. The most common side effects of IVIG administration include renal failure, anaphylaxis, and thromboembolic disease (Table 4–1).

CASE 4

A 35-year-old male is seen by you in the hospital setting after being admitted for pneumonia. Blood cultures reveal *Streptococcus pneumoniae*. The patient was well until 25 years when he began having recurrent infections and developed an autoimmune hemolytic anemia. He also relates frequent sinus infections requiring antibiotics 8–10 times a year. His last bout of pneumonia required a stay in the intensive care unit. You suspect immune deficiency in this individual. What is the most useful test for making the diagnosis in this patient?

A) Complement levels.
B) Immunoglobulin levels.
C) Complete blood count and differential.
D) Bone marrow biopsy.
E) Nitroblue tetrazolium test.

Discussion

The correct answer is B. The clinical picture for this patient is most consistent with common variable immunodeficiency (CVID). CVID, or acquired agammaglobulinemia, is similar to X-linked agammaglobulinemia, but generally has a later age of onset. In addition, it is associated with various gastrointestinal disorders, autoimmune disorders, and malignancy. Immunoglobulin levels are decreased secondary to inadequate B cell differentiation. Therefore, the most useful laboratory for diagnosis of CVID would be serum immunoglobulin levels. The other answers are

Table 4–1 **IMMUNODEFICIENCY SYNDROMES**

Syndrome	Age of Onset	Defect/Laboratory Findings	Manifestations	Organisms
Humoral				
X-linked agamma-globulinemia	Late 1 year but up to 50 years (in very mild disease)	Low IgG, almost undetectable IgM, IgD, IgE and IgA; no B cells	Multiple, recurrent infections (generally start age 6–18 months) especially lung, sinuses, ears, CSF; eventually bronchiectasis and pulmonary insufficiency	*Streptococcus, Haemophilus, Giardia*
Common variable immuno-deficiency	Variable but >2 years and mostly by 30 years; occasionally may occur in those over 30 years of age	Low levels of serum immunoglobulins	Sinus and respiratory infections; GI infections especially *Giardia*; enhanced chance of lymphoma as adult, autoimmune disorders	*Pneumococcus, Haemophilus, Mycoplasma*
Hyper IgM	First 2 years	Elevated IgM, No IgG, IgA, IgE (although few may have very low level IgA, IgE)	Recurrent bacterial infections but also *Pneumocystis, Cryptosporidium, Histoplasmosis*	
IgA deficiency	Not before 6 months; more severe disease presents by 5 years	Low IgA levels, normal immunoglobulins otherwise	Most asymptomatic; may have respiratory tract infections; watch for anaphylaxis with blood product	*Haemophilus,* pneumococcus
Cellular				
Myeloperoxidase deficiency	Variable	Poor phagocytic killing	None except in presence of other defects (eg, diabetes)	*Candidiasis*
Chronic granulomatous disease	Infant, toddler but occasionally in late life	Neutrophil dysfunction measured by nitroblue tetrazolium testing (and other tests)	Recurrent life-threatening illnesses especially pulmonary, hepatic, skin and lymphatic abscesses	*Staphylococcus, Aspergillus*
Leukocyte adhesion deficiency	Early (poor separation of umbilical stump) or outside of the neonatal period if mild disease; those with mild disease rarely have life-threatening illnesse	Poor adhesion of leukocytes to endothelium, etc	Periodontal and dental infections, recurrent infections of skin, upper and lower airways, bowel, perirectal area	*Pseudomonas* and other Gram-negative rods, *Staphylococcus*

(Continued)

Table 4–1   IMMUNODEFICIENCY SYNDROMES (Continued)

Syndrome	Age of Onset	Defect/Laboratory Findings	Manifestations	Organisms
Cellular				
Hyper IgE (Job syndrome)	Newborn to 1 month	Elevated IgE levels, poor leukocyte chemotaxis	Facial abnormalities (hypertelorism; prominent, protruding triangular mandible; broad, somewhat bulbous nose); sczema, mucocutaneous candidiasis, sinus, pulmonary and skin infections	Multiple organisms, but especially *Staphylococcus*, *Haemophilus*, *Candida*
			Recurrent "cold abscesses" in skin secondary to lack of inflammation.	
Wiskott-Aldrich	Early infancy; fatal by 10 years without bone marrow transplant	Low IgM, diminution of cellular immunity ability to respond to polysaccharide capsules	Eczema, thrombocytopenia with purpura, recurrent infections	Encapsulated organisms (Pneumococcal, *Klebsiella*)
Severe combined immunodeficiency	Early, by 6 months; death by 2 years	Leukopenia, no mature T cells, low serum immunoglobulin levels	Colon and lung infections including diarrhea, abscesses	Multiple, including viral
DiGeorge	Early; craniofacial abnormalities, congenital heart disease, chromosomal abnormalities, hypocalcemia	Absent thymus, reduced T3+ cells	Recurrent infections but variable in penetrance; some have normal or near normal immune function	*Pneumococcus*, *Haemophilus*

tests that are aimed at other causes of unexplained immunodeficiency:

Complement levels will be low in patients with immunodeficiency secondary to complement disorders.

Nitroblue tetrazolium test will be abnormal in patients with phagocytic disorders.

Response to vaccines will be muted or absent in humoral immunodeficiency (eg, immunoglobulin deficiency).

Delayed hypersensitivity skin testing (eg, candida, mumps, etc) may indicate a T-cell defect.

Which of the following is the most appropriate treatment plan for this patient?

A) Prophylactic antibiotics.
B) Bone marrow transplantation.
C) Gene therapy.
D) IVIG replacement.
E) No treatment needed.

Discussion

The correct answer is D. The treatment of choice for CVID includes replacement IVIG, especially in this patient who has a history of life-threatening infections. Prophylactic antibiotics (answer A) may be required in addition to IVIG in some patients. Gene therapy (answer C) is not currently possible because the genetic defect has not been identified. Although bone marrow transplantation (answer B) is useful in other immune deficient states, it is not indicated in CVID.

 HELPFUL TIP: Patients with CVID develop lymphoproliferative disorders (eg, non-Hodgkin lymphoma). New adenopathy should be taken seriously.

 QUICK QUIZ: IGA DEFICIENCY

A 37-year-old female is incidentally found to have an IgA level of 3 mg/dL (below the normal range).

What is the most likely clinical picture in this patient?

A) Pyogenic infections.
B) Thrush.
C) Cold abscesses.
D) Aphthous ulcers.
E) No clinical abnormalities.

Discussion

The correct answer is E. IgA deficiency is present is approximately 1:700 whites in the United States and is the second most common immunodeficiency described. Most of these patients are asymptomatic, but some IgA-deficient patients may present with an increased rate of respiratory tract infections.

 HELPFUL TIP: The evaluation of immunodeficiency should NOT stop when IgA deficiency is discovered since IgA deficiency is often asymptomatic and may be accompanied by a more serious form of immunodeficiency.

 QUICK QUIZ: IVIG

Which of the following patients is most likely to develop an anaphylactic reaction in response to the administration of IVIG?

A) A patient with IgA deficiency.
B) A patient with IgG deficiency.
C) A patient with sickle cell anemia.
D) A patient with graft versus host disease.
E) A pregnant patient.

Discussion

The correct answer is A. Patients with IgA deficiency are likely to develop anti-IgG antibodies and thus develop an anaphylactic reaction in response to IVIG (and FFP, for that matter). Patients with IgG deficiency may have a similar problem, but it is much less common.

BIBLIOGRAPHY

Azar AE. Evaluation of the adult with suspected immunodeficiency. *Am J Med.* 2007;120(9):764.

Cooper MA. Primary immunodeficiencies. *Am Fam Physician.* 2003;68(10):2001.

Golden DB. Insect sting anaphylaxis. *Immunol Allergy Clin North Am.* 2007;27(2):261,vii.

Orange JS. Congenital immunodeficiencies and sepsis. *Pediatr Crit Care Med.* 2005;6(Suppl 3):S99.

Quillen DM. Diagnosing rhinitis: allergic versus nonallergic. *Am Fam Physician.* 2006;73(9):1583.

Scurlock AM: Food allergy in children. *Immunol Allergy Clin North Am.* 2005;25(2):369,vii.

5

Nephrology

Jason K. Wilbur

CASE 1

A 49-year-old female with a 5-year history of diabetes mellitus type 2 presents for an initial visit. She has no known complications of diabetes. She takes metformin, glyburide, and aspirin. She does not use tobacco or alcohol. On physical examination, you find a pleasant, obese female in no distress. Her blood pressure is 136/86, pulse 86, respirations 14, and temperature 37°C. As you discuss monitoring of her diabetes, you recommend screening for early kidney disease.

Which of the following approaches is the BEST way to screen for diabetic kidney disease?

A) Obtain a 24-hour urine collection for albumin now and again in 3 years.
B) Obtain a spot urine microalbumin every year.
C) Obtain a spot urine microalbumin/creatinine ratio every year.
D) Obtain a urinalysis every year.
E) Obtain a serum creatinine every year.

Discussion

The correct answer is C. Microalbuminuria, which denotes small amounts of albumin in the urine, is a marker for possible future kidney disease in diabetics (and others). The **best** test to evaluate for microalbuminuria is the urine microalbumin/creatinine ratio. Its advantages include ease of use, relatively low cost, and good correlation with 24-hour urine collections. Since albumin concentration is influenced by urine volume, calculating a ratio between microalbumin and creatinine eliminates the influence of volume and offers improved sensitivity and specificity compared with spot urine microalbumin alone.

Some of you may have chosen answer B. Microalbumin is the classic way to screen. As a practical matter, many physicians use microalbumin alone as a method of screening for urine protein, but this is not the best test. A random spot urine microalbumin/creatinine ratio is normally <30 mg/g. Values above 30 mg/g are consistent with 24-hour measures showing abnormal amounts of albumin. Answers D and E are incorrect because they offer measures of kidney function that simply are not sensitive enough to use for screening purposes.

The patient's microalbumin/creatinine ratio is 42 mg/g. The next step to confirm microalbuminuria is:

A) Repeat urine microalbumin/creatinine ratio.
B) Urine dipstick for protein.
C) 24 hour urine collection for total protein excretion.
D) Serum creatinine.

Discussion

The correct answer is A. Verification by repeat urine microalbumin/creatinine ratio is sufficient for a diagnosis of microalbuminuria, so 24-hour urine collections (answer C) need not be performed for confirmation. Since protein excretion must exceed 300–500 mg per day for a urine dipstick to detect proteinuria, urinalysis (answer B) is not sensitive enough to detect microalbuminuria and cannot be used for confirmation. Serum creatinine elevation (answer D) may be a marker for diabetic kidney disease, but it would develop late in the process.

Which of the following can cause a false-negative microalbumin/creatinine?

A) Vigorous exercise.
B) Fever.
C) Cachexia.
D) Poor glycemic control.
E) Large muscle mass.

Discussion

The correct answer is E. Patients with a large muscle mass have a high rate of creatinine excretion, which may result in a false-negative microalbumin/creatinine ratio (as the urine creatinine goes up, the ratio goes down). Patients with cachexia (answer C) have the opposite problem, with low amounts of creatinine excretion, resulting in **false-positive** microalbumin/creatinine ratio. Fever (answer B), vigorous exercise (answer A), heart failure, and poor glycemic control (answer D) can cause transient microalbuminuria, potentially resulting in **false-positive** microalbumin/creatinine ratios.

* *

Your patient's other laboratory studies reveal the following: hemoglobin A1C 6.4%, serum creatinine 1.4 mg/dL, and normal electrolytes. A month later your patient returns. She reports good blood glucose readings, averaging about 110 before breakfast and about 140 before bed. Her blood pressure is 138/84. Her urine microalbumin/creatinine remains elevated on a second measurement. According to an eye exam yesterday, she has nonproliferative diabetic retinopathy.

Because your patient has type 2 diabetes mellitus and microalbuminuria, you realize that her likelihood of progressing to overt nephropathy is:

A) Almost zero.
B) About half that of a similar patient with type 1 diabetes.
C) Nearly equal to that of a similar patient with type 1 diabetes.
D) More than twice that of a similar patient with type 1 diabetes.
E) Absolutely certain (100% chance).

Discussion

The correct answer is C. Although earlier studies showed a greater progression to overt nephropathy in patients with type 1 diabetes, more recent studies demonstrate a nearly equal rate of progression in types 1 and 2. About 20% to 40% of white patients with type 2 diabetes and microalbuminuria will progress to diabetic nephropathy. The rate of progression to nephropathy in non-white populations is even higher. Overt diabetic nephropathy is characterized by decreased glomerular filtration rate and structural abnormalities in the renal parenchyma that can be identified on biopsy.

What is the most appropriate next step in the evaluation and management of this patient's microalbuminuria?

A) Start an ACEI.
B) Order renal ultrasound with Doppler of the renal arteries.
C) Start insulin.
D) Refer to a nephrologist.

Discussion

The correct answer is A. For at least two reasons, the next step should be initiation of an angiotensin-converting enzyme inhibitor (ACEI) or an angiotensin II receptor blocker (ARB). First, diabetes is known to be a "coronary artery disease equivalent," and your patient has blood pressure in excess of the goal for diabetics (<130/80). Second, she has persistent microalbuminuria. There is no good evidence for the superiority of an ARB over an ACEI. In fact, there is good data to suggest that ARBs do not change cardiovascular outcomes (even though they are renal protective). ACEIs should be the first-choice drugs unless there is a contraindication to their use. Answer B is incorrect because a renal ultrasound is not indicated at this point in time. Answer C is incorrect. Although strict glycemic control reduces the risk of microvascular disease, your patient appears to have relatively good glycemic control, so adding insulin is not a priority. Consultation with a nephrologist (answer D) may be warranted at some time, but it is too early for that.

* *

The patient has a full urinalysis to rule out renal inflammation (eg, nephritis) and overt proteinuria (nephrotic syndrome). The urinalysis is entirely negative.

What further investigations must your patient undergo to eliminate other potential causes of proteinuria?

A) Renal biopsy.
B) Renal ultrasound with Doppler of the renal arteries.
C) ANA, ESR, CRP.
D) All of the above.
E) None of the above.

Discussion

The correct answer is E. No further evaluation is necessary in this patient with microalbuminuria. The combination of diabetic retinopathy (a marker for diabetic renal disease), hypertension (BP >130/80 mm Hg in a diabetic), and abnormal protein in the urine as measured by the urine microalbumin/creatinine ratio is sufficient to make the diagnosis of early diabetic nephropathy. Renal biopsy (answer A) is quite invasive and unlikely to change management. ANA, ESR, CRP (answer C), and ultrasound (answer B) are unlikely to offer new information. If things change (eg, nephritic urine, gross proteinuria, etc), further evaluation may be indicated.

 HELPFUL TIP: Not all kidney disease in a diabetic is caused by diabetes. Diabetic retinopathy and nephropathy go together. But if a diabetic patient with renal disease has no retinopathy, consider other causes of kidney disease.

* *

You continue to follow this patient for several years. Her disease progresses and insulin is eventually required. She is admitted for chest pain, rules out for myocardial infarction, and has a positive stress test. She will need to have a cardiac catheterization.

In addition to holding her metformin, which of the following interventions would be most likely to reduce her risk of developing contrast-induced nephropathy?

A) N-acetylcysteine and IV saline.
B) N-acetylcysteine and mannitol.
C) Sodium bicarbonate and IV saline.
D) Sodium bicarbonate and mannitol.
E) Mannitol and IV saline.

Discussion

The correct answer is C. Sodium bicarbonate (isotonic sodium bicarbonate solution at 3 mL/kg for 1 hour before the procedure and continue at 1 mL/kg for 6 hours after the procedure) has good evidence for benefit with little risk. For patients at risk of contrast-induced nephropathy, including those with creatinine ≥1.5 mg/dL, contrast studies should be avoided if possible, using ultrasound non-contrast MRI or other

modalities. If a contrast study must be done, there are several interventions shown to reduce the risk of contrast-induced nephropathy. First, aggravating medications like NSAIDs should be held. Plenty of hydration, usually with IV saline, should be given if there are no contraindications (eg, heart failure). Nonionic lower osmolality (or even iso-osmolar) contrast agents should be used. N-acetylcysteine has conflicting evidence, but it is still often used along with sodium bicarbonate and IV hydration. The diuretics mannitol and furosemide may be associated with an **increased** risk of nephropathy, and mannitol in particular has an undesirable side effect profile.

 HELPFUL(AND VERY IMPORTANT) TIP: The use of MRI contrast (gadolinium) in patients with renal disease has been associated with a scleroderma-like syndrome. Gadolinium should also be avoided in those with renal disease, if possible.

* *

Upon cardiac catheterization, the patient is found to have several lesions. She undergoes coronary artery bypass grafting and is discharged on aspirin, insulin, simvastatin, lisinopril, metoprolol, furosemide, and nitroglycerin as needed. Her creatinine remains stable at 1.4 mg/dL.

A few months later, you are called to the ED to admit her. She is dyspneic and complaining of a cough. Her vitals show temperature 37°C, pulse 76, respiratory rate 24, and blood pressure 92/46. You note crackles at both lung bases. Her heart rhythm is regular and an S4 is audible. She has JVD of 9 cm and 2+ pitting pretibial edema.

The ECG shows sinus tachycardia. Labs: Troponin-T and CK normal, BUN 70 mg/dL, Cr 2.0 mg/dL, Na 128 mEq/L, K 5.3 mEq/L, HCO_3 19 mEq/L, WBC 14,500 per mm^3, remainder of CBC normal. Urinalysis shows protein and glucose and a specific gravity >1.030, but there are few cells and no casts. Cultures and a chest x-ray are pending.

You suspect that her elevated creatinine is primarily due to which of the following processes?

A) Adverse drug effects.
B) Heart failure or other prerenal cause of renal failure such as dehydration.

C) Sudden progression of diabetic nephropathy.
D) Urinary obstruction.
E) Urinary tract infection.

Discussion

The correct answer is B. Your patient has clinical evidence of congestive heart failure (CHF), including edema and rales. With a BUN/Cr ratio >20 and an elevated urine-specific gravity, she appears to have a prerenal azotemia, likely secondary to insufficient cardiac output.

Answer A is incorrect. Drugs may play a role, but she has been stable on these drugs for quite a few months; therefore, the most likely culprit is CHF. Answer C is incorrect. Sudden increases in BUN and creatinine are probably not due to worsening diabetic nephropathy, although the existence of the disease reduces underlying renal reserve. Answer D is incorrect. Although it has not been eliminated as a cause, urinary obstruction is less likely in this female with urine output and no signs of obstruction. Answer E is incorrect since the urinalysis does not support diagnosis of infection, and CHF explains the overall clinical picture much better.

 HELPFUL TIP: Remember that a BUN/Cr ratio >20 generally indicates a prerenal cause of azotemia. These causes include dehydration and poor renal perfusion (shock such as sepsis, CHF, hypotension, etc). A BUN/Cr ratio <20 is suggestive of intrinsic renal disease or urinary outlet obstruction. Use clinical judgment. These broad generalizations apply to adults.

Which of the following is the most likely cause of her hyperkalemia?

A) Renal tubular acidosis type 1.
B) Renal tubular acidosis type 2.
C) Renal tubular acidosis type 3.
D) Renal tubular acidosis type 4.

Discussion

The correct answer is D. Renal tubular acidosis (RTA) type 4 is due to aldosterone deficiency or resistance to the activity of aldosterone. The most common cause of RTA type 4 is hyporeninemic hypoaldosteronism, which is often seen in diabetic nephropathy. The disorder is recognized by hyperkalemia and mild acidosis in patients at risk for it. RTA types 1 and 2 usually are hypokalemic and these forms of RTA are not associated with diabetes. RTA type 3 is a rare autosomal recessive disorder.

In an effort to REDUCE her serum potassium level (not temporize), you should do which of the following?

A) Temporarily hold her furosemide and ACEI.
B) Increase her furosemide and temporarily hold her ACEI.
C) Administer IV calcium gluconate.
D) Bolus IV normal saline 1–2 L.

Discussion

The correct answer is B. Because ACEI can increase serum potassium, you should stop her ACEI. One approach to lowering her serum potassium is to add a loop diuretic or increase its dose. Switching to IV administration increases the bioavailability of furosemide and may be a useful strategy in hospitalized patients.

Answer A is incorrect because stopping the furosemide may lead to worsening CHF symptoms and worsening hyperkalemia. In hyperkalemia, calcium gluconate (answer C) is used to protect cardiac conduction, but it is not effective for reducing potassium concentrations. A bolus of normal saline (answer D) is contraindicated in a patient with an acute exacerbation of CHF.

Due to reduced creatinine clearance, you should also discontinue:

A) Insulin.
B) Metoprolol.
C) Metformin.
D) Aspirin.
E) Simvastatin.

Discussion

The correct answer is C. Your patient's creatinine increased from 1.4 to 2.0 mg/dL, corresponding to a nearly 50% reduction in creatinine clearance—a rough measurement of glomerular filtration rate. When creatinine clearance decreases, patients on metformin are at higher risk of developing the rare adverse effect of lactic acidosis. There is some evidence that patients with mild CHF or slight elevations in creatinine can safely take the drug, but stopping metformin in renal failure continues to be the standard of care.

HELPFUL TIP: A rough estimate of the creatinine clearance can be calculated using the Cockcroft-Gault formula:

Estimated creatinine clearance = (140 – Age [yr]) (Body weight [kg])/(72 × (Serum creatinine [mg/dL]))

For women, multiply this figure by 0.85. One caveat is that this formula may not reflect early renal injury because of compensatory hypertrophy of the remaining glomeruli. **Normal** for healthy adult is 94 to 140 mL/min for men and 72 to 110 mL/min for women.

 HELPFUL TIP: There is no definitive equation for calculating the glomerular filtration rate (GFR). The abbreviated Modified Diet in Renal Disease (MDRD) calculation is used because it seems to be an accurate representation of kidney function in adults with renal disease. Unlike the Cockcroft-Gault equation, the MDRD makes an adjustment for black race but does not take weight into account. Both equations adjust for gender. Many labs now calculate the MDRD GFR. If you want to calculate it yourself, go to the National Kidney Foundation website at http://www.kidney.org/professionals/KLS/gfr_calculator.cfm.

* *

You administer intravenous furosemide. The night after admission she starts vomiting, and your partner inserts a nasogastric tube, which is left to continuous suction overnight. The next morning, your patient's labs are as follows: BUN 49 mg/dL, Cr 2.0 mg/dL, Na 132 mEq/L, K 3.5 mEq/L, HCO_3 35 mEq/L.

Based on the history and laboratory data provided, you strongly suspect:

A) Metabolic acidosis.
B) Respiratory acidosis.
C) Metabolic alkalosis.
D) Respiratory alkalosis.

Discussion

The correct answer is C. Loss of gastric acid, through emesis or gastric suction, can result in a metabolic alkalosis. Although no pH is available to confirm alkalosis, you are able to infer the diagnosis based on the elevation in serum HCO_3.

 HELPFUL TIP: Diuretics will often cause a hypochloremic "contraction" alkalosis from volume contraction. Watch for this in your patients on a diuretic.

* *

Your patient recovers surprisingly well from her heart failure. Her creatinine returns to near baseline (1.5 mg/dL). You try to re-challenge the patient with an ACEI and then an ARB. However, her hyperkalemia recurs and she is unable to tolerate either of these drugs. With β-blocker and loop diuretic therapy, her average blood pressure is 130/80. At a follow-up visit, you find no signs or symptoms of CHF.

You want to lower your patient's risk of progressing to end stage renal disease.

To reduce proteinuria, which of the following strategies is best?

A) Add isosorbide dinitrate.
B) Add a non-dihydropyridine calcium channel blocker (eg, diltiazem, verapamil)
C) Add a dihydropyridine calcium channel blocker (eg, amlodipine, nifedipine)
D) Restrict protein in the diet.

Discussion

The correct answer is B. Nondihydropyridine calcium channel blockers reduce protein excretion in diabetics with nephropathy and slow the progression of renal disease. Answer A, nitrates, would be effective for angina and will lower blood pressure but do not demonstrate an effect on diabetic nephropathy. The dihydropyridine calcium channel blockers (answer C) do not slow progression to nephropathy to the same degree as some other antihypertensive drugs. The effect of protein restriction (answer D) on diabetic nephropathy has not been well studied, but in one prospective study it did not appear to reduce progression of the disease.

 HELPFUL TIP: For diabetic nephropathy, always start with an ACEI and try to maximize the dose. Full-dose ACEI treatment is associated with improved survival in diabetic nephropathy compared with low-dose ACEI. The dose of ACEI may be limited by serum potassium level or patient blood pressure.

* *

Over the next year, your patient experiences increasing difficulties with glycemic control. Despite your efforts, her proteinuria and serum creatinine increase. As you discuss referral to a nephrologist, she asks about dialysis.

Which of the following statements is TRUE regarding the initiation of hemodialysis in chronic renal failure?

A) Malnutrition is **not** an indication for starting dialysis.

B) There are well-accepted criteria for starting dialysis early in asymptomatic chronic renal failure.

C) You should wait until acute complications of renal failure develop before starting dialysis.

D) Serum creatinine >5 mg/dL requires dialysis.

E) Persistent nausea and vomiting are indications for dialysis.

Discussion

The correct answer is E. In chronic renal failure due to any cause, **absolute clinical indications for initiating dialysis** include persistent nausea and vomiting, pericarditis, fluid overload, uremic encephalopathy, accelerated hypertension, bleeding due to uremia, serum creatinine >12 mg/dL, and severe electrolyte abnormalities. These are potentially life-threatening situations that must be dealt with acutely. Malnutrition is a relative indication that occurs more indolently.

Most nephrologists recommend starting dialysis prior to the development of life-threatening complications listed above. But other than these complications of uremia, there are no criteria to determine when to initiate dialysis.

Guidelines developed by the National Kidney Foundation recommend that benefits and risks of dialysis be considered for patients with a glomerular filtration rate <15 L/min per 1.73 m² (stage 5 chronic kidney disease). It is important to note that there is no evidence that early dialysis reduces morbidity and mortality and that there are many side effects of dialysis (infection, anemia, shunt complications, etc). In some studies early dialysis actually increased morbidity and mortality. Randomized studies of early versus late dialysis are ongoing.

Objectives: Did you learn to . . .

• Screen for microalbuminuria in diabetics?

• Evaluate and treat microalbuminuria and proteinuria in diabetics?

• Identify prerenal renal failure?

• Describe the features of renal tubular acidosis type 4?

• Identify gastric suctioning as a common cause of metabolic alkalosis in the hospital?

• Discuss when to initiate dialysis in a patient with chronic renal failure?

 QUICK QUIZ: ACUTE RENAL FAILURE

You are caring for a 70-year-old male whom you admitted 2 days ago. His initial complaint was chest pain. Immediately after admission, the patient underwent cardiac catheterization with angioplasty and stenting of the left anterior descending coronary artery. Incidentally, a 4.5-cm abdominal aortic aneurysm was discovered. Two days ago, his creatinine was 1.1 mg/dL and BUN 12 mg/dL. This morning his creatinine is 1.6 mg/dL with a BUN of 20 mg/dL. His vital signs are normal. Even though his extremity exam was normal on admission, today he has lower extremity edema, livedo reticularis of the legs, purplish discoloration of several toes, and a 5-mm skin ulcer at the right great toe. Urine output has declined some, but there are few red cells and no white cells on urine microscopy.

Which of the following is the most likely cause of his reduced renal function?

A) Interstitial nephritis.

B) Congestive heart failure.

C) Atheroembolic disease.

D) Sepsis.

Discussion

The correct answer is C. This patient has signs of atheroembolic disease, including evidence of lower extremity occlusive disease (eg, livedo reticularis, cyanosis and ulceration of the toes). You should also strongly consider contrast-induced nephropathy. While some patients with contrast-induced nephropathy will have a dramatic rise in their creatinine, the majority will have a minor elevation that returns to baseline within a short period of time. The BUN/creatinine ratio argues against a prerenal cause for this patient's renal failure (eg, CHF). Normal vital signs make sepsis unlikely. Rhabdomyolysis is a concern when an elderly person has a prolonged surgery. In such cases, ecchymosis or muscle tenderness is often observed.

CASE 2

A 49-year-old African American female with type 2 diabetes, hypertension, and hyperlipidemia returns for a follow-up visit. She has had diabetes for 15 years, and her control has been variable over that time. Now, her glycosylated hemoglobin is 8%. You review her other labs. She has microalbuminuria and diabetic retinopathy. You point out that her renal function has progressively declined, and this alarms her because her mother is on hemodialysis. Her creatinine was 1.2 mg/dL 3 years ago, and now it is 1.9 mg/dL. Her GFR is 36 mL/min/1.73 m². She weighs 100 kg, and her blood pressure is 120/76.

Which of the following is the most appropriate description of her renal function?

A) Stage 1 chronic kidney disease.
B) Stage 2 chronic kidney disease.
C) Stage 3 chronic kidney disease.
D) Stage 4 chronic kidney disease.
E) Stage 5 chronic kidney disease.

Discussion

The correct answer is C. She has stage 3 chronic kidney disease (CKD). Table 5–1 defines the various stages of CKD. Not all patients will progress through all of the stages of CKD. Based on age alone, many elderly patients may be classified as having stage 2 CKD, and they may never progress. Knowledge of a patient's CKD stage is useful in determining how to treat, what drugs to avoid, etc. Also, many experts believe that CKD should be treated as a "coronary artery disease equivalent."

 HELPFUL TIP: Patients with CKD, with or without diabetes, are at increased risk of coronary artery disease, so other risk factors for heart disease should be treated aggressively.

* *

You increase the patient's insulin and lisinopril doses, confirm that she is taking aspirin, and convince her to quit smoking. One month later, your patient returns with typical symptoms of a urinary tract infection (UTI). Her urine culture grows *E. coli* resistant to trimethoprim/sulfamethoxazole but susceptible to all other antibiotics tested.

The most appropriate antibiotic regimen for this patient's UTI is:

A) Ciprofloxacin 250 mg PO every other day for 2 doses.
B) Ciprofloxacin 250 mg PO once.
C) Ciprofloxacin 250 mg PO BID for 3 days.
D) Levofloxacin 750 mg PO daily for 7 days.

Discussion

The correct answer is C. This patient's GFR is 36 mL/min/1.73 m² and her creatinine clearance is 56 mL/min (using the Cockcroft-Gault equation given earlier). Therefore, the usual ciprofloxacin dose of 250 mg PO BID for UTI is safe and appropriate. Less frequent dosing may be required for lesser GFR or creatinine clearance. The important thing here is to recall that CKD may require dosage adjustments for many medications. Numerous drugs are renally cleared, so

Table 5–1 STAGES OF CHRONIC KIDNEY DISEASE

Stage	GFR (mL/min/1.73 m²)	Comments
1	≥90	Defined by evidence of kidney damage (eg, structural damage, albuminuria) with normal GFR
2	60–89	Mild decline in renal function; about 5.4% of U.S. population
3	30–59	Moderate decline in renal function; about 5.4% of U.S. population (same percent as stage 2)
4	15–29	Severe decline in renal function; approaching need for dialysis
5	<15	End-stage disease

it's always prudent to know the GFR or creatinine clearance and check for dosage adjustments before prescribing.

* *

You assume the UTI cleared because you do not hear from her for a few months. Then her sister brings her in acutely for nausea, vomiting, confusion, and generalized weakness. These symptoms began yesterday. The only other thing new with her health is heartburn, which she has been self-treating with increasingly larger amounts of Tums (calcium carbonate), taking "handfuls" over the last few days. Her labs now include: Creatinine 2.5 mg/dL, Calcium 14 mg/dL, HCO_3 30 mEq/L.

The most appropriate treatment for her now includes:

A) Hydrochlorothiazide.
B) Furosemide.
C) Normal saline IV.
D) A and C.
E) B and C.

Discussion
The correct answer is E. Your patient is now presenting with a classic case of milk-alkali syndrome. The diagnosis should be recognized by the triad of hypercalcemia, metabolic alkalosis, and renal insufficiency in combination with the history of typical symptoms (described in the case), and excessive calcium carbonate ingestion. Treatment includes removal of the offending agent and treatment of the hypercalcemia with IV saline (to improve renal perfusion and metabolic alkalosis) and furosemide (since loop diuretics cause renal calcium wasting). Thiazide diuretics result in reabsorption of calcium—the opposite of what you want to achieve in a patient with hypercalcemia.

HELPFUL TIP: Compared to loop diuretics, thiazide diuretics are generally better at lowering blood pressure. However, at a GFR <30 mL/min/1.73 m², thiazides are less effective as antihypertensive agents. For stages 4 and 5 CKD patients, especially those with hypervolemia, consider using a loop diuretic or metolazone instead of a thiazide.

* *

As your patient's renal disease progresses, you find that she has become anemic with a hemoglobin of 10.1 g/dL. She takes a multiple vitamin. Her iron studies are normal, and her screening colonoscopy last year was normal. The anemia is normocytic and normochromic.

If you were to treat her with an erythropoietic agent (eg, erythropoietin or darbepoetin), her target hemoglobin would be:

A) 9–10 g/dL.
B) 11–12 g/dL.
C) 13–14 g/dL.
D) >15 g/dL.

Discussion
The correct answer is B. For patients with CKD and anemia of chronic disease (when other causes of anemia have been ruled out and/or treated), erythropoietic agents should be used to achieve "near normal" or "partially corrected" hemoglobin levels. Most expert panels recommend that hemoglobin levels of 11–12 g/dL be the target for treatment with erythropoietic agents. In addition to the expert guidelines, there is increasing evidence that higher hemoglobin levels are associated with a greater risk of adverse events, including increased risk of mortality. This finding is consistent with a similar finding in cancer patients. When non–chemotherapy-induced anemia in cancer patients is treated with erythropoietic agents, an increased risk of mortality and thromboembolic events has been observed.

 HELPFUL TIP: Several adverse events seen with erythropoietic agents used to correct anemia in CKD include heart failure, uncontrolled hypertension, graft thrombosis, stroke, and death.

Objectives: Did you learn to . . .

- Stage chronic kidney disease?
- Adjust medication doses based on renal function?
- Recognize and treat milk-alkali syndrome?
- Recognize complications of treatment with erythropoietic agents?

CASE 3

A 55-year-old male presents to your office for evaluation of blood in his urine. On further questioning, you find that he underwent some laboratory tests prior to purchasing additional life insurance. He brings in urinalysis results which show 2 + blood on urine dipstick and 2 RBC/HPF. The remainder of the urinalysis and microscopic exam is normal.

After an appropriate history and physical exam, your first step in the evaluation of this urine abnormality is to:

A) Repeat the urinalysis and microscopic exam.
B) Obtain urine for culture.
C) Order a renal ultrasound.
D) Order a CT scan of the abdomen.
E) Order an IVP.

Discussion

The correct answer is A. According to the urinalysis, there is a small amount of blood in the patient's urine, but the number of RBCs is actually normal (<3 RBC/HPF). Your first step should be to repeat the urinalysis and urine microscopic exam to determine if this patient actually meets the criteria for microscopic hematuria (≥3 RBC/HPF on 2 of 3 properly collected urine specimens, according to the American Urological Association).

* *

A urine culture may prove useful later in the evaluation process but is not necessary now. Likewise, ordering ultrasound, CT, or IVP studies is premature because the diagnosis of microscopic hematuria has not been made.

> **HELPFUL TIP:** Kidney stones are a common cause of gross and microscopic hematuria. Remember that 20% of patients with kidney stones will have no blood in their urine and a normal urinalysis. IgA nephropathy is one of the most common intrinsic renal diseases to cause microscopic hematuria; kidney cysts, including polycystic kidney disease, are common causes as well. Neoplastic diseases, specifically bladder cancer and renal cell carcinoma, are sometimes discovered during the investigation of microscopic hematuria.

* *

Further history reveals that the patient smokes 1–2 packs of cigarettes per day. He has a normal blood pressure and the remainder of the physical exam is unrevealing. On 2 urine samples, you find microscopic hematuria, with a positive dipstick and 5 RBC/HPF. There is no gross blood. The rest of the urinalysis is normal, and there are no red cell casts.

In your evaluation of this patient, you include all of the following tests EXCEPT:

A) Urine cytology.
B) CBC.
C) Serum creatinine.
D) CT scan of the abdomen and pelvis with particular note of the kidneys.
E) Renal biopsy.

Discussion

The correct answer is E. In most cases of microscopic hematuria, renal biopsy is not indicated. However, if an intrinsic renal cause of hematuria is suspected, renal biopsy may prove necessary. Intrinsic renal disease is more likely if there is proteinuria, hypertension, elevated serum creatinine, or an active urinary sediment (eg, nephritic; dysmorphic red cells, and red cell casts).

There is no completely standardized evaluation of microscopic hematuria, and recommendations vary depending on the author. However, the recommendations always include serum creatinine and usually include CBC, coagulation studies, and serum chemistries (Table 5–2). Depending on the patient's age, further studies may be indicated. For patients >40 years, you should consider studies to evaluate for urinary tract cancers. Urine cytology has low sensitivity but high specificity for bladder cancer and may be quite useful in conjunction with cystoscopy. Imaging of the urinary system is an absolute requirement in the workup of microscopic hematuria in older patients. CT scan appears to have the greatest sensitivity for detecting masses, but ultrasound, IVP, or the combination of the two may also be employed. Cystoscopy should be considered if the CT scan is normal since CT is poor at visualizing bladder abnormalities.

The U.S. Preventive Services Task Force recommends which of the following screening strategies for detecting microscopic hematuria?

Table 5–2 EVALUATION OF MICROSCOPIC HEMATURIA

After microscopic hematuria has been identified (2 of 3 urine samples with 3 or more RBC/HPF), the AUA recommends the following evaluation:

- Infection identified → treat with antibiotics and repeat urinalysis
- RBC casts, proteinuria, or elevated creatinine → begin evaluation for glomerulonephritis and consider referral to a nephrologist
- No infection or primary renal disease identified in first 2 steps → urine cytology, bladder cystoscopy (if at risk for bladder cancer based on environmental exposures and/or >40 years), and CT scan (helical CT if stones suspected, contrast-enhanced CT if stones not suspected)
- If entire thorough diagnostic evaluation negative → follow-up urinalysis, urine cytology, blood pressure, and serum creatinine every 6–12 months

A) Annual urinalysis after age 50.
B) Urinalysis every 2 years after age 50.
C) Annual urinalysis after age 65.
D) Annual urinalysis in all high-risk patients >65 years.
E) No screening at any age.

Discussion

The correct answer is E. The U.S. Preventive Services Task Force recommends against routine screening for microscopic hematuria to detect urinary tract cancers. In one-time urine specimens in healthy adults, the presence of abnormal numbers of RBCs (≥3 RBCs/HPF) can be as high as 39%. In up to 70% of patients, even after imaging of the upper and lower urinary tract, the source of microscopic hematuria cannot be found. In a low-risk population, the false-positive rate of microscopic hematuria found on urinalysis would be unacceptably high. Also, there is no evidence that early detection of bladder cancer through screening urinalysis improves prognosis.

* *

Your patient returns to discuss his lab and radiology results. His serum creatinine is 1.1 mg/dL, and his CBC, chemistries, and coagulation studies are normal. His urine cytology was negative, as was cystoscopy performed by a urologist. CT scan of the abdomen and pelvis reveals normal size kidneys and no masses, but three stones,

measuring 2–3 mm in diameter, are noted in the left renal pelvis. There does not appear to be any obstruction. Your patient denies any history of renal colic.

Regarding the finding of stones in the left renal pelvis, which of the following interventions is warranted at this time?

A) Observation.
B) Lithotripsy.
C) Ureteral stent placement.
D) Ketorolac and fluids by IV.

Discussion

The correct answer is A. The incidental finding of stones during the evaluation of microscopic hematuria is common. The stones may be the reason for your patient's hematuria. Since the stones are small, they may pass without intervention. Most stones <5 mm in diameter will pass spontaneously. No further intervention is warranted in asymptomatic patients. Answer D is of particular note. Ketorolac (and other NSAIDs) are effective in treating the pain of urolithiasis. However, **fluid is not helpful** in treating acute ureteral colic (unless the patient is dehydrated). Fluid does nothing to push the stone out and probably increases pain. For those of you old enough to remember routine IVPs, remember the 1- and 2-hour delayed films? The body simply shifts the excess fluid to nonobstructed kidney. This is why there is delayed visualization of the kidney on IVP. So, forgo the fluids during renal colic if the patient is euvolemic.

 HELPFUL TIP: Compared to microscopic hematuria, **gross hematuria** is more commonly associated with malignancy and, once confirmed by micro exam, should prompt a thorough evaluation. Benign causes of **microscopic hematuria** in adults include vigorous exercise, menstruation, sexual activity, viral illness, and trauma.

* *

Your patient does well for a year. When you see him next, he presents to your office as a late afternoon add-on and complains of severe abdominal pain that woke him from sleep at 3 a.m. He describes the pain as sharp or crampy, occurring in his left lower quadrant and radiating to the left testicle. Although the pain has waxed and waned, it has not resolved completely. He is also nauseated and has been vomiting. On exam, he is afebrile and tachycardic and has a blood pressure of 110/56. He appears uncomfortable. There is left lower quadrant tenderness but no rebound. His left flank and left costovertebral angle are tender as well.

Your next action is to:

A) Prescribe oral ibuprofen and morphine and arrange follow-up tomorrow.
B) Give IM ketorolac and arrange follow-up tomorrow.
C) Bolus 1L IV saline, administer IV ceftriaxone and arrange follow-up tomorrow.
D) Send him to the ED for pain management, fluids, and possible admission.

Discussion

The correct answer is D. In a patient with known kidney stones presenting with classic findings of urolithiasis, the most likely diagnosis is renal colic due to stones. This patient is nauseated and vomiting frequently and may not do well at home overnight. He may not be able to tolerate oral medications and could become dehydrated. For these reasons the most appropriate action is aggressive pain management, which can be accomplished in the ED. If the patient is unable to keep down oral pain medications after treatment in the ED, admission to the hospital is warranted.

Narcotic analgesics, IV NSAIDs (ketorolac), and IV fluids to maintain normal hydration are all appropriate therapies to institute when your patient is admitted. The role of antibiotics will depend on urinalysis findings, but most cases of acute renal colic do not require antibiotics.

 HELPFUL TIP: Urolithiasis and abdominal aortic aneurysm can have the same presenting symptoms and signs (including hematuria). For that reason, imaging is mandatory in the older individual in whom an abdominal aortic aneurysm is a consideration.

＊ ＊

You admit the patient to the ED, start IV saline, and administer narcotics, NSAIDs (ketorolac), and antiemetics. CT scan shows a 5-mm stone in the proximal ureter. There is no hydronephrosis. Serum electrolytes, BUN, creatinine, and CBC are all normal. Urinalysis: 2 + blood, 1 + leukocyte esterase, trace protein, pH 6, specific gravity 1.025, 20 RBC/HPF, few calcium oxalate crystals, and otherwise normal.

Which of the following is the most appropriate management at this point in time?

A) Add antibiotics to the current therapy.
B) Continue the current therapy and observe.
C) Refer for extracorporeal shock wave lithotripsy.
D) Refer for endoscopic lithotripsy.

Discussion

The correct answer is B. There is no reason to change management at this time. Many 5-mm stones will pass spontaneously. Answer A is incorrect. Although leukocyte esterase is detected on the urine dipstick, there is no compelling evidence of infection (eg, fever, elevated WBC count, etc), so antibiotics are not appropriate. Answers C and D are incorrect. Extracorporeal shock wave lithotripsy (ESWL) is the procedure most commonly used when kidney stones require intervention beyond conservative management. Generally, ESWL is reserved for moderate-sized stones that do not pass with conservative measures. Stones 6–10 mm in diameter located in the proximal ureter or the renal pelvis are often good candidates for ESWL. Complications of ESWL include persistent large fragments of stones and reversible damage to the kidney parenchyma. Also, a ureteroscope may be employed to endoscopically approach the stone, then fragment it and remove it.

 HELPFUL TIP: Stones ≥6 mm will pass spontaneously only 10% of the time and those 4–6 mm 50% of the time. Stones <4 cm pass the great majority of the time. If pain persists or the stone does not pass within 72 hours, consider urologic intervention such as nephrostomy stent placement. Renal injury from obstruction generally does not occur for at least 72 hours.

 HELPFUL TIP: NSAIDs (especially given IV) are as effective as narcotics in controlling the pain of renal colic. The combination of NSAIDs and narcotics may offer even greater pain control. However, due to their antiplatelet effects,

NSAIDs should be discontinued prior to lithotripsy. Patients discharged from the ED with urolithiasis should be placed on an NSAID in addition to a narcotic. This reduces pain and bounce-back visits.

A) Restrict calcium intake.
B) Restrict oxalate intake (eg, leafy green vegetables, chocolate).
C) Increase daily water intake.
D) Reduce meat and fish consumption.
E) Increase consumption of citrus fruits.

Discussion

The correct answer is A. To prevent recurrent urolithiasis, restricted calcium intake was encouraged in the past. Now, moderate calcium intake (1 g/day) is recognized as beneficial and should be encouraged. Patients should take calcium with meals, which will bind oxylate and prevent its absorption. A low-calcium diet permits greater absorption of oxalate in the intestines, possibly leading to hyperoxaluria and an increased risk of urolithiasis.

Increases in urine oxalate greatly increase the risk of stone formation. Restriction of oxalate (answer B) in the diet may help to reduce the risk of recurrent urolithiasis. Unfortunately, oxalate is also the end product of numerous metabolic pathways, and significant reduction in urinary oxalate levels often proves difficult.

Increased fluid intake (answer C) to achieve a urine volume >2 L/day reduces stone formation. Water and citrus juices are traditionally recommended, but most fluids consumed are associated with a positive effect, including drinks with caffeine.

Meat, fish, and poultry are sources of purine, which is metabolized to uric acid. A uric acid crystal can form a pure uric acid stone or serve as a nidus for calcium stone formation. Therefore, a general recommendation to avoid recurrent urolithiasis is to reduce purines in the diet by reducing meat, fish, and poultry consumption (answer D). Urinary citrate inhibits calcium stone formation. Hypocitraturia is a common cause of recurrent urolithiasis. A nonspecific measure to decrease calcium stone formation is to increase citrus fruits in the diet (answer E). Lemonade and orange juice are excellent sources of citrate and can also be used to increase urine volume.

* *

* *

Your patient asks how he can avoid kidney stones in the future.

Which of the following tests will be most useful in determining the treatments that may prevent future stone formation?

A) Urine culture.
B) Stone recovery and analysis.
C) Urinary calcium excretion.
D) Urinary oxalate excretion.
E) Serum uric acid.

Discussion

The correct answer is B. The prevention of further stone formation is aided considerably by knowledge of the stone type. You should always attempt to recover the stone and send it for analysis—unless the patient is a well-known stone-former and the composition of his or her stones is already known.

The other studies listed have value, mostly depending on the stone type. Struvite stones form during bacterial infections of the urinary tract, and a urine culture (answer A) will help direct therapy when these stones are identified. Calcium oxalate stones are most commonly identified, and 24-hour urine collection to determine calcium and oxalate excretion (answer C) can lead to diagnoses of metabolic disturbances (hyperoxaluria and hypercalciuria). Patients with uric acid stones should be evaluated for symptoms of gout and undergo serum uric acid measurements (answer E).

* *

Your patient passes the stone, his pain completely resolves, and he is discharged from the hospital within 24 hours of his admission. The stone is pure calcium oxalate. Studies of his 24-hour urine collection are pending.

In order to reduce his risk of forming more stones, you tell him to incorporate all of the following lifestyle changes EXCEPT:

Results of your patient's 24-hour urine have returned and are as follows (normal values):

Volume 1.6 L

pH 6.5

Creatinine clearance normal

Calcium 410 mg (100–300 mg)

Uric acid 410 mEq (250–750 mEq)

Oxalate 42 mg (7–44 mg)

Citrate 560 mg (100–800 mg)

Magnesium 3.1 mEq (3–5 mEq)

Which of the following medications is most likely to reduce his risk of developing kidney stones in the future?

A) Allopurinol.
B) Potassium citrate.
C) Hydrochlorothiazide.
D) Sodium bicarbonate.
E) Furosemide.

Discussion

The correct answer is C. According to the 24-hour urine studies, your patient has hypercalciuria, suboptimal urine volumes (the goal for urine output in urolithiasis should be 2 L/day or more), and no other abnormalities. Patients with urolithiasis and hypercalciuria benefit from long-term treatment with thiazide diuretics, such as hydrochlorothiazide, which decrease calcium excretion and therefore stone formation.

Furosemide (answer E) increases calcium excretion and has the potential to increase stone formation. Patients with calcium oxalate stones and hyperuricosuria may benefit from allopurinol (answer A). Allopurinol is also useful in treatment of patients with uric acid stones. Patients with uric acid stones and hyperuricosuria may benefit from alkalinization of the urine with sodium bicarbonate (answer D) or potassium citrate (answer B). In general, dietary citrate should be maximized. Oral potassium citrate is indicated for patients with hypocitraturia.

* *

This patient is wondering why he got a kidney stone and whether or not he can expect to get another stone.

All of the following are true EXCEPT:

A) The peak incidence of kidney stones is age 30.
B) Kidney stones are more common in men than in women.
C) The rate of a second kidney stone is 60–80%.
D) He should have an IVP done because this is more sensitive for urolithiasis than is a helical CT.
E) Helical CT, if done, should be done without contrast.

Discussion

The correct answer is D. CT is more sensitive for urolithiasis than is IVP. Additionally, it can give you information about the rest of the abdomen and may find other pathology. The CT also has the advantage of being done without contrast, which reduces the risk of renal damage from the dye used during IVP. Kidney stones are more common in men and have a peak incidence at 30 years. Between 60% and 80% of patients with a kidney stone will suffer a recurrence.

Drugs that can cause or contribute to the formation of urolithiasis include all of the following EXCEPT:

A) Indinavir.
B) Sulfonamide antibiotics.
C) Acetazolamide.
D) Methotrexate.
E) Aspirin.

Discussion

The correct answer is E. Aspirin has not been associated with an increased risk of urolithiasis. Drugs implicated in urolithiasis include: sulfonamide antibiotics, triamterene, acetazolamide, acyclovir, indinavir, theophylline, uricosurics, methotrexate, and vitamins C and D.

Which of these kidney or ureteral stone patients requires hospitalization?

A) Those with high-grade obstruction.
B) Those with intractable pain or vomiting.
C) Those with an associated urinary tract infection.
D) Those with a solitary kidney, transplanted kidney, or in whom the diagnosis is uncertain.
E) All of the above.

Discussion

The correct answer is E. All of the patients listed should be admitted. Stones >6 mm pass only 10% of the time and usually require urologic consultation and admission. Obviously, patients having uncontrollable pain or vomiting will do poorly as outpatients. Renal colic with coexistent infection is a significant problem due to the risk of abscess formation, bacteremia, and renal parenchymal destruction. These patients require IV antibiotics and immediate urologic consultation for admission, particularly in the presence of comorbidity. Patients with solitary or transplanted kidneys or in whom the diagnosis of renal colic is unclear should be admitted for monitoring of renal function and further evaluation.

> **HELPFUL TIP:** The use of an α-blocker (eg, tamsulosin) may help speed up stone passage (NNT = 4). While not yet standard of care, it is another option in patients with particularly large or difficult stones.

Objectives: Did you learn to . . .

- Define microscopic hematuria?
- Evaluate a patient with microscopic hematuria based on risk and differential diagnosis?
- Evaluate and manage a patient with urolithiasis?
- Identify causes of urolithiasis based on the characteristics of the stone?
- Decide when a patient with urolithiasis should be referred for lithotripsy?
- Use strategies to prevent stone formation based on the characteristics of the stone?

CASE 4

A 19-year-old female presents to your office concerned about protein in her urine. On a routine physical examination for employment, a urinalysis showed 2 + protein. She has no urinary symptoms and denies fever, weight changes, and edema. She reports being quite healthy and takes no medications. She does not smoke and has no family history of kidney disease. She is afebrile with a blood pressure of 118/68. Examination is otherwise unremarkable. Repeat urinalysis in the office shows 1 + protein, specific gravity 1.020, pH 6.5, and no blood. The urine microscopic exam is normal.

Which of the following is the most appropriate next action in evaluating this patient?

A) Repeat urinalysis and urine culture.
B) Ultrasound of the kidneys.
C) 24-hour urine collection for protein and creatinine.
D) Random urine protein/creatinine ratio.
E) C or D.

Discussion

The correct answer is E. Your patient already has protein on urinalysis twice. Another urinalysis (answer A) will not help to determine if this is truly a worrisome finding or not. When the remainder of the urinalysis is

normal, urinary tract infection is not likely to cause proteinuria, and urine culture is of low yield in this situation. There is no indication for renal ultrasound at this point (answer B).

Now, with confirmed proteinuria, you need to quantify the protein loss. You should ask the patient to collect urine for 24 hours for protein and creatinine measurements (answer C). Alternatively, random urine protein/creatinine ratios (answer D) correlate well with 24-hour collections and are much easier to obtain. Besides, who wants to lug around a jug of their own urine all day?

> **HELPFUL TIP:** Concentrated or alkaline urine can result in overestimation of urine protein on dipstick.

Which type(s) of protein are detected on a urine dipstick?

A) Albumin.
B) Amino acids.
C) Immunoglobulin light chains.
D) A and B.
E) A and C.

Discussion

The correct answer is A. The urine dipstick detects only large-molecular-weight proteins—generally this means albumin. Amino acids are not detected. Immunoglobulin light chains, such as Bence Jones proteins, are not detected on urine dipstick.

* *

After analysis of her 24-hour urine collection, your patient returns. She has 1.0 g of protein in the 24-hour collection. Creatinine clearance is normal. Serum creatinine, BUN, albumin, glucose, and electrolytes are normal.

Which of the following is the next step in your evaluation and management?

A) Reassure the patient and schedule follow-up urinalysis in 6 months.
B) CT scan of abdomen and pelvis.
C) Measure recumbent urine protein level.
D) Refer for renal biopsy.

Discussion

The correct answer is C. Proteinuria may be either transient or persistent. Transient proteinuria is often due to fever, exercise, or other causes and is not associated with significant kidney disease. Transient proteinuria is found in 7% of women and 4% of men. It often resolves spontaneously, and subsequent urine tests will probably be negative. However, at this point you do not know if this case will be transient or persistent proteinuria.

Orthostatic proteinuria is a common type of transient proteinuria seen in young, healthy persons. Up to 5% of adolescents have orthostatic proteinuria, and young adults may present with it as well. Protein is spilled in the urine when the patient is upright, but not when recumbent.

There are two ways to determine recumbent urine protein: an easy way and a hard way. The easy way is to have the patient void before going to bed, stay supine all night (~8 hours), and collect urine immediately upon waking. This urine is checked for protein/creatinine ratio. Another urine must be checked for protein/creatinine after the patient has been upright. If the upright is abnormal and the recumbent is normal, you have diagnosed orthostatic proteinuria. The hard way involves splitting a 24-hour urine collection. Orthostatic proteinuria is a benign condition that usually resolves as the patient ages, and it require no additional evaluation.

A finding of 1 g of protein in a 24-hour urine collection is abnormal (normal <0.15 g per day), but it does not yet reach the nephrotic range (>3 g per day). Reassuring the patient at this stage is not appropriate. CT scan of the abdomen and pelvis is unlikely to add any new information. Referring for renal biopsy is premature.

* *

The patient collects urine in upright and recumbent positions, and both have abnormal amounts of protein. You refer the patient to a nephrologist who recommends follow-up rather than biopsy. Annual follow-up will include blood pressure, serum creatinine, and spot urine protein/creatinine ratio.

In order to prevent worsening proteinuria, which medication will be your first choice?

A) Amlodipine.
B) Diltiazem.
C) Furosemide.
D) Benazepril.
E) Aspirin.

Discussion

The correct answer is D. Patients with proteinuria tend to respond well to ACEIs. ACEIs have been shown to reduce proteinuria by 35–40%. This effect is true in nondiabetics with proteinuria as well as diabetics. ACEIs appear to be superior to other antihypertensives, including calcium channel blockers (answer B).

Compared to other antihypertensive drugs, dihydropyridine calcium channel blockers, like amlodipine (answer A), appear to be less effective at preventing progression of kidney disease. Furosemide (answer C) would be indicated if your patient develops edema, but loop diuretics should not be used primarily for treatment of hypertension or proteinuria. Aspirin (answer E) may be indicated for protection against coronary artery disease in patients with risk factors, including chronic kidney disease, but is not a primary treatment of proteinuria or hypertension. Remember that NSAIDs can adversely affect renal function.

* *

Unfortunately, over the next few years, your patient develops hypertension. You maximize the dose of benazepril and need to add another drug to control her pressure. Her proteinuria increases to 3.5 g/day, and her plasma creatinine increases to 2.0 mg/dL. She develops edema, and her serum albumin is 2.8 g/dL.

This patient's current clinical condition is most appropriately described as:

A) Hypertensive nephropathy.
B) Acute renal failure.
C) Focal nephritic glomerulonephritis.
D) Nephrotic syndrome.

Discussion

The correct answer is D. While identifying no specific disease state, "nephrotic syndrome" refers to a constellation of signs and laboratory abnormalities. A number of diseases may lead to nephrotic syndrome. When urine protein exceeds 3 g/day, it is often referred to as nephrotic range proteinuria. Complete nephrotic syndrome is characterized by nephrotic range proteinuria, edema, hypertension, hypoalbuminemia, and hyperlipidemia (Table 5–3).

Which of the following findings in urine sediment is associated with nephrotic syndrome?

A) Red cell casts.
B) White cell casts.
C) Oval fat bodies.
D) Uric acid crystals.
E) Granular casts.

Table 5–3   CRITERIA FOR NEPHROTIC SYNDROME

Required for the diagnosis of nephrotic syndrome:
- Albuminuria >3 g/day
- Hypoalbuminemia (serum albumin of <3 g/dL)
- Peripheral edema

Other (nonnecessary) findings:
- Hyperlipidemia
- Thrombotic events

Discussion

The correct answer is C. Urine sediment in nephrotic syndrome is typically bland. There is little cellular matter. Oval fat bodies and fatty casts occur in the urine of patients with heavy proteinuria and hyperlipidemia. **The presence of oval fat bodies in the urine suggests some type of glomerular disease (including nephrotic syndrome).** The one exception is polycystic kidney disease. Remember that fat can also be seen in the urine of patients with fat embolism syndrome.

Red cell casts, the hallmark of glomerulonephritis, are absent in nephrotic urine. White cell casts are associated with interstitial nephritis and pyelonephritis. Uric acid crystals are sometimes seen in gout, hyperuricemia, and urate stone disease. Granular casts are not specific to any particular pathologic process and may be found in acute tubular necrosis, glomerulonephritis, and other renal diseases (Table 5–4).

Nephrotic syndrome is not a specific disease entity but can be the end result of a number of processes.

Which of the following causes nephrotic syndrome?

A) Diabetes.
B) Minimal change disease.
C) Amyloidosis.
D) Systemic lupus erythematosus.
E) All of the above.

Discussion

The correct answer is E. All of the above can be a cause of **nephrotic** syndrome. Remember that many causes of nephrotic syndrome can present initially with **nephritic** urine. Causes of nephrotic syndrome are summarized in Table 5–5.

Table 5–4   URINE SEDIMENT FINDINGS AND ASSOCIATED CONDITIONS

Sediment Finding	Associated Condition
Renal tubular cell casts	ATN, acute glomerulonephritis
Fat bodies, fatty casts	Massive proteinuria (nephrotic syndrome), fat emboli, polycystic kidney disease
Granular casts	Nonspecific—many renal disorders
Hyaline casts	Concentrated urine, diuretic use, normal finding
Red cell casts	Glomerulonephritis, vasculitis (very specific to these)
Waxy casts	Advanced renal failure
White cell casts	Pyelonephritis, acute interstitial nephritis, various glomerular diseases

Which of the following tests is NOT indicated in most patients with nephrotic syndrome?

A) Hepatitis B and C serology.
B) ANA.
C) Serum and urine protein electrophoresis.
D) Antistreptococcal antibodies (eg, ASO titer).
E) CA-125 antigen.

Table 5–5   CAUSES OF NEPHROTIC SYNDROME

- Diabetes
- Amyloidosis
- Systemic lupus erythematosus
- Minimal change disease (Nil disease)
- Diffuse glomerulonephritis
- Membranous nephropathy
- IgA nephropathy
- Postinfectious glomerulonephritis (eg, poststreptococcal GN)
- Membranoproliferative glomerulonephritis
- Various neoplastic diseases (lymphoma, multiple myeloma, lung cancer, etc)
- Preeclampsia
- Familial kidney disease (Alport disease, Fabry disease)
- Focal and segmental glomerulosclerosis
- Medications (NSAIDs)
- Miscellaneous

Discussion

The correct answer is E. Evaluation for cancer should be done if there is a specific reason to believe the patient has a malignancy (weight loss, mass on exam, etc). CA-125 is a marker for ovarian cancer and need not be done routinely. It is not a useful screening test for ovarian cancer. In addition to a thorough history and physical, routine evaluation of patients with nephrotic syndrome (and nephritis and glomerulonephritis) include the following:

- Hepatitis B and C serology
- ANA
- Serum and urine protein electrophoresis
- ASO titer
- Cryoglobulins
- Serum complement levels
- ANCA
- Serum calcium (to rule out sarcoid)
- Antiglomerular basement membrane antibodies

Doing this complete panel will find the cause of the majority of cases of nephritic syndrome. However, do testing systematically based on your clinical suspicion and other associated findings (elevated LFTs, history of strep throat, butterfly rash, etc).

* *

The diagnosis in your patient is unclear despite the workup noted above. It is time to consider a renal biopsy.

Which of the following is an absolute contraindication to renal biopsy?

A) Hypertension.
B) Use of warfarin for atrial fibrillation.
C) Pyelonephritis.
D) Renal cyst.
E) All of the above.

Discussion

The correct answer is C. The presence of renal or perirenal infection is an absolute contraindication to renal biopsy. None of the other answer choices is an absolute contraindication. However, **uncontrollable hypertension, irreversible coagulopathy, multiple bilateral** cysts, hydronephrosis, small kidneys (indicative of chronic, irreversible disease), known renal tumor and lack of consent are all contraindications to renal biopsy.

Which of the following is an indication for renal biopsy?

Table 5–6   INDICATIONS FOR RENAL BIOPSY

- Nephrotic syndrome **without** a systemic etiology found on other testing
- Hematuria from a glomerular source **with** hypertension or increasing creatinine
- Nephritis **without** a systemic explanation (eg, no lupus, drug exposure, etc).
- Suspicion of Wegener granulomatosis or polyarteritis nodosum where other tissue is not available
- Acute or subacute renal failure without another explanation (although history will usually result in a presumptive diagnosis)

A) **Persistent** hematuria in a patient with normal renal function and an otherwise negative workup.
B) **Persistent** low grade proteinuria (1-2 grams per day range) with normal blood pressure and creatinine.
C) Polycystic kidney disease.
D) Nephrotic syndrome likely from diabetes mellitus.
E) **Persistent** low grade proteinuria with elevated blood pressure and/or elevated creatinine.

Discussion

The correct answer is E. Patients with low-grade proteinuria and increasing creatinine and blood pressure should have a renal biopsy in order to determine the etiology of their disease (Table 5–6).

Objectives: Did you learn to . . .

- Evaluate and follow a healthy-appearing patient with proteinuria?
- Define and diagnose orthostatic proteinuria and understand its significance?
- Manage a patient with progressive proteinuria?
- Recognize nephrotic syndrome?
- Identify causes of nephrotic syndrome?

CASE 5

While you are covering the ED, a 62-year-old female you have known for several years presents with her husband. Your patient appears very lethargic and is unable to give a coherent history. Her husband tells you that she began having stomach pain, nausea, and diarrhea 2 days ago. Although she has not been vomiting, she has been unable to drink or eat much due to nausea. She took an afternoon nap and then became difficult to arouse and was breathing faster, so he brought her to the ED. According to her husband, she takes furosemide for edema and albuterol/ipratropium (Combivent) for COPD. She smokes 1 pack of cigarettes per day.

On physical examination, her respiratory rate is 30, pulse 104, blood pressure 112/64, and temperature 37.9°C. She is lethargic and disoriented. Oral mucosa is dry. Her lungs show diminished air movement bilaterally. Her abdomen is diffusely tender, but there is no rebound. Rectal exam is negative for occult blood.

The first laboratory test you have available is a room air arterial blood gas: pH 7.12, $PaCO_2$ 33 mm Hg, PaO_2 80 mm Hg, HCO_3 10 mEq/L, oxygen saturation 92%. Her baseline blood gas is in her medical record, which has been ordered.

This blood gas is most consistent with which of the following processes?

A) Compensated metabolic acidosis.
B) Compensated respiratory acidosis.
C) Poorly compensated metabolic acidosis.
D) Poorly compensated respiratory acidosis.

Discussion
The correct answer is C. This patient is clearly acidotic, as her pH is well below the normal range of 7.35–7.45. Based on the bicarbonate (HCO_3) level and the history of gastrointestinal losses due to diarrhea, you would suspect a metabolic acidosis. In order to have appropriate respiratory compensation, the $PaCO_2$ should fall 1.2 points for every 1.0 point drop in the HCO_3 below the normal level (24 mEq/L). In this case, the HCO_3 is 10 mEq/L (14 points below normal); therefore, the $PaCO_2$ is expected to drop by about 17 (1.2 × 14 = 16.8). However, the $PaCO_2$ is not 23 mm Hg; it is 33 mm Hg (close to the normal range of 35–45). The patient's $PaCO_2$ is too high to appropriately compensate for her metabolic acidosis, and she thus has a poorly compensated metabolic acidosis.

* *

You receive the patient's record and find her baseline blood gas obtained last year for follow-up of her COPD. The ABG then was: pH 7.36, $PaCO_2$ 50 mm Hg, PaO_2 80 mm Hg, HCO_3 28 mEq/L.

You realize now that her acid-base disorder (see discussion above) is:

A) Compenstated metabolic acidosis.
B) Compensated respiratory acidosis.
C) Poorly compensated metabolic acidosis.
D) Mixed metabolic acidosis and respiratory alkalosis.

Discussion
The correct answer is C. In patients with chronic lung disease presenting with an acid-base disorder, it is always important to obtain baseline blood gases for comparison. However, in this case, this new information serves to confirm your previous diagnosis. It appears that your patient has chronic hypercapnia ($PaCO_2$ 50 mm Hg, 10 mm Hg above normal), probably due to her COPD. If you repeat your calculation using her baseline values rather than the accepted normal values, you find:

$$\text{Change in } HCO_3 \text{ from her normal} = 28 - 10 = 18$$
$$\text{Anticipated drop in } PaCO_2 = 1.2 \times 18 = 21.6$$
$$\text{Actual drop in } PaCO_2 = 50 - 33 = 17$$

She is retaining more CO_2 than she should for her degree of metabolic acidosis. She is not compensating well.

* *

While you are providing supportive care, the patient's labs are completed:

Na 134 mEq/L, K 2.1 mEq/L, Cl 112 mEq/L, HCO_3 10 mEq/L, BUN 29 mg/dL, Cr 1.1 mg/dL, Ca 9.1 mg/dL. CBC: WBC 16,100 cells/mm³, Hgb 13.9 g/dL, platelets 167,000 cells/mm³. Urinalysis: specific gravity 1.030, remainder normal. Troponin-T, CK, and liver enzymes are normal.

All of the following may be contributing to hypokalemia in this patient EXCEPT:

A) Hypomagnesemia.
B) Furosemide.
C) Albuterol.
D) Diarrhea.
E) Use of "lite" salt.

Discussion
The correct answer is E. "Lite" salt contains potassium chloride in addition to sodium chloride and thus would contribute to an increase, not decrease, in the serum potassium. Through renal potassium wasting, furosemide and other loop diuretics lower plasma potassium. β-Agonists, such as albuterol, shift potassium

into cells, thereby lowering the plasma potassium. Diarrhea results in direct gastrointestinal losses of potassium.

Other causes of hypokalemia include thiazide diuretics, metabolic alkalosis (often from protracted emesis—although this represents a shift of potassium intracellularly and not a true hypokalemia), hyperaldosteronism, and renal tubular acidosis types 1 and 2. Magnesium depletion promotes potassium loss. Remember that an acidosis should cause the serum potassium to be elevated. Thus, this patient is profoundly hypokalemic.

 HELPFUL TIP: Interesting (but useless) tip: Until 1970, "light salt" contained lithium chloride. You could help grandma's hypertension, knock out her thyroid and treat her mania at the same time!

 HELPFUL TIP: Acidosis will spuriously elevate a patient's potassium. The serum potassium goes up by about 1 mEq/L for every decrease in pH of 0.1. Alkalosis will cause hypokalemia.

* *

You do not have any monitored beds available for this patient.

The most appropriate initial therapy to correct her hypokalemia is to give your patient:

A) KCl 40 mEq PO.
B) KCl 80 mEq PO.
C) KCL 20 mEq/hour IV.
D) KCl 20mEq IV push.
E) KCl 60 mEq/hour IV.

Discussion
The correct answer is C. Remember that this patient is vomiting and lethargic. Thus, oral potassium replacement is not going to work. Couple this with the fact that she is profoundly hypokalemic, and IV replacement becomes the treatment of choice. One should not give more than 20 mEq KCl IV per hour without a monitor. It should be given through a large-bore peripheral IV or a central line. If you chose answer D, you just failed your test—IV push KCl is fatal.

Most commonly, the chloride salt (KCl) is administered to replete potassium stores. In an awake patient

with a functional gastrointestinal tract, oral KCl should be administered. Oral and intravenous bioavailability are very similar, but oral doses >40 mEq are typically not well absorbed from the gastrointestinal tract.

 HELPFUL TIP: There are no reliably reproducible ways to gauge potassium depletion and amount needed to make a patient eukalemic. The best thing to do is start replacing with KCl and monitor serum potassium levels, adjusting the KCl dose as you go. Be careful when ordering potassium replacement: the most common cause of *hyper*kalemia is iatrogenic.

In addition to KCl repletion, which of the following interventions do you initiate now in an attempt to correct the acidosis?

A) Bolus normal saline.
B) Sodium bicarbonate.
C) Bolus 5% dextrose.
D) Intubation and mechanical ventilation.

Discussion
The correct answer is A. Based on the history, exam, and BUN/creatinine ratio, your patient is dehydrated. The first step is to correct the dehydration with intravenous fluids. Normal saline is preferred over dextrose, which might lead to further hyponatremia and hypokalemia. Additionally, **dextrose will not stay intravascular and will actually precipitate a diuresis by making the serum hypotonic.** Answer B is incorrect. There is no good evidence that bicarbonate improves outcomes in metabolic acidosis; correct the underlying problem. In most cases, volume replacement will lead to improvement in acidosis without needing to resort to bicarbonate. Although she is oxygenating well now, if your patient's respiratory condition deteriorates, she may require intubation and ventilator settings could be adjusted to aid in correcting the acid/base disorder.

Objectives: Did you learn to . . .

- Distinguish simple metabolic or respiratory acidosis from mixed acidosis?
- Discuss causes of hypokalemia?
- Manage a patient with metabolic acidosis and hypokalemia?

QUICK QUIZ: RHABDOMYOLYSIS

The primary mechanism by which renal failure occurs in rhabdomyolysis is:

A) Glomerular destruction.
B) Acute tubular necrosis.
C) Interstitial nephritis.
D) None of the above.

Discussion

The correct answer is B. Myoglobin deposits in the renal tubules, causing local damage and ischemia, which results in acute tubular necrosis. Findings in the urinary sediment which support acute tubular necrosis include renal tubular epithelial cells and dark brown casts of granular material ("muddy" brown casts).

> **HELPFUL TIP:** Patients with rhabdomyolysis with CK <5,000 U/L and clear urine are unlikely to develop acute tubular necrosis but should be monitored to assure dropping CK and adequate renal function.

QUICK QUIZ: NEPHROLOGY

Which of the following is/are associated with polycystic kidney disease?

A) Liver cysts.
B) Cerebral aneurysms.
C) Colonic diverticula.
D) Cardiac valvular disease.
E) All of the above.

Discussion

The correct answer is E. All of the above are associated with polycystic kidney disease. Of particular importance is the possibility of cerebral aneurysms leading to subarachnoid hemorrhage.

Adult-onset polycystic kidney disease is inherited in an autosomal dominant fashion, and the term autosomal dominant polycystic kidney disease (ADPKD) is more correct. It is associated with a 5–10% incidence of subarachnoid aneurysm. Patients with ADPKD presenting with a severe headache and/or neurologic symptoms should be evaluated for intracranial hemorrhage. Currently, screening for subarachnoid aneurysms in asymptomatic patients with ADPKD is not recommended.

ADPKD occurs in 1 in every 400–2000 live births. Common extrarenal manifestations of ADPKD include hepatic cysts, cardiac valve disease, colonic diverticula, and abdominal and inguinal hernias. Hypertension occurs in 50% to 70% of patients with ADPKD, and heart disease is the most common cause of death. If this patient has children, they should be screened for ADPKD by renal ultrasound.

QUICK QUIZ: TOO SALTY

A 79-year-old female nursing home resident with moderate dementia presents for worsening confusion over the last 2 days. She just finished antibiotics for a urinary tract infection. You have very little information available when she presents to the ED. However, she has been healthy otherwise and is on no medication (it happens . . . we've heard). Her temperature is 38.1°C, pulse 110, respiratory rate 18, and blood pressure 118/60 mm Hg. She is disoriented and lethargic. Examination of the heart, lungs, and abdomen is unremarkable.

Laboratory studies are as follows: Na 165 mEq/L, K 4.6 mEq/L, Cl 118 mEq/L, HCO_3 28 mEq/L, BUN 31 mg/dL, Cr 1.1 mg/dL. Urine specific gravity is >1.030 and urine osmolality is 700 mmol/kg. Her CBC is normal.

Initial treatment for this patient should be:

A) Normal saline IV.
B) Dextrose 5% IV.
C) Sterile water IV.
D) Loop diuretics.
E) DDAVP.

Discussion

The correct answer is A. Demented or delirious patients with an acute febrile illness may not be able to consume enough free water to avoid hypernatremia. Several mechanisms may be at work: free water loss due to illness, impaired thirst, and inability to respond to thirst due to cognitive or physical impairments.

As with hyponatremia, the hypernatremic patient should not be corrected too quickly. Sudden changes in plasma sodium may result in cerebral edema. Although there are no standardized guidelines to direct the correction of hypernatremia, most authorities recommend a maximal correction of 0.5–1 mEq/L/hour. In this patient who appears hypovolemic, the primary concern is to give volume. The administration of normal saline will allow you to administer volume while lowering her plasma sodium. Dextrose 5% solution may lower the sodium too quickly, especially if used to correct hypovolemia. Sterile water should never be administered IV because it will cause massive local hemolysis.

When patients with hypernatremia have signs of volume overload, a loop diuretic can be added to normal saline in order to reduce plasma sodium. Remember that you will need to continue IV fluid replacement to avoid making the patient more hypernatremic. This patient's kidney function is appropriate for her hypernatremia. She is concentrating her urine, as evidenced by her high urine specific gravity and urine osmolality. Therefore, she does not have diabetes insipidus, which is characterized by large volumes of dilute urine. DDAVP is an appropriate treatment for central diabetes insipidus. You can treat nephrogenic diabetes insipidus by correcting the underlying problem and employing salt restriction and thiazide diuretics (Table 5–7).

 HELPFUL TIP: To calculate the free water deficit in a hypovolemic hypernatremic patient, use the following equation:

Water deficit = 0.6 × weight (kg) × [(plasma Na/140) − 1]

In this patient, assuming a weight of 60 kg:

Water deficit = 0.6 × 60 × [(165/140) − 1] = 6.4 L

Table 5–7 CAUSES OF HYPERNATERMIA

- GI loss of water
- Osmotic diuresis
- Excess exercise and sweating
- Diabetes insipidus

Note: Generally, regulatory mechanisms will maintain a normal serum sodium. However, this requires access for free water. Immobile patients (especially the elderly) are particularly prone to problems because of their limited mobility and inability to independently access water.

CASE 6

A surgical colleague asks you to consult on a patient because of increasing creatinine. A 63-year-old woman was admitted for an elective cholecystectomy. The surgeon had planned to perform it laparoscopically, but some complications led to an open cholecystectomy. The patient remains hospitalized after 3 days due to fevers and delirium. Her current medications are morphine, cefotetan, and acetaminophen as needed. She takes nothing by mouth, but has intravenous fluids (5% dextrose/0.45% saline) running at 100 cc/hour. Plasma studies from the day of surgery and this morning are listed in Table 5–8.

The BUN/Cr ratio on the day of consultation suggests that:

A) Patient is dehydrated.
B) Patient has a prerenal cause of her increased creatinine, such as hypoperfusion.
C) Intrinsic kidney disease is more likely than a prerenal cause.
D) None of the above.

Discussion

The correct answer is C. A BUN/Cr ratio <20 generally indicates an intrinsic renal cause of renal failure (increasing Cr) while a BUN/Cr ratio >20 indicates a prerenal cause such as hypoperfusion (eg, CHF, dehydration).

Which of the following is the most appropriate first step in determining the nature of this patient's elevated creatinine?

A) Give a trial bolus of normal saline.
B) CT scan of the abdomen.

Table 5–8 PLASMA STUDIES

Lab Test	Before Surgery	Day of Consultation
Sodium mEq/L	138	130
Potassium mEq/L	4.5	5.8
Chloride mEq/L	103	105
HCO_3 mEq/L	24	18
BUN mg/dL	15	29
Creatinine mg/dL	1.1	2.0

C) Determine volume of urine output.

D) Obtain urine for culture.

E) Give a trial dose of furosemide.

Discussion

The correct answer is C. Currently, all you know about this patient's kidney function is that it has declined since her admission and that it is not likely from a prerenal cause. It is important to know if this patient is oliguric or has adequate urine output. This is important because it can affect treatment. For example, oliguric or anuric patients may become volume overloaded easily in response to IV fluids. Although hospital measurements of intake and output are often plagued by errors, you should start this evaluation by analyzing the patient's urine output, as well as fluid intake, over the last few days.

Urine culture and CT scan may eventually play a role in your evaluation. The decision to give fluids or diuretics cannot be made until more information is gathered.

 HELPFUL TIP: Relatively small changes in serum creatinine may reflect renal failure. A patient with a baseline creatinine of 0.7 mg/dL has lost **half** her renal function when her creatinine increases to 1.4 mg/dL, even though this number may still be in the normal range.

* *

Vital signs, intake, and output have been recorded by the nurses for each shift since admission and are provided in Table 5–9.

You have now determined that your patient has become oliguric.

Which of the following is most likely to help you narrow the differential diagnosis of renal failure?

A) Calculation of creatinine clearance.

B) Arterial blood gases.

C) CT scan of the abdomen.

D) Fractional excretion of sodium.

E) Furosemide challenge.

Discussion

The correct answer is D. In this patient, you know that her BUN/Cr ratio is <20, pointing you toward intrinsic renal disease. But this ratio is not specific enough to rely upon, and other data are needed. In oliguric renal failure, the fractional excretion of sodium (FENa) is a useful tool to help differentiate prerenal causes of renal failure from intrinsic renal causes. If the FENa is <1%, the kidney is functioning appropriately to conserve sodium and water, and a prerenal cause of failure is more likely. If the FENa is >1%, salt and water losses are excessive, suggesting intrinsic kidney dysfunction. This calculation is only useful in oliguric renal failure (urine output <400 cc/day). Also, FENa may be inaccurate in the elderly, patients receiving diuretics, and in chronic renal failure. The equation used to calculate FENa is:

$$\text{FENa (\%)} = [(\text{Urine Na/Plasma Na})/(\text{Urine Cr/Plasma Cr})] \times 100$$

 HELPFUL TIP: This is easy to remember teleologically. If the FENa is <1%, the kidney is working: it is conserving sodium to try to increase serum volume to better perfuse the kidney. This is what a normal kidney should do. If the FENa is >1%, the kidney is unable to hold on to sodium and therefore is not working.

Table 5–9 VITAL SIGNS, INTAKE, AND OUTPUT

	Day 1 Shift 1	Day 1 Shift 2	Day 1 Shift 3	Day 2 Shift 1	Day 2 Shift 2	Day 2 Shift 3	Day 3 Shift 1	Day 3 Shift 2	Day 3 Shift 3
BP	118/60	117/63	102/57	80/42	92/48	102/67	105/60	102/56	120/79
Pulse	84	82	92	124	117	106	100	102	93
Temp	37.3	37.0	37.7	40.0	39.1	37.1	38.0	36.9	36.8
RR	12	14	13	15	20	18	20	12	12
IV in (cc)	1,800	800	800	800	800	800	800	800	800
Urine out (cc)	1,650	1,000	750	850	600	400	180	100	80

* *

On examination, you find a mildly disoriented female in no acute distress. She has lower extremity and sacral edema. You obtain urine studies, showing a specific gravity of 1.020, pH 6, 3 RBCs/HPF, 2 WBCs/HPF, and muddy brown granular casts. The urine creatinine is 6.5 mg/dL and the urine sodium is 45 mEq/L. You calculate the FENa which turns out to be >1%.

Given the clinical course and urine findings, which of the following is the best diagnosis?

A) Acute tubular necrosis.
B) Acute interstitial nephritis.
C) Vasculitis.
D) Congestive heart failure.
E) Lactic acidosis.

The correct answer is A. Acute tubular necrosis (ATN) is a major cause of acute renal failure in hospitalized patients. ATN is the result of toxic and/or ischemic effects on the kidney tubules. Metabolic derangements in ATN include progressive hyponatremia, hyperkalemia, and metabolic acidosis with a high anion gap, all of which are present in this case. Typically patients with ATN have a FENa >1% and a urine sodium >40 mEq/L. (Remember, the kidney should be retaining sodium to increase its perfusion. This is not happening here. So it is an intrinsic renal problem.) In this case, FENa is 9.9%. Additionally, muddy brown casts (renal tubular cell casts) are often found in the urinary sediment of patients with ATN. All of these findings point to ATN as the cause of renal failure in this patient.

You suspect that ATN in this patient is the result of:

A) Acetaminophen.
B) Hypotension.
C) Intrinsic renal infection.
D) Cefotetan.
E) Any of the above is equally likely.

Discussion

The correct answer is B. As you review the vital signs, intake, and output, you notice that the patient had a hypotensive period associated with tachycardia and fever (day 2, shifts 1 and 2). She then developed progressively lower urine output despite stable IV intake. It is likely that she has had an ischemic insult to her kidneys as a result of hypotension and decreased perfusion. While many medications can cause ATN, cefotetan and acetaminophen are relatively safe. More often, cephalosporins

cause acute interstitial nephritis. Cephalosporins are more likely to cause renal damage when used in higher doses or in combination with aminoglycosides.

 HELPFUL TIP: In addition to hypoxic insult (shock, hypoperfusion, CHF, etc), common causes of ATN include medications such as tacrolimus, various ACEIs, some of the penicillin derivatives, tobramycin, cyclophosphamide, several antirejection drugs, and more.

Which of the following recommendations do you make for this patient's continuing care?

A) Administer dopamine.
B) Increase IV fluids to 200 cc/hour, using 5% dextrose/0.45% saline.
C) Use only electrolyte-free fluids.
D) Administer hydrochlorothiazide.
E) Administer furosemide.

Discussion

The correct answer is E. The treatment of acute renal failure due to ATN is largely supportive. In this oliguric patient with signs of volume overload (remember the edema and the positive fluid balance?), a trial of a loop diuretic is appropriate. Intravenous furosemide dosed at 20–100 mg every 6–12 hours is a reasonable way to start. Blood pressure, urine output, and electrolytes must be monitored closely. Caution must be exercised in the use of fluids. Giving large doses of fluid (200 cc/hour) is likely to result in volume overload since urine output is depressed. When electrolyte-free fluids are administered to a patient whose renal function is impaired, worsening hyponatremia is the likely result. Hydrochlorothiazide is less likely than furosemide to achieve a good diuretic effect in the setting of a low glomerular filtration rate. Dopamine is not effective in the treatment of ATN.

 HELPFUL TIP: Although traditionally taught, an attempt to convert oliguric to nonoliguric renal failure (by flogging the kidneys with diuretics) is not helpful and is possibly harmful. There is a trend towards greater mortality in patients who are treated this way. The decision to give diuretics should be individualized and based on the patient's volume status and response to diuretics.

* *

Your patient has very little response to furosemide. She begins to eat, and you monitor her fluid intake carefully. You match her fluid intake with output, giving normal saline to match her urine output and suspected insensible losses. You treat her hyperkalemia with sodium polystyrene sulfonate (Kayexelate), which is effective. Her BUN and creatinine continue to rise over the next few days and reach 60 mg/dL and 4 mg/dL, respectively. The plasma HCO_3 is 18 mEq/L.

You now recommend:

A) Hemodialysis.
B) Sodium bicarbonate.
C) Strict protein restriction.
D) Continuing to match intake and output.
E) All of the above.

Discussion

The correct answer is D. There is no reason to change your therapeutic approach now. Hemodialysis (answer A) is not necessary. Indications for hemodialysis in this patient might include symptomatic uremia (eg, coma, pericarditis), severe hyperkalemia or acidosis unresponsive to other therapies, and complications of volume overload (eg, pulmonary edema). Sodium bicarbonate (answer B) is used orally in patients with significant acidosis, but many patients can tolerate mild acidosis associated with renal failure. Dramatic protein restriction (answer C) will probably help control uremia, but lower BUN should not be your primary goal. Your patient is recovering from surgery was probably septic. She requires good nutrition to correct the underlying processes which led to ATN in the first place.

 HELPFUL TIP: Renal failure due to ATN typically lasts 7–21 days, with renal function returning as the tubular cells regenerate. However, the course is highly variable and depends on the patient's general health and the length and degree of the initial injury.

The most common cause of death from acute tubular necrosis is:

A) Hemorrhage.
B) Dialysis.
C) Infection.

D) Transfusion reaction.
E) CHF secondary to fluid overload.

Discussion

The correct answer is C. In patients with ATN who die, infection is the usual culprit. It is critical to avoid sepsis in these patients. Also, serious infection resulting in sepsis is a common cause of ATN.

* *

Ten days after her surgery, your patient's urine output increases markedly. Her BUN and creatinine return to their premorbid levels.

Objectives: Did you learn to . . .

- Evaluate a hospitalized patient for renal failure?
- Utilize renal ultrasound in acute renal failure?
- Use urine studies, including urine sodium and FENa, to assist in the diagnosis of acute renal failure?
- Identify acute tubular necrosis?
- Describe common causes of acute tubular necrosis, its treatment, and its prognosis?

CASE 7

While on call, you admit a 75-year-old female for confusion. One month ago, she started hydrochlorothiazide (HCTZ) for hypertension. Her medications include HCTZ 25 mg daily, levothyroxine 0.125 mg daily, aspirin 81 mg daily, sertraline (Zoloft) 50 mg daily, and atorvastatin (Lipitor) 40 mg daily. She has a 50-pack-per-year history of tobacco use and continues to smoke.

On examination, you find an irritable, confused female in no acute distress. Her admission vitals: blood pressure 100/60, pulse 120, respiratory rate 12, temperature 36.1°C, weight 50 kg. Her oral mucosa is dry and she has poor skin turgor. She has clear lungs, an S_4 on heart exam, and no edema. Her neurologic exam is nonfocal.

Laboratory results: Na 110 mEq/L, K 3.0 mEq/L, Cl 70 mEq/L, HCO_3 33 mEq/L , BUN 30 mg/dL, Cr 1.0 mg/dL, glucose 110 mg/dL. Plasma osmolality 220 mmol/kg.

Which of the following statements is true regarding the etiology of her hyponatremia?

A) She has pseudohyponatremia.
B) She has isovolemic hyponatremia.
C) She has hypovolemic hyponatremia.
D) She has hypervolemic hypernatremia.

Discussion

The correct answer is C. The definition of hyponatremia is a plasma sodium concentration below 135 mEq/L. The evaluation of hyponatremia begins with the determination of the validity of the plasma sodium measurement. You must distinguish true hyponatremia from pseudohyponatremia, which can be the result of hyperlipidemia, hyperglycemia, or hyperproteinemia. If pseudohyponatremia is present, the calculated osmolality will be significantly lower than measured osmolality. Your patient's calculated osmolality is determined by the formula

$$Osm = 2(sodium) + Glucose/18 + (BUN/2.7)$$

Her measured osmolarity is 220 mmol/kg, and the agreement between measured and calculated osmolalities rules out pseudohyponatremia.

The next step in the evaluation of hyponatremia is to determine the patient's volume status. This patient has no signs of volume overload, such as edema or crackles, making hypervolemia unlikely. She is tachycardic with a low blood pressure, dry mucous membranes, and a BUN/Cr ratio >20, suggesting she is hypovolemic. Most likely, she has a hypovolemic hyponatremia.

 HELPFUL TIP: When hyponatremia is discovered, investigate alcohol consumption. In patients who drink alcohol excessively and eat very little, "beer drinker's potomania" can develop. These patients have very little dietary solute intake, and hyponatremia is caused by limitation of free water excretion due to low urinary solute excretion (not due to SIADH). Large quantities of beer or alcohol are **not** required. However, low solute intake is.

What further information will help you narrow the differential diagnosis of hyponatremia in this patient?

A) Fractional excretion of sodium (FENa).
B) Urine osmolality and urine sodium concentration.
C) Urine creatinine concentration.
D) Urine potassium and calcium concentration.

Discussion

The correct answer is B. Urine osmolality can be used to distinguish between impaired water excretion and

pathologic water intake (polydipsia). Urine sodium concentration will help determine if the hyponatremia is due to hypovolemia or the syndrome of inappropriate ADH secretion (SIADH). FENa is useful when determining the cause of renal failure in oliguric patients (prerenal versus renal) but does not aid in determining a cause of hyponatremia. Concentration of potassium and calcium is not likely to add any useful information.

* *

You order urine studies. Urinalysis: specific gravity 1.020, pH 5.0, trace protein, 0–1 RBC/HPF, 0–1 WBC/HPF, otherwise negative. Spot urine Na 70 mEq/L and urine osmolality = 700 mmol/kg.

Given the patient's history, urine studies, and hypovolemic status, what is the MOST LIKELY diagnosis?

A) SIADH.
B) CHF.
C) Diuretic-induced hyponatremia.
D) Hyponatremia due to reset osmostat.
E) None of the above.

Discussion

The correct answer is C. **In order to be useful in the diagnosis of hyponatremia, urine studies must be viewed in the context of volume status, plasma osmolality, and electrolyte levels. This patient's labs are consistent with SIADH. However, patients with SIADH should be euvolemic or slightly hypervolemic.** Thus, her labs and clinical picture are most consistent with diuretic-induced hyponatremia.

The appropriate response of the kidney to hypoosmolality is to make maximally dilute urine (retain sodium to correct the hypoosmolality). Thus, the urine should have a specific gravity <1.005 and osmolality <100 mmol/kg. Inappropriately concentrated urine (osmolality >100 mmol/kg) occurs when there is limited excretion of fluid and may be observed in SIADH, CHF, cirrhosis, and renal failure.

This is also reflected in the urine sodium. If the kidneys respond to hyponatremia as expected, urine sodium concentration should be low, typically <20 mmol/L and often <10 mmol/L. In the setting of hypovolemia, if the urine sodium concentration is inappropriately high, something is inappropriately spurring the kidney on to excrete sodium (eg, diuretic use, hypoaldosteronism).

Diuretic use is the most common cause of hypovolemic hypoosmolality, and thiazides are more commonly associated with hyponatremia than are loop diuretics (furosemide, etc). Your patient is hypovolemic and hyponatremic, with a high urine sodium concentration and the history of diuretic use: most likely, her hyponatremia is diuretic-induced.

Answer D, a reset osmostat, requires special note. A reset osmostat, which is responsible for 20% to 30% of hyponatremia, occurs when the patient's body adapts to hyponatremia and gives up trying to correct the problem—the kidneys throw in the towel. Patients with a reset osmostat will present like SIADH (hyponatremia, euvolemia or slight hypervolemia, inappropriately concentrated urine) but will be resistant to treatment. If a patient with apparent SIADH does not respond to usual treatment, consider a reset osmostat. This can be diagnosed by giving a 10–15 mL/kg water load (orally or IV as D5W). Normal patients and those with a reset osmostat should excrete 80% of this in the urine within 4 hours. Patients with SIADH will not excrete this load normally. Since patients with a reset osmostat generally have mild hyponatremia (125–130 mg/dL) and are generally asymptomatic, trying to correct the sodium by limiting water intake is unnecessary and futile. You will only stimulate the patient's thirst and will cause an increase in ADH secretion.

 HELPFUL TIP: When you encounter a patient with hyponatremic hypoosmolality, also look at the plasma potassium concentration. Diuretic use is a common cause of hyponatremia, hypokalemia, hypochloremia, and hypoosmolality occurring simultaneously.

In addition to discontinuing her diuretic, which of the following approaches is the best initial therapy for her hyponatremia?

A) Saline 0.9% 1 L bolus followed by 150 cc/hr.
B) Fluid restriction to 1500 cc/day.
C) Saline 3% at 100 cc/hr for 24 hours.
D) Saline 0.45% at 100 cc/hr for 24 hours.
E) Saline 3% at 60 cc/hr and furosemide 40 mg IV.

Discussion
The correct answer is A. This patient is hypotensive and tachycardic and thus needs volume quickly to address her abnormal vital signs. If this patient was not hemodynamically compromised, you could forgo the fluid bolus. Excessively rapid correction of hyponatremia may lead to pontine myelinolysis.

Sodium concentrations <120 mEq/L are considered severe hyponatremia. Patients with acute, severe hyponatremia are almost always symptomatic as a result of the low sodium. By definition, acute hyponatremia has been present for ≤48 hours and chronic hyponatremia for >48 hours. As discussed, your patient's hyponatremia is due to a diuretic that she started 1 month ago. Therefore, her hyponatremia is more likely to be chronic.

As a general rule, hypovolemic hyponatremia should be corrected by volume infusion, usually with 0.9% (normal) saline. Fluid restriction (answer C), while good treatment for SIADH, is not appropriate in this patient who is already volume depleted; nor is loop diuretic use (answer E) appropriate. Answers C and E will exacerbate the problem. Hypoosmolar solutions, like 0.45% saline (answer D), will lead to more severe hyponatremia. In this question, you must decide between 3% saline and normal saline.

Your patient has chronic hyponatremia, which needs to be corrected more slowly than acute hyponatremia. Chronic hyponatremia should be corrected no faster than 0.5 mEq/hr or 12/day. For significantly symptomatic patients with acute hyponatremia, sodium can be corrected more quickly with maximum increases in plasma sodium concentration of 1 mEq/hr or 20 mEq/day.

In order to determine how quickly sodium concentrations will rise, you must know the concentrations of the solution being infused and the patient's plasma sodium. A liter of saline will affect the serum sodium by the following calculation:

$$\text{Na increase} = \frac{(\text{Solution Na} - \text{plasma Na})}{(\text{Total body water} + 1)}$$

$$\text{Patient's Na} = 110 \text{ mEq/L}$$
$$\text{Na in 3\% saline} = 513 \text{ mEq/L}$$
$$\text{Na in 0.9\% saline} = 154 \text{ mEq/L}$$
$$\text{Total body water} = \text{weight (kg)}$$
$$\times 0.5 \text{ (females) or } 0.6 \text{ (males)}$$

When using 3% saline solution, 1 L will increase the plasma sodium as follows:

$$\text{Na increase} = (513 - 110)/[(50 \times 0.5) + 1]$$
$$= 15.5 \text{ mEq/L}$$

At 100 cc/hr, the plasma sodium will increase at a rate of 1.55 mEq/hr. This correction is too rapid for chronic hyponatremia.

When using normal saline, 1 L will increase the plasma sodium as follows:

$$Na \text{ increase} = (154 - 110) / [(50 \times 0.5) + 1]$$
$$= 1.7 \text{ mEq/L}$$

Therefore, 1 L of normal saline will increase the plasma sodium by 1.7 mEq initially, and 150 cc/hr will increase the plasma sodium by 0.25 mEq/hr, well within the safe range.

In addition to HCTZ, which medication should you discontinue because of its potential role in hyponatremia in this patient?

A) Aspirin.
B) Atorvastatin
C) Levothyroxine.
D) Sertraline.

Discussion

The correct answer is D. Serotonin reuptake inhibitors (SSRIs) and tricyclic antidepressants, among other medications, can stimulate the release of ADH from the pituitary gland, ultimately causing hyponatremia with a SIADH-type presentation. The association between SSRIs and hyponatremia is strong enough to consider measuring plasma sodium levels in elderly patients before and after starting an SSRI. The other medications are not associated with hyponatremia to any significant degree.

* *

Your patient does well, recovers from her hyponatremia, and is discharged. In place of HCTZ, you start an ACEI for hypertension. You next see her a few months later when she starts to have problems with mild confusion. Her family reports that she is definitely not taking any diuretics. Her vitals are normal. Clinically, she appears euvolemic with normal vitals, and her exam is non-focal. Her plasma sodium is 120 mEq/L, creatinine 1.1 mg/dL, plasma osmolality 240 mmol/kg, and urine osmolality 320 mmol/kg. Urinalysis shows specific gravity of 1.030 but is normal otherwise.

In addition to the lab tests already available to you, which of the following laboratory tests is indicated to help to determine the cause of hyponatremia in this patient?

A) CBC.
B) ESR.
C) TSH.
D) Liver enzymes.
E) ADH.

Discussion

The correct answer is C. Hyponatremia with hypo-osmolality and a normal volume status is often the result of SIADH. However, SIADH is a diagnosis of exclusion. Both hypothyroidism and glucocorticoid deficiency present with similar features and should be ruled out. Hypothyroidism is more common, and at a minimum you must check TSH. Of special note is answer E. Most of the time, ADH levels are not helpful in the diagnosis of SIADH because up to 20% of patients with diagnosable SIADH do not have elevated plasma ADH levels. SIADH is diagnosed on clinical grounds, with characteristic lab data and lack of a better explanation.

 HELPFUL TIP: In any given patient with hyponatremia, what makes SIADH likely? All of the following data are used to support the diagnosis of SIADH: decreased plasma osmolality, inappropriately concentrated urine (eg, a urine osmolality of >100 mmol/kg), clinical euvolemia or mild hypervolemia, elevated urine sodium excretion (urine sodium >20 mEq/L), and the absence of diuretic use, hypothyroidism, and adrenal dysfunction.

* *

You order a number of laboratory tests, including TSH, CBC, and electrolytes. In addition to the labs above, abnormal tests include plasma Cl 90 mEq/L, urine Na 50 mEq/L. Thyroid function tests are normal.

As initial treatment, you prescribe:

A) Demeclocycline.
B) Lithium.
C) Saline 0.9% bolus.
D) Furosemide.
E) Water restriction.

Discussion

The correct answer is E. The labs are consistent with SIADH. Water restriction is the mainstay of therapy in SIADH. Free water should be restricted to 1–2 L per day. Demeclocycline and lithium interfere with the activity of ADH at the collecting tubules, but these drugs are reserved for SIADH patients with severe hyponatremia unresponsive to water restriction. Saline infusion corrects hypovolemic hyponatremia, and furosemide is used in hypervolemic hyponatremia (eg, CHF, renal insufficiency). Neither of these conditions is present in this patient. The patient fails water restriction. The NEXT step in the treatment of this patient is:

A) Demeclocycline.
B) Lithium.
C) Sodium chloride tablets.
D) IV urea.
E) None of the above.

Discussion

The correct answer is C. Increasing salt intake and adding a loop diuretic are other ways to treat SIADH in patients who cannot or will not maintain fluid restriction. IV urea, which causes an osmotic diuresis, is the step to use after the sodium chloride tablets. Demeclocycline and lithium should be reserved for patients who fail the other treatments.

> **HELPFUL TIP:** Conivaptan (Vaprisol) is an ADH antagonist that can be given IV for euvolemic hyponatremia. It should be used as a second- or third-line agent. Its potential problems include exacerbations of heart failure, orthostatic hypotension, and hypokalemia.

Objectives: Did you learn to . . .

• Generate a differential diagnosis for hyponatremia?
• Identify medications that are commonly associated with hyponatremia?
• Use urine osmolality to identify impaired renal water handling?
• Calculate sodium correction using different concentrations of saline?
• Diagnose, evaluate, and treat a patient with SIADH?

CASE 8

A 65-year-old male with a new diagnosis of heart failure returns to your office after starting several new medications within the last month. A cardiologist at an academic health center 100 miles away started these medications but never sent a note and neither you nor your patient knows what the drugs are. Over that same time period, he states that he has felt "worse than I did after my heart attack." At first he was just fatigued, but in the last few days, he has developed nausea, vomiting, and body aches.

On examination, his temperature is 37.1°C, pulse 70, respiratory rate 8, and blood pressure 100/58 mm Hg. His lungs are clear, and his abdomen is diffusely tender. When you stand him up to check his blood pressure, he loses consciousness but quickly recovers when placed supine.

Your nurse draws blood, starts an IV, and obtains an arterial blood gas on room air. ABG: pH 7.52, $PaCO_2$ 49 mm Hg, PaO_2 90 mm Hg, and HCO_3 39 mEq/L.

The blood gas is consistent with the diagnosis of:

A) Metabolic alkalosis with respiratory compensation.
B) Respiratory alkalosis with metabolic compensation.
C) Mixed metabolic/respiratory alkalosis.
D) Mixed metabolic alkalosis and respiratory acidosis.

Discussion

The correct answer is A. Your patient appears to have a pure metabolic alkalosis with respiratory compensation. His pH is above the upper limit of normal (7.45), and his plasma bicarbonate is elevated as well. In metabolic alkalosis, you can expect the $PaCO_2$ to rise in proportion to the rise in HCO_3. $PaCO_2$ should increase by 0.5–0.75 times the increase in HCO_3 from baseline (usually 24 mEq/L). In this case the HCO_3 has increased by 15, and the $PaCO_2$ has appropriately increased by 9.

Which of the following urine tests will aid in determining the cause of this patient's metabolic alkalosis?

A) Urine sodium.
B) Urine potassium
C) Urine chloride.
D) Urine bicarbonate.
E) Urine creatinine.

Discussion

The correct answer is C. You can approach the differential diagnosis of metabolic alkalosis by measuring the urine chloride (see next question). The other urine studies are less useful in metabolic alkalosis. An appropriate history and physical as well as plasma tests are required to determine the correct diagnosis and treatment.

* *

You have admitted the patient and are on your way to the hospital to see him when the lab tests return. His plasma studies: Na 140 mEq/L, K 2.5 mEq/L, Cl 94 mEq/L, BUN 18 mg/dL, creatinine 0.9 mg/dL, Ca 8.4 mg/dL, Mg 1.9 mg/dL. Urine studies: specific gravity 1.025, chloride 45 mEq/L (high).

Of the following choices, which is NOT likely to contribute to metabolic alkalosis in this patient?

A) Corticosteroids.
B) Diuretics.
C) Bartter syndrome.
D) Hypokalemia.
E) Vomiting or NG suction.

Discussion

The correct answer is E. This makes intuitive sense. If there is NG suction or vomiting, the patient will be low on chloride and thus will have little in the urine (where it is being reabsorbed.) The rest of the answers will cause an **elevated** urine chloride. With mineralocorticoid excess (aldosterone)(answer A), one excretes potassium. Hypokalemia adversely affects the kidneys' ability to reabsorb chloride. This explains answers C and D. Bartter syndrome is an inherited disorder that essentially mimics the effect of a loop or thiazide diuretic leading to hypokalemia but also an elevated chloride in the urine (Table 5–10).

Table 5–10 CAUSES OF METABOLIC ALKALOSIS DIVIDED BY URINE CHLORIDE LEVELS

Low Urine Chloride (<25 mEq/L)	High Urine Chloride (>40 mEq/L)
Vomiting	Hypokalemia (severe)
Nasogastric suctioning	Diuretics (loop or thiazide; early effect)
Factitious diarrhea	Alkali load
Cystic fibrosis	Bartter/Gitelman syndromes
Low chloride intake	Primary mineralocorticoid excess
Posthypercapnia	
Diuretics (loop or thiazide; late effect)	

* *

You are able to obtain the cardiologist's records and your patient's medications. He started taking captopril, furosemide, and metoprolol in the last month. He also takes aspirin and isosorbide dinitrate.

All of the following are appropriate interventions in this patient EXCEPT:

A) Discontinue furosemide.
B) Administer potassium chloride.
C) Administer hydrochloric acid through an NG tube.
D) Infuse normal (0.9%) saline.
E) Administer ranitidine.

Discussion

The correct answer is C. Chloride-responsive metabolic alkalosis is usually secondary to volume contraction. Your patient has renal salt and water losses due to a diuretic and has gastrointestinal volume losses due to emesis. Physical exam and laboratory findings support hypovolemia. The diuretic should be discontinued and volume should be replaced. An isotonic solution, such as normal saline, is an appropriate choice. However, you must monitor your patient's volume status closely due to his CHF. Because his potassium is low, he requires KCl. An H_2-blocker, like ranitidine, is a good choice for a patient with alkalosis and gastrointestinal illness: it will reduce acid secretion in the stomach (and thus further acid loss) and may offer some symptomatic relief as well.

Hydrochloric acid is an option in severe metabolic alkalosis unresponsive to other therapies. However, it is not given by NG tube. HCl is very corrosive and should only be infused centrally.

* *

Your patient is not responding to the KCl you are administering.

Which of the following electrolytes do you give to aid in repleting his potassium stores?

A) Sodium.
B) Bicarbonate.
C) Calcium.
D) Phosphate.
E) Magnesium.

Discussion

The correct answer is E. Give magnesium before giving more potassium. Although your patient's magnesium is only slightly low and may in fact be normal by some laboratory reference values, continued hypokalemia in the face of KCl repletion may indicate whole-body magnesium depletion. Serum magnesium levels may not accurately reflect whole-body magnesium stores, especially in patients with CHF. Furosemide causes further magnesium wasting. None of the other electrolytes listed is as important to potassium repletion.

* *

With correction of fluid and electrolyte status, your patient recovers quickly. You try to convey to the cardiologist the importance of good communication.

Objectives: Did you learn to . . .

- Identify metabolic alkalosis?
- Utilize urine chloride in the evaluation of metabolic alkalosis?
- Recognize various causes of metabolic alkalosis?
- Recognize the role of hypomagnesemia in treating hypokalemia?

 QUICK QUIZ: HEMATURIA

A 25-year-old male medical student presents with blood in his urine. When asked about this finding, he admits that he was using urine dipsticks at home to check his urine. He has no gross hematuria, just 1 + blood on his urine self-test. He has no symptoms otherwise. His major concern is that his father had a renal transplant at age 30 for Alport syndrome.

Because his father had Alport syndrome, what is the probability that this student has it?

A) Certain (100% chance).
B) 1 in 2.
C) 1 in 4.
D) 1 in 8.
E) Less than 1 in 20.

Discussion

The correct answer is E. Alport syndrome (aka hereditary nephritis) typically presents with microscopic hematuria and progresses to complete renal failure. Alport syndrome has a heterogeneous inheritance pattern: 80% of cases are due to X-linked disease, approximately 15% are autosomal recessive, and approximately 5% are autosomal dominant. Because most cases are X-linked, males are affected more severely and earlier than females. If your medical student's father had Alport syndrome, it was most likely X-linked, and the patient could not possibly have inherited it. However, there is a 5% chance that the father had autosomal dominant disease and then a 50% chance that the trait was passed on to the patient.

CASE 9

A 33-year-old male presents to the ED complaining of shortness of breath and cough of 10-days' duration. He must sleep in a chair due to orthopnea. He has severe fatigue and a mild, diffuse headache. Four days ago, he was seen in an urgent-care clinic and diagnosed with bronchitis. Currently, he is taking erythromycin, a cough suppressant, and a decongestant, but he took no medications prior to his diagnosis of bronchitis. He reports no medical problems or surgeries. He quit smoking 1 year ago and denies alcohol and drug use. He has a strong family history of hypertension. The review of systems is otherwise negative.

On physical examination, his temperature is 36.8°C, pulse 104, respiratory rate 16, and blood pressure 200/118. There are bibasilar crackles with dullness to percussion at the lung bases. The heart, abdomen, and extremities are unremarkable.

His chest x-ray shows cardiomegaly, mild CHF, and bilateral small pleural effusions. An ECG shows sinus tachycardia with left atrial enlargement and left ventricular hypertrophy. Lab results: troponin-T negative, hemoglobin 9.1 g/dL, WBC count and platelets normal, Na 136 mEq/L, K 4.4 mEq/L, Cl 96 mEq/L, HCO_3 19 mEq/L, BUN 108 mg/dL, Cr 11.9 mg/dL, glucose 104 mg/dL, calcium 7.8 mg/dL, albumin 4.0 g/dL.

Which of the following is the most appropriate next step?

A) Prescribe levofloxacin and discharge patient with follow-up the next day.
B) Prescribe furosemide and discharge patient with follow-up the next day.
C) Administer a bolus of normal saline intravenously and admit the patient.

D) Administer furosemide intravenously and admit the patient.

E) Perform thoracentesis for diagnostic purposes.

Discussion

The correct answer is D. The proper disposition of this patient is the hospital. His uremia is quite severe, and he is symptomatic from his renal failure. He needs further diagnostic tests and requires further monitoring. He has signs and symptoms of volume overload, and he may yet respond to loop diuretics. A trial of IV furosemide is reasonable. The initial diagnosis of bronchitis was most likely erroneous and switching to another antibiotic will only perpetuate that error. As he is volume overloaded, you certainly do not want to administer more volume. If you are willing to attribute his pleural effusions to volume overload due to kidney failure, a thoracentesis is not necessary.

How should the low calcium be approached in the ED?

A) Administer calcium gluconate intravenously.

B) Obtain a serum parathyroid hormone level.

C) Monitor for signs and symptoms of hypocalcemia.

D) Obtain an ionized calcium level.

Discussion

The correct answer is C. Currently, your patient does not have signs and symptoms of hypocalcemia; therefore, he does not need calcium replacement in the ED. He should be observed for the development of signs and symptoms. Symptoms are mostly neurologic—generalized seizures, perioral paresthesias, and carpopedal spasms. The two best known signs of hypocalcemia are Chvostek and Trousseau. Chvostek sign is present if a grimace occurs in response to tapping the facial nerve. Trousseau sign is evoked by inflating a blood pressure cuff above the systolic pressure for 3 minutes and observing for hand spasms.

Since you expect that the patient's hypocalcemia is secondary to renal disease and hyperphosphatemia and you will treat him symptomatically, serum PTH level is not required. As you have access to both the total serum calcium level and the serum albumin, you can calculate the corrected calcium. Therefore, it is not necessary to measure ionized calcium. To correct total calcium for decreased albumin, use the following formula:

$$\text{Corrected calcium} = \text{measured calcium} + [0.8 \times \\ (\text{normal albumin} - \text{measured albumin})].$$

 HELPFUL TIP: If the patient does not respond to furosemide, IV nitroglycerin will likely be successful at reducing this patient's pulmonary edema by decreasing preload and afterload.

* *

Your patient is admitted. Initially, his urine output increases slightly with loop diuretics, but then he becomes oliguric. You ask for a nephrology consult to assist in management of this case. The nephrologist plans to place an IV catheter for dialysis and is considering a renal biopsy. If the patient develops bleeding with these procedures, he may have difficulty achieving hemostasis.

Which of the following treatments is LEAST likely to reduce the risk of bleeding in this patient?

A) Hemodialysis.

B) DDAVP.

C) Cryoprecipitate.

D) Platelet transfusion.

Discussion

The correct answer is D. The cause of bleeding dysfunction in uremia appears to be the effect of uremic toxins on platelet function. Giving a uremic patient more platelets—especially when there is no thrombocytopenia—will not improve the situation, as the platelet dysfunction due to uremia will occur with the new platelets as well.

Hemodialysis (answer A) will remove toxins related to uremia, improving platelet function. DDAVP (answer B) is often the first-line treatment in a bleeding patient with uremia. DDAVP is not generally toxic and quickly reduces bleeding time. It acts by causing the release of factor VIII:vWF multimers from endothelial storage sites. Unfortunately, patients rapidly develop tachyphylaxis to DDAVP; once the multimers are depleted from the endothelial cells, DDAVP will not work until these multimers are replaced (usually a process of several days). Cryoprecipitate (answer C) will reduce bleeding time.

In order to reduce the risk of renal osteodystrophy (elevated serum parathyroid hormone with mobilization of calcium from bone), which of the following medications will you prescribe initially?

A) Calcium carbonate.

B) Aluminum hydroxide.

C) Magnesium hydroxide.

D) Sevelamer (Renagel).

E) Vitamin D.

Discussion

The correct answer is A. Calcium carbonate is associated with the least potential toxicity; therefore, it is the initial choice for treating hyperphosphatemia to reduce the risk of renal osteodystrophy. Renal osteodystrophy occurs when parathyroid hormone levels are elevated and bone is mobilized. This occurs because patients with renal failure cannot clear phosphate. The body tries to compensate by increasing parathyroid hormone secretion, which reduces phosphate and increases serum calcium. However, it also is detrimental to bone and leads to demineralization.

Gastrointestinal binding of phosphate requires large doses of a cation such as calcium (2 g/day). You may also consider calcium acetate, which is as safe as calcium carbonate and is a more potent phosphate binder but more expensive. Avoid aluminum and magnesium products in renal failure as these ions accumulate and can cause toxicity.

Sevelamer is a cationic polymer that binds phosphate in the gastrointestinal tract and avoids the problems that can occur with the calcium, magnesium, and aluminum compounds. It is expensive and does not seem to be superior to calcium, so calcium products should be tried first.

Patients with chronic renal failure or end-stage renal disease on dialysis should also receive vitamin D. However, vitamin D causes increased gastrointestinal absorption of phosphate, so it should be given only after hyperphosphatemia has been controlled.

 HELPFUL TIP: Whenever prescribing calcium, have patients take it with meals—otherwise it will not bind phosphate. Also, calcium is absorbed better when taken with food.

 HELPFUL TIP: Cinacalcet (Sensipar) is another option for treating renal osteodystrophy. By mimicking calcium in the parathyroid, it fools the parathyroid into thinking that the serum calcium is normal and thus reduces the output of parathyroid hormone.

Objectives: Did you learn to . . .

● Anticipate complications of renal failure, including hypervolemia, hypocalcemia, platelet dysfunction, and renal osteodystrophy?

CASE 10

A 10-year-old male presents with his mother, who appears very anxious. She reports several episodes of red-brown urine this morning. The patient reports feeling a bit tired, but otherwise has no complaints. At 5 years, he had myringotomy tubes placed bilaterally, but his past medical history is otherwise unremarkable. He takes no medications. On review of systems, he reports a sore throat that resolved completely a few days ago.

On exam you find a pleasant young male in no acute distress. He is afebrile. His blood pressure is 140/94 mm Hg, and he has trace pretibial edema. The remainder of the exam is unrevealing.

All of the following tests are likely to be helpful in the work up of this patient EXCEPT:

A) Urinalysis.

B) Abdominal x-ray.

C) CBC.

D) Plasma electrolytes.

E) BUN and creatinine.

Discussion

The correct answer is B. Abdominal plain films are not useful in almost any situation unless looking for constipation or bowel obstruction. If this patient had a presentation consistent with urolithiasis, an abdominal CT scan may be indicated. All of the other laboratory tests should be ordered.

* *

Urinalysis shows 2 + blood, 2 + protein, specific gravity 1.015, and numerous red blood cells with red cell casts. BUN is 35 mg/dL and creatinine is 1.8 mg/dL. CBC, coagulation studies, and electrolytes are pending.

All of the following should be considered in the differential diagnosis now EXCEPT:

A) Minimal change disease.

B) Henoch-Schonlein purpura.

C) Poststreptococcal glomerulonephritis.

D) IgA nephropathy.

E) Membranoproliferative glomerulonephritis.

Discussion

The correct answer is A. Minimal change disease usually presents with clinical signs and symptoms of nephrotic syndrome and **not gross hematuria.** All of the other diseases are associated with hematuria, either microscopic or gross. Henoch-Schönlein purpura, poststreptococcal glomerulonephritis, IgA nephropathy, and membranoproliferative glomerulonephritis all have more nephritic features with active urinary sediments (dysmorphic red cells, red cell casts, and granular casts, white cells and protein in the urine). Also, these diseases have a similar pathologic process in which immune complexes deposit in the glomeruli, resulting in glomerulonephritis (Table 5–11).

* *

CBC, coagulation studies, and electrolytes are all normal. You are suspicious that he may have had streptococcal pharyngitis that was unrecognized.

Which of the following statements best describes the usual course of poststreptococcal glomerulonephritis?

A) Most patients progress to renal failure.
B) After resolution of the initial episode, recurrent episodes of gross hematuria are common.
C) In most cases, hypertension and uremia subside within 1–2 weeks.
D) In most cases, hypertension is persistent and requires treatment.
E) Adults tend to recover more quickly than children.

Discussion

The correct answer is C. Poststreptococcal glomerulonephritis, characterized by immune complex deposition

Table 5–11 CAUSES OF GROSS HEMATURIA IN CHILDREN

Idiopathic (usually benign with resolution over time)
Urinary tract infection
Trauma
Congenital anomaly
Urethral irritation or trauma
Nephrolithiasis
Sickle cell disease/trait
Coagulopathy
Glomerular disease (eg, poststreptococcal glomerulonephritis)
Malignancy (eg, Wilm tumor)
Medications (eg, hemorrhagic cystitis from cyclophosphamide)

in the glomeruli, is a self-limited disease in most patients. There is a latent period, averaging 10 days, between pharyngitis and the development of hematuria. Recovery is expected in 1–2 weeks. Unlike IgA nephropathy, recurrent episodes of gross hematuria are rare in poststreptococcal glomerulonephritis. Poststreptococcal glomerulonephritis is more common in children and tends to be more severe when it affects adults. Hypertension and uremia resolve relatively quickly, but microscopic hematuria may persist for 6 months.

 HELPFUL TIP: Renal biopsy is rarely indicated in children with nephritic urine and mild renal failure because the differential diagnosis can be narrowed by the clinical presentation and because many of the diseases are self-limited. In more severe cases, renal biopsy may be necessary to diagnose and treat appropriately.

Objectives: Did you learn to . . .

- Evaluate a child with gross hematuria?
- Generate a differential diagnosis for hematuria and proteinuria in a child?
- Describe the usual course of post-streptococcal glomerulonephritis?

CASE 11

The parents of a 2-year-old female bring her in to your office for a week-long history of diarrhea. Initially, her stools were loose and watery, but over the last few days, they have become bloody. The patient has appeared to have abdominal pain on occasions, and her appetite is depressed. Despite bloody diarrhea, her parents attempted to care for her at home until she became more lethargic. They are also worried about some bruising on her extremities.

The nurse takes her vital signs: temperature 37.2°C, pulse 145, blood pressure 88/47, and respiratory rate 40. The patient appears pale, with slight scleral icterus. You note petechiae and purpura on the extremities. Her abdomen is diffusely tender. She responds to commands but appears very lethargic.

While you are arranging her admission to the hospital, some laboratory tests return: Hgb 8 g/dL, Hct 24%, WBC 14,000/mm³, platelets 50,000/ mm³, Na

128 mEq/L, K 3.9 mEq/L, HCO_3 14 mEq/L, BUN 38 mg/dL, creatinine 2.1 mg/dL. The peripheral blood smear shows schistocytes, Burr cells, and grossly reduced number of platelets.

Which of the following is the most appropriate INITIAL management of this patient?

A) Intravenous fluids.
B) Dialysis.
C) Platelet transfusion.
D) Corticosteroids.
E) Antibiotics.

Discussion

The correct answer is A. The proper initial management consists of supportive therapy. This patient has signs of dehydration, which would be expected from the history of prolonged diarrhea. She is hyponatremic, and isotonic (0.9%) saline is the IV fluid of choice. Use 20 cc/kg boluses until her blood pressure stabilizes. This patient may also require an RBC transfusion given her anemia. Although she has had diarrhea, her potassium is currently in the normal range, probably due to decreased glomerular filtration. Given her renal failure, potassium should not be in her IV fluids.

Consideration of dialysis (answer B) is premature. A platelet count of 50,000 is adequate for hemostasis so answer C is incorrect. The schistocytes suggest a microangiopathic hemolytic anemia. Steroids are not generally helpful for this, so answer D is incorrect. Antibiotics (answer E) may (or may not) be beneficial if the patient has bacterial enteritis, but IV fluids should be administered first.

Based on the available information, which of the following is the most likely diagnosis?

A) Thrombotic thrombocytopenic purpura.
B) Hemolytic uremic syndrome.
C) Postinfectious glomerulonephritis.
D) Henoch-Schönlein purpura.
E) Autosomal recessive polycystic kidney disease.

Discussion

The correct answer is B. Hemolytic uremic syndrome (HUS) is the most likely diagnosis. This patient presents with a classic history of uremia and hemolysis preceded by 5–7 days of diarrhea. Patients tend to become oliguric and sometimes anuric.

Answer A is incorrect. Thrombotic thrombocytopenic purpura (TTP) is a related disorder which is rare in children. TTP tends to occur in young adults with women making up about 70% of all cases. In contrast to HUS, patients with TTP may present with the classic pentad: thrombocytopenia, fever, mental status changes, renal insufficiency, and hemolytic anemia. Usually, there is a prodrome of viral illness, but diarrhea occurs only rarely.

Answer C is incorrect. Postinfectious glomerulonephritis usually occurs after pharyngitis or skin infection with group A beta-hemolytic streptococci. Common symptoms include edema and hematuria but not thrombocytopenia or diarrhea. Answer D is incorrect. Henoch-Schönlein purpura is a transient IgA vasculitis following upper respiratory infections in children and adolescents. There should not be an antecedent history of diarrhea. Answer E is incorrect. Autosomal recessive polycystic kidney disease is a rare disorder that presents early in childhood with abdominal masses, hypertension, urinary tract infections, and renal failure.

 HELPFUL TIP: HUS may occur without diarrhea. This subtype of HUS occurs less frequently, is associated with *Streptococcus* infections, and carries a worse prognosis.

From the BLOOD culture, you expect to find:

A) *Shigella* species.
B) *Escherichia coli.*
C) *Streptococcus pneumoniae.*
D) *Haemophilus influenzae.*
E) None of the above.

Discussion

The correct answer is E. Although HUS is the result of bacterial enteritis, the syndrome is not mediated by bacteremia. Instead, the endothelial damage and hemolysis is caused by Shiga toxin, released from *E. coli* and *Shigella dysenteriae.*

All of the following are true regarding Shiga toxin HUS in children EXCEPT:

A) If dialysis is needed, renal function rarely returns.
B) Half or more of the cases occur in the summer months.
C) Ingestion of contaminated meat is a common source of *E. coli* O157:H7 infection.

D) Cattle are the main vectors of *E. coli* O157:H7.

E) Antibiotics do not reduce the risk of HUS in patients with confirmed *E. coli* O157:H7 infections.

Discussion

The correct answer is A. The prognosis of Shiga toxin HUS in children is generally quite favorable, even if renal failure requires dialysis. All the other statements are true. HUS is more common in rural areas and in the summer. Cows are the culprits.

Answer E requires special note. There is controversy over whether or not antibiotics may **increase** the risk of HUS developing in patients with *E. coli* O157:H7 infections; however, it is fairly clear that antibiotics do not reduce the risk. Remember that most cases of bacterial gastroenteritis—*E. coli* O157:H7 included—will clear without antibiotic therapy.

 HELPFUL TIP: Other subtypes of *E. coli* as well as *Shigella* can be responsible for HUS. The absence of the O157:H7 subtype of *E. coli* does not rule out HUS.

Objectives: Did you learn to . . .

- Evaluate and manage a child with hypovolemia and renal failure?
- Construct a differential diagnosis for renal failure in a child?
- Recognize a clinical history and laboratory findings suggestive of hemolytic-uremic syndrome?
- Identify causes of hemolytic-uremic syndrome?

 QUICK QUIZ: ACID-BASE DISORDER

While covering your local ED, a 15-year-old female presents with her father. He reports that he came home from work, found her asleep on the couch, and had difficulty waking her. She is lethargic and complains of nausea, dizziness, and abdominal pain. Apparently, she had muscle aches after gymnastics practice and then took "handfuls" of aspirin to relieve her pain. She was taking 3–4 tablets every hour or 2 today but is not sure about her total ingestion. She denies other ingestions.

On physical examination, her temperature is 39°C, pulse 110, respiratory rate 18, and blood pressure 104/68. She is diaphoretic. The neurologic exam is nonfocal, but she becomes progressively more lethargic during the exam. An arterial blood gas on room air shows pH 7.38, $PaCO_2$ 23 mm Hg, PaO_2 98 mm Hg HCO_3 15mEq/L. Other lab data: Na 140 mEq/L, K 3.1 mEq/L, Cl 101 mEq/L, HCO_3 15 mEq/L, BUN 19 mg/dL, creatinine 1.1 mg/dL.

The arterial blood gas results are best described as:

A) Metabolic acidosis.

B) Metabolic acidosis/alkalosis.

C) Metabolic acidosis and respiratory alkalosis.

D) Metabolic alkalosis and respiratory acidosis.

E) Just dandy! Look at the pH, professor.

Discussion

The correct answer is C. Although the pH is in the normal range, there is an acid-base disorder present. First, there appears to be a metabolic acidosis with an elevated anion gap. The measured HCO_3 is 15 mEq/L, consistent with an acidosis; and the anion gap is 24 (based on the calculation of $Na - [Cl + HCO_3]$, in this case: $140 - [101 + 15] = 24$). This patient has taken an inadvertent overdose of aspirin. In salicylate overdoses, a high anion gap metabolic acidosis is often observed. Since salicylates directly stimulate the CNS respiratory center there is usually a concurrent respiratory alkalosis.

In metabolic acidosis, the $PaCO_2$ should drop by 1.25 mm Hg for every 1 mEq/L drop in HCO_3. In this case, the serum HCO_3 is 9 mEq/L below normal (if the normal is counted as 24), so $PaCO_2$ should be about 29 mm Hg ($40 - [9 \times 1.25]$). However, the measured $PaCO_2$ is 23 mm Hg, indicating the presence of a respiratory alkalosis. Also, the pH is nearly normal despite the presence of a disturbance in measured HCO_3, **which only occurs when a mixed disorder is present.**

Proper treatment of salicylate overdoses includes supportive therapy, urine alkalinization with sodium bicarbonate, and activated charcoal if the patient presents early enough. Dialysis may also be necessary.

 HELPFUL TIP: It is impossible to overcorrect a metabolic abnormality. Thus, a patient with a metabolic acidosis will not become alkalotic or normal unless there is another primary process present (eg, respiratory alkalosis). Likewise, a patient with a respiratory acidosis from the retention of CO_2 will not become alkalotic or normal unless there is a secondary primary process going on (eg, metabolic alkalosis).

QUICK QUIZ: DYSURIA

Your nurse comes to you with a patient request. A 25-year-old female called in to complain of 2 days of burning with urination, urgency to urinate, and increased frequency. She has no fever, nausea, abdominal pain, flank pain, or vaginal discharge. The patient wants to know, "Can't I just get some antibiotics?" She is certain this is a bladder infection, just like the one she had last year. By the way, she is leaving for Europe tomorrow for her honeymoon.

Your response is to:

A) Prescribe ciprofloxacin 250 mg BID for 3 days.
B) Prescribe trimethoprim/sulfamethoxazole BID for 14 days.
C) Ask her to come in for a urinalysis.
D) Ask her to come in for a urine culture.
E) Recommend cranberry juice.

Discussion

The correct answer is A. Although you could argue that the diagnosis of UTI should be confirmed by urinalysis, there is evidence that history alone is sufficiently accurate. If a woman complains of dysuria and increased frequency without vaginal discharge, the likelihood ratio of UTI is about 25 and posttest probability is >90% that she has a urinary tract infection (JAMA 2002;287(20):2701).

Answer C is incorrect. If her urinalysis were completely normal, she may still have an infection and have a false-negative dipstick urine. **Using urine dipstick alone in a woman with urinary symptoms increases the posttest probability to only 81%.** Thus, certain symptoms and historical elements are more useful than urinalysis. For this patient, empiric antibiotic therapy with an appropriate antibiotic (nonrespiratory fluoroquinolone, trimethoprim/sulfamethoxazole, or other) for 3 days is reasonable. Fourteen days of trimethoprim/sulfamethoxazole (answer B) is overkill. Of course, urine culture (answer D) is the gold standard for diagnosing UTI, but she will be in Europe by the time you get the results. There is some evidence that cranberry products may reduce the frequency of recurrent UTI, but cranberry juice (answer E) does not seem to work for treatment. Trials of cranberry products for UTI suffer from high drop-out rates and variability in products and measurements.

HELPFUL TIP: With typical UTI symptoms (eg, dysuria, frequency) and a negative urine culture or no response to antibiotics, consider other causes: interstitial cystitis, chlamydia urethritis, prostatitis (in men), pelvic inflammatory disease (in women), pelvic mass, herpes genitalis, and drugs (eg, diuretics, caffeine, and theophylline).

CASE 12

You are asked to consult on a patient who is hospitalized by an orthopedic surgeon. The patient is a 25-year-old female who has a history of osteomyelitis from an open fracture sustained in a skiing accident. She has recently begun to spike a fever and have a rapid increase in her creatinine.

Medications: Methicillin, Ibuprofen, morphine, Lactated Ringer solution IV 100 cc/hr

Labs: Cr = 3.5 mg/dL, BUN = 25 mg/dL

CBC shows mild eosinophilia

What would you expect to find?

A) FENa >2%, Urine Sodium <20.
B) FENa <1%, Urine Sodium <20.
C) FENa >2%, Urine sodium >40.
D) FENa <1%, Urine sodium >40.

Discussion

The correct answer is C. The patient's BUN/Cr <20 therefore it is likely **not** prerenal disease (and she's receiving volume and has no history of heart failure). Thus, the patient likely has intrinsic kidney disease. This means that the FENa should be >2% and the urine sodium >40 mg/dL. In this scenario, the kidney is not trying to hold on to sodium in an attempt to correct a prerenal cause of increasing creatinine.

* *

The patient's exam shows a diffuse rash and the urine contains white cell casts. There are no red cells in the urine.

The most likely diagnosis is:

A) Acute tubular necrosis.
B) Interstitial nephritis.
C) Renal infarction.
D) Glomerulonephritis.
E) Nephrotic syndrome.

Table 5–12 COMMON DRUGS ASSOCIATED WITH INTERSTITIAL NEPHRITIS

- Penicillins
- Aspirin
- Ciprofloxacin (and likely other fluoroquinolones)
- Allopurinol
- NSAIDs
- Some ACEIs
- Erythromycin

Discussion

The correct answer is B. The combination of fever, rash, mild eosinophilia, exposure to a new drug (methicillin) and white cell casts in the urine essentially makes the diagnosis of interstitial nephritis. Answer A is incorrect. The patient with ATN may have the same FENa and urine sodium as this patient but should have renal tubular cells and/or granular casts in the urine. Also, ATN does not cause fever, eosinophilia, or rash. Renal infarction (answer C) is unlikely in a young patient and the rest of the clinical picture does not fit. Glomerulonephritis (answer D) is a possibility (eg, lupus could cause a rash and fever). However, glomerulonephritis is associated with **red cell casts** and not white cell casts. As you learned above, nephrotic syndrome (answer E) presents with a bland urine (Tables 5–12 and 5–13).

How long after drug exposure does interstitial nephritis generally begin?

A) 2–3 days.
B) 10–14 days.
C) Several months.

Table 5–13 SYMPTOMS/SIGNS/LABORATORY FINDINGS IN ACUTE INTERSTITIAL NEPHRITIS

- Fever
- Rash (variable, may not be seen in all)
- Acute rise in plasma creatinine
- Active urine sediment that includes white cell casts
- Peripheral eosinophilia and urine eosinophils (in most cases)
- Renal tubular acidosis

Note: Interstitial nephritis secondary to NSAIDs may occur without fever, rash, or eosinophilia.

D) A and B.
E) All of the above.

Discussion

The correct answer is E. Patients can develop interstitial nephritis anywhere from 1 day to several months after beginning a drug. Rifampin can often cause interstitial nephritis on day one. Interstitial nephritis can begin within 2–5 days if there has been a prior exposure to the drug, will typically begin within 10–14 days on **first** exposure to a drug, and may delayed for months in the case of NSAID exposure.

 HELPFUL TIP: Patients with interstitial nephritis will often have eosinophils in the urine and peripheral smear, but eosinophils may be absent especially in those with NSAID-induced interstitial nephritis. Treatment is to stop the offending drug. If this doesn't work, steroids or cytotoxic drugs may be needed.

Objectives: Did you learn to . . .

- Recognize the presenting symptoms of acute interstitial nephritis?
- Describe causes and prognosis of interstitial nephritis?

 QUICK QUIZ: SAVE THOSE NEPHRONS!

A 45-year-old male comes to your office to establish care. He reports a history of hypertension treated with verapamil and chlorthalidone. His blood pressure today is 130/78. You order some labs and find that his creatinine is 2.5 mg/dL.

You recommend which strategy to preserve his renal function?

A) Start a low-dose ACEI.
B) Start a high-dose ACEI.
C) Start furosemide.
D) Start amlodipine.

Discussion

The correct answer is A. Even in patients with renal dysfunction as evidenced by elevated creatinine, ACEIs can reduce the rate of progression of renal disease. More importantly, ACEIs can be used safely in patients with stage 4 CKD. Due to the risk of rising creatinine and potassium, ACEIs should be started at a low dose and increased slowly, checking creatinine and potassium levels within 1 or 2 weeks after making a dose adjustment. Furosemide and amlodipine have not been shown to preserve renal function.

 HELPFUL TIP: ACEIs have been shown to be useful in reducing progression of renal disease even when the patient's creatinine is 5.0 mg/dL, but, be very careful in this group.

BIBLIOGRAPHY

Bent S, Nallamothu BK, Simel DL, et al. Does this woman have an uncomplicated urinary tract infection? *JAMA*. 2002;287(20):2701.

Cantarovich F, Rangoonwala B, Lorenz H, et al. High-dose furosemide for established ARF: a prospective, randomized, double-blind, placebo-controlled, multicenter trial. *Am J Kidney Dis*. 2004;44(3):402.

Carroll MF, Temte JL. Proteinuria in adults: a diagnostic approach. *Am Fam Physician*. 2000;62(6):1333.

Grossfield GD, Wolf JS Jr, Litwan MS, et al. Asymptomatic microscopic hematuria in adults: summary of the AUA best practice policy recommendations. *Am Fam Physician*. 2001;63(6):1145-54.

Hou FF, Zhang X, Zhang GH, et al. Efficacy and safety of benazepril for advanced chronic renal insufficiency. *N Engl J Med*. 2006;354:131.

Kellum J, Leblanc M, Venkataraman R. Acute renal failure. *Am Fam Physician*. 2007;76(3):418.

Levey AS, Coresh J, et al. K/DOQI Clinical Practice Guidelines for Chronic Kidney Disease: Evaluation, Classification, and Stratification. Accessed October 20, 2007, at http://www.kidney.org/professionals/kdoqi/guidelines_ckd/toc.htm.

Miller NL, Lingeman JE. Management of kidney stones. *BMJ*. 2007;334(7591):468.

Parsons JK, Hergan LA, Sakamoto K, et al. Efficacy of alpha-blockers for the treatment of ureteral stones. *J Urol*. 2007;177(3):983.

Phrommintikul A, et al. Mortality and target haemoglobin concentrations in anaemic patients with chronic kidney disease treated with erythropoietin: A meta-analysis. *Lancet*. 2007;369:381.

Price CP, Newall RG, Boyd JC. Use of protein:creatinine ratio measurements on random urine samples for prediction of significant proteinuria: a systematic review. *Clin Chem*. 2005;51(9):1577.

Ritz E, Orth SR. Nephropathy in patients with type 2 diabetes mellitus. *N Engl J Med*. 1999;341:1127.

Rose BD, Post TW. *Clinical Physiology of Acid-Base and Electrolyte Disorders*. 5th ed. New York: McGraw-Hill; 2001.

Simerville JA, Maxted WC, Pahira JJ. Urinalysis: a comprehensive review. *Am Fam Physician*. 2005;71(6):1153.

Strippoli GF, Bonifati C, Craig M, et al. Angiotensin converting enzyme inhibitors and angiotensin II receptor antagonists for preventing the progression of diabetic kidney disease. *Cochrane Database Sys Rev*. 2006 Oct 18; (4):CD006257.

Tarr, PI, Gordon, CA, Chandler, WL. Shiga-toxin-producing *Escherichia coli* and haemolytic uraemic syndrome. *Lancet*. 2005;365:1073.

6

Hematology and Oncology

Deborah Wilbur

CASE 1

A 6-month-old male infant presents to your office after his mother notices swelling and ecchymosis over his anterior right thigh. She does not recall any trauma to the area. The mother denies any history of bleeding problems, including during his circumcision. On physical exam the child has a large hematoma over his thigh. There are no obvious bony deformities and the child otherwise looks well. You suspect the child may have an inherited coagulation disorder.

Which of the following statements is NOT TRUE?

A) Child abuse should be included in the differential diagnosis.
B) The child did not bleed during circumcision, so the possibility of hemophilia need not be considered.
C) A careful family history is important in the workup.
D) Coagulation studies (PT, PTT) and CBC should be obtained.

Discussion

The correct answer is B. The absence of bleeding during circumcision does not rule out hemophilia. Up to 50% of hemophiliac patients do not bleed after circumcision. Depending on the severity of factor deficiency, the diagnosis may not be made until the child is very active or even in adulthood, after surgery, etc.

Which of the following statements is TRUE about the patient with a bleeding disorder?

A) Factor deficiencies generally present with mucosal bleeding/petechiae.

B) Hemarthrosis generally reflects a platelet deficiency.
C) Hematomas are usually the result of a factor deficiency.
D) All of the above are true.

Discussion

The correct answer is C. Hematomas are the result of a factor deficiency. Hemarthrosis (answer B) is the result of a factor deficiency as well. Generally, petechiae and mucosal bleeding (answer A) are the result of platelet deficiency (eg, mild von Willebrand disease and thrombocytopenia). Severe von Willebrand disease may present with hemarthrosis and hematomas.

Which of the following is NOT TRUE about hemophilia A?

A) It is an X-linked disorder.
B) It is the result of factor Xa deficiency.
C) It generally leads to hemarthrosis.
D) It occurs most often in males.

Discussion

The correct answer is B. Hemophilia A is an X-lined deficiency of factor VIII which presents with hematomas, bleeding, and hemarthrosis (and not generally mucosal bleeding or petechiae). Deficiency of factor IX, or hemophilia B, is also X-linked but is much less common. Answer D deserves special note. Hemophilia rarely occurs in females but can in two situations: (1) the female patient is a heterozygote who has early inactivation of the second X chromosome during embryogenesis or (2) if both parents are carriers.

> **HELPFUL TIP:** Von Willebrand disease may be autosomal dominant (type I), variable (type II), or autosomal recessive (type III). There is often a family history of factor deficiency or bleeding, but a minority of cases are acquired, often occurring with autoimmune diseases.

Which of the following is indicated when evaluating for a suspected inherited coagulopathy?

A) CBC.
B) PT and PTT.
C) Platelet count.
D) PFA-100.
E) All of the above.

Discussion

The correct answer is E. The PTT is actually the most sensitive test for hemophilia. Answer D deserves special note. The PFA-100 (platelet function assay) tests for (appropriately enough) platelet functioning and will be abnormal in von Willebrand disease. Other qualitative platelet defects are rare, however.

> **HELPFUL TIP:** Treatment for hemophilia is lifelong and should be provided through a designated comprehensive hemophilia treatment center. In addition to factor replacement, treatment can include topical thrombin, desmopressin, or aminocaproic acid and should include genetics counseling, regular follow-up with specialized dentists, and regular physical therapy evaluations to assess for the development of chronic arthropathy.

CASE 2

A 3-year-old female is brought to you by her mother after she is noted to have small pink spots on her lower extremities and bleeding from her gums. She had a cold 2 weeks ago. You note petechiae on her lower extremities and purpura in her oropharynx. The mother and patient deny hematuria, rectal bleeding, or melena. You obtain a CBC, which is normal except for a platelet count of 15,000/mm³. You suspect idiopathic thrombocytopenic purpura (ITP).

Which of the following is the LEAST appropriate treatment for ITP in this child?

A) IVIG.
B) Steroids (eg, prednisone).
C) Platelet transfusion.
D) Splenectomy.

Discussion

The correct answer is C. You do not want to do this because transfused platelets will just be devoured by the same antiplatelet antibodies that have lead to ITP in the first place. **Most patients can simply be observed. The only indication for treatment is bleeding.** All of the treatments have a downside. Splenectomy (answer D) is associated with a risk of sepsis. If possible, delay splenectomy until after the child is >5 years. Steroids (answer B) may cause behavioral problems and long-term problems such as avascular necrosis.

> **HELPFUL TIP:** If the child were ill, sepsis with DIC and TTP–HUS (thrombotic thrombocytopenic purpura—hemolytic uremic syndrome) should also be considered. ITP is most common in children between 2 and 4 years. The condition often resolves without specific therapy: 80% to 90% of pediatric patients are back to normal within a few months, and <20% of children will remain thrombocytopenic for greater than 12 months. Only 0.1% to 0.5% develop intracranial bleeding.

> **HELPFUL TIP:** Do not bother checking for antiplatelet antibodies in those with ITP. Patients **without** ITP may have antiplatelet antibodies and the presence of these antibodies is not predictive of outcome.

CASE 3

Just for the sake of argument, let's say the patient's grandmother presents with a similar clinical picture (petechiae and purpura without other symptoms) and a platelet count of 15,000/mm³. Her CBC, including peripheral smear reviewed by your friendly neighborhood pathologist, is otherwise totally normal. **Her blood type is O negative**. You're thinking ITP (because this is the hematology chapter... and you're smart).

What do you recommend first for this patient?

A) Bone marrow biopsy.
B) Immediate splenectomy.
C) Prednisone.
D) Rho(D) immune globulin (WinRho SDF).
E) Rugby.

Discussion

The correct answer is C. There are two main points to this question: (1) relapses and refractory ITP are common in adults compared to children, so treatment is usually required and (2) Rh **positive** patients with ITP can be treated with Rho(D) immune globulin (answer D). Initial treatment for adults typically includes prednisone 1 mg/kg/day with a slow taper lasting several weeks after patients respond. Intravenous immunoglobulin is another valuable treatment option, particularly when significant bleeding is present. For refractory cases, splenectomy (answer B) is often indicated but is not typically first-line therapy. Patients who require splenectomy should be immunized as early as possible with pneumococcal, meningococcal and *Haemophilus influenzae* B vaccines. Answer E is incorrect because you want patients with thrombocytopenia to avoid trauma, including contact sports. Answer A is incorrect because bone marrow biopsy is not indicated for the work-up of ITP, and a primary bone marrow process is unlikely since the rest of the CBC is normal.

 HELPFUL TIP: Failure of ITP to respond to splenectomy may be due to the presence of an accessory spleen, which can often be identified by a liver-spleen radionuclide study.

CASE 4

A 24-year-old female presents to your office with a bruise on her anterior tibia, which she noticed after bumping into a coffee table. She is G1 P0, at 39 weeks gestation. She has been well during her pregnancy and has had appropriate prenatal care. She has no other medical history, does not smoke or drink alcohol, and takes only prenatal vitamins. Her physical exam is unremarkable with the exception of an 8-cm bruise over her right anterior tibia. She has a normal blood pressure, normal reflexes and no peripheral edema. You obtain the following lab tests: CBC, which demonstrates WBC 9,000/mm^3, hemoglobin 11.8 g/dL, and platelet count 95,000/mm^3; negative urinalysis, normal liver enzymes.

What is your next step?

A) Recommend immediate delivery by cesarean section as the fetus likely has thrombocytopenia as well and is at high risk for intracranial hemorrhage.
B) Recommend immediate delivery by cesarean section as this disorder will likely progress to eclampsia.
C) Recommend close observation, and reassure the patient that this is typically a self-limited condition.
D) Start prednisone, 1 mg/kg per day, and taper slowly over the next 6 weeks.
E) Recommend splenectomy as soon as possible after delivery.

Discussion

The correct answer is C. This patient likely has gestational thrombocytopenia, a condition that occurs in up to 5% of pregnant women. It is characterized by mild thrombocytopenia occurring in late gestation; the platelet count is usually >70,000/mm^3 (two-thirds are between 130,000/mm^3 and 150,000/mm^3). The condition resolves after delivery and is not associated with severe neonatal thrombocytopenia. No specific change in routine obstetrical care is warranted, although the anesthesiologist who places an epidural may want a follow-up platelet count closer to the time of delivery.

 HELPFUL TIP: A platelet count of >20,000–50,000/mm^3 is generally considered adequate for appropriate clotting.

CASE 5

The patient's 22-year-old sister presents to your office for a routine obstetric visit. She says, "We do everything together—even pregnancy!" She is G1 P0 and is at 20 weeks' gestation. She has noticed some spontaneous bruising and gingival bleeding while flossing. She feels well otherwise and has no significant past medical history. She is taking only prenatal vitamins. Her blood pressure is normal. Her CBC is as follows: WBC 6,000/mm^3, hemoglobin 11.2 g/dL, platelet count 15,000/mm^3, and no protein on urine dipstick. She says, "Look! I've even got the same problem as my sister. Oh, well."

You counsel her and initiate therapy including all of the following EXCEPT:

A) Start prednisone 1 mg/kg daily.
B) Tell her that her baby will have a 1 in 10 chance of a transient platelet count <50,000/mm^3 at birth.
C) Tell her that she may need a splenectomy at some point during her pregnancy.
D) Recommend that the baby be delivered by cesarean section.
E) Explain that her baby's platelet count will likely reach its lowest point several days after birth.

Discussion

The correct answer is D. This patient's condition differs from her sister's because more severe thrombocytopenia developed earlier in her pregnancy. This is concerning for ITP. Her child has a 10% chance of being born with a platelet count <50,000/mm^3, with the platelet count reaching its nadir several days after the infant's birth. Despite these statistics, there is no increase in morbidity in the infant delivered by vaginal delivery versus cesarean section.

Because this patient has a significantly low platelet count, treatment should be initiated. If possible, splenectomy should be avoided due to technical problems with surgery on a gravid abdomen. Patients who do require splenectomy also have a higher incidence of infants born with severe thrombocytopenia.

Objectives: Did you learn to . . .

- Obtain a thorough bleeding history?
- Use laboratory testing to assist in the diagnosis of a bleeding disorder?
- Identify common congenital bleeding disorders?
- Identify and treat common acquired bleeding disorders?

QUICK QUIZ: COAGULATION STUDIES

Which of the following conditions should be considered if both PT and PTT are abnormally elevated in a patient noted to be oozing from a surgical incision?

A) Severe liver disease, disseminated intravascular coagulation, factor X deficiency.
B) Heparin effect, von Willebrand disease, factor XII deficiency.
C) Warfarin effect, factor VII deficiency, vitamin K deficiency.
D) All of the above.

Discussion

The correct answer is A. The three factor deficiencies that may prolong both PT and PTT are factors II, V, and X. Both PTT and PT may be prolonged due to severe liver disease and DIC as well. Mild vitamin K deficiency or liver disease generally affects the PT only. Generally, heparin affects PTT, and warfarin affects PT.

CASE 6

A 42-year-old male presents to the ED with a gastrointestinal bleed caused by ibuprofen use, and his hemoglobin is 6.8 g/dL. You decide to transfuse him 2 units of packed red blood cells (PRBC). After 30 minutes of transfusion, the patient complains of dyspnea and back pain. Repeat examination of this patient reveals a diaphoretic man with a pulse of 130 and blood pressure of 88/50. His lung fields are clear.

What is your next step?

A) Stop the blood transfusion and begin normal saline through the IV.
B) Increase the rate of transfusion.
C) Administer acetaminophen 650 mg by mouth.
D) Administer furosemide 40 mg IV.
E) Place a nasogastric tube for lavage.

Discussion

The correct answer is A. The transfusion must be stopped. The patient is exhibiting signs and symptoms of a hemolytic transfusion reaction, which is generally the result of an ABO incompatibility. Patients may exhibit nausea, flushing, dyspnea, oliguria, back pain, and hypotension. Other findings include hemoglobinuria, elevated serum free hemoglobin, reduced haptoglobin, elevated bilirubin, and positive direct antiglobulin (Coombs) test. Hemolytic reactions occur in 1/25,000 blood transfusions and are fatal in 1/100,000. The reaction typically occurs after infusion of approximately 200 mL of blood but can occur after as little as 30 mL. Therapy includes IV saline at a high enough rate to initiate a brisk diuresis and prevent hemoglobin from precipitating in the kidneys causing acute tubular necrosis.

> **HELPFUL TIP:** When you suspect a transfusion reaction, you must assume that the patient has received blood intended for someone else. The blood bank must be notified. A system error may have occurred whereby patient blood samples or transfusion products may have been inadvertently switched. Another patient in the hospital could be at risk

CASE 7

An 18-year-old male arrives in the ED with multiple fractures and a splenic laceration sustained as an unrestrained passenger in a motor vehicle collision. He is admitted to the surgical intensive care unit after splenectomy and is noted to have oozing at his suture sites. He received 22 units of PRBC during the surgery. (You think this is some kind of record, but the surgeon says she's seen worse.)

What is your initial suspicion and how do you manage it?

A) Disseminated intravascular coagulopathy; start heparin 500 units/hr.
B) Disseminated intravascular coagulopathy; transfuse 2 units PRBC and recommend surgical exploration for a retained foreign body.
C) Thrombocytopenia and decreased coagulation proteins secondary to massive transfusion; check PT and PTT and transfuse an 8-pack of platelets plus fresh frozen plasma.
D) Previously undetected hemophilia; measure factor levels to obtain a diagnosis.
E) Aspirin effect from medications ingested prior to the accident; transfuse an 8-pack of platelets.

Discussion

The correct answer is C. The patient has received a massive transfusion, which creates a number of specific complications. "Massive transfusion" has several definitions that vary from study to study. Most common definitions include a transfusion requirement of more

than 10 units of blood in 24 hours or replacement of more than 50% of a patient's blood volume in 12–24 hours. This can lead to dilutional thrombocytopenia, which may require platelet transfusion. Additionally, packed red blood cell units are plasma-poor and coagulation proteins may drop by 10% per unit. Fresh frozen plasma (FFP) transfusions should be considered if the PT or PTT is increased. Giving a fixed number of units of FFP per unit of PRBC transfused (eg, 1:5) is suboptimal. Monitor coagulation studies and transfuse FFP as appropriate. Also, monitor acid-base status, calcium, and potassium levels, as significant metabolic alkalosis (due to citrate), hypocalcemia, and hyperkalemia can result from massive blood transfusions.

> **HELPFUL TIP:** Remember that trauma patients may also have DIC (especially with head trauma), so don't assume that all bleeding with low platelets is dilutional.

> **HELPFUL TIP:** In a nonbleeding patient, the transfusion of 1 unit of PRBC can be expected to raise the hematocrit by 3% to 4% (1 g/dL for Hb).

CASE 8

An 18-month-old male is admitted to the ED after being knocked out of his stroller. The child did not lose consciousness, and had a strong cry. An initial survey demonstrates a 12-kg child, temperature 37.8°C, pulse 160, blood pressure 88/50, and respirations 20. Plain films of the pelvis demonstrate fractures of the superior and inferior pubic rami bilaterally. His initial hematocrit is 28%. You suspect that the source of his anemia is the pelvic fracture. While awaiting a CT scan and the orthopedic team, you place a pelvic binder and type and cross-match the patient for transfusion.

What are your initial transfusion orders?

A) Transfuse an 8-pack of platelets.
B) Transfuse 2 units of PRBC.
C) Transfuse 40 mL of PRBC.
D) Transfuse 1,200 mL of PRBC.
E) Transfuse 120 mL of PRBC.

Discussion

The correct answer is E. The child is 12 kg, and the initial calculation for his transfusion should be 10 mL/kg, or 2.5 mL/kg/hour. This should increase his hemoglobin by 2–3 g/dL.

CASE 9

A 56-year-old male presents to the ED with an acute abdomen, likely from a perforated diverticulum. He is taking warfarin for a DVT that occurred after a total knee arthroplasty. He weighs 65 kg. You are evaluating him for surgery and find the following labs: Hb 14.3 g/dL, platelets 478,000/mm³, INR 3.5, PTT 28 seconds.

Which of the following statements about his preoperative management is correct?

A) Platelet transfusion preoperative will produce the most immediate reduction in risk of bleeding from warfarin.

B) FFP transfusion will produce the most immediate reduction in risk of bleeding from warfarin.

C) Vitamin K administration orally will produce the most immediate reduction in risk of bleeding from warfarin.

D) Vitamin K administration subcutaneously will produce the most immediate reduction in risk of bleeding from warfarin.

E) Cryoprecipitate transfusion will produce the most immediate reduction in risk of bleeding from warfarin.

Discussion

The correct answer is B. The patient would benefit most immediately from the administration of FFP, which contains all the soluble plasma proteins found in whole blood including the vitamin K–dependent factors that are depleted by warfarin. If more sustained reversal is desired, the simultaneous administration of vitamin K is effective. It should be given either orally or IV and not SQ which is less effective. The effects of FFP rarely last 24 hours; the effects of vitamin K are usually not apparent for 12–24 hours. The use of cryoprecipitate will not provide the appropriate factors depleted by warfarin. Cryoprecipitate contains von Willebrand factor, factor VIII, factor XIII, fibrinogen, and fibronectin, but not significant amounts of other factors. Platelet transfusion would not benefit this patient since warfarin does not affect platelet function.

 HELPFUL TIP: Oral administration of vitamin K is the safest, most effective route. It's hard to argue for another route if the oral route is available. Subcutaneous administration is less predictable, and intravenous administration may produce hypotension. If a patient requires immediate anticoagulation after a procedure, the use of vitamin K may make it difficult to achieve a therapeutic INR when the warfarin is restarted.

Objectives: Did you learn to . . .

• Recognize hemolytic transfusion reactions?
• Treat a patient with a massive blood transfusion?
• Appropriately dose packed cells for pediatric patients?
• Treat warfarin-induced hypocoagulability?

CASE 10

A 20-year-old female with acute myeloid leukemia completed her second cycle of consolidation chemotherapy 5 days ago. She presents to the ED with complaints of fatigue and fever. She denies cough, dysuria, abdominal pain, sinus drainage, or redness around her Hickman catheter. Her physical exam reveals a temperature of 38.4°C, pulse 100, blood pressure 120/58, respirations 14. Her exam is otherwise unremarkable, including no redness or tenderness at the Hickman site. Her labs reveal the following: WBC 200/mm³, hemoglobin 9 g/dL, hematocrit 27%, and platelet count 47,000/mm³. Blood cultures have been drawn.

What is your next step, and what is your rationale?

A) Administer IV amphotericin B because a *Candida* urinary tract infection is most likely.

B) Administer IV cefepime because she requires empiric coverage for both Gram-negative and Gram-positive organisms.

C) Administer IV nafcillin because a Gram-positive bacterial infection is most likely and broader antibiotic coverage will encourage growth of resistant bacteria.

D) Administer IV vancomycin and remove the Hickman catheter because she most likely has a catheter infection.

E) Close observation because there is no evidence of infection and she looks well.

Discussion

The correct answer is B. This patient has a neutropenic fever which is a medical emergency. Prompt treatment with broad-spectrum antibiotics has drastically improved the survival of patients with neutropenic fever. Neutropenia is usually defined as neutrophils plus bands (absolute neutrophil count) <500/mm³ or <1000/mm³ when the nadir has not been reached. Most myelosuppressive chemotherapeutic agents produce a reduction in WBCs 4–10 days after completion and nadir at 10–14 days. Fever is defined as a single oral temperature >101°F (38.3°C) or a temperature >100.4°F (38°C) persisting for 1 hour or more. Patients who are at risk for febrile neutropenia should be instructed to notify their physician immediately if they develop fever as defined above.

Broad-spectrum coverage of Gram-positive and Gram-negative organisms, including pseudomonas, is the cornerstone of therapy with specific therapy for any localizing symptoms or risk signs. See Table 6–1 for common antibiotic regimens.

All of the following are accurate statements about neutrophil counts in children EXCEPT:

A) African American children may have a normal absolute neutrophil (ANC) count of 1,000/mm³.

B) Children >6 years should be expected to have a normal ANC of 1,500–8,000/mm³.

C) Neonates typically have a normal ANC of <500/mm³ at birth.

D) Infants typically have 20%–30% neutrophils on WBC differential.

E) Five-year-old children have 50% neutrophils on WBC differential.

Discussion

The correct answer is C. In the pediatric population, neutropenia is typically described as an absolute neutrophil count of <1,500/mm³. Up to 30% of African American children have an asymptomatic ANC of <1,000/mm³ (eg, no increased risk of infection). At birth, neutrophils make up the majority of the WBC differential, and this decreases to 20%–30% after the first few days of life. At 5 years, neutrophils comprise approximately 50% of the differential, and this reaches 70% by puberty.

 HELPFUL TIP: Good prognostic factors in neutropenic fever include age <60 years, absence of comorbid illness such as diabetes or COPD, temperature <39°C, respiratory rate <24/minute, normal blood pressure, absence of confusion, cancer in complete or partial remission, and no personal history of fungal infection or recent antifungal therapy.

Table 6–1   ANTIBIOTIC REGIMENS FOR NEUTROPENIC FEVER

Single Agents		Combinations
Cephalosporins • Cefepime • Ceftazidime	Carbapenem • Imipenem • Meropenem	Aminoglycoside + one of the following: • Cefepime • Ceftazidime • Antipseudomonal penicillin (ticarcillin, piperacillin) • Carbepenem • Extended spectrum quinolone (levofloxacin) if penicillin-allergic
• Add vancomycin if a line infection (cellulitis around line site or bacteremia) is suspected, MRSA is likely, patient is clinically more ill (hypotension, etc), or if no improvement after 3–5 days of empiric therapy.		
• Add antifungal (voriconazole, amphotericin B) if still febrile 4–7 days after starting antibiotics. The risk of fungal infection is increased by this point.		

Adapted from IDSA guidelines (Hughes WT, et al. 2002 Guidelines for the use of antimicrobial agents in neutropenic patients with cancer. *Clin Infect Dis.* 2002;34:730).

HELPFUL TIP: Patients with a neutropenic fever can have any infection seen in normal hosts, but you should also consider IV catheter infections, perirectal infections and abscesses, and necrotizing enteritis (aka "typhlitis"). Remember that they may not have an inflammatory reaction around a catheter site, abscess formation, infiltrate on CXR, or WBCs in the urine because of the neutropenia. The absence of signs or symptoms should not dissuade the physician from starting empiric antibiotic therapy.

CASE 11

A 63-year-old male with a diagnosis of non–small-cell lung cancer, undergoing weekly chemotherapy and radiation to a left upper lobe mass, presents to your office. He complains of dull, nonradiating back pain in the lower thoracic area. He denies trauma or any new activities. He has no associated weakness or paresthesias. He denies difficulties with bowel or bladder function. His past medical history includes COPD, hypertension, and osteoarthritis, and he currently takes an albuterol MDI and hydrochlorothiazide.

What is your initial diagnostic and/or therapeutic approach to this patient?

A) MRI of thoracic and lumbar spine and NSAIDs.
B) Plain films of the thoracic and lumbar spine and COX-2 inhibitor.
C) Plain films of the thoracic spine and NSAIDs.
D) Prescription for physical therapy and NSAIDs.
E) Urinalysis with culture and antibiotics.

Discussion

The correct answer is A. This is not your average back pain. Any patient with active malignancy complaining of back pain should be investigated for metastasis. While a plain film of the spine may be useful, the gold standard is MRI. The real emergency is spinal cord impingement. Spinal cord compression may occur from direct extension of metastatic disease from the vertebrae or extension from retroperitoneal or paravertebral disease. Frequently, the pain predates neurologic symptoms, and because of the potential for severe, adverse outcomes, you want to catch the disease early to prevent chronic impairment.

* *

The patient undergoes MRI of the spine which demonstrates a compressing lesion at L1.

Which of the following is NOT an appropriate therapeutic modality?

A) Decompression surgery.
B) Dexamethasone 10 mg bolus IV, followed by 6 mg every 6 hours.
C) Observation with pain control (eg, with morphine PCA).
D) Radiation therapy to the affected area.

Discussion

The correct answer is B. *C.* Patients with spinal cord compression who have aggressive interventions are more likely to retain function, including ambulation and bowel and bladder control. Steroids will help reduce edema surrounding the tumor and hopefully will relieve pressure on the cord. Radiation (answer D) can often provide symptomatic relief and reduce the likelihood that the tumor will spread locally to impinge on the cord. Surgical decompression (answer A) is another option. If this patient opted for a palliative care approach and had decided upon hospice, answer C might be appropriate, but he is still getting active therapy, and his remaining time could be spent with less pain and better function if one of the other options were chosen.

CASE 12

A 32-year-old female presents to your office with complaints of dyspnea, constipation, menorrhagia, and fatigue that are new over the last few weeks. She has a distant history of Hodgkin disease treated with chemotherapy and radiation to the chest. She has a history of mild asthma, is a smoker, and denies alcohol use. Her physical exam reveals a well-developed woman, who appears comfortable at rest. Her temperature is 36.7°C, pulse 92, blood pressure 120/64, respirations 16, and oxygen saturation of 95% on room air. Her lung exam shows good air movement with occasional end expiratory wheezes. She has no adenopathy and the remainder of her exam is unremarkable. Her CBC with WBC differential is normal.

Which of these diagnoses can be ruled out based on this patient's history?

A) Coronary ischemia.
B) Hypothyroidism.
C) Lung cancer.
D) Relapse of the Hodgkin disease.
E) None of the above.

Discussion

The correct answer is E. Patients with a history of Hodgkin disease and chest radiation are at risk for a wide range of complications—even years after the disease has been successfully treated. Even though 80% of Hodgkin patients have long-term disease-free survival, 1 in 6 patients can be expected to die from late effects of therapy. Although coronary artery disease (answer A) would be extremely unusual in a normal 32-year-old, a patient with a history of chest radiation has a relative risk of coronary disease of 5–10 times that of age-matched controls. Thyroid disease (answer B) is highly likely, with over 50% of patients treated with chest radiation requiring thyroid hormone replacement. A TSH would be adequate screening. There is a high risk for secondary malignancy, including breast cancer, lung cancer (answer C), leukemia, sarcoma, and non-Hodgkin lymphoma. Finally, you should always be concerned about recurrence (answer D).

* *

The patient has a normal chest radiograph and ECG. However, her TSH is markedly elevated, and you start her on levothyroxine. You plan to see her back in 8 weeks for reevaluation and will provide additional counseling at that time.

Which of the following preventive health issues is (are) necessary to address at follow-up?

A) Early intervention by a fertility specialist if the patient desires pregnancy.
B) Smoking cessation.
C) Yearly mammograms.
D) All of the above.
E) None of the above.

Discussion

The correct answer is D. Female patients who were treated for Hodgkin disease with chemotherapy and radiation prior to age 20 have up to a 35% incidence of breast cancer by age 40. The typical latency period is 15 years. National guidelines recommend that annual mammography of Hodgkin's survivors treated with chest irradiation should begin 5–8 years posttreatment, or age 40, whichever comes first. Smokers with a history of Hodgkin disease have a 20-fold increased chance of developing lung cancer when compared to nonsmokers with a history of Hodgkin disease. Also, female patients with Hodgkin disease have a 69% incidence of premature ovarian failure if treated for their cancer before age 29 and up to 96% if treated after age 30. Although these statistics are improving with newer chemotherapy regimens, a patient should seek early referral to a fertility specialist if she desires pregnancy but is unable to conceive.

CASE 13

A 40-year-old male who has just received his first course of chemotherapy for non-Hodgkin lymphoma (NHL) presents to your ED complaining of weakness, cramps, and decreased urine output. He has no other medical problems and takes no medications except for prochlorperazine as needed for nausea. He has been eating and drinking well.

His physical examination reveals a tired-appearing male, with temperature 37.4°C, pulse 90, blood pressure 134/72, respirations 16. His head and neck exam is unremarkable, except for bilateral palpable cervical lymph nodes approximately 2 cm in diameter. His lungs are clear in the upper lung fields with crackles bilaterally at the bases. Muscle strength is normal, and reflexes are 3 + and symmetric. He exhibits 6 beats of clonus at the ankles. Chest radiograph shows evidence of early pulmonary edema.

What is the most likely set of laboratory values you will find for this patient?

A) Potassium 2.3 mEq/L, phosphorus 3.1 mg/dl, uric acid 4 mg/dL, calcium 9 mg/dL.
B) Potassium 2.6 mEq/L, phosphorus 6 mg/dL, uric acid 5 mg/dL, calcium 12 mg/dL.
C) Potassium 6.5 mEq/L, phosphorus 7 mg/dL, uric acid 18 mg/dL, calcium 6 mg/dL.
D) Potassium 6 mEq/L, phosphorus 6.8 mg/dL, uric acid 5 mg/dL, calcium 6.7 mg/dL.
E) Potassium 4.5 mEq/L, phosphorus 3.2 mg/dL, uric acid 9 mg/dL, calcium 8 mg/dL.

Discussion

The correct answer is C. This patient most likely has tumor lysis syndrome, which can occur in a patient with a highly responsive leukemia or bulky lymphomas that is being treated with chemotherapy (it rarely occurs without treatment). Tumor lysis syndrome occurs when there is rapid release of intracellular contents into the bloodstream. **It is characterized by high potassium, high phosphorus, high uric acid, and low calcium.** There may be associated renal failure, arrhythmias, fatigue, muscle cramps, and tetany.

* *

The patient is found to have a creatinine of 8 mg/dL.

What is the most likely cause of this patient's renal failure?

A) Dehydration.
B) Heart failure.
C) Hemoglobinuria.
D) Rhabdomyolysis related to chemotherapy.
E) Uric acid nephropathy.

Discussion

The correct answer is E. Patients with tumor lysis syndrome have renal failure secondary to uric acid nephropathy. This is caused by the precipitation of uric acid in the kidney, and it can be prevented by the use of allopurinol prior to the administration of chemotherapy. Although dehydration (answer A) is not the cause of renal failure, it certainly will exacerbate the situation.

Which of the following is MOST LIKELY to help this patient's current condition?

A) Allopurinol 300 mg orally.
B) Calcium carbonate 500 mg orally.
C) Emergent hemodialysis.
D) IV D5W with 2 amps bicarbonate.
E) IV normal saline 200 mL/hr.

Discussion

The correct answer is C. Answers A and B are incorrect. The horses are already out of the barn, and in fact they're probably over the hills and through the woods. Allopurinol and oral calcium will not help this situation. The patient already has renal failure from his tumor lysis syndrome. While he may benefit from preventive measures, including aggressive hydration (answer D) and allopurinol prior to undergoing chemotherapy, none of these measures is going to help his current renal failure. Additionally, the patient may

develop worsening pulmonary edema if given too much volume with IV fluids (answer E).

While waiting for the hemodialysis to be initiated, you should treat the patient for his hyperkalemia, which may include IV calcium gluconate, insulin and dextrose, and oral sodium polystyrene sulfonate (Kayexalate).

Objectives: Did you learn to . . .

- Recognize and initiate treatment for some oncologic emergencies, including spinal cord compression, tumor lysis syndrome, and neutropenic fever?
- Recognize late complications of cancer and cancer therapy, including distant radiation and chemotherapy?

CASE 14

A 60-year-old male presents to your office with complaints of fatigue, weight loss, episodes of melena, and headache. He has a history of alcoholic cirrhosis, diet-controlled diabetes, and hypertension and currently takes hydrochlorothiazide, enalapril, and monthly testosterone injections. He smokes two packs of cigarettes daily and consumes 6–8 beers nightly. His physical exam reveals an obese, ruddy-faced man with a temperature of 37°C, pulse 90, blood pressure 164/80, and respirations 14. He is found to have a hematocrit of 54%.

Which of the following items in his history is LEAST likely to explain the elevated hematocrit?

A) Alcoholic cirrhosis.
B) Diabetes.
C) Hypertension related medications.
D) Other medications he is currently taking.
E) Smoking.

Discussion

The correct answer is B. Diabetes should not cause an elevated hematocrit. Approach an elevated hematocrit with two questions: (1) Is it due to increased red blood cell mass or decreased plasma volume? (2) Is it primary erythrocytosis or secondary?

This patient has many potential secondary causes of an elevated hematocrit. Alcoholic cirrhosis (answer A) can lead to hepatocellular carcinoma which, along with other malignancies, can result in overproduction of erythropoietin, causing an elevated hematocrit. Diuretics (answer C) decrease plasma volume, causing an apparent elevation of hematocrit. Testosterone injections (answer D) may cause polycythemia. He has a significant smoking history (answer E) that may produce a secondary polycythemia due to tissue hypoxia.

* *

You repeat the patient's CBC, which demonstrates a WBC of 21,000/mm³, hemoglobin 18.7 g/dL, hematocrit 61%, MCV 70 fL (microcytosis), and platelet count 428,000/mm³. His oxygen saturation is 97% on room air. You note that all of his cell lines are increased.

Which of the following signs and symptoms is/are NOT associated with polycythemia vera?

A) Erythromelalgia (burning pain in hands and feet associated with acral paresthesias and color change [erythema, pallor, cyanosis] in the presence of palpable pulses).
B) Plethoric facies.
C) Pruritus, especially after taking a hot bath or shower.
D) Thrombotic events such as Budd-Chiari syndrome (portal vein thrombosis).
E) Wheezing and dyspnea.

Discussion

The correct answer is E. Wheezing and dyspnea are not typical features of polycythemia vera. Of note, the pruritus and erythromelalgia of polycythemia vera often respond to aspirin.

 HELPFUL TIP: Aspirin works by irreversibly inhibiting platelet cyclooxygenase. Cyclooxygenase catalyzes the conversion of arachidonic acid to thromboxane A2. This is an important step in reinforcing platelet activation. The irreversible binding may make the patient prone to prolonged bleeding. Even though the average life of platelets is 8–12 days, there are enough new platelets in the circulation to return bleeding times to normal within 3 days of stopping aspirin (eg, before surgery).

* *

You refer the patient to a hematologist who diagnoses polycythemia vera and recommends treatment, but the patient never follows through. You see him back in clinic 6 months later when he is complaining of worsening fatigue and dyspnea.

Which of the following best explains his symptoms?

A) Development of acute myeloid leukemia.
B) Compression of the diaphragm due to massive splenomegaly.
C) Anemia due to bone marrow fibrosis.
D) All of the above.
E) None of the above.

Discussion

The correct answer is D. Polycythemia vera can progress from the proliferative phase, characterized by splenomegaly, erythrocytosis, and thrombocytosis, to post-polycythemic myeloid metaplasia (PPMM). PPMM is characterized by extramedullary hematopoiesis (manifested by progressive hepatosplenomegaly) and bone marrow fibrosis with pancytopenia.

Three percent of patients treated with phlebotomy alone progress to acute myeloid leukemia. Patients who are well managed typically have a long median survival after diagnosis (>15 years), but a high percentage will have complications, usually related to thrombosis (less commonly from bleeding).

CASE 15

A 30-year-old female presents to your office for a routine visit. She mentions that she was hospitalized 3 months ago for an appendectomy. You review her discharge summary from that hospital stay and note that at the time of surgery, her platelet count was found to be 1,400,000/mm³, which her surgeon felt was most likely reactive. She has no other past medical history. She takes no medications, does not smoke, drinks alcohol only rarely, and exercises 3 times per week. She denies any other changes in her medical history since her last appointment with you, and in fact, has no complaints today. You repeat the CBC, showing WBC 5,000/mm³, hemoglobin 13 g/dL, and platelet count 800,000/mm³.

What is your next step in managing this patient?

A) Anticoagulation with warfarin to a goal INR 2–3.
B) Counseling against becoming pregnant.
C) Initiation of hydroxyurea 500 mg BID.

D) No further evaluation or follow-up necessary.

E) Observation and periodic evaluation of her CBC.

Discussion

The correct answer is E. This patient likely has essential thrombocythemia. Essential thrombocythemia (ET) is the most common myeloproliferative disorder in the United States and is more common in females. The median age at diagnosis is 60 years, but about 20% of patients with ET are diagnosed at age <40 years. Patients with ET have a higher rate of mortality than matched controls due to risk of thrombosis (arterial >venous) and bleeding events. In order to diagnose ET, other causes of thrombocytosis (eg, inflammation, iron deficiency, recent surgery, infection, bleeding, and malignancy) must be excluded. A bone marrow biopsy may be helpful in establishing the diagnosis by demonstrating adequate iron stores and ruling out chronic myelogenous leukemia or myelodysplasia.

Answer A is incorrect. Warfarin is not appropriate prophylactic therapy and would not be used unless the patient had a thromboembolic event. Answer B is incorrect. Although patients with ET have a high rate of spontaneous abortion, the patient can be counseled regarding this risk and aspirin can be considered if the patient has had prior pregnancy loss. Answer C is incorrect. The patient is at low risk for thromboembolic events (platelet count <1.5 million/mm³, young age, no comorbid illness or prior events). Hydroxyurea could be considered if the patient was at high risk or symptomatic.

> **HELPFUL TIP:** The most common cause of an abnormally high platelet count is reactive thrombocytosis, which can result from iron deficiency, infection, inflammation, or malignancy. There is no increased risk in bleeding or clotting in patients with reactive thrombocytosis.

Objectives: Did you learn to . . .

• Recognize symptoms and causes of polycythemia?

• Differentiate between primary and secondary polycythemia?

• Recognize the presentation and implication of essential thrombocythemia?

• Evaluate a patient with an elevated hemoglobin or platelet count?

CASE 16

A 15-year-old female presents to your office with the complaint of fatigue. She has been healthy, takes no medications, and does not smoke or drink alcohol. She is not sexually active. She reports menarche at age 13 and complains of heavy menses in the last year. Her physical examination reveals a well-developed, well-nourished, pale female. You find no hepatosplenomegaly. Her labs reveal a WBC of 6,000/mm³, hemoglobin of 8.9 g/dL, hematocrit of 27%, platelet count 400,000/mm³, MCV 72 fL, RDW 16. You order more laboratory tests.

What are the expected findings in this patient?

A) Increased iron, decreased ferritin, increased total iron binding capacity.

B) Decreased iron, decreased ferritin, decreased total iron binding capacity.

C) Increased iron, increased ferritin, increased total iron binding capacity.

D) Decreased iron, increased ferritin, decreased total iron binding capacity.

E) Decreased iron, decreased ferritin, increased total iron binding capacity.

Discussion

The correct answer is E. This patient likely has iron-deficiency anemia related to her heavy menses. There are three stages of iron deficiency. The first stage is characterized by decreased iron stores in bone marrow, normal hemoglobin, and decreased ferritin. The body can compensate with increased dietary iron absorption. In the second stage, there is decreased erythropoiesis due to lack of available iron. The hemoglobin may be mildly decreased or normal, with decreased serum iron, decreased ferritin, and increased total iron binding capacity (TIBC). The third stage is characterized by anemia in addition to decreased serum iron, decreased ferritin, increased TIBC, and decreased transferrin saturation. Hypochromic microcytic red blood cells are found on peripheral smear. The decrease in serum ferritin is proportional to the decrease in total body iron stores.

> **HELPFUL TIP:** The prevalence of von Willebrand disease in women with menorrhagia ranges from 5% to 20%. Always take a good personal and family bleeding history.

HELPFUL TIP: The level of ferritin to use to diagnose iron deficiency is a matter of debate. In the presence of anemia, a ferritin of <12 ng/mL is 50% sensitive, 99% specific. Using a ferritin of <41 ng/mL is 98% sensitive and 98% specific. Other cutoffs fall in between with regards to sensitivity and specificity. Always consider other causes of anemia such as B_{12} deficiency, folate deficiency, and thalassemia (Table 6–2).

* *

You start iron supplementation therapy in this patient.

Which of the following tests will be the first to indicate that you have instituted appropriate therapy?

A) Increase in hematocrit.
B) Increase in reticulocyte count.
C) Increase in serum free hemoglobin.
D) Decrease in ferritin.
E) Decrease in transferrin saturation.

Discussion
The correct answer is B. The patient's reticulocyte count will increase first—before the hematocrit (answer A). Answer C is incorrect. Only in exceptional circumstances (intravascular hemolysis) will there be free hemoglobin in the blood. Answer D is incorrect because the ferritin is low in iron deficiency anemia and should increase with therapy. Transferrin saturation (answer E) should increase in patients once you start to treat their anemia, but the reticulocyte count increases first.

HELPFUL TIP: Ferritin is not a useful test for iron deficiency in hospitalized patients or in those who are chronically ill. Ferritin is an acute-phase reactant and thus may be elevated in these patients even when the patient has iron deficiency anemia (where the ferritin should be low).

How long should you continue iron supplementation once the patient's labs have normalized?

A) Stop immediately once anemia has resolved.
B) Continue 3–6 months after the anemia has resolved.
C) Continue for 1 year after the anemia has resolved.
D) Indefinite iron supplementation is indicated.

Discussion
The correct answer is B. Continue iron for 3–6 months after the anemia has resolved. Also address the underlying

Table 6–2   CAUSES OF ANEMIA BY RED CELL VOLUME

Low MCV (usually <80 fL)	Normal MCV (usually 80–100 fL)	High MCV (usually >100 fL)
Thalassemias	Acute blood loss	B_{12} deficiency
Iron-deficiency anemia	Early iron deficiency	Folate deficiency
Sideroblastic anemias	Endocrine (eg, hypothyroidism)	Alcohol
Anemia of chronic disease	Anemia of chronic disease	Hypothyroidism
Lead poisoning	Chronic renal insufficiency	Primary bone marrow
	Primary bone marrow disorders	Drug effect
		Liver disease
		Hemolytic anemia

Note: More than one cause of anemia may be present in the same patient. For example, it is not uncommon for a patient with a history of gastric bypass to present with a profound **normocytic anemia** due to both iron deficiency and B_{12} deficiency, which would usually present with microcytic and macrocytic anemia, respectively.

problem, in this patient her heavy periods, which may respond to hormonal contraception.

* *

The patient returns to your office in 2 months but her labs are worse than at first presentation. The patient swears that she has been taking the iron faithfully.

Which of the following can lead to a failure of iron therapy for iron deficiency anemia?

A) Proton pump inhibitors.
B) Incorrect diagnosis.
C) Oral antacids (eg, calcium carbonate).
D) Atrophic gastritis, celiac disease, or *H. pylori* infection.
E) All of the above.

Discussion

The correct answer is E. Anything that neutralizes the stomach pH will interfere with absorption including proton pump inhibitors (PPIs), antacids, and loss of acid-producing cells (eg, pernicious anemia). Other GI diseases (celiac disease, *H. pylori*) can interfere with iron absorption. Tea and some green leafy vegetables can also reduce iron absorption.

 HELPFUL TIP: Vitamin C (supplements or orange juice) enhances iron absorption and should be considered if a patient is not responding to iron therapy. Meat can also increase iron absorption (which we hate to say because one of us [MG] is a vegetarian . . . however, the truth hurts).

 HELPFUL TIP: A widened RDW and an elevated platelet count are typical of iron deficiency anemia. Conversely, the RDW will be normal in thalassemias.

CASE 17

A 24-year-old woman presents for a routine prenatal visit. She is G3 P2 in her second trimester. She has delivered two healthy children by vaginal delivery. The last infant was born 11 months ago. She has no other medical history, does not smoke or drink alcohol, and takes only prenatal vitamins. She states she has been

feeling well except for some fatigue. Her physical exam reveals a gravid woman, slightly pale-appearing, with a temperature of 37°C, pulse 88, blood pressure 110/62, and respirations 14. Her fundal height is appropriate for 22 weeks gestation, and fetal heart tones are auscultated. She has a normal urine dipstick. Her hemoglobin is 9.0 g/dL.

What do you recommend?

A) Start 10 mg elemental ferrous iron orally daily.
B) Encourage the patient to take prenatal vitamins on an empty stomach to increase absorption.
C) Continue present management of the patient and encourage her to get more sleep.
D) Start 200 mg elemental ferrous iron orally daily.
E) Start 1,000 mg elemental ferrous iron orally daily.

Discussion

The correct answer is D. This patient requires iron supplementation, and the usual does is 200 mg per day (usually given as ferrous sulfate 325 mg TID). During pregnancy approximately 300 mg of iron is diverted to the fetus and placenta, while 500 mg is needed to accommodate the expanded blood volume. The World Health Organization defines anemia in a pregnant woman as <11 g/dL. The Centers for Disease Control defines anemia as <11 g/dL in the first and third trimester, <10.5 g/dL in the second trimester. The definition of normal hemoglobin is slightly lower than in a non-pregnant female because plasma volume increases during pregnancy and is out of proportion to the increase in red cell mass, particularly during the second trimester.

* *

The patient returns to your office for her next prenatal visit and mentions that she has had some difficulty taking the iron tablets because of gastrointestinal side effects. She still feels fatigued. You check her hemoglobin, which is 8.8 g/dL. The patient will not agree to take any further iron orally because of the GI side effects. However, she is willing to consider other suggestions.

What is your next step?

A) Encourage the patient to take the iron preparation along with calcium carbonate (Tums) to reduce the gastrointestinal side effects.
B) Continue her prenatal vitamin only and encourage her to eat more red meat.

C) Give iron sucrose 200 mg IV weekly for 4 weeks.
D) Transfuse 2 units of PRBC immediately.

Discussion

The correct answer is C. If oral preparations are **not** tolerated, IV iron preparations are available. Intramuscular preparations are best avoided due **to pain at the** injection site, **skin discoloration, and risk for infection.** Options for **IV replacement include iron dextran and iron sucrose. Iron dextran carries a risk of** anaphylaxis in **0.6%–2.3% of patients and other side effects** in up to **25% of** patients, **including bronchos**pasm, flushing, headache, fever, **urticaria, nausea, vo**miting, hypotension, seizures, my**algia, arthra**lgia, and increased thromboembolic events. **Iron** sucrose has a lower incidence of side effects—typically nausea, constipation, diarrhea, **or** a transient minty taste—and may be given **to patients** who have had **a** previous reaction to **iron dextran.** Answer A is incorrect because calcium will interfere with iron absorption. Answer B is incorrect because she needs more iron than can be provided through prenatal vitamins and her diet. Answer D is incorrect as transfusion carries potential risks that could be avoided if she responds to IV iron replacement.

* *

The patient is reluctant to undergo any intravenous therapy. You counsel her on the effects the anemia may have on her pregnancy.

These effects include all of the following EXCEPT:

A) A pregnant woman has a relative increase in plasma volume, so this degree of anemia is not significant and should not affect her or her fetus.
B) The risk of premature delivery is increased with maternal anemia.
C) The risk of intrauterine growth retardation is increased with maternal anemia.
D) Without therapy, it is likely that her anemia will persist for up to 24 weeks postpartum.
E) There is an increased incidence of infection associated with maternal anemia.

Discussion

The correct answer is A. Anemia in pregnancy is a public health concern because of the increased risk of prematurity and intrauterine growth retardation. There is also an increased risk of infection in both the infant and the mother. Anemia developing during pregnancy is

slow to respond to iron therapy after delivery and may persist for up to 24 weeks.

CASE 18

A 60-year-old male presents for an office evaluation, complaining of fatigue for 6 months. He reports a 30-pound weight loss over the past year, which his wife attributes to the fact that he is constantly chewing on ice and does not have time to eat solid food. His physical exam reveals a well-appearing male with normal vital signs and no discernible abnormalities. A CBC is performed, which demonstrates a WBC 6,000/mm³, hemoglobin 11.8 g/dL, hematocrit 35%, platelets 280,000/mm³, MCV 74 fL (microcytic).

What is your next step in his evaluation and why?

A) Consider addition of oral iron supplementation to his usual medications, as he likely has a dietary iron deficiency.
B) Schedule him for a follow-up appointment in 6 months, as he is generally healthy for a 60-year-old.
C) Evaluate him for thalassemia, because he has a low MCV and no evidence of bleeding.
D) Schedule him for a colonoscopy, as he has microcytic anemia and pica, and you are worried about malignancy.
E) Evaluate his B_{12} and folate stores, as he has a history of using alcohol.

Discussion

The correct answer is D. Any adult patient with microcytic anemia should be evaluated further to clarify the etiology. Iron deficiency is likely given his low MCV and history of pica (chewing on ice—yum!). In this age group, gastrointestinal blood loss is a common cause of microcytic anemia. Colitis, malignancy, or malabsorption from inflammatory disease should be considered in the differential diagnosis. Starting the patient on iron supplementation may improve the patient's hemoglobin but will not help to find the underlying cause. B_{12} or folate deficiency is not likely the sole etiology of this patient's anemia, but mixed anemias can occur.

 HELPFUL TIP: Tailor your workup to the patient's symptoms. If he has symptoms referable to the upper GI tract (eg, dyspepsia, etc), consider an upper GI endoscopy in addition to colonoscopy.

CASE 19

A 52-year-old woman with a history of rheumatoid arthritis is in your clinic for a 1-month follow-up after having an infected knee prosthesis (*Staphylococcus aureus*) removed. You obtain a CBC, revealing a WBC 8,000/mm³, hemoglobin 9.5 g/dL, hematocrit 28%, platelet count 450,000/mm³, and MCV 83 fL. Serum iron levels are low, serum transferrin receptor is normal, while ferritin is increased.

What is the most likely diagnosis?

A) Iron deficiency anemia due to rheumatoid arthritis.
B) Anemia of chronic disease due to rheumatoid arthritis and osteomyelitis.
C) Hemolytic anemia induced by antibiotics.
D) Acute blood loss during surgery.
E) Myelodysplastic syndrome associated with rheumatoid arthritis.

Discussion

The correct answer is B. Anemia of chronic disease (aka anemia of inflammation) is a hypoproliferative anemia that occurs in the setting of chronic infection, inflammation, or malignancy. The anemia is usually mild and characterized by low serum iron, increased ferritin (remember that ferritin is an acute-phase reactant), decreased serum transferrin, normal (or low) serum soluble transferrin receptor level, and decreased transferrin saturation. In addition, the reticulocyte count is typically low, the erythropoietin may be mildly elevated, and the peripheral smear may show hypochromic, microcytic red blood cells or normochromic, normocytic red blood cells.

If differentiation between iron deficiency anemia and anemia of chronic disease is not apparent, a bone marrow biopsy can be obtained to assess iron stores. However, the transferrin receptor can also help differentiate between the two conditions. The transferrin receptor is a transmembrane glycoprotein found on most cells, and is involved in the internalization of iron into cells. **The serum transferrin receptor level is inversely correlated to iron storage levels. Thus, high serum transferrin receptor levels are associated with iron deficiency but not with anemia of chronic disease.** One caveat: the serum transferrin receptor level will also be elevated in states in which there is rapid cell turnover (eg, hemolytic anemia).

However, it should not be checked in this situation so you shouldn't get confused.

CASE 20

A previously healthy 3-year-old child with a history of anorexia and irritability for 3 days is brought to your ED by her mother. On the day of admission, the child is difficult to arouse. Her mother admits that because of financial difficulties, she has been unable to keep up with regular well-child visits to her pediatrician. No one at home is ill, although on detailed questioning, you learn that the child's 6-year-old brother has had some difficulty reaching appropriate developmental milestones and is a fussy eater.

Physical examination reveals a slightly pale-appearing child, who responds to tactile stimuli, but not to voice. Her temperature is 36.8°C, pulse 94, blood pressure 100/56, and respirations 22. Examination of her heart, lungs, and abdomen is unremarkable. Laboratories include a WBC 8,000/mm³, hemoglobin 10 g/dL, platelets 300,000/mm³, MCV 75 fL (microcytic). Her urine dipstick is normal, except for 1+ glucose; there are no ketones in the urine. Her blood chemistries are within normal limits, with the exception of a phosphorous of 2.0 mg/dL. Her peripheral blood smear shows red cells with coarse basophilic stippling.

What is the best working diagnosis at this time?

A) Acute lead poisoning.
B) Anemia of chronic disease.
C) Early diabetic ketoacidosis.
D) Severe iron deficiency anemia.
E) Unrecognized bacteremia secondary to pyelonephritis.

Discussion

The correct answer is A. Lead poisoning should be considered in a child presenting with symptoms of encephalopathy and anemia with basophilic stippling on red blood cells. Anemia of chronic disease (answer B) is incorrect because this illness is acute. DKA (answer C) is incorrect because urine ketones are 99% sensitive for DKA. Answer D is incorrect because there should be no neurologic symptoms associated with iron deficiency anemia. Pyelonephritis (answer E) is incorrect because the patient is afebrile and has a normal white count and negative urine.

HELPFUL TIP: Lead levels >10 micrograms/dL may cause developmental delay, loss of milestones (especially language), encephalopathy, seizures, cerebral edema, and cognitive impairment. CNS effects are especially problematic in children <6 years who have an incomplete blood brain barrier. Lead paint in houses built before the 1970s and use of imported products such as pottery, solder, cosmetics, and crayons (and some toys made in China) provide sources of lead ingestion.

 HELPFUL TIP: **Other symptoms of lead intoxication** include anorexia, decreased activity, irritability, insomnia, hearing loss, peripheral neuropathy, SIADH, decreased renal function, and anemia. **Laboratory findings** may include anemia, signs of hemolysis, coarse basophilic stippling on red blood cells, glycosuria, hypophosphatemia, positive qualitative urine coproporphyrin, and moderate increases in free erythrocyte protoporphyrin.

* *

The patient's lead level is 70 micrograms/dL. Because of your concern about acute lead intoxication and resulting encephalopathy, you decide to admit the child and treat her with dimercaprol.

All of the following are true EXCEPT:

A) Dimercaprol should not be given if the child has a peanut allergy.
B) The child's diet should be monitored for adequate intake of calories, iron, and calcium.
C) The child's sibling should be tested, and arrangements should be made for close follow-up for both children.
D) The dose of dimercaprol should be tripled for patients with G6PD deficiency.

Discussion

The correct answer is D. Dimercaprol is a lead chelator used to treat elevated lead levels. It is administered intramuscularly, is water-insoluble, and must be given in a peanut oil vehicle. **Dimercaprol may cause hemolysis in individuals with G6PD deficiency,** so

these patients should be monitored closely and not receive larger doses. It is important to test siblings of an affected child, because the source of lead is often in the house. Close follow-up of affected children is essential to monitor for increasing blood lead levels after treatment, which may indicate the source of lead has not been removed. The absorption of lead can be made worse by malnutrition, iron deficiency, and poor intake of calcium. Iron deficiency frequently occurs in affected patients and may worsen anemia.

 HELPFUL TIP: A large percentage of lead is absorbed into bone with a half-life >25 years. In periods of physiologic stress, the inert pool of lead can be mobilized and released into the bloodstream, producing signs and symptoms of lead intoxication years after the initial exposure.

CASE 21

A 6-month-old male infant is brought to you for a well-baby checkup. His mother reports that he has had difficulty with feeding, has frequent colds, and is often irritable.

His physical exam reveals a small child, faintly jaundiced. His temperature is 37.5°C, pulse 160, blood pressure 85/50, and respirations 30. His abdomen is soft with palpable splenomegaly. The remainder of the exam is unremarkable. Laboratories reveal a WBC of 13,000/mm³, hemoglobin 9 g/dL, platelets 260,000/mm³, and MCV 60 fL. He is noted to have target cells on peripheral blood smear.

Which one of the following is the most appropriate next step?

A) Order PT/PTT.
B) Order hemoglobin electrophoresis.
C) Transfuse with 1 unit of packed RBCs.
D) Test for G6PD deficiency.
E) Test for sickle cell anemia.

Discussion

The correct answer is B. The clinical and laboratory presentation is consistent with a hereditary hemoglobinopathy, most likely a thalassemia. The splenomegaly, significant anemia, target cells, and the profoundly low MCV are all suggestive of thalassemia. Answer A is incorrect. He has no history of abnormal bleeding, so

PT/PTT would not be indicated. Patients with thalassemia often ultimately suffer from severe iron overload due to repeated transfusions, and so transfusions should be minimized. Answer C is incorrect because the child does not appear to be in distress. G6PD-deficient patients experience episodes of hemolytic anemia. Answer D is incorrect. Peripheral smear review at that time may reveal bite or blister cells, rather than target cells. Answer E is incorrect since the peripheral smear would reveal sickle cells if the patient had sickle disease.

* *

Beta thalassemia major is confirmed by hemoglobin electrophoresis.

Which of the following regarding his management is NOT TRUE?

A) Untreated, mortality may approach 80% by 5 years of age.
B) Frequent blood transfusions may be required.
C) The condition will improve with age.
D) The child is likely to have growth retardation and delayed sexual maturation.
E) Without chelation therapy, there is a high incidence of mortality with this disease.

Discussion

The correct answer is C. Beta thalassemia refers to the disease state in which there are mutations in both genes that code for beta globin. Without treatment, mortality from thalassemia major approaches 80% by 5 years of age. Judicious use of transfusions and concurrent chelation therapy with deferoxamine has reduced long-term complications related to the disease. Deferasirox (Exjade), an oral chelating agent, is also now available. Bone marrow transplant can be curative. Beta thalassemia minor (or beta trait) is much less severe and occurs when only one of the genes is defective.

 HELPFUL TIP: Alpha thalassemia has a more variable course. There are 4 alpha globin genes. If 1 gene is defective, there is a silent carrier state. If 2 genes are defective, there is a mild microcytic anemia. If all 4 genes are defective, intrauterine fetal demise is the rule. Memory aid: **4** looks similar to **A** in "Alpha."

 HELPFUL TIP: Due to the persistence of fetal hemoglobin up to 6 months of age, hemoglobinopathies might not be apparent until that time. Infants may present with pallor, jaundice, irritability, growth retardation, and hepatosplenomegaly.

 HELPFUL TIP: Thalassemias may be erroneously diagnosed as iron-deficiency anemia due to a low MCV. Consider testing for thalassemia in a patient with microcytic anemia, normal or increased iron levels, and appropriate ethnic background (eg, Mediterranean or African descent).

 HELPFUL TIP: In other hemoglobin synthesis related news . . . When you see the middle-aged female with abdominal pain and psychiatric symptoms for the tenth (or twentieth) time, think of acute intermittent porphyria before you make the diagnosis of somatization disorder.

CASE 22

A 72-year-old male is brought to your office because a home health nurse noted he was becoming progressively weaker and more fatigued. The patient was widowed approximately 9 months ago and now lives alone. He has a history of celiac disease for which he follows a strict gluten-free diet, but he has not been eating well. He also has a history of a seizure disorder and takes phenytoin. His review of systems is positive for dyspnea on exertion and mild anorexia. He has no other symptoms. Physical exam reveals a thin, pale-appearing man with normal vital signs. His conjunctivae are pale and his tongue is smooth, with moist mucosa and no oropharyngeal lesions. The remainder of the exam is unremarkable. A CBC reveals a WBC of 4,500/mm^3, hemoglobin 9 g/dL, hematocrit 28%, platelet count 140,000/mm^3, MCV 102 fL, RDW 14, and B$_{12}$ level 900 ng/L (normal).

Which of the following statements is most likely FALSE?

A) The patient may have a high homocysteine level.

B) The patient's condition could be made better with a trial of folate replacement.

C) The patient may have a low red blood cell folate level.

D) The patient's condition will likely require chronic blood transfusions.

E) The patient may have a normal serum folate level.

Discussion

The correct answer is D. This patient likely has folate deficiency, given a normal B_{12}, macrocytic anemia, and risk factors for folate deficiency—old age, poor diet, avoidance of gluten (flour is normally fortified with folate), use of phenytoin, and possible malabsorption due to GI disease (celiac disease in this case, but also any other infiltrating or inflammatory process of the bowel). Dietary deficiency is uncommon in the United States due to supplementation of grain products with folate (remember that this patient has not been eating gluten-containing products). Foods naturally high in folate include melons, bananas, leaf vegetables, asparagus, and broccoli. The recommended intake is 400 micrograms/day, and the body stores approximately a 4-month supply. If he has had recent adequate folate intake, the serum folate level may be normal, but the red blood cell folate will still be low, reflecting the deficiency (think of it as the HbA_{1C} of folate). Red blood cell folate may be low in B_{12} deficiency as well. However, with folate deficiency, homocysteine levels will be high and methylmalonate levels will not be elevated (as they would be in B_{12} deficiency). You must exclude B_{12} deficiency before replacing folate, because folate replacement can reverse the anemia but will permit progression of neurologic effects of B_{12} deficiency.

 HELPFUL TIP: Folate replacement is dosed as 1–5 mg daily. If macrocytic anemia persists, other causes must be considered.

CASE 23

A woman brings her 10-week-old female infant for evaluation. The child is colicky and irritable after feeding. She was born full-term but has not been gaining weight appropriately. The child's sister has sickle-cell trait, so you obtain a hemoglobin electrophoresis, which ultimately demonstrates SS genotype.

Which of the following is NOT TRUE regarding the child's care?

A) The child should remain on prophylactic antibiotics until 5 years due to a high risk of pneumococcal sepsis.

B) The child may develop splenomegaly and lymphadenopathy related to her disease.

C) The disease provides protection against infection with parvovirus.

D) The child may not develop pain crisis until she is older due to protection from fetal hemoglobin (Hg-F).

E) The child is likely to have a delay in puberty.

Discussion

The correct answer is C. The child has homozygous SS sickle cell disease. This child's mother should be counseled regarding the importance of continuing antibiotic prophylaxis until the age of 5 years because her child is at high risk for pneumococcal sepsis. In addition, the development of a parvovirus infection can be life-threatening due to the development of aplastic anemia.

During infancy, children may be noted to have reticulocytosis, hemolytic anemia, and sickling by 10–12 weeks. At 5–6 months, splenomegaly may be noted, and lymphadenopathy may be prominent between 6 months and 5 years. The earliest pain crisis often involves hands and feet (dactylitis), and occurs after the fetal hemoglobin decreases to adult values. This usually does not occur until >4 years. The spleen involutes by 5–8 years. Puberty is delayed by an average of 2.5 years.

 HELPFUL TIP: Sickle trait, the condition in which a patient is heterozygous for hemoglobin S, is associated with a normal life expectancy and no symptoms other than occasional hematuria and inability to concentrate urine. Pain crises are extremely rare, and occur only in the settings of low-oxygen atmosphere (eg, very high altitude) or extreme physical activity (eg, running a marathon).

* *

The child follows regularly with you for years, and she begins to develop more frequent pain crises in college.

She is found to have an elevated C-reactive protein, increased LDH, and decreasing hemoglobin. You explain to her that some measures can be taken to reduce the frequency of pain crises.

These measures include all of the following EXCEPT:

A) Initiation of hydroxyurea therapy.
B) Avoidance of hot showers.
C) Prompt treatment of infections.
D) Adequate hydration and nutrition.
E) Avoidance of emotional stress.

Discussion
The correct answer is B. Two main features of sickle cell disease are shortened RBC survival and vasoocclusion due to poorly deformable RBC membranes. Pain episodes occur due to acute episodes of tissue hypoxemia and micro-infarction. Crises can be precipitated by stress, fatigue, cold weather (not hot showers, which cause problems in multiple sclerosis patients), infection, dehydration, acidosis, and poor nutrition. The use of hydroxyurea promotes increased levels of fetal hemoglobin, and fetal hemoglobin is associated with decreased frequency and severity of pain crises.

 HELPFUL TIP: Acute chest syndrome (ACS) should be suspected when a sickle cell patient presents with fever, cough, chest pain, and pulmonary infiltrates on chest x-ray. ACS may be due to infection or pulmonary infarction. Treatment involves aggressive pain management, antibiotics for respiratory pathogens, supplemental oxygen, cautious hydration, and blood transfusion if the patient is significantly anemic. Exchange transfusion may also be required in more severe cases.

* *

It is 22 years later. Your patient is getting married. She is concerned about significant illness related to her disease. You counsel her regarding the most common causes of morbidity and mortality.

All of the following statements are true EXCEPT:

A) ACS and pain crises are the most common causes for hospital admission for patients with sickle-cell disease.
B) Eighty percent of patients develop cholelithiasis by age 35 years.
C) Strokes may occur in 8% of patients by age 14 years, may be either symptomatic or clinically silent, and tend to be recurrent.
D) Pregnancy should be avoided under any circumstance.

Discussion
The correct answer is D. The average life expectancy in patients with Hb SS is 42 years for men and 48 years for women. Maternal mortality occurs in about 1% of pregnancies. All of the rest are true including cerebrovascular events causing seizures and possible cognitive difficulty early in life. Of particular note, renal failure may be the cause of death in up to 10% of cases. Avascular necrosis and osteomyelitis (as a result of *Salmonella* infection), chronic skin ulcers, and priapism are also common.

Objectives: Did you learn to . . .

- Obtain a thorough history in an anemic patient?
- Use laboratory parameters to identify the etiology of anemia?
- Initiate treatment for various causes of anemia?
- Recognize idiopathic or external causes that may precipitate anemia?
- Identify certain anemias, especially iron deficiency, B$_{12}$ and folate deficiency, thalassemias, and sickle-cell disease, based on clinical and laboratory manifestations?

 QUICK QUIZ: B$_{12}$ DEFICIENCY

A 47-year-old female presents to your office with complaints of tongue soreness, fatigue, and dyspnea with exertion. She denies unusual bleeding, weight loss, fevers, and night sweats. Her past medical history includes hypothyroidism, for which she takes levothyroxine, and she does not drink alcohol or smoke. Physical exam reveals a tired-appearing woman with lemon–yellow-colored skin, temperature 37°C, pulse 110, blood pressure 120/74, and respirations 12. The exam is otherwise unremarkable. A CBC demonstrates a WBC count 4,000/mm³, hemoglobin 9 g/dL, platelet count 140,000/mm³, and an MCV of 105 fL. Her B_{12} level is 100 pg/mL (normal >300 pg/mL) and folate 40 ng/mL.

Which of the following historical elements is LEAST likely to contribute to her condition?

A) History of working as a park ranger in Canada.
B) History of Zollinger-Ellison syndrome.
C) History of hypothyroidism.
D) History of new vegetarian diet started last month.
E) History of gastrointestinal surgery.

Discussion

The correct answer is D. Most likely, this woman has pernicious anemia caused by B_{12} deficiency. Pernicious anemia is caused by immune destruction of parietal cells in the stomach, resulting in decreased absorption of B_{12}. It typically develops in people >40 years and is more common in people of northern European descent or in African Americans, as well as people with type A blood. Laboratory findings include antiparietal cell antibodies in 90% of affected patients (5% of normal individuals) and antibodies to intrinsic factor in 70% of patients. Individuals commonly have other autoimmune diseases such as thyroid disease, diabetes, and vitiligo. Individuals may complain of paresthesias, gastrointestinal symptoms, sore tongue, or weight loss. The lemon-yellow appearance of the skin is due to anemia and mild jaundice.

Other causes of cobalamin (B_{12}) deficiency include gastrectomy, Zollinger-Ellison syndrome (inability to alkalinize the small intestine), blind loop syndrome, bacterial overgrowth from previous surgery, and ingestion of undercooked fish infested with the tapeworm *Diphyllobothrium latum* (found in Canada, Alaska, and the Baltics). Although a strict vegetarian diet can cause B_{12} deficiency, there are sufficient stores to last 3–5 years (in other words, >1 month).

 QUICK QUIZ: DID HE SWALLOW A PENNY?

A 21-year-old college student is brought to the ED by his friends because of bizarre behavior. His friends state that he has been acting a little odd lately, but they are unaware of any drug abuse. He does drink alcohol but

is not known to be a binge drinker. His friends do not know his medical history but state he was taking a prescription drug for a "metabolic disorder," which he stopped several months ago. He is uncooperative, paranoid, and disoriented. You note **brownish pigmentation of his corneas** on physical exam. This may be the first case of Wilson disease you have ever seen.

Regarding this patient, which of the following is NOT TRUE?

A) The patient has likely had episodes of hemolytic anemia in the past.
B) The patient likely has discontinued penicillamine.
C) The patient likely has an elevated ceruloplasmin level on blood test.
D) The patient likely has hepatolenticular degeneration.
E) The patient is at risk for hepatic failure.

Discussiom

The correct answer is C. This patient likely has Wilson disease, which presents with **decreased levels of ceruloplasmin,** increased liver enzymes, and signs of hemolysis (from the direct toxic effect of copper on the cell). Symptoms typically present in the teens and early twenties. Presenting symptoms may include Kayser-Fleisher rings (golden-brown pigmentation of the cornea), hemolytic anemia, or neurologic symptoms, often mimicking psychiatric illness. Treatment of the disease includes life-long therapy with penicillamine or trientine (chelating agents), and should be considered even for asymptomatic individuals known to have the disease.

 QUICK QUIZ: "HOLE-Y BONES"

A 50-year-old male presents to your office with low back pain of 8 weeks duration. He denies any history of trauma or overexertion. He notes the pain is constant and does not improve with positioning. Also, he has noticed some fatigue. He has no past medical history except for an inguinal hernia repair 5 years ago. He does not smoke or drink and takes only ibuprofen for his back pain. He has no other complaints.

Physical exam reveals a well-nourished male with normal vital signs. His neurologic exam is normal. On musculoskeletal exam, he has midline point tenderness over T12. Plain films reveal a compression fracture at T12. A serum total protein level is 9 mg/dL (elevated), but the remainder of an evaluation for endocrine causes of osteoporosis is normal.

All of the following are necessary for the diagnosis of this patient EXCEPT:

A) Bone scan.
B) Serum and urine protein electrophoresis with immunofixation.
C) Bone marrow aspirate and biopsy.
D) Quantitative immunoglobulins.
E) Skeletal survey.

Discussion

The correct answer is A. A spontaneous vertebral fracture in a 50-year-old male is definitely not normal. Multiple myeloma should be considered in patients with this presentation. A bone scan is **not** useful because the lytic lesions characteristic of multiple myeloma do not take up radioisotope.

Multiple myeloma is a clonal disorder of plasma cells. Risk factors include black race, male sex, and advancing age (median age 60–65 years at presentation). Workup for the diagnosis of multiple myeloma requires a serum and urine protein electrophoresis with immunofixation (answer B). This will help to identify a monoclonal protein. Quantitative immunoglobulins (answer D) will help to assess whether this patient has an elevation of immunoglobulins in the range required for the diagnosis of multiple myeloma. A skeletal survey (answer E) and bone marrow biopsy (answer C) complete the diagnostic workup.

CASE 24

On a routine insurance physical, a 55-year-old male was found to have a total protein of 9 g/dL. The remainder of his serum chemistries and his CBC were normal. He is active, feels well, and is not taking any medications. His physical examination is unremarkable. You order a serum and urine electrophoresis with immunofixation and quantitative immunoglobulins. He has a monoclonal spike with 1,400 g/dL of IgG kappa. His other immunoglobulins are within normal limits. A skeletal survey demonstrates no lytic lesions, and his bone marrow aspirate and biopsy demonstrate 6% plasma cells (normal is 1%–4%). After the bone marrow biopsy, the hematologist sends him back to you for follow-up.

What is your next step in the management of this patient?

A) Monitor blood, including serum immunoglobulins, every 3–6 months and, if stable after 1 year, annually thereafter.
B) Monitor blood, including serum immunoglobulins, every 4 weeks.
C) Start on chemotherapy for multiple myeloma.
D) Obtain yearly bone marrow biopsy and skeletal survey.
E) No follow-up is necessary.

Discussion

The correct answer is A. This patient has monoclonal gammopathy of undetermined significance (MGUS), which is found in up to 3% of asymptomatic adults >50 years. A bone marrow biopsy indicating 10% plasma cells is required to make the diagnosis of multiple myeloma; this patient only has 6%. Additionally, this patient has a normal CBC and is asymptomatic (no fatigue, bone pain suggestive of lesions, etc). Thus, this patient has MGUS. Patients with MGUS typically do well, with only 1% per year progressing to multiple myeloma.

Although patients should be reassured of the typically benign nature of this condition, 30% will have complications (multiple myeloma, amyloidosis, other myeloproliferative disorders). After several unchanged immunoglobulin levels and normal CBCs, yearly evaluation should be adequate. Any changes in the patient's condition, such as unexplained anemia, increased immunoglobulin levels, renal insufficiency, or bony pain, should prompt further evaluation. An increase in immunoglobulin does not necessarily mean the monoclonal protein is increasing, and a serum protein electrophoresis and immunofixation should be obtained. Repeat bone marrow biopsy is indicated only if the clinical picture is confusing.

CASE 25

A 63-year-old female presents to your office with complaint of fatigue. She states she felt like she spent the winter taking antibiotics because she developed one infection after the other. Prior to this past winter, she had been well and did not take any prescription drugs regularly. Physical examination demonstrates a slightly pale, thin woman. Her temperature is 37.5°C, pulse 90, blood pressure 120/58, and respirations 12. Her oropharynx demonstrates purpuric lesions. Her abdominal exam shows no organomegaly, and the remainder of the physical exam is unremarkable. You obtain blood tests: WBC 2,100/mm³, hemoglobin 8.4 g/dL, and platelet count 20,000/mm³. A bone marrow aspirate and biopsy are obtained, which demonstrate a hypercellular marrow with 4% blasts, 4% ringed sideroblasts, and megakaryocytes. You talk to the hematologist, who suspects that your patient has a myelodysplastic syndrome.

Which of the following statements is NOT TRUE?

A) The small number of blasts in the bone marrow indicates a better prognosis.
B) The patient cannot have myelodysplastic syndrome because she has pancytopenia.
C) The patient may benefit from administration of erythropoietin.
D) The patient may develop acute myeloid leukemia.
E) The patient's gender may result in a better prognosis.

Discussion

The correct answer is B. Patients with myelodysplastic syndrome **can** be pancytopenic. Myelodysplastic syndrome includes a number of clonal stem cell disorders characterized by dysplasia and ineffective hematopoiesis of one or more cell lines. The disease is typically one of older adults, with a median age of 65 to 70 years at onset; however, a better prognosis is associated with age <60 years and female gender. There is an increased risk of myelodysplastic syndrome in smokers, those exposed to benzene or alkylating agents, and with some hereditary disorders. Prognosis depends on the number of blasts, the number of lineages affected, and cytogenetic abnormalities. Median survival ranges from 10 months to 66 months, and progression to acute leukemia ranges from 6% to 33% of patients, depending on the subtype of MDS.

Depending upon the age and overall performance status of the individual MDS patient, treatment can range from supportive care with blood or platelet transfusions, to treatment with GCSF, to chemotherapeutics such as azacytidine, or even to bone marrow transplantation.

Objectives: Did you learn to . . .

- Identify pancytopenia as a presentation of myelodysplastic syndrome?
- Recognize the presentation of multiple myeloma?

CASE 26

A 49-year-old male presents to your office with complaints of joint pain, fatigue, and increased urination. There is a family history of cirrhosis of the liver, apparently not related to alcohol. He does not take any medications and does not smoke but drinks two glasses of wine each night. Physical examination reveals a thin male with tanned skin and normal vital signs. His heart and lung exams are unremarkable. The abdomen is soft, nontender, and nondistended, and his liver edge is palpable 2 cm below the costal margin. He has tenderness with range of motion in his hips, knees, and MTP joints. The remainder of the exam is unrevealing. Serum electrolytes are normal, but his glucose is 282 g/dL. His transaminases are elevated.

Of the following, what is the most likely diagnosis?

A) Alcoholic hepatitis.
B) Colon cancer.
C) Hemochromatosis.
D) Vitamin B_{12} deficiency.
E) Wilson disease.

Discussion

The correct answer is C. This patient presents with a classic history of hemochromatosis. Symptoms start at age ≥50 years, are initially mild and progress slowly. "Bronze diabetes" (bronze or tan skin color caused by iron deposition accompanied by hyperglycemia) is sometimes noted. Most organs can eventually be involved, but most commonly symptoms are due to liver, cardiac, joint, and testicular involvement. Alcoholic hepatitis (answer A), typically occurs after larger quantities of alcohol are ingested. You would not expect to see some of the other symptoms (eg, of diabetes, arthritis) in relation to alcoholic hepatitis. Colon cancer (answer B) is unlikely to present in this way. Vitamin B_{12} deficiency (answer D) typically presents with anemia and neurologic symptoms. Wilson disease (answer E) is caused by increasing copper concentrations in the body, and patients usually present with progressive liver disease.

Which of the following laboratory values are most consistent with this patient's presentation?

A) Decreased iron, decreased ferritin, decreased transferrin saturation.

B) Decreased iron, decreased ferritin, increased transferrin saturation.

C) Increased iron, decreased ferritin, increased transferrin saturation.

D) Increased iron, increased ferritin, decreased transferrin saturation.

E) Increased iron, increased ferritin, increased transferrin saturation.

Discussion

The correct answer is E. All of these iron studies are elevated in patients with hereditary hemochromatosis. A normal person maintains approximately 3–4 g of iron in the body. Normal individuals absorb about 1 mg/day of iron (10% of what is ingested), which is precisely balanced with loss through sweat, sloughing of cells, and gastrointestinal losses. In hereditary hemochromatosis, 2–4 mg of iron is absorbed daily, resulting in the accumulation of approximately 1 g of excess iron per year. This accumulates in tissues, and patients may ultimately develop symptoms. The diagnosis of hereditary hemochromatosis should be considered in patients with elevated iron, ferritin, and transferrin saturation levels.

* *

The patient's diagnosis is confirmed, and you counsel him regarding his disease.

All of the following statements are true EXCEPT:

A) This is an autosomal dominant disease.

B) Affected females typically present later in life due to increased iron losses.

C) Patients may benefit from phlebotomy even after development of symptomatic disease.

D) Patients are susceptible to unusual infections.

E) Patients are at high risk for hepatocellular carcinoma.

Discussion

The correct answer is A. Hereditary hemochromatosis is an autosomal recessive disorder. Approximately 10% of whites are heterozygous, and 5/1,000 are homozygous for the gene mutation. Individuals are at increased risk for infections due to *Listeria*, *Vibrio vulnificus* (sorry, no sushi!), and *Yersinia enterocolitica*. Affected females may present later in life due to increased iron losses from menstruation, pregnancy, and lactation. Men are affected more commonly than women. Treatment includes phlebotomy or chelation therapy if phlebotomy is contraindicated. Patients should be monitored closely for development of hepatoma, since therapy does not reduce the risk of hepatocellular carcinoma once cirrhosis is present. Family members should be screened for the disease so they can be started on therapy early, in order to prevent the development of cirrhosis.

 HELPFUL TIP: Other causes of iron overload include thalassemia, sideroblastic anemia, and frequent blood transfusions.

CASE 27

A 56-year-old male undergoes a laryngoscopy. In an outdated move that is generally not recommended now, his doctor used extra doses of benzocaine spray (like gallons of the stuff) to overcome a strong gag reflex. The patient tolerated the procedure well, but afterwards he started to have cyanosis around the lips. You are now seeing him in the ED, and he has a bluish discoloration of his lips and fingertips and is complaining of a headache. You administer oxygen by nasal canula with no improvement in his cyanosis. You draw venous blood for labs, and find that it has an unusual chocolate color.

All of the following statements are true about this patient EXCEPT:

A) A measured arterial blood gas will demonstrate a normal PaO_2.

B) The pulse-oximeter will show a high-normal oxygen saturation.

C) The patient may require therapy with methylene blue.

D) The patient should not be treated with methylene blue if he has a history of G6PD deficiency.

E) Additional doses of benzocaine can be lethal.

Discussion

The correct answer is B. This patient has methemoglobinemia, which was likely a reaction to the benzocaine spray. Methemoglobinemia results when iron in hemoglobin is oxidized from the ferrous to the ferric state and the hemoglobin becomes incapable of binding and transporting oxygen.

In a normal patient, <1% of hemoglobin is found in the methemoglobin form. Depending on the percentage of methemoglobin, presentations will vary. At **10%–20%,** patients present with cyanosis refractory to oxygen. The arterial blood gas may show a normal PaO_2 with low oxygen saturations, because oxygen cannot be released from the hemoglobin molecule. When methemoglobin levels are **>30%,** patients present with headache, dizziness, dyspnea, and tachypnea. At **>50%,** patients develop stupor and obtundation, and **>70%** may be lethal. Certain drugs such as nitroprusside, sulfonamides, some local anesthetics, and acetaminophen have been found to cause methemoglobinemia.

Treatment for methemoglobinemia is methylene blue. However, patients with G6PD deficiency should not be given methylene blue, and hyperbaric oxygen therapy should be considered instead. Remember, when patients have been exposed to cyanide, you want to **cause** methemoglobinemia. The exact mechanism by which this protects against cyanide is unknown, since patients begin to improve prior to the presence of methemoglobinemia.

 HELPFUL TIP: Children with diarrhea may develop methemoglobinemia although it is rarely clinically significant.

CASE 28

A 16-year-old African American male presents to your office with complaints of progressive fatigue and dyspnea over the last few days. He also has some mild upper respiratory symptoms which are being treated with sulfamethoxazole-trimethoprim (a plague on the house of his doctor who treats a URI with antibiotics). On examination, you find a well-nourished male in no distress. He is afebrile but slightly tachycardic. You note mild scleral icterus and pallor of the palmar creases, but the remainder of the exam is unremarkable. A CBC shows normal WBC count and platelets, with hemoglobin 10.2 g/dL. On peripheral smear, "bite cells" and rare Heinz bodies are reported. The LDH and bilirubin are elevated and the serum haptoglobin is low, but the other serum chemistries are normal.

Which of the following is the most likely diagnosis?

A) Hereditary spherocytosis.

B) Glucose-6-phosphate dehydrogenase (G6PD) deficiency.

C) Sickle cell disease (homozygous).

D) Sickle cell trait (heterozygous).

E) Iron-deficiency anemia.

Discussion

The correct answer is B. The most likely cause of this patient's anemia is G6PD deficiency. He likely has a hemolytic anemia, as evidenced by the elevated LDH, bite cells, elevated bilirubin, low haptoglobin and the acute onset of symptoms. Heinz bodies are inclusions in red cells seen on peripheral smear within the first few days of an oxidative stress in patients with G6PD deficiency. Bite cells are formed as the red cells pass through the spleen and the Heinz bodies are removed. The other diagnoses are less likely. Hereditary spherocytosis (answer A) is caused by an inherited defect in the red cell membrane, and episodes of hemolytic anemia may be brought on by environmental stress. However, patients generally have a baseline anemia, and spherocytes should be seen on peripheral smear. Sickle cell disease and trait are discussed in more detail elsewhere in this chapter. This patient does not have sickle cells on the peripheral smear. Iron deficiency anemia (answer E) does not generally present acutely and is not associated with findings of hemolysis.

 HELPFUL TIP: G6PD deficiency is the most common inherited red blood cell enzyme defect, affecting 10% of the black male population. It occurs more commonly in African and Mediterranean populations.

＊ ＊

Hemolytic anemia in G6PD deficiency is caused by oxidative stress on red cells, most commonly as the result of infection or administration of certain drugs.

Which of the following can precipitate a hemolytic crisis in G6PD deficiency?

A) Sulfa antibiotics.

B) Fava beans.

C) Nitrofurantoin.

D) Some antimalarial drugs.

E) All of the above.

Discussion

The correct answer is E. All of the above can cause a hemolytic crisis in G6PD deficiency. Multiple other drugs can be involved as well including vitamin C, salicylates, isoniazid, phenytoin, etc.

 HELPFUL TIP: Fresh fava beans aren't worth the bother. First you have to shell them and then *peel each and every bean*. After all that work, you just end up with a hemolytic crisis if you have G6PD deficiency. Get the canned ones.

Which of the following is the most appropriate intervention for this patient with G6PD deficiency at this point?

A) Admit to the hospital and observe.
B) Admit to the hospital and transfuse 2 units of packed red cells.
C) Recommend supportive care and follow-up in a few days.
D) Recommend splenectomy and refer to a general surgeon.

Discussion

The correct answer is C. The hemolytic anemia of G6PD deficiency is self-limited and will resolve. This is because in most cases of G6PD deficiency, only about 25% of the RBCs (the older cells) are susceptible to oxidative stress. Severe episodes should be treated in the hospital setting, but most episodes can be managed as an outpatient. Patients should be educated on the drugs and stressors that may precipitate an episode of hemolytic anemia. Splenectomy may limit hemolysis in patients with more severe disease.

Objectives: Did you learn to . . .

- Recognize disorders of iron metabolism?
- Describe symptoms and signs of hemochromatosis?
- Recognize complications related to iron overload?
- Identify clinical and laboratory manifestations of G6PD deficiency and describe its management?

 QUICK QUIZ: TOO MANY LYMPHOCYTES

A 72-year-old male presents to your office for follow-up after a recent hospitalization for pneumonia. He is now 6 weeks out and feels well. But while he was in the hospital, he had an increased WBC with lymphocytosis. You repeat his CBC and find a WBC of 18,000/mm³, with 80% lymphocytes, hemoglobin of 14 g/dL, and a platelet count of 200,000/mm³. You review office records from a visit 1 year ago and find a WBC of 14,000/mm³ with 76% lymphocytes. You send his peripheral blood for flow cytometry, which is consistent with a diagnosis of chronic lymphocytic leukemia (CLL).

Which of the following statements about this patient is NOT TRUE?

A) This patient is at risk for the development of hemolytic anemia.
B) This patient is at risk for serious infection.
C) This patient is likely to experience a relatively benign disease course.
D) This patient should be started on chemotherapy.
E) This patient may develop "B symptoms" (fever, night sweats, weight loss).

Discussion

The correct answer is D. CLL is characterized by progressive accumulation of long-lived lymphocytes. It is more common in men and tends to be a disease of older adults (median age at diagnosis 65 years); however, up to 20% of cases occur in patients <60 years. Diagnosis is made if a patient has >5,000/mm³ mature-appearing lymphocytes in the blood and 30% lymphocytes on bone marrow biopsy. With the use of immunophenotyping, bone marrow biopsy is not necessary for diagnosis, but may be useful for prognosis.

This patient has a low-stage CLL and does not require immediate treatment with chemotherapy. He should be monitored every 6–12 months or sooner if he develops symptoms, such as infections, fatigue, bulky lymphadenopathy, or bleeding. Patients with CLL are at risk for developing autoimmune diseases, including hemolytic anemia, autoimmune thrombocytopenia, pure red cell aplasia, and autoimmune neutropenia.

 QUICK QUIZ: TOO MANY NETUTROPHILS

A 46-year-old woman presents to your office for a preoperative evaluation. She is planning an elective hysterectomy for painful, bleeding uterine fibroids. She has no significant past medical history. Her review of systems is positive only for sweats that she suspected were related to the onset of menopause, although her menses are still regular. Her physical examination is unremarkable except for a palpable spleen tip. You obtain a CBC, showing WBC count of 50,000/mm³, hemoglobin 11 g/dL, platelet count 350,000/mm³. On her peripheral blood smear, she has mostly neutrophils and bands, with some metamyelocytes, myelocytes, and basophils as well.

All of the following are likely to be true EXCEPT:

A) The patient has an underlying infection with leukemoid reaction.
B) The patient has a balanced translocation between chromosome 9 and 22.
C) The patient produces an abnormal tyrosine kinase protein.
D) The patient will likely develop progressive leuko-cytosis, fevers, anemia, and thrombocytopenia if untreated.

Discussion

The correct answer is A. Although a leukemoid reaction is a possibility, it would be unusual to see a full range of maturation of myeloid cells (eg, metamyelo-cytes, myelocytes) in the peripheral blood along with increased basophils and a palpable spleen. Rather, this patient likely has chronic myelogenous leukemia (CML), which is a clonal myeloproliferative disorder, characterized by the "Philadelphia chromosome" (translocation between chromosomes 9 and 22), which encodes for an abnormal tyrosine kinase protein (answer C). This is the target for the tyrosine kinase inhibitors, such as imatinib (Gleevec), which have resulted in significant improvement in survival.

Patients with CML typically present between 40 and 60 years of age. Up to 40% of patients are asymptomatic at presentation. Others complain of weight loss, fatigue, abdominal pain, night sweats, and fever.

QUICK QUIZ: ACUTE LEUKEMIA

You have a febrile 37-year-old male with a very high WBC count, most of which are blasts. Most likely, he has an acute leukemia. A bone marrow has not yet been done, and it is unknown if this is an acute myeloid leukemia or an acute lymphoblastic leukemia.

Which of the following statements is NOT TRUE?

A) The patient's fever is likely due to the leukemic cells, and antibiotics should be started only if you identify a specific infection.
B) The patient is at risk for tumor lysis syndrome and should be started on allopurinol.
C) Aggressive inpatient chemotherapy is required for both the treatment of acute myeloid leukemia and acute lymphoblastic leukemia.
D) You should consult a hematologist/oncologist as soon as possible.

Discussion

The correct answer is A. Patients with acute leukemia and fever should be cultured, and antibiotics should be started as soon as possible since a fever is often the result of a concurrent infection. These patients should be kept well hydrated and given allopurinol (answer B) to prevent tumor lysis syndrome, as this can occur even without chemotherapy if the tumor burden is high enough. Treatment for acute leukemias requires intensive chemotherapy (answer C) and should be started as soon as possible, so prompt evaluation by a hematologist/oncologist is imperative (answer D).

CASE 29

A 65-year-old male who is on ticlopidine is brought into the ED. Last night he was complaining of a headache, fever, and numbness on the right side of his face. This morning, he was acting erratically. His physical examination demonstrates a confused male, with a temperature of 39°C, pulse 110, blood pressure 180/94, respirations 14. He has a few petechiae on his palate. He is tachycardic and lungs are clear to auscultation bilaterally. His abdomen is soft, without organomegaly. His neurologic examination is difficult to complete because of his inability to cooperate. Laboratories include WBC 6,000/mm³, hemoglobin 8.4 g/dL, and platelets 50,000/mm³. Schistocytes are noted on a peripheral blood smear.

All of the following may be expected in this patient EXCEPT:

A) Creatinine of 3.2 mg/dL.
B) LDH of 640 IU/L.
C) Elevated haptoglobin.
D) Elevated indirect bilirubin.
E) Negative direct antiglobulin test (direct Coombs).

Discussion

The correct answer is C. An elevated haptoglobin would suggest the absence of active hemolysis. The presence of schistocytes suggests ongoing microangiopathic hemolysis, in this case due to thrombotic thrombocytopenia purpura (TTP). TTP is classically described by a pentad of findings: microangiopathic hemolytic anemia (suggested by schistocytes on peripheral smear), thrombocytopenia, fever, renal insufficiency, and mental status changes. Not all 5 features need to be present for diagnosis, but your patient seems to have the pentad. The negative direct antiglobulin test (direct Coombs) (answer E), suggests that the hemolytic anemia is not due to an autoimmune process. Note that the patient is on ticlopidine, one of the drugs that can cause TTP. Clopidogrel can also cause TTP although much less commonly.

> **HELPFUL TIP:** Schistocytes are the result of intravascular trauma to RBCs. Any microangiopathic hemolytic anemia can result in schistocytes as can other intravascular trauma such as that secondary to artificial heart valves, HELLP syndrome, malignant hypertension, some malignancies, transjugular intrahepatic portosystemic shunts (TIPS), eclampsia, etc.

* *

Therapy with plasma exchange has reduced the mortality rate from 90% to <25%. Other treatments may include glucocorticoids and splenectomy in refractory cases. Platelet transfusion should be avoided as it can worsen the patient's condition.

Which of the following laboratory findings would you expect to see in this patient with TTP?

A) Normal PT/INR.
B) Elevated PTT.
C) Elevated fibrin degradation products.
D) Low level of fibrinogen.

Discussion

The correct answer is A. Patients with TTP should have a normal PT/INR. This is important because TTP can be confused with DIC, in which the PT/INR should be elevated and fibrinogen should be low. In TTP, thrombosis is secondary to platelet activation and not activation of the coagulation cascade. Thus,

PT/PTT/INR, factor levels, fibrinogen and fibrin degradation products are normal.

* *

Your patient is started on plasma exchange. You note that he has not had any change in his hemoglobin or platelet count, and his renal function is worsening.

Which of the following may mimic TTP and should be considered in a poorly responsive patient?

A) Rocky Mountain spotted fever.
B) Disseminated aspergillosis.
C) Disseminated malignancy.
D) Malignant hypertension.
E) All of the above.

Discussion

The correct answer is E. When patients are poorly responsive to therapy, an alternative diagnosis should be sought. In female patients, preeclampsia or HELLP syndrome can mimic TTP. Autoimmune disease (eg, systemic lupus erythematosus, scleroderma), malignant hypertension, and disseminated malignancy may also mimic TTP. Infections that can be confused with TTP include Rocky Mountain spotted fever, disseminated aspergillosis, cytomegalovirus sepsis, and group B streptococcal sepsis.

CASE 30

A 23-year-old female goes to emergency cesarean section after she is noted to have placental abruption. She is G1 P0 at term and has no other significant medical history. After the delivery, you note that she is still having brisk vaginal bleeding and oozing from her venipuncture sites. You obtain laboratories: WBC 9,000/mm³, hemoglobin 8.2 g/dL, platelet count 80,000/mm³, INR 2.4, PTT 22 seconds, and fibrinogen 80 mg/dL (normal 190–420 mg/dL). Fibrin degradation products are elevated. A CBC at admission was normal.

Which of the following statements is NOT TRUE?

A) The patient may benefit from platelet transfusion.
B) The patient may benefit from cryoprecipitate transfusion.
C) The patient may benefit from FFP transfusion.
D) The patient may benefit from crystalloid infusion.

Discussion

The correct answer is A. This patient is exhibiting signs of disseminated intravascular coagulopathy (DIC), which is characterized by the disordered regulation of normal coagulation. It can be precipitated by a number of conditions resulting in excess thrombin generation and secondary activation of the fibrinolytic system. Thrombin also activates platelets, causing platelet aggregation and consumption. Antithrombin is consumed in this process as well.

Treatment is directed at correcting the underlying cause of DIC whenever possible. Patients may benefit from platelet transfusion (answer A) to maintain a platelet count above 20,000/mm³, but **transfusion at higher levels can worsen platelet aggregation.** Transfusion of FFP (answer C) will replace consumed factors. Patients with low fibrinogen levels will benefit from transfusion of cryoprecipitate. The use of heparin is controversial and newer products may soon replace heparin for treatment of this syndrome. If used, heparin is typically given at low doses (500 U/h) in order to try to block activation of the coagulation system and ongoing consumption of fibrinogen and platelets. It may also be considered if there are prominent thrombotic complications. The use of crystalloid (answer D) to maintain blood pressure may prevent further stimulation of DIC.

 HELPFUL TIP: Laboratory findings in DIC include low platelets, prolonged PT/INR, normal or prolonged PTT, low fibrinogen, and increased fibrin degradation products. D-dimer and thrombin time are also increased, antithrombin may be low, and peripheral blood smear will reveal schistocytes. An elevated D-dimer isolation is not helpful since D-dimer is elevated in many states, including DVT/PE.

Objectives: Did you learn to . . .
- Recognize the clinical presentation of TTP?
- Treat a patient with TTP?
- Develop a differential diagnosis for a patient with microangiopathic anemia?
- Distinguish DIC from TTP?

CASE 31

A 22-year-old female college student presents to your office with complaints of an enlarged cervical lymph node and sore throat. She has felt feverish on and off for several weeks but never measured her temperature. She is afebrile today, a rapid strep test is negative, and you treat her symptomatically. You ask her to return if her symptoms do not resolve within 2–4 weeks.

She returns 4 weeks later. The sore throat has resolved; however, she now complains of intense pruritus and sweats at night. The cervical lymph node now measures 3 cm. The remainder of her physical examination is negative.

What is the most appropriate next step?
A) Direct laryngoscopy.
B) Empiric antibiotic trial.
C) Lymph node biopsy.
D) MRI of the neck.
E) Observation for another 4 weeks.

Discussion

The correct answer is C. The prolonged (>1 month) presence of a large (>1 cm) lymph node deserves a biopsy. MRI of the neck (answer D) and laryngoscopy (answer A) may be indicated depending on the biopsy results. Empiric antibiotic therapy (answer B) is inappropriate and unlikely to be helpful, as you have no source of primary infection. Further observation (answer E) will delay the diagnosis.

* *

You obtain a lymph node biopsy that is consistent with nodular sclerosing Hodgkin disease.

Which of the following statements is NOT TRUE?
A) The patient has B symptoms.
B) The lymph node biopsy probably shows Reed-Sternberg cells.
C) Further staging is necessary.
D) Chemotherapy is useless in treatment of this patient.
E) Her prognosis with standard therapy is very poor.

Discussion

The correct answer is D. Chemotherapy regimens for Hodgkin disease have resulted in response rates of over 90%, with fewer long-term complications than prior regimens. Although it is well known, Hodgkin is an uncommon disease, with about 8,000 cases occurring each year in the United States. It is a disease of young people, occurring typically in patients in their twenties. Patients often present with lymphadenopathy. Symptoms known as "B symptoms" (answer A) include weight loss, fever, and drenching night sweats. Other symptoms may include pruritus, diffuse pain after consuming alcoholic beverages, and symptoms related to the development of a mediastinal mass. Reed-Sternberg cells (answer B) are typically seen on biopsy in Hodgkin disease. After a diagnostic lymph node biopsy, further staging (answer C) includes CT scans, bone marrow biopsy, and routine labs.

 HELPFUL TIP: Non-Hodgkin lymphoma (NHL) is increasing in incidence and is more common than Hodgkin disease. Risk factors for NHL include HIV infection and advancing age.

Objectives: Did you learn to . . .

- Recognize presentation of a patient with Hodgkin disease?
- Describe "B symptoms"?

CASE 32

A 34-year-old female presents to your office with calf pain and swelling. She denies trauma to the leg. She has no other significant medical history and takes only oral contraceptives. She smokes a half-pack of cigarettes daily but does not drink alcohol. Her physical examination is also unremarkable, with the exception of swelling and tenderness of the left calf. A lower extremity Doppler study demonstrates a new thrombus occluding the common femoral vein.

Which of the following would NOT be appropriate in this patient?

A) Start the patient on warfarin to maintain an INR of 2–3.
B) Have the patient scheduled for placement of an inferior vena cava filter.
C) Discontinue hormonal contraceptives.
D) Encourage the patient to stop smoking.
E) Obtain further history of her family.

Discussion

The correct answer is B. This patient has an acute DVT and risk factors for developing a DVT, including smoking, and hormonal contraceptive use. You

should start her on heparin (or low-molecular-weight heparin) and warfarin with a goal INR of 2–3. Heparin should be used for at least 5 days and overlapped with therapeutic doses of warfarin that have reached the target INR for at least 4 days. She should be anticoagulated for at least 3 months. Encourage her to stop smoking and to find an alternative form of birth control. Obtain family history to assess her risk of having an inherited thrombophilia.

 HELPFUL TIP: Workup of an inherited or acquired thrombophilia is controversial because the treatment of the patient is not likely to change. When a thromboembolic event is unprovoked, it is probably prudent to screen the patient. When there is a provoked event (eg, surgery, prolonged immobilization, pregnancy, oral estrogen), the role of such a workup is less well defined.

* *

The patient returns 3 months later. She has been relatively easy to anticoagulate (somebody has to be, right?), maintaining a stable INR. She stopped smoking and knows to avoid hormonal contraception. She has learned some family history: her mother had a DVT and her maternal aunt died of a pulmonary embolus. Now, the patient wants to know how this new information will affect her long-term care. You decide to screen her for thrombophilia.

Which of the following sets of tests may be performed while she remains on warfarin?

A) Factor V Leiden mutation, antithrombin, prothrombin gene mutation.
B) Factor V Leiden mutation, prothrombin gene mutation, antiphospholipid antibodies.
C) Homocysteine, protein C, antithrombin.
D) Protein C, protein S, antithrombin.
E) All of the above.

Discussion

The correct answer is B. There are 7 types of thrombophilia for which you might initially test: factor V Leiden mutation, antithrombin deficiency, prothrombin gene mutation, protein C deficiency, protein S deficiency, antiphospholipid antibody syndrome, and hyperhomocystinemia. Not all causes of thrombophilia can be tested while on anticoagulant therapy. Factor V Leiden gene mutation, prothrombin gene mutation, homocysteine, and antiphospholipid antibodies are not affected by warfarin. However, warfarin can reduce protein C and S levels (giving false-positive test results) and increase antithrombin levels (giving a false-negative result).

Factor V Leiden mutation is the most common cause of inherited thrombophilia, being found in 3% to 6% of non-black blood donors. Antithrombin deficiency (previously known as antithrombin III) is less common, occurring in 1/1,000 to 1/5,000 individuals. The homozygous condition is fatal in utero. Heterozygotes have a 30% chance of developing a thromboembolic event by age 30.

Protein C deficiency occurs in 1/200 to 1/300 people; however, fewer than 1/1,000 heterozygotes develop venous thromboses. Protein S deficiency is estimated to occur in 0.03% to 0.13% of persons and has a clinical presentation similar to protein C deficiency. The prevalence of prothrombin gene mutation varies widely and occurs most commonly in persons of southern European descent. Unlike the other thrombophilias discussed, antiphospholipid antibody syndrome is an acquired disorder that is associated with arterial as well as venous thromboembolic events. Finally, hyperhomocystinemia is associated with the development of venous thrombosis and atherosclerotic heart disease.

 HELPFUL TIP: The major risk factor for having another DVT is having the first DVT. This trumps all of the thrombophilia tests in determining your patient's subsequent risk.

CASE 33

A 19-year-old gravid female presents during her second trimester and complains of left calf swelling. With the help of Doppler studies, you diagnose her with a DVT.

Which of the following statements is true?

A) DVT occurs most commonly in the right lower extremity in pregnant women.

B) DVT is common in pregnancy due to increased venous stasis and increased levels of fibrinogen, factor VIII, and VWF.

C) Anticoagulation should be avoided in pregnant women due to fetal risks.

D) Anticoagulation with heparin produces no risk to the fetus or mother.

E) DVT is most common in the third trimester.

Discussion

The correct answer is B. DVT, and the broader category of venous thromboembolism (VTE), occurs 2–4 times more often in pregnant women compared to non-pregnant controls. Increased risk is found with cesarean delivery versus vaginal delivery. The majority of DVTs occur in the **left** lower extremity of pregnant women, likely caused by the compression of the left iliac vein by the right iliac artery as they cross. The increased incidence of VTE is multifactorial, including: increased levels of fibrinogen, factor VIII, and VWF; increased venous stasis; increased venous distension secondary to increased estrogen; and anatomic distortion related to the gravid uterus.

VTE occurs **equally during all three trimesters**, but increased lower extremity swelling is frequently seen in normal patients during the third trimester, making the diagnosis less obvious. Treatment of VTE with anticoagulation is more difficult in a pregnant woman. Warfarin crosses the placenta and has teratogenic effects in addition to increased risk of fetal bleeding. Heparin and danaparoid do not cross the placenta, but are associated with a 2% risk of maternal bleeding. Heparin carries the risks of heparin-induced thrombocytopenia with thrombosis, osteoporosis, and bleeding at the uteroplacental junction. Dosing of unfractionated heparin is difficult during pregnancy, and low-molecular-weight heparin is probably the best choice for anticoagulation. Heparin and warfarin are safe for lactating mothers.

CASE 34

A 52-year-old female presents to the ED with shortness of breath and respirophasic chest pain. She has been on warfarin for atrial fibrillation. Despite her anticoagulation, you suspect pulmonary embolism (PE) and obtain a spiral CT scan, which shows a thrombus in the right pulmonary artery. Prior to the initiation of any therapy, her coagulation studies return and show INR 2.8 and PTT 49 seconds.

Which of the following is the most appropriate next step?

A) Test the patient for antiphospholipid antibodies.
B) Place an inferior vena cava filter.
C) Repeat the INR and PTT since the patient's sample was probably contaminated with heparin.
D) Confront the patient about her noncompliance with warfarin.

Discussion

The correct answer is A. Patients who have a new VTE while on appropriate anticoagulant therapy should be evaluated for antiphospholipid antibody syndrome. This patient has a prolonged PTT, which is suspicious for an antiphospholipid antibody. She was an outpatient prior to having her blood drawn and was not taking heparin, so contamination with heparin (answer C) is unlikely (although heparin causes an increase in the PTT). The increased INR suggests that the patient has been compliant with her warfarin (answer D). Cava filters (answer B) are rarely useful unless the patient is at high risk from anticoagulation. Development of VTE is increased with long-term use of cava filters, and there is no long-term benefit seen with the use of vena cava filters.

 HELPFUL TIP: Previously, retrospective studies resulted in the recommendation that patients with an antiphospholipid antibody and VTE be maintained at an INR of 3–4. This recommendation has changed with newly available prospective data, and these patients should have a target INR of 2.5.

 HELPFUL TIP: Genetic testing is available for warfarin sensitivity that can help predict which patients will need higher (or lower) doses of warfarin to maintain adequate anticoagulation. However, these tests are very expensive and contribute little to patient care.

CASE 35

A 50-year-old male is admitted to the hospital with a fractured tibia after a motor vehicle collision. You are asked to assist in his perioperative management. The patient is generally healthy but is taking warfarin for a DVT that he developed after a total knee arthroplasty

3 weeks ago. His INR is 1.8, and he is scheduled for open reduction/internal fixation tomorrow.

Which of the following statements is FALSE?

A) The patient has an approximate 50% risk of recurrent VTE without appropriate therapy.
B) The patient has high risk of mortality with a recurrent VTE.
C) Heparin should be started preoperatively.
D) Heparin should be continued postoperatively.
E) Resumption of warfarin alone postoperatively is adequate anticoagulation.

Discussion

The correct answer is E. Perioperative management of a patient with recent VTE is complicated. While there are established guidelines for VTE prophylaxis depending on the type of surgery planned, this patient already has an active thrombotic event. Answer E is a false statement because discontinuing warfarin may result in a "rebound" hypercoagulable state, and surgery creates a prothrombotic state.

Patients who have a VTE within 1 month of surgery have a 50% risk of a second VTE if not treated aggressively with anticoagulation. These recurrent events carry a mortality rate of approximately 6%. Such patients should be placed on heparin before and after surgery. Starting warfarin after surgery decreases the risk of bleeding but is less effective at preventing VTE immediately postoperatively, so heparin should be employed as well. Patients with a VTE within 1–3 months before a scheduled surgery should be considered for postoperative heparin therapy, while a VTE >3 months before the scheduled surgery should not pose significant additional risk, and established prophylaxis guidelines should be followed.

Objectives: Did you learn to . . .

• Obtain an appropriate history in a patient with clotting?
• Recognize common inherited and acquired hypercoaguable risk factors?
• Describe anticoagulation approaches in perioperative care?
• Recognize the risks of venothromboembolism in the pregnant patient?
• Identify a patient presenting with antiphospholipid antibodies and understand the management of such patients?

BIBLIOGRAPHY

Abramson N, Melton B. Leukocytosis: Basics of clinical assessment. *Am Fam Physician.* 2000;62(9):2053.

Allen GA, Glader B. Approach to the bleeding child. *Pediatr Clin North Am.* 2002;49(6):1239.

American College of Chest Physicians. The Seventh ACCP Conference on Antithrombotic and Thrombolytic Therapy. *Chest.* 2004;126(suppl).

Bain BJ. Diagnosis from the blood smear. *N Engl J Med.* 2005;353:498.

Bitran, J. *Expert Guide to Oncology.* Philadelphia: American College of Physicians—American Society of Internal Medicine; 2000. (A good, readable overview).

Brandhagen DJ, Fairbanks VF, Baldus W. Recognition and management of hereditary hemochromatosis. *Am Fam Physician.* 2002;65(5):853.

George JN. Thrombotic thrombocytopenic purpura. *N Engl J Med.* 2006;354:1927.

Killip S, Bennett JM, Chambers MD. Iron-deficiency anemia. *Am Fam Physician.* 2007;75(5):671.

O'Connell TX, Hortia TJ, Kasravi B. Understanding and interpreting serum protein electrophoresis. *Am Fam Physician.* 2005;7(1):105.

Sunga AY, et al. Care of cancer survivors. *Am Fam Physician.* 2005;71(4):699.

Useful Web Sites

Sponsored by the American Society of Hematology, including links to many blood disease Web sites.
www.hematology.org

Information on general hematology/oncology subjects and laboratory testing, also general medicine.
www.hematology.org

Everything you want to know about platelets.
w3.ouhsc.edu/platelets/index.html

Sponsored by the American Society of Clinical Oncology for physicians.
www.asco.org

Everything about myeloma; sponsored by the Multiple Myeloma Research Foundation.
www.multiplemyeloma.org

Web site for patients living with cancer; sponsored by American Society of Clinical Oncology.
www.plwc.org

7

Gastroenterology

Ottar Bergmann

CASE 1

A 43-year-old female complains of a burning pain in the retrosternal area. Her symptoms started about 2 years ago and responded initially to self-medication with antacids or histamine2 receptor antagonists (H$_2$-blockers). However, within the last 4 months, she has had daily problems. She wakes up frequently in the middle of the night with retrosternal, burning pain, radiating to her neck. She also notices frequently an acidic taste in her mouth. While antacids help somewhat, they provide only transient relief. She has otherwise been healthy. She currently takes up to 4 tablets of cimetidine (200 mg) per day and uses antacids. She denies tobacco or alcohol use. Her physical examination is normal.

What additional question is MOST important to address first?

A) Does she have problems swallowing?
B) Does she have *H. pylori* infection?
C) Does she have liver enzyme abnormalities?
D) Does she have diarrhea?

Discussion

The correct answer is A. You need to make sure there are no high-risk associations such as dysphagia, weight loss, etc. The patient has typical symptoms of gastroesophageal reflux. There is a high prevalence of gastroesophageal reflux disease (GERD) in the United States, so performing extensive studies on every patient with symptoms of GERD would be extremely costly. Fortunately, typical symptoms of GERD are sensitive

and specific to the disease. Epidemiologic studies show that the presence of heartburn and regurgitation on a weekly basis is diagnostic of GERD with a sensitivity and specificity greater than 90%. Further assessment may be warranted if warning symptoms, such as dysphagia or weight loss, coexist. In the absence of such red flags, further testing is not necessary.

 HELPFUL TIP: The link between *H. pylori* and GERD is poorly defined. There is no good evidence to support eradication of *H. pylori* for the treatment of GERD.

* *

The patient denies any warning symptoms. Based on this information, you assume that this patient has GERD.

You recommend:

A) Barium swallow study.
B) Esophageal manometry.
C) Endoscopy.
D) Ambulatory pH study of the esophagus.
E) Trial of omeprazole and lifestyle modifications.

Discussion

The correct answer is E. The sensitivity and specificity of classic symptoms (approximately 90%) allows for the diagnosis of GERD without additional studies. Testing is less sensitive for GERD with the sensitivity of tests varying between 50% and 70%. Many patients have a false-negative esophagogastroduodenoscopy (EGD). Diagnostic studies are needed in patients with warning symptoms, complications, cases refractory to conventional therapy or prior to surgery for reflux disease. The main concern is the association between gastroesophageal reflux and adenocarcinoma of the esophagus. Metaplasia of the epithelium ("Barrett esophagus") may lead to the development of dysplastic changes and ultimately cancer. Screening for the presence of Barrett esophagus in patients with GERD is low yield. Additionally, it is not feasible to perform endoscopies in the 20% of the adult population in the United States with GERD. The patient described in this scenario has a low likelihood of Barrett esophagus (see below); therefore, current evidence argues against further invasive testing in her.

While H$_2$-blockers should still be first-line treatment in patients with GERD, this patient has already failed cimetidine. Starting a proton pump inhibitor (PPI), like omeprazole, is the next step and is preferred as first-line therapy in patients with severe symptoms. Lifestyle modifications should be made including: weight loss (if overweight); avoidance of carbonated beverages, caffeine, excessive alcohol, and large or late-evening meals; avoidance of anticholinergics, calcium channel blockers, NSAIDs and sedative drugs; smoking cessation; and elevation of the head of the bed using 6-inch blocks.

 HELPFUL TIP: Most patients with GERD will have negative endoscopic findings, known as nonerosive reflux disease (NERD)—really, we didn't make this one up. Symptoms do not correlate well with the presence or degree of esophageal inflammation or erosion.

* *

Your patient is willing to try the PPI you prescribe, but she also wants to know about surgery for GERD that her friend had.

Regarding surgery for GERD, you can tell her:

A) Bloating and inability to belch do not occur with antireflux surgery; her friend is probably suffering a psychosomatic illness deeply rooted in her childhood belch-punishment-shame cycle.

B) Antireflux surgery should be thought of as first-line because it is vastly superior to medical therapy.

C) Years after antireflux surgery, many patients will require medication for GERD symptoms.

D) Fundoplication results in impaired lower-esophageal sphincter function.

E) None of the above.

Discussion

The correct answer is C. Surgery may be an option in select patients with reflux disease. The usual indications for antireflux surgery include failure of medical therapy to control symptoms and failure of medical therapy to prevent complications (eg, stricture, pneumonia, etc). The most commonly performed surgery is fundoplication, in which the lower esophageal sphincter is wrapped to enhance its competency. While fundoplication will alleviate symptoms in 80% to 95% of patients, there is progressive loss of effectiveness over time (only 40% are without medication after 10 years). Adverse effects of surgery include persistent dysphagia (requiring additional interventions in 3%–7%), gas, bloating, and inability to belch.

* *

After a trial of PPI therapy your patient continues to have symptoms. You review lifestyle modifications with her, and she assures you that she has made these changes. You refer her for upper endoscopy (EGD). The esophageal biopsy is consistent with the visual report, which shows Barrett esophagus.

All of the following are true regarding Barrett esophagus EXCEPT:

A) Males are more likely to have Barrett esophagus than females.

B) Barrett esophagus is caused by a change in the esophageal mucosa from columnar to squamous.

C) Barrett esophagus occurs in 10% to 15% of patients with erosive esophagitis.

D) Barrett esophagus increases the risk of adenocarcinoma by up to 30-fold.

E) Patients with Barrett esophagus should undergo periodic screening EGD.

Discussion

The correct answer is B. Barrett esophagus is diagnosed histologically when esophageal mucosal metaplasia has occurred **and the usual squamous epithelial cells**

have changed to columnar epithelium. Risk factors for Barrett include long-standing reflux, male gender (6:1 male:female preponderance), middle age, tobacco use, and white race. Barrett esophagus occurs in 10%–15% of patients with erosive esophagitis, and it dramatically increases the risk of esophageal adenocarcinoma (30-fold). However, the absolute risk of adenocarcinoma is still small, about 0.2%–2% annually. Surveillance for Barrett depends on the level of dysplasia found on initial exam, and guidelines exist that dictate the frequency with which repeat EGD should be performed.

 HELPFUL TIP: Prokinetic agents, like metoclopramide (Reglan), can be useful in the treatment of GERD. In addition to promoting stomach emptying, metoclopramide increases gastroesophageal sphincter tone.

 HELPFUL TIP: Complications of chronic GERD include erosive esophagitis, peptic stricture, and adenocarcinoma of the esophagus. However, the absence of heartburn symptoms does not rule out reflux-related complications since approximately one-fourth of patients with peptic stricture and one-third of those with adenocarcinoma of the esophagus had no heartburn prior to diagnosis. Barrett esophagus can regress with adequate treatment of GERD.

Objectives: Did you learn to ...

- Describe the diagnosis and management of GERD?
- Use H$_2$-blockers and PPIs in the management of GERD?
- Recognize complications of GERD and risk factors for Barrett esophagus?

CASE 2

A 53-year-old female comes to your office complaining of chest pain and problems swallowing. She says food seems to hang up in the retrosternal area. This started several years ago and has progressed gradually and now occurs at least twice per week. Generally, only solid foods cause problems. She has become very careful, taking only small bites and chewing them well before swallowing. Should she experience problems, she has found that drinking additional liquids alleviates her symptoms within minutes. She does not regurgitate food and has not lost weight.

What is the symptom this patient is complaining of?

A) Dysphagia.
B) Globus sensation.
C) Odynophagia.
D) Aerophagia.
E) None of the above.

Discussion

The correct answer is A. Dysphagia, from the Greek *dys* (with difficulty . . . as opposed to *Dis* which is a city in Dante's Hell . . . . what were you thinking?) and *phagia* (to eat), is the sensation that food is being hindered in its passage from the mouth to the stomach. Odynophagia (answer C) is pain upon swallowing, aerophagia (answer D) is swallowing of air, and globus sensation (answer B) is a perception of a lump or fullness in the throat that is relieved temporarily by swallowing.

 HELPFUL TIP: Aerophagia is a common and underdiagnosed cause of abdominal symptoms. Patients will complain of belching associated with abdominal bloating, especially after meals. It is not uncommon for patients to mention that they have to loosen their belt after meals. Aerophagia is exacerbated by gum-chewing (which causes frequent swallowing of air), eating quickly, and smoking. Aerophagia can be mitigated by eating more slowly, avoiding carbonated beverages, etc.

What information is important when evaluating this patient with dysphagia?

A) When the sensation first occurs in relation to swallowing.
B) What medications the patient is taking.
C) Whether solids or liquids are affected.
D) The patient's HIV status.
E) All of the above.

Discussion

The correct answer is E. Taking a careful history is key to evaluating the patient who presents with dysphagia.

Some of the important questions include:

1. When does the sensation first occur in relation to swallowing? Is it oropharyngeal dysphagia or esophageal dysphagia?

2. What types of food produce the symptoms? Solids, liquids or both? If solids are involved there could be a stricture. If only liquids are involved, it suggests an esophageal motility disorder.

3. What is the temporal progression of symptoms? Dysphagia to both solids and liquids from the beginning suggests a motility disorder of the esophagus. If dysphagia initially involves only solids and only later progresses to involve liquids, it suggests a mechanical obstruction.

4. Are symptoms progressive or intermittent? Progressive dysphagia suggests a carcinoma, or a peptic stricture, while intermittent dysphagia points to a lower esophageal ring. Motility disorders may be progressive (usually achalasia or scleroderma) or intermittent (usually diffuse esophageal spasm or nonspecific motility disorders).

5. Review of systems? Important elements include heartburn, weight loss, hematemesis, coffee ground emesis, anemia, regurgitation of food particles, and respiratory symptoms.

6. Coughing or choking after swallowing? Regurgitation of food through the nose? These findings suggest aspiration and/or oropharyngeal dysphagia.

7. How rapid is the symptom progression? Rapid progression of symptoms suggests malignancy.

8. Are there other significant illnesses present? Specifically, does the patient have HIV/AIDS, neurologic disorders, GERD, etc?

9. Is there a prior history of surgery or radiation to the gastrointestinal tract?

10. What medications is the patient using?

* *

A complete review of systems and physical examination are unrevealing.

Which of the following is the BEST test to arrive at a diagnosis in this patient?

A) Barium swallow.
B) Esophageal manometry.
C) Esophagogastroduodenoscopy.
D) Ambulatory pH study of the esophagus.
E) Diagnostic trial of a high-dose PPI.

Discussion

The correct answer is C. Visualization of the esophagus is critical in patients with dysphagia. This can be done by either endoscopy or barium swallow. Your patient presents with esophageal dysphagia for solids, which is most consistent with a structural problem, such as a stricture, web, or neoplasm. Endoscopy is the best diagnostic study to evaluate the esophageal mucosa as it allows one to obtain biopsies and perform endoscopic interventions such as dilations, if indicated. While many authorities may recommend a barium swallow first, it does not let one obtain a biopsy or perform an intervention if warranted. Should the endoscopy come back negative, esophageal manometry (answer B) may be useful as it will help determine if a motility disorder is the cause of symptoms. While a diagnostic trial with PPIs (answer E) is an appropriate strategy in patients with noncardiac chest pain, the presence of an alarm symptom, such as dysphagia, requires further testing. An ambulatory pH study (answer D) does not help in defining the etiology of the dysphagia.

 HELPFUL TIP: Many patients have breakthrough pain at night even when on a PPI. This is because PPIs act only on cells that have been activated (such as by a meal). Try adding an H_2-blocker at nighttime for patients having breakthrough pain.

* *

The patient returns from her endoscopy. According to the report, she had severe esophagitis with confluent erosions in the distal esophagus. During the physical examination, you find the skin changes shown in Figure 7–1. When you ask about these, the patient reports a history of bluish fingertip discoloration with cold temperatures. She also complains that her fingers feel "tight" at times.

With this new information, which of the following diagnoses are you considering?

A) CREST syndrome.
B) Esophageal adenocarcinoma.
C) Metastatic colonic adenocarcinoma.
D) Sicca syndrome.
E) Peptic ulcer disease.

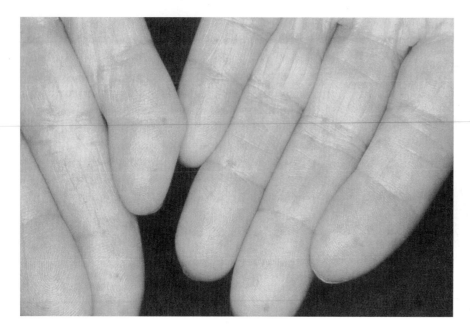

Figure 7–1

Discussion

The correct answer is A. CREST is an acronym for a syndrome that includes **c**alcinosis cutis, **R**aynaud phenomenon, **e**sophageal dysmotility, **s**clerodactyly, and **t**elangiectasias. Figure 7–1 (see also color section) shows telangiectasias on the palmar digital pad. Up to 60% of patients with CREST have erosive esophagitis. Dysphagia is common and is due to esophageal stricture and/or dysmotility.

Given her endoscopic physical exam findings that indicate the patient likely has CREST syndrome, what treatment do you suggest?

A) H₂-blocker.
B) PPI.
C) Open fundoplication.
D) *H. pylori* eradication.
E) Laparoscopic fundoplication.

Discussion

The correct answer is B. Severe reflux and dysphagia are hallmarks of CREST syndrome. The esophagus may be amotile with impaired function of the lower esophageal sphincter. The barrier to acid reflux and the motor clearance of refluxing material are affected, requiring chronic and potent acid suppressive medications, such as PPIs. Answer A, H₂-blocker, is less likely to provide a benefit since H₂-blockers are less potent than PPIs. Surgery is **relatively contraindicated**, as the poor contractile function of the esophagus may not generate enough force to overcome a barrier created

by fundoplication (answer C) or other interventions (and thus food will not move into the stomach). *H. pylori* treatment (answer D) has no role in the management of this illness. In real life, as opposed to a board exam, CREST syndrome is an uncommon cause of dysphagia. Other causes of esophageal dysphagia are listed in Table 7–1.

 HELPFUL TIP: A cause of dysphagia is eosinophilic esophagitis. The classic adult patient presents with dysphagia to solids to the extent that it may cause food impaction. Children often present with feeding problems (aged 2 years), recurrent vomiting (aged 8 years) and chronic abdominal pain (aged 12 years). Association with childhood asthma is strong and dietary elimination therapy may be helpful in children. Treatment in adults involves swallowing inhaled corticosteroids (fluticasone), montelukast, and in severe cases, systemic steroids. Systemic eosinophilia is rare.

Objectives: Did you learn to …

• Differentiate dysphagia from other gastrointestinal symptoms?
• Take an adequate history to evaluate the etiology of dysphagia?

Table 7–1 CAUSES OF ESOPHAGEAL DYSPHAGIA

Mechanical Lesions: Intrinsic	Mechanical Lesions: Extrinsic
Benign tumors	Aberrant subclavian
Caustic esophagitis/stricture	artery
Radiation esophagitis/stricture	Cervical osteophytes
Peptic esophagitis/stricture	Enlarged aorta
Eosinophilic esophagitis	Enlarged left atrium
Diverticula	Mediastinal mass
Malignancy	Post-spinal surgery
Post-GI surgery	
Rings and webs	
Foreign bodies	
Motility Disorders	
Achalasia	
Chagas disease	
(*Trypanosoma cruzi*)	
Diffuse esophageal spasm	
Hypertensive lower esophageal	
sphincter	
Nonspecific esophageal motility	
disorder	
Nutcracker esophagus	
Scleroderma	

- Describe different types of dysphagia and identify various causes of dysphagia?
- Recognize that CREST syndrome is a cause of dysphagia?

 QUICK QUIZ: REGURGITATION

You see a 61-year-old female in your office with complaints of halitosis, regurgitation of undigested food 4 hours after eating, and heartburn. She also feels that the food is sticking in her throat.

What is the MOST LIKELY cause of her symptoms?

A) Schatzki ring.
B) Zenker diverticulum.
C) Achalasia.
D) Foreign body.
E) Esophageal web.

Discussion

The correct answer is B. Late regurgitation of undigested food is pathognomic for Zenker diverticulum.

A Zenker diverticulum is an out-pouching of esophageal mucosa that is acquired and typically becomes symptomatic in middle age or later in life. The diagnosis is confirmed by lateral view of a barium swallow. The other diagnoses listed can cause dysphagia and regurgitation, but are less likely. Schatzki ring (answer A) is a lower esophageal mucosal ring that can catch food and cause dysphagia. Achalasia (answer C) results from a loss of innervation of the lower esophagus and generally occurs in young and middle-aged adults. Patients with achalasia typically have dysphagia with solids and liquids. Foreign body (answer D) should be diagnosable by history. Elderly adults, children, and patients with psychiatric disease are at highest risk for foreign body in the esophagus. Esophageal web (answer E) is caused by a thin layer of mucosa across the esophageal lumen and presents much like a Schatzki ring.

CASE 3

A 32-year-old female presents with 3 years of intermittent gastrointestinal complaints after eating. She describes epigastric pressure and bloating after food intake. Her weight is stable. She denies heartburn, vomiting, diarrhea, constipation, or blood in her stools. She takes only a multivitamin and she has not tried any specific remedies. The physical examination is normal.

What is the MOST LIKELY diagnosis given the information above?

A) Pyrosis.
B) Peptic ulcer disease (PUD).
C) Non-ulcer dyspepsia.
D) Stomach cancer.

Discussion

The correct answer is C. Non-ulcer dyspepsia is an ill-defined condition characterized by the presence of recurring intermittent symptoms of epigastric discomfort and fullness with other associated symptoms in the absence of mucosal lesions or other structural abnormalities of the GI tract. Non-ulcer dyspepsia is also known as functional dyspepsia, as there are no identifiable structural or anatomic abnormalities of the GI tract. Although approximately 20% of the general population has non-ulcer dyspepsia, only about 20% of these seek medical attention. Pyrosis (answer A) is the same as heartburn; this patient has no complaints of heartburn. PUD or stomach cancer of 3 years' duration would usually be accompanied by other systemic symptoms (such as fatigue, weight loss, or death—is that a systemic symptom?), which the patient denies. In general, the history and physical exam do not allow you to rule out PUD, but young patients without alarm symptoms can be treated empirically without extensive investigation, as the risk of underlying serious pathology is low.

Which of the following symptoms WOULD NOT be a normal symptom of non-ulcer dyspepsia?

A) Fullness.
B) Early satiety.
C) Belching.
D) Intolerance to eggs.

Discussion

The correct answer is D. Intolerance to eggs is not a symptom of non-ulcer dyspepsia. What have you got against eggs? The editors like eggs, poached if possible. Non-ulcer dyspepsia is characterized by all the other answer choices and includes symptoms such as abdominal distention, borborygmi (ie, grandpa's tummy gurgling heard across the room at Thanksgiving), epigastric or substernal pain, anorexia, nausea, vomiting, and abdominal tenderness. Although there are several proposed pathophysiologic mechanisms by which non-ulcer dyspepsia may occur, food intolerance is not one of them.

What is the most appropriate next step in this patient?

A) Obtain *H. pylori* antibodies.
B) Obtain an abdominal ultrasound examination of liver, biliary tree, and pancreas.
C) Obtain a detailed dietary history.
D) Obtain an upper gastrointestinal x-ray series.
E) Refer for gastroscopy.

Discussion

The correct answer is C. Does this seem to be a contradiction to the previous question?. Although food intolerance does not cause non-ulcer dyspepsia, the symptoms of the two types of disorders overlap. The prevalence of selective carbohydrate malabsorption syndromes, high-intake of lactose- and fructose-containing food and beverages may contribute to GI symptoms in a significant number of patients. Therefore, the history should always contain a detailed assessment of dietary habits. A more extensive workup

is not necessary at this time as the patient is <55 years and has no alarm symptoms. While infection with *H. pylori* causes gastritis and peptic ulcers, several controlled studies demonstrated no consistent benefit of *H. pylori* eradication in dyspeptic patients without ulcers.

 HELPFUL TIP: If you choose to test and treat for *H.pylori*, the preferred testing strategy is 13C urea breath test or stool antigen test (see case later in this chapter).

* *

You obtain a detailed dietary history, suggesting a potential contribution of fructose intolerance and excessive carbonated beverage intake (it's those 5 Giant Gulp soft drinks a day). Her symptoms persist despite appropriate adjustment of food intake. Then, you choose to start the patient on a PPI. One week later, your nurse receives a call from your patient with complaints of severe abdominal pain and diarrhea. She has **not** noticed blood in her stool. In addition, she has developed left lower quadrant pain that often precedes defecation and is alleviated by passing a bowel movement.

What is the best next step?

A) She is having withdrawal from the soft drinks. Add back the fructose and the 2,000 Kcals.
B) Check fasting gastrin level.
C) Antibiotic therapy for bacterial overgrowth.
D) Discontinuation of the PPI.
E) Therapeutic trial of an antidiarrheal.

Discussion

The correct answer is D. Diarrhea is a common adverse effect of PPIs which occurs in at least 5%–7% of patients. Discontinuation leads to a rapid resolution in the majority of cases. While reduced stomach acidity from PPIs or H₂-blockers may result in bacterial colonization of the proximal gastrointestinal tract, the early onset and severity of symptoms described argue against bacterial overgrowth as the etiology of this patient's symptoms. While PPIs can elevate gastrin levels, the hypergastrinemia seen is not comparable to levels seen in Zollinger-Ellison syndrome, which can also cause diarrhea. Stool studies and empiric therapy with antidiarrheals may be considered if discontinuing the PPI does not improve symptoms.

 HELPFUL TIP: No drugs have good evidence to support their use in non-ulcer dyspepsia. PPIs and H_2-blockers are often used. Prokinetic agents may be helpful. In the United States this is metoclopramide. Cisapride has been removed from the market secondary to cardiac arrhythmias (QT prolongation with torsade de pointes).

Which of the following is TRUE of the natural history of non-ulcer dyspepsia?

A) Most patients will not have symptom-free periods, instead having constant dyspepsia.
B) Most patients improve with placebo treatment.
C) Most patients will go on to develop ulcers.
D) Spontaneous resolution of symptoms is rare.

Discussion

The correct answer is B. Up to 60% of patients in placebo controlled trials respond to placebo, making it difficult to prove efficacy of medications. As the above number suggests, spontaneous resolution of symptoms is common, while many patients will have a chronic, intermittent course characterized by symptom-free periods. Most patients will not develop serious pathology.

 HELPFUL TIP: For non-ulcer dyspepsia, general management strategies are reassurance by the physician and the avoidance of repeated diagnostic testing. Patients should make appropriate lifestyle modifications (avoid tobacco, caffeine products, and alcohol) and limit or avoid aggravating medications (NSAIDs). Patients should chew their foods slowly and eat more frequent, small meals. Finally, if there is underlying psychiatric morbidity, relaxation training or treatment of specific diseases can be helpful.

Objectives: Did you learn to . . .

- Diagnose and manage non-ulcer dyspepsia?
- Appreciate the natural history of non-ulcer dyspepsia?
- Recognize diarrhea as a side effect of PPIs?

CASE 4

A 56-year-old female comes to the ED after a sudden episode of hematemesis. She describes a vague abdominal discomfort in the epigastric area that started about 4 days prior to presentation. Yesterday, she had 2 bowel movements that were dark, sticky, and foul-smelling. She woke up nauseated and has twice vomited a small amount of bright red blood. She also feels dizzy. Because of knee pain related to skydiving 1 week ago (she says, "It was a blast—do it before you die or die doing it!"), she started taking 5 tablets of naproxen twice a day. She takes no other medicines and denies any significant past medical history.

On physical exam, you find a pale, uncomfortable, but alert patient. She has tachycardia (108 beats/min) and a drop in blood pressure from 116/72 mm Hg supine to 93/65 mm Hg standing. Her abdomen is flat with hypoactive bowel sounds. You note epigastric tenderness but no rebound or guarding. There is melena on rectal examination.

Which of the following steps will be LEAST helpful now?

A) Admission to the hospital.
B) Immediate treatment with an intravenous H_2-blocker.
C) Referral for emergent endoscopy.
D) IV access and fluid resuscitation.
E) Laboratory tests including hemoglobin, coagulation studies, and blood type and cross-match.

Discussion

The correct answer is B. The patient has symptoms and clinical findings of a hemodynamically significant upper GI tract bleed. Although she is walking and talking just fine, fluid administration and hospital admission with close monitoring in an intensive care environment are indicated. A baseline hemoglobin and hematocrit should be obtained. **However, a normal hemoglobin does not exclude a significant acute bleed, as hemodilution (in the absence of IV fluids) requires several hours.** Given the presentation, a blood transfusion may become necessary in the future; therefore, blood should be sent for to type and cross-match. Early endoscopy should be performed to identify the cause of her bleeding, and endoscopic therapy should be undertaken if appropriate. Treatment with H_2-blockers does not affect the rate of bleeding; these medications do not increase the gastric pH enough to enhance coagulation.

Recent studies have demonstrated that intravenous PPIs do decrease the risk of rebleeding in high-risk patients by increasing gastric pH to enhance coagulation. However, these studies combined a PPI with endoscopy.

> **HELPFUL TIP:** Orthostatic vital signs are not very useful. Many hypovolemic patients are **not** orthostatic and many patients who are euvolemic **have** orthostatic changes (eg, patients on antihypertensives, the elderly, etc). Use orthostatic vital signs to confirm your clinical suspicion but do not use them as an absolute guide to the patient's volume status.

* *

Indications for surgery for peptic ulcer bleeding include:

A) Hemodynamic instability despite vigorous resuscitation (>3 units blood transfusion) **or** continued slow bleed with a transfusion requirement exceeding 3 units per day.
B) Failure of endoscopy to stop the bleeding.
C) Recurrent significant hemorrhage after initial stabilization with fluids and endoscopy.
D) Shock associated with recurrent hemorrhage.
E) All of the above.

Discussion

The correct answer is E. All of the answer choices are indications for surgical management. Relative indications for surgery include: rare blood type or difficult cross-match, refusal of transfusion, shock on presentation, advanced age, severe comorbid disease, and a bleeding chronic gastric ulcer. Randomized studies have shown that if endoscopic hemostasis is successful and the patient rebleeds, a second endoscopy has better outcome than surgery. If available, interventional radiology can often successfully stop bleeding and prevent the need for surgery, but controlled trials are lacking.

* *

The patient undergoes endoscopy, which shows a small duodenal ulcer in the bulb with a visible vessel in the ulcer base. Gastric biopsies show chemical gastropathy and no evidence of *H. pylori*. After endoscopic treatment, the patient recovers nicely. Then, 3 months later,

she returns to your office for a follow-up evaluation. She is asymptomatic and continues taking a PPI. Her physical examination is normal. Laboratory tests show normal hemoglobin.

What is the best next step?

A) Repeat endoscopy to document healing and rule out malignancy.
B) Upper gastrointestinal x-ray series to document healing.
C) Switch to an H$_2$-blocker.
D) Discontinue acid-suppressive medication.
E) *H. pylori* antibody test.

Discussion

The correct answer is D. While nonhealing ulcers may be due to a neoplasm, the majority of **duodenal** ulcers are benign. Therefore, neither endoscopic nor radiologic documentation of healing is necessary. Patients with uncomplicated and small (<1 cm) duodenal or gastric ulcers who have received adequate treatment for *H. pylori* or NSAID-induced ulcer do not need long-term therapy directed at ulcer healing as long as they are asymptomatic following therapy. Antisecretory drugs can be discontinued after 4–6 weeks in these patients. Serology for *H. pylori* will not be helpful in this patient. First, histology is as sensitive as other tests for *H. pylori* infection and the patient's biopsies were negative for *H. pylori*. Second, **serologic testing does not tell us if the patient is currently infected.** Many patients have antibody positivity as long as a year after treatment.

> **HELPFUL TIP:** PPIs are not benign drugs and have been associated with (1) increased risk of hip fracture in the elderly, (2) increased risk of pneumonia, (3) increased risk of *C. difficile* colitis, and (4) diarrhea as noted above. Stop them as soon as possible.

> **HELPFUL TIP:** Sensitivity of serologic testing for *H. pylori* is 90%–100%. Breath testing is 88%–95% sensitive with most false negatives the result of the use of antibiotics and antacids, including H$_2$-blockers and PPIs. Make sure the

patient has been off antibiotics for at least a month prior to testing and has not taken acid suppressors for 2 weeks prior to testing. This also holds true for CLO testing. Stool antigen testing is now available to help with the noninvasive documentation of *H. pylori* infection or eradication.

* *

Three weeks later, the patient contacts your office again. She developed recurrent knee pain after mowing her lawn.

Which of the following treatments is the safest way to manage her pain?

A) Acetaminophen 1,000 mg three times daily.
B) Ibuprofen 400 mg three times daily combined with ranitidine 150 mg twice daily.
C) Celecoxib (Celecoxib) 200 mg twice daily.
D) Ibuprofen 400 mg three times daily combined with sucralfate 1 g four times daily.
E) Naproxen 500 mg twice daily.

Discussion
The correct answer is A. Given her prior GI bleeding, she fits the profile of a high-risk patient and should not receive NSAIDs without appropriate prophylaxis. Acetaminophen does not cause bleeding and should be the first choice analgesic in patients with a history of GI bleeding. Another, but less desirable, option is to use a PPI with an NSAID. Another option is misoprostol given with an NSAID. It is as effective for ulcer prophylaxis as a PPI, but side effects of diarrhea have limited widespread use of this combination.

Answer C, celecoxib, requires special note. Despite years (and millions of $$$$) of marketing, celecoxib and other COX-2 inhibitors are not indicated for analgesia in patients at risk for GI bleeding. They carry the same FDA labeling for GI irritation as do nonselective NSAIDs. Some COX-2 inhibitors have reduced GI toxicity in the short term compared to other NSAIDs; however, they can still cause ulcers in the GI tract. The GI risk with celecoxib is comparable to that of ibuprofen when used long term. So, do not assume that celecoxib is safe from a GI perspective.

 HELPFUL TIP: Nonacetylated salicylates like diacetylsalicylic acid (Salsalate) and choline magnesium trisalicylate (Trilisate) are less likely to cause GI bleeding in comparison with other NSAIDs. Ibuprofen, nabumetone (Relafen), and etodolac (Lodine) are among the safer of the traditional NSAIDs. Piroxicam, a very long-acting NSAID with significant enterohepatic circulation, has been associated with a higher risk of GI complications than other NSAIDs. Ketorolac is even worse.

 HELPFUL TIP: COX-2 inhibitors have been found to carry an increased risk of cardiovascular events, and therefore Valdecoxib (Bextra) and Rofecoxib (Vioxx) have been removed from the market. Celecoxib is still available with a warning about cardiovascular side effects and should be used with caution in older patients and patients with cardiovascular risk factors. COX-2 inhibitors should be avoided in patients with cardiovascular diseases. Note that low-dose aspirin negates any GI benefit from the COX-2 inhibitors. Other NSAIDs now carry a black box cardiovascular disease warning.

All of the following patients are considered to be at higher risk of NSAID-induced gastrointestinal bleeding EXCEPT:

A) Patients on high doses of NSAIDs.
B) Patients >60 years.
C) Patients concurrently taking glucocorticoids.
D) Patients concurrently taking anticoagulants.
E) Male patients.

Discussion
The correct answer is E. The risk of NSAID-induced GI toxicity is greater with increasing age, higher dose and longer use of NSAIDs, **female gender**, serious systemic illnesses, and concurrent use of certain other medications (eg, anticoagulants, glucocorticoids, other NSAIDs).

What is the risk of suffering a clinically significant GI event on NSAIDs?

A) 1%–4% per year.
B) 5%–10% per year.
C) 15%–20% per year.
D) 25%–30% per year.
E) 45%–50% per year.

Discussion

The correct answer is A. The risk of a clinically significant NSAID-related GI event, including gastrointestinal bleeding, perforation, or obstruction, is about 1%–4% per year.

 HELPFUL TIP: Rebound acid-hypersecretion can lead to symptom recurrence if potent antisecretory agents, such as PPIs, are stopped abruptly. It is recommended to step down PPIs to H$_2$-blockers prior to cessation. However, H$_2$-blockers can cause rebound acid-hypersecretion, also. So, consider tapering these drugs as well.

* *

Your patient returns with recurrent epigastric pain. She vehemently denies any aspirin or NSAID use. She has not been smoking tobacco or drinking alcohol. **Repeat endoscopy reveals several new ulcers.** Biopsy for *H. pylori* is again negative.

Which of the following would be the most appropriate laboratory test to obtain in order to discover an etiology for her ulcers?

A) Vasoactive intestinal peptide.
B) Gastrin.
C) Glucagon.
D) Somatostatin.
E) None of the above.

Discussion

The correct answer is B. A screening test for gastrinoma is warranted in a patient who has recurrent or refractory ulcers. Zollinger-Ellison syndrome is the state in which there is acid hypersecretion secondary to increased gastrin production, usually from a gastrin-producing tumor (gastrinoma). Up to 1% of patients with PUD have a gastrinoma. Serum gastrin levels should be obtained with the patient fasting **and off PPIs as they will increase gastrin levels.** If the serum gastrin is elevated, further investigations will need to

be performed. Other reasons to consider obtaining a serum gastrin level include: ulcers in unusual locations, multiple ulcers, family history of ulcers, and ulcers associated with reflux esophagitis.

Answer A is incorrect. Vasoactive intestinal peptide (VIP) works to suppress acid secretion. VIPomas do occur (they're actually tumors and not related to VIP patients calling you at all hours), but they are associated with watery diarrhea and hypokalemia—not ulcers. Glucagon (answer C) will not be effective here. Glucagon oversecretion results in glucose intolerance, anemia, and skin changes. Somatostatin (answer D) is a hormone that inhibits the secretion of gastrin and thus would be protective vis-à-vis ulcers. Somatostatin-secreting tumors are very rare.

 HELPFUL TIP: NSAID-induced ulcers can occur in the stomach, duodenum, and occasionally in the small bowel and colon. However, NSAIDs are more frequently found to be the cause of gastric ulcers (up to 30%) compared to duodenal ulcers (up to 20%).

Objectives: Did you learn to . . .

- Describe the epidemiology of peptic ulcer disease?
- Appreciate the role of NSAID use in peptic ulcer disease?
- Manage an acute gastrointestinal bleed?
- Identify patients at high risk for NSAID-induced gastrointestinal toxicity?
- Describe Zollinger-Ellison syndrome and determine when to test for it?

 QUICK QUIZ: GI BLEEDING

Isolated bright red hematemesis (eg, no tachycardia, no fever, etc) which occurs after several bouts of vomiting or dry heaves is referred to as:

A) Boerhaave tear.
B) Mallory-Weiss tear.
C) Cameron lesion.
D) None of the above.

Discussion

The correct answer is B. A Mallory-Weiss tear occurs after repeated trauma to the lower esophageal and gastric mucosa from forceful retching. This can be differentiated from a Boerhaave tear (answer A) by the (generally) self-limited nature of the bleeding and the absence of other symptoms. A Boerhaave tear is of a similar etiology but occurs in the esophagus and is associated with mediastinitis, fever, shock, and death if intervention is not forthcoming. Cameron lesions (answer C) are small ulcers in patients with hiatal hernia, are usually an incidental finding, and are thought to be caused by rubbing of the stomach against the diaphragm as the hernia slides. They can bleed, but the history given above is classic for a Mallory-Weiss tear.

 QUICK QUIZ: ABDOMINAL PAIN

A 35-year-old female presents to your clinic with complaints of onset of severe mid-epigastric pain and vomiting following meals. Between meals she is asymptomatic. This has been going on for the past 2 years ever since she purposefully lost 25 pounds to attain a healthy weight for her height. Unfortunately, she has continued to lose weight because of the postprandial pain and vomiting. On her exam you notice a mid-epigastric bruit.

The most likely diagnosis is:

A) Aortic aneurysm.
B) Atherosclerotic disease of the celiac trunk.
C) Superior mesenteric artery syndrome.
D) Chronic pancreatitis.
E) None of the above.

Discussion

The correct answer is C. This is a typical history and physical exam for superior mesenteric artery (SMA) syndrome. SMA syndrome is more likely to occur in a patient who has lost significant weight, resulting in thinning of the mesenteric fat pad. Here is the pathophysiology: the superior mesenteric artery runs above the duodenum and becomes stretched and partially occluded in response to meals (as the stomach and duodenum expand), leading to mesenteric ischemia and food aversion. SMA syndrome can be diagnosed using Doppler ultrasound to demonstrate increased velocity of blood in the SMA. Aortic aneurysm (answer A) and atherosclerotic disease of the celiac trunk (answer B) are unlikely in a young patient. Chronic pancreatitis (answer D) should not be associated with a bruit.

CASE 5

A 54-year-old male comes to your office for his annual physical. He is taking naproxen for a recent ankle injury. Based on your recommendation last year, he started taking 1 aspirin (81 mg) daily. He does not take any other medications. He exercises regularly, does not smoke, and drinks 1 glass of wine every day. Your examination is completely normal, except for a test for occult fecal blood that is positive.

What is the next best step?

A) Upper endoscopy.
B) CBC.
C) Colonoscopy.
D) A and B.
E) B and C.

Discussion

The correct answer is E. Current recommendations suggest screening for colorectal cancer in all patients >50 years. Testing for fecal occult blood is one of the accepted methods. However, it should only be performed as screening test in asymptomatic individuals. The use of aspirin and/or NSAIDs and foods such as undercooked meat may increase the number of false-positive tests and should be avoided. However, once you have a Guaiac positive stool, you must proceed to colonoscopy in a patient >50 years. A CBC is also important to determine if the patient is anemic. Since the patient currently has no symptoms referable to upper GI pathology, evaluation of the upper GI tract should only be considered if the colonoscopy is negative.

 HELPFUL TIP: Iron causes stool to darken. So do iron supplements cause false-positive Guaiac tests? No. Guaiac tests rely on the presence of hemoglobin in the stool, not iron. Do not blame a positive Guaiac on an iron supplement.

* *

The patient's records indicate that he underwent a colonoscopy 3 years ago. Three small adenomatous polyps were found. He also had scattered diverticula in the sigmoid.

Based on this new information, which strategy do you recommend?

A) Colonoscopy now.
B) Colonoscopy in 5 years.
C) Yearly tests for fecal occult blood.
D) Yearly tests for fecal occult blood and colonoscopy in 7 years.
E) Colonoscopy in 7 years.

Your answer is:

A) In 3 months.
B) In 1 year.
C) In 3 years.
D) In 5 years.
E) In 10 years.

Discussion

The correct answer is A. Adenomatous polyps, such as this patient had, are considered precancerous. Recommended follow-up of an adenomatous polyp is by colonoscopy every 3–5 years. So, he did not have a truly negative colonoscopy (no adenomatous polyps) 3 years ago. Plus, you are not doing the colonoscopy in this case for screening; it is diagnostic. You may find another source of his bleeding. If his previous colonoscopy were completely normal, you could argue for stopping the aspirin and NSAIDs and following up with serial fecal occult blood tests. In this alternative scenario, persistently positive Guaiac tests would lead to colonoscopy as well.

HELPFUL TIP: Adenomatous colon polyps, either pedunculated or sessile, are associated with transformation to cancer. Hyperplastic polyps are considered benign.

HELPFUL TIP: U.S. Preventive Services Task Force recommends routine screening for colorectal cancer, starting at 50 years for average-risk patients (this does NOT apply to high-risk patients—positive family history, known adenomatous polyps, etc). Any of the following modalities is acceptable: annual fecal occult blood testing (FOBT) alone; annual FOBT with sigmoidoscopy every 5 years with or without dual contrast barium enema every 5 years; colonoscopy every 10 years.

* *

The patient underwent colonoscopy. The report from the endoscopist shows 1 small sessile adenomatous polyp in the sigmoid colon that was completely removed. The patient wants to know when he needs another colonoscopy.

Discussion

The correct answer is D. The current **postpolypectomy** surveillance guidelines recommend the following:

1. No polyps or only rectal hyperplastic polyps; repeat in 10 years.
2. 1–2 tubular adenomas <1 cm in size with only low-grade dysplasia; repeat colonoscopy in 5 years.
3. 3–10 tubular adenomas, or villous features or high grade dysplasia; surveillance in 3 years.
4. Patients with >10 adenomas should be screened more frequently and familial colon cancer syndromes should be considered.
5. If a sessile polyp is removed in piecemeal fashion, repeat exam in 3 months to ensure complete removal.
6. If prep is not good, repeat colonoscopy at earliest convenience.

Patients presenting with hereditary nonpolyposis colorectal cancer (HNPCC) or "Lynch syndrome" are more likely than patients with sporadic colon cancer to have which of the following findings?

A) Left-sided colon cancers.
B) Late-age-onset of colon cancer.
C) Multiple colon cancers diagnosed simultaneously.
D) An unusual desire to visit Lynchburg, Tennessee.

Discussion

The correct answer is C. Patients with HNPCC (Lynch syndrome) are at increased risk of developing colon cancer. About 2%–3% of colon cancers occur in patients with Lynch syndrome. Transformation from an adenoma to cancer is faster in patients with Lynch syndrome. In addition, many of the neoplasms are located in the right colon, so answer A is incorrect. Compared to sporadic colon cancer patients, those with Lynch syndrome are younger at the time of diagnosis, more frequently present with multiple colon tumors, and are more likely to have extracolonic tumors—especially endometrial cancer. This is a genetic disorder, and the occurrence of colorectal and/or **endometrial** cancer in three relatives <50 years should suggest HNPCC. The current recommendation is to perform surveillance colonoscopies at least every 3 years in these patients.

Objectives: Did you learn to . . .

- Describe the limitations of fecal occult blood testing?
- Choose the appropriate tests and screening and surveillance intervals for colorectal neoplasias?
- Learn how family and personal history of colorectal neoplasia affects screening and surveillance strategy?

CASE 6

A 28-year-old graduate student comes to your office complaining of diarrhea. About 6 months ago, she noted a sudden onset of loose stools. Although she initially attributed these symptoms to stomach flu, her problem has persisted. She currently has about 4–6 loose bowel movements per day with nighttime defecations. She has not seen blood in her stool. In addition, she complains of cramps located in the left and occasionally right lower abdomen. The cramps are made worse with food intake and often are associated with a need to defecate. She has lost about 8 kg unintentionally within the last 3–4 months. She denies any travel or antibiotic use. On physical examination, you notice some tenderness in the right lower quadrant. You see a painless anal fissure in the anterior commissure, and by the appearance, you judge that the fissure is probably chronic in nature.

What do you recommend as the next step in the evaluation and management of this patient?

A) Loperamide.
B) Referral to a holistic clinic for a colonic cleansing regimen.
C) Check titers of atypical ANCA.
D) Colonoscopy.
E) Botulinum toxin injection into the area of the anal fissure.

Discussion

The correct answer is D. The patient's history and physical findings with a painless, anteriorly located anal fissure are consistent with Crohn disease. The best next step in her evaluation is colonoscopy with inspection of the terminal ileum. You may want to do some stool testing before colonoscopy; and testing for *Giardia*,

C. difficile toxin, and other pathogens would be reasonable. But of the choices presented, colonoscopy is the best option. Answer A is incorrect because this is long-standing with weight loss; symptomatic control is fine but we need to figure out what is going on with this patient. Answer B is incorrect. She has diarrhea—her colon is already clean. Answer C, serologic testing, is a reasonable choice but not the best. Crohn disease is associated with antibodies against saccharomyces (ASCA), while ulcerative colitis (UC) patients are more often positive for antineutrophil cytoplasmic antibodies (ANCA). However, the sensitivity of these tests is only about 60%. Moreover, there is about a 20% overlap (eg, ANCA positive in Crohn), raising further questions about the overall usefulness of these tests. Answer E is incorrect. Fissures are one of the anal manifestations of Crohn disease and should be approached by treating the underlying disease rather than using surgical techniques, botulinum injection, etc. Botulinum injections, nitroglycerin ointment, and nifedipine have all been used for anal fissures with success, but you need to diagnose this patient and address the underlying disease.

 HELPFUL TIP: In Crohn disease, about 25% of patients have disease confined to the colon. Another 40% have disease in the ileum and cecum, and 30% have disease confined to the small bowel. The remainder has more diffuse disease and/or disease in the proximal gastrointestinal tract.

* *

The patient has a colonoscopy performed which is diagnostic of Crohn disease. The following year, she consults you because of an ulcer on her lower extremity. About 2 weeks prior to presentation, she noted an area of redness on her left shin. Although she initially attributed this to a banal injury, it ulcerated within the next 3 days and continues to worsen despite application of topical antibiotics. You notice a deep ulcer with undermined, violaceous borders measuring about 1.5 cm in diameter. There is an erythematous margin surrounding the lesion.

Based on these findings, which approach do you recommend?

A) Wide excision with at least 1-cm margin.
B) Debridement.
C) Intravenous antibiotics.
D) Wound culture followed by targeted antimicrobial therapy.
E) Biopsy followed by immunosuppression.

Discussion

The correct answer is E. The findings described above suggest pyoderma gangrenosum (PG), an idiopathic ulcerating skin disease that is often associated with inflammatory bowel disease. Although PG is more common in severe cases of IBD, the course usually **does not** follow the course of IBD. Controversy remains if the lesion should be biopsied as it has pathergy (worsens with trauma). This is a judgment call since PG can be confused with skin cancer. Treatment for PG is with either topical or systemic immunosuppression. Complete excision and debridement are **contraindicated** as they will only increase the ulcer size.

Which of the following is TRUE regarding the pathophysiology and history of Crohn disease?

A) Crohn is a genetic disorder, transmitted in an autosomal dominant fashion.
B) Crohn is a relapsing/remitting disease, and 30% of patients will improve spontaneously.
C) Patients with Crohn rarely progress to disease requiring surgery.
D) Maintenance therapy with glucocorticoids will reduce the rate of recurrence of Crohn.
E) Gastrointestinal fistulae and abscesses are rare complications of Crohn.

Discussion

The correct answer is B. Crohn and UC are both relapsing/remitting diseases. Up to 30% of initial exacerbations of Crohn will remit without any intervention. While there is a genetic component to IBD (up to a 100-fold increase in risk among first-degree relatives with IBD), no single, autosomal dominant gene has been identified. Answer C is incorrect because half or more of patients with Crohn will ultimately require some sort of surgery. Answer D is incorrect. Unfortunately, chronic glucocorticoid administration does not lower the rate of relapse. There are many complications of IBD (see next question), and gastrointestinal abscesses and fistulae occur with a relatively high frequency (2%–40%) in Crohn disease.

 HELPFUL TIP: Although considered a disease of young adults, there is a second peak of inflammatory bowel disease in adults >70 years.

Extraintestinal features of IBD include all of the following EXCEPT:

A) Alopecia.
B) Arthritis.
C) Sclerosing cholangitis.
D) Uveitis.
E) Cholelithiasis.

Discussion

The correct answer is A. Alopecia is not an extraintestinal manifestation of IBD. Arthritis related to IBD (enteropathic arthritis) is fairly common and usually migratory in nature, involving the large joints. Spondyloarthropathy may also be seen. Sclerosing cholangitis and autoimmune hepatitis can occur and may be fatal. Eye disease may include uveitis and episcleritis. Importantly, the main treatment for extraintestinal manifestations is to treat the IBD. IBD spondyloarthropathy and pyoderma gangrenosum are important exceptions, as these do not always improve with treatment of the underlying IBD.

 HELPFUL TIP: Toxic megacolon is a potentially deadly complication of IBD that should be suspected in a patient with IBD who presents with fever, abdominal pain, and shock. Also consider other causes of intestinal obstruction.

* *

Returning to your patient, you next see her in the ED, where she presents with fever, abdominal pain, and bloody diarrhea. She is tachycardic and slightly hypotensive but alert and oriented. You suspect a relapse of her Crohn disease.

All of the following are important aspects of her management at this time EXCEPT:

A) Surgical consultation.
B) Intravenous access and fluid administration.
C) Glucocorticoids.
D) Thalidomide.
E) Metronidazole.

Discussion

The correct answer is D. Thalidomide has been used as chronic therapy for IBD, but it is not indicated in the acute setting. The patient should be stabilized, and this includes IV access and fluid resuscitation. An exacerbation (or relapse) of IBD can be treated with glucocorticoids in the acute setting, and antibiotics are often helpful. It appears that metronidazole has beneficial effects that are not solely due to its antimicrobial properties. In this patient, who may have an abscess or obstruction, further evaluation (eg, labs, abdominal CT, etc) and surgical consultation are necessary.

Which of the following is indicated in the long-term treatment of inflammatory bowel disease?

A) Azathioprine.
B) Methotrexate.
C) 5-ASA moieties.
D) Loperamide.
E) All of the above.

Discussion

The correct answer is E. All the answer choices are indicated for the treatment inflammatory bowel disease. Of special note are the 5-ASA drugs (eg, Pentasa, Asacol). These have fewer side effects than sulfasalazine and are the initial drugs of choice for maintenance once control of symptoms has been obtained. Systemic steroids (eg, prednisone) are useful acutely to induce remission but should be tapered and stopped as soon as possible. Additional drugs for treatment of IBD include cyclosporine, 6-MP (6-mercaptopurine), infliximab, and adalimumab (just say Humira, it's much easier), among others. Antidiarrheal drugs such as loperamide are useful to control symptoms. However, be sure to avoid antidiarrheal drugs in patients who may have impending toxic megacolon.

* *

Due to cost considerations, your patient would like to try sulfasalazine.

Which of the following is an absolute contraindication to the use of sulfasalazine?

A) Sulfa allergy.
B) Aspirin allergy.
C) Anemia.
D) A and B.
E) B and C.

Discussion

The correct answer is D. Sulfasalazine contains both sulfa and salicylate moieties and therefore is contraindicated in patients with sulfa or aspirin allergy.

Which of the following is LEAST likely to be a complication of infliximab (Remicade, an anti-TNF-alpha antibody) therapy for IBD?

A) Sepsis.
B) Headache.
C) Abdominal pain.
D) Diarrhea.
E) Anemia.

Discussion

The correct answer is E. Anemia generally will improve with the treatment of IBD. Anemia in IBD is often due to a combination of iron deficiency and anemia of chronic disease, but IBD can cause an autoimmune hemolytic anemia as well. All of the rest are common—or particularly severe in the case of sepsis—complications of infliximab. In fact, ongoing infection is an absolute contraindication to the use of infliximab.

All of the following characteristics differentiate UC from Crohn disease EXCEPT:

A) The risk of colon cancer is greater in UC than in Crohn.
B) Histologically, UC appears as transmural disease, whereas Crohn involves only the mucosal and submucosal layers.
C) UC almost always involves the rectum, whereas Crohn may or may not.
D) In UC the diseased segments are continuous, whereas "skip" areas of healthy bowel are seen in Crohn.

Discussion

The correct answer is B. Histologically, UC involves only the mucosa and submucosal tissue, while Crohn is transmural. All of the other statements are true. UC involves the rectum in 95% of cases and advances proximally.

 HELPFUL TIP: Medical and surgical treatments for UC and Crohn are similar. Patients with long-standing UC with frequent relapses are candidates for colectomy.

HELPFUL TIP: IBD increases the risk of colon cancer, so more frequent and earlier colonoscopies are recommended. Recommendations vary, but most recommend colonoscopy every 1–2 years in patients with UC after 8 years with disease. Screening in those with Crohn is less well established.

 HELPFUL TIP: Indications for surgery for IBD include perforation, obstruction, massive hemorrhage, toxic megacolon, and severe and persistent disease that impairs function or quality of life. Surgical resection should be considered for intolerable extracolonic disease including arthritis and skin lesions. Ankylosing spondylitis (secondary to Crohn disease) and liver dysfunction do not respond to colectomy.

Objectives: Did you learn to . . .

- Diagnose inflammatory bowel disease?
- Differentiate Crohn disease from ulcerative colitis (UC)?
- Manage a patient with inflammatory bowel disease?
- Recognize extraintestinal manifestations and complications of inflammatory bowel disease?

CASE 7

A 52-year-old female has complaints of abdominal pain, bloating, and constipation. Her symptoms started about 5 years ago and became more bothersome within the last 6 months. She describes a dull pain in the left lower abdomen. This pain is alleviated by passing gas or having a bowel movement. The pain is generally related to eating, and she has had intermittent diarrhea and constipation with constipation predominating. Two years ago, she underwent a screening colonoscopy, which was normal. Her review of systems is notable for a weight gain of about 5 pounds within the last 3 years. She is taking only a multivitamin daily. Her physical examination is normal.

Which is the best next step?

A) Defecogram.
B) Barium enema.
C) Anorectal manometry.
D) TSH level.
E) Colonoscopy.

Discussion

The correct answer is D. The patient's presentation with pain and constipation meets criteria for constipation-predominant irritable bowel syndrome (Table 7–2). This patient underwent colonoscopy for screening 2 years prior to presentation, so further evaluation for colon cancer (answers B and E) can be delayed unless there is another indication. Secondary causes of constipation, such as hypothyroidism, medication side effects, or hypercalcemia, should be ruled out as appropriate. Therefore, a TSH level should be obtained prior to deciding on additional diagnostic or therapeutic steps. Anorectal manometry (answer C) and defecogram (answer A) are unnecessarily invasive procedures, and neither will help you to determine that this patient has irritable bowel syndrome.

* *

The patient is euthyroid. Hypercalcemia and other electrolyte abnormalities have been ruled out. Because she does not use medications other than the multivitamin, you decide to initiate treatment for irritable bowel syndrome (IBS). Based on available evidence, you suggest using fiber supplements.

What do you tell your patient to expect?

A) Complete resolution of her symptoms.
B) Increase in stool frequency and stool volume with less need for straining.
C) Increase in stool frequency but worsened abdominal pain.
D) Decrease in abdominal pain and bloating.
E) Enlightenment and absolute bliss.

Table 7–2   ROME III CRITERIA FOR IRRITABLE BOWEL SYNDROME

Continuous or recurrent abdominal pain or discomfort, at least 3 days per month in the last 3 months, with symptoms starting at least 6 months prior to diagnosis, and associated with at least 2 of the following:

- Relief with defecation
- Change in stool frequency
- Change in stool form

Adapted from Longstreth GF, et al. Functional bowel disorders. *Gastroenterology.* 2006;130:1480.

Discussion

The correct answer is B. Although there is not much evidence for its efficacy, the mainstay of therapy for IBS is fiber. Fiber supplements increase stool volume and frequency and soften stools, thereby alleviating symptoms of constipation. While bowel habits can be successfully changed with bulking agents for constipation or loperamide for diarrhea-predominant IBS, pain is generally not affected by these measures. Increased fiber intake may transiently worsen some symptoms due to fermentation and generation of gas, potentially resulting in flatulence or bloating. Answer E requires special note. Bliss and enlightenment can only occur with proper colon purging procedures provided at a very expensive resort!

 HELPFUL TIP: IBS has a relatively good prognosis, and up to 60% of patients improve on placebos in trials, making it hard to show benefit of any treatment. There is no increase in mortality, and symptoms usually improve over time.

* *

The patient returns to your office. Her constipation did indeed improve. However, she continues to have pain, unchanged in nature.

What do you suggest?

A) Docusate sodium 100 mg three times daily.
B) Hyoscyamine 0.125 mg every 6 hours as needed.
C) Nifedipine 10 mg three times daily.
D) Lorazepam 0.5 mg every 8 hours as needed.

Discussion

The correct answer is B. Despite a large number of trials on the treatment of IBS, only a few of the published studies recruited sufficiently large sample sizes to determine superiority of an intervention compared to placebo. Currently available evidence supports the use of spasmolytic agents, such as the anticholinergic hyoscyamine (Anaspz, Levbid, and others), and tricyclic antidepressants. **Both classes of drugs can exacerbate constipation, which needs to be considered in this patient.** Lorazepam and other drugs with abuse potential should be avoided.

Tegaserod (Zelnorm) has been removed from the market because of cardiovascular side effects but is available on a compassionate use protocol for women with constipation-predominant IBS who have failed other treatments. Alosetron (Lotronex) was approved for diarrhea-predominant IBS, removed from the market due to ischemic colitis, and rereleased under a protocol similar to Zelnorm.

 HELPFUL TIP: Tailor therapy to the patient. Most patients with IBS have either constipation-predominant or diarrhea-predominant disease. For diarrhea-predominant disease, try modifying the diet and using traditional antidiarrheals and anticholinergics.

 HELPFUL TIP: Some patients with constipation-predominant IBS will respond to oral SSRI medications such as fluoxetine or paroxetine which seem to increase bowel transit times.

Objectives: Did you learn to . . .

- Evaluate a patient with constipation?
- Diagnose and manage irritable bowel syndrome (IBS)?

CASE 9

A 32-year-old male has complaints of fatigue and episodic abdominal pain. His pain is located in the periumbilical region and the left lower quadrant. It is cramp-like in nature and is associated with flatulence and diarrhea. Passing gas alleviates his symptoms. He notes that milk and other dairy products worsen his symptoms. His weight has remained stable. His prior medical history, family and social history and physical examination are unremarkable. Laboratory tests reveal hemoglobin of 11.5 g/dL and a normal blood glucose and TSH.

What is the most appropriate next step in your evaluation?

A) Lactose breath test.
B) Dietary trial of strict lactose avoidance.
C) Enteroclysis.
D) Colonoscopy.
E) Tissue transglutaminase antibody titer.

Discussion

The correct answer is B. The patient's symptoms are consistent with lactose intolerance. He may have malabsorption secondary to lactose intolerance which may be partially responsible for his anemia. If his symptoms resolve with a trial of a lactose-free diet, you have your diagnosis. Further follow-up should include rechecking his CBC and perhaps other studies, such as stool for occult blood, to evaluate the anemia. If these symptoms are new, he could have a secondary form of lactase deficiency (eg, Crohn disease or bacterial overgrowth) or a coincidental problem with the absorption of this carbohydrate.

* *

The patient tries a lactose-free diet but this is of no benefit and his abdominal cramping and diarrhea continue. You are considering additional diagnoses now.

Which of the following is UNLIKELY in this patient?

A) Bacterial overgrowth syndrome.
B) Gluten-sensitive enteropathy.
C) *Giardia lamblia*.
D) *Clostridium difficile*.
E) Whipple disease.

Discussion

The correct answer is E. It is unlikely that this patient has Whipple disease, which is a result of an infection with *Tropheryma whippelii*. Whipple disease is associated with nondeforming arthritis, weight loss, fever, diarrhea, etc. All of the other answer choices are possibilities in this patient. Bacterial overgrowth syndrome (answer A) presents with bloating, diarrhea, dyspepsia, and possible malabsorption and weight loss. It can occur as a result of bowel dysmotility, chronic pancreatitis, etc. Gluten-sensitive enteropathy (nontropical or celiac sprue) (answer B) presents with similar symptoms including malabsorption. *Giardia* infection (answer C) can be chronic and presents with gas, diarrhea, and occasionally constipation. *Clostridium difficile* infection (pseudomembranous colitis) (answer D) can also be chronic in nature with chronic diarrhea and blood loss.

* *

You continue to work up this patient's diarrhea with stool cultures, stool for *C. difficile* toxin, direct immunofluorescence analysis for *Giardia* and *Cryptosporidium*, and 3 stools for ova and parasites. All of the studies are negative. You now turn your attention to possible bacterial overgrowth syndrome.

The best test(s) for bacterial overgrowth syndrome is (are):

A) Quantitative stool culture.
B) Stool leukocytes.
C) 72-hour fecal fat.
D) [14-C] D-xylose breath test.
E) B and D.

Discussion

The correct answer is D. The D-xylose breath test takes advantage of the fact that the bacteria responsible for bacterial overgrowth syndrome (Gram-negative aerobes) catabolize D-xylose. The breath test measures radioactive CO_2 that is formed as a result of bacterial breakdown of radioactive D-xylose. The glucose breath test, in which glucose is administered to the patient and breath hydrogen is measured, is also helpful and commonly used. However, it is less sensitive and specific than the D-xylose test and has a 30%–40% false-negative rate. Workup of bacterial overgrowth syndrome should also include an upper GI endoscopy and possible small bowel biopsy. GI hypomotility, small bowel dilatation or small bowel diverticula support the diagnosis of bacterial overgrowth syndrome. Stool culture (answer A) will not help diagnose bacterial overgrowth. Stool leukocytes (answer B) are not useful in general and do not have a good correlation with infectious causes of diarrhea (high false-positive and false-negative rates). Fecal fat collection (answer C), is useful in documenting fat malabsorption syndromes, including those secondary to severe pancreatic insufficiency (eg, cystic fibrosis with >90% pancreatic dysfunction) and short bowel syndrome.

 HELPFUL TIP: An option to diagnose bacterial overgrowth is empiric treatment for 7–10 days with medications to cover aerobes and anaerobes (cephalexin plus metronidazole, TMP/SMX plus metronidazole, amoxicillin/clavulanate). Definitive treatment may require surgical intervention to shorten the bowel, resect diverticula, etc.

* *

This patient's D-xylose test is negative and you consider the possibility of gluten-sensitive enteropathy (celiac disease).

The BEST test for the diagnosis of gluten-sensitive enteropathy is:

A) Antiendomysial antibodies.
B) Tissue transglutaminase antibodies.
C) Antigliadin antibodies.
D) Radiolabeled wheat flour absorption test.
E) None of the above.

Discussion

The correct answer is B. Tissue transglutaminase antibodies are sensitive and specific for severe gluten-sensitive enteropathy but may be falsely negative in mild-to-moderate cases. Antiendomysial IgA antibodies (answer A) are also relatively sensitive and very specific for gluten-sensitive enteropathy. The definitive test (gold standard) is a small bowel biopsy and should be considered if your clinical is suspicion is high and the patient has negative antibodies. Patients with positive antibodies should also have and endoscopy; the diagnosis should be confirmed by endoscopy and biopsy before committing the patient to a gluten-free diet for life.

 HELPFUL TIP: Up to 1:200 whites living in the United States may be affected with gluten-sensitive enteropathy.

* *

The results of the patient's tissue transglutaminase test are positive. You educate him about gluten-sensitive enteropathy (celiac disease) and have an endoscopy performed. A small bowel biopsy demonstrats blunted villi with a significant increase in intraepithelial lymphocytes, consistent with gluten-sensitive enteropathy. With a gluten-free diet, the patient experiences a significant increase in his energy level. Two years later he comes for a routine visit. He has gradually reintroduced some wheat products into his diet and tolerates this very well.

What do you recommend?

A) Resume gluten-free diet.
B) Continue dietary challenge and repeat examination in 6 months.
C) Repeat small bowel biopsy.
D) Check tissue transglutaminase antibody titer.
E) Avoid wheat, but try barley or rye products.

Discussion

The correct answer is A. Although there are no data on the benefit of a long-term gluten-free diet in patients who can tolerate small amounts of gluten, two factors argue for continuing a gluten-free diet. First, many patients will have subclinical nutrient deficiencies if they reintroduce gluten. Patients with gluten sensitive enteropathy should be screened for osteoporosis and take a multivitamin. Second, there is some data that patients who reintroduce gluten show an increase in mortality from GI lymphoma despite tolerance of the gluten. This is especially true in pediatric patients where deficiencies may lead to stunted growth.

 HELPFUL TIP: With a gluten-free diet, antibodies (tissue transglutaminase, antigliadin, antiendomysial) often return to normal levels.

 HELPFUL TIP: Patients with gluten-sensitive enteropathy must be compulsive about their diet. Rice, corn, and soybean-based flours are safe to consume. Oats are often contaminated with wheat.

Objectives: Did you learn to ...

- Evaluate a patient with diarrhea?
- Recognize clinical manifestations of gluten-sensitive enteropathy?
- Manage a patient with gluten-sensitive enteropathy?

CASE 10

A 22-year-old previously healthy male reports a 3-day history of explosive and watery diarrhea. He is having up to 6 bowel movements per day. He recalls eating at a new Mexican restaurant 5 days ago. His head sinks a little low as he recalls drinking a "fishbowl-sized" margarita—or **thinks** he remembers drinking it! He denies fever, blood in his stool, or recent travel. Other people ate the same food but he is the only one who is sick. His vital signs are normal (including supine and standing blood pressures), and the remainder of the physical exam is remarkable only for mild, diffuse abdominal tenderness.

What is the most likely diagnosis?

A) Celiac sprue.
B) Viral gastroenteritis.
C) Lactose intolerance.
D) Small bowel bacterial overgrowth.
E) *Clostridium difficile* colitis.

Discussion

The correct answer is B. This is always a dilemma. It can be difficult to differentiate acute gastroenteritis from food poisoning. What makes gastroenteritis more likely is that there is no clustering of cases among people who ate the same food. With only 3 days of symptoms, answers A, C, and D would be premature. Without recent antibiotic exposure, answer E would be unlikely in an otherwise healthy male.

 HELPFUL TIP: Acute diarrhea is increased frequency or decreased consistency of stool lasting less than 3 weeks. In textbooks, diarrhea is often approached by pathophysiologic mechanism: secretory, inflammatory (exudative), osmotic, and disordered motility. In practice this approach is not as useful as considering causes. Table 7–3 lists causes of acute and chronic diarrhea.

Table 7–3 DIFFERENTIAL DIAGNOSIS FOR DIARRHEA

Acute diarrhea
- Bacteria (eg, *Campylobacter, Salmonella, Clostridium*)
- Viruses (eg, Norwalk, rotavirus)
- Parasites (eg, *Giardia*)
- Protozoa (especially in HIV)
- Medications
- Anything that causes chronic diarrhea

Chronic diarrhea
- Inflammatory (eg, IBD, radiation enteritis)
- Osmotic (eg, gluten-sensitive enteropathy, lactase deficiency)
- Secretory (eg, Zollinger-Ellison syndrome, villous adenoma)
- Disordered motility (eg, irritable bowel syndrome, overflow from fecal impaction)

What is the MOST appropriate diagnostic or therapeutic step to perform now?

A) Order a CBC.
B) Order electrolytes.
C) Order stool examination for ova and parasites.
D) Recommend hydration and antidiarrheals as needed.
E) Order an abdominal film.

Discussion

The correct answer is D. No workup is needed for a mild case of acute diarrhea, because such cases are usually self-limited. Generally, the history and physical exam should provide the diagnosis and indicate need for further workup. Further workup and treatment is indicated if the patient has severe or bloody diarrhea, dehydration, systemic toxicity, or severe pain.

* *

You treat the patient with oral rehydration and prochlorperazine for some nausea and he does well. He returns to see you a few weeks later after a trip to Mexico. He liked that fishbowl-sized margarita so much he decided to go for an original (remember that we live in a college town . . . . this could easily be true!). He has diarrhea that began a couple of days after his arrival in Cancun and has now been present for 5 days. He has had frequent, watery diarrhea with nausea but no vomiting. He has noticed no blood in the stool. He was very careful to avoid salads and water but did have some ice in a soft drink.

The most likely organism in this patient is:

A) *Salmonella*.
B) *Shigella*.
C) Enterotoxigenic *E. coli*.
D) Enterohemorrhagic *E. coli*.
E) *Campylobacter*.

Discussion

The correct answer is C. Entero**toxigenic** *E. coli* is the most common cause of traveler's diarrhea in patients traveling to Mexico. Entero**hemorrhagic** *E. coli* (answer D) is less likely and should be associated with bloody diarrhea. The other answer choices are much less likely to be causes of traveler's diarrhea.

In which of the following organisms is antibiotics CONTRAINDICATED?

A) *Campylobacter*.
B) *Shigella*.

C) *Clostridium difficile.*
D) *E. coli* subtype O157:H7 (enterohemorrhagic *E. coli*)

Discussion

The correct answer is D. The use of antibiotics in patients with shiga toxin producing *E. coli* (*E. coli* subtype O157:H7 and others, the enterohemorrhagic *E. coli*) may increase the risk of developing hemolytic uremic syndrome. The use of antibiotics is indicated in *Campylobacter*, and *Clostridium*. For *Clostridium difficile*, metronidazole is the drug of choice with vancomycin a more expensive alternative that should be reserved for unresponsive disease. **Fluoroquinolones are no longer recommended as first-line treatment in travelers' diarrhea from South East Asia because of resistance. The current CDC recommendation is azithromycin.**

HELPFUL TIP: Many physicians would not treat a patient with *Shigella* unless that patient is clinically ill (eg, fever). Treatment with antibiotics is **relatively** contraindicated in *Salmonella* because it prolongs the carrier state. Use your judgment of the clinical scenario in treatment of the patient who is particularly ill.

HELPFUL TIP: The above recommendations are for immunocompetent adults. In those who are immunosuppressed (eg, HIV), are frail or have coexisting disease, more liberal criteria for treatment can be used.

Which of the following is (are) appropriate for the treatment of this patient's traveler's diarrhea (remember, he has no vomiting)?

A) Oral rehydration.
B) Antidiarrheals.
C) Eat any food (eg, no need for a bland diet with slow advancement).
D) All of the above.
E) None of the above.

Discussion

The correct answer is D. This patient has nonbloody diarrhea and no systemic signs, so it should be safe to treat him with antidiarrheal agents (eg, loperamide) (answer B) and avoid antibiotics. Oral rehydration (answer A) is the rule unless a patient is too nauseated or has some other reason that he cannot take adequate fluids by mouth. Patients (including children) should eat anything they can tolerate (answer C). The concept of "gut rest" is passé and leads to increased bowel permeability and more persistent diarrhea. **Lactose deserves special note.** The American Academy of Pediatrics has changed their recommendations about lactose in diarrhea. They recommend withholding lactose **only** in children <3 months. This seems to be the age group in which transient lactase deficiency occurs.

HELPFUL TIP: *Klebsiella oxytoca* can produce an antibiotic-related diarrhea that is indistinguishable from *Clostridium difficile*. In those with a negative stool for *Clostridium* antigen, consider: (1) false-negative test (some of the newer strains of *Clostridium* are not detected by traditional stool antigen) or (2) *Klebsiella oxytoca* or (3) the *C. difficile* toxin degenerates rapidly at room temperature (no toxin may be detectable after 2 hours of exposure to room temperatures) or (4) ELISA tests generally only test for Type A antigen. The patient may have an antigen Type B-producing strain **or** there may be a mutation of antigen Type A.

Objectives: Did you learn to . . .

- Evaluate a patient with acute diarrhea?
- Treat acute diarrhea?
- Recognize different causes of diarrhea?

CASE 11

A 49-year-old male comes to your office requesting testing for hepatitis C. He recently attended his 25-year college reunion where he heard from a mutual acquaintance that an old friend was seriously ill with cirrhosis due to hepatitis C. The patient became very concerned because he had partied with this friend during a brief period of experimentation with injection drugs while in college. The patient is otherwise healthy and denies any symptoms except for occasional fatigue after a long day at work. Physical examination of the patient is unremarkable. There are no stigmata of chronic liver disease.

Which of the following is the most appropriate course of action?

A) Check a quantitative HCV PCR ("viral load").
B) Order a recombinant immunoblot assay (RIBA).
C) Order HCV antibody test (enzyme immunoassay).
D) Order a qualitative HCV PCR.
E) Order ALT and AST.

Discussion

The correct answer is C. The sensitivity and specificity of the present-day HCV antibody test are excellent; thus, this is the best test to perform in this situation. Rarely, patients with immunologic impairment, such as HIV infection, have HCV viremia without detectable antibody, but this would not be a concern in this otherwise healthy patient. Quantitative HCV PCR (answer A) is not a reliable means for diagnosing HCV infection because currently used methods are insensitive at low levels of viremia; thus, infection cannot be ruled out if the level of HCV viremia is below the lower limit of detection of the test. The RIBA (answer B) was developed as a confirmatory test at a time when the specificity of first-line antibody tests was suboptimal. Because of the improved specificity of present-day antibody testing, the RIBA is now rarely used. **Qualitative** HCV PCR (answer D) is the most sensitive test for the presence of HCV RNA, with a limit of detection that is lower than that of quantitative PCR. It is useful to establish the presence of viremia, but is more expensive than antibody testing and thus not a first-line test. Many patients with chronic HCV infection have normal liver enzymes and can still have progressive disease; therefore, in a high-risk patient, ALT and AST (answer E) are not appropriate for screening for HCV.

* *

The patient returns several weeks later to discuss his test results. His HCV antibody test is positive. A liver panel obtained that day shows an ALT of 48 IU/L (normal range, 0–20) and an AST of 39 IU/L (0–31). His albumin and total bilirubin are within normal limits. He is extremely anxious about his liver.

To determine the degree of liver disease, your next step is to:

A) Obtain a liver-spleen scan to assess for evidence of cirrhosis.
B) Reassure the patient that his mild liver test abnormalities rule out cirrhosis.

C) Refer for percutaneous liver biopsy.
D) Order abdominal ultrasound with Doppler to assess for evidence of cirrhosis.
E) Obtain abdominal CT to assess for evidence of cirrhosis.

Discussion

The correct answer is C. Having established that the patient has hepatitis C with elevated liver enzymes, the next step is to determine the severity of his liver disease. Although his liver function tests are reassuring, it does not exclude the possibility of advanced fibrosis or even well-compensated cirrhosis. Although the argument has been made that not all patients with chronic hepatitis C require liver biopsy, it is the only direct means to evaluate the extent of liver injury. You would not be incorrect to order imaging (answer D) in addition to the liver biopsy.

* *

The patient agrees to a liver biopsy, which is scheduled for the following week. Nonetheless, he is still very concerned about his situation and asks what you think the chances are that he already has cirrhosis.

With regard to the development of progressive liver disease in hepatitis C, all of the following are true EXCEPT:

A) Approximately 20% of patients with chronic HCV infection will develop serious liver disease.
B) Heavy alcohol use is a risk factor for development of serious liver disease.
C) Acquisition of HCV infection after the age of 40 years is associated with increased risk of developing serious liver disease.
D) HCV genotype impacts on the probability of developing end-stage liver disease.
E) Males are more likely than females to develop serious liver disease.

Discussion

The correct answer is D. Although a minority of persons infected with HCV develop serious liver disease, the likelihood of progression is difficult to predict in an individual patient. Nonetheless, male gender, heavy alcohol use, and acquisition of HCV infection after age 40 years are associated with increased risk of progressive liver disease; however, genotype is not.

HELPFUL TIP: Patients who have a persistently normal ALT, acquire hepatitis C <35 years, are female, do not drink alcohol, and have minimal or no fibrosis on liver biopsy are unlikely to progress to end-stage liver disease.

* *

The patient is concerned that he may transmit the virus to his wife or children. They are tested and are found to be negative for HCV antibody. He is relieved but asks for advice to prevent infecting them. You counsel him on the transmission of HCV.

All of the following are true statements about transmission of HCV EXCEPT:

A) No change in sexual practices is recommended for couples in a long-term monogamous relationship in which one partner is HCV+ and the other HCV–.

B) The use of condoms is recommended for couples in a long-term monogamous relationship in which one partner is HCV+ and the other HCV–.

C) Hepatitis C is not spread by hugging, sneezing, or sharing a drinking glass.

D) Household members of persons infected with HCV should not share items that might be contaminated with small amounts of blood such as razors or nail clippers.

E) Parenteral exposure to infected blood is a major route of transmission of HCV.

Discussion

The correct answer is B. HCV is spread by parenteral contact with infected blood. In contrast to hepatitis B, sexual transmission of HCV is inefficient and appears to be a minor route of spread. Additionally, the efficacy of latex condoms in preventing disease is not known. **The NIH and the USPHS do not recommend condom use for patients in a stable, long-term, and monogamous relationship. That said, using condoms will likely reduce an already low risk even further.**

* *

The patient's liver biopsy shows mild-moderate inflammatory activity and portal and periportal fibrosis (stage 2). He is relieved to find out that he does not have cirrhosis, but remains very concerned about his hepatitis and wants to do everything possible to "get rid of" the hepatitis C. He asks about treatment for his HCV.

You tell him which of the following?

A) Combination therapy with interferon and ribavirin results in sustained virologic responses (SVR) in 40%–70% of patients treated.

B) Combination therapy with interferon and ribavirin can cause numerous side effects including cytopenias, flu-like symptoms, worsening of autoimmune conditions, depression, and hemolytic anemia.

C) The HCV genotype is a strong predictor of response to treatment.

D) All of the above.

Discussion

The correct answer is D. Combination therapy with interferon and ribavirin is the standard treatment of HCV. The HCV genotype is a major factor determining the likelihood of achieving sustained virological response (SVR)—**although not the likelihood of progression to end-stage liver disease.** Genotype 1 (including 1a and 1b) is the most difficult to clear, while genotypes 2 and 3 are the most responsive to treatment. Stage of fibrosis is also a factor, with patients with stages 3 and 4 (bridging fibrosis and cirrhosis) being less likely to achieve SVR. Higher baseline viral levels also tend to predict poorer response to treatment. Combination therapy is expensive and is associated with significant toxicities. The major concerns with ribavirin are hemolytic anemia and teratogenicity, while the interferons (standard or the long-acting pegylated forms) have a long list of potential side effects, of which neuropsychiatric problems, such as depression and irritability, are often the most troublesome.

Objectives: Did you learn to . . .

- Evaluate a patient at risk for hepatitis C?
- Understand the natural history of the disease process in hepatitis C?
- Describe the transmission of hepatitis C?
- Discuss treatment issues for a patient with hepatitis C?

CASE 12

A 24-year-old female comes to your office with the complaint of fatigue for the past month. Despite getting 8–9 hours of sleep each night, she becomes easily fatigued and often has to push herself to get through her work. She has also had a poor appetite and has lost about 3 pounds over this period. She reports that she was told that she had hepatitis when she was about

10 years old but does not recall what type. She is otherwise healthy and takes no medications. The patient is a graduate student from China. She is single and uses neither tobacco nor alcohol. She has no history or percutaneous exposures or blood transfusion. Her grandfather died of liver cancer.

Physical examination reveals a thin, tired-appearing woman. The liver edge is palpable 2 cm below the right costal margin and is slightly tender. There are no ascites, splenomegaly, or cutaneous stigmata of chronic liver disease.

Laboratory studies are remarkable for mild anemia (hemoglobin 9.1 g/dL). Liver tests reveal elevated aminotransferases (ALT 289 IU/L, AST 158 IU/L), albumin 3.2 g/dL, total bilirubin 1.5 mg/dL (normal 0.2–1.0 mg/dL).

Diagnostic possibilities include:

A) Hepatitis A.
B) Hepatitis B.
C) Hepatitis C.
D) Autoimmune hepatitis.
E) All of the above.

Discussion

The correct answer is E. Constitutional symptoms such as fatigue and anorexia can be seen with any form of acute or chronic liver disease; thus, they are not helpful in establishing a differential diagnosis. The first priority is to rule out infectious hepatitis including hepatitis A, B, and acute hepatitis C. Autoimmune hepatitis deserves consideration, particularly in female patients. Although HCV infection is a world-wide problem, HBV infection is endemic in Asia and Africa, and the possibility of chronic hepatitis B also warrants special attention in this patient.

Appropriate laboratory studies at this point include which of the following?

A) Quantitative HCV PCR.
B) HB$_s$Ag (hepatitis B surface antigen).
C) Anti-hepatitis A antibodies (IgG and IgM).
D) B and C.
E) All of the above.

The correct answer is D. The quantitative HCV PCR is not a useful test for diagnosing HCV infection. HCV antibody testing would be a better choice. If the HCV antibody test and the rest of the evaluation are negative, **acute** HCV infection might be considered. In that case, a qualitative HCV PCR would be useful on the assumption that the patient has not been infected long enough to have a detectable HCV antibody. Both HB$_s$Ag and anti-HAV are useful tests in this patient. HB$_s$Ag is helpful to assess for HBV infection (acute and chronic) and anti-HAV antibodies will rule out acute hepatitis A infection. A positive total anti-HAV (positive IgG) with a negative IgM would indicate past infection, while a positive IgM would suggest acute HAV infection. Table 7–4 interprets the HBV antigens (Ag) and antibodies (Ab).

* *

The patient's results show a positive HB$_s$Ag, positive total anti-HAV with no IgM detected, and negative anti-HCV antibody. You phone her to discuss these results, but her roommate tells you that the patient had to return to China unexpectedly because her mother had become ill.

Four months later, she returns for a follow-up visit. She tells you that she took an herbal medicine while she was back in China and has been feeling much better recently. Her HB$_s$Ag remains positive, but her liver

Table 7–4   HEPATITIS B VIRAL SEROLOGIES FOR DIFFERENT PHASES OF INFECTION

Antigen/Antibody	Acute	Chronic	Recovered	Vaccinated/Immune
HB$_s$Ag	+	+	–	–
HB$_e$Ag	+	+	–	–
Anti-HBsAb	–	–	+	+
Anti-HB$_c$Ab	+ (IgM)	+ (IgG)	+ (IgG)	–
Anti-HB$_e$Ab	–	+/–	+	–
HBV DNA	+	+/–	+/–	–

KEY: HBs = surface antigen or antibody, HB$_c$ = core antigen or antibody, HB$_e$ = "e" antigen or antibody; Ag = antigen; Ab = antibody.

enzymes, albumin, and total bilirubin are now completely normal.

Appropriate actions at this time include:

A) Treatment with interferon-alpha 5 million units daily for 16 weeks.
B) Order hepatitis B_e antigen, anti-HB_e, and HBV DNA level.
C) Begin periodic screening for hepatocellular carcinoma with ultrasound and alpha-fetoprotein (AFP).
D) A and C
E) B and C

Discussion

The correct answer is E. The hepatitis B_e antigen reflects viral replication. Loss of HB_eAg (with or without conversion to anti-HB_e antibody positivity) indicates decreased viral replication and less of a risk of progression to cirrhosis. Loss of HB_eAg may occur spontaneously; it is also the therapeutic endpoint of antiviral treatments for HBV infection (interferon, lamivudine, adefovir). If she is negative for HB_eAg and is anti-HB_e antibody positive (anti-HB_e^+) or has low or undetectable levels of HBV DNA, she has a low level of viral replication and will not benefit further from antiviral treatment.

Her liver panel should be monitored periodically, as should the AFP and ultrasound. Even asymptomatic HBV carriers with minimal liver disease are at risk for hepatocellular carcinoma and screening recommended in chronic HBV carriers (men >40 years, women >50 years, in those with a family history of HCC, in cirrhotic patients, and in those of African ancestry >20 years). Your patient has a positive family history of HCC.

* *

The patient returns to discuss the results of her tests. Laboratory results show that she is negative for HB_eAg and is anti-HB_e positive. Her HBV DNA is undetectable using an unamplified assay. AFP is within limits and abdominal ultrasound is unremarkable. She continues to feel well. She tells you that she will be getting married in 2 months. She asks you what can be done to prevent her fiancé and future children from becoming infected with HBV.

All of the following are accurate responses to her question EXCEPT:

A) No special precautions need to be taken because she has undetectable HBV and is therefore not infectious.
B) If her fiancé has not been immunized against HBV, he should be tested and vaccinated if not immune.
C) If her fiancé is not immune to HBV, they should use barrier contraceptives (eg, condoms) until he has completed his HBV vaccination series.
D) She should cover any open cuts or scratches with a bandage and clean up any blood spills with bleach.
E) Administration of hepatitis B immune globulin (HBIG) and HBV vaccination begun immediately after birth is 95% effective in preventing perinatal transmission of HBV.

Discussion

The correct answer is A. Although patients with higher levels of HBV DNA are more infectious than those with lower levels of viral DNA, the risk of transmission in the latter case is not zero. In the case of this patient, undetectable HBV DNA indicates a level of HBV DNA that falls below the limit of detection of an unamplified assay (on the order of 10^5 copies/mL). Precautions should be taken to prevent sexual or household transmission to her fiancé (use of condoms, immunization if required, etc) and to her future children (HBIG and HBV vaccination).

Objectives: Did you learn to . . .

- Generate a differential diagnosis for patients with abnormal liver enzymes?
- Identify patients at risk for hepatitis B?
- Use the various hepatitis B antigens and antibodies to determine a patient's infection status?
- Describe the route of transmission of hepatitis B?

 QUICK QUIZ: HEPATITIS C

All of the following are significant side effects of interferon therapy for hepatitis C EXCEPT:

A) Depression.
B) Hypoglycemia.
C) Aggression and homicidal behavior.
D) Myalgias.
E) Leukopenia.

Discussion

The correct answer is B. Interferon therapy is fraught with adverse effects including those listed above. Flu-like symptoms of myalgias, malaise, fever, chills, headache, and weight loss are particularly common.

CASE 13

A 73-year-old male comes to your office with complaints of abdominal and ankle swelling, decreased energy, and poor appetite for the past 2 months. He dates the onset of his symptoms to a reaction to penicillin given for dental work. He claims the antibiotic made him sick with nausea and malaise. He took it only for a few days, but the symptoms have persisted and worsened since that time. He says that before taking the penicillin, he was in excellent health, walked 3 miles per day, and helped his neighbors with their yard work. Now he is too weak and tired to care even for his own yard.

His past medical history is remarkable for coronary artery bypass surgery done 6 yrs ago. He also recalls having "yellow jaundice" (as opposed to the purple kind) when he was stationed in Korea. He has no significant family history. He drank a bit on the weekends when he was in the service but has drunk very little alcohol in the past 50 years. He also quit smoking about 50 years ago. His medications are aspirin 81 mg daily and ibuprofen 600 mg as needed for knee pain caused by degenerative joint disease.

Diagnostic considerations suggested by the history should include which of the following?

A) Adverse drug reaction to penicillin.
B) Malignancy.
C) Cirrhosis.
D) Congestive heart failure.
E) All of the above.

Discussion

The correct answer is E. The patient's history of abdominal and lower extremity swelling suggests fluid overload. Penicillin is known to cause interstitial nephritis and secondary nephrotic syndrome which can lead to fluid retention. Sources of fluid overload besides the kidneys should be considered in this patient, including liver and heart disease. Intra-abdominal malignancies, specifically with liver involvement, can cause ascites. He is on an NSAID which can cause fluid retention although rarely to this degree.

Physical examination reveals a fragile-appearing elderly man with temporal wasting. The jugular venous pressure is not elevated. The lungs are clear to auscultation. The heart sounds are regular, with no murmurs or gallops. The abdomen is protuberant with bulging flanks. Shifting dullness is present. The liver edge is palpable about 1 cm below the right costal margin and is nontender. The spleen is not palpable. There is 2+ ankle edema bilaterally and scattered telangiectasias on skin exam. He has no asterixis.

Which of the following findings would you expect on laboratory exam?

A) Elevated hemoglobin and hematocrit (17.5 gm/dL and 55%).
B) Decreased platelet count of 80,000/mm^3.
C) Elevated serum albumin.
D) BUN/Cr ratio of <20.
E) All of the above.

Discussion

The correct answer is B. This patient likely has portal hypertension given his ascites and stigmata of liver disease (spider angiomata/telangiectasias). Blood is shifted towards the spleen because of the increased portal pressure (the blood, like the rest of us, likes the path of least resistance). This shifting of blood to the spleen leads to the spleen removing platelets and thrombocytopenia.

* *

Diagnostic paracentesis is performed and approximately 50 mL of clear light yellow fluid are obtained.

Appropriate laboratory studies on the ascitic fluid include which of the following?

A) pH.
B) Gram stain.
C) Albumin.
D) Lactate.
E) Triglycerides.

Discussion

The correct answer is C. The ascitic fluid albumin is needed to calculate the serum-ascites albumin gradient (SAAG), which is helpful to distinguish between ascites resulting from portal hypertension from ascites due to other causes. Lactate and pH have been proposed as markers for spontaneous bacterial peritonitis but have proven to be unreliable. The yield of Gram stain in diagnosing spontaneous bacterial peritonitis is very low because bacteria counts are rarely high enough to allow detection by this method. Consequently, a cell count showing ≥250 polymorphonuclear leukocytes/mm³ is presumptive evidence of spontaneous bacterial peritonitis. Measurement of triglycerides is useful to confirm chylous ascites; however, in the absence of grossly milky-appearing fluid, there is no need to perform this test.

 HELPFUL TIP: In addition to total protein and albumin, all ascitic fluid should be sent for cell count and cultures. Other studies should be ordered as indicated.

* *

Ascitic fluid total protein is 2.5 g/dL with an albumin of 1.9 g/dL. A liver panel reveals normal aminotransferases, normal bilirubin, serum albumin 3.3 g/dL and alkaline phosphatase 147 IU/L. Electrolytes, BUN, and creatinine are within normal limits.

Which of the following is the most accurate interpretation of these results?

A) The serum-ascites albumin gradient is 1.7, which is consistent with portal hypertension as its cause.
B) The serum-ascites albumin gradient is 1.7, which rules out portal hypertension as its cause.
C) The serum-ascites albumin gradient is 1.4, which is consistent with portal hypertension as its cause.
D) The serum-ascites albumin gradient is 1.4, which rules out portal hypertension as its cause.

Discussion
The correct answer is C. In the past, ascitic fluid was classified as a transudate or an exudate using a total protein concentration of >2.5–3 g/dL as a cutoff. In contrast to pleural effusions, this categorization was not helpful in determining the etiology of the ascites, since many cases of portal hypertension (which is expected to cause "transudative" ascites) produce ascitic fluid total protein levels that are in the "exudative" range. Thus, the serum-ascites albumin gradient (SAAG) was developed, which has better diagnostic accuracy. The SAAG is the difference between the serum albumin and the ascitic fluid albumin, or 3.3–1.9 = 1.4. **A SAAG of ≥1.1 indicates portal hypertension with 97% accuracy.** Remember this by associating high SAAG with high pressure in the portal system.

 HELPFUL TIP: Ascites from any cause of portal hypertension will have a high SAAG. Portal hypertension is most commonly caused by cirrhosis, which in turn can be caused by many diseases. Aside from cirrhosis, portal hypertension also may result from schistosomiasis, sarcoidosis, portal vein thrombosis (Budd-Chiari syndrome), congenital hepatic fibrosis, CHF, myxedema, etc. Causes of a low SAAG include: serositis from connective tissue disorders, nephrotic syndrome, pancreatic-related ascites, and peritoneal carcinomatosis among others.

In addition to a complete evaluation to determine the cause of his portal hypertension, which of the following is (are) are appropriate action(s) now?

A) Refer the patient to a nutritionist for instruction on a 2-g sodium diet.
B) Discontinue ibuprofen and prescribe a COX-2 selective inhibitor for arthritis.
C) Prescribe spironolactone 100 mg daily and furosemide 40 mg daily.
D) A and C.
E) A, B, and C.

Discussion
The correct answer is D. The initial approach to the management of ascites caused by portal hypertension is sodium restriction and diuretics. Sodium restriction is difficult for most patients, and counseling by a nutritionist (answer A) may improve compliance. The majority of patients will **not** have an adequate response to sodium restriction alone, so begin diuretics at the outset. Spironolactone, an aldosterone antagonist, (answer C) is useful because portal hypertension is a state of hyperaldosteronism. Spironolactone tends to cause hyperkalemia, an effect that can be mitigated by the coadministration of furosemide. Once-daily doses are appropriate for initial therapy; adjustments are made based on the patient's electrolytes, renal function, and response to treatment. NSAIDs should be avoided, due to sodium retention. **COX-2 selective inhibitors have no advantage over nonselective NSAIDs in this regard.** Other approaches to the patient's knee pain should be considered, including intraarticular injections, acetaminophen (up to 2 g daily is likely safe in cirrhosis) and narcotics, provided encephalopathy is not a problem.

* *

A few months later, your patient comes to the ED "feeling sick." He complains of diffuse abdominal pain and swelling, stating that his abdomen feels tense. On examination, you find a pale, uncomfortable male with a temperature of 38.3°C. The remainder of his vital signs are normal. His abdomen is tense and distended. Again, you note shifting dullness. His abdomen is diffusely tender and his bowel sounds are hypoactive. You perform a paracentesis which shows 400 polymorphonuclear leukocytes/mm³.

What is the most appropriate next step in the evaluation and treatment of this patient?

A) Discharge to home with increased doses of spironolactone and furosemide.
B) Discharge to home with amoxicillin and the same doses of diuretics.
C) Perform a large-volume paracentesis for symptomatic relief and discharge to home.
D) Admit to the hospital and start IV ceftriaxone.
E) Admit to the hospital and place a peritoneal tube for drainage.

Discussion

The correct answer is D. This patient meets criteria for spontaneous bacterial peritonitis (≥250 polymorphonuclear leukocytes/mm³ in the ascites fluid) and has clinical findings to suggest infection. This patient could become unstable quickly, so discharge from the ED is not recommended. Increasing doses of diuretics and/or large-volume paracentesis may be required, but these interventions should be considered only in the setting of hospital admission. Broad-spectrum antibiotics are the standard of care for spontaneous bacterial peritonitis, and intravenous third-generation cephalosporins are typically the first-line agents in hospitalized patients. Fluoroquinolones have been used to decrease the frequency of spontaneous bacterial peritonitis episodes. Amoxicillin (answer B) is not sufficient. **Albumin dose of 1.5 g/kg on day 1 followed by 1 g/kg on day 3 reduces the chance of renal failure and death and should be given to all patients with SBP.**

Send the ascites for cell count and culture culture. Blood cultures, CBC, and serum chemistries should be obtained as well. Consider imaging the abdomen with ultrasound or CT. Further tests should be ordered as indicated.

 HELPFUL TIP: The most common organisms in spontaneous bacterial peritonitis include *Streptococcus pneumoniae*, *Escherichia coli*, and *Klebsiella*.

Objectives: Did you learn to . . .

• Generate a differential diagnosis for ascites?
• Analyze ascitic fluid to determine potential causes of ascites?
• Initiate treatment for a patient with ascites?
• Diagnose and manage spontaneous bacterial peritonitis?

CASE 14

A 42-year-old male with known hepatitis C who is also a heavy drinker presents to your office because of increasing confusion. He hasn't noticed much of anything (hey, most of his life has been like this . . .), but his family has noticed that he is somewhat confused and on occasion difficult to wake up. He has a known history of end-stage liver disease. He is supposed to be on a low-protein diet but decided that it was time to go on a low-carbohydrate diet to "lose that gut" (he even found himself a "low carb" beer). So, he has increased his intake of protein.

Which of the following is NOT a common cause of hepatic encephalopathy?

A) GI bleeding.
B) Constipation.
C) High-carbohydrate diet.
D) Up-regulation of GABA receptors.

Discussion

The correct answer is C. High-carbohydrate diets are not associated with hepatic encephalopathy. Alternatively, high-protein diets are associated with hepatic encephalopathy as is up-regulation of GABA receptors in the CNS (answer D). Similarly, a GI bleed (answer A) delivers a large protein load to the GI tract. **A patient with hepatic encephalopathy should be evaluated for a GI bleed.** Other causes of acute hepatic encephalopathy include constipation (answer B), sedative use (eg, benzodiazepines), hypokalemic metabolic alkalosis, etc.

HELPFUL TIP: An elevated ammonia level is associated with hepatic encephalopathy although there is not a direct linear correlation between serum ammonia level and mental status.

* *

You decide to admit the patient to the hospital for treatment of his hepatic encephalopathy.

Which of the following is NOT part of the treatment of hepatic encephalopathy secondary to alcohol use?

A) Lactulose.
B) Polyethylene glycol (eg, GoLYTELY, MiraLax).
C) Oral antibiotics.
D) Fluid and electrolyte management.

Discussion

The correct answer is B. Polyethylene glycol plays no role in the treatment of hepatic encephalopathy. Although it makes intuitive sense that it would work since lactulose works, this is not the case. The mechanism of action of lactulose is dependent on bacterial metabolism of lactulose into lactic and acetic acids. This reduces the pH of the colon leading to precipitation of nonabsorbable ammonia in the colon which reduces serum ammonia levels. Enemas (soap suds, etc), may help acutely by removing colonic contents. Answer C is of particular note. Oral antibiotics (neomycin, metronidazole, and others) should be reserved for patients who do not respond to lactulose. Their efficacy is more limited.

* *

The patient does well on the regimen of lactulose and oral metronidazole.

What other problems do you need to worry about in this patient?

A) Elevated PTT.
B) Elevated PT/INR.
C) Thrombocytopenia.
D) A and B.
E) All of the above.

Discussion

The correct answer is E. Patients with end-stage liver disease tend to have a lack of vitamin K-dependent clotting factors (and thus elevated PT and PTT) and have thrombocytopenia due to shunting of blood from the liver to the splanchnic bed because of elevated portal pressures.

* *

It turns out that this patient has also been drinking again, but he made it through his hospital stay without going through withdrawal. He is ready to discharge from the hospital.

Which of the following is (are) indicated for this patient at the time of discharge, if is hemodynamically stable?

A) Nadolol.
B) Isosorbide dinitrate.
C) Pentoxifylline.
D) Oral vitamin K.
E) All of the above.

Discussion

The correct answer is E. All of the answer choices are indicated in the further treatment of this patient. Nadol (answer A) and isorbide dinitrate (answer B) will reduce portal pressures and reduce the risk of variceal bleeding. Pentoxifylline (answer C) has antitumor necrosis factor activity and a decrease in mortality when used acutely (in the first 4 weeks after an event of alcoholic hepatitis). Vitamin K (answer E) is indicated because of liver failure-induced coagulopathy.

* *

The patient does relatively well and abstains from alcohol. In addition to the medications noted above, you have the patient on spironolactone and furosemide and a low-salt diet to reduce edema and ascites. He seems to be following your instructions but returns to the clinic because of increasing dyspnea, abdominal distention, and pain. On exam, he has no peritoneal signs but obviously has massive ascites. You are considering a large-volume paracentesis in your office.

Which of the following statements best reflects the current thinking on large-volume paracentesis?

A) Patients who have more than 4 L of fluid removed should receive IV albumin.
B) There is no consistent data with regards to the use of albumin in large-volume paracentesis.
C) Under no circumstance should more than 5 L of ascites be removed at one time.
D) Given this patient's dyspnea, large-volume paracentesis is contraindicated.
E) None of the above is true.

Discussion

The correct answer is B. It is unclear who needs albumin replacement. Answer A is incorrect. There is clearly no need for albumin in patients who have less than 5 L of fluid removed. However, for patients who have more than 5 L of fluid removed, the standard of care is replacement with albumin although the data are limited. Answer C is incorrect. In some studies, up to 10 L of ascitic fluid has been removed (don't try this one at home . . .). Answer D is incorrect. Respiratory compromise is one reason to do a large-volume paracentesis. Removal of fluid will help with diaphragmatic excursion and may help with the resolution of pleural effusions.

* *

You perform a large-volume paracentesis, and the patient feels better. In the meantime, he has had a variceal bleed and has been hospitalized yet again. He needs something else done, and you refer him for a transjugular intrahepatic portosystemic shunt (TIPS) procedure to help reduce portal pressures, prevent the re-accumulation of ascites, and hopefully prevent further bleeding.

Which of the following statements best reflects the status of TIPS?

A) TIPS is ineffective in controlling acute variceal bleeding.
B) TIPS unequivocally improves survival from end-stage liver disease.
C) TIPS is associated with an increased risk of hepatic encephalopathy.
D) Once placed, TIPS remains effective for at least 3 years.
E) None of the above is true.

Discussion

The correct answer is C. TIPS is clearly associated with an increased risk of hepatic encephalopathy. Answer A is incorrect. TIPS is **effective** in controlling variceal bleeding. Answer B is incorrect. There may be some survival **disadvantage** to TIPS. However, the data is equivocal. Answer D is incorrect because TIPS shunts tend to clot and may need to be evaluated for patency by Doppler if ascites reaccumulates or other symptoms occur.

 HELPFUL TIP: Over-diuresis can lead to hepatorenal syndrome which is characterized by increasing BUN and creatinine and oliguria. Sepsis, GI bleeding, etc can also lead to hepatorenal syndrome.

Objectives: Did you learn to . . .

- Recognize causes of hepatic encephalopathy and identify patients at risk?
- Manage a patient with hepatic encephalopathy?
- Discuss risks and benefits of TIPS and large-volume paracentesis?

 QUICK QUIZ: AUTOIMMUNE LIVER DISEASE

Which of the following is a marker for primary biliary cirrhosis?

A) Antimitochondrial antibodies.
B) Anti-smooth muscle antibodies.
C) Alpha-1 antitrypsinase.
D) Polyclonal antibodies on serum protein electrophoresis.

Discussion

The correct answer is A. Antimitochondrial antibodies (AMA) are found in primary biliary cirrhosis (95% sensitive and 98% specific). Anti–smooth-muscle antibodies (answer B) are found in autoimmune hepatitis. **Reduced levels** of alpha-1 antitrypsinase (answer C) are found in hepatitis from alpha-1 antitrypsin deficiency (surprise!). Polyclonal antibodies (answer D) are found in autoimmune hepatitis.

 HELPFUL TIP: The diagnosis of sclerosing cholangitis is made by cholangiography with strictures and dilatation of intrahepatic and/or extrahepatic ducts.

CASE 15

A 31-year-old male comes to your office for evaluation of "abnormal liver tests." He changed jobs 2 months ago and, as part of his evaluation for disability insurance, a panel of blood work was done. He shows you a lab report with elevated total bilirubin (2.1 mg/dL) with normal direct bilirubin. The AST, ALT, GGT, albumin, and alkaline phosphatase are normal. A CBC obtained at that time was unremarkable.

The patient feels generally well. When you ask about jaundice, he recalls that when he was sick with the flu while in college, his roommate told him that he "looked a little yellow." He went to the student health service a few days later when he felt better and was told there was nothing to be concerned about. The patient's past medical history is otherwise unremarkable. He drinks 6–8 beers/week and takes ibuprofen once or twice a month for knee pain.

Physical examination is unremarkable. A repeat liver panel shows a total bilirubin of 1.7 mg/dL with normal direct bilirubin and normal AST, ALT, and alkaline phosphatase. CBC and reticulocyte count are also normal. A blood smear, LDH, and haptoglobin are normal.

The most likely diagnosis is:

A) Crigler-Najjar syndrome type I.
B) Choledocholithiasis.
C) Gilbert syndrome.
D) Hemolytic anemia.
E) Occult acetaminophen abuse.

Discussion

The correct answer is C. Gilbert syndrome is the most common inherited disorder of bilirubin metabolism, affecting up to 5% of whites. It is characterized by isolated mild unconjugated hyperbilirubinemia, with serum bilirubin levels usually <3 mg/dL. However, bilirubin levels in patients affected with Gilbert syndrome can increase with fasting or during febrile illnesses, though rarely exceeding 6 mg/dL. Crigler-Najjar syndrome type I (answer A) is a rare disorder leading to severe unconjugated neonatal jaundice and neurologic impairment due to kernicterus. Both choledocholithiasis (answer B) and acetaminophen hepatotoxicity (answer E) would be unlikely to cause an isolated increase in unconjugated bilirubin; the LFTs should be elevated with these. The normal blood smear, reticulocyte count, normal LDH, and normal haptoglobin make significant hemolysis (answer D) unlikely. Therefore, this presentation is most consistent with Gilbert syndrome.

The most appropriate next step is:

A) Recommend genetic testing for mutations in uridine diphosphoglucuronate glucuronosyltransferase 1A.
B) Recommend family screening.
C) Abdominal ultrasound.
D) Reassurance.
E) Liver biopsy.

Discussion

The correct answer is D. Persistent elevations in unconjugated bilirubin with normal liver enzymes and lack of evidence for hemolysis are sufficient to make a diagnosis of Gilbert syndrome, and more sophisticated tests are not required. It is worthwhile to counsel patients about this to avoid unnecessary genetic testing (answer A) of family members, but there is no need for screening (answer B) for this benign condition. Gilbert syndrome is not a cause of liver disease; thus, ultrasound (answer C) and biopsy (answer E) are not indicated.

* *

Several months later, the patient's older sister comes to see you. She had gone to a local health fair where screening laboratory tests were done. She received notification that her liver tests were abnormal and that she should see a doctor about this. She recalled her brother mentioning something about a familial problem causing liver test abnormalities and wonders if this is the same thing her brother has.

The patient is 39 years old. Her general health is good, although she wishes she could lose weight. She says she has been 30–40 pounds overweight for at least 10 years and is now at her heaviest weight ever. She relates that both of her maternal grandparents were overweight and diabetic, as is her mother. She is not taking any medications except for a multivitamin daily. She drinks no alcohol and is a nonsmoker, and she denies any risk factors for viral hepatitis.

Physical examination reveals an obese woman. Blood pressure is 138/88; BMI is 35 kg/m². There is no scleral icterus or other cutaneous stigmata of chronic liver disease. The examination of the heart and lungs is unremarkable. The abdomen is protuberant. The liver edge is palpable about 3–4 cm below the right costal margin and is slightly tender to palpation. There is no splenomegaly and no evident ascites.

Her liver panel from the health fair 3 months ago shows the following: ALT 87 IU/L (normal range, 0–20), AST 53 IU/L (0–31), alkaline phosphatase 110 IU/L (30–115), total protein 7.8 g/dL (6.0–8.0), albumin 4.2 g/dL (3.3-5.0), total bilirubin 0.9 mg/dL (0.2–1.0), direct bilirubin 0.1 mg/dL (<0.2).

Appropriate steps at this time include all of the following EXCEPT:

A) Repeat the liver panel.
B) Counsel the patient that her labs suggest Gilbert syndrome.
C) Counsel the patient that her labs suggest some type of problem other than Gilbert syndrome.
D) Recommend a serologic evaluation to assess for chronic viral and autoimmune hepatitis if the liver test abnormalities persist.

Discussion

The correct answer is B. Gilbert syndrome is defined by isolated unconjugated hyperbilirubinemia. This patient's pattern of liver test abnormalities with aminotransferase elevations clearly indicates a different type of problem. If these abnormalities persist, an evaluation for causes of chronic aminotransferase elevations is warranted. Chronic viral hepatitis and autoimmune hepatitis would be among the diagnostic considerations. As evidenced by the apparent hepatomegaly and tenderness on physical examination, an imaging study of the liver is indicated.

* *

The repeat liver panel is remarkable for ALT 129 IU/L, AST 76 IU/L. The other tests are normal. HB$_s$Ag and HCV antibody are negative. Antinuclear and anti–smooth-muscle antibodies are <1:40 (normal). The ultrasound examination shows an enlarged liver with increased echogenicity, suggestive of diffuse fatty infiltration.

Regarding nonalcoholic fatty liver disease, all of the following are true EXCEPT:

A) It is frequently associated with one or more features of the metabolic or insulin resistance syndrome.
B) It is more common in men than women.
C) The histologic features can closely mimic those of alcoholic hepatitis.
D) It may cause cirrhosis in a minority of patients.
E) There is no therapy that has been proven to be effective.

Discussion

The correct answer is B. Nonalcoholic fatty liver disease (NAFLD) is more common in women and is among the most common causes of elevated liver enzymes. NAFLD refers to a spectrum of histologic findings that range from simple steatosis to an aggressive injury pattern that may include hepatocyte ballooning, inflammation, Mallory bodies, and fibrosis. These latter findings are also characteristic of alcoholic liver disease; thus, it is important to obtain an accurate alcohol history in patients in whom they are present. NAFLD often occurs in association with obesity, dyslipidemia and/or glucose intolerance, hypothyroidism and occurs more commonly in women than men. Although most patients with NAFLD will not develop progressive liver disease, a minority are at risk to develop cirrhosis. Female gender and the presence of diabetes increase the risk of progression to cirrhosis. Although a variety of medications have been evaluated, none has been clearly shown to be beneficial.

All of the following are appropriate actions EXCEPT:

A) Obtain a fasting lipid panel.
B) Obtain fasting serum glucose.
C) Recommend a very–low-calorie diet (300 kcal/day) with a goal of reducing her BMI to the normal range.
D) Consider obtaining a liver biopsy.

Discussion

The correct answer is C. There is no proven benefit to weight loss in NAFLD. However, weight loss and addressing underlying metabolic illnesses (diabetes, hypothyroidism) is a good idea. Modest weight loss may be sufficient to improve liver enzymes even if the patient does not attain ideal body weight. Rapid weight loss may be counterproductive in the setting of NAFLD, as mobilization of peripheral fat stores may worsen hepatic steatosis. The role of liver biopsy (answer D) remains controversial in patients with risk factors and imaging studies consistent with NAFLD and a negative evaluation for other potential causes of chronic liver enzyme abnormalities. Although the biopsy is useful to confirm the diagnosis and provide information regarding the severity of the injury, it is unlikely to alter management. Many hepatologists recommend that biopsy be deferred for 6–12 months, pending a trial of lifestyle modification.

 HELPFUL TIP: Limited data suggests metformin is useful in NAFLD. It is worth a try. Statins have also been used with some success as have the "glitazones." Remember that the glitazones may cause CHF and other cardiac events.

Objectives: Did you learn to . . .

• Evaluate a patient with abnormal liver tests?
• Recognize the clinical and laboratory presentation of Gilbert syndrome?
• Describe findings of NAFLD?
• Manage a patient with "benign" liver disease?

QUICK QUIZ: GI BLEED

Which of the following has shown a decrease in mortality from variceal GI bleeding?

A) Vasopressin.
B) Somatostatin/octreotide.
C) Band ligation of varices.
D) TIPS.
E) C and D.

Discussion

The correct answer is E. TIPS and ligation of varices via an endoscope show a decrease in mortality. Although medical treatment may benefit the patient by reducing bleeding, there is no evidence that vasopressin (answer A) or somatostatin (answer B) decrease mortality. Vasopressin may show an increase in mortality because of associated GI ischemia. Somatostatin reduces rebleeding but does not affect mortality.

CASE 16

A 70-year-old female presents to the ED with the complaint of midepigastric pain associated with vomiting. It started approximately 12 hours ago and now she notes vomiting, fever, and myalgias. Her vital signs are blood pressure 110/70, pulse 115, and temperature 38.5°C. On exam the patient is quite tender in the midepigastric region with guarding and some rebound. Her past history is significant for lone atrial fibrillation and a seizure disorder for which she is taking phenytoin.

Your next steps in the diagnosis of this patient should include all of the following EXCEPT:

A) Chest radiograph.
B) CBC.
C) Liver enzymes.
D) Abdominal CT with contrast.
E) Amylase.

Discussion

The correct answer is D. An abdominal CT is not indicated in this patient as part of the initial workup. An upright chest radiograph (answer A), is the best plain radiograph for finding free abdominal air and is indicated for this reason. Additionally, the etiology of abdominal pain may also include pneumonia and other thoracic pathology that may be evident on a chest radiograph. Liver enzymes (answer C), amylase (answer E), and CBC (answer B) are indicated since midepigastric pain with fever can be related to pancreatitis, acute cholecystitis, etc.

* *

The laboratory results are as follows: elevated AST and ALT (mild), normal amylase, mildly elevated WBC count (13.5×10^3 cells/mm^3), elevated GGT.

The accurate interpretation of these results is:

A) The patient does not have pancreatitis.
B) The elevated GGT is specific for biliary outlet obstruction.
C) The elevated AST and ALT may indicate biliary outlet obstruction.
D) None of the above.

Discussion

The correct answer is C. Early in the course of biliary outlet obstruction (eg, biliary colic, common duct stone), the AST and ALT may be mildly elevated. Answer A is incorrect because the amylase is only 80% sensitive for pancreatitis. Twenty percent of patients with pancreatitis have a normal amylase—a false-negative test. Answer B is incorrect because GGT is nonspecific. GGT is an inducible enzyme and can be elevated in response to alcohol and various medications including phenytoin.

 HELPFUL TIP: In alcohol-related liver disease, the AST is generally 2× the ALT.

* *

The patient has a history of atrial fibrillation and is not on anticoagulation (because she has "lone atrial fibrillation" as defined by the new criteria; see Chapter 2, Cardiology). You are concerned that there may be bowel ischemia caused by an embolism.

Which of the following is true of mesenteric thrombosis and bowel ischemia?

A) Patients generally have guarding and rebound early in the course.
B) The pain is out of proportion to the exam and patients may have a normal initial exam.
C) A serum lactate level is helpful and specific for the diagnosis of bowel ischemia.
D) The best study to diagnose this disease entity is CT with contrast.

Discussion

The correct answer is B. Patients with small bowel ischemia from either embolism or mesenteric thrombosis will generally present with severe abdominal pain and an exam that is unremarkable. Late in the course there will be guarding, rebound, and other peritoneal signs as the bowel perforates. Early in the course of the illness, severe pain with a relatively benign exam is consistent with the presentation of bowel ischemia. Answer A is incorrect for the reasons stated above. Answer C is incorrect because the serum lactate can be elevated in a number of states, not just bowel ischemia. Abdominal pain plus lactic acidosis should raise the suspicion that there may be bowel ischemia. Answer D is incorrect because radiographic findings on CT scan are present in approximately 65% of patients with mesenteric thrombosis/embolism. The **best** study remains angiography.

* *

Since the patient's exam includes guarding and rebound you put the diagnosis of bowel ischemia lower in your list of possibilities. Based on the elevated WBC count and elevated ALT and AST, you order an ultrasound of the right upper quadrant which shows evidence of a common duct stone. There is thickening of the gallbladder wall but no pericolic fluid noted. You decide that there is a mild cholecystitis and want to admit the patient to the hospital. This patient needs to be started on antibiotics.

Which antibiotic is the most appropriate choice for this patient?

A) IV clindamycin.
B) IV vancomycin.
C) IV gentamicin.
D) IV ampicillin/sulbactam.

Discussion

The correct answer is D. The most appropriate antibiotic for this patient is ampicillin/sulbactam (Unasyn). The main organisms that need to be covered are Gram-negative organisms and anaerobes (*E. coli, Enterococcus, Klebsiella,* and *Enterobacter*). Ampicillin/sulbactam will cover all of these organisms. Answer A is incorrect because clindamycin, although it covers Gram-positive organisms and anaerobes, does not cover most Gram-negative organisms. Additionally, many enterococci are resistant. Answer B is incorrect because vancomycin covers only Gram-positive organisms.

Answer C is incorrect because gentamicin does not cover anaerobic organisms. Other antibiotic options for treating this patient include cefotetan and cefoxitin.

* *

The patient is admitted to the hospital. She is treated with ampicillin/sulbactam and pain medication.

The next step for this patient is:

A) Percutaneous T-tube placement to drain the gallbladder.
B) 2 weeks of IV antibiotics followed by cholecystectomy.
C) ERCP with sphincterotomy.
D) Lithotripsy.

Discussion

The correct answer is C. The patient should have an endoscopic retrograde cholangiopancreatography (ERCP) with sphincterotomy in an attempt to retrieve the stone in her common bile duct. Answer A is incorrect because in this healthy patient, percutaneous drainage would be a third-line procedure. Answer B is incorrect because the patient has a closed abscess (the gallbladder blocked by a stone) which requires drainage. If the patient had cholecystitis **without** obstruction, prolonged antibiotics followed by cholecystectomy would be an option. **In patients with cholecystitis without obstruction outcomes are overall better with an early cholecystectomy.** Answer D is incorrect and would be a less desirable approach than is ERCP with sphincterotomy.

 HELPFUL TIP: Studies have demonstrated improved outcome in patients with severe gallstone pancreatitis and/or cholangitis that receive early (within 72 hours after admission) ERCP with biliary sphincterotomy.

* *

The ERCP is successful but the patient develops worsening pain in the midepigastric region.

Which of the following is the most common adverse consequence of ERCP?

A) Pancreatitis.
B) Contrast allergy.
C) Perforation.
D) Bleeding.

Discussion

The correct answer is A. Of the complications listed, pancreatitis is the most common, with an incidence of approximately 5% of patients after ERCP. Elevations in pancreatic enzymes (mostly not significant) occur in up to 75% of patients post-ERCP. The less common complications in order of descending incidence are: bleeding, perforation, sepsis, contrast allergy (rare).

* *

Although you suspect that this patient has pancreatitis secondary to the ERCP, you consider other potential causes of pancreatitis.

All of the following are causes of pancreatitis EXCEPT:

A) Viral infection.
B) HMG-CoA reductase inhibitors (eg, atorvastatin).
C) Alcohol.
D) Indinavir.
E) Spider bites.

Discussion

The correct answer is E. The venom of a scorpion bite can result in pancreatitis, but spider bites are not known to do so. The most common causes of acute pancreatitis are ethanol ingestion, biliary tract disease, and endoscopic procedures with biliary tract disease which is the most common cause in the United States. Answer A is true. Common viruses that can cause pancreatitis include HIV, hepatitis viruses, EBV, and Coxsackie viruses. Answers B and D are true. Many drugs can cause pancreatitis: of note are didanosine (DDI), some diuretics, some NSAIDs, some antibiotics (Table 7–5).

* *

You check laboratory studies and the patient does indeed have worsening pancreatitis from the ERCP. The surgeon on the case recommends against using morphine and would rather use meperidine in this patient.

All of the following are true statements EXCEPT:

A) There is no evidence that meperidine is superior to morphine even in gallbladder and pancreatic disease.
B) Meperidine is more likely than morphine to cause seizures in this patient.
C) Meperidine is more likely than morphine to cause confusion and agitation in elderly patients.
D) When used in combination with an SSRI, morphine is more likely to cause a serotonin syndrome than is meperidine.

Table 7–5   DRUGS ASSOCIATED WITH PANCREATITIS

Drugs with Definite Association	Drugs with Probable Association
Thiazide diuretics	Acetaminophen
Sulfonamides	Salicylates
Azathioprine/ 6-Mercaptopurine	Metronidazole
Furosemide	Nitrofurantoin
Estrogens	Erythromycin
Tetracycline	NSAIDs
Valproic acid	ACE inhibitors
Pentamidine	Methyldopa
Valproic acid	Steroids
Dideoxyinosine	

Discussion

The correct answer is D. Meperidine (and tramadol) may cause a serotonin syndrome when combined with an SSRI. This is not a problem with morphine. The rest of the answer choices are true statements. There is no evidence to support the tradition that meperidine is superior to morphine in biliary or pancreatic disease (answer A). Meperidine is metabolized into normeperidine which can cause agitation and seizures (answers B and C). In general, then, morphine is a much cleaner drug than meperidine to use for pain management.

* *

You have the patient's pain managed well with morphine.

Which of the following treatments is ROUTINELY indicated in pancreatitis?

A) NG tube with intermittent suction.
B) H$_2$-blockers (eg, cimetidine) or PPIs (eg, lansoprazole).
C) IV antibiotics.
D) NPO order.

Discussion

The correct answer is D. The routine treatment of pancreatitis includes making the patient NPO, IV fluids, and pain management. Answer A is incorrect because there is no indication for an NG tube in the patient who is not vomiting. Answer B is incorrect because H$_2$-blockers or PPIs do not change the outcome in pancreatitis. Answer C is incorrect unless there is evidence of infection (eg, fever) or necrotizing pancreatitis.

 HELPFUL TIP: Prophylactic antibiotics should be used in patients with necrotic pancreatitis. Antibiotics are not helpful in patients with simple pancreatitis.

* *

You make the patient NPO. However, over the 2 days, the patient's condition worsens. She begins to vomit and has increased pain as well as tachycardia and fever. The patient wants to know what her chances of surviving this bout of pancreatitis are.

All of the following are part of Ranson criteria EXCEPT:

A) Age.
B) WBC on admission.
C) Hematocrit at 72 hours.
D) Glucose on admission.

Discussion

The correct answer is C. The hematocrit at **48 hours** is one of the Ranson criteria. The criteria are listed in Table 7–6.

 HELPFUL TIP: The Ranson criteria are neither sensitive nor specific for severe pancreatic disease and cannot be completed before 48 hours of hospitalization. The Apache II score accounts for blood pressure, oxygenation, temperature, respiratory rate, creatinine, GCS, etc, and is a better predictor of survival. A HCT of 44% or greater at admission and failure to decrease at 24 hours is also an excellent predictor of necrotizing pancreatitis and multi-organ failure.

* *

The patient developed a fever and vomiting, so you begin IV antibiotics and place an NG tube. Since the patient is vomiting and it appears that it will be a protracted course, the patient will need nutrition.

The BEST way of providing nutrition for this patient is:

Table 7–6 RANSON CRITERIA

On admission	• Age >55 years • WBC >16,000 • Glucose >200 • LDH >350 • AST >250
At 48 hours	• Hematocrit reduction by >10% • Bun increase of >5 • Calcium <8 • Po_2 <60 • Base deficit >4 • Fluid sequestration of >6 liters

Mild pancreatitis is defined by presence of 1-3 Ranson criteria; mortality increases with the presence of 4 or more.

A) Feeding via the NG tube.
B) Central Venous Nutrition (CVN, TPN).
C) Clear liquid diet.
D) Peripheral nutrition with 10% dextrose and lipids.

Discussion

The correct answer is B. Nutrition is critical for inpatients because of increased metabolic demand. The best choice for this patient is CVN. Answer A is incorrect because you want to avoid food in the stomach. Answer C is incorrect for the same reason. Answer D is better than giving enteric feeding but will not provide amino acids, vitamins, or enough calories.

 HELPFUL TIP: **Enteral nutrition is preferred over CVN for pancreatitis** as long as the feeding is done below the ligament of Treitz. Jejunal feeding does not stimulate pancreatic enzymes and is associated with fewer complications than is CVN.

Which of the following is NOT a complication of CVN?

A) Infection.
B) Cholestasis.
C) Hypoglycemia.
D) Ileus.

Discussion

The correct answer is D. Infection, cholestasis, and hypoglycemia can all be a result of CVN. Hypoglycemia generally occurs when stopping CVN because of increased levels of circulating insulin. This can be mitigated by tapering CVN or administering IV dextrose.

* *

Since the patient has continued to do poorly, you order a CT scan of the abdomen which shows evidence of a pseudocyst.

Which of the following is NOT true about a pancreatic pseudocyst?

A) Pseudocysts occur in 10% of patients with pancreatitis.
B) Pseudocysts can be drained by forming a fistula with the stomach endoscopically.
C) Pseudocysts can lead to the formation of arterial pseudoaneurysms which can cause severe bleeding.
D) Open drainage is the preferred method of treatment.
E) Not all pseudocysts require drainage.

Discussion

The correct answer is D. The formation of a fistula with the stomach using an endoscope is the preferred method of drainage. The one major contraindication to endoscopic treatment is a pseudoaneurysm. Injury to an artery can cause significant bleeding which is difficult to control.

 HELPFUL TIP: CT scan can be used to look for a pseudoaneurysm before endoscopic drainage. An aneurysm should be suspected in these circumstances: evidence of an upper GI bleed, a drop in the hematocrit, or a sudden expansion of the pseudocyst.

Objectives: Did you learn to . . .

• Recognize and diagnose mesenteric thrombosis?
• Identify causes of acute pancreatitis?
• Diagnose and manage a patient with acute pancreatitis?
• Manage the complications of pancreatitis?
• Use parenteral nutrition in a hospitalized patient?
• Describe the principles of narcotic choice in parenteral pain management?

 QUICK QUIZ: GALLSTONES

A 40-year-old female presents to you with gallstones found on a "full body CT scan" performed at Live4Ever Imaging Technologies, Inc. She is anxious that she will become sick like her sister who had emergent cholecystectomy for her gallstone pancreatitis. She asks you if she should have her gallbladder removed. She is asymptomatic and her liver enzymes are normal.

Which of the following should you recommend?

A) Laparoscopic cholecystectomy because of family history of severe gallstone pancreatitis.
B) Ultrasound to confirm gallstones and to check for common bile duct stones.
C) No treatment or follow-up is needed unless she develops symptoms.
D) ERCP with sphincterotomy to allow stones to pass without obstructing common bile duct or compressing pancreatic duct.
E) Recheck liver enzymes and if elevated recommend cholecystectomy.

Discussion

The correct answer is C. Asymptomatic gallstones do not need special attention since 70%–80% remain asymptomatic. Only 2%–3% of patients will present with acute cholecystitis or other complications and therefore prophylactic cholecystectomy is not indicated. American Indians have high risk of stone-associated gallbladder cancer and are an exception to this rule. Diabetics or sickle-cell disease patients have higher risk of complications from gallstones but still should not have the gallbladder removed if asymptomatic. Family history of complication from gallstones is not an indication for prophylactic cholecystectomy.

CASE 17

A 58-year-old female with type 2 diabetes mellitus presents to your clinic with complaints of nausea, vague epigastric abdominal pain, bloating, early satiety, and intermittent vomiting for 3 weeks. Her past medical history is significant for hypertension and hyperlipidemia, and her diabetes is complicated by retinopathy and neuropathy. She is on metformin and glyburide for her diabetes, lisinopril for her hypertension, and simvastatin for hyperlipidemia. She takes a daily aspirin as well. She is afebrile and not ill-appearing on exam. She has mild epigastric tenderness without rebound or guarding. Bowel sounds are normal and there is no abdominal distention. Labs show normal CBC and differential count, and HbA1c is 9.4%. Her weight is 95 kg and was 90 kg 1 year ago. You suspect diabetic gastroparesis.

Which statement is FALSE for diagnosis of gastroparesis?

A) On scintigraphy (gastric emptying study) >50% of the standard meal present in the stomach at 2 hours suggests gastroparesis.

B) On scintigraphy >10% of the standard meal at present in the stomach at 4 hours suggests gastroparesis.

C) EGD looking for evidence of food after an uncontrolled restaurant meal is a good test for diagnosing gastroparesis.

D) Gastroparesis can be diagnosed by exhaled radiolabeled CO_2 measurement.

Discussion

The correct answer is C. Looking for retained gastric contents at an unspecified time after an unspecified ingestion is **not** the way to diagnose gastroparesis. The most widely used test for diagnosing gastroparesis is radionucleotide scan. The patient is given standardized meal containing 99 m technetium sulfur colloid in low-fat eggs, and nuclear activity is measured at 2 hours and 4 hours. If radioactivity in the stomach is >50% at 2 hours or >10% at 4 hours, the patient is considered to have delayed gastric emptying. You can do a liquid phase gastric emptying study if you suspect dumping syndrome, but it is not necessary to evaluate for gastroparesis. Radiolabeled CO_2 breath test (answer D) correlates well with nuclear scintigraphy (answers A and B) and is easier to perform in the community setting. However, a radiolabeled CO_2 breath test requires normal small bowel, pancreas, liver, and lung function.

* *

You order a radionucleotide gastric emptying study, and it shows that 75% of the meal was present in the stomach at 2 hours and 20% at 4 hours. You diagnose gastroparesis.

The best long-term treatment option for the patient is:

A) Cisapride.

B) Domperidone.

C) Erythromycin.

D) Metoclopramide.

E) Improved glucose control.

Discussion

The correct answer is E. The treatment of diabetic gastroparesis is often difficult and frustrating for patients and clinicians. Although not proven in prospective trials, most experts believe improved glucose control with dietary and lifestyle modification is the key to long-term success in diabetic gastroparesis. All of the above-listed medications (answers A–D) have shown benefit in the short term to reduce symptoms associated with diabetic gastroparesis. Cisapride was removed from the market in the United States because of prolongation of the QT interval. Domperidone is not available in the United States but is used in other countries for gastroparesis. Erythromycin and metoclopramide are effective and available. However, both can cause cramps, and erythromycin can cause nausea while metoclopramide may cause tardive dyskinesia or dystonia. Other macrolides are not effective.

* *

You add insulin to the diabetic regimen in an attempt to tighten glucose control and prescribe metoclopramide 5 mg 30 minutes before meals.

In addition to this you recommend all of the following dietary and lifestyle modifications EXCEPT:

A) Increase dietary fiber.

B) Change from 4 large to 6 small meals daily.

C) Moderate exercise.

D) Decrease dietary fat.

E) ADA 1800 kcal diet.

Discussion

The correct answer is A. In patients with gastroparesis, fiber and raw vegetables can form gastric bezoars (phytobezoar) which are commonly seen on endoscopy. Bezoars cause early satiety and bloating and add to the symptom burden of gastroparesis. If a bezoar is found, it can be dissolved using cellulase (Kanalase) or N-acetylcysteine orally. More frequent, smaller meals help with symptoms, and moderate exercise can be helpful but excessive exercise may slow gastric emptying. Your patient is gaining weight, so it is important to reinforce the ADA diet. Fat slows gastric emptying; therefore, dietary fat should be reduced to less than 40 g/day.

Which of the following medications can exacerbate preexisting gastroparesis?

A) Fluoxetine.

B) Oxycodone.

C) Angiotensin-converting enzyme inhibitors.

D) Metformin.

E) Insulin.

Discussion

The correct answer is B. Oxycodone and all narcotics reduce GI motility and are rarely tolerated by patients with gastroparesis. This can be clinically challenging, and attention to the cause of pain and alternative management options should be explored. Fluoxetine does not have significant effects on gastric motility, but tricyclic antidepressants and other drugs with anticholinergic activity do and are not good options for pain syndromes in gastroparesis. ACE inhibitors do not affect GI motility. Although metformin is associated with GI side effects, it does not affect GI motility. Insulin has no adverse effect on GI motility. Other medications that reduce gastric emptying are dopaminergic agents, antiadrenergic antihypertensives, calcium channel blockers, and anticholinergic agents. All drugs known to affect gastric motility should be stopped prior to obtaining a gastric emptying study.

 HELPFUL TIP: The last resort in severe, unremitting gastroparesis with weight loss and brittle diabetic control can be to place percutaneous endoscopic jejunostomy. The patient is then placed on jejunal feedings temporarily while diabetic control and nutritional balance is regained (if possible).

Objectives: Did you learn to . . .

- Diagnose gastroparesis?
- Identify medications that can exacerbate gastroparesis?
- Manage gastroparesis?

 QUICK QUIZ: GI BLEED

You admit a 65-year-old female with end-stage renal disease on hemodialysis because of recurrent episodes of melena requiring transfusions. She is anemic with low ferritin, iron, and iron saturation. The gastroenterologist performs an upper and lower endoscopy without any bleeding source found. A capsule enteroscopy shows multiple small angiodysplasias throughout the small bowel, without any large, endoscopically treatable lesions.

Your patient is discharged after a blood transfusion. Her hemoglobin is 11 g/dL. At follow-up 1 month later, her hemoglobin is 9 g/dL. The patient is on maximum doses of erythropoietin with dialysis and is still having guaiac-positive stools. She refuses to take oral iron because of constipation.

Which of the following is the best next step in management of this patient?

A) Prescribe iron dextran or sucrose IV with dialysis to maintain her iron stores.
B) Try to prevail upon the gastroenterologist to repeat endoscopy and treat any angiodysplasia lesions that can be reached.
C) Prescribe octreotide.
D) Order a Meckel scan.
E) Prescribe estrogen-progesterone.

Discussion

The correct answer is A. This is an appropriate situation for the administration of iron IV. It is safer than blood transfusions and can be given on an outpatient basis during hemodialysis. There are rare occurrences of anaphylaxis with iron dextran, and a test dose should be given. Some reports suggest iron sucrose is safer. Repeat endoscopies (answer B) with treatments of angiodysplasias may help but should be adjunctive therapy to maintenance of iron stores. The scope only reaches the proximal jejunum and the patient has lesions throughout the small bowel. Octreotide (answer C) has been reported in case series to have a beneficial effect, but no randomized trials have been performed and it cannot be recommended at this time. A Meckel scan (answer D) would be redundant as another cause has been found and the patient does not fit the age group. Hormone replacement therapies (answer E) initially seemed effective at reducing bleeding from angiodysplasia but randomized trials failed to show benefit.

 HELPFUL TIP: Angiodysplasias are commonly missed and are associated with age, end-stage renal disease, aortic stenosis and hereditary telangiectasias (autosomal dominant) and are more likely to bleed in patients on long-term anticoagulation and antiplatelet therapies. Other commonly missed lesions include Cameron lesions (small ulcers caused by rubbing of hiatal hernia sac against diaphragm) and peptic ulcer disease.

HELPFUL TIP: Capsule endoscopy of the small bowel using a small camera can be helpful if a small-bowel follow-through does not show a source of bleeding. Other possibilities include tagged red blood cell scan and angiography which are only really useful in overt bleeding. The tagged RBC scan needs 0.1 mL/min bleeding rate and angiography requires 0.5 mL/min bleeding rate to detect bleeding sites.

QUICK QUIZ: GI BLEED

A 30-year-old female presents to your clinic with complaint of intermittent blood on toilet paper for 3 years. She says she always has been constipated and takes polyethylene glycol (Miralax) on regular basis. She has no family history of colorectal cancer and is asymptomatic and has no weight loss. On exam, she does not appear anemic and abdominal exam is normal. Rectal exam is normal and nontender. Anoscopy is normal.

What is the most appropriate action?

A) Reassurance.
B) Anusol suppositories 3 times/week for 6 weeks; follow-up as needed.
C) Flexible sigmoidoscopy.
D) Colonoscopy.
E) Anorectal manometry.

Discussion

The correct answer is C. Patients reporting persistent blood per rectum without lesions seen on anoscopy should be referred for endoscopic evaluation. Colon cancer is rare in this age group but can happen. The symptom of red blood per rectum suggests that the cause could be found distal to descending colon and likely in the rectum. If there is only a single episode of bleeding, some would argue for a more conservative approach in patients <50 years without other alarm symptoms (constitutional symptoms or change in bowel habits).

In this young patient, a full colonoscopy (answer D) is not necessary unless there is a strong family history of colorectal cancer or other symptoms suggestive of colitis such as urgency, weight loss, or diarrhea. Anorectal manometry (answer E) is not useful in the evaluation of rectal bleeding. Anusol suppositories (answer B) can be helpful to reduce pain associated with hemorrhoids, but if bleeding is the only symptom, fiber supplements and stool softeners are sufficient. If the patient is >50 years with rectal bleeding, full colonoscopy is indicated.

CASE 18

A 73-year-old male comes to your office with the complaint of 3 days of left lower quadrant abdominal pain. He has felt cold and clammy at times but has not checked his temperature. He has had no nausea, vomiting, or diarrhea. The pain does not worsen after meals, but his appetite has been poor since this started. On review of systems, he reports increased urinary frequency and urgency for the same amount of time. He has had no surgeries on his abdomen. He has diabetes mellitus type 2 and is on glipizide. He also takes aspirin 81 mg per day. He has always declined screening colonoscopy, stating, "If it ain't broke, don't fix it"—apparently a way of life. On exam he is in no distress with blood pressure 125/75 mm Hg, pulse 90, respirations 15, temperature 38.5°C. His heart sounds are normal, and his chest is clear bilaterally. He has moderate left lower quadrant tenderness without rebound tenderness or guarding. There is no abdominal distention or organomegaly. Bowel sounds are normal, and the rectal exam is normal without stool in ampulla. Urinalysis is normal.

What is the most likely diagnosis?

A) Ischemic colitis.
B) Colon cancer with large bowel obstruction
C) Irritable bowel syndrome.
D) Pyelonephritis.
E) Diverticulitis.

Discussion

The correct answer is E. Diverticulitis is the most likely cause of the patient's pain. Fever associated with acute onset abdominal pain located in left lower quadrant makes this pain likely due to diverticulitis. Diverticulitis can occur in any part of the colon. Ischemic colitis (answer A) can present with abdominal pain in this location but is usually associated with bloody diarrhea, so it is less likely. Irritable bowel syndrome (answer C) almost never presents in this age group, is not associated with fevers, and is a chronic condition, not acute. Pyelonephritis (answer D) was a possibility until the urine dipstick returned normal. Urinary symptoms are common in diverticulitis because of bladder irritation. Colon cancer with large bowel obstruction (answer B) would present with severe abdominal pain and distention. In obstruction, bowel sounds are typically hyperactive with intermittent rushing.

* *

The most appropriate next step in the workup of the patient is:

A) CT scan of abdomen and pelvis with triple contrast.
B) Surgical consult.
C) Gastroenterology consult.
D) Abdominal ultrasound.
E) Colonoscopy.

Discussion

The correct answer is A. CT scan is very sensitive and specific for diverticulitis and can simultaneously evaluate for other causes of abdominal pain. CT scan is indicated if the patient has peritoneal signs or mass suggesting diverticular abscess formation. In a patient who has previously documented attacks with none of the above symptoms, empiric treatment is appropriate. Surgical and/or GI consults (answers B and C) may be indicated but are premature at this point. Abdominal ultrasound (answer D) can diagnose diverticulitis and/or abscess, but it is less sensitive than CT scan. Colonoscopy (answer E) is indicated only in the acute setting if obstruction is present or if colitis is thought to be more likely. In the setting of acute diverticulitis the risk of perforation during colonoscopy is increased, and colonoscopy is preferably delayed until inflammation has subsided.

 HELPFUL TIP: In the absence of a CT scanner, it is reasonable to admit a patient with a classic history of diverticulitis, give IV antibiotics, and perform serial abdominal exams. If the patient improves rapidly, you can schedule colonoscopy when the attack has resolved. If the patient worsens, he goes immediately to a center that has a CT scan and a surgeon (do not pass go, do not . . . you get the idea).

* *

You get the CT scan the same day and have the patient return to your office to discuss the results. The CT scan shows inflammation in the sigmoid colon with some outpouching structures suggesting diverticulosis.

There is a 1.5-cm fluid collection posterior to the sigmoid colon suggesting pericolonic abscess. No other findings were noted, and the colon above sigmoid appeared normal. No free air was seen.

Which of the following is the most appropriate next step in management?

A) CT-guided drainage of the abscess.
B) Surgical consult for immediate diverting colostomy and abscess drainage.
C) Admission with IV antibiotics and serial abdominal exams.
D) Discharge to home on levofloxacin and metronidazole.
E) GI consult for endoscopic ultrasound guided transcolonic drainage of abscess.

Discussion

The correct answer is C. This patient should be admitted for IV antibiotics. Mild attacks of diverticulitis can be managed on an outpatient basis. Your patient has a small abscess that requires inpatient therapy. In addition, he is immunosuppressed by his diabetes, and all immunosuppressed patients with diverticulitis should be admitted for IV antibiotics since they are more likely to develop complications and need surgery. Answer A is incorrect. It is reasonable to ask the radiologist if this abscess can be drained but the likely answer is no, because it is very small and is posterior to colon. Answer B is incorrect. The patient does not have peritoneal signs and the abscess will likely will respond to IV antibiotics. Thus, immediate surgery is not indicated. As discussed above, colonoscopy (and by extension endoscopic ultrasound) is relatively contraindicated in the setting of acute diverticulitis. Answer E is incorrect. No gastroenterologist has been found crazy enough to try to drain abscesses by a transcolonic approach to our (and Pubmed's) knowledge. Perhaps the emerging Natural Orifice Transluminal Endoscopic Surgeons (NOTES) will attempt this in the future but not on our patient today. (We didn't make this one up—they have been doing cholecystectomies via a transvaginal approach.)

 HELPFUL TIP: Antibiotic regimens for diverticulitis must include both Gram-negative and anaerobic coverage. Some common regimens include ciprofloxacin + metronidazole, ampicillin sulbactam, amoxicillin clavulanate, ampicillin + gentamicin + clindamycin, ceftriaxone + metronidazole.

* *

The patient is admitted and he responds to IV antibiotics and supportive measures. A repeat CT scan 2 weeks later shows resolution of the abscess. The gastroenterologist performs colonoscopy 2 months after the attack and confirms left-sided diverticulosis with otherwise normal colonoscopy.

Which of the following statements is true about this patient's prognosis?

A) When the patient has his second attack of uncomplicated diverticulitis, a resection of the diseased segment is always indicated (sigmoid colectomy).
B) 50% of patients will have a repeat attack within 5 years.
C) He has 20%–30% chance of perforation of diverticulitis in 2 years.
D) He has 30% chance of diverticular bleeding in next 2 years.
E) 33% of patients will have a second attack.

Discussion

The correct answer is E. Only 33% of patients with an episode of diverticulitis will have a second episode. There is no set rule for the number of attacks needed before partial colectomy is indicated. The commonly used rule of 3 attacks is not based on prospective evidence. The decision has to be individualized, but the tendency is to operate on healthy young people with frequent attacks while opting for observation of elderly patients with comorbidities (even if they have more than 3 attacks). Perforation of diverticulitis is rare and occurs in only 5%–10% of patients within 2 years of the initial event. Diverticular bleeding happens in 3%–5% of patients with diverticulosis and the risk is not increased with diverticulitis; if bleeding occurs during an episode of presumed diverticulitis, other diagnoses should be strongly considered.

* *

On a weekend call 6 months later your patient presents to the ED after experiencing sudden onset of bright red blood per rectum mixed within stools. He has passed 5 stools in 3 hours and the last one had blood clots. He feels dizzy but has not passed out. He stopped taking his aspirin after his last illness, but otherwise his health and medications are unchanged. His abdomen is nontender and bowel sounds are normoactive. Rectal exam reveals fresh blood on the glove but no masses in rectum. Hemoglobin is 10 g/dL, and you place 2 large-bore IVs and admit him to the hospital. He has no more bowel movements overnight, his hemoglobin is 8.2 g/dL the next morning, and he is feeling well. You assume that the bleeding was diverticular.

Which of the following statements is TRUE?

A) Urgent colonoscopy is needed to localize and treat the lesion.
B) Colonoscopy is needed but can be done on an outpatient basis.
C) Tagged RBC scan followed by angiography is indicated to prevent rebleeding.
D) No further workup is indicated at this point.
E) Sigmoid colon resection is indicated because of the dogmatic diverticular duo (diverticular bleed and diverticulitis).

Discussion

The correct answer is D. The patient has classic presentation of diverticular bleeding with rapid onset and spontaneous resolution of bleeding (75% stop spontaneously). The patient underwent colonoscopy recently and the only finding was diverticulosis. Since the patient has stopped bleeding, colonoscopy (answer A) is unlikely to help in the management of his condition and urgent surgical resection (answer E) is unnecessary as well. For the same reason, colonoscopy does not need to be done as outpatient (answer B). If the patient had continued to bleed, there would be 2 approaches for managing this patient and both are acceptable. The first approach is to perform rapid colonic lavage by placing an NG tube and giving 6 liters (1.5 gallons) of polyethylene glycol (GoLytely) over 4 hours and perform colonoscopy to try to find the bleeding site and treat it. Often multiple blood-filled diverticuli are seen, and the source of the bleed cannot be identified. The second approach is to perform a tagged RBC scan (answer C) to confirm active bleeding, followed by selective angiography to identify the bleeding vessel and embolize it. The approach taken depends on the local expertise available. Without treatment, 25% of patients eventually rebleed and of those who rebleed, 50% will have a third bleed.

Objectives: Did you learn to . . .

- Identify signs and symptoms of diverticulitis?
- Appreciate the natural history of diverticular disease?
- Manage complications of diverticular disease?

BIBLIOGRAPHY

Baron TH, Morgan DE. Acute Necrotizing Pancreatitis; current concepts. *NEJM.* 1999;340(18):1412.

Bytzer P, Talley, NJ. Dyspepsia. *Ann Intern Med.* 2001;134:815.

Chan FK, Leung, WK. Peptic-ulcer disease. *Lancet.* 2002; 360:933.

Ferzoco LB, Raptopoulos V, Silen W. Acute diverticulitis. *NEJM.* 1998;338(21):1521.

Heidelbaugh JJ, Bruderly M. Cirrhosis and chronic liver failure: part I. Diagnosis and evaluation. *Am Fam Physician.* 2006;74(5):756.

Heidelbaugh JJ, Sherbondy M. Cirrhosis and chronic liver failure: part II. Complications and treatment. *Am Fam Physician.* 2006;74(5):767.

Lanza FL. A guideline for the treatment and prevention of NSAID-induced ulcers. Members of the Ad Hoc Committee on Practice Parameters of the American College of Gastroenterology. *Am J Gastroenterol.* 1998;93:2037.

Lee LA, Robinson M, Katz PO, et al. Updated guidelines for the diagnosis and treatment of gastroesophageal disease. *American J Gastroenterol.* 1999;94(11):S1.

Longstreth GF, Thompson WG, Chey WD, et al. Functional bowel disorders. *Gastroenterology.* 2006;130:1480.

Flamm SL. Chronic hepatitis C virus infection. *JAMA.* 2003;289:2413.

Rockey DC. Occult gastrointestinal bleeding; primary care. *NEJM.* 1999;341(1):38.

Smith DS, Ferris CD. Current concepts in diabetic gastroparesis: Therapy in practice. *Drugs.* 2003;63(13):1339.

Swaroop VS, Chari ST, Clain JE. Severe acute pancreatitis. *JAMA.* 2004;291:2865.

Tack J, Talley NJ, Camilleri M, et al. Functional gastroduodenal disorders. *Gastroenterology.* 2006;130:466.

Trate DM, Parkman, HP, Fisher, RS. Dysphagia: evaluation, diagnosis and treatment. *Prim Care.* 1996;23:417.

United States Preventive Services Task Force. Screening for Colon Cancer. 2002. Accessed November 20, 2007, at http://www.ahrq.gov/clinic/uspstf/uspscolo.htm.

Yamada, T, Alpers DH, et al. *Handbook of Gastroenterology.* Philadelphia: Lippincott Williams & Wilkins, 1998.

Infectious Diseases

8

Margo Schilling

CASE 1

An increasing number of patients with fevers and respiratory tract infections have filled your waiting room this December. Many patients report that they have sick family members. You have not been paying attention to the local school attendance rates but know that many of your nursing home's staff members are home ill.

What additional information might you use to determine if influenza is in your community?

A) Public health lab reports of an increase in local influenza activity.

B) CDC reports of regional influenza activity.

C) A report of a positive influenza culture in the community.

D) An increase in the number of influenza-like illnesses seen in your practice in recent days.

E) All of the above.

Discussion

The correct answer is E. Any of this information will increase the likelihood that patients will present with influenza. From October to May the Influenza Branch of the Centers for Disease Control and Prevention (CDC) collects and reports information regarding national influenza activity via a Web site (http://www.cdc.gov/flu/weekly/fluactivity.htm).

* *

The CDC annually publishes recommendations for administering influenza vaccine to the American public.

The CDC recommends vaccination for all of the following groups EXCEPT:

A) Health-care workers.

B) Nursing home residents.

C) Egg-allergic, febrile neonates.

D) Diabetics.

E) The elderly.

Discussion

The correct answer is C. Children ≤6 months (including neonates, obviously) should not be vaccinated, nor should children who are febrile. The other contraindications to influenza vaccination are a known hypersensitivity to eggs or to other components of the influenza vaccine.

 HELPFUL TIP: Vaccinate all individuals >6 months. All health-care personnel and persons at high risk for complications of influenza should receive annual influenza vaccination. There are two forms of vaccine available: trivalent inactivated influenza vaccine and live, attenuated influenza vaccine. Live attenuated influenza vaccine (ie, FluMist) is indicated only for healthy, nonpregnant persons aged 2–49 years, including health-care workers.

* *

You have determined that there is an influenza outbreak in the community.

What intervention(s) is/are most appropriate now for all your *unvaccinated*, frail nursing home

patients who have no symptoms of febrile respiratory illness?

A) Antiviral prophylaxis with oseltamivir.
B) Antiviral prophylaxis with amantadine.
C) Influenza immunization.
D) A and C given together.
E) B and C given together.

Discussion

The correct answer is D. Persons at high risk for complications of influenza can still be vaccinated after an outbreak of influenza has begun in the community, but development of antibodies in adults can take up to 2 weeks. **Chemoprophylaxis should be considered for persons at high risk during the time from vaccination until immunity has developed.** Answer A alone might be appropriate for individuals who have a contraindication to vaccination and wish to protect themselves from influenza. Answer B is incorrect because influenza A is increasingly resistant to M2 drugs (amantadine, rimantadine), and influenza B has never been sensitive. Answer C, vaccination alone, can be used in individuals **without** known high-risk conditions (chronic disorders including asthma, diabetes, renal dysfunction, immunodeficiency, or cardiovascular disease) but is inadequate for those who are institutionalized and the chronically ill. These higher risk patients also need to be covered by oseltamivir until immunity has developed (2 weeks).

* *

At the peak of the outbreak, many of your office staff have not yet received the influenza vaccine this season. Your office manager is watching the bottom line, and she asks you to develop an intervention to prevent absenteeism among employees who have **direct patient contact**.

Your best recommendation is to:

A) Not offer any intervention.
B) Offer to **vaccinate** any employee who has not received the influenza vaccine this season.
C) Offer antiviral **prophylaxis** to any employee who has not received the influenza vaccine this season.
D) Offer to **vaccinate** any employee who has not received the influenza vaccine this season **and provide antiviral drugs** for 2 weeks until vaccine response is complete.
E) Pass out masks and hand wipes to every patient with a cough who enters the clinic.

Discussion

The correct answer is D. To reduce the spread of virus to persons at high risk during community outbreaks, antiviral chemoprophylaxis of unvaccinated health-care workers who have direct and frequent contact with patients at high risk for complications of influenza infection can be considered. **This is not a substitute for vaccination, and all health-care workers should be immunized.**

 HELPFUL TIP: Sensitivity and specificity of rapid diagnostic tests for influenza (70%–75% and 90%–95%, respectively) are lower than viral culture. **Resistance of influenza A to oseltamivir has been rising.** In outpatients, reserve this drug for those who have a positive rapid diagnostic test and present within 48 hours of symptom onset. The benefit is limited to a 24-hour reduction in symptoms after 5 days of treatment. This benefit is in those with Influenza A; the benefit is less in Influenza B.

* *

The director of nursing at your community nursing home calls about an outbreak of febrile respiratory infections. In the last 24 hours, 3 patients have become ill in the dementia care unit. All residents of the home were vaccinated with the current year's influenza vaccine in November. Several of the aides have not been vaccinated and 2 recently left work after complaining of feeling tired, feverish, and achy.

You suspect an influenza outbreak and take the following actions EXCEPT:

A) Quarantine the nursing home and restrict access to visitors, new admissions, and ill staff.
B) Hospitalize all patients suspected of having influenza.
C) Limit the interaction of ill residents with well residents.
D) Administer antiviral prophylaxis to all well residents.
E) Provide influenza vaccine to any unvaccinated residents.

Discussion

The correct answer is B. Moving sick patients risks spread of the infection to the hospital. In addition to measures above, employees should be assigned to one work area only to prevent spread via employees.

Activities, visits and gatherings in central common areas should be curtailed during the outbreak.

 HELPFUL TIP: Influenza vaccine is approximately 50% effective in nursing home patients. Still, there is some herd immunity and vaccination is recommended as the primary way to prevent an influenza outbreak.

* *

Your 97-year-old patient was one of the first recognized flu cases in the nursing home almost 2 weeks ago. She was improving, but now she has a productive cough, low-grade fever, and confusion.

You should:

A) Initiate treatment with amantadine for influenza A infection.

B) Obtain a viral culture and use the results to decide if you need to treat with oseltamivir or rimantadine.

C) Perform a thorough exam and obtain CXR, oxygen saturation, CBC, and urinalysis.

D) Give ceftriaxone 1 g IM daily for 5 days.

Discussion

The correct answer is C. Infection in the elderly may present with confusion alone. **Fever may not be a prominent symptom of infection in frail or immunocompromised individuals.** Answer A is incorrect. There is resistance to amantadine that makes it a suboptimal drug choice for Influenza A. Additionally, she is now **2 weeks out** from her diagnosis, making antiviral therapy useless. Answer B is incorrect for the same reason. Additionally, a culture will take days to come back. Answer D is incorrect. Empiric antibiotics are not indicated, specifically IM injections in a patient without more evidence of bacterial infection. Pursuing a diagnosis is critical. Additional evidence might confirm pneumonia, and empiric antibiotic therapy would be warranted.

 HELPFUL TIP: The most common cause of bacterial pneumonia complicating influenza is *Streptococcus pneumoniae*. *Staphylococcus aureus* pneumonia (usually uncommon in the community) is an important entity during influenza outbreaks and generally presents with more severe symptoms.

Objectives: Did you learn to . . .

- Describe methods to detect influenza in the community, outpatient office practice and health-care facilities?
- Identify appropriate interventions to halt the transmission of influenza in community and health-care influenza outbreaks?
- Lead a successful influenza prevention program in a health-care setting?
- Prescribe influenza antivirals appropriately?

CASE 2

An 80-year-old female fell, broke her hip, and underwent intraoperative repair with pinning of the fracture. She developed a local infection at the site of the repair and was treated with a 10-day course of oral clindamycin. She is transferred to the nursing home for rehabilitation and has developed loose, watery stools. Today when you visit her she reports feeling diffuse abdominal discomfort and has had 10 bowel movements. She is very concerned because she cannot work with the therapist and risks losing her Medicare benefit for skilled nursing.

You plan to do the following:

A) Begin loperamide (Imodium) as needed to prevent diarrhea during the therapy sessions.

B) Obtain stool specimens for *Clostridium difficile* toxin.

C) Obtain an abdominal CT scan looking for evidence of obstruction.

D) Ask the GI physician to perform emergency endoscopy for evaluation of lower GI bleed.

E) Obtain stool specimens for ova and parasites.

Discussion

The correct answer is B. *Clostridium difficile* is the most common bacterial cause of infectious diarrhea in the United States. Although other causes of diarrhea are possible, the most cost-effective approach in this patient would be stool assay for *C. difficile* repeated on 2–3 specimens (to improve sensitivity) prior to any other more invasive procedure. The assay for *C. difficile* cytotoxin is approximately 75% sensitivity (enzyme immunoassay). There are several subtypes of toxin, some of which are not detected by this assay. The most common inducing antibiotics are clindamycin, fluoroquinolones and broad-spectrum cephalosporins. Although symptomatic therapy is important, answer A is incorrect because antiperistaltic agents should be avoided in patients with *C. difficile*.

* *

A stool specimen reveals the presence of *C. difficile* toxin A.

Treatment of this patient should include:

A) Metamucil to bulk up her stools.
B) Lactose restriction and acidophilus milk products.
C) Metronidazole 500 mg orally three times daily for 10 days.
D) Vancomycin 250 mg orally four times daily for 10 days.
E) No treatment is indicated without culture and sensitivity results.

Discussion

The correct answer is C. Treatment includes supportive care, discontinuation of the offending antimicrobial agent, and initiation of oral metronidazole 250 mg 4 times daily or 500 mg TID for 10 days. Metronidazole is preferred over vancomycin because of the nearly identical efficacy/relapse or reinfection rates, lower cost, and lower theoretical risk of promotion of acquisition of vancomycin-resistant *Enterococcus faecalis* (VRE).

Risk factors for *Clostridium difficile* infection in nursing home patients include:

A) Advanced age.
B) Recent acute hospitalization.
C) Treatment with broad-spectrum antibiotic therapy.
D) Long-term residence in a chronic care facility.
E) All of the above.

Discussion

The correct answer is E. Risk factors for acquisition of *Clostridium difficile* infection in nursing home patients are similar to that of hospitalized patients and include hospitalization, advanced age, gastrointestinal surgery/procedures and antibiotic exposure. PPI use has also been recognized as a risk factor for *C. difficile.*

 HELPFUL TIP: Infection control precautions for those with *C. difficile* include patient isolation, contact precautions and the use of 1/10 dilution of bleach for cleaning environmental contamination. Handwashing is more effective than alcohol-based products at reducing transmission of spores via health-care workers' hands.

 HELPFUL TIP: *C. difficile* diarrhea and colitis can be caused by **any** antibiotic, including metronidazole and vancomycin. The probability of diarrhea seems highest with clindamycin. Fluoroquinolones are increasingly associated with *C. difficile* infection, including a highly toxigenic strain.

* *

Failure to resolve *C. difficile*-associated diarrhea after a 10-day course antibiotic therapy is common. Your patient's diarrhea has persisted.

The most reasonable treatment approach is to:

A) Repeat a course of oral metronidazole.
B) Treat with a course of oral vancomycin.
C) Treat with a course of IV vancomycin.
D) A or B.
E) B or C.

Discussion

The correct answer is D. Relapse is very common. Approximately 20% of patients have a recurrence of symptoms within 1 week of completing therapy. These patients usually respond to retreatment with either metronidazole or vancomycin. IV vancomycin (answer C) is **ineffective** treatment for *C. difficile* because vancomycin dose not enter into the GI tract from the vascular space.

 HELPFUL TIP: *C. difficile* toxin degrades at room temperature. A stool that has been at room temperature for 2 hours will likely be negative for *C. difficile* toxin even though the toxin was initially present. A newly identified cause of *C. difficile* negative pseudomembranous colitis is *Klebsiella oxytoca*. Consider this if stool studies are negative for *C. difficile*. A positive stool culture is not diagnostic of pseudomembranous colitis. *C. difficile* is a normal gut flora. You need a positive toxin to make the diagnosis of *C. difficile*-associated diarrhea or pseudomembranous colitis.

HELPFUL TIP: The use of probiotics seems to help prevent *C. difficile* colitis and may prevent recurrences. **In particularly recalcitrant cases, stool transplants have been done.** Patients are given healthy stool via NG tube to reestablish normal GI flora.

Objectives: Did you learn to . . .

● Recognize the presentation of *C. difficile* infection?
● Identify risk factors for the development of *C. difficile* colitis?
● Treat patients with initial and recurrent *C. difficile* infections?

CASE 3

You are called to the ED to examine a 40-year-old male with fever and headache. His past history is remarkable only for a splenectomy secondary to trauma at 10 years. He is not allergic to any antibiotics. Upon exam you note that he has meningeal signs. Nondilated fundal exam shows sharp disc margins, and he is neurologically intact with a nonfocal exam.

The most appropriate action is:

A) Obtain a head CT so that you can proceed safely with lumbar puncture.
B) Order IV penicillin as you prepare to perform lumbar puncture.
C) Perform a lumbar puncture immediately and begin antibiotic therapy empirically.
D) Order IV erythromycin as you prepare to perform lumbar puncture.
E) Order IV vancomycin and IV ceftriaxone as you wait for the CBC. If the CBC is abnormal you will do the LP.

Discussion

The correct answer is C. Once you suspect bacterial meningitis, rapid diagnostic evaluation and emergent treatment are imperative, including lumbar puncture and blood cultures. **If lumbar puncture is going to be delayed, give appropriate empiric antimicrobial and adjunctive therapy without delay.** Head CT (answer A) is necessary only in individuals who are immunocompromised (HIV/AIDS, are receiving immunosuppressive drugs, transplant recipients), have a history of CNS disease (brain tumor, stroke, etc),

develop new onset seizures, display papilledema on exam, or have an abnormal/focal neurologic deficit or abnormal level of consciousness. Antibiotics for a 40-year-old male should cover *Neisseria meningitidis* and *Streptococcus pneumoniae*, and would include vancomycin and ceftriaxone (answer E). However, answer E is incorrect because you never wait for a CBC to determine if a patient needs an LP. The decision to do an LP is a clinical one.

 HELPFUL TIP: The standard of care for suspected meningitis is to administer antibiotics within 30 minutes of the patient presenting to the ED. Draw the blood cultures and give the antibiotics. You will not change the culture results if you give a single dose of antibiotics prior to CT scan. However, it is considered prudent to do the LP within 2 hours of administering IV antibiotics.

* *

Results of the CSF obtained after lumbar puncture are as follows: cloudy, WBC count 5,000 cells/mm³, 95% neutrophils, glucose 20 mg/dL, Gram-positive cocci in pairs.

The most likely pathogen is:

A) *Streptococcus pneumoniae*.
B) *Listeria monocytogenes*.
C) *Staphylococcus aureus*.
D) *Neisseria meningitidis*.
E) *Pseudomonas* species.

Discussion

The correct answer is A. Gram-stain examination of CSF may permit rapid identification of the causative organism in bacterial meningitis with a sensitivity of 60%–90%. Prior antibiotic therapy (eg, a partially treated meningitis—not a single dose of antibiotics in the ED) may reduce the sensitivity by 20%. The likelihood of a positive Gram stain is highest in cases of *Streptococcus pneumoniae*. Approximately 33% of *Listeria monocytogenes* meningitis cases demonstrate a positive Gram stain.

An adjunctive therapy that has demonstrated improved neurologic outcomes in pneumococcal meningitis is:

A) Dexamethasone.
B) Activated Protein C.
C) Vasopressors.
D) CSF shunt implantation.
E) Monoclonal antibody directed against the capsule antigen of the bacterium.

Discussion

The correct answer is A. The Infectious Disease Society of America (IDSA) guideline recommends adjunctive dexamethasone to be administered to all adult patients with pneumococcal meningitis. No other adjunctive therapy has proven benefit. Patients should receive standard supportive therapies in an intensive care setting. Complications, if they occur, usually develop within the first 2–3 days of therapy. Complications include sepsis, mental status changes, electrolyte abnormalities, etc.

Highly resistant *Streptococcal pneumoniae* infections of the CNS should be treated with:

A) Third-generation cephalosporin.
B) Vancomycin and a third-generation cephalosporin.
C) High-dose penicillin G.
D) Ampicillin.
E) Vancomycin, gentamycin, and rifampin.

Discussion

The correct answer is B. Vancomycin should be combined with a third-generation cephalosporin (eg, ceftriaxone or cefotaxime) for highly resistant pneumococcus. Do not use vancomycin alone; it does not cover Gram-negative organisms. The newer generation fluoroquinolones have enhanced in vitro activity against *S. pneumoniae* and may be used as alternative agents. **Fluoroquinolones are not recommended unless the patient cannot tolerate or is allergic to standard drugs.**

 HELPFUL TIP: Resistance to penicillins (and others) is noted by the MIC. For penicillin, highly resistant pneumococcus has an MIC of >2 microgram/mL, intermediate resistance is 0.12–1 microgram/mL while sensitive is <0.06 microgram/mL.

 HELPFUL TIP: The combination of Kernig and Brudzinski signs carries a sensitivity of 5% and a specificity of 95%. The great majority of patients do not manifest these signs when they have meningitis, and they are useless to rule out meningitis. The sensitivity and specificity of nuchal rigidity (stiff neck) is 30% and 68%, respectively. In adults the classic triad of headache, stiff neck, and altered mental status was found in only 46%, with 85% having fever, 70% having neck stiffness, and 67% having mental status changes.

 QUICK QUIZ: MENINGITIS

What is the most common bacterial cause of meningitis in college-aged patients who live in dormitories?

A) *N. meningitidis.*
B) *S. pneumococcus.*
C) *L. monocytogenes.*
D) *H. influenzae.*
E) *E. coli.*

Discussion

The correct answer is A. Although *S. pneumococcus* is the most common cause of bacterial meningitis in the adult population in the United States, *N. meningitidis* remains the leading cause of bacterial meningitis in adolescents and is particularly prevalent in the setting of dormitory living (eg, college or military). The presence of petechial (or purpuric) rash in the lower extremities and pressure points is typical of *N. meningitidis*. The advent of vaccination has made *H. influenzae* a less common cause. *L. monocytogenes* is more prevalent in adults >50 years, infants, and immunocompromised individuals. *E. coli* is a common cause for meningitis in neonates and infants but is very uncommon in adolescents and adults.

Objectives: Did you learn to . . .

- Diagnose meningitis?
- Identify the most likely causative organism based on epidemiology and patient characteristics?
- Describe proper use of empiric antibiotics and steroid therapy for bacterial meningitis?

QUICK QUIZ: SPLEENLESS IN SEATTLE

Patients undergoing elective splenectomy should receive all of the following EXCEPT:

A) Pneumococcal polysaccharide vaccine (Pneumovax).
B) *H. influenzae* type B conjugate vaccine.
C) Influenza vaccine.
D) Meningococcal vaccine.
E) Oral polio vaccine.

Discussion

The correct answer is E. Oral polio vaccine is no longer recommended in the United States. All patients undergoing elective splenectomy should receive preoperative vaccination against encapsulated organisms at least 14 days prior to splenectomy; this includes vaccines against *S. pneumoniae*, meningococcus, and *H. influenzae* type B (all encapsulated bacteria). It is also reasonable to offer influenza vaccination annually at the appropriate time. Splenectomized individuals should be re-immunized against pneumococcus at 5-year intervals. Patients who have undergone splenectomy need to be educated about seeking prompt medical attention for fever.

CASE 4

A 74-year-old female presents to your office for a complete physical. As part of the routine labs you obtain a urinalysis (although there is no recommendation for a screening urinalysis for any nonpregnant patients). On further questioning, she has had stress urinary incontinence for a number of years, which is unchanged. She reports no fevers, hematuria, dysuria, flank pain, or other symptoms. The urinalysis shows 10–20 WBC/hpf and is nitrite positive on dipstick. A culture of the urine shows 100,000 cfu/mL of *Escherichia coli*.

How should you treat this patient?

A) Trimethoprim-sulfamethoxazole DS 1 tab PO BID for 10 days.
B) Erythromycin 500 mg PO q 6 hours for 14 days.
C) Ampicillin 250 mg PO q 6 hours for 10 days.
D) Ceftriaxone 1 g IM every day for 3 days.
E) No antibiotic treatment is indicated.

Discussion

The correct answer is E. A positive urine culture in an asymptomatic patient (eg, asymptomatic bacteriuria) should not be treated with antibiotics. Asymptomatic bacteriuria is a common finding, especially in elderly females, persons with indwelling catheters, and institutionalized individuals. Treatment does not reduce the incidence of symptomatic infection. Treatment also does not reduce mortality in frail elderly patients, and does not improve **chronic** urinary incontinence symptoms. Persistent asymptomatic bacteriuria does not result in renal insufficiency or the development of hypertension.

Which statement is TRUE of asymptomatic bacteriuria?

A) The finding of pyuria in a urinalysis distinguishes urinary tract infection from asymptomatic bacteriuria and guides treatment decisions.
B) The prevalence of asymptomatic bacteriuria in women is unrelated to age, function, or hormonal status.
C) Asymptomatic bacteriuria need not be treated in the pregnant patient.
D) None of the above.

Discussion

The correct answer is D. None of the statements is true. Answer A is incorrect because the finding of pyuria with low numbers of white blood cells in a urinalysis specimen is nonspecific, common, and frequently unrelated to infection. Answer B is incorrect because the prevalence of asymptomatic bacteriuria in women increases with age, declining functional capabilities, and institutionalization. More than 10% of community-dwelling women >65 years and up to 50% of elderly women in nursing homes will have asymptomatic bacteriuria on screening urinalysis. Answer C is incorrect because pregnancy is one state in which treating asymptomatic pyuria/bacteriuria is indicated. The risk of infection from asymptomatic bacteriuria is high in pregnant patients.

 HELPFUL TIP: Bacteriuria necessitates treatment in individuals with the following conditions: urinary tract obstruction (functional or anatomic), nephrolithiasis, pregnancy, planned urinary instrumentation, and children with vesicoureteral reflux (although treatment of children with vesicoureteral reflux has been challenged recently).

HELPFUL TIP: Not all pyuria is caused by UTI. Other pathogenic causes of pyuria include vaginitis (infectious and atrophic), urethritis (*Chlamydia trachomatis*, *Neisseria gonorrhoeae*), and genital herpes infections.

* *

Several years later, the same patient is now 80 years old and is admitted to a nursing home. Her initial TB skin test with 5–tuberculin-unit injection of purified protein derivative (PPD) was interpreted as 0 mm diameter of induration after 48 hours.

What is your next step?
A) Repeat the PPD now.
B) Repeat the PPD in 2 weeks.
C) Repeat the PPD in 1 year.
D) Declare the patient free of TB.
E) Obtain a chest x-ray.

Discussion
The correct answer is B. Because the prevalence of a positive PPD (Mantoux test) doubles between the first and second tests in initial nonresponders, the U.S. Public Health Task Force recommends a 2-step PPD by the Mantoux method for screening high-risk populations (eg, individuals living in nursing homes). If the first PPD is negative, a second test should be performed approximately 2 weeks later in order to detect the "booster phenomenon." Individuals admitted to a nursing home with a positive PPD and no symptoms of active TB may be presumed to have a distant history of infection.

 HELPFUL TIP: False-positive PPDs can be due to BCG vaccine and infection with other mycobacteria. **However, patients who are 1 year or more out from their BCG vaccine should be treated as though they are true responders.** False-negatives occur when immunity is impaired. If you suspect impaired immunity, use *Candida* and/or mumps controls.

* *

A second PPD 2 weeks later is interpreted again as 0 mm diameter of induration after 48 hours. You reassure the patient that her tuberculin test is negative.

In this patient, what most accurately represents a positive tuberculin skin test?
A) Erythema 5 mm in diameter.
B) Induration 5–10 mm in diameter.
C) Erythema of 10 mm in diameter.
D) Induration 10 mm in diameter.
E) Erythematous induration of any size.

Discussion
The correct answer is D. Here is the bottom line:
1. Routine screening is not recommended for low-risk patients (eg, community-dwelling individuals from a low-risk country). Screen only the following: contacts of those with TB, HIV infected patients, IV drug users, those with predisposing factors to TB infection (diabetes, immunosuppressive drugs, lung cancer, etc), foreign-born individuals arriving in the U.S. within the last 5 years, health-care workers, nursing home and other institutionalized individuals, homeless individuals.
2. Measure the induration and not the erythema.
3. The definition of a positive PPD changes with the population tested (Table 8–1).

 HELPFUL TIP: Whole-blood interferon gamma assay (QuantiFERON-TB Gold test) is FDA approved for use in any situation in which the PPD is currently employed. It is more expensive and should not be the front-line screening test but may help in situations in which the PPD result is questionable.

* *

One year after admission to the nursing home, the patient presents to you to interpret her annual PPD. The diameter of induration is 12 mm by your exam. The patient denies cough, weight loss, fever, or chills.

The most appropriate next step is to:
A) Obtain a chest radiograph and, if normal, initiate isoniazid 300 mg and pyridoxine for 9 months.
B) Obtain a chest radiograph and, if normal, observe the patient annually for signs of active TB (weight loss, cough, fever, etc).
C) Obtain a chest radiograph and, if abnormal, initiate isoniazid 300 mg once daily and pyridoxine for 9 months.

Table 8–1   INTERPRETATION OF PPD SKIN TESTS

Diameter of Induration:	Positive in These Situations:
5–10 mm	Chest x-ray consistent with past or current infection; HIV positive; recent close contact of individual with active TB
≥10 mm	Institutionalized individuals; IV drug users; immunocompromised states other than HIV; children <4 years; children exposed to high-risk adults, health-care workers
≥15 mm	Individuals without risk factors; these are people who probably should not have been tested in the first place (eg, the general public without any exposure to TB)

and multiple drug regimens should be initiated in patients with signs and symptoms of active disease based on clinical history, exam, and radiographic findings.

 HELPFUL TIP: If active TB is diagnosed, appropriate therapy should be initiated with a 3- or 4-drug regimen for 6–8 weeks followed by continuation therapy with a simpler regimen. A number of regimens are available, and all include isoniazid and rifampin. INH alone is never appropriate for active TB. First-line drugs include: isoniazid, rifampin, pyrazinamide, and ethambutol. Second-line drugs include levofloxacin, streptomycin, and others. Regimens vary by location and local resistance patterns. Contact your local health department.

D) Obtain a chest radiograph and, if abnormal, observe the patient annually for signs of active TB.

E) Obtain sputum specimens for AFB stains and mycobacterial culture and sensitivity testing; and initiate therapy with isoniazid, pyridoxine, pyrazinamide, and rifampin for 6 months.

Discussion

The correct answer is A. The patient lives in a high-risk setting (nursing home). The results of her Mantoux test 1 year ago suggest that she was not infected with *Mycobacterium tuberculosis* at that time. She has newly converted—probably caused by exposure to an active case of TB. **The risk of developing active disease following TB infection is greatest in the first 2 years following infection. The risk/benefit ratio favors prophylactic therapy with isoniazid (INH) for the patient who has converted within the last 2 years, as long as there is no sign of active disease and the chest x-ray is negative.**

Answer B is incorrect because a negative chest x-ray does not mean that you can forego prophylactic therapy. Answer C is incorrect because an abnormal chest radiograph must be followed with collection of sputum specimens for acid-fast bacilli (AFB) staining and culture. Answer E is incorrect because a chest radiograph is necessary to evaluate all patients with a positive Mantoux skin test. Sputum specimens should be collected

Which of the following are risk factors for developing active TB?

A) Renal failure.
B) Diabetes.
C) Age > 65 years.
D) HIV infection.
E) All of the above.

Discussion

The correct answer is E. Risk factors associated with developing active TB include advancing age, immunocompromised state including immunosuppressive drugs, and comorbid illnesses such as renal failure and diabetes mellitus. Additional risk factors include low socioeconomic status, smoking, and migration from an area with high prevalence of TB.

* *

The patient's son is somewhat distraught that she has TB. He asks if she should have received a vaccine before coming into this nursing home.

Regarding the bacillus Calmette-Guérin (BCG) vaccine, which of the following statements is true?

A) Foreign-born individuals who received the BCG vaccine should never have a PPD administered.
B) The BCG vaccine is most efficacious for older adults, and children benefit much less from the vaccine.

C) A PPD in an individual with a remote history of BCG vaccine, but no skin test following vaccine administration, should be interpreted as if the BCG had not been given.

D) The BCG vaccine is made from killed *Mycobacterium tuberculosis*.

Discussion

The correct answer is C. The PPD should be interpreted the same way in those who have and those who have not had BCG. Answer D is incorrect. The BCG vaccine is made from attenuated *Mycobacterium bovis*. Answer B is incorrect. BCG is most efficacious in children but protection from the vaccine wanes over several years. Even in children, it is a poor vaccine, protecting children from TB approximately 50% of the time. Individuals vaccinated with BCG should still be evaluated by PPD (if appropriate), and an increase in induration >10 mm (<35 years) or >15 mm (>35 years) from baseline is considered positive.

* *

Prior to starting INH, you measured the patient's aminotransferase levels, which were normal. Now, 3 months into treatment, her alanine aminotransferase (ALT) is 42 IU/L (about twice the upper limit of normal).

Your next step is to:

A) Stop her INH since she has had a few months of treatment.

B) Continue the INH as scheduled and follow up with clinical and laboratory monitoring.

C) Switch to rifampin and pyrazinamide.

D) Refer her to a hepatologist for liver biopsy.

E) Start her on milk thistle.

Discussion

The correct answer is B. While liver injury is a significant problem with isoniazid, the drug need not be stopped unless the liver enzymes rise to >3 times the upper limit of normal. Others would suggest that even then the drug can be continued and that only signs and symptoms of hepatitis (fatigue, anorexia, nausea, and vomiting) along with further liver enzyme elevations should prompt discontinuation of the drug. Answer A is incorrect because she should have 9 months of prophylactic therapy. Answer C is incorrect because rifampin and pyrazinamide have potentially more hepatotoxicity than INH! Answers D and E are

incorrect. Neither liver biopsy nor milk thistle (touted for its benefit in liver disease) is likely to be useful.

* *

In an odd turn of events, you learn that your patient did a little time in a Russian prison in the 1980s. She mentioned something about a misunderstanding with the KGB. You ponder the problem of drug-resistant TB and are relieved that she does not have active TB.

A major factor in the development and spread of drug-resistant TB is:

A) Poor hand hygiene.

B) Inadequate treatment regimens.

C) Rats, mice, and other rodents.

D) Advancing age.

Discussion

The correct answer is B. A major factor in the emergence and spread of drug-resistant TB is inadequate treatment of active TB, either through noncompliance or inappropriate treatment regimens. The incidence of drug-resistant TB has been declining in the United States but is increasing elsewhere in the world. Answer C is incorrect. Transmission of TB from animals is not an issue in the United States although *Mycobacterium bovis* was a common infection transmitted by cow's milk in the past. Answer D is incorrect. Older patients often have reactivation of previous TB infection or activation of latent TB infection from many years ago, and as such they are less likely to have been exposed to partial or inadequate drug therapy.

 HELPFUL TIP: There is drug-resistant TB, multidrug-resistant TB (MDR-TB), and extensively drug-resistant TB (XDR-TB). The differences among them are:

Drug-resistant TB is resistant to one of the first-line drugs (INH, rifampin, ethambutol, streptomycin, pyrazinamide).

MDR-TB is resistant to at least INH and rifampin and possibly more drugs.

XDR-TB is resistant to at least INH, rifampin, fluoroquinolones, and aminoglycosides or capreomycin or both.

Objectives: Did you learn to . . .

- Distinguish between asymptomatic bacteriuria and symptomatic urinary tract infection in terms of diagnosis and treatment?
- Interpret tuberculin skin test results?
- Describe the BCG vaccine and how patients who receive it should be approached?
- Recommend appropriate treatment for a positive PPD?
- Recognize complications of isoniazid therapy?
- Define and recognize the importance of drug-resistant TB?

CASE 5

A 37-year-old female with a history of mitral valve prolapse and mitral regurgitation presents for evaluation. She reports no symptoms of shortness of breath or exercise intolerance. In the next year she plans to undergo health-screening procedures, including dental exams for routine cleaning and filling of several caries, pelvic exam with removal of an intrauterine device (IUD), and colonoscopy.

According to the American Heart Association (AHA) 2007 Guidelines on the Prevention of Infective Endocarditis, what should she receive prior to these procedures?

A) Amoxicillin 2 g PO.
B) Azithromycin 500 mg PO.
C) Clindamycin 600 mg PO.
D) Nothing.

Discussion

The correct answer is D. In 2007 there were major changes to the AHA guidelines on infective endocarditis prevention. The one change that would seem to affect the greatest number of patients in primary care practices is the downgrading of mitral valve prolapse with regurgitation, which is no longer considered a high-risk condition. If the patient had a condition for which prophylaxis was warranted, the other regimens (Answers A, B, and C) are options depending on the patient's allergies, etc.

* *

According to the AHA 2007 Guidelines on the Prevention of Infective Endocarditis, which of the following conditions is NOT a high-risk

condition for the adverse outcome of infective endocarditis?

A) Bioprosthetic aortic valve.
B) Mechanical aortic valve.
C) Congenital heart disease completely repaired with prosthetic material.
D) Bicuspid aortic valve.
E) Previous history of infective endocarditis.

Discussion

The correct answer is D. The 2007 AHA guidelines recommend antibiotic prophylaxis for conditions considered to be high risk for adverse outcomes of infective endocarditis. High-risk conditions include prosthetic valves (bioprosthetic homograft and allograft valves and mechanical valves), previous infective endocarditis, and complex cyanotic congenital heart disease.

 HELPFUL TIP: Moderate-risk conditions for which prophylaxis is **not** indicated include acquired valvular dysfunction, such as rheumatic heart disease, hypertrophic cardiomyopathy, bicuspid aortic valve, and mitral valve prolapse with auscultatory evidence of valvular regurgitation and/or thickened leaflets.

 HELPFUL TIP: Infective endocarditis is more likely to result from transient bacteremia that occurs with routine dental care at home (eg, brushing and flossing) than from dental, GI, and GU procedures. Good oral hygiene to lower the risk of bacteremia is more important than prophylactic antibiotics.

If the patient has a mechanical aortic valve, appropriate endocarditis prophylaxis includes:

A) Ampicillin IV 2 hours prior to **colonoscopy** if biopsy of lesions is anticipated.
B) Ampicillin IV 2 hours prior to **pelvic exam and IUD removal**.
C) Amoxicillin PO 2 hours prior to routine dental **cleaning**.
D) Amoxicillin PO 2 hours prior to any **injection of local anesthesia and filling of caries**.
E) All of the above.

Discussion

The correct answer is C. For high-risk conditions (eg, mechanical aortic valve), antibiotic prophylaxis is recommended by the AHA prior to cleaning of teeth and removal of plaque. The risk of endocarditis is highest for dental procedures that might traumatize the oral mucosa, such as tooth extractions, periodontal procedures, and cleaning of teeth with removal of adherent plaque. Answers A, B, and D are incorrect. Prophylaxis is not recommended prior to these procedures. The risk of endocarditis is low for procedures such as lower GI endoscopy and pelvic exam with IUD removal because the microorganisms likely to cause transient bacteremia following these interventions are not capable of adhering to cardiac valve tissues. Antibiotic prophylaxis is not recommended for restorative dental procedures (eg, fillings).

* *

All of the evaluations, including the dental exam, seem to go well. However, 1 month later, she returns to see you for gradually worsening fever, malaise, and night sweats. You are concerned that she may have developed infective endocarditis.

The evaluation of a patient suspected of having subacute bacterial endocarditis includes all of the following EXCEPT:

A) Three sets of blood cultures obtained at 1-hour intervals within the first 24 hours of assessment.
B) Auscultation of chest for evidence of new or changing murmur.
C) Transthoracic or transesophageal echocardiogram.
D) Spiral chest CT.
E) Electrocardiogram.

Discussion

The correct answer is D. Spiral chest CT is not indicated in the diagnosis of subacute bacterial endocarditis. History is important because onset of infection can sometimes be related to a recent dental extraction, IV drug abuse, or invasive medical procedure. Symptoms generally begin insidiously and may include weakness, fatigue, fever, night sweats, arthralgias/myalgias, and hematuria. Echocardiography (answer C) is indicated. The yield for visualization of vegetations for transthoracic echocardiography is 60%–77% and increases to 96% with transesophageal echocardiography. A prolongation of the PR interval on an electrocardiogram (answer E) may suggest involvement of the cardiac conduction system and abscess.

* *

You examine the patient carefully and find that she is febrile and slightly tachycardic.

You look for signs of infective endocarditis, focusing on all of the following EXCEPT:

A) Osler nodes.
B) Painless erythematous macules on the palms and soles.
C) Splinter hemorrhages.
D) Painless nodules over bony prominences.
E) Roth spots.

Discussion

The correct answer is D. Physical exam findings of endocarditis include intermittent fever; petechiae; conjunctival hemorrhage; splinter hemorrhages under the nails; erythematous painful nodules on the fingers, palms, and soles (Osler nodes); fundic hemorrhages (Roth spots); painless erythematous macules on the palms and soles (Janeway lesions); and new diastolic murmur. Answer D is not a physical exam finding in infective endocarditis. Painless nodules over bony prominences are observed in rheumatic fever and are one of the Jones criteria.

 HELPFUL TIP: Laboratory evaluation in endocarditis may be remarkable for anemia, leukocytosis, elevated erythrocyte sedimentation rate, and microscopic hematuria.

Which of the following is (are) included in the major criteria of the modified Duke criteria for endocarditis?

A) Positive blood cultures.
B) Janeway lesions (painless macules on palms and soles).
C) Echocardiographic evidence of valvular vegetation.
D) A and B.
E) A and C.

Discussion

The correct answer is E. The modified Duke criteria were developed to provide clinicians with standardized criteria for the diagnosis of endocarditis. They have been validated by pathologic examination and are more sensitive than other endocarditis criteria systems (Table 8–2).

Table 8–2 DUKE CRITERIA FOR BACTERIAL ENDOCARDITIS

Definite endocarditis is established by the presence of 2 major criteria and at least 1 minor criterion. Probable endocarditis is established by the presence of 1 major and 1 minor criterion, or 3 minor criteria.

Major Duke criteria	New valvular regurgitation Echocardiographic evidence of vegetations 2 positive blood cultures of an organism known to cause endocarditis Single blood culture or antibody evidence of *Coxiella burnetti* (Q fever)
Minor Duke criteria (not an exhaustive list but the most common manifestations)	Fever Vascular phenomena (eg, Janeway lesions, splinter or conjunctival hemorrhages, septic emboli) History of predisposing illness (eg, IV drug abuse, heart lesion, artificial valve) Immunologic phenomena (eg, glomerulonephritis, Osler's nodes)

 HELPFUL TIP: Remember this about blood cultures—more is better. The sensitivity of blood cultures for endocarditis and bacteremia is directly related to the **amount** of blood taken for culture and the number of cultures drawn. Three sets of blood cultures are recommended for suspected endocarditis, and at least 20 mL should be drawn for each culture. Timing of blood cultures is less important, but sick patients should have the cultures drawn in rapid succession (eg, over 1 or 2 hours).

* *

You draw a CBC, which shows leukocytosis with a left shift. Chest x-ray and urinalysis are unrevealing. You draw blood cultures and admit her to the hospital and start antibiotics. The next morning, 2 blood cultures are reported to grow Gram-positive cocci in clusters. You start IV vancomycin and order a transesophageal echocardiogram. The echocardiogram shows a small vegetation on her mitral valve. Blood cultures return showing methicillin-sensitive *Staphylococcus aureus*.

What is the most appropriate treatment for this patient now?

A) Nafcillin 2 g IV q 4 hours for 4–6 weeks.
B) Penicillin G 2 million units IV q 2 hours for 4–6 weeks.
C) Vancomycin 1 gram IV q 12 hours for 1 week.
D) Ceftriaxone 1 gram IV q 24 hours for 2 weeks.
E) Levofloxacin 500 mg IV q 24 hours for 4–6 weeks.

Discussion

The correct answer is A. Nafcillin is the drug of choice for the treatment of methicillin-sensitive *S. aureus* endocarditis. Answer C is incorrect. Vancomycin should be reserved for patients with penicillin allergy or patients with methicillin-**resistant** *S. aureus*. This answer is also incorrect because the duration of 1 week is inadequate treatment for endocarditis. Neither ceftriaxone (answer D) nor levofloxacin (answer E) is appropriate therapy for staphylococcal endocarditis.

 HELPFUL TIP: **Patients who have a sensitive organism do better with nafcillin than with vancomycin.** Save vancomycin for MRSA or other resistant organisms.

* *

While hospitalized, the patient develops symptoms of heart failure and worsening mitral regurgitation by echocardiogram. The heart failure is managed medically, but the regurgitation is now categorized as "severe." She has had 3 days of antibiotics.

Which of the following is the most appropriate course of action?

A) Complete 6 weeks of antibiotics and manage her heart failure medically for the foreseeable future.
B) Complete 6 weeks of antibiotics and manage her heart failure medically; plan for valve replacement after 6 weeks of antibiotics.
C) Refer her for emergent valve replacement surgery.
D) Refer her for immediate coronary catheterization.
E) None of the above.

Discussion

The correct answer is B. Progressive heart failure and worsening valvular function are indications for surgery. It is generally preferable to complete the course of antibiotics first if the patient's heart failure can be medically managed. Thus, answer C is incorrect. Answer D is incorrect, because there is no indication for coronary catheterization.

 HELPFUL TIP: Other indications for surgery in cases of endocarditis include: multiple embolic events, infections that are difficult or impossible to treat adequately with medications (eg, fungal infections), cardiac conduction abnormalities caused by infection, persistent bacteremia, partially dehisced prosthetic valve, and perivalvular infection (eg, cardiac abscess, fistula).

Which of the following organisms is MOST LIKELY to cause infective endocarditis?

A) *Escherichia coli.*
B) *Streptococcus viridans.*
C) *Proteus mirabilis.*
D) None of the above.

Discussion

The correct answer is B. *Streptococcus viridans* is the most likely organism to cause endocarditis. Organisms typically found causing endocarditis are *S. aureus*, *Streptococcus viridans*, enterococci (aerobic, Gram-positive organisms in chains that are GI or vaginal flora), *Streptococcus bovis*, and HACEK organisms (*Haemophilus* species, *Actinobacillus actinomycete comitantes*, *Cardiobacterium hominis*, *Eikenella* species, and *Kingella kingae*). Gram-negative organisms, such as *E. coli* and *P. mirabilis*, are infrequent causes of infective endocarditis.

Objectives: Did you learn to . . .

• Determine who is an appropriate candidate for infective endocarditis prophylaxis?
• Recognize signs and symptoms of infective endocarditis?
• Diagnose infective endocarditis?
• Prescribe appropriate treatment for infective endocarditis?

CASE 6

A 10-year-old child presents with complaints of intense itching, worse at night, since the first week of school.

He has numerous excoriations in the interdigital web spaces, wrists, and anterior axillary folds. His infant sister has recently developed intensely pruritic linear lesions on her palms, soles, face, and scalp. Their mother works in a nursing home and has developed pruritus and reddish-brown nodular lesions in her axillae and perineum that have persisted several months after she treated herself with a lotion that was provided at her place of work.

The most likely ectoparasite affecting this family is:

A) Head lice (pediculosis).
B) Chiggers (mites).
C) Ticks.
D) Fleas.
E) Scabies.

Discussion

The correct answer is E. Scabies' mites (*Sarcoptes scabiei*) burrow into the epidermis, lay eggs, and hatch larvae in cycles of 3–4 days. The most notable clinical symptom is intense pruritus that is worse at night. The typical lesion is small, erythematous, and papular and may resemble eczema in quality and distribution. Approximately 7% of individuals develop a nodular variant (like the mother in this case). Transmission is typically by direct contact and infestations may appear as epidemics in institutions like nursing homes. The organism may be spread by fomites as well, although to a lesser extent. Young children and infants often have involvement of palms, soles, face, and scalp. A clinical diagnosis may be made in the setting of pruritic rash, typical distribution, and multiple family members affected.

What is the next best step in this case?

A) Removal of the individual organisms.
B) Tetracycline 10 mg/kg divided TID for all affected family members.
C) Single-dose oral ivermectin 200 micrograms/kg, repeated in 2 weeks for all affected family members.
D) Symptomatic treatment with topical steroids and oral antihistamines.
E) Single-dose oral ivermectin 200 micrograms/kg repeated in 2 weeks for the mother; one application of 5% permethrin cream for all other family members for 8–14 hours, followed by showering.

Discussion

The correct answer is E. Permethrin cream is the topical medication of choice, but the failure rate is high. Answer B is incorrect because tetracycline is not helpful in this situation and should be avoided in children. Answer C is incorrect because oral ivermectin should be avoided in infants (<15 kg) due to concerns about increased penetration of the blood-brain barrier. Ivermectin, an antihelmintic medication, is indicated for adults with nodular disease (like the mother in this case), in epidemic settings, and for treatment of scabies crustosa. Answer D is incorrect because scabies should be treated with specific therapy rather than simply symptomatic therapy.

> **HELPFUL TIP:** All family members should be treated, regardless of the presence or lack of symptoms. Microscopic exam of a skin scraping may identify the mite but has poor sensitivity. Other viable treatment alternatives include crotamiton 10% solution, precipitated sulfur in petroleum, and lindane (avoid lindane in children <2 years).

* *

You successfully treated the whole family. They are now comfortable, happy, and confident in your abilities. The mother returns with her daughter, who is now 3 years old, with a new complaint. The child has complained of her "bottom" hurting, a symptom that her mother has interpreted to mean perineal pain. The pain is worse at night and the child has awakened several nights complaining of vaginal pain. The mother thinks that she may have a bladder infection, but there are no urinary symptoms. In the office, the patient complains only of "itchy butt" and her exam is normal.

What is the next best step in diagnosis of this problem?

A) Reassurance that this is "just a stage."
B) Vaginal speculum exam with cultures.
C) "Scotch tape" test.
D) Stool collection for ova and parasites.
E) Referral to a pediatric behavioral disorders specialist.

Discussion

The correct answer is C. The presentation is consistent with pinworm (*Enterobius vermicularis*) infection.

Clinical manifestations of pinworm infection are related to the life cycle of the parasite, in which the adult worm resides in the colon, exits the anus at night, lays eggs in the perianal skin, and may also infest the female genitourinary tract. Typical symptoms include pruritus ani, vulvitis, vaginal pain, poor sleep, and—rarely—abdominal pain. The diagnostic test of choice is the "Scotch tape" test. Clear cellophane tape is wrapped around a tongue depressor, sticky side up, and used to sample the perianal area first thing in the morning before bathing. Multiple specimens should be obtained and stored in a refrigerator (good thing OSHA has no jurisdiction in the home). The tape is then examined microscopically for the characteristic ova.

* *

Your "Scotch tape" test is a success, proving your clinical suspicions.

The best intervention is to:

A) Treat the patient with mebendazole 100 mg PO once, repeat in 2 weeks, and encourage good hand-washing for the whole family.
B) Treat the patient and the entire family with mebendazole 100 mg PO daily for 14 days.
C) Treat the patient and the entire family with mebendazole 100 mg PO once, and repeat in 2 weeks.
D) Treat the patient with metronidazole 500 mg PO once, and repeat in 2 weeks.

Discussion

The correct answer is C. As with scabies, the entire family should be treated. Mebendazole is the agent of choice, although other antiparasitic agents may also be used. Metronidazole (answer D) is not used for helminthic infections but is effective against protozoal infections, including amebiasis and trichomoniasis.

Objectives: Did you learn to . . .

- Diagnose and treat scabies infestations?
- Diagnose and treat pinworm infections?

 QUICK QUIZ: FEVER

A 54-year-old construction worker with no significant travel history presents with a fever. He developed the fever 4 weeks ago **and has been febrile each day**

since. He saw another doctor recently. He was evaluated but received no antibiotics or other treatment. His evaluation, including history, physical exam, CBC with differential, urinalysis, serum chemistries, and chest x-ray, has been unrevealing. Today his temperature is 38.5°C.

What tests should be included in the MINIMUM evaluation of this patient's fever?

A) ESR, rheumatoid factor, ANA, tuberculin skin test, blood cultures, abdominal CT scan.

B) Lumbar puncture, chest CT scan, colonoscopy, PSA.

C) Bone scan, urine culture, blood cultures, chest CT scan.

D) Abdominal CT scan, blood cultures, PSA, stool cultures.

E) Blood cultures, urine culture, spinal fluid culture, stool culture.

Discussion

The correct answer is A. This patient has a fever of unknown origin (FUO). FUO in adults is defined as fever >38.3°C of at least 3 weeks' duration with no obvious cause despite extensive evaluation. In older adults, collagen-vascular diseases, such as giant cell arteritis and rheumatoid arthritis, are more likely sources of FUO; thus, rheumatologic tests are appropriate. Infections are the most common source of FUO in children and young adults. The most common infections include TB and abscesses. The abdominal CT scan is to evaluate for occult abscess and malignancy.

> **HELPFUL TIP:** The most common malignancies to present with FUO are lymphoma, leukemia, renal cell carcinoma, and hepatoma. A CT scan of the abdomen should detect these, except leukemia. Table 8–3 lists causes of FUO.

CASE 7

A 45-year-old male physician who has returned from an early summer fishing vacation in rural North Carolina presents for a febrile illness. He reports a 5-day history of fever, malaise, headache, and vomiting. Today he has developed a nonpruritic rash that began on his extremities and has spread to his body. On exam he has a fever of 38.3°C with a pulse of 120 and otherwise normal vitals. The rash is maculopapular and generalized, involving his palms and soles. Oral mucosa is dry but intact, and the exam is otherwise nonspecific.

Table 8–3 PARTIAL LIST OF ETIOLOGIES OF FUO

Infections
- TB
- Lyme disease
- HIV
- Endocarditis
- Dental abscess
- Abdominal/pelvic abscess
- CMV
- Epstein-Barr virus

Malignancies
- Metastatic cancer
- Lymphoma
- Leukemias
- Renal cell carcinoma

Autoimmune Conditions
- Polymyalgia rheumatica
- Rheumatoid arthritis
- Inflammatory bowel disease
- Lupus
- Vasculitides

Drug-induced Fever

Factitious Fever

Venous Thrombosis

Sarcoidosis

What is the most appropriate next step?

A) Reassurance and symptomatic treatment.

B) CBC, electrolytes, BUN, creatinine.

C) Blood cultures.

D) Dermatology referral.

E) Admission to the ICU.

Discussion

The correct answer is B. This man is sick (pulse of 120, dry oral mucosa, headache, vomiting). A CBC and electrolytes may give us an indication of the degree of dehydration and help us narrow the differential (bacterial versus viral, etc).

We would be amiss to reassure or refer this patient (answer A). Blood cultures (answer C) may be useful but the results will be delayed.

* *

The test results return quickly. CBC shows mild thrombocytopenia but is normal otherwise. BUN and creatinine are at the upper limits of normal, and the electrolytes are normal.

The most likely diagnosis is:

A) Chicken pox.
B) Syphilis.
C) Parvovirus B19.
D) Rocky Mountain spotted fever.
E) Human monocytic ehrlichiosis.

Discussion

The correct answer is D. Rocky Mountain spotted fever (RMSF) is a tick-borne (dog or wood tick) disease caused by *Rickettsia rickettsii*. It presents with a prodrome of fever and headache several days before the onset of the characteristic rash—a maculopapular eruption that begins at the wrists and ankles and spreads centrally. Despite its name, RMSF is endemic in the southeastern United States, the Atlantic states, and the northern Rocky Mountains. Laboratory manifestations of RMSF are generally nonspecific: mild thrombocytopenia (rarely becoming severe), hyponatremia, azotemia, elevated transaminases, and prolonged PTT and PT.

Answer B is incorrect because the secondary stage of syphilis is characterized by a generalized maculopapular rash, which affects the palms and soles, and is **not** associated with systemic symptoms. Answer E is incorrect. Human monocytic ehrlichiosis is caused by *Ehrlichia chaffeensis* and presents with a fever and nonspecific flu like symptoms (headache, fever, myalgias, chills, cough).

Rarely a rash, maculopapular or petechial, is seen. Thus, it may be easily confused with RMSF. Patients are often leukopenic and thrombocytopenic. If you think you have a case of RMSF but there is no rash, consider human monocytic ehrlichiosis (sometimes called "Rocky mountain **spotless** fever") (Table 8–4).

What is the appropriate next step for this patient?

A) Obtain serologic studies and await results while treating symptomatically.
B) Obtain skin biopsy and await results while treating symptomatically.
C) Obtain serologic studies and start doxycycline 100 mg PO BID.
D) Obtain skin biopsy and start levofloxacin 500 mg PO daily.
E) Hospitalize and start ceftriaxone 1 g IV daily until fever has resolved.

Discussion

The answer is C. Early treatment is essential. Individuals treated after 5 days of symptoms have poorer outcomes than those treated earlier. Awaiting serologic studies is inappropriate and treatment should not be delayed. The drug of choice in the treatment of RMSF is doxycycline 100 mg PO BID for 14 days. **This is true for children as well.** Pregnant women should be

Table 8–4 TICK-BORNE ILLNESSES

Disease	Etiologic Agent	Geographic Distribution	Clinical Findings
Babesiosis	*Babesia* species	New England, upper Midwest, California	Fever, sweats, myalgias, arthralgias, red urine, hemolytic anemia (most severe cases occur in splenectomized patients); similar to malaria in that there are periodic fever spikes
Human monocytic ehrlichiosis	*Ehrlichia chaffeensis* and *ewingii*	South, Midwest	Fever, headache, myalgias (similar to RMSF but no rarely a rash)
Lyme disease	*Borrelia burgdorferi*	Northeast, upper Midwest	Erythema migrans, myalgias, arthralgias, arthritis, fever, headache
RMSF	*Rickettsia rickettsii*	Southeast, Atlantic coast states	Fever, headache, GI symptoms, maculopapular rash, myalgias
Tularemia	*Francisella tularensis*	South, Midwest	Fever, headache, cough, myalgias, GI symptoms, tender lymphadenopathy with rare skin ulceration

treated with chloramphenicol. Agents such as penicillin, fluoroquinolones, and cephalosporins are inappropriate in this situation.

Objectives: Did you learn to ...

- Identify and diagnose Rocky Mountain spotted fever?
- Initiate treatment of Rocky Mountain spotted fever?
- Recognize other tick-borne illnesses?

 QUICK QUIZ: HAND INFECTIONS

A 27-year-old male carpenter presents with pain, redness, and swelling of the distal aspect of the right index finger. He reports getting a splinter in the site 2 days ago while working. The pain is now so severe that he cannot work. On examination, the patient is afebrile. The right index fingertip is extremely tender, and there is an area of fluctuance at the palmar aspect of the finger. All of the redness and warmth are distal to the proximal interphalangeal joint.

What is the most appropriate diagnosis?

A) Paronychia.
B) Felon.
C) Whitlow lesion.
D) Tenosynovitis.

Discussion

The correct answer is B. A felon is an abscess of the distal fingertip, most commonly occurring in the index finger and thumb. It can be distinguished from paronychia (answer A) because a felon is located in the fat pad of the finger and not the tissue around the nail. Often, an area of fluctuance is palpable. A felon can spread quickly and can involve the periosteum and bone. Appropriate management includes x-ray of the finger (to rule out osteomyelitis), antibiotics, and incision and drainage. Answer C is incorrect because a whitlow lesion results from inoculation of broken skin of the hand with type 1 or 2 herpes simplex virus. The whitlow lesion is often typical of herpes (vesicles on erythematous papules) but can also be confused with paronychia or felon if at the distal finger. Answer D is incorrect. Tenosynovitis should not involve the distal aspect of the digit without affecting the rest of the tendon sheath.

CASE 8

The Smith family presents to your office in December seeking travel vaccines for a trip to Nigeria. John (34) and Jane (35) Smith have two children, Jack (7) and Jill (5). They will be in Nigeria for a month and will be living in a suburb of Lagos, Nigeria's largest city, and expect to take sightseeing trips into less developed areas. John has no previous medical problems. Jane is currently taking venlafaxine (Effexor) for depression and is known to have a sulfa allergy. Jack has had occasional bouts of reactive airway disease and also has a sulfa allergy. Jill is healthy. Everyone in the family is up to date on all routine North American vaccines.

Which of the following parasitic organisms will they NOT be at risk to contract?

A) *Plasmodium ovale.*
B) *Plasmodium falciparum.*
C) Dengue fever.
D) *Entamoeba histolytica.*

Discussion

The correct answer is C. Dengue fever (aka "break bone" fever) is a viral infection cause by Flavivirus. It is most common in Asia but also occurs in Africa. Patients typically present with fever, headache, retro-orbital pain, leukopenia, and thrombocytopenia. The sine qua non of "break bone fever" is severe myalgias and arthralgias, hence the name "break bone fever." More mild forms do occur without the severe myalgias, etc. Generally, Dengue fever is self-limited unless the patient develops hemorrhagic complications which may be fatal. *Plasmodium falciparum* (answer A) and *P. ovale* (answer B) are two species of malaria parasites. *P. falciparum* tends to produce more severe infections that can be rapidly fatal in patients naive to malaria. *E. histolytica* (answer D) is the intestinal protozoan parasite responsible for amebiasis.

* *

You provide the Smith family with general information on health risks they might face during their stay in Nigeria.

Regarding the prevention of bites from potentially infectious mosquitoes and other insects, you tell them that:

A) Bed nets add little additional protection.
B) Bed nets are essential and should be used by the whole family.
C) Bed nets are useful, but quickly degrade when coated with the insecticide permethrin.

D) Bed nets are useful against large insects such as tsetse flies, but the tiny mosquitoes of West Africa can easily penetrate most netting.
E) The use of bed nets makes insect repellent and window screens obsolete.

Discussion

The correct answer is B. Bed nets clearly reduce morbidity and mortality from insect-borne disease, and well-maintained nets are effective against any insect species. Bed nets are more effective when coated with the topical insecticide permethrin. While effective, bed nets are meant to be used in addition to other antiinsect measures, such as screens on windows and doors and repellent applied to the skin.

* *

Mr. Smith asks for advice on the use of insect repellent.

What do you recommend?

A) Any repellent will do. Just use the cheapest.
B) Pleasant-smelling repellents, such as Avon Skin-So-Soft, are as effective as any DEET-containing formulation.
C) Use repellent with DEET concentrations of at least 50% for the children since their protection is so vital.
D) The addition of permethrin insecticide applied to the skin will enhance any other repellent's efficacy.
E) DEET-containing and Picaridin repellents are safe and are the most efficacious insect repellents available, but avoid DEET concentrations >30% in children.

Discussion

The correct answer is E. Repeated experiments clearly show DEET and Picaridin-containing repellents to be the most effective for deterring insect bites and these are the two recommended by the CDC. Picaridin-containing insect repellents do not cause neurotoxicity. Answer C is incorrect. The American Academy of Pediatrics recommends ≤30% DEET for use in children, due to a slight risk of toxicity seen in frequent applications over a long period of time. Answer D is incorrect. DEET should be applied to clothing rather than to skin in order to reduce the risk of toxicity. Adults can use any concentration, but 30% is usually sufficient for most situations. Answer B is incorrect. Avon brand Skin-So-Soft is a more cosmetically pleasing product, but controlled experiments show that the

effect against mosquitoes lasts a mere fraction of the duration of DEET compounds. Permethrin insecticide, when applied to clothes, tents, and bed nets, is synergistic with insect repellent, but permethrin itself is not formulated for use as an insect repellent on skin.

 HELPFUL TIP: Picaridin, which is now available in the United States, was developed in the 1980s and is as, or more, effective than DEET. It is recommended by both the World Health Organization and the CDC to prevent mosquito-borne diseases, including malaria.

* *

Mrs. Smith reports that her friends get sick with diarrhea every time they travel abroad. She would like to prevent this.

Which of the following is (are) true about traveler's diarrhea?

A) Enterotoxigenic *E. coli* (ETEC) is the most common cause of this condition.
B) Even carefully avoiding the consumption of tap water or unwashed vegetables may not be sufficient to prevent the disease.
C) Fluoroquinolones can help to cure this condition rapidly but are contraindicated in pregnancy and young children.
D) The use of loperamide is effective in reducing the duration of symptoms but is contraindicated in children <2 years.
E) All of the above are true.

Discussion

The correct answer is E. In most parts of the world, including Africa, ETEC is the most common cause of traveler's diarrhea. Although it is advisable to avoid tap water, unwashed foods, and raw foods, these measures are usually insufficient to completely eliminate the risk of contracting the disease. A traveler may drink only bottled liquids, but might forget that the ice in the glass is made from tap water. Although the disease is self-limited, a single dose of ciprofloxacin 750 mg will usually significantly shorten the course of symptoms. A patient's symptoms can be further shortened by adding loperamide, which is safe in the absence of bloody stools (dysentery). Loperamide is potentially toxic to infants and toddlers.

HELPFUL TIP: The answer for the board examination is: Use a fluoroquinolone for traveler's diarrhea. **The CDC no longer recommends fluoroquinolones for traveler's diarrhea because of resistance. The current recommendation is to use azithromycin for traveler's diarrhea.**

* *

The children in the family have been immunized against hepatitis B, but the parents have not. The parents start the vaccine series for hepatitis B, and everyone gets hepatitis A and yellow fever vaccines.

Which other region-specific vaccine(s) should be provided?

A) Dengue fever.
B) Cholera.
C) Japanese encephalitis.
D) Meningococcus.
E) All of the above.

Discussion

The correct answer is D. Nigeria is located in the heart of the "meningitis belt," a collection of countries in central and western Africa prone to seasonal epidemics of meningococcal meningitis. These epidemics may affect thousands and usually occur during the dry season, from January to April. Japanese encephalitis, a mosquito-borne disease similar to West Nile virus, occurs only in parts of Southeast Asia and China, and the vaccine is not necessary for travel to Africa. There are no licensed cholera or dengue fever vaccines in the United States. Typhoid vaccine would also be indicated for travel to Nigeria.

HELPFUL TIP: The CDC maintains a user-friendly and up-to-date travel Web site at http://wwwn.cdc.gov/travel/default.aspx. Always check here first to ensure you are giving the right vaccines.

* *

Finally, you discuss the medication options for malaria prophylaxis.

Which of the following is true?

A) Mefloquine (Larium) is relatively contraindicated for Jane due to her history of psychiatric illness.

B) Doxycycline would be a safe and effective option for the whole family.
C) Although malaria is resistant to chloroquine in many parts of the world, it can still be used for prophylaxis in West Africa.
D) Atovaquone/proguanil (Malarone) is contraindicated for Jane and Jack due to their sulfa allergy.
E) A month is too long a time to use malaria prophylaxis safely; recommend against it.

Discussion

The correct answer is A. Mefloquine is an effective, once-a-week prophylaxis for malaria. However, it carries a significant risk of CNS side effects, including vivid or disturbing dreams. There have been case reports of the medication inducing psychosis, therefore the drug is relatively contraindicated for patients with a history of psychiatric illness (such as Jane Smith). Doxycycline (answer B) may be a good option for the parents, but is contraindicated in children because of their age and risk of tooth discoloration. Answer C is incorrect. Malaria throughout Africa, India, Southeast Asia, and South America is now assumed to be resistant to chloroquine. Atovaquone/proguanil (answer D) is relatively contraindicated in patients with G6PD-deficiency due to a risk of hemolysis, but it does not contain sulfa. One month is a reasonable duration of therapy for malaria prophylaxis. When taking longer courses ($\geq$6–12 months), the side effects of the medications may outweigh the benefits. In the case of chloroquine, irreversible retinal toxicity may occur.

* *

The Smith family thanks you for your help and leaves for Africa. Two weeks into their trip, Mrs. Smith calls you from Nigeria with the news that Jack (7) has fallen ill with a febrile illness. He has a mild cough and abdominal pain but no vomiting, diarrhea, or rash. He has had cyclic fevers and significant headache. She says that she knows of a medical clinic there with an American doctor, but they rely on local medications. You remind her that it is very difficult to diagnose Jack over the phone.

What is your advice?

A) His illness is most likely a viral syndrome; treat him with oral fluids and acetaminophen.
B) He cannot have malaria, as he has not been in Africa long enough.
C) Avoid local health care at all costs; they cannot treat this problem.

D) Seek local health care, but remind her that Jack is likely allergic to sulfadoxine-pyrimethamine (Fansidar), a common local therapy for malaria.

E) Even if Jack has malaria, he will likely recover with symptomatic therapy only.

Discussion

The correct answer is D. Although Jack may have any viral illness, the most likely diagnosis is malaria. The incubation period for malaria is 7–10 days, so 2 weeks is a long enough exposure to contract the disease. Malaria is so common in sub-Saharan Africa that in many places the word for fever is the same as the word for malaria. Local physicians have extensive experience treating it, and local medical care should be the first course of action. The first-line drug given locally will often be sulfadoxine-pyrimethamine (Fansidar), but this contains sulfa and would be contraindicated for Jack.

 HELPFUL TIP: Although malaria may be benign for an adult living in Africa who has had it multiple times, it can be fatal rapidly in young children and visitors who have never experienced malaria and thus have no immunity.

* *

Weeks pass, and you hear nothing more until you are called to the acute care clinic, where Jack Smith has been brought in by his parents for fever and lethargy. Jack had been treated in Lagos, Nigeria, for his previous febrile illness with an unknown medication, and he subsequently recovered. The Smith family completed their stay in Africa, and then returned home. Jack was apparently well until 10 days after returning home, when he developed rapid onset of a fever and shaking chills. He also had complaints of generalized abdominal pain and watery, nonbloody diarrhea. The parents treated him at home for a day with ibuprofen and acetaminophen, but he seemed to worsen. He became lethargic, stopped drinking and eating, and the fever continued.

Upon exam, Jack appears drowsy and listless but is arousable. He does not respond to questions about current symptoms, but cooperates with an exam. Findings are: temperature 39.1°C, pulse 136, blood pressure 100/50, respiratory rate 24. His neck is supple with mild lymphadenopathy. He is tachycardic with a mild flow murmur. His abdomen is nontender with a palpable

spleen. No rash or petechiae are noted. The rest of the exam is unremarkable. A recurrence of malaria is suspected.

What is the best method for confirming this diagnosis?

A) Blood culture.

B) Malaria serology.

C) Malaria antigen test.

D) Thin and thick blood smears.

E) Stool ova and parasite.

Discussion

The correct answer is D. Malaria is usually diagnosed by blood smear. The thick blood smear is the more sensitive screening test, and the thin blood smear is used to identify the species of parasite. The antigen test (answer C) is a rapid and sensitive test that can be done in any lab (does not require the expertise associated with reading blood smears), but it lacks specificity. The blood smear (answer D) remains the gold standard. Malaria serology (answer B) and cultures (answer A) are used only in experiments and are not helpful for diagnosis of an individual patient. PCR-based testing has excellent sensitivity and specificity but is expensive and not widely available. The malaria parasite cannot be identified in stool (answer E).

* *

You begin intravenous fluids and arrange hospital admission. The relevant laboratory tests are drawn and sent, including CBC, blood cultures, tests for malaria, chemistry profile, blood type and screen, and urinalysis. A lumbar puncture is performed and the CSF is normal. In the meantime, the laboratory calls with the report that *Plasmodium falciparum* has been identified.

What antimicrobial should be chosen as initial therapy?

A) PO hydroxychloroquine (Plaquenil), since many hospitals do not stock chloroquine.

B) PO mefloquine (Larium).

C) PO quinine.

D) IV quinidine, since IV quinine is not generally available in the U.S.

E) IV atovaquone/proguanil (Malarone).

Discussion

The correct answer is D. Since this patient is ill and not tolerating oral intake, an IV route for malaria treatment is indicated. IV atovaquone/proguanil does not now exist, so the only available option is quinine. But IV quinine is not available in the United States, so its isomer, quinidine (the antiarrhythmic), is used instead. In patients from chloroquine-sensitive zones (currently Central America and the Middle East), treatment with chloroquine is acceptable. Hydroxychloroquine is an option if chloroquine is not available.

* *

Despite a frightening hospital course that included generalized seizures, hypoglycemia, hematuria, renal insufficiency, and an exchange transfusion, Jack eventually recovers completely. The Smith family thanks you for your help.

Objectives: Did you learn to . . .

- Identify important elements of a patient's travel plans and unique risks when providing counseling for overseas travel?
- Identify preventative measures for malaria, including chemoprophylaxis and insect bite avoidance?
- Diagnose traveler's diarrhea and describe its prevention and treatment?
- Recognize the signs and symptoms of malaria, describe methods of diagnosis, and initiate therapy?

 QUICK QUIZ: CRITTERS

A family comes to see you because the two children, aged 7 and 4 years, have developed itchy scalps. The parents seem unaffected. So far, they have not tried any treatments. On examination of both children, you find erythematous papules on the occiput and small white eggs firmly attached to the hair shaft about 1 cm from the scalp.

The most appropriate treatment is:

A) Application of 1% permethrin cream to all family members for 10 minutes followed by rinsing; combing out all nits with a special louse comb; and decontaminating affected garments and bed linens.

B) Elimination of animal or fomite sources of infestation and use of insect repellents.

C) Removal of any adherent organisms and doxycycline for 14 days.

D) Application of 5% permethrin cream to all family members for 8–14 hours, followed by showering.

Discussion

The correct answer is A. These are head lice. Pediculosis infestations of the hair and scalp are usually asymptomatic but can present with itching. The diagnosis is made by demonstration of the louse or nits, which fluoresce a pale blue under a Wood light. Treatment with topical agents such as permethrin cream for 2 applications and wet-combing to remove nits is recommended by the CDC. Ivermectin may be effective in cases of resistant organisms. It is reasonable to recommend washing clothing and bedclothes of an infested person, but head lice do not survive off the scalp longer than 48 hours. The other answers are treatments appropriate for chiggers (mites) and fleas (answer B); ticks (if also associated with a tick-borne illness) (answer C); scabies (answer D).

CASE 9

A 19-year-old female college student presents to student health services with "the flu." She has noted a fever of 38.9°C and myalgias. She is treated with symptomatic care and discharged back to her dormitory. Three hours later her roommate finds her lethargic and difficult to arouse, so she calls 911. On exam her blood pressure is 70/30 with a pulse of 145. Her neck is supple but she is lethargic and complaining of severe muscle aches. She denies headache. There is a fine macular rash over her abdomen.

The most important historical factor(s) in this case is (are):

A) History of splenectomy.
B) Use of tampons.
C) History of acetaminophen overdose.
D) A and B.
E) All of the above.

Discussion

The correct answer is D. Answer A is correct since patients with a splenectomy can get sick rather rapidly from pneumococci and other encapsulated bacteria. Answer B is correct because this patient may have toxic shock syndrome, which is related to the use of tampons. Answer C is incorrect for two reasons. First, shock is not a prominent feature (if it occurs at all) in acetaminophen overdose. Second, acetaminophen overdose is not associated with a rash.

* *

The patient is able to give you additional history that she does not use tampons and has not taken any medication except for occasional acetaminophen and ibuprofen in recommended doses.

On the basis of this information you decide that:

A) It is unlikely that this is toxic shock syndrome given that she does not use tampons.
B) The combination of acetaminophen and ibuprofen in this patient with the flu has led to hypotension.
C) Because she is immunocompetent and has her spleen intact, this cannot be sepsis since it started so quickly.
D) Toxic shock, a major problem in the 1980s and early 1990s, no longer occurs since the advent of less absorbent tampons.
E) None of the above.

Discussion

The correct answer is E. Answer A is incorrect because up to 50% of cases of toxic shock occur as the result of staphylococcal infections unrelated to tampons. These may be ingrown toenails, infected abrasions, etc. Answer B is incorrect. Acetaminophen and ibuprofen are frequently combined without difficulty. Answer C is incorrect. Splenectomized patients are more prone to sepsis from encapsulated organisms, but the fact that the patient has a spleen does not grant invincibility. Sepsis obviously occurs in the normal host as well. Answer D is incorrect. Although absorbent tampons are a major culprit in toxic shock syndrome, as noted above, there are other causes. Thus, toxic shock syndrome is not going away anytime soon.

The organism(s) responsible for toxic shock syndrome is (are):

A) *Staphylococcus.*
B) *Haemophilus influenzae.*
C) *Streptococcus.*
D) A and B.
E) A and C.

Discussion

The correct answer is E. There are two types of toxic shock syndrome, one caused by *Staphylococcus* and the other by *Streptococcus*. There are subtypes that make the toxin responsible for toxic shock syndrome. Not all strains of these bacteria make the toxins (called exotoxins), and only certain hosts are thought to be susceptible. Most patients with streptococcal toxic shock are bacteremic, whereas those with staphylococcal toxic shock are not.

Which of the following would you NOT expect to find on laboratory testing?

A) Creatinine of 2.0 mg/dL (normal 1 mg/dL).
B) Elevated ALT/AST.
C) Platelets of 450,000/mm³.
D) Elevated CPK.

Discussion

The correct answer is C. The platelet count should be <100,000/mm³. The other findings are representative of the multisystem dysfunction that categorizes toxic shock syndrome.

* *

Your patient is a bit more alert. A second set of vitals shows: blood pressure 72/44, pulse 140, respirations 24, temperature 39°C. Labs are pending.

What is the best next step in the care of this patient?

A) Start IV nafcillin.
B) Place two large bore IV lines and start aggressive fluid replacement.
C) Start IV dopamine.
D) Give a single dose of IV dexamethasone.
E) Transfuse 2 units of packed red cells.

Discussion

The correct answer is B. Treatment is mainly supportive. She is in shock. Two large bore IV lines should be placed with fluids running wide open, and dopamine (or other pressor) should be available if her pressure does not improve rapidly.

Answer A is of special note. Patients with classic toxic shock syndrome (staphylococcal) are not septic. Therefore, while an antistaphylococcal drug is important (as is locally treating the site of infection with incision and drainage, toenail removal, etc), the antistaphylococcal drug is not to treat sepsis. The patient should receive an antibiotic because you presume there is a localized infection somewhere. Answers D and E are incorrect because neither steroids nor blood products is currently indicated.

Objectives: Did you learn to . . .

- Identify signs and symptoms of toxic shock syndrome?
- Describe the pathophysiology of toxic shock syndrome?
- Initiate management for a patient with sepsis and toxic shock syndrome?

QUICK QUIZ: THE UNPRONOUNCEABLE DRUGS

Which of the following has been found to be useful in both Gram-positive and Gram-negative sepsis?

A) High-dose steroids.

B) Low-dose steroids.

C) Drotrecogin alfa (yes, it is alfa . . . activated protein C, Xigris).

D) Adalimumub (antitumor necrosis factor alpha, Humira).

E) Anti–Gram-negative endotoxin.

Discussion

The correct answer is C. Drotrecogin alfa is useful in sepsis and is likely to be beneficial in patients with more severe illness. To add to the confusion, it is **not** useful in patients with an APACHE II score of <25. There is an increased risk of hemorrhage, including intracranial hemorrhage, with drotrecogin alfa. When the APACHE II score is <25, the risk outweighs the benefit. Answers A and B are incorrect. Steroids shown no benefit in most patients with sepsis. However, it is not unreasonable to check patients for adrenal dysfunction (not an uncommon finding with sepsis) and treat those patients with adrenal insufficiency with physiologic doses of steroids. High-dose steroids are counterproductive and there is an increase in mortality. Answer D is incorrect. The antitumor necrosis factors (eg, infliximab, etanercept, and adalimumab) predispose to sepsis. Anti–Gram-negative endotoxin (answer E) had promise, but large trials failed to find a significant benefit.

BIBLIOGRAPHY

Annane D, Bellissant E, Cavaillon JM. Septic shock. *Lancet.* 2005;365:63.

Boutin RD, et al. Update on imaging of orthopedic infections. *Orthop Clin North Am.* 1998;29:41.

Bratton RL, Corey R. Tick-borne disease. *Am Fam Physician.* 2005;71(12):2323.

Centers for Disease Control and Prevention. Section on Traveler's Health. Accessed November 4, 2007, at http://wwwn.cdc.gov/travel/default.aspx.

Couch RB. Prevention and treatment of influenza. *N Engl J Med.* 200;343:1778.

Fihn SD. Clinical practice. Acute uncomplicated urinary tract infection in women. *N Engl J Med.* 2003;349(3):259.

Frieden TR, Sterling TR, Munsiff SS, Watt CJ, Dye C. Tuberculosis. *Lancet.* 2003;362:887.

Hirschmann JV. Fever of unknown origin in adults. *Clin Infect Dis.* 1997;24:291.

Lew DP, Waldvogel FA. Osteomyelitis. *N Engl J Med.* 1997;336:999.

Lo Re V 3rd, Gluckman SJ. Travel immunizations. *Am Fam Physician.* 2005;71(12):2254.

Mylonakis E, Calderwood, SB. Infective endocarditis in adults. *N Engl J Med.* 2001;345:1318.

Nichol KL, Nordin JB, Nelson DB, et al. Effectiveness of influenza vaccine in community-dwelling elderly. *N Engl J Med.* 2007;357:1373.

Schroeder MS. *Clostridium difficile*-associated diarrhea. *Am Fam Physician.* 2005;71(5):921.

Wendel K, Rompalo A. Scabies and pediculosis pubis: an update of treatment regimens and general review. *Clin Infect Dis.* 2002;35:S146.

Wilson W, Taubert KA, Gewitz M, et al. Prevention of infective endocarditis: guideline from the American Heart Association. *Circ.* 2007;116(15):1736.

9

HIV/AIDS

Mark A. Graber and Jason K. Wilbur

The antiretroviral treatment of HIV/AIDS (HAART) has become increasingly complex. This chapter focuses on the primary care aspects of HIV/AIDS including initial evaluation, drug adverse effects, and infectious disease prophylaxis.

CASE 1

A 23-year-old male presents to your clinic with complaints of sore throat, fever, and body aches. He reports that the illness began about 1 week ago and has persisted despite therapy with NSAIDs, acetaminophen, and sore-throat lozenges. He has not sought medical advice for this condition previously. He denies cough, abdominal pain, nausea, or vomiting, but reports a persistent headache. His past medical and surgical history is unremarkable. The patient smokes about 1 pack of cigarettes a week, drinks alcohol occasionally and denies use of other drugs, including intravenous use. He is heterosexual, and has had 16 sexual contacts in the past year. He does not use condoms.

On exam his vital signs are: T 38.9°C; P 112; BP 115/68; R 20. General: well-nourished male who appears uncomfortable. Head, ears, eyes, and nose are unremarkable. The patient has pharyngitis and enlarged tonsils with exudates. There is diffuse cervical lymphadenopathy, but the neck is supple. There are enlarged nodes in his axilla and inguinal areas as well. The spleen is palpable and nontender. The rest of the exam is unremarkable.

In addition to a throat culture, blood count, and Mono Spot, an appropriate laboratory test to rule out the acute retroviral syndrome is:

A) HIV-1 antibody by ELISA and Western blot.
B) HIV-1 antibody by rapid detection method.
C) HIV-1 p24 antigen or HIV viral load by PCR.
D) CD4 T lymphocyte count.
E) Sperm centrifuge for viral culture.

Discussion

The correct answer is C. This patient may have an acute retroviral syndrome, which occurs very early in the infection and is characterized by a mononucleosis-like illness that can last a couple of weeks. Since the antibody to HIV will not develop for at least 55 days after infection and the retroviral syndrome typically occurs before then, a test for HIV antibody (answer A), including rapid-detection methods (answer B), will most likely be negative (unless the patient was previously infected with HIV and the current illness is something else, such as lymphoma). The p24 antigen and PCR viral load, however, become positive as soon as detectable levels of the virus develop in the serum (approximately 10 days after infection), and will be positive in patients symptomatic with the retroviral syndrome. The p24 antigen may be falsely negative in up to 10% of patients with acute HIV infection. The CD4 count (answer D) is not a reliable way to diagnose HIV infection; it can become depressed with any acute illness or may be normal in early HIV disease. Culture of

318

semen (answer E) is not an accepted form of clinical diagnosis.

 HELPFUL TIP: The p24 antigen and viral load are **not** the tests of choice in the diagnosis of **chronic** HIV infection because of significant false-positives and false-negatives when the HIV load is low.

* *

After appropriate treatment and adequate counseling, follow-up is arranged for this patient. He returns to the office 2 months later with no complaints or symptoms. A complete history and physical are performed. The patient has mild cervical lymphadenopathy and no other findings. Laboratory studies are ordered and show:

WBC: 3,200 cells/mm³

Chemistry Panel (normal)

Anti-HIV ab (+)

Hct: 42%

Liver enzymes (normal)

Platelets: 185,000 cells/mm³

CD4 lymphocytes: 645 cells/mm³

HIV viral load: 5,000 copies/mL

What other baseline studies should now be ordered?

A) PPD.
B) RPR.
C) *Toxoplasma* antibody.
D) Hepatitis B and C antibody.
E) All of the above.

Discussion

The correct answer is E. During the initial assessment of an HIV-infected individual, all of these studies are important. A positive PPD (>5 mm in an individual infected with HIV) warrants INH and pyridoxine therapy for 9 months. Since patients who have a sexually transmitted infection (STI) are at risk for another STI, screening for syphilis with an RPR is good practice. The same rationale applies for Hepatitis B and C, which can be acquired via the same routes as HIV. *Toxoplasma* is a common CNS parasitic infection in HIV-infected patients, and a negative initial *Toxoplasma*

antibody may prove useful in evaluation of later disease. Prophylaxis is indicated for *Toxoplasma* Ab (+) patients with a CD4 count <100 cells/mm³.

* *

The patient is counseled appropriately about all the results.

What is the most important factor to determine when to start highly active anti-retroviral therapy (HAART)?

A) A rising viral load.
B) A decrease in CD4 count.
C) The development of an opportunistic infection.
D) The patient's willingness and ability to comply with the difficult regimens involved.
E) An undetectable viral load (<50 copies/mL).

Discussion

The correct answer is D. The decision to start HAART is a difficult one that must be done very carefully and on an individual basis. There is much controversy over the best time to start therapy. The most important consideration is the willingness of the patient to strictly adhere to complicated medical regimens. **Poor compliance guarantees the development of resistance, hampers treatment of the patient in later stages, and risks the spread of resistant strains to other patients.** If a patient is ready, the CD4 count is used to determine the optimum time for treatment (based on 2002 World Health Organization [WHO] guidelines). At CD4 counts >350 cells/mm³, the risk for disease progression is outweighed by the risk of toxicity of the drugs. At CD4 counts <200 cells/mm³, less immune reconstitution is seen, so ideally, therapy should be started when the CD4 count is between 200 and 350 cells/mm³. These numbers represent general rules in treatment, and other compelling indications may dictate variations in the approach to treating a specific individual. Evidence does not support using the viral load as an independent determinant of initiating therapy.

 HELPFUL TIP: Most sources recommend initiation of treatment **immediately** for a patient who is identified during the acute retroviral syndrome. These patients have very high viral loads and acute treatment may be helpful. This benefit wanes unless the patient continues HAART.

Besides considering HAART and stressing the importance of partner notification, what other intervention should be offered at this stage?

A) Pneumococcal and hepatitis B vaccines.
B) Trimethoprim/sulfamethoxazole (TMP/SMX) DS 1 tab/day for the prevention of *Pneumocystis jiroveci* pneumonia.
C) Azithromycin 1,250 mg per week for the prevention of *Mycobacterium avium* complex (MAC).
D) Fluconazole 100 mg per day for the prevention of cryptococcal meningitis.

Discussion

The correct answer is A. Adequate immunizations at a clinical stage when the patient is likely to benefit from the vaccines (CD4 >500 cells/mm³) are important. **Live vaccines, such as the MMR, should be avoided in immunocompromised persons, generally considered those HIV-infected persons with a CD4 count <200 cells/mm³.** TMP/SMX for PCP is indicated when the CD4 count is <200 cells/mm³. Azithromycin is indicated for MAC prophylaxis when the CD4 count is <50 cells/mm³. Fluconazole is used for chronic suppression after the treatment of cryptococcal meningitis or for the treatment of esophageal candidiasis. It is not currently used as prophylaxis; there is no survival benefit to prophylaxis for cryptococcal meningitis (Table 9–1). Current labs include: WBC 4,500 cells/mm³; Plts 128,000 cells/mm³; Hb 10.1 g/dL; MCV 110 fL; Hct 29.8%.

* *

After consultation with an HIV specialist, the patient elects not to start therapy at this time and is scheduled for follow-up with regular checks of his viral load and CD4 count. After 1 year, the patient's lab values have changed: CD4 lymphocytes 220 cells/mm³; viral load: 110,000 copies/mL In the past year, he has been treated

Table 9–1 RECOMMENDED PROPHYLAXIS IN HIV + PATIENTS

CD4+ Count	Organism	Recommended Prophylaxis
<200	Pneumocystis	TMP/SMX or Dapsone
<100	Toxoplasmosis	TMP/SMX
<50	Mycobacterium Avium Complex (MAC)	Azithromycin or rifabutin

three times for lobar pneumonia and once for oral candidiasis (without esophageal disease).

Does this patient meet the CDC case definition for the acquired immune deficiency syndrome (AIDS)?

A) No, because he has not had an AIDS-defining illness.
B) No, because his CD4 count is >200 cells/mm³.
C) No, because he has been diagnosed with HIV infection for only 1 year.
D) Yes, because he has had recurrent (>2 episodes) of lobar pneumonia.
E) Yes, because his viral load is >100,000 copies/mL.

Discussion

The correct answer is D. The 1993 Revised CDC HIV classification system requires a case of HIV infection be reported as AIDS if the CD4 count is <200 cells/mm³ OR the patient develops an AIDS defining illness. These AIDS defining illnesses include *esophageal* (not oral) candidiasis, cryptococcal infection, invasive cervical cancer, tuberculosis, HIV wasting disease, and *recurrent pneumonia*. Other infections, Kaposi sarcoma, and certain lymphomas may also define AIDS in an HIV infected person. Duration of infection and viral load are not currently criteria.

Table 9–2   CASE 1, LAB RESULTS

	January	**March**	**May**
CD4 count	204 cells/mm³	178 cells/mm³	180 cells/mm³
Viral Load	5,500 copies/mL	<500 copies/mL	<500 copies/mL

* *

The patient is started on nelfinavir (Viracept) plus Combivir (lamivudine and zidovudine). He does well with the treatment, and tolerates the medications. On a later routine follow-up, he reports mild fatigue, but is otherwise well. His lab results over several visits are listed in Table 9–2. Current labs also include: WBC 4,500 cells/mm³; Hb 10.1 g/dL; Hct 29.8%; Plts 128,000 cells/mm³; MCV 110 fL.

What changes, if any, should now be made to the patient's regimen?

A) The patient has failed HAART treatment, and the drug regimen should be changed.

B) The patient has suffered a severe adverse effect (anemia) from the drug regimen and all three drugs should be changed.

C) The patient is doing well, but needs B_{12} and folate supplementation due to his macrocytic anemia.

D) The patient has failed to reconstitute his immune system (CD4 count still <200 cells/mm³), so one of his drugs should be changed.

E) The patient is doing well and his regimen should be continued. The macrocytic anemia is an expected and manageable side effect of zidovudine.

Discussion

The correct answer is E. The patient's viral load is suppressed, which is the primary goal of HAART. The patient has not suffered any major adverse reactions. The macrocytic anemia is typical for patients on zidovudine, and should be followed regularly. It is usually mild, but can become severe on occasion. Criteria for changing drug regimens include: <1 $\log_{10}$ reduction of viral RNA by 8 weeks (eg, 100,000 to 10,000 is a 1 $\log_{10}$ reduction), failure to depress viral RNA to undetectable levels by 6 months, repeated detection of viral RNA after initially achieving undetectable levels, persistent decline in CD4 counts (on at least

2 measurements), or significant clinical deterioration. When changing drug regimens, it is important to change all 3 drugs if possible, to impair the development of resistance.

* *

The patient's HAART regimen is maintained, and he continues to do well. He misses his next 2 appointments, and returns to clinic 6 months later. He reports taking all of his medications but complains of a 10-pound unintended weight loss. He notes increased frequency of night sweats but no fevers. A physical exam is unremarkable except for a gaunt appearance and temporal muscle wasting. His lab results show:

CD4 count: 78 cells/mm³

Viral load: 6,400 copies/mL

CBC: WBC 2,400 cells/mm³

Hb: 9.8 g/dL

Platelets: 145,000 cells/mm³

MCV: 112 fL

Repeat CD4 count and viral load 2 weeks later shows:

CD4 count: 82 cells/mm³

Viral load: 7,100 copies/mL

What changes, if any, should be made now to the patient's regimen?

A) The patient has failed HAART treatment and all 3 drugs should be changed.

B) Since his anemia has persisted, the patient is assumed to have suffered a severe adverse affect from the zidovudine component of Combivir, so it alone should be changed.

C) The patient is doing well on his current regimen, but needs B_{12} and folate supplementation due to his macrocytic anemia.

D) The viral load is not >50,000 copies/mL, so the current regimen should be continued.

E) The patient is doing well and his regimen should be continued. The macrocytic anemia is an expected and manageable side effect from the zidovudine component of the Combivir.

Discussion

The correct answer is A. The patient has failed HAART based on several criteria, including the reemergence of detectable viral RNA after it had been completely suppressed and a falling CD4 count (see explanation of previous question, above). All 3 drugs should be changed.

* *

The patient's regimen is changed to Indinavir (Crixivan), Stavudine (d4T), and Didanosine (ddI). He is counseled appropriately on their use and the importance of maintaining regular clinic visits, and scheduled for follow-up in two months. After only 2 weeks, however, the ED calls because the patient has arrived there complaining of sudden onset severe right flank pain. The pain radiates from the right flank to the groin. The patient also reports hesitancy, urgency, and dark urine. On exam, he is writhing on the gurney, moaning in pain. He has significant right costovertebral angle tenderness and moderate right upper quadrant tenderness to deep palpation. The rest of the exam is unremarkable.

After adequate analgesia, what tests should be ordered next?

A) CD4 count and viral load.
B) Amylase, lipase, liver enzymes, and right upper quadrant ultrasound to evaluate for gallbladder pathology due to therapy with stavudine (d4T).
C) Amylase, lipase, liver enzymes, and a computerized tomography (CT) scan of the abdomen to evaluate pancreatitis due to therapy with didanosine (ddI).
D) Urinalysis, creatinine, amylase, lipase and CT of the urinary tract to evaluate for renal stones caused by indinavir.
E) Complete blood count and surgical consult to consider appendicitis.

Discussion
The correct answer is D. Based on his symptoms and signs, it is most likely that this patient has developed a renal stone due to indinavir use. This occurs in approximately 7% of patients within the first 4 months of therapy. The drug may be continued afterwards, but approximately 50% of patients are likely to suffer a recurrence. Pancreatitis can be caused by many drugs, including didanosine (ddI). Didanosine can cause pancreatitis in up to 9% of patients. Both didanosine and stavudine (d4T) have been associated with peripheral neuropathy, but neither is typically associated with biliary disease. Appendicitis is an important consideration

in anyone with severe abdominal pain, but it is unlikely in this patient, given the presentation. A viral load or CD4 count would not add any information to the work-up of the patient's current symptoms.

* *

The patient was treated appropriately and recovered. His current drug regimen was continued. Unfortunately, he was subsequently lost to follow-up. Attempts to contact him by phone and mail went unanswered.

* *

Approximately 2 years later, this patient presents to the clinic complaining of severe shortness of breath. Between gasps, he reports that he stopped taking all of his HIV-related medication (including HAART and chemoprophylaxis) about 6 months ago. Prior to that, he had found the medications increasingly difficult to take because of side effects and a lack of economic resources. He was treated at a health-care facility in another state 4 months ago for a persistent fever that responded to therapy for *Mycobacterium avium* complex (MAC).

This current illness began 3 days ago as a fever and mild cough. He noticed significant dyspnea with even mild exertion. His illness progressed, and today he has shortness of breath at rest. His chest hurts bilaterally, worse with inspiration. He has continued fevers and night sweats. He denies hemoptysis, sputum production, nausea, vomiting, or abdominal pain. Physical exam reveals the following vital signs:

T 39°C

BP 90/60

P 135, RR 38

Oxygen saturation 78% (RA)

The patient is in severe respiratory distress, in the tripod position. Neck exam reveals bilaterally enlarged lymphadenopathy. The patient is tachycardic, and there are no murmurs appreciated on heart exam. The lung exam shows diffuse rales and tachypnea. The abdomen is nontender. The remainder of the exam is unremarkable. He does not respond to oxygen and becomes more unresponsive.

Aside from respiratory isolation, what should be done next?

A) Sputum culture.
B) Bronchoalveolar lavage (BAL) for direct immunofluorescence (DFA).

C) Intravenous fluids and rapid sequence intubation.
D) Oxygen, furosemide, and nitroglycerin.
E) Chest x-ray, blood count, CD4 count, and viral load.

Discussion

The correct answer is C. This patient is in extremis—in severe distress and impending respiratory failure. He is also hypotensive and tachycardic and must be stabilized before any further workup is done. Oxygen, furosemide and nitrates are useful treatments for congestive heart failure, but this is unlikely in such a young person. *Pneumocystis jiroveci* pneumonia (PCP) is a more likely diagnosis that explains all the findings.

* *

After appropriate resuscitation, laboratories and a chest x-ray are obtained. You suspect *Pneumocystis jiroveci* pneumonia (PCP).

Laboratory results are:

WBC 3,400 cells/mm^3

Hb 11 g/dL

Platelets 180,000 cells/mm^3

Creatinine 2.4 mg/dL

LDH 1,280 IU/L

PT 12.4 sec, PTT 27 sec

Liver enzymes normal

ABG: pH 7.56, PaCO$_2$ 23 mm Hg, PaO$_2$ 72 mm Hg (on 100% FiO$_2$)

Sputum and blood cultures are pending.

What should be the initial antibiotic therapy?

A) 4 drug antituberculosis regimen.
B) Azithromycin or levofloxacin IV.
C) TMP-SMX IV.
D) TMP-SMX IV, preceded by corticosteroids.
E) No antibiotics initially; just wait for the culture results.

Discussion

The correct answer is D. This patient is acutely ill, and likely has PCP. Steroids (40 mg BID for 5 days followed by 40 mg QD for 11 days) decrease the mortality in patients with severe PCP (PaO$_2$ <70 on room air). The best antibiotic for PCP is TMP-SMX (trimethoprim/sulfamethoxazole). Pentamidine IV may be used in cases of sulfa allergy, but it has been associated with hypotension and hypoglycemia. Although the classic chest x-ray appearance for PCP is bilateral interstitial infiltrates, it can present differently (as in this case). Initially normal x-ray exams are not uncommon. **Because the infecting organism is not known with certainty, it is reasonable to add empiric therapy for bacterial pneumonia with azithromycin and/or levofloxacin.** PCP does not grow in standard cultures; it can be seen with silver stain on bronchoalveolar lavage or with direct fluorescent assay.

* *

The patient is admitted to the ICU and given antibiotics. His condition seemed to stabilize, until 4 hours into his ICU stay. At that time, his respiratory rate on assist-control ventilation dramatically increases from 18 to 42. Peak airway pressures according to the ventilator are >60 cm of H$_2$O, when they were <30 cm H$_2$O previously. Breath sounds are absent on the right side of the chest, and the trachea is deviated to the left. Heart sounds are audible, but tachycardic. Neck veins are distended bilaterally.

What is the next appropriate step BEFORE a repeat chest x-ray is taken?

A) Give Versed 2mg IV for sedation, the patient must be very anxious.
B) Pull the ET tube back 1–2 cm, as it is likely in the right mainstem bronchus.
C) Perform a blind pericardiocentesis, as the patient is developing tamponade.
D) Insert a large Angiocath into the left second intercostal space to relieve the tension pneumothorax on the left.
E) Insert a large Angiocath into the right second intercostal space to relieve the tension pneumothorax on the right.

Discussion

The correct answer is E. This patient has developed a dreaded complication of PCP, a pneumothorax. The organism, *Pneumocystis*, was so named for its propensity to cause blebs (cystis) in the lung tissue (pneumo). Since the patient was receiving positive-pressure ventilation, a tension pneumothorax developed and requires immediate needle decompression. This should be done without waiting for a portable chest x-ray. When the pneumothorax is later confirmed, a tube thoracostomy may be performed under controlled conditions.

* *

Despite aggressive ICU care, this patient continues to deteriorate. After a prolonged stay with multiple secondary infections, he remains ventilator-dependent and unconscious. Next of kin agree to withdraw life support and the patient dies.

Objectives: Did you learn to . . .

- Identify the signs and symptoms of the acute retroviral syndrome?
- Use appropriate tests for diagnosis of HIV infection?
- Evaluate a patient with HIV and monitor that patient's progress?
- Review the preventative health measures important in patients with HIV infection?
- Understand the guidelines for initiating and changing highly active anti-retroviral therapy (HAART)?
- Recognize some of the more common medications used to treat HIV and their side effects?
- Recognize some of the more common opportunistic infections in HIV patients?

CASE 2

A 32-year-old female presents to the office seeking prenatal care. Her last normal menstrual period began 2$\frac{1}{2}$ months before her visit. She believes that she is pregnant and has tested positive with a home pregnancy test. She has been pregnant twice before, with one living child and one spontaneous abortion (G3 P1). She is married to the father of the children. She has no health problems but does smoke a half-pack of cigarettes per day. She also admits to occasional alcohol use (1 drink every 2 weeks). She denies oral or intravenous drug use.

In addition to prenatal vitamins with iron, you recommend:

A) Quitting smoking.
B) Confirming the home pregnancy test with a serum HCG in your lab.
C) HIV testing and counseling.
D) A and C.
E) All of the above.

Discussion

The correct answer is D. Smoking during pregnancy is associated with lower birth weight and pre-eclampsia, and smoking in the house with a young child is associated with respiratory diseases, especially asthma. Although confirming pregnancy by examination (uterine size or fetal heart tones) and/or urine HCG is

appropriate, serum HCG is unnecessary and expensive. When used correctly, home pregnancy tests are highly sensitive and specific. HIV testing and counseling should be routinely offered to all women seeking prenatal care, regardless of their particular social situation. Routine testing for HIV in expectant females has dramatically reduced the HIV prevalence in children in developed countries. Vertical transmission of HIV is a major problem in Africa and other developing regions of the world. Remember that testing for HIV antibodies is not enough—the patient must understand the purpose and implications of the test. Pre- and post-test counseling is always included with the blood draw.

 HELPFUL TIP: The CDC now recommends (or dictates, depending on your perspective) universal HIV testing for all individuals between 13 and 64 years "in all health-care settings. If, after testing 1,000 patients, the prevalence of discovered HIV is <1 in 1,000 in your practice, you can stop testing your population." (*MMWR* September 22, 2006/55[RR14];1). On the bright side, the CDC states that special consent is NOT necessary prior to testing for HIV (a patient's general consent for medical care should be enough), and the CDC promotes "opt-out" testing "(telling all patients that they should be screened for HIV and allowing them to decline or opt-out)."

* *

You counsel the patient and order the HIV test. Her pregnancy is confirmed, but she is found to be ELISA positive for HIV and Western blot positive for HIV.

What does this mean?

A) She has been infected with HIV in the last month.
B) She has a false-positive test for HIV.
C) She has antibodies to HIV and must be immune.
D) She has been infected with HIV longer than 1 month ago.
E) Not enough information to judge: order a p24 antigen and RNA PCR.

Discussion

The correct answer is D. The ELISA is the highly sensitive "screening" HIV antibody test, and the Western Blot is the highly specific "confirmatory" test. A positive result for both is a reliable indication for the presence of HIV antibody and indicates infection at some point in the past. Since it can take 4 weeks or more for the generation of antibodies, recent infections may not test positive. Viral p24 antigen or the RNA PCR can detect HIV before the seroconversion (development of antibodies). Immunity to HIV is very rare. Some patients test positive for the antibody, but the disease does not progress as expected. These individuals have been and are being studied in hopes of identifying a molecular site for an HIV vaccine.

* *

Your patient is understandably upset by the news of this test result. She is most concerned about her unborn child.

What should you tell her?

A) Her child is almost certainly also infected.
B) A therapeutic abortion at this point is the only humane thing to do.
C) With proper therapy, the risk of transmission to the child can be lowered to <5%.
D) With proper therapy, the risk of transmission to the child can be lowered to 15%.
E) Despite proper therapy, the risk of transmission remains at 25%.

Discussion

The correct answer is C. Although it is possible for HIV to infect the unborn fetus, the large majority of transmission from mother to child occurs caused by exposure to the mother's blood at the time of birth. The first antiretroviral protocol for reducing this rate of transmission used zidovudine (ZDV) therapy alone, and succeeded in lowering the rate from 25% to 8.3%. There are numerous options now, depending upon when the mother presents for prenatal care (if at all). Ideally, the mother should be well suppressed (undetectable viral load) on combination anti-retroviral therapy (HAART). This, combined with perinatal therapy for the newborn, lowers the transmission risk to <2% (one study found a 1.4% transmission rate!). If the mother presents for the first time just prior to delivery or in the case of very limited resources (as in Africa), one option is nevirapine (Viramune). A single dose to the mother (200 mg PO) given at the onset of labor and a single dose to the infant 48–72 hours after birth is as effective as 7 days of ZDV or 7 days of ZDV plus 3TC to both mother and child.

* *

Your patient is somewhat relieved that her baby can be protected, and wants to know what can be done to treat her. She feels fine, and would rather not take medications unless she had to. Some additional laboratory tests are ordered, with the following results:

CD4 count: 756/mm^3

HIV viral load: 50,000 copies/mL

Hb: 11.2 g/dL

BUN/Cr: 11 mg/dL / 0.7 mg/dL

What should you tell her about HAART in pregnancy?

A) To minimize the risk of transmission to her child, she should start triple antiretroviral therapy as soon as possible.
B) Antiretroviral medications are teratogenic and should be avoided at all costs during pregnancy, except just before delivery.
C) Since her CD4 count is normal and she feels well with no sign of opportunistic infections, starting HAART is not indicated.
D) Her renal function makes HAART relatively contraindicated.
E) Her hemoglobin level makes HAART relatively contraindicated.

Discussion

The correct answer is A. The risk of vertical transmission of HIV increases with the following: high maternal viral load, low maternal CD4 count (most important), high clinical disease stage, lack of maternal use of antiretrovirals, increasing duration of ruptured membranes, and vaginal delivery (versus cesarean section, but only if no maternal therapy had been given previously). Therefore, HAART should be considered in all pregnant women, despite their current clinical stage of disease. In nonpregnant women, therapy is often reserved until CD4 counts drop, viral load is very high, or clinical symptoms are apparent. But the goal here is to prevent transmission to the child. Most antiretroviral medications are safe (or presumed to be safe) in pregnancy. Clearly, the benefit of preventing morbidity from HIV infection outweighs the risk of most medications. Although the patient's hemoglobin is low, it does not preclude her from taking therapy. Her renal function is normal, so it should not be an issue.

* *

The patient is started on HAART and tolerates her regimen well. Repeat laboratory results at a return visit are as follows:

CD4 count: 692/mm^3

HIV viral load: 5,000 copies/mL

Hb: 10.9 g/dL

Her HAART seems to be effective. Her viral load has decreased by 1 log$_{10}$.

What do you recommend regarding *Pneumocystis jiroveci* **pneumonia (PCP) prophylaxis?**

A) She should begin prophylaxis with TMP-SMX immediately because PCP in pregnancy can be particularly severe.

B) She should begin PCP prophylaxis with inhaled pentamidine because TMP-SMX is contraindicated in pregnancy.

C) PCP prophylaxis is not indicated since her CD4 count is >200/mm^3

D) PCP prophylaxis is not a major concern for pregnant patients.

Discussion

The correct answer is C. PCP is particularly severe in pregnant patients, but prophylaxis is not generally indicated for CD4 counts >200 cells/mm^3. TMP-SMX is associated with hyperbilirubinemia in newborns, but is still indicated for PCP prophylaxis. Oral dapsone is another option, as is inhaled pentamidine.

* *

She continues her antiretroviral therapy and remains well controlled. Her viral load never becomes undetectable (always the goal with HAART), but she remains healthy and maintains her normal CD4 count. As the due date approaches, you discuss delivery plans with the patient.

Which of the following is (are) true regarding the delivery?

A) A cesarean section (C-section) is likely to reduce the risk of transmission to her infant.

B) A C-section is indicated because this patient's viral load remains >1,000 copies/mL despite HAART.

C) A C-section should be performed at 38 weeks' gestation, prior to the onset of labor.

D) Peripartum ZDV should be given to the mother and infant.

E) All of the above.

Discussion

The correct answer is E. If a patient achieves effective suppression with HAART (undetectable viral load), the risk of transmission is minimal, and the mode of delivery should depend on the preferences of the mother and the other usual obstetric factors. If, as in this patient's case, the viral load remains >1,000 copies/mL, the CDC recommends delivery by C-section. When performed at 38 weeks, prior to the onset of labor, the relative risk of transmission is reduced by 50%. Perinatal ZDV, as discussed, may help reduce the risk of transmission. Also, the premature rupture of membranes (PROM) should be addressed promptly in HIV-infected mothers. Children born to mothers >4 hours after rupture are twice as likely to acquire HIV.

* *

The patient delivers a healthy, 3-kg male infant via C-section. The postpartum course is uneventful. Blood taken from the infant at day 1 and at 2 weeks both test positive for HIV antibodies.

What does this mean?

A) The infant is infected with HIV.

B) Although technically HIV positive, the infant's infection status is unclear from the information given.

C) Maternal HIV antibodies are expected to be circulating in the infant, but it can be assumed that no transmission of infection took place.

D) A positive test at day 1 is expected due to maternal antibodies, but a repeat positive at 2 weeks indicates infant antibody production and is evidence of infection.

E) None of the above.

Discussion

The correct answer is B. All children born to HIV-positive mothers will initially be HIV-positive as well (and may continue to test positive for up to 15 months). For at least the first 6 months of an infant's life, he or she depends on maternal antibodies acquired across the placenta. Therefore, the standard HIV antibody test is not the proper method to assess for maternal-fetal transmission. Nor will waiting 2 weeks make any difference.

How should the HIV status of the infant be determined?

A) Serial HIV antibody tests: a four-fold drop in titer can be considered negative.

B) p24 antigen testing in the first 48 hours of life.

C) Viral load by PCR in the first 48 hours of life.

D) Viral load by PCR at 48 hours, 4 weeks, and 4 months.

E) p24 antigen and PCR viral load on cord blood samples.

Discussion

The correct answer is D. The best test to perform in the neonate is viral load by PCR. A positive viral load in the first 48 hours indicates in-utero transmission. When transmission occurs during delivery (the most common scenario), the viral load at 48 hours is negative (the patient is in the initial stages of the infection and has not produced sufficient viral copies to be detected). However, the viral load may be detectable at 2–6 weeks, so repeating the viral load on more than one occasion is recommended. Remember that a positive test should be confirmed before starting treatment.

Answer A is incorrect. HIV antibody testing is useless in infants, and quantified titers are not typically generated. Answer B is incorrect because the p24 antigen is less specific and less sensitive than the viral load. Answer E is incorrect. Tests done on the cord blood may be contaminated with maternal blood and do not give an accurate assessment of the infant's status.

What should you advise your patient about breast-feeding her son?

A) HIV is not transmitted by breast milk.

B) HIV is transmitted by breast milk, but the benefits of breast-feeding outweigh the risk of transmission.

C) HIV is transmitted by breast milk, but her son will be protected from serious infection due to maternal antibodies in the breast milk.

D) HIV is transmitted by breast milk, and breast-feeding should be avoided if possible.

E) None of the above.

Discussion

The correct answer is D. Postpartum transmission of HIV from mother to child occurs in 10%–14% of breast-feeding mothers. This is not a major problem in developed nations, where there is reliable access to formula. HIV-positive mothers should be discouraged from breast-feeding. The recommendations may be different in developing areas of the world, where mother's milk may the only clean source of nutrition available to the infant. In many developing nations, the benefit of breast-feeding outweighs the risk of HIV transmission because of inadequate access to good nutrition and risk of diarrheal illnesses. The World Health Organization (WHO) suggests that "when replacement feeding is acceptable, feasible, affordable, sustainable and safe" bottle-feeding is the best option (http://www.who.int/child-adolescent-health/NUTRITION/HIV_infant.htm).

* *

Despite the best efforts of your patient and the physicians and nurses participating in her care, her child tests positive by PCR for HIV at 4 weeks and 4 months.

Which of the following is true about the use of HAART in children?

A) Treatment should be initiated immediately for all children as soon as HIV infection is diagnosed.

B) Because they are just little adults with relatively big heads compared to their torsos, treatment indications for children and adults are the same.

C) HAART is highly toxic in children and treatment should be reserved until the child's life is in immediate danger from HIV-related complications.

D) No one knows the best approach, but treatment is recommended in most children and should be given to infants <1 year.

E) Treatment indications for children are similar to those for adults, but monotherapy is preferred over combination therapy.

Discussion

The correct answer is D. The ideal therapy for children has yet to be defined, but a few general principles are assumed based on limited trials, observation of the natural history of HIV in children, and extrapolation from adult data. Children tend to demonstrate very high viral loads early in life when they lack the normal immunological control of viral replication. Furthermore, children may suffer early and severe neurologic and developmental injury due to HIV infection. The CD4 count is used in adults to monitor the degree of immune system suppression, but in children the CD4 starts fairly high and decreases normally throughout the first 4 years of life. Therefore, therapy should be strongly considered for a child <1 year, a child with very high viral loads, and a child in which adherence can be assured. HAART can be more difficult to choose and adjust in children because there is a limited number of pediatric (non-pill) formulations and a lack of data about long-term efficacy and safety. Combination therapy can effectively and safely suppress viral load and stimulate immunologic reconstitution. Monotherapy is **not** recommended.

Which of the following statements regarding the natural history of HIV complications in children is true?

A) Hepatobiliary complications, such as AIDS cholangiopathy, are more common in children.
B) Kaposi sarcoma frequently occurs in young children.
C) Focal brain lesions in children are almost always due to toxoplasmosis.
D) Many children show cognitive and motor deficits, but frank AIDS dementia is uncommon.
E) Lymphocytic interstitial pneumonitis is more common in adults than in children.

Discussion

The correct answer is D. Twenty-five percent of children with HIV infection demonstrate some cognitive and motor deficits. They face problems with verbal expression, attention deficits, hyperactivity, and hyperreflexia. Lymphocytic interstitial pneumonitis (LIP) is characterized by diffuse reticulonodular infiltrates and hilar lymphadenopathy and occurs in up to 40% of children with perinatally acquired HIV. LIP is very rare in adults. Kaposi sarcoma is associated with a herpes virus infection and is very rare in children. Toxoplasmosis, usually presenting as focal mass brain lesions, is a reactivation of previous infection, and is therefore also very rare in children. Hepatobiliary complications are more common in adults than in children, but the reason for this is unclear.

What should you recommend for this infant regarding PCP prophylaxis?

A) Prophylaxis is unnecessary because children do not get PCP.

B) Prophylaxis is unnecessary if the child's CD4 count is >200 cells/mm^3.
C) Prophylaxis is unnecessary until the child reaches 1 year.
D) Prophylaxis with TMP-SMX is contraindicated in infants <6 months because of the risk of hyperbilirubinemia.
E) Prophylaxis with TMP-SMX as the first-line agent should be initiated at 4 weeks because the highest risk for PCP in children is at 3–6 months.

Discussion

The correct answer is E. PCP in children has a peak onset at 3–6 months and often carries a poor prognosis. TMP-SMX is still the first-line agent and can be started safely at 4 weeks. If this drug is not tolerated, dapsone or aerosolized pentamidine are acceptable alternatives. Remember that CD4 counts in children are naturally higher, starting at 1,500/mm^3 in infants and decreasing to adult levels by 6 years. Due to the naïve nature of young children's immune systems, PCP can occur in infants despite a "normal" CD4 count.

* *

The child tolerates his HAART very well and demonstrates a consistently suppressed viral load. He gets further follow-up by a pediatric infectious disease specialist. The mother returns to you for further care. She had been taking the previously prescribed HAART, but quit all her medications 3 months ago because she had forgotten to take a couple of doses and did not want to "screw things up." Her latest laboratory results show the following:

CD4 count: 254 cells/mm^3

HIV viral load: 50,000 copies/mL

(Previously: CD4 count: 692/mm^3; HIV viral load: 5,000 copies/mL)

What do you tell her now?

A) She should have continued to take the medications because now the HIV has a "foothold" and it will be much harder to treat.
B) It would not have mattered if she took the medications or not. Her disease is progressing as expected.
C) With the degree of drop seen in her CD4 count, the virus must be resistant, and further HAART is futile.

D) She should have continued the medications, even if she was missing doses. A little of antiretroviral activity is better than nothing.

E) She did the right thing by stopping the medications. If a patient is not able to comply fully, it is better not to take any HAART at all.

Discussion

The correct answer is E. Starting HAART is a very difficult and serious decision and should be made after careful and complete counseling. If taken intermittently, HAART can quickly become ineffective. Patients who miss frequent doses of HAART are likely to have a more precipitous course to their HIV infection. Once multidrug resistance develops, it can be difficult to find an effective regimen to slow disease progression.

 HELPFUL TIP: ZDV, 3TC, and abacavir (Ziagen) are available in a combination taken as 1 pill BID (Trizivir). This is easy for patients to follow.

* *

She agrees to try Trizivir BID and does well. She suffers only moderate diarrhea, and repeat labs show an improvement in her viral load: CD4 count: 261 cells/mm³; HIV viral load: 7,000 copies/mL.

* *

You explain that if her viral load continues to fall and becomes suppressed (undetectable), she can expect a rebound in her CD4 count. You use this office visit as an opportunity to catch up on preventative medicine. On one prior occasion 6 years ago, she had an abnormal Pap smear result that was returned to normal after a repeat exam and colposcopy. Prior to her diagnosis of HIV, she had never been diagnosed with a sexually transmitted infection (STI). A pelvic exam today reveals a normal appearing cervix. A sample for Pap smear is collected and sent to pathology.

How often should this patient get screened for cervical cancer with Pap smear?

A) Cervical cancer is inevitable, so you should recommend prophylactic radical resection.

B) She must be tested every 6 months, regardless of results of this Pap smear.

C) If she has 2 negative Pap smears 6 months apart and a normal CD4 count, she may be screened per the usual guidelines for HIV-negative women.

D) She may be tested per the usual guidelines for HIV-negative women.

E) She has almost no chance of developing cervical cancer and screening may be discontinued.

Discussion

The correct answer is C. Human papilloma virus (HPV), implicated as a cause of cervical cancer, has a higher prevalence and demonstrates a more aggressive course in women with HIV infection. If the patient has a relatively normal CD4 count and has had 2 normal smears at 6-month intervals, PAP smears can be done at 1-year intervals. **If the patient has a CD4 count <200 cells/mm³, screening every 6 months is recommended.** Any detection of cervical intraepithelial neoplasia (CIN) is treated the same as with HIV-negative women. It is not unusual for multiple STIs to be transmitted together, so consider testing for other STIs when obtaining a Pap smear.

 HELPFUL TIP: Any STI causing genital ulcers (eg, herpes) increases the risk of transmission of HIV.

 HELPFUL TIP: Male circumcision can reduce the rate of HIV transmission by 50% in high-risk populations (eg, in some populations in Africa).

Besides increased risk of aggressive HPV and a high rate of menstrual disorders, how does the natural history of HIV infection in women differ from that in men?

A) Women have a lower rate of progressive multifocal leukoencephalopathy (PML) and bacterial pneumonia.

B) Women are more likely to present with oral thrush and recurrent genital candidiasis.

C) Women with the same level of medical care as men have significantly shortened survival.

D) HAART is more effective and better tolerated in women.

E) Most women in the U.S. acquire HIV from same-sex partners.

Discussion

The correct answer is B. The natural history of HIV infection in women and men is very similar. Women with the same level of access to medical care have similar survival rates to men, and HAART is equally effective (and hazardous) in both sexes. Women more often present with recurrent, refractory vaginal candidiasis, oral thrush, PML, and bacterial pneumonias. The majority of women in the United States who have HIV have acquired it from heterosexual contact. The second largest route of exposure for U.S. women is intravenous drug use. Females who have sex with other women are at low risk of contracting HIV; the opposite is true for men who have sex with other men. Worldwide, heterosexual contact is by far the most common means of transmission.

Objectives: Did you learn to . . .

- Interpret HIV antibody and viral load tests?
- Evaluate the risk of vertical transmission of HIV?
- Reduce the risk of vertical transmission of HIV?
- Interpret HIV tests in the neonatal period?
- Use HAART in children?
- Identify several differences in the clinical manifestations of HIV in women and children?

CASE 3

A 39-year-old female who works as a nursing assistant in your hospital comes into the ED looking quite upset. About 30 minutes earlier, she was helping to move a patient with known HIV when his IV was pulled out and he bled. Several drops of blood got on her hands, but she washed them immediately and thoroughly. On exam, she has intact skin on the hands, no signs of trauma, and no residual blood on her.

The most appropriate action to take is:

A) Reassure her that her risk of contracting HIV for this event is almost zero.
B) Obtain HIV antibody testing.
C) Start her on HAART for prophylaxis.
D) Have her return in 6 weeks for HIV antibody testing.
E) B and D.

Discussion

The correct answer is A. Fortunately, HIV is not the most efficient virus when it comes to spreading itself.

Health-care workers are at risk of contracting HIV when working with HIV-infected patients, but exposure to infected bodily fluid must occur through a percutaneous route or contact with a mucous membrane or non-intact skin. Even percutaneous exposure (eg, open bore needle) with HIV-infected blood carries a transmission rate of only about 0.3%, and the mucous membrane exposure to HIV-infected blood carries a 0.09% risk. Therefore, contact of an infected patient's blood with intact skin is very low risk.

* *

The patient is reassured that her risk of contracting HIV is negligible. She looks a little sheepish when she tells you, "In all the commotion I knocked over the urinal and spilled the patient's urine on my leg." She changed clothes and washed her leg. You inspect her and find some eczema in the area where the urine was spilled.

Now, you recommend that she:

A) Not worry, as the risk of transmission from this event is negligible.
B) Start zidovudine for 4 weeks for prophylaxis.
C) Be tested for HIV by viral load.
D) Start HAART.

Discussion

The correct answer is A. Your patient now has an area of nonintact skin, which is a concern. However, urine is not considered infectious unless it is grossly bloody. Other bodily fluids not considered infectious: feces, vomitus, sputum, tears, sweat, nasal secretions, and saliva. Any visibly bloody fluids, blood, semen, and vaginal secretions are all considered infectious. Other bodily fluids not already mentioned (eg, CSF, amniotic fluid) should be considered potentially infectious.

 HELPFUL TIP: If HIV post-exposure prophylaxis is deemed necessary, 2 or 3 drug regimens should be started as soon as possible and continued for 4 weeks. There are many options for prophylaxis with various advantages and disadvantages; one of the most commonly used is zidovudine and lamivudine (Combivir).

Objectives: Did you learn to . . .

- Identify when a health-care worker is at risk for contracting HIV?

BIBLIOGRAPHY

Branson BM, Handsfield HH, Lampe MA, et al. Revised recommendations for HIV testing of adults, adolescents, and pregnant women in health-care settings. *MMWR* Recomm Rep 2006;55(RR-14):1.

Khalsa AM. Preventive counseling, screening, and therapy in the patient with newly diagnosed HIV infection. *Am Fam Physician* 2006;73:271.

Oleske J, for the Working Group on Antiretroviral Therapy and Medical Management of HIV-Infected Children. Guidelines for the Use of Antiretroviral Agents in Pediatric HIV Infection. Accessed December 4, 2007, at http://aidsinfo.nih.gov/contentfiles/PediatricGuidelines.pdf

Perlmutter BL, Glaser JB, Oyugi SO. How to recognize and treat acute HIV syndrome. *Am Fam Physician* 1999; 60:535.

Public Health Service Task Force. Recommendations for Use of Antiretroviral Drugs in Pregnant HIV-Infected Women for Maternal Health *and* Interventions to Reduce Perinatal HIV Transmission in the United States. Accessed December 4, 2007, at http://aidsinfo.nih.gov/contentfiles/PerinatalGL.pdf.

Panlilio AL, Cardo DM, Grohskopf LA, et al. Updated U.S. Public Health Service Guidelines for the Management of Occupational Exposures to HIV and Recommendations for Postexposure Prophylaxis. *MMWR* Recomm Rep 2005;54(RR-9):1.

Mark A. Graber

CASE 1

A 27-year-old female presents to the office with the chief complaint of chronic fatigue for 4 months. She reports a 17-pound weight gain over the last 3 months, despite a decreased appetite. She also complains of depression, increased sleep, a disturbing lack of energy, hair loss, and cold intolerance. Her past medical history is unremarkable, and she takes no medications. She has never had any surgeries.

Which of the following physical exam findings would be expected?

A) Tachycardia.
B) Exophthalmos.
C) Fine tremor.
D) Peripheral sensory loss.
E) Delayed relaxation in reflexes.

Discussion

The correct answer is E. The history given is consistent with a hypothyroid state. Symptoms of hypothyroidism include thinning hair, dry skin, a hoarse, deep voice, bradycardia, and a prolonged relaxation in the reflexes. Tachycardia (answer A) and a fine tremor (answer C) are typical of hyperthyroidism, and exophthalmos (answer B) is characteristic of Graves disease (one specific cause of hyperthyroidism). Proximal muscle weakness may occur in hypothyroidism, but sensory loss (answer D) is not typical (although hypothyroidism can contribute to carpal tunnel syndrome).

How can the diagnosis of hypothyroidism best be confirmed?

A) Elevated thyroid-stimulating hormone (TSH) level.
B) Low TSH level.
C) Thyroid biopsy.
D) Radionucleotide scan.
E) Serum thyroglobulin.

Discussion

The correct answer is A. The TSH is the most sensitive test for both hypo- and hyperthyroidism, and changes in the TSH can precede abnormalities in serum thyroxine (best measured as free T_4) level. An elevated TSH occurs when the pituitary detects insufficient thyroid hormone production, and TSH production is shut off when an excess of thyroid hormone is circulating. If the pituitary produces insufficient TSH, a low TSH (answer B) will result despite inadequate T_4. Therefore, adding serum free T_4 to a TSH assay is required to demonstrate hypothalamic or pituitary hypothyroidism (eg, in the case of a pituitary adenoma). Because these disorders are rare, and often suggested by other clues in the history and physical, TSH alone is usually sufficient for initial screening for thyroid disease. A biopsy (answer C) is used to evaluate thyroid masses and nodules. Radionucleotide scan (answer D) is used in the evaluation of thyroid masses and can differentiate functioning adenomas from carcinomas and benign cysts. The serum thyroglobulin measurement (answer E) is used to monitor thyroid carcinoma (**not** the initial screening).

* *

Her laboratory results are listed in Table 10–1.

Table 10–1 LABORATORY RESULTS

Complete Blood Count	Chemistry
WBC: 4,500 cells/mm³	Na: 132 mEq/L
Hb: 11g/dL	K: 3.9 mEq/L
Hct: 32%	Cl: 101 mEq/L
Plts: 206,000 cells/mm³	CO_2: 22 mEq/L
	Glucose 115 mg/dL
TSH: 22.3 uIU/mL (0.27–4.20)	
Free T_4: 0.56 ng/dL (0.93–1.70)	

What is the MOST likely cause of this patient's disease?

A) Autoimmune hypothyroidism.
B) Iatrogenic hypothyroidism.
C) Tuberculosis infiltration of the thyroid gland.
D) Non-functioning pituitary adenoma.
E) Congenital hypothyroidism.

Discussion

The correct answer is A. Autoimmune hypothyroidism (Hashimoto thyroiditis) is the most common cause of hypothyroidism in areas where there is adequate iodine. If this patient had a pituitary adenoma causing hypothyroidism, the TSH (as well as the free T_4) would be low, since the pituitary is the source of TSH. Congenital hypothyroidism causes a severe mental retardation and constellation of other signs. It is tested for at birth as part of routine neonatal screening. Tuberculosis is a rare cause of hypothyroidism, but is the most common cause of adrenal failure worldwide.

 HELPFUL TIP: Outside the United States, iodine deficiency is the most common cause of hypothyroidism in the world. An estimated 2 billion individuals are iodine-deficient although not all are hypothyroid.

How should this patient be managed?

A) I¹³¹ administration.
B) Surgical excision of thyroid gland.
C) Start synthetic levothyroxine at 25 micrograms PO QD, and recheck symptoms and TSH in 2 months.
D) Start synthetic levothyroxine at 200 micrograms PO QD, and recheck symptoms and TSH in 2 months.
E) Start synthetic levothyroxine at 25 micrograms PO QD, and double every week until the patient experiences weight loss, tremor, and poor sleep.

Discussion

The correct answer is C. The patient is deficient in thyroid hormone and needs supplementation. Two strategies may be considered: (1) start with levothyroxine 25 micrograms daily and titrate up every 1–2 months until the TSH is in the normal range, or (2) start with full-dose therapy based on weight (1.6 micrograms/kg daily) and adjust based on TSH in 1–2 months. Either option is appropriate in young, otherwise healthy adults. **Older patients (>65 years) or those with multiple comorbidities should be started at a low dose (25 micrograms daily).** If the patient is titrated up to 200 micrograms of levothyroxine and does not seem to be responding, the diagnosis needs to be reconsidered or the patient's compliance needs to be carefully assessed. **Iron and food decrease the absorption of levothyroxine (L-thyroxine) by as much as 40%.** It usually takes 6–8 weeks for the body's endocrine response and TSH to reach a steady state. The goal of therapy is a euthyroid state with the patient experiencing neither hyper- nor hypothyroid symptoms.

 HELPFUL TIP: Answers A and B are treatments for **hyper**thyroidism. Surgical excision and radioablation with I¹³¹ are approaches to the treatment of Graves disease. Both can result in iatrogenic hypothyroidism that requires life-long thyroid hormone therapy.

 HELPFUL TIP: We generally recommend starting synthetic levothyroxine at a low dose for two reasons. First, titrating the dose up will ensure that you do not overshoot. Second, if patients are started at 100 micrograms (a common final dose), it can cause metabolic stress, especially in the elderly, resulting in angina, atrial fibrillation, etc.

* *

Your patient is started on 25 micrograms L-thyroxine (Synthroid) and is scheduled to return in 2 months. At follow-up, she reports a general improvement in symptoms but is not "back to normal." She reports continued constipation, a lack of energy, and feeling depressed. She has not lost any additional weight and reports a thickening of her hair. Laboratory results are as follows:

TSH: 11.8 uIU/mL (0.27–4.20)

Free T$_4$: 0.75 ng/dL (0.93–1.70)

What adjustments, if any, should be made to her regimen?

A) None; she will continue to improve at the current dose.

B) Increase the dose to 50 micrograms per day, and recheck in 2 months.

C) Increase the dose to 200 micrograms per day, and recheck in 2 months.

D) She is becoming hyperthyroid, so cut the dose to 12.5 micrograms per day, and recheck in 2 months.

E) L-thyroxine is ineffective in this patient. Change her to desiccated thyroid tissue (eg, Armour Thyroid).

Discussion

The correct answer is B. This patient has improved from her initial presentation, but she is clinically and chemically (elevated TSH) still hypothyroid. The half-life of thyroxine is about 1 week, so she has had plenty of time to reach steady state. It is doubtful that her thyroid levels will change much after 2 months on this dose, so it is time to increase her dose. Since you started with a low dose, doubling of the dose is a reasonable increase that is unlikely to make her hyperthyroid. Answer E is of special note. Desiccated thyroid is generally avoided due to variability in concentration of thyroid hormone content.

 HELPFUL TIP: Poor compliance is the most common reason for failure of medical therapy. Other causes include malabsorption, drug interactions (rifampin, amiodarone), drug-food interactions, or drugs that reduce absorption (iron, sucralfate).

Which of the following can result from over-suppression of the TSH (eg, iatrogenic hyperthyroidism)?

A) Renal failure.

B) Pulmonary fibrosis.

C) Hirsutism.

D) Osteoporosis.

E) Loss of secondary sex characteristics.

Discussion

The correct answer is D. Hyperthyroidism, either iatrogenic or endogenous, causes osteoporosis. For this reason, it is important to monitor the TSH and ensure that the patient is not overreplaced.

Objectives: Did you learn to . . .

• Recognize the presentation of hypothyroidism and its most common causes?

• Identify common physical exam findings consistent with hypothyroidism?

• Describe the basic medical and laboratory management of patients with hypothyroidism?

CASE 2

A 32-year-old male presents to the office complaining of severe anxiety. For the last 4 months, he has had difficulty sleeping, progressively worsening nervousness, a 25-pound weight loss, and constant feeling of "too warm." He feels "shaky" and has difficulty concentrating. He denies diarrhea, but reports having normally-shaped stools 4–5 times per day, more than usual for him. The patient denies neck or eye discomfort, and has not noticed any neck swelling. He admits to smoking a half pack of cigarettes per day, a habit that he started recently to "help him calm down." He denies alcohol or illicit drug use. His only medication is an antihistamine for seasonal allergies. He has no other significant medical history. His mother, who died 3 years ago from coronary artery disease, had a "thyroid problem," but he doesn't know any more details.

Physical exam reveals an anxious young adult male. He has a noticeable resting tremor. You note mild exophthalmos, conjunctival injection, and lid lag. His thyroid is diffusely, mildly enlarged and a bruit is audible over the gland. The cardiac exam reveals tachycardia with a flow murmur. The rest of the exam is unremarkable.

What is the most likely diagnosis?

A) Viral thyroiditis.

B) Graves disease.

C) Anaplastic thyroid carcinoma.

D) Hyperactive thyroid adenoma.

E) Surreptitious thyroid hormone ingestion.

Discussion

The correct answer is B. This is a classic presentation of Graves disease. The family history, the symptoms and signs of hyperthyroidism (especially the diffusely enlarged goiter with a bruit), and the exophthalmos are all typical. Conjunctival infection is also frequently noted. Answer A is unlikely. Viral thyroiditis can cause hyperthyroidism and a goiter, but the thyroid gland is usually tender. Also, viral thyroiditis will likely not last 4 months, but is usually self-limited to a few weeks. Anaplastic carcinoma is a devastating disease with a dismal prognosis: the thyroid gets very large very quickly, but the disease does not present with hyperthyroidism. A hyperactive adenoma and surreptitious ingestion of thyroid hormone would not cause a goiter or exophthalmos.

 HELPFUL TIP: 75% of patients with viral thyroiditis will progress from 2 weeks of hyperthyroidism to 3–6 months of hypothyroidism that is also self-limited. The hyperthyroid phase is best treated with NSAIDs, β-blockers, and prednisone if needed.

Which of the following tests is most SPECIFIC for Graves disease?

A) Antithyrotropin receptor antibody.

B) Antithyroglobulin antibody.

C) Antithyroid peroxidase antibody.

D) Markedly suppressed TSH.

E) A and C.

Discussion

The correct answer is A. Graves disease is an autoimmune process, and lymphocytes in the thyroid gland itself are responsible for a large amount of the thyroid autoantibodies produced. Although several types of antibodies can be tested, antithyrotropin receptor antibody is the most specific. Antithyrotropin receptor antibody is found in 80% to 95% of patients with Graves disease and in essentially no other condition (although it may be elevated in 10% to 20% of those with other forms of autoimmune thyroiditis). Antithyroglobulin antibodies (answer B) are found in Graves disease, autoimmune thyroiditis, some patients with type 1 diabetes, and in up to 20% of the general population. Antithyroid peroxidase antibody (answer C) is elevated in Graves disease, autoimmune thyroiditis, type 1 diabetes, some pregnant patients, etc.

* *

Your patient's laboratory results are as follows: complete blood count is normal and TSH is undetectable.

How should the patient be treated acutely?

A) Propanolol and propylthiouracil (PTU) started immediately.

B) Control the patient's symptoms with propanolol now, then start PTU when the patient feels better.

C) Iodine (Lugol solution).

D) Radioablation with I^{131}.

E) Thyroidectomy.

Discussion

The correct answer is A. There is no need to wait before starting propylthiouracil (PTU) or the alternative methimazole (Tapazole), which block production of thyroid hormone. PTU is a better choice in those with significant symptoms because it will also partially block the peripheral conversion of T_4 (inactive) to T_3 (active form). Propanolol is helpful for controlling the symptoms of hyperthyroidism (tachycardia, tremor, etc). Iodine will provide further substrate for the body in the production of thyroid hormone and should not be given unless a thyroid-blocking agent has been started. Iodine is useful during thyroid storm to prevent the release of stored thyroid hormone, but it is given one hour after PTU or methimazole. Radioablation is used for patients who prove refractory to medicine or have poor compliance. Thyroidectomy is rarely used for Graves in current medical practice because of the ease and efficacy of radioactive iodine administration (except in the case of pregnancy and a few other unusual cases).

Which of the following is a possible side effect of PTU therapy?

A) Granulocytopenia.

B) Aplastic anemia.

C) Elevated liver transaminases.

D) Inhibition of fetal thyroid gland.

E) All of the above.

Discussion

The correct answer is E. All of the above are known side effects of antithyroid drugs (thioamides). Granulocytopenia occurs in about 0.5% of patients and is a sudden, idiosyncratic reaction. **Classically, patients present with a severe sore throat. If you have a patient on PTU with a sore throat, check a CBC.** Aplastic anemia may occur but is rare. For these reasons, patients starting these medications should have a baseline CBC. Mild, transient elevation of the liver transaminases is common, and the drug should be discontinued if the level is greater than three times normal. Both PTU and methimazole cross the placenta and will inhibit the fetal thyroid, increasing the risk for congenital hypothyroidism. The risk to a fetus posed by the drugs is less than the danger posed by a mother with accelerating hyperthyroidism, so the medications should be used even during pregnancy if indicated. PTU is regarded as slightly safer in pregnancy. Nonetheless, you should use the smallest dose possible. If a pregnant patient is not controlled with PTU, consider surgical thyroidectomy.

 HELPFUL TIP: Avoid radioactive iodine treatment during pregnancy since it will affect the fetus as well.

* *

Your patient complies with the recommended regimen, and improves. He is not symptomatic at a return visit in 2 months, and his eye pathology has not progressed. After 6 months of good control, the patient elects to have cosmetic eye surgery to repair his exophthalmos. A preoperation physical is unremarkable.

Laboratory findings prior to surgery are as follows:

WBC: 7,200 cells/mm^3

TSH: 0.2 uIU/mL (low)

Free T$_4$: 3 ng/dL (high)

Hb: 12.3 g/dL

Hct: 37%

Plts: 240,000 cells/mm^3

After an uneventful surgery, you are called to the postanesthesia room by the oculoplastics surgeon. She reports that the patient has become very anxious and has a sinus tachycardia of 165. A quick review of the chart reveals no known allergies, no personal or family history of reactions to anesthesia, and the only medication is PTU (propanolol had been discontinued 2 months earlier due to lack of symptoms).

Physical exam shows T 39.8°C, BP 98/25, RR 34, P 166. The patient is agitated but alert and in acute distress. He is tachypneic, tremulous, and is unable to carry on a conversation. He seems confused and distracted. The skin is diaphoretic and flushed. His mucous membranes are dry, and his surface veins are flat; there is no JVD. His heart is tachycardic with a flow murmur. Pulmonary exam reveals diffuse rales. Reflexes are brisk, his mental status is as noted above, but the rest of the neurologic exam is unremarkable.

What is the cause of this patient's symptoms and signs?

A) The patient became fluid overloaded during the surgery due to excessive hydration.

B) The patient has neuroleptic malignant syndrome.

C) The patient has thyroid storm induced by the stress of surgery.

D) The patient has an allergic reaction to isoflurane.

E) The patient has endocarditis and suffered a valve rupture.

Discussion

The correct answer is C. The syndrome of thyroid storm is characterized by fever, tachyarrhythmias, altered mental status, and high-output cardiac failure. It is induced by a major stress (infection, surgery, myocardial infarction, etc) in a patient with underlying hyperthyroidism (usually undiagnosed). This patient, although **clinically** well controlled, had a **low TSH and high free T$_4$ prior to surgery,** suggesting he may have suffered a recurrence of disease or had stopped taking his medications. The patient is not fluid overloaded, as evidenced by his clinically dry status (intravascular depleted → dry mucous membranes, flat neck veins); thus answer A is incorrect. The pulmonary edema (rales) is due to high output failure. Neuroleptic malignant syndrome (NMS) and a reaction to isoflurane both present with altered mental status and hyperthermia (due to increased metabolic activity). Although this patient is hyperthermic, his cardio-pulmonary status would be unusual with NMS or an allergy to isoflurane. Also, the patient is not currently taking neuroleptics and has no family history of anesthesia problems (an isoflurane reaction is often familial). A ruptured valve due to endocarditis would fit the patient's clinical picture, but he had no fever preceding the surgery. For endocarditis to progress to valve rupture, it must be long-standing, and there is nothing in the presurgical evaluation or history to suggest this.

Which of the following is (are) NOT a sign/symptom of thyroid storm?

A) Hypothermia.
B) Right upper quadrant pain.
C) Diffuse muscle weakness.
D) Atrial fibrillation.
E) Hypomania, confusion, other CNS signs and symptoms.

Discussion

The correct answer is A. Patients with hyperthyroidism will generally be hyperthermic. The other answer choices are true statements. Right upper quadrant pain (answer B) results from liver congestion secondary to high-output congestive heart failure.

> **HELPFUL TIP:** Thyroid storm is a clinical diagnosis. Even though most patients will have an elevated T_3 and free T_4, there is no laboratory level of these hormones that defines thyroid storm. A clinical diagnosis is made based on hyperthermia, tachycardia, CNS dysfunction, and signs and symptoms of peripheral hyperthyroidism.

> **HELPFUL TIP:** A pheochromocytoma can be confused with hyperthyroidism. Both include tachycardia, possible hypertension, etc. Serum catecholamines **are normal** (certainly high normal—but normal) in thyroid storm. Catecholamines will be elevated with a pheochromocytoma.

How should this patient now be treated?

A) Aggressive fluid hydration, cooling measures, benzodiazepines, and dantrolene.
B) Fluid hydration, cooling measures, beta blockade (IV propranolol), PTU, corticosteroids, then iodine 1 hour later.
C) Fluid hydration, dopamine drip, and antibiotics; consult cardiovascular surgery immediately.
D) Hold fluids; administer nitroglycerin drip and furosemide; consider an intraaortic balloon pump.
E) Fluid hydration, aspirin, antibiotics, and corticosteroids.

Discussion

The correct answer is B. This is the appropriate management for thyroid storm in the correct sequence of therapies. This patient is in extremis (hypotensive and tachycardic) and needs fluid hydration, despite his pulmonary edema. Cooling measures address his hyperthermia, and beta blockade (propranolol) will improve his high-output failure (and reduce the pulmonary edema). Corticosteroids help block release of thyroid hormone and decrease peripheral conversion of T_4 to T_3. Additionally, corticosteroids will treat any underlying adrenal insufficiency. PTU prevents thyroxine synthesis and conversion of T_4 to T_3. This must be given before iodine. The iodine blocks any further release of thyroid hormone. Answer A is the appropriate management of neuroleptic malignant syndrome. Answer C is an appropriate approach for valve rupture from endocarditis. Answer D describes the management of severe heart failure. Answer E describes essential steps in the treatment of sepsis. The inclusion of corticosteroids would be appropriate if adrenal insufficiency were suspected.

> **HELPFUL TIP:** In patients with hyperthyroidism, diarrhea is a sign that can presage thyroid storm.

* *

Your patient is treated appropriately and eventually recovers. He continues on PTU and propanolol and remains in good control.

Objectives: Did you learn to . . .

- Identify the more common causes of hyperthyroidism?
- Recognize the presentation of Graves disease?

- Manage hyperthyroidism and describe the indications and risks of each treatment option?
- Recognize and treat thyroid storm?

QUICK QUIZ: THYROID TESTS

You are seeing a 45-year-old female in your office. As part of a routine blood panel, the patient's TSH is noted to be elevated at 7.2 uIU/mL (normal 0.27–4.20 uIU/mL). She has a normal free T_4 and is asymptomatic.

The best option is to:

A) Start levothyroxine at a low dose to normalize the TSH.
B) Begin T_3 at a low dose.
C) Reassure the patient and have her follow up for repeat thyroid studies.
D) Begin a workup for central hypothyroidism.
E) None of the above.

Discussion

The correct answer is C. There is convincing evidence that in **asymptomatic** patients with a mildly elevated TSH (generally <10 uIU/mL) and normal free T_4 do not benefit from treatment in terms of quality of life, etc. Treated patients tend to have more symptomatic anxiety. The term for this condition (asymptomatic, TSH between 5 and 10, and normal free T_4) is subclinical hypothyroidism. Follow-up thyroid studies are indicated, although the interval may differ based on the clinician's judgment.

There is controversy regarding what to do about subclinical hypothyroidism, but most experts and consensus guidelines recommend that patients have their TSH levels monitored rather than start treatment. Of note, many patients will have transient changes in their thyroid hormone levels due to comorbid illness, viral thyroiditis, etc. The thing to do is recheck rather than start treatment.

QUICK QUIZ: THYROID MEDICATIONS

The patient in the previous Quick Quiz becomes overtly hypothyroid and you start her on levothyroxine. Her TSH and free T_4 are all within normal limits. She requests a prescription for T_3 because she still feels tired and is gaining weight.

Your response is:

A) Write a prescription for T_3 (Cytomel).
B) Inform her that no well done study demonstrates T_3 to be of any help.
C) Give IM haloperidol and lorazepam.
D) Refer to a specialist.

Discussion

The correct answer is B. Although there is anecdotal evidence cited by patients, no well done study has shown an advantage to T_3. Her symptoms are likely caused by depression, excess calorie intake, deconditioning, insomnia.

QUICK QUIZ: THYROID TESTS

A 52-year-old male is being seen in your clinic for weight loss, tachycardia, and anxiety. You suspect hyperthyroidism and decide to check blood work. The patient has a low TSH suggestive of hyperthyroidism but has a normal free T_4.

The most likely explanation of this patient's symptoms and laboratory findings is:

A) He has pituitary dysfunction with a pending central hypothyroidism.
B) He has an isolated T_3 hyperthyroidism.
C) He likely has Addison disease.
D) He is taking aspirin which interferes with the assay for free T_4.
E) He it taking aspirin which interferes with the assay for TSH.

Discussion

The correct answer is B. Five percent of patients with hyperthyroidism have an isolated T_3 hyperthyroidism. If you suspect hyperthyroidism and the patient has a low TSH but a normal free T_4, check a T_3-RIA. It is worth noting that TSH is more sensitive than free T_4 for thyroid dysfunction.

QUICK QUIZ: HYPERTHYROIDISM

Which of the following cause(s) hyperthyroidism?

A) Lithium.
B) Amiodarone.
C) Peginterferon alfa-2a.
D) Phenytoin.
E) B and C.

Discussion

The correct answer is E. Amiodarone and Peginterferon alfa-2a can cause hyperthyroidism. Lithium (answer A) and phenytoin (answer D) cause hypothyroidism. Amiodarone (answer B) is interesting because it can cause **hyper**thyroidism or **hypo**thyroidism. It has multiple effects on the thyroid gland and on metabolism of T_4 and T_3, which can result in **hypo**thyroidism. It carries a huge iodine load, which can result in **hyper**thyroidism. Between 2% and 30% of patients taking amiodarone will have thyroid dysfunction. Amiodarone is highly lipophilic and may have a half-life as long as 100 days, resulting in toxicity long after the drug is stopped.

CASE 3

A 45-year-old female presents to the office with complaint of a "ball in my neck." She noticed a lump in her anterior neck approximately 1 month ago. She is not sure if it has increased in size. She has not noticed any other lumps or masses. She denies dysphagia, odynophagia, neck pain, cough, weight loss, fever, chills, sweats, or a change in bowel habits. She also denies any hyperthyroid or hypothyroid symptoms. She is premenopausal, and her cycles are regular. She has been treated for diabetes for 6 years, which is well controlled with glyburide 5 mg daily. In 1993 she immigrated to the United States from Kiev, Ukraine, where she had lived for most of her life. She has no family history of thyroid or other endocrine disorders, but several of her relatives in Kiev have been diagnosed with various cancers.

Which of the following factors from her history INCREASES the likelihood that the nodule is malignant?

A) Nodule not increasing in size.
B) No regional adenopathy.
C) Age >40 years.
D) Female.
E) History of possible radiation exposure.

Discussion

The correct answer is E. This patient lived in Kiev, near the Chernobyl nuclear power plant during and after the reactor accident in 1986. She was exposed to radiation and, like her family members, is at significantly increased risk for cancer, specifically thyroid malignancies. Other factors from the history and physical that suggest a

malignant etiology include: a nodule >2 cm or increasing in size, dysphagia, hoarseness, regional lymphadenopathy, a fixation to the surrounding tissues, male gender, age <40 years, and family history.

 HELPFUL TIP: There are many cancer survivors walking around who received radiation to the neck (eg, mantle radiation for Hodgkin lymphoma). These patients are at increased risk of developing thyroid cancers.

* *

Physical exam reveals an obese female in no acute distress. Her head, eye, nose, and oral exams are normal. She has a 2-cm firm nodule on the right pole of the thyroid. The nodule moves along with the other subcutaneous structures upon swallowing. She has no lymphadenopathy. The remainder of the exam is normal.

Which of the following next steps would most likely yield a definitive diagnosis?

A) Thyroid ultrasound.
B) Fine-needle aspiration.
C) Thyroid scan (Tc^{99}).
D) Serum thyroglobulin level.
E) Serum calcitonin level.

Discussion

The correct answer is B. Fine-needle aspiration (FNA) is a biopsy technique that can conclusively prove or disprove the presence of neoplasm and should be considered for all thyroid nodules and cysts. Answer A is incorrect because an ultrasound would determine if the mass is cystic or not, but it will not exclude malignancy for a solid nodule. A thyroid scan (answer C) identifies whether a nodule is actively processing thyroid hormone ("functional" or "hot") or is not metabolically active ("nonfunctional" or "cold"). A "hot" nodule may cause hyperthyroidism, is **usually** nonmalignant ("hot is not") and can be treated with I^{131}. A cold nodule is either an adenoma or a malignancy and a biopsy is mandated. A serum thyroglobulin (answer D) is the tumor marker for thyroid carcinoma and should be drawn before thyroidectomy. It has no value as a diagnostic test in the initial evaluation before malignancy is determined but can be followed as a marker. Serum calcitonin levels (answer E) are elevated in the case of medullary carcinoma, but would have low yield in the initial evaluation.

* *

A tissue diagnosis reveals probable papillary carcinoma. A serum thyroglobulin level, TSH, basic chemistries, a blood count, and a blood type are ordered.

What should be done next?

A) Observe the nodule for 1 month.
B) Computerized tomography (CT) of the head and neck with contrast.
C) Radiation therapy with I^{131}.
D) Radiation therapy with external beam radiation.
E) Suppression of TSH levels with thyroxine.

Discussion

The correct answer is B. Surgery for removal of the tumor is the most appropriate next step, but a CT scan is indicated to delineate the extent of the neoplasm. Radiotherapy with I^{131} (answer C) is used after surgery for metastatic disease. External beam radiation (answer D) is not used for thyroid cancers except for the palliative therapy of anaplastic carcinoma. Because these tumors are TSH responsive, suppression of TSH level **following surgery** for papillary carcinoma is achieved with thyroxine (usually 2.2–2.5 micrograms/kg—a fairly high dose) (answer E).

> **HELPFUL TIP:** The most common thyroid cancer is papillary carcinoma. Medullary carcinoma may be associated with an elevated calcitonin and other endocrine malignancies (eg, multiple endocrine neoplasia type 2).

Objectives: Did you learn to . . .

- Recognize the major risk factors influencing the development and prognosis of thyroid carcinomas?
- Evaluate a thyroid nodule?
- Describe the management of papillary carcinoma, the most common of the thyroid cancers?
- Recognize and briefly describe the other types of thyroid cancer?

CASE 4

A 78-year-old female is brought to the ED because of strange behavior. According to her family, she has been more sleepy and weak throughout the last week. She is acting withdrawn and depressed and seems to respond to nonexistent external stimuli. When asked about her depression, she reports she is sad because a man in a clown suit who trains poodles keeps telling her she is going to die. She complains of abdominal cramps and blames it on "being plugged up," and her family reports she has had no bowel movement for 2 days. She also notes chronic bone pain in her hips and back.

A physical exam is notable only for a 3-cm irregular mass in her right breast. The patient denies noticing the mass before. Her neurologic exam is normal, except for her apparent confusion.

What finding would you expect from an ECG?

A) Peaked T waves.
B) Diffuse ST-segment elevations.
C) Long QT interval.
D) Short QT interval.
E) Second degree Mobitz II block.

Discussion

The correct answer is D. This patient likely has **hypercalcemia,** probably from an undiagnosed metastatic breast cancer. The ECG in a patient with significant hypercalcemia will show a short QT interval. **Hypo**calcemia is associated with a long QT interval (answer C), which can occasionally lead to arrhythmias due to an R on T phenomenon. Hypercalcemia produces symptoms in the central nervous system (confusion, psychosis, depression), gastrointestinal system (abdominal pain, cramps, constipation), kidneys (nephrolithiasis, polyuria, renal insufficiency), and musculoskeletal system (weakness, myopathy, osteoporosis). To remember the symptoms of hypercalcemia, use the rhyme "stones, bones, moans, groans, with psychiatric overtones." Peaked T waves (answer A) are associated with hyperkalemia. Diffuse ST-segment elevations (answer B) is a finding in pericarditis. The Mobitz II block (answer E) may develop for a variety of reasons, including ischemia and digitalis toxicity, but it is not associated with a particular electrolyte abnormality.

Which of the following tests should now be done?

A) Electrolytes, including a calcium level.
B) Complete blood count.

C) TSH.

D) Chest x-ray.

E) All of the above.

Discussion

The correct answer is E. The differential diagnosis for altered mental status in an elderly individual is relatively large, and many more tests might be appropriate. In addition to hypercalcemia, hyponatremia, and hypernatremia are possibilities in this case. This patient has several symptoms of hypothyroidism, so a TSH is critical. Rarely, hyperthyroidism may present in the elderly with lethargy rather than hyperkinetic activity—a presentation known as apathetic hyperthyroidism. Infections are common causes of altered mental status in the elderly. A complete blood count may reveal an elevated white blood cell count, a left shift, or anemia. The chest x-ray may detect a subclinical pneumonia or, more likely in this case, a mass from metastatic cancer.

* *

Your patient's calcium level is reported as 15.3 mg/dL (elevated).

What is the next step in her treatment?

A) Moderately aggressive normal saline hydration.

B) IV chlorthalidone administration.

C) IV calcitonin administration.

D) IV bisphosphonate infusion.

E) Gallium nitrate infusion.

Discussion

The correct answer is A. Before any diuretic can be given, adequate hydration with normal saline must be ensured. Decreasing the body's volume with a diuretic in the presence of hypercalcemia will only increase the relative concentration of calcium in the serum. A normal saline infusion will also increase urinary calcium excretion by inhibiting proximal tubular sodium and calcium reabsorption. This can be followed by a loop diuretic, usually IV furosemide, to enhance calcium excretions (be sure to keep up with IV fluids so as not to cause dehydration). Intravenous bisphosphonate infusion should then be started and will lower the calcium level over 2–4 days. Saline and furosemide can be used in the mean time to keep the calcium level under control. Calcitonin (answer C) has a limited duration of action and can be used in emergencies where saline and furosemide are ineffective. Gallium nitrate (answer E)

is an older treatment that has fallen out of favor with the advent of the reliable and safe bisphosphonates (answer D). It can still be used in refractory cases. Answer B is of special note. Chlorthalidone and other thiazide diuretics **increase** calcium levels and are contraindicated.

* *

The patient is treated appropriately for her hypercalcemia and her mental status improves. A biopsy of her breast mass is done and reveals an infiltrating ductal carcinoma. A bone scan reveals diffuse metastatic disease.

Which of the following statements about the mechanism for malignancy associated hypercalcemia is (are) TRUE?

A) Decreased bone reabsorption increases the serum calcium.

B) Secretion of osteoclast-inhibiting factors increases the serum calcium.

C) Secretion of PTH-like substances increases the serum calcium.

D) Direct erosion of bone by tumor cells never plays a role.

E) All of the above.

Discussion

The correct answer is C. Malignancy increases the serum calcium level by secreting osteoclast-**activating** (not inhibiting as in answer B) factors and PTH-like substances. This leads to increased bone reabsorption (not decreased as in answer A) and retention of calcium by the kidneys, which elevates the serum calcium. Answer D is incorrect because direct erosion of bone by tumor cells contributes to the release of calcium from the bones (and predisposes the patient to fractures). The neoplasms most commonly associated with hypercalcemia are cancers of the breast, lung, prostate, and kidney, as well as multiple myeloma and a few other hematologic cancers.

* *

Your patient's cancer cannot be cured.

How can her chronically elevated calcium level be managed?

A) Oral glucocorticoids.

B) Oral phosphates.

C) Oral bisphosphonates.

D) All of the above.

Discussion

The correct answer is D. Glucocorticoids decrease intestinal calcium absorption, but in and of themselves can lead to bone density loss and an increased risk for fractures. Oral phosphates can decrease intestinal calcium absorption and bone re-absorption of calcium. Bisphosphonates, as previously discussed, decrease the serum calcium and increase bone density.

Objectives: Did you learn to . . .

- Recognize neoplastic causes of hypercalcemia?
- Identify presenting symptoms of hypercalcemia?
- Understand the mechanisms underlying hypercalcemia in malignancy?
- Initiate emergency treatment for symptomatic hypercalcemia?

CASE 5

A 42-year-old male presents to the office for routine follow-up of his hypertension. He denies any complaints. He has primary hypertension, for which he takes benazepril 20 mg PO daily and hydrochlorothiazide 25 mg PO daily. The patient takes no other medications. His vital signs are as follows: BP 135/70, P 72, R 18, T 98.6°F. The physical exam is completely normal. His laboratory test results are listed in Table 10–2.

You consider what you know about hypercalcemia.

Which of the following is responsible for spuriously elevated serum calcium?

A) Pseudo-potassium transport.
B) Fever and active metabolic state.
C) Use of alendronate or risedronate.

Table 10–2 LABORATORY RESULTS

Complete Blood Count	Chemistry	
WBC: 8,9000 cells/mm³	Na: 140 mEq/L	BUN: 12 mg/dL
Hb: 12 g/dL	K: 3.6 mEq/L	Cr: 0.9 mg/dL
Hct: 36%	Cl: 110 mEq/L	Ca 12.8 mg/dL
Plts: 245,000 cells/mm³	CO₂: 24 mEq/L	

D) Prolonged application of the tourniquet while drawing blood.
E) All of the above.

Discussion

The correct answer is D. Prolonged application of the tourniquet or a high-calcium meal before a blood draw can both cause a spuriously elevated serum calcium. Approximately 50% of patients have a normal calcium when it is checked a second time. So, the next step after finding an elevated calcium is to repeat the test. Answer C will cause a low calcium level. Answer A doesn't exist that we know of.

* *

Assuming you repeat the lab value and it remains elevated, your next step is:

A) A bone scan for occult cancer.
B) Immediate dialysis.
C) Nothing, since the patient is asymptomatic.
D) Discontinue the hydrochlorothiazide and recheck calcium in 2 weeks.
E) Discontinue the benazepril and recheck potassium in 2 weeks.

Discussion

The correct answer is D. This patient has hypercalcemia. Asymptomatic hypercalcemia is not uncommon on routine screening examinations. It should be addressed because it is always abnormal and can be treated early before any symptoms develop. In this patient, the most likely cause is hydrochlorothiazide. Thiazide drugs increase the renal reabsorption of calcium. Angiotensin-converting enzyme (ACE) inhibitors may cause hyperkalemia but are usually not associated with hypercalcemia. An investigation for occult cancer may be indicated in this patient's future, but it is reasonable to address the potential adverse drug effect first. Dialysis is not indicated.

* *

The patient stops taking the hydrochlorothiazide and returns for a laboratory draw in 2 weeks. The calcium level is now 12.9 mg/dL.

What should you do next?

A) Wait another month and recheck before taking any other action.
B) Order a 24-hour bisphosphonate infusion.
C) Perform prostate and testicular exam for masses, chest x-ray, and iPTH (parathyroid hormone level).

D) Perform prostate and testicular exam for masses, CT of the chest, abdomen, and pelvis, and bone scan.

E) Perform prostate and testicular exam for masses, chest x-ray, then reassure patient if normal.

Discussion

The correct answer is C. In this patient, it is reasonable to rule out primary hyperparathyroidism while also checking for other obvious causes. A chest x-ray will rule out significant lung masses and sarcoidosis. A testicular and prostate exam for masses is important so that **large** tumors in these organs do not go unnoticed (remember that a digital rectal exam is neither sensitive nor specific for prostate cancer). An elevated PTH in the presence of a calcium level >12 mg/dL confirms the diagnosis of hyperparathyroidism. The test for **intact** parathyroid hormone (iPTH) will not cross-react significantly with the PTH-like hormone produced by neoplasms. Unless the history or physical is suspicious for lymphoma, or some other occult neoplasm, a pan-body scan is a waste of money and exposes the patient to unnecessary radiation. It is not necessary now to acutely lower the calcium level because the cause has not been identified and the patient is asymptomatic (Table 10–3).

* *

The patient's complete exam is normal as is the chest x-ray. The PTH level is twice the upper limit of normal.

How should this patient be treated?

A) Immediate CT of the chest, abdomen, and pelvis.

B) Intravenous bisphosphonate infusion.

C) Daily dialysis until the calcium level is normal.

D) Referral for parathyroidectomy.

E) Referral for thyroidectomy.

Discussion

The correct answer is D. This patient has primary hyperparathyroidism. He has an elevated parathyroid hormone in the presence of hypercalcemia. This is usually caused by a functional parathyroid adenoma and is best treated in otherwise healthy patients with a parathyroidectomy. This can be done without significant loss of thyroid tissue. In elderly patients with mild hyperparathyroidism and asymptomatic hypercalcemia, medical management is an option. If the patient had a low or normal PTH level, occult cancer should be considered (check for PTH-like hormone in the serum), and a bone scan or body CT (answer A) may be warranted. Although bisphosphonates (answer B) will

Table 10–3 CAUSES OF HYPERCALCEMIA

Pseudohypercalcemia

Excessive calcium intake

Hypervitaminosis D

Hyperparathyroidism (primary and secondary)

Hyperthyroidism

Malignancy

Hypervitaminosis A

Adrenal insufficiency

Pheochromocytoma

Rhabdomyolysis

Familial hypocalciuria

Immobiliation

Medications

   Lithium

   Megestrol

   Methyltestosterone

   Mycophenolate

   Tacrolimus

   Tamoxifen

   Theophylline (toxicity)

   Thiazides

lower the serum calcium and may be used in an emergency, a parathyroidectomy is curative. Dialysis (answer C) is not indicated in this patient. Answer E is incorrect because you want to remove the parathyroid glands, not the thyroid. If you chose answer E, you were probably reading to fast.

* *

Your patient undergoes a parathyroidectomy and is discharged from the hospital. The pathology report on the removed tissue confirms the presence of a parathyroid adenoma and no malignancy. He returns for his first postoperative appointment 1 week later, and he is complaining of weakness. He says that the day after the surgery he felt fine, but has progressively gotten weaker "all over" since that time. Last night, he was kept awake by recurrent muscle spasms in his legs and arms. He denies fever, chills, nausea, or vomiting. He says he is eating, drinking, and passing urine as normal. He has had no hematuria or dysuria.

His vital signs are: BP 140/80, P 88, R 18, T 98°F. On physical exam, he appears anxious. Just after taking the patient's vital signs, his left arm develops a muscle spasm and an involuntary flexion of the wrist that lasts for about 20–30 seconds. Tapping the cheek just anterior to the tragus causes the ipsilateral face to twitch. The rest of cranial nerve exam is normal. His neck wound is healing well, with minimal erythema and no tenderness. The rest of the physical exam is unremarkable.

What is the cause of this patient's symptoms?

A) He suffers from vitamin D deficiency.
B) This patient has MEN II and also has a pheochromocytoma.
C) Too much parathyroid tissue was removed during the surgery.
D) The stress of the surgery precipitated thyrotoxicosis.
E) The stress of the surgery precipitated the onset of multiple sclerosis.

Discussion

The correct answer is C. This patient likely has hypocalcemia due to excessive removal of parathyroid gland tissue. This is a rare, but unfortunate, complication of parathyroid gland removal and is usually detected in the immediate postoperative course. The patient's physical exam demonstrates Chvostek sign (tapping over the facial nerve elicits a twitch) and Trousseau sign (carpopedal spasm after placement of a blood pressure cuff). Vitamin D deficiency, although a cause of hypocalcemia, is unlikely to develop so quickly. The usual cause of vitamin D deficiency is malabsorption, but there is nothing in the patient's history to suggest this. There is nothing to suggest MEN II (multiple endocrine neoplasia II: hyperparathyroidism, medullary thyroid carcinoma, and pheochromocytoma). There is also nothing here to suggest pheochromocytoma (episodic diaphoresis, labile blood pressure, recurrent palpitations, and near-syncope). There is no clinical evidence of thyrotoxicosis (tachycardia, tremor, etc).

* *

Calcium and albumin levels are sent, as well as a complete blood count and routine chemistry panel. The results are listed in Table 10–4.

Does this patient have hypocalcemia?

A) No, the serum calcium level is normal.
B) No, the serum calcium level when corrected for the albumin is normal.
C) Yes, because the serum (calcium × phosphate) product is >20.

Table 10–4   LABORATORY RESULTS

WWBC: 6,700 cells/mm³	Na: 140 mEq/L	
Hct: 13 g/dL	K: 4.0 mEq/L	Ca: 5.1 mg/dL
Hb: 40%	Cl: 110 mEq/L	P: 4.2 mg/dL
Plts: 213,000 cells/mm³	CO₂: 24 mEq/L	Mg: 2.0 mEq/L
BUN: 12 mg/dL	Cr: 0.8 mg/dL	Albumin: 3.0 g/L

D) Yes, because the serum calcium level is still low when corrected for albumin.
E) Insufficient information to determine.

Discussion

The correct answer is D. The patient's calcium level is low, even after correcting for the hypoaluminemia. To correct for albumin, add 0.8 mg/dL to the serum calcium level for each 1 g/L the albumin is <4. Corrected serum calcium = [(4 − albumin) × 0.8] + measured serum calcium. Here the equation is

$$[(4 - 3) \times 0.8] + 5.1 = 5.9 \text{ mg/dL}$$

When evaluating hypocalcemia it is prudent to check a BUN and creatinine to rule out renal failure as a cause (from renal osteodystrophy; see Chapter 5 for more information).

 HELPFUL TIP: If you don't want to correct for albumin, check for ionized calcium. An ionized calcium will also be useful in patients with monoclonal gammopathy or multiple myeloma. Occasionally, these proteins can also bind calcium.

How should this patient now be treated?

A) Calcium gluconate 1 g by rapid IV push.
B) Correct his hypomagnesemia with IV MgSO₄.
C) Correct his hyperphosphatemia with phosphate-binding antacids.
D) Calcium carbonate 1–4 g with vitamin D PO daily.
E) No therapy, as the calcium level will correct itself.

Discussion

The correct answer is D. The patient now requires oral calcium supplementation, usually with vitamin D to stimulate absorption. He will likely require it life-long. This patient has neither hypomagnesia nor hyperphosphatemia. If he had, correcting either would also raise the serum calcium. Answer A is of special note. IV calcium gluconate or calcium chloride can be used in this situation. But they should not be given by rapid IV push but rather by slow push over a couple of minutes.

Objectives: Did you learn to . . .

- Describe the evaluation and treatment for primary hyperparathyroidism?
- Recognize the signs and symptoms of hypocalcemia and hypercalcemia?
- Recognize the causes of hypercalcemia and hypocalcemia?
- Evaluate and treat hypocalcemia?

CASE 6

A 36-year-old female presents to the office with complaint of difficulty losing weight. She seeks a prescription drug to aid in efforts to lose unwanted weight she has been gaining for 2 years. She has tried every fad diet, but nothing seems to help. She tries to exercise regularly, but manages only walking a couple of miles each week. A nutritional history reveals that she is eating a sensible low-fat diet. Her past medical history includes hypertension treated with medications for the last 3 years and non–insulin-dependent diabetes mellitus for the last year. She also has been seeing a psychiatrist over the last 6 months for emotional lability, which she attributes to anxiety over her inability to get pregnant. The patient takes glyburide 5 mg PO daily and benazepril (Lotensin) 40 mg PO daily. A review of systems reveals thinning hair, irregular menses, delayed wound healing, and infertility.

What dietary advice can you offer this patient now?

A) She is eating right, she just needs to exercise more.
B) Low-fat diets are ineffective, she needs to reduce her carbohydrate intake.
C) She has failed lifestyle modifications and appetite suppressant medications are indicated.

D) She is likely depressed, and needs to continue psychiatric therapy and probably should start treatment with an SSRI.
E) Reserve any dietary advice at this time, as she first needs a medical workup.

Discussion

The correct answer is E. The patient's symptoms of weight gain and associated findings on review of systems (emotionally labile, thinning hair, infertility, irregular menses, and delayed wound healing) suggest a secondary cause, most likely an endocrine abnormality.

 HELPFUL TIP: Did you notice that she is trying to get pregnant and is on an ACE inhibitor? ACE inhibitors are teratogenic and contraindicated in pregnancy.

* *

A physical exam reveals the following:

Vitals: P 88, BP 155/94, R 20, T 37.7°C

General: Middle-aged female with obese body and thin extremities

HEENT: Thinning hair, round facies, hirsutism

Back: Buffalo hump noted

Skin: Hyperpigmentation, abdominal striae

The rest of the physical exam is unremarkable.

Based on this patient's history and physical exam, what diagnosis is most likely?

A) Hypothyroidism.
B) Hyperthyroidism.
C) Cortisol excess secondary to chronic steroid therapy.
D) Cortisol excess secondary to an endogenous process (Cushing disease).
E) Cortisol deficiency secondary to autoimmune adrenal insufficiency.

Discussion

The correct answer is D. This patient has the classic symptoms and signs of Cushing *syndrome*, or cortisol excess. This may result from corticosteroid therapy (the most common cause), ectopic ACTH production from neoplasms of the lung, pancreas, kidney, etc, adrenal neoplasms producing cortisol, or ACTH production from a pituitary neoplasm (termed Cushing *disease*). Her condition is unlikely resulting from steroid therapy, as this should have been revealed in her medical history. At this point in the evaluation, it is not clear what the source of ACTH is, only that there is excess ACTH being produced.

* *

Laboratory findings are as follows: Na 142 mEq/L, K 2.9 mEq/L, Cl 112 mEq/L, CO_2 30 mEq/L, BUN 14 mg/dL, Cr 1.1 mg/dL, Glucose 210 mg/dL, 24-hour urinary free cortisol: 115 micrograms (normal: <100 micrograms)

Based on these findings, a dexamethasone suppression test is ordered. The patient is given huge, supratherapeutic dexamethasone for 2 days, and then serum ACTH is drawn, and another 24-hour urine collection is done. The results are: serum ACTH, normal; 24-hour urinary free cortisol, 78 micrograms (normal).

What is the source of this patient's cortisol excess?

A) An ACTH-producing tumor.
B) A cortisol-producing adrenal tumor.
C) Surreptitious use of oral steroids.
D) Not enough information to determine.

Discussion

The correct answer is A. When the patient was given exogenous steroids during the test, there was a partial suppression of cortisol production (mild decrease in 24-hour urinary free cortisol). But more important, the serum ACTH level remained normal despite the high steroid load. It should have been low in the presence of dexamethasone or any exogenous steroid, which acts to shut off ACTH production in the normal patient.

Normal mechanisms provide negative feedback on the pituitary gland (the source of ACTH) when cortisol levels are high. If ACTH is still being produced despite a high steroid load, there must be an ACTH-producing neoplasm somewhere in the body—either ectopic production from a lung, renal, or pancreas cancer, or an ACTH-producing pituitary tumor which has escaped normal regulatory feedback mechanisms (eg, increased steroids cause decreased ACTH).

 HELPFUL TIP: In a cortisol-producing adrenal neoplasm, the high endogenous steroid doses effectively suppress ACTH production because the pituitary is functioning. The urinary

free cortisol remains high (the tumor produces cortisol independent of any hormonal control). However, since the pituitary is functioning, the baseline ACTH would is low to begin with.

* *

On physical exam, the patient has a visual field cut.

What is the best next step in this patient's evaluation?

A) Ultrasound of kidneys to assess for masses and adrenal flow.
B) CT scan of the brain to rule out metastatic lesions and assess pituitary size.
C) CT scan of the adrenals to evaluate for adrenal neoplasms.
D) MRI of the pancreas to evaluate for neoplasms.
E) MRI of the pituitary gland to evaluate for a neoplasm.

Discussion

The correct answer is E. The previous studies strongly suggest Cushing syndrome and the visual field cut suggests a pituitary source of the ACTH (eg, ACTH-producing tumor of the pituitary gland). An MRI of the pituitary is the best means to confirm this. CT scan (answers B and C) may suggest enlargement of the sella turcica (where the pituitary gland sits), but it is insensitive for detecting abnormalities in the pituitary, especially microadenomas. If the MRI is negative, the more rare case of ectopic ACTH production from occult cancer must be considered, and a body CT scan is indicated. This patient's studies do not suggest the presence of an adrenal tumor.

Objectives: Did you learn to . . .

- Recognize the common presenting signs and symptoms of Cushing syndrome?
- Identify the causes of cortisol excess and how they are best evaluated?

CASE 7

JFK, a 38-year-old male, presents to the office with the chief complaint of weakness. He reports that he lacks the energy to complete his previously busy work schedule and has cut his hours back the last 2–3 weeks, which has recently become a financial hardship. JFK also reports poor appetite and a 20-pound weight loss over the last month. He has had alternating periods of diarrhea and constipation. He reports feeling faint often and has come near to passing out after standing up quickly a few times. This is different for him from baseline. He has no previous medical or surgical history. He denies medications or allergies. He reports that several relatives on his mother's side have had "thyroid problems."

The results of a physical exam follow:

Vitals: BP 85/38, P 85, R 20, T 37°C

General: Well-developed male in no acute distress

HEENT: Hyperpigmentation of buccal mucosa

Thyroid exam: Normal

Neuro: 5-/5 strength in both upper and both lower extremities; weakness is more pronounced in the proximal muscles; cranial nerve, sensory, reflexes, and cerebellar examination are normal

Skin: Hyperpigmentation of the elbows, knuckles, knees, and the palmar creases; no edema

What is the most likely cause of this patient's symptoms?

A) Hyperthyroidism.
B) Hypothyroidism.
C) Adrenal gland hyperactivity.
D) Adrenal insufficiency.
E) Depression.

Discussion

The correct answer is D. Several clues point in this direction. First, the hyperpigmentation found at stress/crease points on the peripheral skin suggest the diagnosis of adrenal insufficiency. The low blood pressure and orthostasis are also more likely to be seen in adrenal insufficiency.

This patient has a number of symptoms consistent with both depression (answer E) and hypothyroidism (answer B), but his physical exam suggests another diagnosis. A patient with depression and no underlying medical cause would have a normal physical exam. A patient with hypothyroidism may have a slightly low blood pressure, but not markedly low as in this patient. The heart rate in symptomatic hypothyroidism is usually low. Hypothyroidism may also cause changes in the hair, skin, and thyroid gland that are not seen here.

Finally, the patient's reflexes are normal, rather than delayed. There is nothing in this case to suggest hyperthyroidism (answer A) or cortisol excess (answer C).

* *

Laboratory results are:

Na: 129 mEq/L (low)

BUN: 18 mg/dL

Cr: 0.7 mg/dL

K: 5.4 mEq/L (high)

Glucose: 65 mg/dL (low)

Cl: 96 mEq/L

TSH: 4.2 micrograms×IU/mL

HCO_3: 22 mEq/L

Hb: 11 g/dL

Based on the above, what other laboratory test should be ordered?

A) Cosyntropin stimulation test.
B) Random serum cortisol.
C) Bone marrow biopsy.
D) Plasma renin.
E) Ultrasound of kidneys to measure their size.

Discussion

The correct answer is A. The laboratory chemistry results (hyperkalemia, hyponatremia, and hypoglycemia) strongly suggest a mineralocorticoid deficiency. A cosyntropin stimulation test uses synthetic ACTH to try to induce a burst of cortisol secretion. No increase in the serum cortisol in response to the cosyntropin suggests that the adrenal glands are unable to respond to the body's mineralocorticoid and glucocorticoid needs. A positive cosyntropin test makes the diagnosis of adrenal insufficiency. A random serum cortisol (answer B) is unlikely to be helpful, as cortisol levels normally fluctuate widely throughout the diurnal cycle. Plasma renin (answer D) is used in the evaluation of mineralocorticoid excess (hyperaldosteronism). Ultrasound of kidneys (answer E) is not likely to be helpful. Even in the case of adrenal insufficiency, the kidneys are unlikely to change in size. Although an ultrasound may show small, shrunken adrenals that have been destroyed by tuberculosis infection, a CT scan is a better tool for assessing the adrenals. Bone marrow biopsy (answer C) is way off base. This patient has no indication for a bone marrow biopsy.

* *

You receive further laboratory results:

Random serum cortisol: 12 micrograms/dL (normal ≥20 micrograms/dL)

Serum cortisol 1 hour after 0.25 mg cosyntropin IV: 13.5 micrograms/dL (the rise in cortisol is expected to be >7micrograms/dL)

What is the most likely underlying cause of this patient's condition?

A) Autoimmune disease.
B) Invasive carcinoma.
C) Meningococcal septicemia.
D) Sarcoidosis.
E) Tuberculosis.

Discussion

The correct answer is A. All the conditions listed are known causes of primary adrenal insufficiency, and all cause this disorder by destruction of the adrenal glands. This results in a lack of adrenal hormone secretion and a blunted response of the adrenals to ACTH—hence, the minimal rise of cortisol despite administration of synthetic ACTH (cosyntropin). A cortisol rise of <7 micrograms/dL (in response to cosyntropin) with a baseline cortisol <20 micrograms/dL is suggestive of primary adrenal insufficiency. Autoimmune destruction is the most common cause in North America, and invasion of the adrenals by tuberculosis is the most common cause worldwide.

* *

Without measuring the serum ACTH or 24-hour urine ACTH level, it is possible to differentiate between primary (lack of adrenal response to ACTH) and secondary (lack of ACTH) adrenal insufficiency.

Which of the following suggests primary adrenal insufficiency (eg, adrenal destruction) rather than secondary?

A) Elevation of cortisol by cosyntropin test of >7 micrograms/dL.
B) Presence of hyperpigmentation on physical exam.
C) Presence of neuropathy on physical exam.
D) Predominant symptoms of depression.
E) Evidence of hyponatremia.

Discussion

The correct answer is B. Hyperpigmentation occurs only in primary adrenal insufficiency because the pituitary is intact and the ACTH level is high, as are levels of melanocyte-stimulating hormone. An elevation of cortisol >7micrograms/dL during the cosyntropin test (answer A) suggests an intact adrenal system with a pituitary problem. Hyponatremia (answer E) and depression (answer D) are symptoms common to all causes of adrenal insufficiency. Neuropathy (answer C) is not a common finding in adrenal insufficiency.

 HELPFUL TIP: Patients with primary adrenal insufficiency **may** present with low serum sodium and high serum potassium (although many have normal electrolytes). This is primarily because of loss of the aldosterone system. Patients with secondary adrenal insufficiency (eg, pituitary cause) have intact adrenal glands and therefore intact aldosterone. Thus, they generally have normal electrolytes and less dehydration, hypotension, etc.

How should this patient now be treated?

A) Prednisone 60 mg PO for 5 days, then slowly tapered over 2 weeks.
B) Cosyntropin 0.5 mg SC daily indefinitely.
C) Corticosteroids (prednisone 5 mg or hydrocortisone 15 mg) daily indefinitely.
D) Corticosteroids (prednisone 5 mg or hydrocortisone 15 mg) daily plus mineralocorticoid (fludrocortisone 0.1 mg) daily indefinitely.
E) Adrenal transplant.

Discussion

The correct answer is D. This patient requires chronic corticosteroid supplementation, and, because he has primary adrenal insufficiency, he also requires mineralocorticoid supplementation. Cosyntropin treatment would have no effect since the adrenals are not functioning. A short burst of prednisone is important if this patient experiences a sudden stressor, such as an infection, but it is not the primary therapy. Medical therapy is fairly effective, so adrenal (or renal) transplant is not a usual treatment option.

* *

JFK is treated appropriately and, after 4 weeks, is feeling much better, has regained most of his lost weight, and feels well enough to invade Cuba. He no longer suffers spells of lightheadedness or depression. To celebrate his new good health, he and a blond starlet go out for lavish seafood dinner, including fresh steamed oysters. Within 8 hours of the meal, JFK develops severe cramping abdominal pain and profuse watery diarrhea. He tries to treat himself at home with Pepto-Bismol and oral fluids, but gets progressively weaker. After 12 hours of intestinal symptoms, he calls for an ambulance because he is too weak to stand.

Upon presentation in the ED, these are the findings:

Vital signs: P 130, BP 70/20, R 30, T 38°C

General: Diaphoretic, ill-appearing male in severe distress

HEENT: Dry mucous membranes

Heart: Tachycardia

Chest: Mostly clear to auscultation

Abdomen: Diffuse tenderness, no masses

Rectal: Heme negative stool

Skin: Poor turgor, but no petechiae or purpura

After establishing adequate intravenous access, what should be done next?

A) Order a chest x-ray.
B) Start "renal-dose" dopamine through a peripheral line.
C) Give 2 liters normal saline by bolus.
D) Start normal saline at 125 cc/hour.
E) Give levofloxacin 500 mg IV.

Discussion

The correct answer is C. This patient is severely volume depleted and needs crystalloid immediately. All other treatments, although they may be done eventually, are secondary.

* *

Fluid is run in quickly and he remains hypotensive.

What should have been done simultaneously for this patient when the fluids were started?

A) Intubation by rapid sequence and mechanical ventilation.
B) Administration of a phenylephrine drip.
C) Administration of 4-mg dexamethasone IV.
D) Administration of 100-mg hydrocortisone IV.
E) C or D.

Discussion

The correct answer is E. This patient has adrenal insufficiency and requires additional "stress doses" of steroids in times of severe physical stress (eg, infection, trauma, chest pain). The steroids he takes regularly for his disease may not be sufficient during these periods, precipitating addisonian crisis. Without this additional treatment, the patient may experience intractable hypotension and possibly death.

 HELPFUL TIP: If you suspect adrenal insufficiency crisis, start steroids immediately even if you do not have laboratory confirmation. Dexamethasone is an option for treatment, and it will not interfere with the cortisol assay when doing a cosyntropin stimulation test.

Objectives: Did you learn to . . .

- Recognize the presentation of adrenal insufficiency?
- Evaluate a patient with adrenal insufficiency?
- Treat a patient chronically for adrenal insufficiency and when in adrenal crisis?

 QUICK QUIZ: DIABETES DIAGNOSIS

Which is the most appropriate laboratory test to use for the initial diagnosis of diabetes mellitus?

A) 1-hour oral glucose tolerance test.
B) Fasting blood glucose.
C) Anti–beta-cell antibodies.
D) 3-hour oral glucose tolerance test.
E) Glycosylated hemoglobin (HbA_{1c}).

Discussion

The correct answer is B. Fasting blood glucose testing is preferred to any oral glucose tolerance test due to ease of performance, convenience for patients, and cost. Anti–beta-cell antibody testing is indicated for differentiating type 1 from type 2 diabetes, not in the initial diagnostic phase. The hemoglobin A_{1c} (glycosolated hemoglobin or HbA_{1c}) test has not yet been sufficiently standardized for use as a diagnostic test; its main use is in monitoring glycemic control in patients with diabetes. Obviously, a patient with a very high HbA_{1c} has diabetes. However, patients may have mild diabetes with a relatively normal HbA$_{1c}$. Thus, the fasting or random blood sugar is still critical to the diagnosis of diabetes.

QUICK QUIZ: DIABETES DIAGNOSIS

Which of the following statements is FALSE?

A) The diagnosis of diabetes can be made if a fasting blood sugar is ≥126 mg/dL **or** a random blood sugar is >200mg/dL in a patient with symptoms (polyuria, polydipsia); the glucose level must be confirmed on a different day.

B) Impaired fasting blood glucose is defined as a fasting level of 100–125 mg/dL.

C) Patients with diabetes type 1.5 (also known as latent autoimmune diabetes in adults or slowly progressing type 1) are generally thin.

D) Patients with diabetes type 1.5 comprise approximately 20% of patients diagnosed with diabetes type 2.

E) Patients with diabetes type 1.5 manifest significant insulin resistance.

Discussion

The correct answer is E (which is a false statement). Patients with diabetes type 1.5 **do not** have insulin resistance. Diabetes type 1.5 (also known as latent autoimmune diabetes in adults or slowly progressing type 1) is a relatively new concept. Type 1.5 patients have adult-onset diabetes similar to type 2 patients. However, type 1.5 patients are generally thin, not hypertensive, and do not have the rest of the constellation of disease in diabetes type 2 (low HDL, high triglycerides). Generally, they need insulin relatively early in the course of their treatment although they initially respond to oral hypoglycemic agents. The other answer choices are true statements. Note the criteria for making the diagnosis of diabetes mellitus in answers A and B.

HELPFUL TIP: The American Diabetes Association has determined that a blood sugar of 100mg/dL is now "prediabetes" and represents "impaired fasting glucose." The authors think calling a normal blood sugar prediabetes is absurd. So does the European Diabetes Epidemiology Group which advocates use of the original 110 mg/dL as impaired fasting glucose. Remember that the risk of diabetes is continuous along all fasting blood glucose levels, with no clear-cut point for increased risk of end-organ disease.

CASE 8

You are called to the ED to see a 17-year-old male brought in by his parents who found him at home in his room. He is lethargic, but not unconscious or comatose. He is unable to give a coherent history. His parents state that they have been concerned because the patient has been losing weight in the last two months, and acting more tired than usual. They are worried that he might be abusing drugs, but have not found any drugs or drug paraphernalia in the home. They have observed no other signs of illness. The family history is positive for hypertension in multiple family members, and the patient's mother has hyperlipidemia. There is no family history of kidney or liver disease, heart attacks or strokes, diabetes, or cancer.

Your exam discloses the following:

Vital signs: Temp 36.9°C, pulse 125, BP 98/54, respirations are deep with a rate of 28

Mental status: Lethargic, arouses to pain; nonverbal

HEENT: Mucous membranes dry, tongue fissured; fruity aroma on breath

Neck: Supple, no masses

Lungs: Clear to auscultation throughout, no wheezes or stridor

Heart: Regular rapid rate, no murmur or gallop

Abdomen: Soft, mild generalized tenderness without guarding or rebound; no masses or organomegaly

Extremities: Skin turgor is poor

Test results are as follows:

ECG: Sinus tachycardia, otherwise normal

Portable CXR: No infiltrates or other abnormalities seen

Hemogram: Hb 17.9 g/dL; WBC 16,200 cells/mm³, predominantly neutrophils; platelets 650,000 cells/mm³

Electrolytes: Sodium 131 mEq/L, potassium 5.7 mEq/L, chloride 97 mEq/L, bicarbonate 10 mEq/L

Renal: BUN 63 mg/dL, creatinine 1.8 mg/dL, glucose 635 mg/dL

Hepatic: Transaminases, bilirubin, alkaline phosphatase, gamma-GT all normal

ABG (room air): pH 7.2; pCO$_2$ 27 mm Hg; PO$_2$ 101 mm Hg, Bicarb 10mEq/L

Serum ketones: Positive

You diagnose diabetic ketoacidosis with dehydration >10% and admit the patient to the ICU. As the first stage of therapy you wish to replace the lost fluid volume.

Which of the following regimens is the most appropriate?

A) 5% dextrose in 0.45% (half-normal) saline to run at 150 cc/hour.

B) 0.45% (half-normal) saline with 20 mEq potassium/liter, to run at 150 cc/hour.

C) 0.9% (normal) saline 1 L to infuse as quickly as possible.

D) 0.9% (normal) saline with 20 mEq potassium/liter to run at 1000 cc/hour.

E) 5% dextrose in 0.225% (quarter-normal) saline with 20 mEq potassium/liter to run at 1000 cc/hour.

Discussion

The correct answer is C. Initial volume replacement should be with isotonic saline infused at a rapid rate (in the absence of cardiac disease) until the volume deficit is corrected.

Answer D is of special note. In general, potassium should be added to the **second liter** of fluid unless the patient is already hypokalemic on the first blood gas (getting a potassium, glucose, and sodium on the first blood gas is good policy). Potassium replacement is essential even in the hyperkalemic patient, as correction of the ketoacidosis leads to a rapid shift of potassium into the intracellular compartment. Remember that an acidosis artificially increases the serum potassium by shifting potassium extracellularly. See Chapter 5, Nephrology for more on acidosis, alkalosis, and the effects on potassium. Answer D is incorrect because you would like the first liter to infuse as quickly as possible in DKA and not over an hour. Besides, 20 mEq of potassium IV in 1 hour should not be routine and only given if the patient is on cardiac monitors.

 HELPFUL TIP: Urine ketones are >99% sensitive for diabetic ketoacidosis. Checking serum ketones is superfluous in most cases.

Which of the following regimens is most appropriate for this patient?

A) Subcutaneous NPH insulin, 1 unit/kg; repeat as necessary.

B) IV regular insulin, 5 unit IV bolus, followed by constant infusion at 0.1 U/kg/hour; adjusted as needed.

C) Subcutaneous regular insulin, 0.5–1 unit/kg; adjust dose by fingerstick blood glucose results.

D) Intramuscular regular insulin, 5–10 units hourly; adjust dose by fingerstick blood glucose results.

Discussion

The correct answer is B. A bolus of intravenous regular insulin, followed by a constant infusion, adjusted to reduce the blood glucose level by 50–75 mg/dL/hour is the appropriate therapy. This may frequently require <0.1 U/kg/hour but this is a good place to start. Intramuscular insulin administration is an alternative, but absorption is unreliable, especially in hypotensive patients. Long-acting insulins and subcutaneous insulin administration have no place in the initial management of diabetic ketoacidosis.

 HELPFUL TIP: Although conventional, the bolus of 5 units of regular insulin is unnecessary and does not change outcomes. Starting a drip of regular insulin is the critical step here.

Which of the following types of insulin can be administered IV?

A) NPH insulin.

B) Lantus insulin.

C) Lente insulin.

D) Ultralente insulin

E) None of the above.

Discussion

The correct answer is E. The only insulin that can be administered IV is regular insulin.

* *

The patient's status improves, and you recheck his blood sugar. His glucose is now 200 mg/dL and his insulin drip is still at 5 units per hour. His pH is 7.30 with a bicarbonate level of 14 mEq/L.

Because his glucose has almost normalized, your decision now is to:

A) Administer bicarbonate in order to finish correcting the pH.
B) Decrease the rate of the insulin infusion to 2 units per hour.
C) Add 10% dextrose to his treatment.
D) Consider the addition of an oral hypoglycemic agent.
E) None of the above.

Discussion

The correct answer is C. This patient is still acidotic and will need continued insulin to reverse his catabolic state. Thus, the appropriate treatment is to increase the amount of sugar he is getting. Remember, diabetic ketoacidosis is not primarily a result of too much sugar but rather of too little insulin. Answer A is incorrect. **Bicarbonate plays no role in the treatment of diabetic ketoacidosis no matter what the pH**. The administration of bicarbonate prolongs acidosis and ketosis and produces a paradoxical CNS acidosis. Additionally, it shifts the oxygen dissociation curve to reduce oxygen delivery to the tissue. **The only predictor of cerebral edema in children treated for DKA is the administration of bicarbonate.** So, there is no need to restrict fluids in children being treated for DKA (although this does **not** mean you should overhydrate them).

The common causes of diabetic ketoacidosis include all of the following EXCEPT:

A) Missed insulin.
B) Infection.
C) Myocardial infarction.
D) Dietary indiscretion.
E) Metabolic stress.

Discussion

The correct answer is D. Dietary indiscretion does not generally precipitate DKA. DKA is a state caused by a lack of insulin rather than by increased intake of carbohydrates. Certainly dietary indiscretion will complicate glucose control but it will not precipitate DKA. All of the other answer choices can cause DKA.

Which of the following statements is FALSE:

A) The Somogyi phenomenon occurs when a patient's blood sugar becomes elevated and there is a reactive hypoglycemia.

B) Patients who are being treated appropriately for DKA may have an increase in serum ketones during treatment.
C) There is no correlation between the WBC count and the presence of infection in patients with DKA.
D) Glucagon is an inappropriate treatment for patients with alcoholic hypoglycemia.

Discussion

The correct answer (and false statement) is A. The Somogyi phenomenon occurs when a patient becomes **hypo**glycemic (often in the middle of the night) and there is a reactive **hyper**glycemia from adrenergic outpouring. Often, patients will have an elevated morning blood sugar and will increase their evening NPH. This may be counterproductive if the problem is the Somogyi phenomenon. Symptoms of Somogyi phenomenon include night sweats and vivid, sometimes disturbing dreams. The other answer choices are true statements. Beta-hydroxybutyrate is metabolized to acetoacetic acid which will increase serum ketone measurements (answer B). Answer C is true since patients in DKA generally have an elevated WBC count, and leukocytosis in this setting cannot be relied upon as a sign of infection. Answer D is true because patients with alcoholic hypoglycemia have exhausted their glycogen stores and are generally NAD deficient and thus have impaired gluconeogenesis. Thus, glucagon will not work. Another group on which glucagon will not work is the infant or child who becomes hypoglycemic overnight and has a seizure in the morning. They have already depleted their stores of glucagon.

 HELPFUL TIP: Consider the possibility of a silent myocardial infarction in a diabetic patient who is generally well controlled but suddenly has elevated blood sugars.

 HELPFUL TIP: Twenty percent of patients with DKA have "normoglycemic" DKA with a blood sugar <300 mg/dL.

* *

This patient presents to your clinic 4 months after his hospitalization. He has noted postprandial fullness, reflux, and occasional vomiting. You do a gastric emptying study which shows delayed gastric emptying.

Which of the following drugs is (are) appropriate for treating this patient's delayed gastric emptying?

A) Omeprazole.
B) Metoclopramide.
C) Ranitidine.
D) Erythromycin.
E) B and D.

Discussion

The correct answer is E. Both metoclopramide and erythromycin speed gastric emptying. A third drug, cisapride, is available on compassionate use protocol. It was removed from the general market secondary to prolonged QT and subsequent torsade de pointes. **Diabetic gastropathy is somewhat reversible with good glucose control.** The higher the sugar, the worse the stomach empties.

Objectives: Did you learn to . . .

- Diagnose a patient with diabetic ketoacidosis (DKA)?
- Initiate therapy in DKA?
- Identify causes of DKA?
- Describe the Somogyi phenomenon?
- Prescribe treatment for diabetic gastroparesis?

QUICK QUIZ: DIABETES PREVENTION

Which intervention has been shown to be MOST EFECTIVE in preventing or delaying the onset of type 2 diabetes mellitus in patients with impaired fasting glucose or impaired glucose tolerance?

A) Dietary modifications and increased activity.
B) Early glipizide treatment.
C) Early metformin treatment.
D) Intensive fitness training.
E) Weight loss >25% of baseline.

Discussion

The correct answer is A. Metformin has demonstrated some benefit in delaying progression to diabetes mellitus but is less effective than diet and activity

modifications. The studies showing benefit from lifestyle modifications used much less aggressive targets for weight loss and activity level than the 25% listed in answer E. Thus, answer E is incorrect. No other medication has demonstrated benefit in retarding the progression to diabetes from impaired fasting glucose or impaired glucose tolerance.

QUICK QUIZ: DIABETES PREVENTION

Which of the following interventions has NOT been shown to prevent loss of vision in patients with type 2 diabetes?

A) Laser photocoagulation therapy.
B) Aspirin.
C) Tight glycemic control.
D) Tight blood pressure control.

Discussion

The correct answer is B. Aspirin has not demonstrated benefit in the Early Treatment Diabetic Retinopathy Study. All the other answer choices have been shown to retard the development of diabetic retinopathy or prevent its progression to visual loss.

CASE 9

You are seeing a new patient in your office. He is a 47-year-old male with a presenting complaint of fatigue for several months. He denies fever, rigors, cough, nausea, or diarrhea. He has lost about 10 pounds. Upon questioning him you discover that he is also having nocturia most nights and is thirsty all the time. He has asthma, for which he uses an albuterol metered-dose inhaler occasionally; he has no other chronic medical problems and takes no other medications on a regular basis. He has a family history of diabetes, hypertension, and heart disease. He smokes about 1 pack per day, and he works as a teacher at the local high school. He is aware of no occupational exposure to toxins.

Physical exam reveals the following: Temp 37°C, BP 135/83, Pulse 72, BMI 38kg/m². Aside from obesity, the remainder of the exam is normal.

Laboratory test results reveal the following: normal CBC, BUN/Cr, electrolytes.

You ask him to return to the office the next day for fasting lab tests, which reveal the following: Fasting blood glucose: 131 mg/dL, HbA$_{1c}$: 7.5%

Does this patient have diabetes?

A) Yes; he has an elevated fasting glucose.

B) Probably; he needs a second fasting glucose to confirm the diagnosis.

C) No; his fasting glucose is not >140 mg/dL.

D) Yes; he has the classic symptoms of diabetes: fatigue, weight loss, and thirst.

E) Probably not; his HbA$_{1c}$ is not >8%.

Discussion

The correct answer is B. The ADA criteria for the diagnosis of diabetes require 2 fasting blood glucose measurements ≥126 mg/dL on different days. Because of inadequate standardization, the HbA$_{1c}$ is not useful in making an initial diagnosis of diabetes.

If another fasting blood glucose level is elevated, what further study must be done to confirm the diagnosis of diabetes and determine whether the patient has type 1 or type 2 diabetes?

A) C-peptide level.

B) Anti-islet cell antibodies.

C) Serum insulin level.

D) Anti-insulin antibodies.

E) None of the above.

Discussion

The correct answer is E. This patient's age, history, examination, and laboratory findings are consistent with the diagnosis of type 2 diabetes mellitus. None of the other studies listed needs to be performed. However, if questions remain about the type of diabetes (which will then affect therapy, prognosis, follow-up, etc), you may perform further studies. In type 1 diabetes, the C-peptide level (a marker of endogenous insulin production) is low. If the level is equivocal, give a glucose load (eg, large meal) and see if it goes up. If it goes up, the diagnosis is likely type 2. Anti-islet cell antibodies are present in 80% of type 1 diabetics and are diagnostic of type 1 diabetes. The serum insulin level (answer C) is generally not helpful. Answer D is incorrect because anti-insulin antibodies have a low sensitivity.

 HELPFUL TIP: Anti-GAD (anti-glutamic acid decarboxylase) antibodies are present in 70% of patients with type 1 diabetes at the time of diagnosis.

The pathologic factors involved in type 2 diabetes in adults include:

A) Pancreatic beta cell destruction through a yet undetermined infectious process.

B) The production of anti-insulin antibodies that cause precipitation of insulin/antibody complexes.

C) Resistance to the effects of insulin at peripheral tissues and a relative insulin deficiency which is progressive over time.

D) An autosomal-dominant process, with the diabetes gene located on the long arm of chromosome 18.

E) Too much exercise and a complete lack of a "beer gut."

Discussion

The correct answer is C. Type 2 diabetes is the result of the development of insulin resistance at the peripheral tissues (eg, fat and muscle cells) and a relative lack of insulin compared to the increasing amount that the body requires. Answer A is incorrect. Autoimmune destruction of beta cells in the pancreas is responsible for causing diabetes type 1. Answer B is just plain incorrect. Answer D is incorrect, but there is a strong genetic component to type 2 diabetes. The genetic factors that cause type 2 diabetes in adults have not been completely elucidated, but there does not appear to be a single gene transmitted in an autosomal-dominant fashion. However, there is an entity called maturity-onset diabetes of the young, which is an uncommon cause of type 2 diabetes but is genetically determined in an autosomal dominant fashion. Answer E is incorrect because lack of exercise, weight gain, dietary factors, and truncal obesity ("beer gut") predispose individuals to the development of type 2 diabetes.

* *

You obtain a second fasting blood glucose 2 days later, and it is 145 mg/dL. You meet with the patient and his wife to go over the test results and explain the diagnosis of diabetes. Given his age, habitus, and lack of exercise, you are certain that this patient has type 2 diabetes. You provide some basic education on the nature of diabetes, its natural history, and what can be done to manage it.

What is the most important next step for this patient?

A) Initiation of insulin therapy.

B) Initiation of an ACE inhibitor.

C) Referral to an endocrinologist.

D) Diabetic education classes.

Discussion

The correct answer is D. A general education program which includes information on diet, disease management, and the family's role in successful diabetes care is the most important intervention listed. Although specialist consultation may be useful in complex diabetic patients or in those who are not responding to treatment, generalist physicians can, and do, provide the majority of care to patients with diabetes. Insulin therapy is not indicated at this point. An ACE inhibitor may or may not be helpful depending on the patient's blood pressure and urine protein.

Which of this patient's other conditions does NOT have a direct impact on his diabetes?

A) Asthma.
B) Elevated blood pressure.
C) Smoking.
D) Obesity.
E) Elevated LDL cholesterol.

Discussion

The correct answer is A. Asthma does not have a direct impact on his diabetes, but taking systemic corticosteroids for an exacerbation will complicate his diabetes management. Hypertension and hyperlipidemia have been shown to increase the risk of microvascular complications in type 2 diabetes. Smoking is an additional risk factor for coronary heart disease. Obesity is common in type 2 diabetes; even a modest weight loss can lead to significant improvements in blood glucose and lipid profiles.

* *

You find that the patient's blood pressure is elevated (systolic pressure ≥130 or diastolic pressure ≥80 mmHg).

Which class of medications is the best choice for initial therapy of hypertension in diabetics?

A) ACE inhibitors.
B) Calcium channel blockers.
C) Loop diuretics.
D) Vasodilators.
E) β-Blockers.

Discussion

The correct answer is A. ACE inhibitors have demonstrated renal protection in type 1 and type 2 diabetics. Patients with microalbuminuria and hypertension will benefit from an ACE inhibitor. Angiotensin receptor blockers (ARBs) are a good alternative in the patient with microalbuminuria if an ACE inhibitor is not tolerated. ARBs, although they decrease proteinuria, do nothing

to reduce adverse cardiovascular outcomes (see Chapter 5, Nephrology). Vasodilators (answer D) and calcium channel blockers (answer B) are not considered first-line agents for the treatment of hypertension. Loop diuretics (eg, furosemide) (answer C) are not indicated for the primary treatment of hypertension in diabetics (or anyone else). Answer E, β-blockers, is incorrect because these drugs are no longer recommended as first-line therapy in the treatment of essential hypertension.

* *

After 3 months of dietary therapy and lifestyle modifications, the patient returns to see you. Although he has been adherent to the recommendations given by you and the diabetes education staff, his HbA$_{1c}$ remains elevated at 8.7%. You decide to begin pharmacologic therapy.

Which medication is the MOST appropriate first-line therapy for an obese patient with type 2 diabetes?

A) A glitazone (Avandia, Actos).
B) A sulfonylurea.
C) Insulin.
D) Metformin.
E) Sitagliptin (Januvia).

Discussion

The correct answer is D. Metformin does not cause weight gain (unlike most other treatments for diabetes) and thus is the drug of choice in obese patients. It is effective, inexpensive, well-tolerated by most patients, and has very little risk of hypoglycemia. Studies comparing effects on end-organ disease show better outcomes with metformin than with traditional sulfonylureas. Sulfonylureas are also effective and well-tolerated, but have a significant risk for hypoglycemia. All other oral drugs are best considered second-line agents.

Answer E is of special note. Sitagliptin is the first of a class of drugs ("gliptins") that block the degradation of the body's endogenous incretin, which helps to lower blood sugar. It should be used as an add-on if traditional hypoglycemic agents are not effective. It tends to cause weight loss.

 HELPFUL TIP: In addition to the gliptins which help prevent the breakdown of endogenous incretins, incretin mimetics are being developed. The first of these mimetics is exenatide (Byetta). It is given by subcutaneous injection and is weight neutral or may even cause weight loss.

Metformin should NOT be used in which class of patients?

A) Patients with COPD.
B) Patients with impaired renal function.
C) Patients with leukemias or lymphomas.
D) Postmyocardial-infarction patients with normal systolic function.
E) Thin patients.

Discussion

The correct answer is B. Patients with renal disease are at a higher risk of lactic acidosis, the most severe complication of metformin therapy. **There is little or no evidence that metformin causes lactic acidosis; it is a theoretical risk.** Patients with pulmonary or neoplastic diseases may take metformin unless they also have severe hepatic or renal failure. Postmyocardial-infarction patients may use metformin as long as they do not have congestive heart failure, but metformin should be held for 48 hours for contrast studies.

* *

After 6 months on a modified diet and metformin, your patient returns for a fasting lipid profile. You obtain the following results:

Total Cholesterol: 209 mg/dL

LDL Cholesterol: 132 mg/dL

HDL Cholesterol: 47 mg/dL

Triglycerides: 153 mg/dL

What is the appropriate course of action now for the management of this patient's lipid profile?

A) No action is necessary, as all these values are acceptable.
B) Institute statin therapy to reduce LDL to <100 mg/dL.
C) Revise his diet to include more stringent restrictions on fat intake.
D) Institute nicotinic acid therapy to reduce total cholesterol and increase HDL cholesterol.

Discussion

The correct answer is B. Patients with diabetes have a risk of cardiovascular disease equal to that of patients with preexisting cardiovascular disease; they require lipid-lowering therapy to reduce the LDL to <100 mg/dL. Although a more stringent diet may reduce LDL levels to some degree, a diet becomes more difficult to maintain as it becomes more stringent, and the failure rates increase. Statin (HMG CoA reductase inhibitor) therapy is the first choice for lowering LDL cholesterol in patients without contraindications to this class of drugs. Nicotinic acid is a second-line drug, although it may be useful in patients who cannot tolerate statins and require lowering of LDL cholesterol and triglycerides.

Which one of the following is NOT a risk factor for lower-extremity amputation in patients with diabetes?

A) Diabetic retinopathy.
B) Bony deformity of the feet or ankles.
C) CRP level.
D) Abnormal monofilament testing for sensory function.
E) Severe nail pathology.

Discussion

The correct answer is C. An elevated CRP is not a known risk factor for amputation, but CRP may be elevated if there is lower-extremity infection present. The risk of amputations or ulcers is increased in patients who have had diabetes for ≥10 years, are male, have a history of poor glucose control, or have evidence of microvascular complications of diabetes. Bony deformities, loss of protective sensation, and severely dystrophic toenails are also risk factors for amputation.

* *

At the next visit, you review the patient's medical record and try to ensure that he is up to date on his preventive health care.

Which of the following is NOT true regarding preventive services in diabetics?

A) Patients diagnosed with type 2 diabetes should have a dilated eye exam at the time of diagnosis.
B) Patients with type 1 diabetes should have a dilated eye exam at the time of diagnosis if they are >12 years, or have had type 1 diabetes for 5 years.
C) Patients with type 1 diabetes should have a urine microalbumin checked every 6–12 months after age 12.
D) A urine microalbumin should be checked at least yearly in all patients with type 2 diabetes.
E) A foot examination using a 10-g nylon microfilament should be done at every visit.

Table 10–5 DIABETES SCREENING RECOMMENDATIONS

Diabetes mellitus type 1:   Urine microalbumin starting at age 12 and then every 6–12 months, dilated eye exam 5 years after diagnosis and then yearly, HbA_{1c} every 6 months, foot check and blood pressure screening every visit.

Diabetes mellitus type 2:   Eye exam at time of diagnosis and then yearly, urine microalbumin at the time of diagnosis and then every 6–12 months, HbA_{1c} every 3 months, foot and blood pressure check at every visit.

Discussion

The correct answer is B. Patients with type 1 diabetes should have an eye exam **5 years** after the diagnosis and yearly thereafter. Age at the time of diagnosis is not a factor in determining when an eye exam should be done. See Table 10–5 for current diabetes screening recommendations.

* *

Unfortunately, this patient follows the "rule" of type 2 diabetes and ends up on multiple medications. When he returns to your clinic a few months later, he has complaints of shortness of breath and lower-extremity edema.

Which of the following drugs (alone—not in combination with other drugs) is the most likely cause of this patient's edema, shortness of breath, and possible heart failure?

A) Metformin.
B) Glyburide.
C) Rosiglitazone.
D) Lisinopril.
E) Insulin.

Discussion

The correct answer is C. The "glitazones" tend to cause edema as one of their major side effects. They are contraindicated in patients with a history of CHF. Some drug combinations can cause edema, including the combination of glimepiride and metformin.

 HELPFUL TIP: There are FDA warnings about CHF and adverse cardiovascular events with the glitazones.

* *

Because of the problem with edema, you decide to change this patient to a sulfonylurea, and you choose to start glyburide. The patient does well on this for several weeks but is then found unconscious in his home with a blood sugar of 20. He is rapidly revived by the paramedics with an amp of D50. You are called to see the patient in the ED. He is currently awake, conversant and eating ("a great excuse for a couple of cookies, Doc"). He would like to go home since he is back to his baseline.

Which of the following is TRUE about patients with hypoglycemia?

A) Patients with type 1 diabetes on NPH insulin should be admitted for observation after a hypoglycemic episode.
B) Patients with type 2 diabetes controlled with insulin should be admitted for observation after a hypoglycemic episode.
C) Patients on metformin have a higher risk of hypoglycemia than those taking only a sulfonylurea.
D) Patients on oral hypoglycemic agents should be admitted for observation after a hypoglycemic episode.
E) All of the above are true.

Discussion

The correct answer is D. Patients on an oral hypoglycemic agent should be admitted for observation. because of the somewhat erratic absorption of oral hypoglycemic agents and their prolonged effect. The patient may have an additional episode of hypoglycemia for up to 36–48 hours after the initial episode. This is not true of patients on NPH insulin, who are using a drug that is relatively short-acting. One of the benefits of metformin is that it rarely (if ever) causes hypoglycemia. The main action is to reduce gluconeogenesis and release of glucose from the liver (although it also improves skeletal muscle use of glucose).

* *

While you were on vacation, one of your partners has started this patient on a β-blocker for its cardioprotective and antihypertensive effects. The patient wants to know if this may have prevented him from noticing the signs and symptoms of hypoglycemia.

Your response is that:

A) β-Blockers reduce patients' ability to recognize hypoglycemia and the drug should be stopped.

B) β-Blockers reduce patients' ability to recognize hypoglycemia but the benefits are worth it.

C) β-Blockers do not decrease patients' ability to recognize hypoglycemia to any great degree.

D) ACE inhibitors are better drugs because they do not contribute to hypoglycemia in diabetics.

E) None of the above.

Discussion

The correct answer is C. β-Blockers do not interfere significantly with patients' ability to recognize hypoglycemia. The problem that contributes to unawareness of hypoglycemia in diabetics is the rate of glucose drop (a slow drop is less likely to be noticed) and autonomic insufficiency (patients cannot respond with tachycardia, sweating, etc to the outpouring of andrenergics). Answer D is incorrect. ACE inhibitors, like β-blockers, are associated with hypoglycemia in diabetics.

* *

You advise the patient to carry a source of glucose with him at all times and everybody has a happy outcome.

CASE 10

Your patient's 22-year-old daughter, Lulu, is also your patient. She has recently become pregnant for the first time and comes to you concerned about the possibility of "pregnancy diabetes," in view of her father's condition.

What is the best INITIAL test for the presence of gestational diabetes?

A) Fasting blood glucose (FBG).

B) Random blood glucose.

C) 100-gram oral glucose tolerance test (OGTT).

D) 50-gram glucose challenge test (GCT).

E) HbA_{1c}.

Discussion

The correct answer is A. An elevated FBG, repeated on a second day, is sufficient to make the diagnosis of diabetes in pregnant women. The same diagnostic criterion is used: FBG ≥126 mg/dL. As with diabetes in general, random blood glucose levels are not relied upon for diagnosis, so answer B is incorrect. **The GCT is the preferred screening test for pregnant patients who do not have fasting hyperglycemia.**

The OGTT is used to confirm gestational diabetes in women who have an abnormal GCT result. HbA_{1c} is not used in the diagnosis of gestational diabetes.

* *

Lulu's father has developed persistent hyperglycemia despite being on maximal doses of metformin and glyburide. He is willing to begin insulin therapy, but wants to give himself as few injections as possible.

Which of the following regimens would be best for him?

A) A single injection of insulin glargine (Lantus) at bedtime.

B) A single injection of 70/30 NPH/regular insulin at bedtime.

C) A baseline injection of insulin glargine at bedtime, and up to 3 injections of short-acting insulin with meals.

D) Two-thirds of the total daily insulin dose (divided two-thirds NPH and one-third regular) in the morning, and the remainder (divided fifty-fifty, NPH and regular) in the evening.

Discussion

The correct answer is A. Because of its slow release, insulin glargine provides a steady-state insulin level throughout 24 hours and is less likely to cause nocturnal hypoglycemia. Other prolonged-action options are insulin detemir and ultralente insulin. A single injection of 70/30 insulin (answer B) is a reasonable alternative, but should be given at dinnertime, not at bedtime. Multiple daily insulin injections (answer C) may be necessary for type 1 diabetes, but rarely are needed for type 2 diabetes. The combination of NPH and regular (answer D), involves 2 injections daily, and may be complicated to remember or administer. If you are trying to start with the simplest possible regimen, choose something like A.

* *

Your patient is hospitalized for acute diverticulitis and requires urgent partial colectomy.

Which of the following statements regarding the management of diabetes in hospitalized patients is TRUE?

A) Hyperglycemia in the hospital has minimal if any effect on outcomes of myocardial infarction.

B) A standardized sliding-scale insulin regimen is adequate to control hyperglycemia in all hospitalized diabetic patients.

C) Insulin requirements will be lower for acutely ill hospitalized diabetic patients.

D) Metformin should be discontinued in seriously ill hospitalized patients.

E) A calorie-restricted clear liquid ADA diet is an appropriate choice for refeeding diabetic patients after gastrointestinal surgery.

Discussion

The correct answer is D. It is true that one should consider discontinuing metformin in severely ill, hospitalized patients due to contrast studies, changes in fluid balance, changes in glomerular filtration rate, etc. Answer A is incorrect. Hyperglycemia is associated with worse outcomes in hospitalized patient with cardiac disease or who are in the intensive care unit. Answer B is incorrect. Sliding-scale regimens, if used at all, should be individualized to each patient, rather than prescribed as a standardized regimen. Recent studies show that a sliding scale is not the best way to control blood sugars in hospitalized patients. Continuing a "normal" insulin regimen is best, using supplemental insulin as needed. Answer C is incorrect. The stress of acute illness and surgery will likely increase insulin requirements in most diabetics, not decrease them. Answer E is incorrect. A clear liquid ADA diet implies the elimination of both simple and complex carbohydrates and fats; soluble protein is usually not palatable. A restricted-calorie full liquid diet is more appropriate.

 HELPFUL TIP: It is under debate if an elevated blood sugar in the hospital is responsible for unfavorable outcomes in hyperglycemic patients. It is likely that the elevated glucose is a marker for metabolic stress and thus for sicker patients. Tight control of sugars has not improved outcomes in these patients.

Objectives: Did you learn to . . .

- Recognize diagnostic criteria for diabetes?
- Differentiate diabetes mellitus type 1 from type 2?
- Evaluate a patient with new-onset type 2 diabetes mellitus?
- Identify risk factors for complications of diabetes?
- Initiate oral therapy in diabetes?
- Manage a patient on insulin?
- Manage diabetes in the hospital setting?
- Evaluate a pregnant patient for gestational diabetes?

 QUICK QUIZ: GLUCOSE MONITORING

How often should a patient with type 2 diabetes on oral hypoglycemic agents measure his or her blood glucose?

A) Once or twice a week, at varying times during the day.

B) Four times daily, before meals and at bedtime.

C) Twice a day, fasting and 2 hours after a meal.

D) Once or twice a day, fasting and before a meal.

E) Routine blood sugars are not indicated on a daily basis for patients with type 2 diabetes.

Discussion

The correct answer is E. Daily measurements of fingerstick sugars in patients on oral hypoglycemic agents do nothing to improve glycemic control. In these patients, we are not reacting to daily fluctuations in glucose control but rather making changes in response to the HbA_{1c}. Occasional random sugars are not unreasonable to get a general idea about glycemic control. **Patients with type 2 diabetes on insulin (and all patients with type 1 diabetes) should measure their blood glucose at least daily, and ideally twice a day, regardless of the presence or absence of symptoms.**

 QUICK QUIZ: DIABETES MEDICATIONS

Which of the following medications for diabetes is notable for its association with the development of pancreatitis?

A) Exenatide (Byetta).

B) Sitagliptan (Januvia).

C) Metformin.

D) Glyburide.

E) A and B.

Discussion

The correct answer is A. Exenatide (Byetta), the injectable incretin mimetic, has been associated with the development of pancreatitis.

CASE 11

A 32-year-old female presents to your office with major complaint of "hypoglycemia." She reports that 2–3 hours after a meal she gets nauseated, shaky, and irritable. When she wakes up in the morning, she feels well even though she eats dinner at about 5:00 p.m., does not eat any snacks afterwards, and generally does not have breakfast until 8:00 a.m.

You can tell her that:

A) She likely has an insulinoma.
B) She likely will have normal blood sugars when she feels shaky.
C) Hypoglycemia does not exist as an entity in this form and she likely has anxiety.
D) She likely has "fasting" hypoglycemia.
E) None of the above.

Discussion

The correct answer is E. Answer A is incorrect because a patient with an insulinoma should be hypoglycemic after a 15-hour fast (5:00 p.m.–8:00 a.m.). Answers B and C are incorrect . . . . . because she is hypoglycemic. Answer D is incorrect. The patient does not have symptoms of fasting hypoglycemia, which occur 4–6 hours (or longer) after the last meal.

This patient may have **postprandial hypoglycemia** which occurs 2–4 hours after eating. The process leading to postprandial hypoglycemia is: the patient has a large meal with simple carbohydrates, the serum insulin level increases in response but overshoots, and the patient becomes transiently hypoglycemic for 15–20 minutes 2–4 hours after eating. This is associated with adrenergic outpouring in an attempt to correct the problem. It is the adrenergic outpouring that causes the symptoms of tremor, nausea, etc.

All of the following are associated with postprandial hypoglycemia EXCEPT:

A) Early diabetes.
B) Diuretics.
C) Alcohol intake.
D) Postgastrectomy syndrome.
E) β-Blockers.

Discussion

The correct answer is B. Diuretics tend to increase the blood sugar a bit. In addition to the list above, aspirin, ACE inhibitors, pentamidine, and renal failure may be associated with postprandial hypoglycemia.

You advise this patient to do all of the following EXCEPT:

A) Increase the amount of simple carbohydrates with her meals.
B) Increase the amount of complex carbohydrates with her meals.
C) Eat smaller, more frequent meals.
D) Use propantheline to delay gastric emptying.
E) None of the above is correct.

Discussion

The correct answer (and what you would not want to do) is A. The problem is caused at least in part by a high intake of simple carbohydrates, leading to a rapid and high peak of the blood sugar followed by an excessive release of insulin. Thus, one would want to decrease the amount of simple carbohydrates in the diet. Alternatively, all of the rest may be helpful in treating hypoglycemia.

Answer D is of special note. Delaying gastric emptying (using an agent like propantheline, an anticholinergic/antispasmodic) leads to a lower blood sugar peak and thus less insulin production. This will often help the problem, especially in a patient with a dumping syndrome or in the patient who is postgastrectomy.

 HELPFUL TIP: For insulinoma, watch the patient during a **controlled** fast during which the patient is observed and can be treated for hypoglycemia if necessary. If you are considering self-induced hypoglycemia with insulin (eg, factitious hypoglycemia), measure the C-terminal peptide. This will be **low** if the patient is being administered exogenous insulin because pancreatic insulin production will be shut off in response to hypoglycemia (remember that it will also be low in patients with type 1 diabetes).

Objectives: Did you learn to . . .

- Evaluate a patient with possible hypoglycemia?
- Treat a patient with postprandial hypoglycemia?
- Identify causes of hypoglycemia?

CASE 12

A 24-year-old female presents to the office with complaint of amenorrhea. Six months ago, her menses became irregular and light. For the last 4 months, she has not had a period at all. This is causing her distress, as she worries constantly about becoming pregnant. She does desire to have children someday, but not now. She has run multiple home pregnancy tests, all of which have been negative. Last week, she developed clear leakage from her nipples, and is now convinced she is pregnant and that the home pregnancy tests must be faulty. She requests that you perform "a real pregnancy test."

Which of the following may cause her amenorrhea?

A) Emotional stress.
B) Pregnancy, despite multiple negative tests.
C) Thyroid dysfunction.
D) Pituitary tumor.
E) All of the above.

Discussion

The correct answer is E. The differential diagnosis for amenorrhea is rather broad, but includes all of the above diagnoses. The most common cause in a woman of childbearing age is, of course, pregnancy. Although urine-based pregnancy tests have become very sensitive (able to detect as little as 20 IU/mL of β-hCG), the patient may have been using the tests incorrectly and was getting false negative results. Other causes of amenorrhea include hypothyroidism, strenuous exercise or anorexia, emotional stress, pituitary tumor, medications (eg, phenothiazines, dopaminergic agents, chemotherapy, estrogens, etc), and end-organ (ovarian) failure or agenesis. See Chapter 16, Obstetrics and Women's Health for a discussion of amenorrhea.

* *

Additional patient history reveals menarche at age 12, no previous pregnancies, and no previous history of menstrual irregularities. She participates in low-impact exercise regularly and does not engage in long-distance running or other demanding endurance sports. Review of systems reveals frequent mild headaches, the aforementioned nipple discharge, but no visual disturbances or symptoms of hypothyroidism.

Physical exam demonstrates a well-developed, well-nourished (not obese or excessively thin) adult female. She has appropriate secondary sex characteristics, no hirsutism, and a normal thyroid gland to palpation. Galactorrhea is noted on breast examination. The pelvic exam is normal, with appropriately developed external genitalia, vagina, and cervix. The uterus is palpable and small, and the ovaries are not palpable or tender.

In addition to a serum β-hCG and a TSH, what other test(s) should be ordered?

A) Karyotype, to evaluate for testicular feminization and Turner syndrome.
B) Adrenal MRI, to evaluate for adrenal hyperplasia.
C) Prolactin level, to evaluate for pituitary dysfunction.
D) All of the above.
E) None of the above.

Discussion

The correct answer is C. A prolactin level is an essential component of this evaluation. A prolactinoma is the most common form of pituitary adenoma, and it can cause secondary amenorrhea, galactorrhea, and infertility (or impotence in men). Expansion of the mass in the sella turcica may cause headaches or visual field defects (bitemporal hemianopsia), but the tumors are often too small to have any local effects. Adrenal hyperplasia is unlikely in the patient because of a lack of virilizing characteristics from androgen excess (such as hirsutism). Adrenal imaging (answer B) is not usually the first step in the diagnosis of this disorder (24-hour urine collection for cortisol and 17-OHS is indicated if adrenal hyperfunction is suspected). A karyotype (answer A) is not indicated in this patient because she has secondary amenorrhea, or amenorrhea that has developed after a period of time of normal menses. Patients who complain of never having a menstrual cycle are considered to have primary amenorrhea, which may be evidence of either Turner syndrome (XO genotype) or complete androgen insensitivity (aka testicular feminization, which has an XY genotype with end-organ resistance to testosterone, resulting in a female phenotype). Both cases result in ovarian agenesis and, therefore, no menstrual cycles.

* *

You obtain laboratory tests, and the results are as follows:

TSH 3.1 IU/mL (0.27–4.20), β-hCG undetectable, Prolactin 150 ng/mL (3.4–24.1)

What is the best next step in this patient's evaluation?

A) Reassure patient that stress is causing her lack of periods and she will improve when she learns to deal with her life.
B) No additional tests at this time, but return in 2 weeks for a repeat prolactin level.
C) Admit the patient to the hospital as start bromocriptine therapy STAT.
D) MRI brain to evaluate for pituitary mass.
E) Refer patient for neurosurgical intervention.

Discussion

The correct answer is D. This patient has a high prolactin level and symptoms of prolactin excess. In the absence of medications causing an elevated prolactin (phenothiazines, narcotics, estrogens, etc) and a normal TSH, this prolactin result is virtually diagnostic for a prolactinoma. Imaging is indicated regardless of visual symptoms. A visual field exam by confrontation is insensitive for a minor loss of field. If she had a mild elevation in prolactin (up to 2 times the upper limit of normal), and no other symptoms/signs, repeating the level over several visits would be appropriate (answer B); and if the elevated level persisted, imaging and medical therapy should then be considered. If the level remains elevated, imaging and medical therapy should then be considered. Neurosurgical intervention (answer E) is not immediately indicated, since a trial of medical therapy should be done.

* *

This patient undergoes a MRI, which shows a 1.3-cm pituitary mass.

How should this mass be treated?

A) This is a microadenoma, and the result can be ignored.
B) This is a microadenoma, and medical therapy with a dopamine agonist is indicated.
C) This is a macroadenoma, so medical therapy is futile, and the patient should be referred for surgery.
D) This is a macroadenoma, but medical therapy with a dopamine agonist should still be attempted.
E) This is a macroadenoma, which tends to be self-limited, so therapy can be held for 6 months when a repeat scan will be done.

Discussion

The correct answer is D. A pituitary tumor <1 cm is considered a microadenoma, and tumors ≥1 cm are considered macroadenomas. Treatment implications are slightly different. In both cases, medical therapy with a dopamine agonist (eg, bromocriptine, cabergoline, etc) is indicated. Successful shrinkage of macroadenomas is possible with this therapy. Remember that the secretion of prolactin is under a negative feedback loop. As CNS dopamine levels go up, prolactin levels go down. As dopamine levels go down, prolactin levels go up.

* *

The patient is started on bromocriptine, and is scheduled for follow-up in 3 weeks. She returns earlier than scheduled due to severe nausea and lightheadedness. No other new symptoms have occurred. The patient's vital signs are normal, but the systolic blood pressure decreases by 20 mm Hg and the pulse increases by 20 beats/minute upon standing.

Aside from a bolus of intravenous fluids, how should you address this problem?

A) This is a common side effect from bromocriptine. Decrease or stop the bromocriptine, and consider another type of dopamine agonist, such as cabergoline.
B) Admit her to the hospital and arrange for a STAT head CT scan to rule out bleeding from the pituitary adenoma.
C) Repeat the pregnancy test.
D) She is having an anaphylactic allergic reaction. Administer epinephrine and diphenhydramine immediately.
E) She has failed medical therapy and must be referred for neurosurgical intervention.

Discussion

The correct answer is A. The most common side effects of dopamine agonists are nausea, postural hypotension, and difficulty concentrating. These symptoms tend to be lessened when lower doses are used and the dose is increased very slowly. Cabergoline tends to be better tolerated than bromocriptine.

* *

The patient is able to tolerate cabergoline, and continues the medication for 6 months. During this time, the prolactin level decreases slowly. She has had resumption of her menses. A repeat MRI is done after 6 months and shows a marked decrease in size of the adenoma. The patient has reached that magical inflection point in life where she recognizes that her own mortality is inevitable, and she desires to get pregnant "as soon as I can." She wants to know if she should have surgery to remove the adenoma.

What is (are) the indication(s) for transsphenoidal pituitary surgery?

A) Failure to respond to dopamine agonists.
B) Failure to tolerate dopamine agonists.
C) Treatment of large adenoma in a patient who desires pregnancy, despite efficacy of medical therapy.
D) A and B.
E) All of the above.

Discussion

The correct answer is E. Surgery should be reserved for those patients who fail to respond to or cannot tolerate medical therapy. Note that visual field defects are not a specific indication for surgery, since medical therapy can be effective in decreasing the size and related local effects of the tumor. If a patient desires pregnancy and has a large mass (>3cm), surgery may be considered as an adjunct to medical therapy. During pregnancy, there is a physiological increase in the size of the pituitary gland. If the patient becomes pregnant (without a prior reduction in tumor size) and discontinues the agonist for the duration of pregnancy, the adenoma may increase to a clinically important size before delivery.

 HELPFUL TIP: Bromocriptine and cabergoline are classified as category B for pregnancy risk (in other words, they are generally considered safe). These medications can be continued during pregnancy, but a careful risk-benefit analysis and discussion between patient and physician must occur before making treatment decisions.

* *

The patient wants to know how long she should be on cabergoline or bromocriptine and when a trial off of the medication is indicated.

You let her know that:

A) Patients with a pituitary adenoma have to be on medication chronically to suppress the tumor.

B) A trial off of a dopamine agonist should be done at 6 months.

C) Dopamine agonists can be stopped at 1 year and tumor shrinkage will be sustained.

D) Prolactin levels can be allowed to rise after menopause without problem unless visual symptoms or other local symptoms develop.

E) None of the above.

Discussion

The correct answer is D. Dopamine agonists can be stopped at menopause. Follow-up can be done using blood levels of prolactin. If prolactin levels rise, an MRI can be done to see if the adenoma is becoming larger. If not, there is no reason to treat the adenoma in postmenopausal patients. Answer A is incorrect. A trial off of medications at 1 year is reasonable. If prolactin levels remain under control, there is no need to continue medication. Answers B and C are incorrect. A trial off of drugs should be tried at 1 year (not 6 months). Tumors recur in a large number of cases, so patients may need chronic treatment.

Objectives: Did you learn to . . .

- Generate a list of potential causes of secondary amenorrhea?
- Evaluate a patient with secondary amenorrhea?
- Diagnose and treat hyperprolactinemia secondary to a pituitary prolactinoma?

CASE 13

A 39-year-old female presents to the office with complaint of amenorrhea. She has had normal menses until 8 months ago, when they became infrequent and then stopped. She insists she cannot be pregnant, because she denies sexual activity "in years." She believes she is going through "the change" but wants to know why she is reaching menopause at a much earlier age than other women she knows. On review of systems, she complains of headaches "for years" and recent onset of weakness and fatigue. She also complains of arthritis in the hip and knees, something she attributes to "getting old." She reports that her hands are swollen, and her rings do not fit any more. She denies other complaints.

On physical exam, vitals are normal. The patient is an adult female of average height, with a noticeably large jaw and hands. Her hair is thick and course, and hirsutism is present. Her thyroid gland is slightly enlarged, but regular in shape. No bruit or tenderness is present. The point of maximal impulse is displaced laterally, but the heart rhythm is regular with no murmurs. The rest of the exam is normal.

What is the most appropriate next step?

A) Reassure the patient that menopause is a normal process and offer estrogen replacement therapy for symptomatic relief (but warn the patient about risks of long-term use).

B) Tell the patient you suspect depression and offer a regimen of counseling combined with serotonin-reuptake inhibitor (SSRI) therapy.

C) Although she is likely depressed, tell the patient she may have a thyroid disorder at least contributing to the problem and recommend measuring her TSH level.

D) Although she is likely depressed, tell the patient she may suffer from growth hormone (GH) excess, and recommend sending a serum insulin-like growth factor-I (IGF-I) level.

E) None of the above.

Discussion

The correct answer is D. This patient represents a classic presentation of acromegaly due to GH excess, and the best single test for this is the IGF-I level. Although GH levels will often be elevated, the IGF-I does not vary from hour to hour and is not dependent on food intake, as is the case with GH. An elevated GH after a glucose load is also very suggestive of GH excess. Acromegaly of adult onset (after fusion of the long bones) does **not** result in increased height, but does cause coarsening of facial features, prognathism, and thickening of the feet and hands. These changes can be very subtle, and there is generally a lag of 12 years before diagnosis. Comparing older photographs of the patient to her current appearance may be a clue (a driver's license photograph may be a convenient source). Patients with acromegaly also develop hypertrophy of certain organs (such as the thyroid and heart) and may present with congestive heart failure due to cardiomyopathy. Eighty-five percent of females with acromegaly have at least some menstrual dysfunction and 60% are amenorrheic.

> **HELPFUL TIP:** Premature ovarian failure is defined as menopause at ≤40 years (2 standard deviations below the mean).

* *

The patient's IGF-I is elevated, and her TSH is normal. An MRI is performed which reveals a pituitary mass slightly <1 cm in diameter.

What is the most effective therapy for this condition?

A) Weekly anti-IGF-I antibody infusions.
B) Bromocriptine therapy.

C) Transsphenoidal pituitary resection.
D) Somatostatin analogs (such as octreotide).
E) Pegvisomant (growth hormone receptor antagonist).

Discussion

The correct answer is C. Acromegaly is caused by a GH-secreting pituitary tumor. Surgery is the treatment of choice for patients with a microadenoma (<1 cm in diameter) or for patients with a macroadenoma that appears to be fully resectable. Somatostatin analogs (answer D) and pegvisomant (Somavert) (answer E) may be useful adjuncts to surgery, and are an option for patients who are not surgical candidates. Bromocriptine (answer B) is not very effective, and only about 10% of acromegaly patients will achieve normal IGF-I levels with bromocriptine. Cabergoline (a similar medication) seems to work in about half of patients. Cabergoline has an advantage over somatostatin analogs in that it can be taken orally. Radiation is also an option for therapy, especially for those patients who are not surgical candidates and do not tolerate or do not respond to medical therapy. Anti-IGF-I antibody (answer A) if it existed as a medication would not have an effect on a GH-secreting tumor. But it does not exist. It's a made-up answer, so it's wrong.

Objectives: Did you learn to . . .

- Recognize signs and symptoms of growth hormone (GH) excess?
- Evaluate and manage a patient with GH excess?

QUICK QUIZ: GROWTH HORMONE

A boy of 6 years is brought into the office by his concerned mother because he is "growing too slowly." She has noticed that he is significantly shorter than his classmates at school, and she wants something done about it. She heard a report on the nightly news about a new medication that makes children grow taller and insists on getting it for her son. Both parents want their son to play in the NBA or NFL and believe he will not make it unless he "gets a lot taller really soon." She informs you that if you don't prescribe this "growing pill," she will find someone who will. You believe this mother is in need of some education about GH deficiency.

What are the APPROVED indications in children and adolescents for GH replacement therapy?

A) GH deficiency.
B) Growth failure due to chronic renal insufficiency, intrauterine growth retardation, Turner syndrome, and Prader-Willi syndrome.
C) An adolescent male who wishes to play basketball but is only 5 foot 9 inches.
D) A and B.
E) All of the above.

Discussion

The correct answer is D. GH replacement is specifically approved for GH deficiency and growth failure due to chronic renal insufficiency, intrauterine growth retardation, Turner syndrome, and Prader-Willi syndrome. It has been approved for use in "idiopathic short stature" (>2 standard deviations below the mean height for age). Not all patients with GH deficiency require GH replacement, because not all will suffer the negative end-organ effects, such as marked short stature, growth failure, hypoglycemia in infancy, and central distribution of body fat.

 HELPFUL TIP: As with acromegaly, insulin-like growth factor 1 (IGF-1) should be checked when considering short stature secondary to pituitary failure. It is also important to check IGF-binding protein-3 levels. Low levels of IGF-binding protein-3 may cause problems with binding of IGF to the proper receptors.

 HELPFUL TIP: Even when used appropriately, GH results in an average increase in adult height of a couple of inches.

 QUICK QUIZ: DIABETES

Which of these drugs can be used in patients with type 1 or type 2 diabetes?

A) Nateglinide (Starlix).
B) Pramlintide (Symlin).
C) Precose (Acarbose)
D) Glimepiride (Amaryl).
E) A and B.

Discussion

The correct answer is B. Pramlintide is a synthetic analogue of amylin, which is secreted by the body along with insulin. This drug (1) prolongs gastric emptying, leading to lower spike in serum glucose, (2) suppresses postprandial glucagon secretion (again lowering blood sugars), and (3) suppresses hunger leading to lower calorie intake. **It is used only in patients who are already on insulin but can be used for both type 1 and type 2 diabetes.** Nateglinide (Starlix) is a meglitinide which releases glucose from the pancreas similar to sulfonylureas. Precose (Acarbose) is an alpha-glucosidase inhibitor which prevents the conversion of starches to simple sugars in the GI tract and thus slows absorption of glucose from the GI tract. Glimepiride (Amaryl) is a sulfonylurea.

BIBLIOGRAPHY

American Diabetes Association. Clinical practice recommendations 2007. *Diabetes Care*. 2007;30(Suppl 1):S3.

Atkinson MA, Eisenbarth GS. Type 1 diabetes: new perspectives on disease pathogenesis and treatment. *Lancet*. 2001;358:221.

Bakris GL. A practical approach to achieving recommended blood pressure goals in diabetic patients. *Arch Intern Med*. 2001;161:2661.

Ben-Shlomo A. Acromegaly. *Endocrinol Metab Clin North Am*. 2001;30(3):565.

Brody SC, et al. Screening for gestational diabetes: a summary of the evidence for the US Preventive Services Task Force. *Obstetrics & Gynecology*. 2003;101(2):380.

Carroll MF. A practical approach to hypercalcemia. *Am Fam Physician*. 2003;67(9):1959.

Cooper DS. Hyperthyroidism. *Lancet*. 2003;362(9382):359.

Findling JW. Diagnosis and differential diagnosis of Cushing's syndrome. *Endocrinol Metab Clin North Am*. 2001; 30(3):729.

Finklestein BS. Effect of growth hormone therapy on height in children with idiopathic short stature: a meta-analysis. *Arch Pediatr Adolesc Med*. 2002;156(3):230.

Ginsberg J. Diagnosis and management of Graves' disease. *CMAJ*. 2003;168(5):575.

Grozinsky-Glasberg S, Fraser A, Nahshoni E, et al. Thyroxine-triiodothyronine combination therapy versus thyroxine monotherapy for clinical hypothyroidism: meta-analysis of randomized controlled trials. *J Clin Endocrinol Metab*. 2006;91:2592.

Harris R, et al. Screening adults for type 2 diabetes: a review of the evidence for the US Preventive Services Task Force. *Ann Int Med*. 2003;138:215.

Hueston WJ. Treatment of hypothyroidism. *Am Fam Physician.* 2001;64(10):1717.

Kearns AE. Medical and surgical management of hyperparathyroidism. *Mayo Clin Proc.* 2002;77(1):87.

Kim N. Evaluation of a thyroid nodule. *Otolaryngol Clin North Am.* 2003;36(1):17.

Mann JI. Diet and risk of coronary heart disease and type 2 diabetes. *Lancet.* 2002;360:783.

Nieman LK. Medical therapy of Cushing's disease. *Pituitary.* 2002;5(2):77.

Norris SL, Engelgau MM, Venkat Narayan KM. Effectiveness of self-management training in type 2 diabetes: a systematic review of randomized controlled trials. *Diabetes Care.* 2001;24(3):561.

Ten S. Clinical review 130: Addison's disease 2001. *J Clin Endocrinol Metab.* 2001;86(7):2909.

11

Rheumatology

Philip N. Velderman and Rebecca S. Tuetken

CASE 1

A 43-year-old female nurse who works in the renal transplant service presents with complaint of body aches and stiffness, worse in the morning. She further describes a low-grade fever and pain in her hands, feet, and left knee. She feels that her grip strength is diminished. These symptoms started rather abruptly 2 weeks ago and have not responded to acetaminophen.

She is an outdoor activities enthusiast and has camped with her husband and daughters for 3 of the last 5 weekends. She remembers that one week they could not go because her 8-year-old daughter had a fever, mild diarrhea, abdominal pain, and a skin rash ("legs, arms, and especially face were red and warm, and she seemed 'flushed' all the time"). Her daughter's symptoms resolved in a few days, she did not see a doctor, and no one else was sick.

Her past medical history is as follows: gravida 2, para 2 (term vaginal deliveries); occasional migraine headaches responding to abortive therapy with "triptans." She takes no other medications. Family history is significant for heart disease. Review of systems is negative in detail.

On physical examination, her temperature is 37.6°C, BP 112/68 mm Hg, and pulse 88 bpm. She is unable to close her hands completely. Although your exam is somewhat limited by pain, there appears to be swelling of all metacarpophalangeal (MCP) and proximal interphalangeal (PIP) joints. You detect a bulge sign (indicating effusion) upon examining the left knee. Also, you notice mild erythema over the MCPs.

If found on physical exam, which of the following would be LEAST helpful in narrowing the differential diagnosis?

A) Bilateral metatarsophalangeal (MTP) joint swelling and tenderness.
B) Painless oral ulcerations, with clean edges.
C) Firm, slightly tender subcutaneous nodules at the olecranon bursae.
D) A "bull's eye" rash in the right axilla.
E) Icterus and tender hepatomegaly.

Discussion

The correct answer is A. This patient presents with a picture of a polyarticular inflammatory arthritis of unclear etiology. While important to note, metatarsophalangeal joint swelling would not add much to the picture of subacute, symmetrical, small joint polyarthritis that you have already found on your examination.

Your differential diagnosis will include acute viral arthritis, specifically parvovirus B19 (due to the daughter's history of acute illness resembling erythema infectiosum), coxsackievirus, hepatitis B (answer E, liver exam findings will be useful), and HIV. Also on your differential will be Lyme disease (answer D, the "bull's eye" rash of erythema migrans), rheumatoid arthritis (RA) (answer C, presence of rheumatoid nodules), and other inflammatory disorders (answer B, painless ulcerations associated with systemic lupus).

* *

Upon further examination, she has no rash. You detect bilateral pain and swelling of MTPs 3 and 4. There are no oral ulcerations and no lymphadenopathy. She is not icteric, and her abdomen is diffusely, mildly tender. There is no hepatomegaly. You decide to order some blood tests.

If positive, which of the following serologic tests would be MOST helpful in ruling in a specific diagnosis?

A) Positive antinuclear antibody (ANA).
B) Elevated white count.
C) Positive parvovirus B19 IgG and IgM.
D) Positive urinalysis for white blood cells.
E) Elevated ESR and CRP.

Discussion

The correct answer is C. The presence of IgM antibodies to parvovirus B19—or rising titers of IgG antibodies—indicates acute viral infection, which may present with symptoms and signs seen in this patient. Answer A, an ANA, will not help you rule in a diagnosis now. Although the ANA is a highly sensitive test, it is not specific and has a low positive predictive value. Answers B D, and E are important findings but do not lead you toward a specific diagnosis.

HELPFUL TIP: Although ANA, RF, ESR, and CRP may be useful in confirming a clinical diagnosis and assessing disease activity, these tests have **poor specificity** and may be positive in a variety of disease states. Anti-CCP antibodies are specific for RA, their sensitivity is 70% and therefore may be negative in RA. Even though a negative ANA rules out systemic lupus (SLE), a positive ANA without a clinical diagnosis is meaningless. RF helps gauge prognosis (seropositive vs. seronegative) in RA, but has very limited value as a diagnostic test. False-positive RF can be found in Wegner granulomatosis, many viral infections, primary lung disease, sarcoid, primary liver disease, and other autoimmune diseases. ESR and CRP may support the clinical impression of inflammatory disease, but they are nonspecific.

* *

Her lab results return as follows:

Hepatitis B: Surface antibody positive, surface antigen negative

CMV: IgG positive, IgM negative

Parvovirus: IgG positive, IgM negative

Rheumatoid factor: 1:160 (positive ≥1:40)

Anti-CCP antibody: 64 units (strong positive: 40–59 units)

ANA: Negative

ESR: 58 mm/hour

Which of the following is the most appropriate next step in the diagnosis and management of this patient?

A) Bilateral hand x-rays.
B) CT of the chest.
C) Smith antibody, DsDNA, complement levels.
D) Start piroxicam 10 mg PO BID and follow up in 4–5 weeks.
E) Start prednisone 60 mg PO QD and follow up in 4–5 weeks.

Discussion

The correct answer is D. The best next step is an expectant approach, using first NSAIDs, then possibly low-dose prednisone for what could still be a self-limited disease (eg, viral arthritis). Investigation of other organ involvement should be included as part of her initial evaluation. It is appropriate to obtain CBC, liver function tests, electrolytes, BUN, creatinine, and UA (to rule out glomerulonephritis).

Answer A is incorrect. She has only a descriptive diagnosis now: symmetrical small joint polyarthritis. She is presenting fairly early after the onset of symptoms, so it is unlikely that hand x-rays will provide any significant findings. Answer B is incorrect. Without further symptoms, signs, or risk factors for lung cancer (eg, causing pulmonary osteoarthropathy), a CT scan is inappropriate. Answer C is incorrect. She has no other symptoms of lupus and also had a negative ANA, so further testing for lupus (Smith antibody, DsDNA (aka anti-native DNA antibodies), complement levels) is not appropriate. Answer E is incorrect. Although an argument may be made for low-dose steroids (eg, prednisone 10–20 mg QD), 60 mg is too high a dose given

Table 11–1 CRITERIA FOR THE DIAGNOSIS OF RHEUMATOID ARTHRITIS

Four of the 7 criteria must be present, and at least 1 of the first 4 must be present for at least 6 weeks.
- Morning stiffness in and around joints, lasting >1 hour
- Arthritis of three or more joint areas involved simultaneously
- Arthritis of at least one area in a wrist, metacarpophalangeal (MCP), or proximal interphalangeal (PIP) joint
- Symmetric arthritis involving the same joint areas
- Rheumatoid nodules
- Positive serum rheumatoid factor
- Erosions or periarticular osteopenia on PA hand and wrist radiographs

her clinical presentation. **This patient cannot yet be diagnosed with RA since the definition requires that symptoms be present for at least 6 weeks** (Table 11–1).

 HELPFUL TIP: RA typically has an insidious onset with a fluctuating course; however, a minority of patients (approximately 33%) will experience rapid onset, over days to weeks.

* *

She returns in 4 weeks and is now about 7 weeks into her illness. She reports a moderate response to your intervention, but now she has 1–2 hours of morning stiffness. She continues to complain of pain in her hands and feet, with poor grip. She had to take time off from work during the last week. On exam, she has persistent swelling of MCPs 2–5 bilaterally and MTPs 3 and 4 bilaterally. You observe swelling in the left wrist and both knees. However, now she has no erythema and seems less tender.

What additional findings on exam are UNLIKELY to assist you in making a specific diagnosis?

A) Pleural rub auscultated on lung exam.
B) Firm, slightly tender subcutaneous nodules at the olecranon bursae.

C) Faint pink rash over chest, which is not visible 15 minutes later.
D) Reduced passive flexion in left knee.
E) Left foot drop.

Discussion

The correct answer is D. Limitation of passive movements of the knees is indicative only of knee effusion (or pain), which you have already observed, and is not specific for any particular etiology. She responded modestly to piroxicam but clearly still has arthritis. The clinical picture is now consistent with a chronic, persistent arthritis, and viral disease is less likely. It now becomes necessary to look for clues as to the type of disease.

Answer A is helpful in narrowing the diagnosis. Diagnostic criteria for lupus include serositis, which may be detectable as a pleural rub on auscultation of the lungs (also, look for malar rash, discoid lesions, alopecia, and oral ulcerations). Although not part of the diagnostic criteria for the disease, RA may also present with pleuritis or pericarditis. Rheumatoid nodules (answer B) are included in the diagnostic criteria for RA. A salmon-colored, evanescent macular rash (answer C) would lead you to consider adult Still disease. (Still disease (aka juvenile rheumatoid arthritis [JRA]) presents with an evanescent rash, intermittent fever and arthritis. "Adult onset" Still disease has its onset after age 16.) A finding of isolated foot drop (answer E) may be the result of mononeuritis multiplex, a feature of vasculitides and paraneoplastic syndromes.

 HELPFUL TIP: It is unusual for parvovirus B19 to cause symptoms for 6 weeks. However, in 10% of affected adults the virus can cause prolonged joint pain. An increase in IgG titer or positive IgM would support the diagnosis of parvovirus infection.

* *

Your patient comes in to discuss the following lab results:

Parvovirus: IgG titer unchanged and IgM negative
Negative HIV
Rheumatoid factor: 1:160 (positive)
ESR: 62 mm/hour (elevated)
CRP: 1.2 mg/dL (elevated)

A detailed joint exam reveals the presence of firm, mildly tender subcutaneous nodules over the olecranon bursae. You suspect RA and want to order the appropriate lab tests.

You order all of the following investigations EXCEPT:

A) AST, ALT, alkaline phosphatase.
B) CBC.
C) BUN, creatinine.
D) Uric acid.
E) Hand x-rays.

Discussion

The correct answer is D. Uric acid levels are unlikely to be helpful and are not indicated at the time of diagnosis of RA. With symmetrical polyarthritis in typical locations, findings suggestive of rheumatoid nodules, and a positive RF, the diagnosis of seropositive RA seems secure. Evaluations of liver, renal, and hematological function are necessary, both to assess systemic involvement of RA and to determine baseline function prior to the cytotoxic therapy she will ultimately require. Hand x-rays are necessary now for a baseline evaluation, and they will be used to document disease progression on future examinations.

* *

Once the laboratory results are back, you decide that she needs further therapy.

Which of the following should be your short-term goal?

A) Continue piroxicam but double the dose.
B) Start prednisone 20 mg PO QD and refer for physical therapy.
C) Start prednisone 20 mg PO QD and hydroxychloroquine 200 mg PO BID.
D) Start prednisone 20 mg PO QD, hydroxychloroquine 200 mg PO BID, and methotrexate 10 mg PO weekly.
E) Start prednisone 20 mg PO QD, vitamin D 800 IU PO daily, calcium 600 mg PO BID, hydroxychloroquine 200 mg PO BID, and methotrexate 10 mg PO weekly, and refer for occupational therapy.

Discussion

The correct answer is E. Unfortunately, your patient has features that portend a poor prognosis: a large number of joints involved, presence of rheumatoid nodules, elevated ESR and CRP, positive RF, and anti-CCP antibody. Other extraarticular manifestations of RA, such as pleuritis, pericarditis, and vasculitis, are also associated with a poorer prognosis.

In all cases of RA, and especially in those with a poor prognosis, disease-modifying antirheumatic drugs (DMARDs) should be instituted promptly. Evidence indicates that methotrexate is the DMARD of choice, but combination therapy (methotrexate plus hydroxychloroquine or sulfasalazine) or triple therapy (methotrexate, hydroxychloroquine, and sulfasalazine) improves outcomes over methotrexate alone. Low-dose prednisone is indicated for immediate symptomatic relief. Occupational therapy referral is helpful in identifying and treating functional impairment due to RA. Vitamin D 800 IU per day and calcium 600–800 mg BID should be initiated with prednisone therapy to help prevent steroid-induced osteoporosis. Evaluation of bone density (DEXA scan) and a bisphosphonate (eg, alendronate, risedronate) should also be initiated if >5mg of prednisone is to be used for >3 months.

Since your patient is starting methotrexate, you caution her to avoid which of the following?

A) Aspirin.
B) Sulfonamide antibiotics.
C) Ibuprofen.
D) Folate.
E) Penicillin antibiotics.

Discussion

The correct answer is B. Methotrexate is a folate antagonist; it prevents the conversion of folic acid into the active form, reduced folate cofactors. Antifolate medications, such as sulfonamide antibiotics, must be avoided in patients taking methotrexate; the combination may result in pancytopenia. Supplemental folate, 1 mg daily, reduces the adverse effects of methotrexate. Patients with RA are often treated with aspirin or NSAIDs in combination with methotrexate. Penicillin antibiotics can be administered safely with methotrexate.

 HELPFUL TIP: Pharmacy programs often warn about concomitant use of NSAIDs and methotrexate, as well as aspirin and methotrexate. These warnings are most relevant to high-dose methotrexate used to treat cancer, not the lower doses used for inflammatory arthritis.

* *

Initial hand x-rays demonstrate mild periarticular osteopenia. Liver function tests, urinalysis, CBC, BUN, and creatinine are normal. She returns after 6 weeks, very pleased with your treatment, and has returned to work full-time. She tells you that she still has problems with opening jars and has about 45 minutes of morning stiffness, "but nothing like it was."

What is the BEST course of action to follow now?

A) Continue her current therapy and follow up in 6–12 months with transaminases, RF, and hand x-rays.

B) Continue her current therapy and follow up in 3–4 months with transaminases, RF, and hand x-rays.

C) Continue her current therapy and follow up in 3–4 months; arrange for monthly BUN, creatinine and CBC; and schedule for an annual ophthalmology exam.

D) Continue her current therapy and arrange for monthly transaminases and CBC; schedule for an annual ophthalmology exam; and begin a slow prednisone taper.

E) Instruct her to discontinue methotrexate, taper the prednisone dose, and continue hydroxychloroquine; arrange follow-up in 1 year.

Discussion

The correct answer is D. She seems to be responding to therapy, and a 3-month trial on her current medications (during which the MTX dose may be increased) is indicated. A slow prednisone taper should be initiated once the DMARD therapy becomes effective. Guidelines for monitoring her DMARD regimen require monthly transaminases and CBC for methotrexate and an annual eye exam to assess for hydroxychloroquine-related retinal toxicity. Hand x-rays are recommended at 2-year intervals. Answer E is clearly incorrect: DMARD therapy reduces her risk of joint destruction and disease progression, and it should not be discontinued.

* *

At her next visit 3 months later, she feels better. Prednisone is now 5mg per day. Although she still has difficulty opening jars, she now has <30 minutes of morning stiffness and almost no pain. On exam she has no rash, and her nodules are unchanged. She now has swelling over MCPs 2–4 on the right and 2–3 on the left. Her grip is still somewhat weak but improved. Laboratory data shows an ESR of 28 mm/hour, CRP 0.7 mg/dL, and normal transaminases and CBC.

Which of the following is the most appropriate next step?

A) Increase methotrexate to 25 mg a week and refer to rheumatology.

B) Stop methotrexate and switch to leflunomide 20 mg per day.

C) Increase prednisone to 60 mg QD.

D) Discontinue all medications except methotrexate.

E) Discontinue methotrexate, taper prednisone, and continue hydroxychloroquine.

Discussion

The correct answer is A. Despite her initial response, she has evidence of ongoing inflammatory activity by history and exam. According to published guidelines, consultation with a rheumatologist is now indicated—if it had not been sought sooner. She has had a good, initial response to methotrexate. Further benefit may be gained with increasing the methotrexate dose. However, she may need addition of a biologic agent. Answer B is incorrect. Since she had an initial response to methotrexate, it would be wise to further increase the methotrexate dose, rather than substitute another agent (leflunomide). Answer C is incorrect. Doses of prednisone this high are not indicated for RA. Answers D and E are incorrect. Discontinuing or reducing medication is inappropriate.

 HELPFUL TIP: DMARDs should be started within 3 months of the diagnosis of RA.

* *

This patient wants to get pregnant.

You can tell her that:

A) Symptoms remit in 70% of women when they get pregnant.

B) It is inappropriate to get pregnant while on methotrexate.

C) RA is a contraindication to pregnancy.

D) Prednisone cannot be taken during pregnancy.

E) A and B.

Discussion

The correct answer is E. Answers A and B are true. RA is an autoimmune disease, and it tends to remit during pregnancy when the woman is relatively immunosuppressed.

Methotrexate is class X for pregnancy and is used in ectopic pregnancy to arrest fetal growth. Women and men on methotrexate should use an effective form of contraception, and continue contraception for 3 months after stopping methotrexate. Answer D is incorrect because prednisone is often used to control RA during pregnancy, when methotrexate is contraindicated.

* *

The patient is also concerned about her future. She enjoys running and other activities.

You can let her know that:

A) RA tends to be unremitting and progresses without any remissions to involve almost all joints in all patients.
B) Ninety percent of the joints that will be involved will be involved during the first year.
C) Patients with RA have the same life expectancy as the general public.
D) Joint replacement therapy will not help symptoms of RA since RA is a synovial process.
E) Renal involvement is common with RA and is a major source of morbidity and mortality.

Discussion

The correct answer is B. Ninety percent of the joints that will eventually be involved with RA are involved during the first year. Answer A is incorrect. Patients can go into spontaneous remission—up to 40%, of whom 10% have long-term remissions and up to another 30% have an intermittent course with remissions and exacerbations. Additionally, drugs can induce a remission. Answer C is incorrect. RA reduces the life expectancy as much as 10 years. Answer D is incorrect. Joint replacements may be helpful. The life span of an artificial joint may be 15 years. Thus, replacement should not be undertaken lightly in a young (or any) patient. Answer E is incorrect. Renal disease is a rare complication of RA. It can be a result of some of the medications used for RA. Table 11–2 lists the joints involved in RA.

Objectives: Did you learn to . . .

- Describe an appropriate diagnostic strategy for polyarthritis?
- Develop a differential diagnosis for polyarthritis?
- Develop a management strategy for RA?
- Identify the uses and adverse effects of medications used to treat RA?

Table 11–2 JOINTS INVOLVED IN RHEUMATOID ARTHRITIS

- MCPs 90–95%
- Wrist 80–90%
- PIPs 65–90%
- Knees 60–80%
- MTPs 50–90%
- Shoulders 50–60%
- Ankle/subtalar 50–80%
- Cervical spine (esp C1-2) 40–50%
- Hips 40–50%
- 1Elbow 40–50%
- Temporomandibular 20–30%

QUICK QUIZ: ARTHRITIS IN CHILDHOOD

A concerned mother brings in her 2-year-old son with a history of fever for 1 week. She had expected the fever to resolve by now and is worried. According to his mother, the patient also has a rash, poor appetite, and lethargy. On exam, he looks ill and his temperature is 39.0°C. There is a diffuse, erythematous, macular rash and peeling skin on the fingertips. The oropharynx is injected and the tongue is bright red with white papillae. Cervical lymph nodes are enlarged and tender.

You suspect which of the following diagnoses?

A) Rheumatic fever.
B) Parvovirus B19 infection.
C) Kawasaki syndrome.
D) Juvenile idiopathic arthritis.
E) Varicella infection.

Discussion

The correct answer is C. Kawasaki syndrome is an acute vasculitis of unknown etiology (although multiple infectious agents are suspected) most often seen in children. Kawasaki syndrome presents with a polymorphous rash, conjunctival injection, mucous membrane involvement (eg, "strawberry" tongue), cervical lymphadenopathy, and extremity findings of erythema and desquamation. The usual treatment is aspirin and IVIG. Steroid therapy is controversial and should be reserved for patients in whom two or more courses of IVIG have failed. There may be cardiac involvement with coronary artery aneurysm formation.

Answer A is incorrect. Rheumatic fever, which is rare in developed countries, is recognized by the Jones criteria. The major Jones criteria consist of polyarthritis, carditis, Sydenham chorea, erythema marginatum, and subcutaneous nodules. Answer B is incorrect. Children are generally less ill-appearing with parvovirus B19 infection (fifth disease). Answer D is incorrect. Juvenile idiopathic arthritis, would be unusual at such a young age, and its presentation is similar to adult-onset disease. Answer E is incorrect because this is obviously not varicella.

CASE 2

A 62-year-old male whom you have followed for hypertension for several years presents with complaints of worsening fatigue and aching in his back, shoulders, and neck. He was first seen by your partner for the same complaints 1 month ago. He was then diagnosed with myofascial neck and back pain and prescribed acetaminophen. The use of scheduled acetaminophen has not helped much, and the patient believes that his fatigue is now more severe.

Further history reveals that your patient has experienced stiffness of the neck and shoulders each morning for over 30 minutes. He occasionally has difficulty getting out of bed. Physical examination reveals a temperature of 37.7°C with normal BP and pulse. There is no evidence of synovitis of the hands, wrists, and elbows. Active range of motion in the neck and shoulders is slow but full. There is tenderness to palpation of the shoulders, upper back, and neck, but no apparent muscle atrophy.

Which of the following is the most appropriate next step in the diagnosis of this illness?

A) Obtain an erythrocyte sedimentation rate (ESR) and C-reactive protein (CRP).
B) Obtain a urinalysis.
C) Prescribe a diagnostic trial of steroids.
D) Order a rheumatology panel, including antinuclear antibodies (ANA), uric acid, ESR, CRP, and rheumatoid factor (RF).
E) Perform shoulder radiograph.

Discussion

The correct answer is A. This patient's presentation is consistent with the diagnosis of polymyalgia rheumatica (PMR). Elevations of ESR and/or CRP contribute further evidence to such a diagnosis and are useful in following the treatment of PMR. Although a urinalysis

(answer B) may be important in some rheumatologic illnesses (eg, lupus, Behçet syndrome, Wegener granulomatosis, etc), PMR is not likely to be associated with renal disease. A trial of steroid therapy (answer C) may be appropriate, but an ESR should be obtained first to further clinch the diagnosis. All we know now is that he has bilateral shoulder and neck pain, which could be from a disc disease, syringomyelia, etc. Answer D is incorrect: a rheumatology panel will typically include tests that are not indicated, and positive results can be misleading. In the absence of small joint symptoms or exam findings, an RF is not indicated. Likewise there is no history to suggest an ANA-related disorder. A positive ANA occurs in many rheumatic disorders and is sometimes found in normal individuals. Likewise, RF is positive in many rheumatic and inflammatory disorders. Answer E is incorrect. This patient does not need shoulder radiographs. In a patient with bilateral shoulder pain and neck pain, a neck radiograph may be more useful than shoulder imaging. Neck radiographs help to evaluate for cervical canal narrowing and degenerative disc disease, which may result in pain and neurologic findings in the upper extremities. An MRI of the neck might be useful if cervical spine disc disease or a syrinx were suspected. Diagnostic criteria for PMR are listed in Table 11–3.

 HELPFUL TIP: Patients with PMR often have a low-grade fever and a normocytic anemia.

The sensitivity of an elevated ESR in the diagnosis of polymyalgia rheumatica/temporal arteritis is:

A) 100%
B) 95%

Table 11–3 CRITERIA FOR DIAGNOSIS OF PMR

- Age ≥50 years
- Pain/aching for at least 1 month involving 2 of the following areas: neck, shoulders/proximal arms, and pelvic girdle
- Morning stiffness
- ESR >40 mm/hour
- Exclusion of other potential causes of the symptoms except giant cell arteritis

C) 85%

D) 75%

E) 65%

Discussion

The correct answer is C. Up to 15% of patients with PMR or temporal arteritis have a false-negative ESR (a normal ESR). Using ESR and CRP together is 97%–99% sensitive for temporal arteritis. Double false negatives of ESR and CRP are uncommon but do occur. In the patient in whom PMR/temporal arteritis is suspected but in whom there is a normal ESR and/or CRP, biopsy is still recommended. In those suspected of PMR, a trial of steroids is recommended.

 HELPFUL TIP: PMR is uncommon in non-white populations. The mean age of onset is approximately 70 years (patients must be >50 years to diagnose). Women are affected twice as often as men.

* *

You order radiographs of the neck, which demonstrate mild degenerative disease. A CBC is unremarkable, except for a mild thrombocytosis. The ESR is 80 mm/hour. You relate these findings to the patient and tell him that your presumptive diagnosis is polymyalgia rheumatica.

Which of the following is the most appropriate initial treatment in this case?

A) Naproxen 500 mg BID.

B) Prednisone 20 mg QD and aspirin 81 mg QD.

C) Aspirin 650 mg BID.

D) Prednisone 50 mg QD.

E) Referral to physical therapy.

Discussion

The correct answer is B. Steroids are the treatment of choice in PMR. Doses of prednisone 10–20 mg QD usually control the disease. Higher doses (up to 30 mg per day) should be tried if there is no response in 1–2 weeks. If the patient fails to respond to steroids, the diagnosis of PMR should be reconsidered. Answer A is incorrect because although NSAIDs may effectively treat mild symptoms of PMR, they will not prevent the potential vascular complications of giant cell arteritis (GCA; aka temporal arteritis). Answer C is incorrect. When added to prednisone, low-dose aspirin, 81 mg per day, decreases the risk of vision loss in temporal arteritis. However, high dose aspirin therapy, without steroids is not recommended. Answer E is incorrect. Since patients usually respond quickly to steroids, physical therapy is not necessary—although you could hardly be faulted for employing physical therapy as part of your overall treatment approach.

* *

You prescribe prednisone 20 mg QD, aspirin 81 mg daily, and calcium and vitamin D supplementation. Your patient presents for follow-up 4 weeks later, reporting that he is greatly improved. On examination, there is no muscle tenderness with range of motion or joint inflammation. His ESR is 20 mm/hour. You believe that the patient's disease is now in remission.

Which of the following is the most appropriate next step in his management?

A) Discontinue prednisone and initiate naproxen.

B) Continue the current dose of prednisone for the next 12 months.

C) Continue the current dose of prednisone for the next 6 months.

D) Taper prednisone by 2 mg every 2 weeks to reach the minimum effective dose.

E) Taper prednisone by 10 mg over 2 weeks and then discontinue the dose.

Discussion

The correct answer is D. Relapse of PMR occurs more frequently when steroids are abruptly discontinued or tapered too quickly. However, because of complications associated with steroid therapy, the dose should be reduced as soon as possible; therefore, maintaining prednisone 20 mg QD for 6–12 months is inappropriate. The usual recommendation is to reduce the dose of prednisone by 10% every 1–2 weeks until the minimum effective dose is reached. While tapering the steroid dose, the patient should be monitored with an ESR every 2–4 weeks. If symptoms worsen, the steroid dose should be increased slightly to achieve symptomatic control. If the ESR is ≥40 mm/hour and the patient is asymptomatic, consider continuing the same dose of steroid until the ESR normalizes, then continue the taper. However, an isolated elevation in ESR without symptoms is not a reason to increase the steroid dose.

Which of the following is true regarding the prognosis of PMR?

A) PMR is associated with an increased risk of mortality.

B) Most patients with PMR will require steroid therapy for life.

C) Up to 50% of patients who initially have a successful remission will experience a relapse while tapering prednisone.

D) A relapse of PMR requires high-dose steroids (prednisone 50 mg QD) for successful treatment.

Discussion

The correct answer is C. Relapses occur in 30–50% of patients after induction of a remission and should be treated by resuming or increasing prednisone. Usually, successful treatment of a relapse requires increasing the prednisone dose by a few milligrams. Answer A is incorrect. Although the pathogenesis of PMR is incompletely understood, it has features in common with vasculitides, including potential vascular complications of giant cell arteritis. However, PMR is not associated with an increase in mortality. Answer B is incorrect because PMR is a self-limited disease, and most patients recover within a few months to a few years. Thus, patients require steroids for 6 months to 2 years, but steroid therapy is typically not lifelong. Relapse of PMR after prednisone has been successfully stopped is seen in about 20% of cases, and can occur up to years later.

* *

Your patient does well and is able to taper off steroid therapy. Three months after stopping steroids, he presents to the ED one night. His shoulder and neck pain and stiffness have returned, as well as severe fatigue and feeling feverish. He has lost 5 pounds in 2 weeks. He is now experiencing frequent left-sided headaches. Finally, he is most concerned about a new visual disturbance starting today. He notes that he has a hole in his vision. On physical examination, there is a prominent, tender vessel palpable at the left temporal area. Funduscopic exam of the left eye shows a pale disc with blurred margins. The remainder of the neurologic exam is normal. The ESR is 70 mm/hour.

Which of the following is the most likely diagnosis for the visual symptoms?

A) PMR.

B) Stroke.

C) GCA (Giant Cell Arteritis AKA Temporal Vasculitis).

D) Multiple sclerosis.

E) Acute angle-closure glaucoma.

Discussion

The correct answer is C. Many of the patient's symptoms can be explained by PMR (answer A), but visual symptoms do not occur with this disease. GCA is a related diagnosis that is commonly seen in conjunction with PMR. Some authors believe PMR and GCA are different presentations of the same disease process. With the new symptoms of localized headache and tenderness of the temporal artery and the previously known findings consistent with PMR, this patient meets diagnostic criteria for GCA (Table 11–4). The visual symptoms described are typical of GCA and can occur acutely or chronically. Answers B, D, and E are incorrect. This patient's vision loss is less likely to be due to stroke, multiple sclerosis, or angle-closure glaucoma. Vision loss in multiple sclerosis is attributable to optic neuritis, which is associated with pain and presents initially in a younger population. Acute angle-closure glaucoma is associated with eye pain and redness. The lack of other symptoms makes stroke less likely.

 HELPFUL TIP: The initial visual loss in temporal arteritis is peripheral whereas the initial vision loss in macular degeneration is central. This makes sense. GCA causes an ischemic neuropathy secondary to involvement of the retinal artery by vasculitis. The further from the artery, the poorer the perfusion.

Table 11–4 DIAGNOSTIC CRITERIA FOR GIANT CELL ARTERITIS

Three of the following must be present:
- Age ≥50 years at onset of symptoms
- New localized headache
- Temporal artery tenderness or decreased pulsation
- ESR ≥50 mm/hour
- Temporal artery biopsy findings consistent with vasculitis

Which of the following is the most appropriate initial management of this patient?

A) Withhold treatment for now and arrange for temporal artery biopsy within 48 hours.
B) Refer to a neurologist as soon as possible.
C) Refer to an ophthalmologist as soon as possible.
D) Initiate prednisone 20 mg QD, and refer for temporal artery biopsy.
E) Admit and administer methylprednisolone 1 g IV.

Discussion

The correct answer is E. In patients with severe symptoms of GCA, such as vision loss, admission to the hospital and prompt treatment with intravenous steroids is warranted. Thus answer A is incorrect. You do not want to withhold treatment from this patient whose vision is at risk (see Helpful Tip below). Answers B and C are incorrect for the same reason. Answer D is incorrect because a dose of 20 mg of prednisone is not going to be effective in temporal arteritis (GCA). When symptoms of vision loss occur, aspirin 81 mg daily and intravenous methylprednisolone 1 gram daily for 3 days, followed by aspirin and prednisone 40 to 60 mg daily is the standard of care. In comparison with PMR, higher doses of steroids are necessary to treat GCA. In the absence of vision loss, prednisone doses of 40–60 mg QD are usually required to relieve symptoms. A 3-day course of daily IV methylprednisolone, 1 gram, either as outpatient or inpatient, may be considered for patients without vision loss who have biopsy-confirmed disease. One study showed that the overall duration of corticosteroid therapy is reduced when IV therapy is used in early disease. Answer E is the correct choice: a higher percentage of patients show improved vision when treated with intravenous steroids in comparison with oral steroids.

* *

Six years after his diagnosis of GCA, your patient has experienced several remissions and relapses. Although he has been able to discontinue steroids on occasion, he is taking prednisone 5 mg QD with good symptomatic control. On a night when you are on call, your patient presents to the ED with tearing substernal chest pain radiating to his back. He is alert but anxious and diaphoretic. His left radial pulse is diminished compared to the right. His heart rate is 120 bpm, and his blood pressure is 92/56 mm Hg.

Which of the following studies will confirm the most likely diagnosis?

A) Chest radiograph.
B) Chest CT.
C) ECG.
D) ABG.
E) Troponin-T.

Discussion

The correct answer is B. Your patient's symptoms are classic for a dissecting thoracic aortic aneurysm, which is often mistaken for a myocardial infarction. Thoracic aortic aneurysm is a late complication of GCA; aortic aneurysms generally occur an average of 6–7 years after the initial diagnosis of GCA. Thoracic aortic aneurysms occur 17 times more often in patients with GCA compared to the general population. The diagnosis of thoracic aortic aneurysm is confirmed by CT scan of the chest, echocardiogram, or angiogram. A chest radiograph may show a widened mediastinum. However, this is a nonspecific finding and the mediastinum is negative in 25% of those with an aortic dissection. While the other studies listed should be done, none of them is going to make the diagnosis of a dissecting aneurysm for you.

 HELPFUL TIP: Temporal artery biopsy is vital to the accurate diagnosis of GCA. Characteristic giant cell inflammation pathology can be seen for up to 4 weeks after initiating high dose corticosteroids. However, **corticosteroid therapy should never be delayed for fear of reducing the inflammatory findings on the temporal artery biopsy.**

 HELPFUL TIP: In addition to initiation of steroids in PMR or GCA, start calcium 1200–1500 mg daily and vitamin D 400–800 IU daily for osteoporosis prevention. Aspirin 81 mg per day, if not contraindicated, reduces the risk of vision loss and possibly stroke in these patients. In patients with GCA, an annual chest radiograph is recommended to evaluate for thoracic aortic aneurysm.

Objectives: Did you learn to . . .

- Describe the appropriate evaluation, including physical exam and laboratory test, of diffuse pain in the older patient?
- Recognize the diagnostic criteria for PMR and GCA?
- Describe the appropriate management, including medical therapy, of PMR and GCA?
- Identify complications of PMR and GCA?

QUICK QUIZ: OSTEOARTHRITIS

The preferred initial therapy for elderly patients with arthralgia due to osteoarthritis is which of the following?

A) NSAIDs.
B) COX-2 inhibitors.
C) Acetaminophen.
D) Combination narcotic analgesics.
E) Early joint replacement.

Discussion

The correct answer is C. Because of greater risk of gastrointestinal and renal toxicity in the elderly, NSAIDs should be avoided in this population. COX-2 inhibitors are more expensive than traditional NSAIDs and likely have little advantage in terms of GI toxicity. The best initial choice for osteoarthritis pain in the elderly (and almost everybody, for that matter) is acetaminophen with doses scheduled 3–4 times per day. Combination narcotic analgesics are employed when acetaminophen alone does not suffice and NSAIDs are contraindicated. Although elderly patients should be considered candidates for joint replacement, it is not appropriate as the initial therapy.

> **HELPFUL TIP:** Other treatments for osteoarthritis that have demonstrated benefit for short-term pain control include topical capsaicin cream, topical NSAIDs, intraarticular steroid injection, and intraarticular hyaluronan injection. Glucosamine, with or without chondroitin, has not shown benefit in rigorous trials. None of these treatments has demonstrated clinically significant, long-term benefit.

CASE 3

A 27-year-old male graduate student presents to the ED on a Monday night with an acutely swollen left knee. He admits to "wild partying" over the weekend, and though he got "rather drunk" Saturday night, he is sure that the knee was fine then. However, when he woke up this morning, he noticed the knee was swollen and painful. By early afternoon, he had difficulty bearing weight. He denies fever but feels tired.

He reports a history of juvenile idiopathic arthritis (JIA; previously known as juvenile rheumatoid arthritis [JRA]), and has had ankle and knee swelling previously, but not to this degree. He took prednisone intermittently, as well as hydroxychloroquine and methotrexate, for his JIA until age 18. He then continued on hydroxychloroquine until 8 months ago, when he stopped it because he felt fine. He denies any other medical problems. He smokes only when drinking.

What other information from the history would be most helpful in establishing the diagnosis?

A) Sexual history, including sexual orientation, practices, and last contact.
B) History of gout or pseudogout (calcium pyrophosphate dihydrate disease).
C) History of intravenous drug use.
D) A and B.
E) All of the above.

Discussion

The correct answer is E. All of these points are important in the history. While the patient is generally too young to have gout or pseudogout, a history of either of these diseases in a patient with monoarticular arthritis might change your approach. Although there are several etiologies possible for this patient's presentation, the most critical to identify and treat is septic arthritis. As such, the history and exam should focus on those clues that point towards an infectious etiology and its source. The clinician must also consider noninfectious inflammatory arthropathies.

* *

Your patient is heterosexual and thinks he had intercourse Saturday night but his memory is somewhat blurry. He denies a history of gout and intravenous drug use. He complains of poor sleep and feeling stiff in the mornings and evenings lately.

What findings on physical exam would be LEAST helpful in determining the diagnosis?

A) A few vesiculopustular lesions on the back.
B) Swollen, tender, non-erythematous metacarpophalangeal (MCP) joints.
C) Nontender hepatomegaly.
D) Diastolic murmur at the right sternal border.
E) Whitish discharge from the tip of penis.

Discussion

The correct answer is C. Although nontender hepatomegaly is important to notice and may indicate presence of liver disease, it is unlikely to help identify the etiology of this patient's arthritis. Hepatitis B arthritis usually presents as a symmetric polyarthritis, although it can be migratory or additive (sequential joints becoming involved without resolution in the initial joints). The other answer choices are helpful in making a diagnosis. Sexual history (answer A) is helpful because a vesiculopustular rash occurs in disseminated gonococcal infections. History of gout (answer B) is helpful because the presence of other swollen joints should prompt consideration of noninfectious inflammatory arthritis, and the swelling of the MCPs may be a clue for active RA. Diastolic murmur (answer D) is helpful because a diastolic murmur is always abnormal and may be a clue for endocarditis (which may seed joints causing infectious arthritis). Finally, penile discharge (answer E), can result from acute gonorrheal infections.

* *

On exam, vitals show the following: pulse 112 bpm, temperature 38.2°C, and normal BP. He has no other swollen joints, no skin rash, no penile discharge, and no heart murmur. You palpate a smooth, nontender liver edge 2 cm below the costal margin; it percusses to 15 cm. You note mild cervical lymphadenopathy and whitish pharyngeal exudates.

Which of the following is the most appropriate next step in the management of this patient?

A) Order hepatitis serologies.
B) Order blood cultures, pharyngeal cultures, and abdominal ultrasound.
C) Administer ceftriaxone 1 gm intravenously and inject the knee with triamcinolone.
D) Perform knee aspiration.
E) Prescribe prednisone 20 mg PO QD and arrange consultation with a rheumatologist.

Discussion

The correct answer is D. The most important next step in evaluating acute monoarthritis is joint aspiration, which will allow differentiation between inflammatory and noninflammatory disease. Although blood and pharyngeal (as well as urethral) cultures should also be sent in this case, obtaining these studies must not supplant joint aspiration. A liver ultrasound may be required to evaluate hepatomegaly, but again should not delay joint aspiration. In this case, hepatitis serologies (specifically hepatitis B and C) are important but not urgent, as these results will not affect management in the acute setting. Without determining whether the arthritis is infectious, it would be inappropriate—and potentially hazardous to the patient—to start treatment. Answers C and E are incorrect because you would not want to give steroids—especially intraarticular steroids—to a patient with an infected joint. Analysis of the synovial fluid will aid in determining the appropriateness of treating with antibiotics or anti-inflammatory medications.

 HELPFUL TIP: CBC, sedimentation rate, and CRP are not useful in diagnosis of a septic joint. While they may be somewhat sensitive, they are hopelessly nonspecific. You have to tap the joint regardless!

* *

You have obtained blood cultures, pharyngeal cultures, and urethral cultures. A metabolic profile, CBC, and hepatitis B and C serologies are pending. Knee aspiration yields 45 cc of turbid, blood-tinged fluid.

You send the synovial fluid for all of the following studies EXCEPT:

A) Cell count and differential.
B) Crystal analysis.
C) Culture.
D) Glucose and protein.
E) Gram stain.

Discussion

The correct answer is D. In contrast to analysis of some other bodily fluids (eg, CSF, pleural fluid, ascitic fluid), chemistry analysis on synovial fluid is of little diagnostic value. Low glucose levels in synovial fluid are associated with the degree of inflammation but not its cause.

Likewise, synovial protein levels do not help differentiate between types of arthritis. Cell count with differential, Gram stain, and cultures should be routine when suspecting infection; crystal analysis is also part of the standard examination.

* *

The synovial fluid analysis reveals the following: 50,000 WBC/mm^3, 95% polymorphonuclear cells, and no crystals. Gram stain shows Gram-negative diplococci. The same Gram stain findings are obtained from the urethral, but not the pharyngeal, swab. Cultures are pending.

Which of the following studies will be most important to the OVERALL care of this patient?

A) HIV testing and RPR.
B) Chest x-ray.
C) ANA and RF.
D) Uric acid.
E) ESR and CRP.

Discussion

The correct answer is A. His presentation is very suggestive of disseminated gonococcal infection with acute arthritis, and the presence of diplococci is virtually diagnostic. Therefore, the clinician must also consider the presence of other sexually transmitted diseases and screen the patient appropriately. Assays for hepatitis B and C have been sent, and tests for chlamydia, HIV, and syphilis should now be performed. Also, the patient must be counseled regarding safe sexual practices (eg, condom use, abstinence). In this setting, the other studies are less relevant to his overall health.

 HELPFUL TIP: Gonococcus is cultured from the joint fluid only 50% of the time in patients with gonococcal arthritis. Thus, a PCR of the joint fluid and urethral cultures should be done if gonococcus is suspected but not identified initially.

Which of the following is the most appropriate treatment plan for this patient?

A) Ceftriaxone 1 g IV once, followed by cefixime 400 mg PO bid for 14 days. Follow-up in 7 days.
B) Admit to hospital, administer ceftriaxone 1 g IV QD, and perform repeat knee aspirations.

C) Admit to the hospital and administer intravenous and intra-articular ceftriaxone 1 g QD.
D) Ciprofloxacin 500 mg PO BID for 14 days. Follow-up in 7 days.
E) Penicillin G 4 MU IV once, followed by amoxicillin 500 mg PO TID for 14 days. Follow up with a rheumatologist.

Discussion

The correct answer is B. To ensure the best outcome, this patient should be admitted for monitoring and repeated joint aspiration. Purulent fluid tends to collect rapidly in the joint spaces in patients with septic arthritis, necessitating frequent drainage until antibiotics begin to reduce the inflammation. Most patients with gonococcal arthritis respond to needle aspiration, but arthroscopic or open debridement is occasionally necessary. Because intravenous antibiotics have good penetration into synovial fluid, intraarticular antibiotics are not recommended. When culture, PCR, and sensitivity results become available, antibiotic therapy should be tailored to the sensitivities.

 HELPFUL TIP: The initial antibiotic of choice in gonococcal arthritis is ceftriaxone, administered intravenously. In patients with drug allergies or other contraindications prohibit the use of ceftriaxone, intravenous spectinomycin is an acceptable alternative. Remember that there is now fluoroquinolone-resistant gonococcus. Because of this, fluoroquinolones are no longer recommended as treatment for gonorrhea.

* *

Within 48 hours, your patient shows signs of improvement. His knee appears much better, there is no recurrent effusion, and he is afebrile. He wants to leave the hospital. By the way, his chlamydia PCR turned up positive.

Which of the following management strategies do you recommend?

A) Continue the hospital admission and ceftriaxone 1 g IV QD.
B) Discharge with ciprofloxacin 500 mg PO BID.
C) Discharge with penicillin V 500 mg PO TID.

D) Discharge with cefixime 400 mg PO BID and doxycycline 100 mg PO BID.
E) Daily emergency center visits for ceftriaxone 1 g IV QD.

Discussion

The correct answer is D. Because the patient is improving, continued hospitalization and intravenous antibiotics are not needed. Thus, answer A is incorrect. Without knowing the antibiotic sensitivities of the gonococcus, you should assume that it is penicillin resistant, thus answer C is incorrect. Once local and systemic signs are resolving, you can safely discharge the patient with oral antibiotic therapy, using cefixime 400 mg BID (or an acceptable alternative based on culture and susceptibilities) to complete a 7–14-day course. In cases of gonococcal infection, you should presumptively treat for concurrent chlamydia infection. Although ciprofloxin (answer B) is correct for the treatment of gonococcus, it is not the best choice for this patient. Answer D provides treatment for chlamydia as well.

 HELPFUL TIP: Septic arthritis occurs most often in large joints, such as the knee and hip. Factors that predispose a patient to septic arthritis include: advancing age (>80 years), RA, joint prostheses, recent joint surgery, diabetes, and skin infection.

What is the incidence of mortality in septic arthritis?

A) 0.5%
B) 5%
C) 10%
D) >15%

Discussion

The correct answer is C. Incidence of mortality in septic arthritis is 10%. Up to 33% of individuals having persistent joint problems, such as limited range of motion, pain, and swelling. Note that the mortality does not result from the infection alone but rather to a combination of the underlying illness (eg, immuno-suppression) plus the infection.

Objectives: Did you learn to. . .

- Describe the appropriate evaluation of monoarthritis?
- Appropriately manage a patient with septic arthritis?
- Identify risk factors for septic arthritis?
- Recognize the prognosis of septic arthritis?

CASE 4

A 55-year-old male presents to your office complaining of severe left knee pain of 2 days' duration. Although he was also out partying over the weekend, he went home early He denies any previous history of knee pain or arthritis. He has felt feverish over the last 2 days. He recalls a similar episode of pain in his right great toe 2 years before, but the pain resolved in a few days and he did not seek medical attention. His has hypertension treated with chlorthalidone but is otherwise healthy. He drinks about a case of beer per week. His family history is remarkable for arthritis.

Physical examination reveals an uncomfortable-appearing obese male in no acute distress. His temperature is 37.9°C, BP 168/98 mm Hg, and pulse 84 bpm. The left knee is red, warm, and diffusely tender with a palpable effusion.

Which of the following is the most appropriate next step to accurately diagnose this condition?

A) Radiograph of the affected knee.
B) CBC.
C) Uric acid level.
D) Knee aspiration and synovial fluid analysis.
E) Diagnostic steroid injection.

Discussion

The correct answer is D. The diagnostic study of choice in monoarthritis is synovial fluid analysis. Synovial fluid analysis allows the clinician to determine whether there is an inflammatory, infectious, or crystalline cause of the arthritis. Answer A is incorrect. Radiographs are typically not helpful acutely in inflammatory arthritis (but would be indicated if there was trauma or suspicion of tumor). A CBC (answer B) and uric acid level (answer C) are useful when infection or gout is suspected. However, neither of these labs results will be diagnostic. Steroid injection (answer E) must be avoided in monoarthritis until the possibility of infection is eliminated.

* *

You successfully aspirate 5 cc of clear yellow synovial fluid from the left knee. While the patient is waiting, the laboratory reports the following findings: 5,000 WBC/mm^3, Gram stain negative for bacteria, needle-shaped negatively birefringent crystals are noted.

These synovial fluid findings are most consistent with which of the following diagnoses?

A) Osteoarthritis.
B) Septic arthritis.
C) Calcium pyrophosphate dihydrate disease ("pseudo-gout").
D) Gout.
E) None of the above.

Discussion

The correct answer is D. Monosodium urate crystals of gout are needle-shaped as seen in this patient's synovial fluid (a memory aid for this: Being stuck with a needle hurts—so does gout). Calcium pyrophosphate dihydrate crystals are rod-, square-, or rhomboid-shaped and positively birefringent in polarized light. Thus, the synovial fluid findings given above are most consistent with gout. Answer B is incorrect. Normally, synovial fluid contains <180 WBC/mm^3, but it is considered noninflammatory if there are <2,000 WBC/mm^3. Low WBC counts are seen in the synovial fluid of osteoarthritic joints. Synovial fluid containing ≥2,000 WBC/mm^3 is consistent with an inflammatory process. When there are >100,000 WBC/mm^3, the monoarthritis is considered septic until proven otherwise. Table 11–5 lists diagnostic criteria for gout.

 HELPFUL TIP: Serum uric acid is often normal during an acute attack of gout; thus, you cannot rely on serum uric acid levels alone to diagnose gout.

 HELPFUL TIP: A polarizing microscope is not required to see crystals in synovial fluid! Look under a standard light microscope for either needle-shaped (uric acid) or rhomboid/square (calcium pyrophosphate) crystals.

Table 11–5 DIAGNOSTIC CRITERIA FOR ACUTE GOUT

Presence of characteristic urate crystals in the joint fluid or tophus proved to contain urate crystals by chemical means or polarized light microscopy or presence of 6 of the following 12 phenomena:

- More than 1 attack of acute arthritis
- Maximal inflammation developed within 1 day
- Attack of monoarticular arthritis
- Joint redness observed
- First metatarsophalangeal joint painful or swollen
- Unilateral attack involving first metatarsophalangeal joint
- Unilateral attack involving tarsal joint
- Suspected tophus
- Hyperuricemia
- Asymmetric swelling within a joint (radiograph)
- Subcortical cysts without erosion (radiograph)
- Negative joint fluid culture for microorganisms during attack of joint inflammation

Criteria as set forth by the American College of Rheumatology.

In general, all of the following are risk factors for gout EXCEPT:

A) Tobacco use.
B) Alcohol use.
C) Obesity.
D) Diuretic use.
E) Family history.

Discussion

The correct answer is A. Tobacco use is not associated with gout. Your patient exhibits many of the risk factors for gout, which include: male sex, obesity, high-protein diet, high social class, use of diuretics (loop or thiazide), alcohol, and family history.

 HELPFUL TIP: Many individuals with hyperuricemia do **not** develop gout or nephrolithiasis; asymptomatic hyperuricemia should not be treated with uric acid–lowering agents.

Which of the following is the NEXT step in the management of this patient's acute flare?

A) Prescribe allopurinol.
B) Prescribe acetaminophen.
C) Discontinue chlorthalidone.

D) Prescribe naproxen.

E) Therapeutic joint aspiration.

Discussion

The correct answer is D. An acute attack of gout should be treated initially with NSAIDs, such as naproxen or indomethacin. The doses prescribed should be at the upper limit for the particular NSAID (eg, naproxen 500 mg TID). Earlier treatment is associated with greater relief of symptoms and shorter duration of the acute event. Other first-line agents are steroids and colchicine. Narcotic pain medication is also appropriate. Answer A is incorrect. Allopurinol is indicated for prophylaxis of gout when hyperuricemia is documented, but its use in the acute setting is inappropriate. Initiation of allopurinol may cause or worsen exacerbations of gout. Answer B is incorrect because acetaminophen lacks the antiinflammatory properties of NSAIDs and is less effective. Discontinuing chlorthalidone (a thiazide diuretic) (answer C) may reduce uric acid levels over time but is not likely to improve symptoms in the acute setting. Joint aspiration (answer E) is not therapeutic in gout but may be helpful in pseudogout.

 HELPFUL TIP: Oral or intraarticular steroid administrations are options for patients who have contraindications to NSAIDs, who have failed NSAID therapy, or who have more severe attacks. Steroids are as efficacious as NSAIDS and have fewer side effects. They are replacing NSAIDS as first-line in gout therapy. Narcotic pain medication may be needed as an adjunct to an antiinflammatory.

* *

You start an NSAID. He returns in a few days to discuss his labs and x-rays. A radiograph of the left knee demonstrates an effusion but is otherwise unremarkable. His uric acid level is 10.1 mg/dL (the upper limit of normal for your lab is 7.2 mg/dL). CBC, creatinine, sodium, and potassium are normal. You instruct the patient to reduce his alcohol intake and try to lose weight to decrease his risk of gout attacks and for overall health.

* *

Your patient returns after 1 year. He has been using naproxen frequently and recalls 5 acute attacks of gout in the last year.

Which of the following regimens is most likely to reduce the frequency of gout attacks?

A) Twice-daily colchicine.

B) Daily allopurinol.

C) Daily probenecid.

D) Twice-daily colchicine and daily allopurinol.

E) Daily probenecid and allopurinol.

Discussion

The correct answer is D. Low doses of colchicine administered twice daily have been shown to reduce the frequency of gout attacks 75%–85%. This patient also has hyperuricemia and is likely to benefit from lowering his uric acid level. Remember that the initiation of allopurinol may precipitate or worsen an acute attack of gout. Therefore, allopurinol should be initiated only with concurrent use of colchicine or an NSAID.

Probenecid is a uricosuric agent that also reduces the frequency and severity of acute gout attacks. Although probenecid can be used in conjunction with allopurinol, there are interactions between these two medications that require close monitoring: probenecid accelerates excretion of allopurinol, and allopurinol may increase the half-life of probenecid. Thus, this combination is generally not a good idea. An attempt should be made to lower uric acid to 6–7 mg/dL with one medication before combining two uric acid–lowering agents.

 HELPFUL TIP: Although colchicine is recommended as prophylaxis when allopurinol is initiated, it should be discontinued within 6 months due to the potential side effects of GI irritation, diarrhea, and myopathy.

All of the following are side affects of allopurinol EXCEPT:

A) Aseptic meningitis.

B) Rash.

C) Leukopenia.

D) Fever.

E) GI disturbance.

Discussion

The correct answer is A. Additional side effects include elevated liver enzymes, glomerulonephritis, aplastic anemia, and vasculitis. Not a pretty drug.

HELPFUL TIP: Probenecid should be avoided in patients >60 years because of concern about renal function.

* *

It is 9 years later; the patient has not followed up in that time. He returns, noting 9 years of acute intermittent gout attacks. ("Of course I took my medication, Doc.") He presents with complaint of pain in his knees and feet that has been present for several months. He has also developed swelling and pain in his hands. The pain is less intense than his attacks of gout, but occurs in the same areas and never completely resolves between attacks. He has no morning stiffness, no muscle complaints, and no other systemic complaints. You find diffuse edema of both hands and palpable tophi on the knees.

Which of the following is the most likely cause of his current symptoms?

A) RA.
B) Osteoarthritis.
C) Gout.
D) PMR.

Discussion

The correct answer is C. This patient has a long history of acute intermittent gout. After years of acute attacks, patients with gout may develop a form of the disease called **chronic tophaceous gout,** in which the intercritical periods are no longer free of pain. There is no clinical association between gout and the other rheumatic conditions mentioned and, therefore, no reason to suspect that another rheumatic disorder is causing the chronic pain.

HELPFUL TIP: Hyperlipidemia occurs in 80% of patients with gout—check lipids.

HELPFUL TIP: The first metatarsophalangeal (MTP) joint is affected in 90% of patients with gout, and the initial attack involves the first MTP joint in 50%.

CASE 5

Citing your compassion and attention to detail, your patient refers a friend he met at Gouty Retirees in Love with Life (GRILL). This friend is a 65-year-old male who reports a history of joint swelling, pain, and redness, usually involving his knees, wrists, and hands; he has never had first MTP joint involvement. Although he has never had a joint aspiration performed, he has been treated for gout for 5 years. He takes his medication faithfully but has found allopurinol unhelpful. He is currently asymptomatic, but uses ibuprofen for acute attacks. The joint exam is unremarkable, without joint effusion—but he is currently asymptomatic.

Which of the following studies is most appropriate for this patient?

A) "Diagnostic" knee injection with steroids.
B) CBC.
C) Rheumatoid factor.
D) Radiographs of the knees and wrists.
E) Serum uric acid.

Discussion

The correct answer is D. The initial evaluation should include radiographs of the affected joints, which may give clues to the diagnosis. Radiographs may reveal osteophyte formation typical of osteoarthritis, subchondral cysts and chondrocalcinosis typical of calcium pyrophosphate dihydrate deposition disease (CPPD), or erosions with an overhanging edge typical of gout. Chondrocalcinosis is most often seen in the knees and triangular fibrocartilage of the wrists.

An injection of steroids (answer A) might help relieve symptoms, but will not be diagnostic. A CBC (answer B) is nonspecific and will not be helpful. Rheumatoid factor (answer C) will not be helpful given this patient's symptoms, which are not suggestive of RA. Also, rheumatoid factor may be present in inflammatory arthritides other than RA, and so will not be helpful. Uric acid (answer E) is not diagnostic, but if normal during the intercritical period, it might provide evidence against the diagnosis of gout.

HELPFUL TIP: The crystals of gout (uric acid) and pseudogout (calcium pyrophosphate) can be seen in synovial fluid during intercritical periods. If there is an effusion even in the absence of acute symptoms and you are thinking gout or pseudogout, tap that joint!

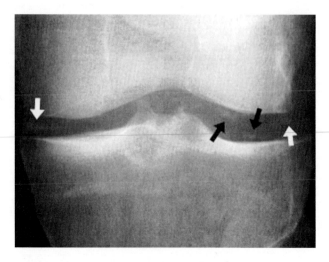

Figure 11–1   Chondrocalcinosis of the knee joint.
(Note arrows highlighting calcification.)

* *

Radiographs of your patient's knee demonstrate chondrocalcinosis (Figure 11–1). Examination of synovial fluid from the knee shows positively birefringent, rhomboid crystals consistent with CPPD (pseudogout).

Which of the following do you recommend to decrease his risk of recurrent acute attacks of pseudogout?

A)   Serial joint aspiration.
B)   Daily allopurinol.
C)   Twice-daily colchicine.
D)   Serial intra-articular steroid injections.
E)   Chondroitin sulfate.

Discussion

The correct answer is C. Pseudogout is diagnosed by the presence of CPPD crystals (described above) in synovial fluid and/or typical x-ray findings (basically, chondrocalcinosis). Although prophylaxis is more predictably successful in gout, colchicine 0.6 mg BID has been shown to reduce the frequency of pseudogout attacks in CPPD. NSAIDs or colchicine may be used in acute attacks. Answers A and D are incorrect. While joint aspiration and steroid injection may be helpful during acute attacks, they play no role in prophylaxis. Answer B is incorrect. Since CPPD is not caused by abnormalities in uric acid metabolism, allopurinol has no role in the management of pseudogout. Answer E is incorrect because chondroitin sulfate does not appear to be useful in osteoarthritis, let alone pseudogout.

CPPD (pseudogout) is associated with which of the following?

A)   Hypothyroidism.
B)   Hyperparathyroidism.
C)   Amyloidosis.
D)   Hemochromatosis.
E)   All of the above.

Discussion

The correct answer is E. All of the above are associated with pseudogout. Additional associated conditions include hypophosphatemia and hypomagnesemia. For this reason, order the following studies in patients newly diagnosed with CPPD: thyroid-stimulating hormone, calcium, phosphate, magnesium, transferrin saturation, and alkaline phosphatase.

 HELPFUL TIP: Precipitants of gout and pseudogout (CPPD) include trauma, surgery, severe medical illness, and alcohol overindulgence.

Objectives: Did you learn to . . .

• Evaluate recurrent monoarthritis?
• Describe the diagnostic implications of synovial fluid findings?
• Define diagnostic criteria for gout and calcium pyrophosphate dihydrate deposition disease?
• Manage a patient with gout and describe adverse effects of the medications used to treat gout?
• Implement appropriate therapy for calcium pyrophosphate dihydrate deposition disease?

 QUICK QUIZ: CRYOGLOBULINEMIA

Cryoglobulinemia, a vasculitic disease caused by antibodies that precipitate in cold temperatures, is most often caused by which of the following viral infections?

A)   HIV.
B)   Hepatitis B.
C)   Hepatitis C.
D)   Parvovirus B19.

Discussion

The correct answer is C. Hepatitis C is found in 80% of vasculitis patients associated with mixed cryoglobulinemia.

Although up to 50% of patients with hepatitis C have cryoglobulins, only a minority of patients have clinical vasculitis. Because of the increasing prevalence of hepatitis C, cases of cryoglobulinemia will most likely increase. As to the other answers, hepatitis B and parvovirus B19 infection may cause a symmetric polyarthritis. HIV is less commonly a cause of cryoglobulinemia but is associated with reactive arthritis. The symptoms of mixed cryoglobulinemia associated with HCV infection typically include arthralgias, fever, renal disease, palpable purpura, and neuropathy.

CASE 6

A 13-year-old male presents to your office with his father. The patient has complaints of pain in his wrists, elbows, and knees bilaterally. He has felt fatigued and has been unable to work his summer job as a busboy at his father's restaurant. He reports intermittent fevers and an evanescent rash that appears during febrile episodes but is short-lived. All of these symptoms have emerged in the last 6 weeks, after a weeklong backpacking trip in Minnesota. He has no significant past medical history. His only medication is acetaminophen daily for joint pain. He denies tobacco use, alcohol use, and sexual activity.

The differential diagnosis should include all of the following EXCEPT:

A) Lyme disease.
B) JIA.
C) PMR.
D) Viral illness.

Discussion

The correct answer is C. The diagnosis of PMR can be made in individuals >50 years. Juvenile idiopathic arthritis (JIA) is a chronic arthritis of childhood that can present in a variety of ways, but must include arthritis of one or more joints, lasting 6 weeks or more, with symptom onset <16 years. Lyme disease has several presentations, presenting with arthritis early or late in the course. Many viral illnesses can result in arthralgias and/or arthritis. Any of the diseases listed may have associated symptoms of fatigue, malaise, headache, and myalgias. One factor that makes Lyme disease a likely diagnosis is the history of being outdoors in an endemic area (90% of Lyme disease in the United States occurs in New York, New Jersey, Connecticut, Rhode Island, Massachusetts, Pennsylvania, Wisconsin, and Minnesota).

Which of the following findings on physical examination would be more consistent with Lyme disease than JIA?

A) Bell palsy.
B) Temperature ≥38°C.
C) Rash.
D) Lymphadenopathy.
E) A and C.

Discussion

The correct answer is A. All of the other findings are seen in both Lyme disease and JIA. Neurologic symptoms, including Bell palsy (answer A) and meningitis, may occur with Lyme disease but not JIA. Rash (answer C) is present in both diseases but differs substantially. The characteristic rash of Lyme disease is erythema migrans. The rash of JIA is macular, salmon-pink, and brought on by heat. Erythema migrans occurs in approximately 80% of patients with acute Lyme disease. The lesion is often described as "targetoid," a red circular rash with central clearing. However, most patients do not have the classic lesion. Rather, they present with a mildly to brightly erythematous patch in the axilla or belt line, where the tick bite occurs. The tick itself is rarely seen. Erythema migrans is usually not painful or pruritic. Both Lyme disease and JIA may have associated systemic findings, including fever and lymphadenopathy, so neither answer B nor D is a good discriminator.

 HELPFUL TIP: Twenty percent of patients with Lyme disease will not have a rash. Classically, erythema migrans is observed at the site of the tick bite, but it can occur at sites distant from the tick bite.

* *

Physical examination reveals a thin male in no acute distress. His temperature is 37.3°C, pulse 100 bpm, and BP 120/70 mm Hg. Small, nontender, mobile lymph nodes are palpable in the neck and axillae. There is a large, warm, erythematous patch with central clearing at the patient's left axilla. There is limited range of motion in his right wrist and left elbow. An effusion is palpable at the left knee, which is diffusely tender.

If you were to aspirate the patient's knee, which of the following would you expect to find in the synovial fluid?

A) >100,000 WBC/mm³.
B) Predominance of eosinophils.
C) Monosodium urate crystals.
D) Spirochetes.
E) Predominance of polymorphonuclear cells.

Discussion

The correct answer is E. This patient is presenting now with classic features of Lyme disease. If synovial fluid is obtained in a patient with Lyme arthritis, analysis of the fluid reveals leukocytes, most commonly polymorphonuclear cells. Answer A is incorrect. If the synovial fluid has >100,000 WBC/mm³, you should consider septic arthritis. Answer B is incorrect because eosinophils are not the predominant cell in synovial fluid of Lyme arthritis. Answer C is incorrect because monosodium urate crystals are observed in gout—an unlikely cause of this patient's joint complaints. Answer D is incorrect. *Borrelia burgdorferi* spirochetes, the causative organism in Lyme disease, are not usually observed in the synovial fluid. Lyme arthritis is thought to be an autoimmune reaction rather than a direct effect of the spirochete.

* *

You strongly suspect Lyme disease and decide not to aspirate the knee effusion.

Which of the following is true regarding laboratory tests for Lyme disease?

A) Serologic tests are reliable within 1 week of the tick bite.
B) Serologic tests are useful in screening for Lyme disease.
C) Blood cultures remain positive for *B. burgdorferi* for months after the tick bite.
D) Serologic tests remain positive for up to 10 years after antibiotic treatment.
E) The diagnosis of Lyme disease is based on serologic tests.

Discussion

The correct answer is D. Serologic tests for Lyme disease can remain positive for up to 10 years, and in some cases 20 years after exposure. Thus, serologic tests alone are not diagnostic of active Lyme disease. Answer E is incorrect. The diagnosis of Lyme disease is clinical with laboratory tests used to confirm the diagnosis. A positive ELISA test is not adequate to make the diagnosis

of Lyme disease. Positive or equivocal ELISA tests should be confirmed with Western blot analysis. Answer A is incorrect. Serologic assays may be falsely negative early in infection. Answer B is incorrect. Because of the high false-positive rate, serologic assays should not be used as a screening tool in the general population. Answer C is incorrect. Positive blood cultures for *B. burgdorferi* are rarely obtained. When cultures do grow *B. burgdorferi*, it is only early in the disease. Cultures of skin biopsied from the erythema migrans lesion are more likely to be positive.

For this patient, whose weight is 50 kg and who has no known allergies, which course of therapy is safest and most efficacious?

A) Amoxicillin, 500 mg PO TID for 1 week.
B) Ceftriaxone, 2 g IM, single dose.
C) Doxycycline, 100 mg PO BID for 4 weeks.
D) Levofloxacin, 250 mg PO QD for 2 weeks.
E) Erythromycin 250 mg PO QID for 4 weeks.

Discussion

The correct answer is C. Recommended therapy for Lyme arthritis (without neurologic disease) is 4 weeks of either amoxicillin 500 mg TID, doxycycline 100 mg BID, or cefuroxime axetil 500 mg BID. This patient is old enough to take doxycycline, which is contraindicated in children <8 years because it causes tooth discoloration. Answer A is incorrect because the duration of amoxicillin prescribed here is too short. If this patient were younger and doxycycline was contraindicated, a 4-week course of amoxicillin or cefuroxime would be the preferred therapy. Ceftriaxone (answer B) is prescribed when neurologic abnormalities are present (such as Bell palsy or meningitis), and it must be dosed daily for 2–4 weeks. Levofloxacin (answer D) is not indicated for Lyme disease. Treatment with erythromycin for 4 weeks (answer E), while an acceptable alternative, appears to be less efficacious.

 HELPFUL TIP: There is no known resistance of *B. burgdorferi* to standard antibiotic regimens.

* *

Several hours after starting antibiotics, your patient's father calls to reports worsening symptoms of fever, shaking, and dizziness.

You recognize this condition as which of the following?

A) An allergic reaction to the antibiotic.
B) *B. burgdorferi* sepsis.
C) Secondary bacterial infection.
D) A cytokine-mediated reaction to the antibiotic-mediated killing of spirochetes (Jarisch-Herxheimer reaction).
E) The expected, natural course of Lyme disease.

Discussion

The correct answer is D. A Jarisch-Herxheimer reaction occurs in 5%–15% of patients treated with antibiotics for Lyme disease. (Remember syphilis? Lyme is also a spirochete disease.) The reaction is mediated by the release of cytokines and occurs within hours of initial administration of antibiotics. In Lyme disease, the reaction is self-limited and usually resolves within a day. Only supportive treatment is necessary, and antibiotics should be continued. Answer A is incorrect because this reaction is not typical of a drug allergy. Answer B is incorrect because *B. burgdorferi* does not cause sepsis. Answer C is incorrect because it is unlikely that a secondary bacterial infection has occurred so quickly. Answer E is incorrect because this does not represent the natural history of Lyme disease (Table 11–6).

Table 11–6 STAGES OF LYME DISEASE

Early localized disease	
(Stage I)	Occurs days to a month after the tick bite and includes erythema migrans, fatigue, fever, malaise, myalgias, arthralgia, arthritis, headache, and lymphadenopathy. Except for erythema migrans, it can be confused with a viral illness.
Early disseminated disease	
(Stage II)	Occurs weeks to months after the tick bite; 5–10% have cardiac manifestations (atrioventricular block of any degree, myocarditis/pericarditis, and heart failure) and 10–15% have neurologic manifestations (see below).
Late disease	
(Stage III)	Occurs months to years after the tick bite and includes myalgias, arthralgias, fatigue, polyarthritis, and neurologic symptoms (encephalopathy, cognitive dysfunction, and peripheral neuropathy).

 HELPFUL TIP: Lyme disease symptoms typically improve a few days after starting antibiotics.

* *

It seems that there is an epidemic of Lyme disease in your office. Your partner has a patient who relates a history and exam identical to your patient's, but also complains of palpitations. An ECG was obtained, which showed complete heart block with a ventricular rate of 70. The patient is being admitted to the hospital.

What is your advice on the most appropriate intervention?

A) Initiate antibiotic therapy.
B) Initiate antiarrhythmic therapy.
C) Consult a cardiologist for electrophysiologic studies.
D) Consult a cardiologist for temporary pacemaker placement.
E) A and D.

Discussion

The correct answer is E. This patient should have antibiotics started and he should be hospitalized for cardiac monitoring. Patients with Lyme carditis (not typical Lyme disease) most often present with atrioventricular conduction abnormalities, ranging from first-degree to complete heart block. Aside from typical features of early Lyme disease, many patients are asymptomatic. When a patient presents with a high-degree heart block, cardiac monitoring is warranted, and appropriate intravenous antibiotic therapy is the treatment of choice. After instituting antibiotics, the heart block resolves within days to weeks. In this patient with complete heart block, admission and possible temporary pacemaker are also indicated.

* *

Since he spends much of his free time hunting deer in Minnesota your patient's father is worried about contracting Lyme disease.

What do you recommend for primary prevention of Lyme disease?

A) Weekly tick checks.
B) *N,N*-diethyl-*m*-toluamide (DEET) application prior to hunting.

C) Daily doxycycline when in endemic areas.
D) Lyme vaccine.
E) Kill as many deer as possible in order to reduce the risk of Lyme disease transmission to humans.

Discussion

The correct answer is B. Primary prevention is best accomplished with the use of insect repellents when in endemic areas. When in endemic areas, tick checks should be performed daily (not weekly as in answer A). A tick that has been attached for <24 hours is not likely to transmit *B. burgdorferi*. Unfortunately, *Ixodes ricinus*, the tick that transmits Lyme disease is very small and difficult to see. Answer C is incorrect. There is no role for routine prophylactic antibiotics. However, if a tick bite from the appropriate species is noticed, a single dose of doxycycline 200 mg administered orally reduces the risk of erythema migrans. The dose should be administered within 72 hours of a known *Ixodes ricinus* bite. Answer D is not an option for this patient. In 2002, the vaccine was removed from the U.S. market because of low demand. When the vaccine was available, antibody titers tended to wane quickly and protection was not complete. After the administration of 3 vaccinations, the efficacy of the vaccine to prevent Lyme disease was 76% at best. Answer E is just plain wrong. The white-footed field mouse, not the white-tailed deer, is the major reservoir of *B. burgdorferi* bacteria.

CASE 7

Your young patient's mother presents with diffuse aching and stiffness worsened by cold weather and stress. She recalls being treated for Lyme disease 2 years ago. The physical examination is remarkable for tender points bilaterally at the occiput, trapezius, lateral epicondyle, gluteus, and knee. There is no redness, swelling, or synovial thickening at the knees and elbows.

You suspect that her symptoms are caused by which of the following?

A) Chronic Lyme disease.
B) Osteoarthritis.
C) Fibromyalgia.
D) RA.

Discussion

The correct answer is C. Fibromyalgia is a diagnosis of exclusion, but compared to the other choices, the history and exam findings are most consistent with this diagnosis. If the patient was successfully treated for Lyme disease, she is unlikely to present with late-stage disease. Fibromyalgia may occur coincidentally after treatment for Lyme disease, but it is not due to ongoing infection and does not respond to antibiotics. Many patients who think that they have chronic Lyme disease are suffering from depression, fibromyalgia, etc.

 HELPFUL TIP: If Lyme meningitis is suspected, confirm by analysis of cerebrospinal fluid. Lyme meningitis must be treated with intravenous ceftriaxone or penicillin G.

Objectives: Did you learn to . . .

- Describe the appropriate evaluation of polyarthritis?
- Diagnose Lyme disease?
- Describe the stages of Lyme disease?
- Implement appropriate therapy for Lyme disease?
- Discuss preventive strategies for Lyme disease and describe some of the complications of the disease?

CASE 8

A 42-year-old female who was referred by an orthopedic surgeon presents to your office with multiple joint complaints. The orthopedist has seen her for left knee pain, intermittent swelling, occasional "clicking and locking," present for about 10 years. After knee radiograph and exam, the orthopedist diagnosed a chronically damaged meniscus, but he wants the patient evaluated by you for her other joint complaints.

Laboratory data included with her records show an ANA 1:40 (speckled pattern) and an ESR 20 mm/hour. The patient moved to the United States from Guam 4 years ago. She reports poor sleep and feeling quite depressed. She feels that she has no friends, and she has had trouble adjusting to the colder weather. You notice she has a bottle of water with her and upon your specific questioning she states, "I have to sip some water throughout the day. I've done this for the last 15 years because my mouth gets so dry." She denies problems with skin rash, cavities, swallowing, and eye pain. She does not use artificial tears.

Which of the following findings in this patient is the most likely to be a sign of inflammatory arthritis?

A) Spider angiomas (telangiectasia) on the back and abdomen.

B) A positive "bulge sign" on left knee exam.

C) Presence of 16/18 fibromyalgia tender points, with nontender control points.

D) Incomplete, weak left grip.

E) Presence of a holosystolic murmur at the left sternal border, without radiation.

Discussion

The correct answer is D. Although her symptoms are suggestive of fibromyalgia and depression, it is critical to differentiate between an inflammatory and a noninflammatory condition, especially since other inflammatory disorders (eg, SLE, RA, Sjögren syndrome) masquerade as fibromyalgia. An incomplete, weak grip in an otherwise healthy young woman is suggestive of synovitis, which can be further assessed by careful small joint exam. When synovitis is present, it is always abnormal and suggests an inflammatory arthritis, requiring further evaluation.

Answer A is incorrect because telangiectasias on the abdomen and trunk are typically related to liver disease, while those found on hands and nail beds are associated with scleroderma and other rheumatic diseases. Answer B is incorrect. A positive knee "bulge sign" (swelling of the knee joint that bulges inferiorly when compressed superiorly), indicates fluid in the left knee joint. But from the patient's history and your orthopedic colleague's determination, this finding is chronic and mechanical in nature. Answer C is incorrect. The presence of 16/18 tender points would argue for fibromyalgia but would not help to differentiate between inflammatory and noninflammatory disorders. Answer E is incorrect. A holosystolic murmur, localized to the left sternal border and present in a healthy young woman, is nonspecific and most likely functional. If there were other signs and symptoms of cardiac disease, the murmur might indicate a more serious disorder.

* *

On physical examination, you find a "bulge sign" on the left knee, but no other joint swelling. She has 16/18 tender points and normal range of motion and strength. The neurologic exam is grossly normal, except for poorly defined numbness and pain to touch on the left side of her face. You also notice a mildly tender, hard, nodular swelling behind the angle of the mandible on the left in the area of the parotid gland. Her oral mucosa appears dry. Her conjuctiva are mildly, symmetrically injected.

All of the following studies and interventions are appropriate EXCEPT:

A) CBC, transaminases, uric acid, ESR, C-reactive protein (CRP).

B) Anti-SS-A (Ro), anti-SS-B (La), anti-double-stranded DNA, rheumatoid factor, serum protein electrophoresis.

C) Prescribe trazodone 50 mg PO QHS and recommend aerobic exercises.

D) Prescribe prednisone 20 mg PO QD, with calcium and vitamin D supplements.

E) Maxillofacial MRI.

Discussion

The correct answer (and the thing to avoid right now) is D. Although prednisone may be used to treat symptoms of autoimmune diseases, the diagnosis is not secure now, and initiating steroid therapy exposes the patient to potentially unnecessary risk. She has findings of Sjögren syndrome—red (possibly dry) eyes, dry mouth, and enlarged parotid glands. However, the differential of mass in the parotid gland must include malignancy (eg, lymphoma), sarcoidosis, and other autoimmune diseases.

Answers A and B are appropriate laboratory tests that may help assess other organ involvement of Sjögren syndrome and aid in confirming the diagnosis. Other potential manifestations of Sjögren syndrome include generalized vasculitis, interstitial lung disease, cirrhosis, peripheral and cranial neuropathies, possibly thyroid disease, and renal disease leading to proteinuria and renal tubule dysfunction. Although not listed as an option, chest radiograph may also be helpful, assessing for findings associated with the diseases on your differential: Sjögren (interstitial lung disease), sarcoidosis (adenopathy and interstitial disease), and lymphoma (adenopathy). Answer E is important because although parotid enlargement may be seen in Sjögren, it is usually symmetrical and nontender. An imaging study is appropriate to evaluate for neurovascular compromise and to rule out a neoplastic process. Answer C is important because her symptoms of fibromyalgia may respond to trazodone and exercise, and these low-risk interventions are appropriate at this juncture.

* *

She starts trazodone and exercise and feels better. The tests you order return as follows: negative SSA, SSB, and Ds-DNA; elevated rheumatoid factor (RF); no monoclonal protein on SPEP but diffusely elevated globulins. A chest x-ray is normal. Her ESR is 35 mm/hour and CRP 0.5. A maxillofacial MRI shows an enlarged left parotid, with an ill-defined $2 \times 3 \times 1.5$-cm dense signal in the center, and there was no neurovascular compromise.

What is the most appropriate NEXT STEP in the management of this patient?

A) Continue your current management and adopt a watchful waiting approach.
B) Refer for biopsy of the left parotid.
C) Initiate prednisone 20 mg PO QD, with calcium and vitamin D.
D) Refer for lip biopsy.
E) Perform a gallium scan.

Discussion

The correct answer is B. Even though her presentation is suggestive of Sjögren syndrome, the presence of a mass-like formation on MRI is concerning for lymphoma, and further evaluation (eg, biopsy) is required. Additionally, the negative SSA and SSB, while not excluding Sjögren, will make a biopsy necessary for diagnosis. Although a lip biopsy (answer D) may be diagnostic of Sjögren, the parotid biopsy should be done first due to the presence of a mass. The elevated RF and polyclonal gammopathy are consistent with Sjögren, and the ESR may be elevated due to increased globulins. Gallium scan (answer E), used in the past for diagnosis of lymphoma, has poor sensitivity and specificity.

* *

Results of the parotid gland biopsy report read as follows: "Lymphocytic infiltrate, no malignant cells noted." You then order flow cytometry, and it has no markers for lymphoma. Her biopsy scar has healed nicely, and she has no pain or numbness. You believe that she probably has Sjögren syndrome.

What would you do next?

A) CT chest/abdomen/pelvis.
B) Start prednisone 20 mg PO QD, with calcium and vitamin D.
C) Recommend sugarless lemon drops and artificial tears as needed and continued trazodone and exercise.
D) Refer for lip biopsy.

Discussion

The correct answer is C. Lemon drops stimulate saliva production that will help her dry mouth. Artificial tears may also be indicated for dry eyes. Your working diagnosis now is Sjögren, and definitive diagnosis by lip biopsy is not likely to alter your therapy. Since she has responded to trazodone and exercise and there is no evidence of systemic involvement, no further antiinflammatory therapy (answer B) is warranted. If she were to develop arthritis or other signs of systemic involvement (eg, cognitive dysfunction or peripheral neuropathy), prednisone would be an option. Further workup for lymphoma, such as CT scanning (answer A), is not warranted. However, she will require active surveillance, because patients with Sjögren carry an increased risk of developing lymphoma.

> **HELPFUL TIP:** Sicca symptoms (dry eyes and mouth) are extremely common, especially in the elderly, and should be confirmed by objective physical findings. Definitive diagnosis of Sjögren syndrome relies on the presence of anti-SS-A or anti-SS-B antibodies or histopathologic gland findings on minor salivary gland (lip) biopsy.

CASE 9

Once again, your diagnostic and therapeutic abilities have earned you a well-deserved referral. Your patient is pleased with the way things are going with her Sjögren syndrome. She refers her 46-year-old sister-in-law to you. The sister-in-law reports having been diagnosed with fibromyalgia several months ago. She takes only acetaminophen and codeine as needed for pain.

Which of the following is the BEST option for treating fibromyalgia?

A) Tramadol (Ultram).
B) Hydromorphone (OxyContin).
C) Acetaminophen with codeine.
D) Nortriptyline (Pamelor).
E) Fluoxetine (Prozac) or another SSRI.

Discussion

The correct answer is D. Of those listed, the tricyclic antidepressant (TCA) nortriptyline is the best treatment option. Narcotics (answers A, B, and C) can be used but are third- or fourth-line after TCAs. However, patients may develop tolerance so that narcotics become less effective over time. Fluoxetine will benefit depression, which can be associated with fibromyalgia, but it is not the best choice for the treatment of fibromyalgia. NSAIDs, good sleep hygiene, and low-impact exercises are other appropriate therapies for fibromyalgia.

 HELPFUL TIP: Fibromyalgia is a common yet poorly understood syndrome characterized by diffuse chronic pain accompanied by other somatic symptoms, accompanied by poor sleep, fatigue, and stiffness, in the absence of identifiable disease. In order to diagnose fibromyalgia, 11 of 18 trigger points must be tender (Figure 11–2), symptoms must be present for at least 3 months, and other rheumatic conditions must be excluded. There is a female predominance in fibromyalgia; approximately 75% of patients are women.

All of the following are associated with fibromyalgia EXCEPT:

A) Irritable bowel syndrome and other GI findings.
B) Subjective fullness/swelling of hands and feet.
C) Paresthesias.
D) Fatigue.
E) Night sweats.

Discussion
The correct answer is E. Night sweats are not associated with fibromyalgia. All of the other answer choices are associated with fibromyalgia. Additional symptoms of fibromyalgia include headaches, depression, sleep disturbance (which may be the etiology), and urethral spasm with dysuria and urgency.

Objectives: Did you learn to . . .

• Describe the appropriate evaluation of polyarthralgia and sicca symptoms?

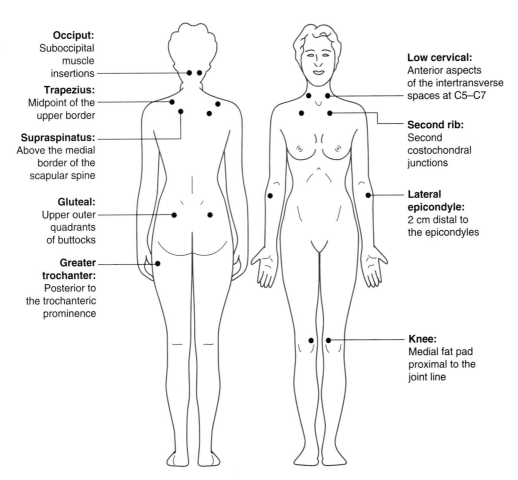

Figure 11–2   Tender points in fibromyalgia.

- Define diagnostic criteria for fibromyalgia and Sjögren syndrome?
- Implement appropriate therapy for fibromyalgia and Sjögren syndrome?

 QUICK QUIZ: OSTEOARTHRITIS

All of the following systemic diseases are secondary causes of osteoarthritis EXCEPT:

A) Diabetes.
B) Hemochromatosis.
C) Hyperparathyroidism.
D) Amyloidosis.

Discussion

The correct answer is A. One of the most common secondary causes of osteoarthritis is previous joint trauma. Systemic diseases that can lead to osteoarthritis include hemochromatosis, hyperparathyroidism, and amyloidosis. Diabetes is not a cause of osteoarthritis, although the two diseases often coexist: obese patients are prone to both diseases.

CASE 10

A 25-year-old Asian American female presents to your office with complaint of bifrontal headaches, occurring intermittently over the last year. Also, she complains of fatigue that seems to be slowly worsening. Over the last 2–3 months she has developed generalized joint pain and stiffness. The remainder of the history, including a detailed review of systems, is unremarkable.

On physical examination, you find a thin female in no acute distress. She is afebrile with a blood pressure of 110/62 mm Hg and a pulse of 72 bpm. The joint exam shows full range of motion and no swelling. There is mild anterior cervical lymphadenopathy. Close inspection of her skin reveals erythema of the malar eminences and the nose laterally, with involvement of the nasolabial folds. You note flaking and scaling in the eyebrows.

The RASH is most characteristic of which of the following diagnoses?

A) Dermatomyositis.
B) Systemic lupus erythematosus.
C) Seborrheic dermatitis.
D) Psoriasis.

Discussion

The correct answer is C. The classic rash of systemic lupus erythematosus is the malar, or "butterfly," rash with erythema over the malar eminences, bridging over the base of the nose. However, the nasolabial folds are spared. Involvement of the nasolabial fold characteristically occurs in seborrheic dermatitis. In dermatomyositis, facial lesions have a reddish-purple (heliotrope) hue. Flat-topped, violaceous papules over the knuckles (Gottron papules) are classic features of dermatomyositis. The typical lesions of psoriasis include erythematous papules and plaques with silvery scales.

Which of the following diagnoses or descriptions most accurately describes your patient's disease process now?

A) Fibromyalgia.
B) Somatoform disorder.
C) Polyarthritis.
D) Polyarthralgia.
E) RA.

Discussion

The correct answer is D. Your patient complains of pain in multiple joints but has no findings of inflammation of the joints; therefore, the designation of "polyarthralgia" fits best at this time. Inflammation of multiple joints is termed "polyarthritis." You do not have enough information now to make any of the other diagnoses.

* *

You screen for depression and anxiety and find neither. You recommend acetaminophen for joint pain and headaches and encourage her to exercise regularly. She returns 2 months later feeling worse. She has severe fatigue and joint pain, most commonly involving her hands and knees. She has taken a leave of absence from her job as a high school English teacher. New symptoms include sores in her mouth and chest pain, which is worse with inspiration. On exam you note the presence of a cardiac friction rub. There is diffuse tenderness to palpation of both knees and a small effusion apparent in the left knee. Her left hand demonstrates slow, incomplete grip. The facial rash is barely noticeable. There are 2 nontender ulcerations of the oral mucosa. The remainder of the examination is unchanged from her previous visit.

Her disease process and current findings are most suggestive of which of the following diagnoses?

A) Lymphoma.
B) Systemic lupus erythematosus.
C) Fibromyalgia.
D) Reactive arthritis.

Discussion

The correct answer is B. Although she does not meet all the criteria for a diagnosis of systemic lupus erythematosus (SLE), this presentation is more consistent with SLE than any of the other answer choices. Several findings point toward SLE: arthritis, cardiac friction rub (presumably due to pericarditis), and painless oral ulcers.

* *

You recognize that your patient may be at higher than normal risk for developing SLE.

All of the following groups have a higher incidence of SLE than the general population EXCEPT:

A) Family members of patients with SLE.
B) Females.
C) Asian Americans.
D) African Americans.
E) Whites.

Discussion

The correct answer is E. Compared to other groups, whites have a lower risk of SLE. The peak incidence of SLE occurs in the third to fifth decades of life. Women are 5–10 times more likely than men to be diagnosed with SLE. First-degree relatives of individuals with SLE are at higher risk as well. Twin studies have shown a 25%–50% concordance rate among monozygotic twins.

* *

You consider that this might represent drug-related lupus, but your patient denies using any medications except acetaminophen.

In drug-related lupus, you expect to see all of the following EXCEPT:

A) Negative ANA.
B) Rapid resolution of symptoms after discontinuing the drug.

C) Polyarthralgia.
D) Negative anti-dsDNA.

Discussion

The correct answer is A. Patients with drug-induced lupus will generally have a positive ANA. However, it can be differentiated from SLE by a negative anti-dsDNA. Drug-related lupus presents with a lupus-like syndrome. The most common features are arthralgias, myalgias, fatigue, malaise, and low-grade fever. Pericarditis and pleuritis are occasionally present. Skin, renal, and neurologic involvement are rare.

* *

Drugs that are associated with drug-induced lupus include all of the following EXCEPT:

A) Hydralazine.
B) Methyldopa.
C) Isoniazid.
D) Quinidine.
E) Trimethoprim-sulfamethoxazole.

Discussion

The correct answer is E. Trimethoprim-sulfamethoxazole is associated with Stevens-Johnson syndrome, not drug-induced lupus. Other drugs that are associated with drug-induced lupus include procainamide, penicillamine, chlorpromazine, and minocycline.

* *

Your patient returns with a painful, swollen left knee, and she wants to do something about it. You also discuss the following laboratory test results: WBC 5,100 cells/mm^3, Hb 11.0 g/dL, platelets 309,000 cells/mm^3; BUN 10 mg/dL, creatinine 1.0 mg/dL; ESR 77 mm/hour; ANA 1:1280 with a nucleolar pattern; urinalysis 1 + protein, otherwise negative; chest x-ray shows no cardiomegaly and normal lung fields; ECG shows normal sinus rhythm. You believe that your patient has SLE.

Which of the following management plans do you suggest to the patient?

A) Start ibuprofen 600 mg PO TID and refer to a rheumatologist (3–6-month wait).
B) Start prednisone 20 mg PO QD and hydroxychloroquine 400 mg PO QD, schedule for follow-up in 1 month, and refer to a rheumatologist (3–6-month wait).

C) Start methotrexate 10 mg PO weekly, prednisone 60 mg PO QD, and hydroxychloroquine 400 mg PO QD, and schedule follow-up in 1 month.

D) Start prednisone 60 mg PO QD and refer to a rheumatologist (3–6-month wait).

E) Start ibuprofen 600 mg PO QD and adopt a watchful waiting approach with follow-up in 6 months.

Discussion

The correct answer is B. Your patient now meets diagnostic criteria for SLE, according to the American College of Rheumatology. **Note that a positive ANA is only one of the criteria and is not required for the diagnosis of lupus.** Prompt treatment of her symptoms is important. NSAIDs, such as ibuprofen, are useful in treating arthralgias, mild arthritis, and mild pleurisy and pericarditis. In this case, oral (or perhaps intraarticular) steroids are indicated for immediate symptomatic relief of her arthritis, and a low to moderate oral dose should be used (20 mg rather than 60 mg). Vitamin D and calcium supplements should be prescribed with the steroids. Methotrexate can be used in recurrent, persistent arthritis. In the event of more serious renal, hematologic, or neurologic disease, high-dose steroids are employed. Hydroxychloroquine may provide relief of musculoskeletal and constitutional symptoms and may also have a steroid-sparing effect. Ideally, this patient should also be referred to a rheumatologist, but appropriate treatment should be started first. Close follow-up is necessary because of the potential adverse effects of these medications (eg, diabetes with prednisone). Table 11–7 lists the diagnostic criteria for SLE.

* *

Over the next year, your patient does very well. She establishes a relationship with a rheumatologist and is in remission when she sees you next. She is interested in becoming pregnant and wishes to seek your advice prior to trying to conceive. Fortunately, she has been able to discontinue prednisone and continues to tolerate hydroxychloroquine.

With regard to pregnancy and SLE, your patient is at higher risk for all of the following EXCEPT:

A) Premature birth.

B) Infertility.

C) Intrauterine fetal demise.

D) Spontaneous abortion.

Discussion

The correct answer is B. Women with SLE have a greater risk of premature birth, spontaneous abortion,

Table 11–7 DIAGNOSTIC CRITERIA FOR SYSTEMIC LUPUS ERYTHEMATOSUS

SLE requires the presence of 4 of the 11 findings below, not necessarily occurring at the same time.

1. Malar rash
2. Discoid rash
3. Photosensitivity
4. Oral ulcers (usually painless)
5. Arthritis (involving 2 or more peripheral joints)
6. Serositis (pericarditis or pleuritis)
7. Renal disorder (proteinuria >0.5 g per day or cellular casts)
8. Neurologic disorder (seizures or psychosis)
9. Hematologic disorder (hemolytic anemia, leukocyte count <4,000/mm^3, lymphocyte count <1,500/mm^3, or platelet count <100,000/mm^3)
10. Positive ANA
11. Immunologic disorder (anti-DNA, anti-Smith, or antiphospholipid antibodies, or a false-positive serologic test for syphilis)

Adapted from the American College of Rheumatology.

and intrauterine fetal demise compared with otherwise healthy women. However, these patients appear to have comparable rates of fertility. Pregnancy outcomes are best when the patient is in remission 6–12 months before conception. Pregnancy appears to have a variable affect on SLE, with some patients experiencing exacerbations of the disease.

* *

Now that she is considering pregnancy, her rheumatologist wishes to perform further serologic testing.

Which of the following antibodies will be most important in predicting problems with the fetus?

A) Anti-dsDNA.

B) ANCA.

C) Anti-Smith.

D) Anti-SSA (anti-Ro).

Discussion

The correct answer is D. The fetuses of women who have SLE with anti-SSA (anti-Ro) antibodies are at increased risk of spontaneous abortion, congenital heart block, and neonatal lupus. The fetus may become subject to passively acquired autoimmunity, as anti-SSA and anti-SSB (anti-La) antibodies appear to cross the placenta, damaging fetal tissue. Cardiac conduction abnormalities are the most serious problem, most often presenting in the second trimester. The most common conduction defect is complete heart block. Although cardiac conduction abnormalities do not reverse spontaneously, the noncardiac findings of neonatal lupus typically resolve by 6 months of age.

* *

Your patient does well with her pregnancy but develops recurrent DVTs in the subsequent few years. You wish to evaluate her for antiphospholipid antibody syndrome.

Which of the following results would you expect to find in a patient with antiphospholipid antibody syndrome?

A) Elevated PT/INR.
B) Low PT/INR.
C) Elevated aPTT.
D) Shortened bleeding time.
E) High-fibrin degradation products.

Discussion
The correct answer is C. Even though they are prone to clotting, patients with antiphospholipid antibody syndrome have a paradoxically elevated aPTT. If this abnormality does not correct in vitro with addition of normal serum, it is presumptive evidence of antiphospholipid antibody syndrome. In addition to venous thrombus formation, women with antiphospholipid antibody syndrome are likely to have late fetal demise and multiple spontaneous abortions.

 HELPFUL TIP: Antiphospholipid antibody syndrome is caused by 3 separate types of antibodies: anticardiolipin antibodies, lupus anticoagulant, and anti-β_2 glycoprotein I antibodies. These can be detected by direct assay, but there is only an 85% concordance between the presence of antiphospholipid antibody syndrome and laboratory detection of the causative antibodies.

 HELPFUL TIP: Only about 10% of patients with lupus have antiphospholipid antibodies.

Which of the following statements is (are) true?

A) Patients with anticardiolipin antibodies should be treated prophylactically even if they have never had a clot, in order to prevent the development of clots.
B) Percent factor II activity is an appropriate way to monitor the response to heparin in patients with antiphospholipid antibody syndrome.
C) Antifactor Xa should be used to monitor the activity of enoxaparin if monitoring is required.
D) A and C
E) B and C.

Discussion
The correct answer is E. Both B and C are true statements. Since patients with antiphospholipid antibody syndrome have an elevated aPTT, this value cannot be used to monitor anticoagulation with standard heparin. Percent factor II activity is the most appropriate way to monitor these patients if they are on standard heparin. Anti-factor Xa is used to monitor anticoagulation with enoxaparin. You will see anti-factor Xa used more; we now know that the "one dose fits all" administration of the low-molecular-weight heparins is not entirely true. Answer A is incorrect because there is no evidence that prophylactic treatment reduces complications. After a patient has had a thrombotic event, or has another indication, she needs anticoagulation.

 HELPFUL TIP: Unfractionated heparin, low-molecular-weight heparin, and aspirin are used in the treatment of antiphospholipid antibody syndrome in pregnancy. Warfarin is FDA Class X and is teratogenic. However, the use of warfarin during pregnancy from week 13 through the middle of the third trimester is safe and is gaining in popularity.

Which of the following drugs used to treat lupus is associated with macular damage, corneal opacities, and ciliary muscle dysfunction?

A) Azathioprine.
B) Prednisone.
C) Hydroxychloroquine.
D) Cyclophosphamide.
E) Methotrexate.

Table 11–8 TOXICITIES ASSOCIATED WITH MEDICATIONS USED TO TREAT SLE

- NSAIDs: gastrointestinal bleeding, renal dysfunction, hypertension
- Steroids: diabetes, hypertension, hyperlipidemia, osteoporosis, cataract formation, weight gain, infections
- Hydroxychloroquine: macular damage, ciliary muscle dysfunction, corneal opacities, myopathy
- Azathioprine: infections, myelosuppression, hepatotoxicity
- Cyclophosphamide: infections, myelosuppression, hemorrhagic cystitis
- Methotrexate: infections, myelosuppression, hepatic fibrosis

Discussion

The correct answer is C. Hydroxychloroquine is associated with macular damage, corneal opacities, and ciliary muscle dysfunction, and its use requires yearly eye exams. SLE drugs and side effects are listed in Table 11–8.

Objectives: Did you learn to . . .

- Identify clinical manifestations of systemic lupus erythematosus (SLE)?
- Define diagnostic criteria for SLE?
- Recognize the waxing and waning course of SLE?
- Implement appropriate treatment for the patient with SLE?
- Recognize adverse effects of medications used in the treatment of SLE?
- Describe some characteristics of antiphospholipid antibody syndrome?

CASE 11

A 22-year-old white female presents to your office with the chief complaint of "blue fingers." She reports a history of intermittent bluish discoloration of the fingertips on both hands when they are exposed to cold temperatures. Although she believes the symptoms are worse now, she cannot recall how long they have been present. She has never had ulcers on her fingers or toes.

With no further information, what is the most likely explanation for these digital color changes?

A) Atherosclerotic disease of the extremities.

B) Acrocyanosis.

C) Scleroderma.

D) Physiologic response to cold.

Discussion

The correct answer is D. All we know now is that this patient's fingers turn blue upon exposure to cold. This is a normal physiologic response—vasoconstriction in response to cold. Answer A is incorrect. Peripheral vascular disease is the result of atherosclerotic disease of the extremities and typically occurs in older individuals; manifestations include claudication and skin ulceration. Answer B is incorrect. Raynaud phenomenon must be distinguished from acrocyanosis, which is a rare vasospastic disorder of persistent coldness and bluish discoloration of the hands and feet (not just fingers and toes), which may follow a viral infection. Answer C is incorrect. Scleroderma by itself does not cause blue fingers.

 HELPFUL TIP: Over 80% of cases of Raynaud phenomenon that present to a primary care physician's office are due to an exaggerated physiologic response to cold or emotional distress. Although Raynaud phenomenon occurs in most patients with scleroderma (90%–95% of patients with scleroderma have Raynaud phenomenon), the converse is not true. Thus the presence of Raynaud phenomenon is not synonymous with the presence of scleroderma.

 HELPFUL TIP: Buerger disease (thromboangiitis obliterans) is strongly associated with tobacco abuse and presents with distal small vessel ischemia and symptoms that are similar to Raynaud phenomenon. It eventually progresses to infarction of tissue, frequently requiring digit amputation.

* *

Further history reveals that the patient uses no medications. She has been healthy all of her life. Her mother and aunt have had blue fingers in cold temperature, too. She denies tobacco use. The review of systems is unremarkable.

All of the following are expected findings in patients with primary Raynaud phenomenon EXCEPT:

A) Symmetric involvement of the hands.
B) Well-demarcated cyanosis.
C) Digital ulcerations.
D) Normal ESR.

C) Blood viscosity testing.
D) ANA.
E) A trial of drug therapy.

Discussion

The correct answer is C. Primary Raynaud phenomenon is diagnosed when other causes of Raynaud have been eliminated. Primary Raynaud phenomenon is not typically destructive, and digital ulcerations generally occur when the phenomenon is secondary to some other disease process (eg, scleroderma, SLE). Primary Raynaud is almost always symmetric. Raynaud phenomenon can be differentiated from a normal response to cold temperatures by the demarcation between pale or cyanotic fingertips and normal-appearing skin. A normal response to cold may include mottling, with indistinct borders between pale and purple-colored skin, and paresthesias of the involved area. In Raynaud patients, the distal-most portion of the involved digit is pale or cyanotic, and the transition to normal skin color is abrupt. Since primary Raynaud is not caused by an inflammatory condition, markers of inflammation such as the ESR are usually normal.

> **HELPFUL TIP:** Nailfold capillary microscopy (NCM) can be used to examine the nailfold capillaries of patients with Raynaud phenomenon. NCM involves placing a drop of oil (a drop of surgical lubricant works well) on the cuticle of one or more digits and visualization of the nailfold capillaries through an ophthalmoscope set at 40 diopters (40 green). Usually the ring fingers (or symptomatic fingers) are examined. Normal capillaries are symmetric, nondilated loops. Distorted, dilated, or absent capillaries suggests secondary Raynaud.

* *

You perform a physical examination, including nailfold capillary microscopy, which is normal. There is currently no discoloration of the fingers.

What is the next most appropriate step in the evaluation and management of this patient?

A) Cold provocation.
B) Doppler ultrasound of the extremities.

Discussion

The correct answer is E. Since she is symptomatic, a trial of drug therapy is warranted. Cold provocation (answer A) is not recommended, as the diagnosis is based on a convincing history of episodic cyanosis. The results of cold provocation are inconsistent. Doppler ultrasound (answer B) might be useful if you were considering large vessel disease from atherosclerosis, etc. However, it is not likely to be helpful in this patient. Blood viscosity testing (answer C) is not something that is done routinely. An ANA (answer D) will be low yield in this case. Based on her age, symmetric involvement, lack of ulcerations, and absence of other symptoms, this patient most likely has primary Raynaud phenomenon unrelated to an underlying disease. A secondary cause (eg, scleroderma) is more likely with any of the following: patients ≥30 years; attacks are asymmetric or associated with skin ulcers; there are symptoms suggestive of systemic involvement (eg, arthralgias, dyspnea, reflux, weight loss). If you are concerned about a secondary Raynaud, an ANA would then be indicated.

> **HELPFUL TIP:** Most patients with secondary Raynaud will develop symptoms of their underlying autoimmune disease within a few years of onset of Raynaud.

* *

After reviewing the diagnosis with your patient, you make several recommendations to help reduce the frequency of attacks: avoid cold temperatures, reduce emotional stress, and avoid tobacco and medications that cause vasoconstriction (eg, sympathomimetic drugs).

Your patient returns 10 months later with new complaints. Both hands are swollen, stiff, and painful. She complains of multiple joint aches and fatigue despite sleeping well. Her appetite is normal, and she has no GI complaints. Although she has no rash, she complains of itchy hands (surely a sign of cancer, she thinks). On exam, you note that there is diffuse, nonpitting edema of her fingers and hands. She has difficulty making a fist. She has no skin findings. Her CBC is normal. Her ANA is strongly positive with a nucleolar pattern.

Which of the following is the most likely explanation of these findings?

A) Raynaud phenomenon
B) RA.
C) Scleroderma.
D) CREST syndrome.

Discussion

The correct answer is C. This patient is now presenting with symptoms of scleroderma (aka systemic sclerosis). Scleroderma encompasses a heterogeneous group of conditions, which are variable in severity but share a common pathophysiologic mechanism—fibrosis of the skin and other organs. The pathology of scleroderma also involves small vessel vasculopathy, a process that leads to Raynaud phenomenon and ischemia of other tissues. Scleroderma may affect the joints, skin, lungs, kidneys, heart, and gastrointestinal system. Fifty percent of patients with scleroderma have depression.

A positive ANA can be helpful when you suspect scleroderma based on clinical findings. ANA by indirect immunofluorescence will report nuclear staining pattern. Centromere or nucleolar patterns are most highly associated with systemic sclerosis, but other patterns (such as speckled) are also seen. Patients with systemic sclerosis may have a negative ANA.

These findings are more than you would see with Raynaud; thus, answer A is incorrect. Diffuse swelling and stiffness is present rather than specific synovitis, so rheumatoid arthritis (answer B) is incorrect. CREST syndrome (answer D) is a type of systemic sclerosis: **C**alcinosis cutis, **R**aynaud phenomenon, **E**sophageal dysmotility, **S**clerodactyly, **T**elangiectasia. Your patient does not have all of the findings of CREST syndrome.

 HELPFUL TIP: Further diagnosis and categorization of scleroderma can be accomplished with the aid of more specific serologic tests, which are less readily available (eg, anticentromere—if ANA done by ELISA—or Scl-70 antibodies). Treatment is mainly symptomatic, though immunosuppressive therapies are showing promise in the long-term management of organ-threatening disease, such as interstitial lung disease.

* *

Because of the digital ulcers you observed and the increased pain of her Raynaud attacks, you decide to prescribe medication for Raynaud phenomenon.

Which of the following is the BEST therapy for reducing the frequency of attacks of Raynaud?

A) Amlodipine 5 mg daily.
B) Nifedipine 10 mg as needed.
C) Nitroglycerin 2% ointment daily.
D) Diltiazem 30 mg as needed.
E) Prazosin 1 mg twice daily.

Discussion

The correct answer is A. All of the medications listed are helpful treatments when Raynaud phenomenon does not respond to conservative measures. The most appropriate choice is daily amlodipine. Dihydropyridine calcium channel blockers, like amlodipine, have been shown to reduce the frequency of attacks by approximately 50% compared with placebo. They must be scheduled, rather than used as needed (thus answer B is incorrect). Diltiazem is not as effective as the dihydropyridine calcium channel blockers. In systemic sclerosis, the benefit of calcium channel blockers is often offset by their exacerbation of GERD. In these patients, ACE inhibitors or angiotensin receptor blockers (ARBs) show benefit for Raynaud, do not exacerbate GERD, and may protect against scleroderma renal crisis. Topical vasodilators like nitroglycerin have a role if calcium channel blockers are not effective or the patient cannot tolerate them. There is less evidence that prazosin is effective, but alpha-antagonists have a role if other therapies are unsuccessful. Sildenafil (a phosphodiesterase inhibitor) appears to promote healing of digital ulcers.

Which of the following is NOT indicated for acute ischemic crisis related to Raynaud phenomenon?

A) Aspirin.
B) β-Blocker.
C) Nifedipine.
D) Digital or wrist nerve block.
E) Topical nitroglycerin.

Discussion

The correct answer is B. β-Blockers are not indicated in the treatment of an ischemic crisis related to Raynaud phenomenon. β-Blockers cause peripheral vasoconstriction and may worsen the problem. Peripherally, beta **agonists** cause vasodilatation. Thus, when a β-blocker is used, the patient ends up with an unopposed alpha-adrenergic response, which worsens vasoconstriction. All of the other therapies are useful in acute ischemic crisis. Of particular note is answer D. A nerve or wrist block with lidocaine effectively causes a sympathectomy, leading to decreased vascular tone. Sildenafil appears to be beneficial in healing ischemic ulcers and for acute ischemic crisis.

 HELPFUL TIP: Raynaud phenomenon may be secondary to connective tissue disease, cancer, some chemotherapeutic agents, exposure to toxins (eg, polyvinyl chloride), trauma, or entrapment syndromes such as thoracic outlet and carpal tunnel syndromes. History and physical examination must focus on evaluation of these potential causes.

Objectives: Did you learn to . . .

- Identify complications of Raynaud phenomenon and diseases associated with it?
- Develop a strategy for the prevention and treatment of symptoms of Raynaud phenomenon?
- Recognize clinical features of scleroderma?

CASE 12

A 17-year-old male presents to your office with a history of low back pain worsening over the past few months. He recalls having intermittent back pain for at least 1 year. The pain does not radiate. He runs cross-country and track without exacerbating his back pain. He denies fevers, weight loss, weakness, incontinence, and history of trauma. He is unaware of any family history of back pain. He is otherwise healthy.

What further information will help you differentiate between potential causes of his back pain?

A) Relief with acetaminophen.
B) Morning stiffness.
C) Relief with rest.
D) A and C.
E) B and C.

Discussion

The correct answer is E. Determining the pattern of the pain is critical. Inflammatory causes of back pain are characterized by morning stiffness and improvement with activity. In contrast, degenerative back disease causes pain that is exacerbated by activity and relieved with rest. Inflammatory back pain typically presents in younger patients; degenerative back pain typically presents between 30 and 40 years. Acetaminophen and other analgesics may relieve pain from either category of disease and so will not help you narrow the diagnosis.

 HELPFUL TIP: In a young patient with back pain, consider fractures (eg, spondylolysis, a bilateral pars defect), infection, disc disease, and osseous malignancies.

* *

On further questioning, your patient reports morning stiffness and pain that improves with stretching. Activity does not seem to aggravate his back but inactivity does. He has had no penile discharge, rash, or conjunctivitis and denies diarrhea or other GI symptoms. On physical examination, your patient is surprised to find it impossible for him to touch his toes, which he had been able to do a few months ago in track practice. Range of motion in the neck, arms, and legs is normal. A focused neurologic exam is normal. There is mild, diffuse tenderness over the lumbosacral spine and with percussion over the sacroiliac joints.

The history and physical exam are most consistent with a diagnosis of:

A) Reactive arthritis (formerly Reiter syndrome).
B) Osteoarthritis of the lumbar spine.
C) Degenerative disc disease.
D) Ankylosing spondylitis.
E) Vertebral body tumor.

Discussion

The correct answer is D. The history and exam are most consistent with ankylosing spondylitis, a seronegative (RF negative) spondyloarthropathy. Ankylosing spondylitis is the most common form of spondyloarthropathy and is thought to have a prevalence of 1% in white populations. There is a 5:1 male-to-female ratio. In addition to historical features mentioned in the previous question discussion, there is often a family history of ankylosing spondylitis in patients ultimately diagnosed with the disease.

Answer A is incorrect. Reactive arthritis occurs in reaction to an infection (*Chlamydia* urethritis, GI infection, etc.) and presents with mono- or oligo-arthritis, usually of the joints in the leg. This patient's age makes osteoarthritis and degenerative disc disease less likely, so answers B and C are incorrect. Also, he has no neurologic findings that you might expect with disc degeneration. Malignancy is associated with constitutional symptoms (fever and weight loss), neurologic involvement, and steadily worsening pain that is not relieved by activity—none of which are present in this case. Physical examination findings of spondyloarthropathies are listed in Table 11–9.

Which of the following is the BEST test to confirm the diagnosis of ankylosing spondylitis?

A) ANA.
B) Lumbar spine radiographs.
C) HLA-B27.
D) ESR.
E) Sacroiliac joint radiographs.

Discussion

The correct answer is E. The hallmark of ankylosing spondylitis is sacroiliitis on pelvic radiographs. Although there are no universally accepted criteria for diagnosing spondyloarthropathies, x-ray evidence of sacroiliitis in the setting of a consistent clinical picture is sufficient to diagnose ankylosing spondylitis. Unfortunately, in early ankylosing spondylitis, x-rays are often inconclusive. MRI is more sensitive for detecting early sacroiliitis, but the cost may be prohibitive. The other answer choices are incorrect. Ankylosing spondylitis is not associated with a positive ANA. Lumbar spine x-rays may be useful in ruling out other conditions and do show some changes in ankylosing spondylitis but may miss early disease. HLA-B27, a class I human leukocyte antigen gene, is present in about 90% of white patients and 50%–80% of nonwhite patients with ankylosing spondylitis and is

Table 11–9 PHYSICAL FINDINGS IN THE SPONDYLOARTHROPATHIES

- Limited range of motion in the spine
- Tenderness at the sacroiliac joints
- Tenderness at tendon insertions, particularly the Achilles tendon and plantar fascia synovitis
- Anterior eye symptoms (anterior uveitis in 30–40%)

generally associated with spondyloarthropathies. However, HLA-B27 is not specific. It is present in many normal individuals as well and is of very little diagnostic value. ESR is slightly elevated in most cases of spondyloarthropathy, but again it is not specific.

* *

Lumbar spine x-rays show squaring of the vertebral bodies. Pelvic x-rays identify mild symmetric sacroiliitis. You are now confident of the diagnosis of ankylosing spondylitis.

Which of the following management plans is best for this patient?

A) Aspirin, 650 mg PO QID (or ZORprin or other extended-release aspirin BID) and physical therapy referral.
B) Naproxen 500 mg BID and physical therapy referral.
C) Orthopedic referral for early surgical consideration.
D) Prednisone 40 mg QD and fitting for a back brace.
E) Naproxen 500 mg BID and fitting for a back brace.

Discussion

The correct answer is B. NSAIDs are the mainstay of medical therapy for active phases of spondyloarthropathy. Patients generally experience significant relief from NSAIDs, and any additional benefit from systemic steroids is questionable. Sulfasalazine is a second-line drug. Aspirin tends to be less effective in these patients. Thus, answer A is incorrect. The management of ankylosing spondylitis should also include an exercise regimen designed specifically for the patient, and physical therapy may play a key role. The use of braces is not helpful and may exacerbate the patient's symptoms. Orthopedic surgery becomes necessary only in cases of advanced ankylosing spondylitis when kyphosis or peripheral joint symptoms becomes severe.

* *

After 3 months of physical therapy and NSAIDs, your patient returns. He has noticed minimal benefit, and now you find limitation of his neck range of motion.

What is the most appropriate next step in the evaluation and management of this patient?

A) Discontinue naproxen and switch to indomethacin 50 mg TID.
B) Begin methotrexate 15 mg per week and folic acid 1 mg QD.
C) Begin prednisone 60 mg QD.
D) MRI of the cervical spine.
E) Continue naproxen and refer to rheumatology.

Discussion

The correct answer is E. The patient is losing range of motion despite NSAID therapy. Referral to a rheumatologist to consider anti-TNF therapy (eg, infliximab [Remicade]) is the best next step. Anti-TNF agents can halt disease progression and often improve range of motion in early disease. Answer A is incorrect. Switching NSAIDs may provide some minor additional benefit but is unlikely to arrest disease progression. Answer B is incorrect. Methotrexate may be beneficial for the peripheral arthritis of spondyloarthropathies, but not for the axial skeleton disease. Answer C is incorrect since systemic steroids have no value in treating spondyloarthropathies. Local corticosteroid injections are often beneficial for enthesopathy and peripheral arthritis. Answer D is incorrect. MRI of the cervical spine will show inflammatory changes of the spine but will not change your management.

* *

The patient fails to keep his rheumatology appointment and returns to you 1 year later. He is taking over-the-counter naproxen. His neck is very stiff, with even less range of motion. He relates that he has been having crampy abdominal pain, and loose stools with bloody mucus. He is having dyspnea with mild exertion. On exam his neck range of motion is worse, back flexion is limited with straightening of his lumbar lordosis.

What is the next most appropriate step in the evaluation and management of this patient?

A) Discontinue naproxen.
B) Check CBC with differential and iron panel.
C) Consult gastroenterology for EGD and colonoscopy.
D) Consult rheumatology and tell patient he must keep his appointment.
E) All of the above.

Discussion

The correct answer is E. The patient now appears to have enteropathic arthritis in association with inflammatory bowel disease. NSAIDs can exacerbate inflammatory bowel disease, so discontinue the naproxen (answer A). A CBC and iron panel (answer B) will likely reveal iron deficiency anemia, which would explain the patient's dyspnea on exertion. Subspecialty evaluations by a gastroenterologist (answer C) and rheumatologist (answer D) are indicated both to confirm the diagnosis and to help with long-term disease management. Anti-TNF agents like infliximab and adalimumab—but not etanercept—are beneficial for both the spondyloarthropathy and inflammatory bowel disease in enteropathic arthritis.

 HELPFUL TIP: Patients with a spondyloarthropathy unresponsive to NSAID treatment benefit from anti-TNF-alpha drugs, such as infliximab, adalimumab or etanercept. Referral to a rheumatologist and early initiation of anti-TNF therapy can improve and maintain axial skeleton mobility.

 HELPFUL TIP: The most common spondyloarthropathies are ankylosing spondylitis, psoriatic arthritis, enteropathic arthritis, and reactive arthritis (including Reiter syndrome). These are pathogenically similar diseases that may be difficult to differentiate in early stages, but lack of differentiation does not affect therapy.

Enteropathic arthritis occurs frequently in patients with inflammatory bowel disease, and has features in common with ankylosing spondylitis, including inflammatory back pain and sacroiliitis.

Objectives: Did you learn to . . .

- Recognize clinical manifestations of spondyloarthropathies, particularly ankylosing spondylitis?
- Differentiate between types of spondyloarthropathies?
- Develop an appropriate evaluation for the patient presenting with inflammatory back pain?
- Appropriately manage a patient with ankylosing spondylitis?

 QUICK QUIZ: SPONDYLOARTHROPATHIES

Which of the following is NOT a characteristic of reactive arthritis?

A) Conjunctivitis.
B) Keratoderma blenorrhagicum.
C) HLA-B8.
D) Urethritis.
E) Arthritis.

Discussion

The correct answer is C. Reactive arthritis is associated with HLA-B27 and not HLA-B8 (which is found in sclerosing cholangitis). All of the other choices are seen with reactive arthritis, including keratoderma blenorrhagicum, which is a rash found especially on the soles of patients with reactive arthritis. The urethritis is generally due to *Chlamydia trachomatis*.

> **HELPFUL TIP:** The onset of reactive arthritis is less insidious than that of ankylosing spondylitis, with some patients presenting with an acute illness that includes fever, acute joint swelling, and rash (keratoderma blenorrhagicum). Generally, reactive arthritis resolves within 12 months. Antibiotics are not effective as treatment (although they may be indicated for the underlying infection).

CASE 13

A 52-year-old female presents to your office for an initial visit with complaint of mild pain and weakness in her hips and thighs. The symptoms have been present for months. About 2 years ago another doctor diagnosed her with psoriasis because of a rash on her hands and elbows, which has since resolved. Otherwise, she reports being relatively healthy and taking no medications. She is a smoker. She has had no recent health screening. On physical exam, her vitals are normal. She has considerable difficulty getting out of her chair. Her strength is symmetrically diminished in the quadriceps and hip flexors. The rest of the exam is unremarkable.

Which of the following diagnostic tests do you order first?

A) Muscle biopsy.
B) Electromyography (EMG).
C) TSH.
D) ANA.
E) Troponin-T.

Discussion

The correct answer is C. Hypothyroidism (along with many other diseases) can cause a proximal muscle weakness. A muscle biopsy or EMG study is premature before evaluation for myopathy with serum enzyme levels (CK, aldolase). Answer D, an ANA, is not likely to be helpful. Autoimmune diseases, such as polymyositis and dermatomyositis, cause myopathy, but ANA is not specific for these diseases. Although CK-MB may be elevated in patients with myopathy, troponin-T (answer E) is an enzyme relatively specific to cardiac muscle and should be normal.

* *

You order TSH and CBC, which are normal. ESR, CK, and AST are elevated. An EMG demonstrates abnormalities of the paraspinal muscles. Your patient returns to discuss her test results and complains that her psoriasis is back. There are violaceous plaques on her knuckles and elbows and around her eyes.

You recommend the following management plan for the disease:

A) Ultraviolet light therapy.
B) Topical steroids.
C) Oral steroids.
D) Topical emollients.

Discussion

The correct answer is C. This patient now has findings that support a diagnosis of dermatomyositis. To diagnose idiopathic inflammatory myopathy, such as dermatomyositis or polymyositis, certain criteria must be present. This patient has 3 of these criteria plus skin changes consistent with dermatomyositis. Violaceous plaques on the knuckles are commonly called Gottron's papules. Similar lesions are often observed over pressure points (eg, elbows). Because dermatomyositis is a systemic condition, treatment should likewise be systemic. Local topical therapies do not treat the disease, and oral steroids are typically the first-line agents. Hydroxychloroquine is helpful when the rash does not respond to corticosteroids. Addition of immunosuppressive drugs, such as methotrexate or azathioprine, may be indicated. Table 11–10 lists criteria for diagnosis of dermatomyositis and polymyositis.

Table 11–10 DIAGNOSTIC CRITERIA FOR POLYMYOSITIS AND DERMATOMYOSITIS

Three of four are required:
• Elevated muscle enzymes (CPK and aldolase)
• Symmetrical proximal muscle weakness
• Abnormal EMG
• Consistent findings on muscle biopsy

Skin findings must be present in order to diagnose dermatomyositis.

* *

You diagnose dermatomyositis.

Which of the following tests and exams should now be ordered?

A) Pap and pelvic exam, CA-125 and pelvic ultrasound.
B) Screening mammogram.
C) Chest radiograph.
D) Fecal occult blood screening.
E) All of the above.

Discussion

The correct answer is E. Adult-onset dermatomyositis has a strong association with malignancy; the risk is up to 6 times greater than in the general population. Upon diagnosing dermatomyositis, a thorough history and physical exam must be performed. All patients should undergo age-appropriate cancer screening tests (eg, Pap smear, fecal occult blood testing, mammography, etc). Other tests recommended include CBC, metabolic profile, liver function tests, urinalysis, and chest x-ray—especially important in smokers. Since the patient is >50 years, colonoscopy is indicated.

 HELPFUL TIP: The association of dermatitis with GI malignancy, especially colon cancer, is particularly strong. You may consider an alpha-fetoprotein, given this association. Some suggest CA-125 in all women with dermatomyositis, as well as a pelvic ultrasound to rule out ovarian cancer.

 HELPFUL TIP: Other causes of proximal muscle weakness include alcohol use, muscular dystrophy, medications (eg, penicillamine, HMG-CoA reductase inhibitors), Cushing syndrome, viral infections, and diabetes mellitus. The list goes on, including myasthenia gravis, Eaton-Lambert syndrome, etc.

Objectives: Did you learn to . . .

- Recognize symptoms and signs of dermatomyositis and polymyositis?
- Describe how inflammatory myopathies are evaluated and diagnosed?

- Appreciate the relationship between malignancy and inflammatory myopathy?

 QUICK QUIZ: OSTEOARTHRITIS

Compared with rheumatoid arthritis, osteoarthritis has a **greater** predilection for which of the following joints?

A) MCPs.
B) DIPs.
C) Knees.
D) Wrists.

Discussion

The correct answer is B. Osteoarthritis tends to affect the DIP and PIP joints in the hand, sparing the MCPs; whereas rheumatoid arthritis affects the MCPs and spares the DIPs. Both disease processes may involve the knees and wrists.

BIBLIOGRAPHY

Abeles AM, et al. Narrative review: the pathophysiology of fibromyalgia. *Ann Intern Med*. 2007 May 15;146(10): 726.

Garcia-De La Torre I. Advances in management of septic arthritis. *Rheum Dis Clin North Am*. 2003;29(1):61.

Harris ED, et al, eds. *Kelley's Textbook of Rheumatology*. 7th ed. Philadelphia: Elsevier Saunders, 2005.

Hayes EB, Piesman J. How can we prevent Lyme disease? *N Engl J Med*. 2003;348(24):2424.

Hinton R. Osteoarthritis: diagnosis and therapeutic considerations. *Am Fam Physician*. 2002;65(5):841.

Khan MA. Update on spondyloarthropathies. *Ann Intern Med*. 2002;136:896.

Klippel JH, Crofford LJ, Stone JH, et al, eds. *Primer on the Rheumatic Diseases*. 12th ed. Atlanta: Arthritis Foundation, 2001.

Margaretten ME, Kohlwes J, Moore D, Bent S. Does this adult patient have septic arthritis? *JAMA*. 2007; 297:1478.

Parikh M, et al. Prevalence of a normal C-reactive protein with an elevated erythrocyte sedimentation rate in biopsy-proven giant cell arteritis. *Ophthalmology*. 2006 Oct;113(10):1842.

Salvarani C, Cantini F, Boiardi L, et al. Polymyalgia rheumatica and giant-cell arteritis. *N Engl J Med*. 2002; 347(4):261.

Steere AC. Lyme disease. *N Engl J Med*. 2001;345(2):115.

Subcommittee on Rheumatoid Arthritis Guidelines, American College of Rheumatology. Guidelines for the management of rheumatoid arthritis. *Arth Rheum*. 2002; 46(2):328.

Wigley FM. Raynaud's phenomenon. *N Engl J Med*. 2002; 347(13):1001.

12

Orthopedics and Sports Medicine

Scott A. Frisbie and Mark A. Graber

CASE 1

A 5-year-old boy presents with acute onset of left anterior thigh and hip pain that began 2 days ago with no known prior trauma. He reports that it initially "loosened-up" after he had been out of bed for a few hours but has become worse again by afternoon. His pain is exacerbated by weight bearing and active or passive range of motion. His mother notes that he had a cold 7–10 days ago, but has been asymptomatic until he complained of pain 2 nights ago. She also notes that he has had a low-grade fever. He has no other significant constitutional symptoms and appears to be in some pain, but otherwise he appears well.

Based on the information obtained thus far, which of the following is the most likely diagnosis?

A) Osteomyelitis.
B) Rheumatic fever.
C) Slipped capital femoral epiphysis (SCFE).
D) Legg-Calve-Perthes disease (LCPD).
E) Transient (toxic) synovitis.

Discussion

The correct answer is E, transient (toxic) synovitis (aka transient tenosynovitis). This presentation is classic for transient synovitis, a condition most commonly presenting in the 2- to 6-year age range and more commonly seen in boys (male to female ratio of 2–3 to 1). It often is preceded by a viral respiratory infection although numerous studies have failed to demonstrate a specific viral or bacterial agent. Physical exam reveals

a limp or refusal to walk and complaint of pain over the groin and/or proximal thigh. There is pain with ROM testing, especially during abduction. Most children will be afebrile with a temperature of ≤38°C.

Appropriate diagnostic workup might include which of the following?

A) Joint aspiration.
B) Plain film radiographs.
C) ESR.
D) CBC with differential.
E) All of the above.

Discussion

The correct answer is E. All of the above may be appropriate as transient synovitis is a diagnosis of exclusion. Patients with mild symptoms may be observed without further investigation. However, if the pain is significant, if ROM is significantly impaired, or if the temperature is >37.5°C, further diagnostic workup is indicated. Laboratory findings consistent with transient synovitis include: clear joint fluid aspirate, normal CBC, and a mildly increased ESR. Blood cultures, ASO titer, bone scan, and MRI may be of benefit to rule out other possibilities (eg, septic arthritis, rheumatic fever, SCFE, etc). **It is of extreme importance to differentiate transient synovitis from septic arthritis. There is no combination of physical findings and laboratory tests short of joint fluid that will confirm that this is transient tenosynovitis.** It requires clinical judgment; decide which patients you are worried enough about that you want to commit them to hip joint aspiration.

HELPFUL TIP: Septic arthritis is an orthopedic emergency and commonly presents with a more elevated temperature, general malaise, pronounced pain—often with spasm and guarding. Generally, you will also have an elevated WBC and ESR **although neither these nor fever are good enough indicators to rule out a septic joint by their normality or absence.** Joint fluid will have numerous WBCs. Blood cultures are positive in 30–40% of patients.

What is the most appropriate treatment for this patient with transient synovitis?

A) Open fixation.
B) Immobilization.
C) Antibiotics.
D) Surgical decompression.
E) None of the above.

Discussion

The correct answer is E. Conservative treatment is warranted: the appropriate initial treatment is rest and observation. Transient synovitis generally responds well to oral NSAIDs (eg, ibuprofen). Home care is acceptable; however, admission is indicated if the diagnosis is equivocal or if significant pain management is required. For septic arthritis, prompt administration of an intravenous antibiotic—directed at the most likely infecting pathogen and altered as necessary based on culture results—is indicated. Surgical irrigation of the joint is often necessary and early orthopedic consultation is needed.

Objectives: Did you learn to . . .

- Recognize the clinical presentation of transient synovitis?
- Differentiate transient synovitis from septic arthritis?
- Treat a patient with transient synovitis?

CASE 2

A 6-year-old white male is brought in by his parents because he has complaint of pain in his hip and anterior thigh. He is walking much less than usual since the pain began about 4 weeks ago. You order a plain radiograph, which shows mild sclerosis with some increased density of the femoral head. An MRI is ordered, which the radiologist interprets as "demonstrating osteonecrosis of the femoral head."

What is the most likely diagnosis in this patient?

A) Osteomyelitis.
B) Septic arthritis.
C) SCFE (Slipped Capital femoral epiphisis).
D) LCPD (Legg-Calve-Perthes disease).
E) Sickle cell anemia.

Discussion

The correct answer is D. LCPD is idiopathic osteonecrosis of the femoral head. It is unilateral in 90% of patients, and the typical age range is 4–8 years, but 2- to 12-year-olds may present with the disease. Answer A is an incorrect because there should be evidence of osteomyelitis on MRI. Answer B is discussed in the previous case. Answer C, SCFE, generally occurs in obese children (usually male) who are in early adolescence. Answer E, sickle-cell anemia, can cause osteonecrosis of the femoral head, but the disease is rare in whites. LCPD is less common in blacks.

Which of the following factors MOST affects the outcome in patients with LCPD?

A) Age at onset of illness.
B) Findings of subchondral fractures or fragmentation.
C) Early appropriate treatment.
D) Severity of pain and ability to bear weight.
E) Bilateral involvement.

Discussion

The correct answer is A. In comparison with older children, younger children have a longer time for remodeling to occur via molding of the femoral head within the acetabulum; and therefore, younger children have less flattening of the femoral head.

Which of the following is the best initial treatment for this patient?

A) Joint replacement.
B) Osteotomy.
C) Rest and traction.
D) None of the above.

Discussion

The correct answer is C. The initial treatment for a patient with LCPD includes rest, traction, and the use of an abduction brace. The objectives are to increase ROM in the hip and to reduce the risk of significant deformity. In general, patients should be seen by a specialist. Answer A is incorrect because joint replacement is not an option. Answer B is incorrect. Although osteotomy may be used, it is reserved for older children and patients who are not progressing well with conservative therapy. LCPD is difficult to treat because of the long duration of treatment and activity restrictions required. Periods of rest with traction, casting or bracing, and surgical intervention may be indicated over 1–2 years of treatment and observation. Even with the best of care, prognosis is fair with need for total hip replacement for approximately 50% of patients by middle age due to severe degenerative arthritis.

Objectives: Did you learn to . . .

- Recognize the clinical presentation of LCPD?
- Manage a patient with LCPD?
- Identify when a patient with LCPD should be referred for further evaluation?

CASE 3

A 15-year-old female cross-country runner presents to your clinic with the chief complaint of knee pain. She describes a gradual increase in her symptoms during the first 3 weeks of the season. She wants to run varsity this year and has done extra running and hill training after practice each day. She describes anterior knee pain in the patellar region with little or no swelling, but complains of crepitus and pain exacerbated by stair climbing and running.

The most likely diagnosis for the condition described is:

A) Osgood-Schlatter disease.
B) Chondromalacia patellae.
C) Patellofemoral pain syndrome.
D) Femoral stress fracture.

Discussion

The correct answer is C. Patellofemoral pain syndrome is a common overuse syndrome seen more frequently in runners and female athletes. Patellofemoral syndrome may involve lateral subluxation or mal-tracking within the femoral groove caused by vastus medialis weakness. Mal-tracking may be observed clinically and subluxation may be seen on plain films using a Merchant view. Osgood-Schlatter disease (answer A) is also related to overuse but is 2–3 times more common in males, particularly in athletes engaging in repetitive jumping. Pain is well localized to the tibial tubercle. Radiographic evidence of fragmentation of the epiphysis or heterotropic ossification anterior to the tubercle may be seen but is not necessary for diagnosis. Chondromalacia patella (answer B) is softening of the articular cartilage of the patella as seen on arthroscopy and may be a result of long-term patellofemoral dysfunction. This is a surgical diagnosis and the term should be avoided clinically.

What is the preferred treatment for this female runner?

A) Arthroscopic debridement.
B) Decreased activity level and quadriceps strengthening.
C) Evaluation for "female athlete triad."
D) Casting or immobilization.
E) Corticosteroid injection.

Discussion

The correct answer is B. Quadriceps strengthening is usually initiated by resisted straight leg raises to minimize patellofemoral compressive forces. NSAIDs and cross-training may also be of benefit. Consider physical therapy referral for exercise instruction and trials of therapeutic modalities such as orthotics. Recalcitrant cases and patients with recurrent dislocation/subluxation should be referred to orthopedics for consideration of surgical intervention.

* *

Three months later, the patient presents with complaint of knee pain over the medial knee joint. Again, this pain is exacerbated by knee flexion. Your exam shows tenderness about 1 cm medial to the patella with palpable fullness in the area.

The most likely diagnosis is:

A) Osteosarcoma.
B) Medial collateral ligament strain.
C) Plica syndrome.
D) Patellofemoral pain syndrome.
E) Meniscal tear.

Discussion

The correct answer is C. This is the typical presentation of plica syndrome. The plica is a synovial remnant that did not resorb properly during development. It can be irritated, chronically or subacutely, especially in sports that require repeated flexion of the knee (rowing, cycling, running). Treatment includes rest, ice, quadriceps strengthening, and NSAIDs. If conservative management fails, steroid injection or arthroscopy may alleviate the symptoms.

 HELPFUL TIP: The plica should be palpable. A medial/inferior plica is the most common (between the patella and the medial joint line). It can also occur laterally and either above or below the midpole of the patella.

Objectives: Did you learn to . . .

- Identify patellofemoral syndrome?
- Generate a differential diagnosis for knee pain?
- Recognize plica syndrome?

CASE 4

A mother brings her 18-month-old son in for well-child check. Her main concern today is that he seems to walk "bow-legged." He has been somewhat pigeon-toed since he could pull himself up and cruise along walls and furniture at home. On exam you find the child's feet to be pointing inward. The foot is flexible and looks normal. The patellae are in a neutral position facing directly forward.

What is the most likely diagnosis in this patient?

A) Cerebral palsy.
B) Excessive femoral retroversion.
C) Forefoot varus.
D) Internal tibial torsion.
E) Bilateral developmental dysplasia of the hip (DDH).

Discussion

The correct answer is D. This represents a case of intoeing (pigeon-toeing), which is often caused by internal tibial torsion. Internal tibial torsion is characterized by a flexible, normal foot, with the patellae in a neutral position. The condition can be diagnosed by examining the child on his knees. Normally, there should be approximately 30 degrees of external rotation of the feet in this position. With internal tibial torsion, the toes will be pointing inward. Additionally, when the child is sitting with legs dangling over a table, the lateral malleolus will be anterior to the medial malleolus, which is the opposite of what is normally observed. Finally, the hips must be normal in order to confirm this diagnosis. Answer A is incorrect because you would expect other findings in a patient with cerebral palsy. Answer B is incorrect. Femoral retroversion is synonymous with "out-toeing," which is the opposite of intoeing. Excessive femoral **anteversion** can be a cause of intoeing. Answer C is incorrect because the foot exam does not show varus deformity. Finally, E is incorrect.

What is the treatment of choice for this child?

A) Referral for bilateral osteotomy.
B) Shoe modification and bracing.
C) Physical therapy referral.
D) Serial casting.
E) Reassurance and watchful waiting.

Discussion

The correct answer is E. Spontaneous resolution is the norm for most intoeing and out-toeing deformities. Most will spontaneously correct by age 7 or 8. Children who continue to have difficulty with persistent trips and falls or grossly unsightly gait beyond this time may benefit from a rotational osteotomy. Children with neuromotor disorders and cerebral palsy are more likely to require surgical intervention.

 HELPFUL TIP: Another cause of intoeing is femoral torsion which is diagnosed by placing the patient prone with the hips in neutral and knees flexed to 90 degrees. Feet are rotated away from midline to measure internal rotation (anteversion). For external rotation (retroversion), place one hand on the buttocks and move one leg through midline until the pelvis begins to tilt. Normal external rotation is 45 degrees, and normal internal rotation is 35 degrees. Rotation greater than these is considered excessive if it is accompanied by a limited ROM in the opposite direction. When a patient with femoral torsion is seated with legs dangling, the patellae will not face forward (they face inward for intoeing and outward for out-toeing).

Objectives: Did you learn to . . .
- Evaluate and manage intoeing and out-toeing in children?

CASE 5

A 13-year-old male presents to the clinic with his mother for difficulty walking. He is unsure of when the problem first began, but has noticed it getting worse over the last week. It has forced him to stop playing sports. He reports a dull pain in the left hip but denies trauma. On examination, you find an obese male in no distress. There is loss of internal rotation at the left hip joint. When his hip is flexed to 90 degrees, this loss of ROM is more pronounced.

What is the most likely diagnosis in this case?
A) Developmental dysplasia of the hip.
B) Septic arthritis.
C) SCFE (Slipped Capital femoral epiphisis).
D) LCPD (Legg-Calve-Perthes disease).
E) Juvenile rheumatoid arthritis.

Discussion
The correct answer is C. SCFE occurs most commonly in active, overweight, adolescent males. Shear forces across the relatively weak physis causes displacement. **Slippage is generally gradual, but may occur acutely.** Mean age at presentation is 12 years for females (range 10–14 years) and 13 years for males (range 11–16 years). Endocrinopathies should be considered in those presenting atypically or outside the typical age range. Watch for development of a similar process in the contralateral hip over time.

Which of the following is the FIRST study you order to confirm the diagnosis?
A) AP and frog-lateral radiographs.
B) CT scan.
C) MRI.
D) ESR.
E) None; physical exam is sufficient.

Discussion
The correct answer is A. Radiographs of the hip should demonstrate displacement of the femoral head, which can then be classified as mild, moderate, or severe. Answers B and C are incorrect because the radiograph is diagnostic in most cases. Answer D is incorrect because SCFE is not an inflammatory condition. Answer E is incorrect because imaging should be obtained in order to confirm the diagnosis and rate the severity.

The treatment of choice for this patient is:
A) Antibiotics.
B) Immobilization.
C) Physical therapy.
D) Surgical decompression.
E) Surgical fixation.

Discussion
The correct answer is E. The goals of treatment of SCFE are to prevent further slippage, promote closure of the physis, and to minimize the risk of osteonecrosis or chondrolysis. These goals are best accomplished through referral to an orthopedic surgeon and surgical fixation. Answers B and C are incorrect because they delay definitive therapy and will not produce the desired result. Answers A and D are incorrect because SCFE is not an infectious process.

Objectives: Did you learn to . . .
- Recognize the clinical presentation of a child with SCFE?
- Evaluate an adolescent with hip pain?
- Treat a patient with SCFE?

CASE 6

A worried mother presents with her 4-year-old son for evaluation of lower extremity pain. She reports the boy has complained of some vague bilateral leg pains over the past several weeks after vigorous physical activities. She became alarmed after he had awakened the past 2 nights crying in pain. The boy reports the pain is hardly noticeable during the day. Recently, the pain has been in the bilateral distal thighs; however, his mother notes times of unilateral pain. The boy and his mother both deny constitutional symptoms now or over the past several weeks. Examination reveals an afebrile, well-developed male in no distress. The musculoskeletal exam is normal.

The most likely diagnosis for the condition described above is?

A) Ewing sarcoma.
B) Growing pain.
C) Kohler disease.
D) Leukemia.
E) Osteochondritis desiccans.

Discussion

The correct answer is B. Growing pain is a diagnosis of exclusion, although history and physical exam usually suffice for excluding more serious diagnoses. It is a condition of unknown etiology, but is thought by some to be a result of overuse/overactivity on an immature musculoskeletal system. It is most frequently seen in otherwise healthy, active children aged 2–5, with some older children affected as well. Pain is commonly bilateral or/and localized to the calf, but may be felt at the ankle, knee, or thigh. Pain may be felt during the day after vigorous activities but is more common in the evening or causing awakening at night. Presentation with constitutional symptoms should lead to radiographic and/or metabolic workup.

Which of the following should you entertain when a patient presents with typical growing pain?

A) Osteomyelitis.
B) Tumor.
C) Juvenile rheumatoid arthritis.
D) All of the above.
E) None of the above.

Discussion

The correct answer is D. It is important to consider other potential causes of what would appear to be growing pain. Although you may not find it necessary to perform laboratory or radiologic studies, you should keep these and other diagnoses in mind when taking your history and performing your exam. Remember, growing pain is a diagnosis of exclusion.

 HELPFUL TIP: Severe or persistent pain during the day is **not** "growing pain." By definition, growing pain occurs primarily at night and is better during the day.

Treatment for growing pain includes:

A) Reassurance, rest, and short-term use of NSAIDs.
B) Amputation.
C) Chemotherapy and radiation.
D) Casting and bracing followed by physical therapy.
E) Staging of the disease is required prior to initiation of therapy.

Discussion

The correct answer is A. This is pretty obvious. Do not do anything drastic for a benign condition!

* *

The same boy returns with his mother years later. He is now 12 years old and requires a physical examination for junior high school sports. You plan to evaluate him for scoliosis.

Which of the following screening methods is the most sensitive for detecting scoliosis?

A) Observe the patient from the front with a loose-fitting shirt on. Measure the difference in shoulder height.
B) Observe the patient from **behind,** with shirt off, while he bends forward at the waist. Look for elevation of the ribs or paravertebral muscle mass on one side.
C) Observe the patient from the front, with shirt off, while he bends forward at the waist. Look for elevation of the ribs or paravertebral muscle mass on one side.
D) Observe the patient from the **side,** with shirt off, while he bends forward at the waist. Look for elevation of the ribs or paravertebral muscle mass on one side.

Discussion

The correct answer is B, which is known as the "forward bending test." This test is more sensitive than the other methods described. The forward bending test is accomplished by having the patient bend at the waist with feet together and hands hanging free. Observe the patient from behind and note any elevation of the ribs or paravertebral muscle mass on one side. The elevation should be measured in degrees (inclinometers are available), and an inclination of 5 degrees or more should be evaluated further. Answers A, C, and D are incorrect because they are **not** accepted methods of screening for scoliosis.

HELPFUL TIP: Routine screening for scoliosis is a recommendation "D" by USPSTF. Routine scoliosis screening is **not** recommended. It may be appropriate in patients who have noticed pain or some other abnormality.

HELPFUL TIP: Scoliosis is a lateral curvature of the spine, usually accompanied by rotation and generally occurring in the thoracic or lumbar areas. It can occur with excessive kyphosis (posteriorly convex curvature) or lordosis (anteriorly convex curvature).

* *

On forward bending test, you find slight elevation of the left paravertebral muscles mass, which you estimate to be 7 degrees. The remainder of the examination is normal. You decide to obtain radiographs which show 12 degrees of angulation (Cobb angle).

This patient's scoliosis is most likely:

A) Congenital.
B) Idiopathic.
C) Related to a tumor.
D) Secondary to infection.

Discussion

The correct answer is B. Most scoliosis that develops during adolescence is idiopathic. When there is no pain, fever, weight loss, or other warning signs (eg, neurologic symptoms), the curvature is unlikely to be due to tumor or infection. Congenital scoliosis (answer A) typically presents earlier in life.

The most appropriate initial management plan for this patient includes:

A) Bracing.
B) Observation.
C) Physical therapy.
D) Surgery.

Discussion

The correct answer is B. In an otherwise healthy patient with a curvature measured at less than 20 degrees, observation is appropriate. Answer C is incorrect because

physical therapy and exercise regimens do not seem to limit the progression of scoliosis. Answers A and D are incorrect because bracing and surgery are typically not warranted for this degree of scoliosis. Repeat examination and possibly repeat radiographs are warranted, but if the scoliosis remains stable and mild, the patient is not likely to experience any significant progression of disease with aging.

HELPFUL TIP: Bracing for scoliosis should be limited to those with idiopathic scoliosis and 20–40 degrees of angulation. Bracing is effective only if the child is still growing and <1 year past menarche if female.

Objectives: Did you learn to . . .

- Consider a broader differential diagnosis in a patient presenting with typical "growing pain"?
- Initiate conservative treatment for a patient with growing pain?
- Screen a patient for scoliosis?
- Develop an approach to the adolescent with scoliosis?

CASE 7

A 5-year-old girl recently recovered from chickenpox presents with her mother for evaluation of left leg pain and refusal to walk. The mother reports that the child has complained of worsening pain over the last 4–5 days. She started to limp noticeably yesterday and refused to walk this morning. Also, the mother reports general malaise and subjective fever. The child complains of pain over the distal thigh and knee. The mother has not seen any swelling of the knee, and the patient denies trauma.

Exam reveals a pleasant 5-year-old female who appears uncomfortable, but nontoxic and in no acute distress. Her temperature is 38.5°C. The left **distal thigh** (not the hip joint) is painful to palpation, and slightly warm. The knee joint has no effusion and the range of motion is full with only mild discomfort on knee motion. There is no hip joint involvement.

What is the most common bacterial pathogen associated with this patient's condition?

A) Group A *Streptococcus*.
B) Group B *Streptococcus*.

C) *Haemophilus influenzae.*
D) *Staphylococcus aureus.*
E) None of the above. This is not an infection.

Discussion

The correct answer is D. The acute nature of the symptoms, presence of fever, and minimal involvement of the joint makes osteomyelitis the most likely diagnosis. Additionally, osteomyelitis is associated with chickenpox in children. *S. aureus* is the most common cause of acute osteomyelitis in normal hosts in all age groups. *H. influenzae* (answer C) is less common since immunizations were begun; however, until culture results are available, it should be covered empirically in children aged 6 months to 4 years who have not yet completed their immunization series. Group B *Streptococcus* (answer B) and enteric rods are seen in neonates and should also be covered empirically in that population until culture results are available.

 HELPFUL TIP: *Pseudomonas aeruginosa* is commonly associated with osteomyelitis in the setting of a puncture wound.

The most common organism causing osteomyelitis in patients with sickle cell disease is:

A) *Neisseria gonorrhoeae* (gonococcus).
B) Polymicrobial.
C) *Salmonella* species.
D) *Staphylococcus aureus.*
E) *Streptococcus* species.

Discussion

The correct answer is C. *Salmonella* species are responsible for up to 85% of bone and joint infections in patients with a history of sickle cell disease. *Staphylococcus*, which is responsible for the majority of bone infections in the "normal" population, is responsible for less than 25% of infections in patients with sickle-cell disease.

 HELPFUL TIP: In most childhood cases of osteomyelitis, infection occurs as the result of hematogenous spread rather than by direct contamination.

Identification of the pathogen in a case of osteomyelitis is typically made by:

A) ASO titer.
B) Blood culture.
C) Joint aspiration, culture, and Gram stain.
D) Pathology report following open biopsy.

Discussion

The correct answer is B. A blood culture will reveal the offending organism in 40%–50% of cases. Joint aspiration is not typically indicated unless there is strong evidence of joint involvement. After 7–10 days, osseous changes may be seen on plain film radiographs, MRI, and bone scan. If changes are identified and a neoplastic process is ruled out, aspiration at the site of periosteal elevation and bony destruction should be considered if a pathogen has not yet been identified by blood culture. ASO titer (answer A) would not be helpful here. Surgical biopsy (answer D) may be required if blood cultures do not reveal a pathogen and the patient is not responding appropriately to empiric antibiotics.

 HELPFUL TIP: Treatment of osteomyelitis requires up to 4–6 weeks of antibiotics. Surgical debridement is usually (if not always) required as well.

Objectives: Did you learn to . . .

- Diagnose osteomyelitis in a child?
- Identify common pathogens involved in osteomyelitis?
- Treat a patient with osteomyelitis?

 QUICK QUIZ: ORTHOPEDIC INFECTIONS

The most common organism causing septic arthritis in the teenage years is:

A) *Neisseria gonorrhoeae* (gonococcus).
B) Polymicrobial.
C) *Salmonella* species.
D) *Staphylococcus aureus.*
E) *Streptococcus* species.

Discussion

The correct answer is A. Gonococcus is the most common organism isolated from the joints of sexually active, teenaged individuals.

CASE 8

A 2-year-old child presents to your office with his mother. He has not been using his right arm. According to the mother, the child was unwilling to leave the sandbox and a tug-of-war ensued with the mother eventually picking the child up by his forearm.

What abnormality are you likely to see on a radiograph of this child?

A) Dislocation at the wrist between the radius and ulna and the carpal bones.
B) Dislocation of the shoulder.
C) Fracture in the midshaft of the radius and ulna.
D) Dislocation at the elbow of the olecranon.
E) No abnormality will likely be seen on radiograph.

Discussion

The correct answer is E. This case is typical of "nursemaid elbow," a subluxation of the radial head. The radiograph is generally normal. The other answer choices are incorrect.

The appropriate treatment for subluxation of the radial head is:

A) Surgical.
B) Closed reduction using finger traps and weights.
C) Closed reduction using the Stimson technique.
D) Supination of the forearm and then flexing the arm at the elbow.
E) None of the above.

Discussion

The correct answer is D. There are a number of techniques for reducing a subluxed radial head, and many different movements may accomplish your goal. The classic technique is supinating the forearm followed by flexing the elbow. You should feel the reduction take place with a "click" at the elbow. Another option is pronating the forearm and flexing at the elbow: Either technique will work.

> **HELPFUL TIP:** The patient with nursemaid elbow should be using the arm normally within minutes. If the child still refuses to use the extremity after adequate observation, reconsider your diagnosis and whether the reduction was successful. Note that many will spontaneously reduce while radiographs are being done.

> **HELPFUL TIP:** When dealing with pediatric orthopedics, remember that child abuse is in the differential diagnosis. Determine that the reported mechanism of the injury is consistent with the findings on exam and radiograph.

* *

After successful reduction, you see the same 2-year-old child a month later presenting to your clinic with the parents who state that the child has been crying and has refused to walk after tripping over a toy several hours ago. You examine the child and find no signs of abuse. A schematic drawing of the resulting radiograph is shown in Figure 12–1.

Your approach at this point is to:

A) Consult Child Welfare because this is almost always abuse.
B) Consult orthopedics for casting and further treatment
C) No treatment necessary for this fracture in a 2-year-old.
D) A and B.

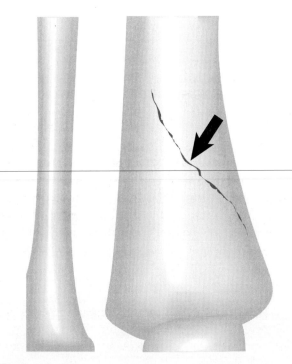

Figure 12–1

Discussion

The correct answer is B. This is a typical "toddler fracture" which consists of a spiral fracture of the tibia usually from insignificant rotational trauma (eg, running and falling with a twisting motion). There should not be an associated fibular fracture. Answer A is incorrect because this type of fracture is not usually from abuse. A midshaft fracture would more likely be from abuse. Answer C is incorrect because this fracture needs to be treated.

Objectives: Did you learn to . . .

● Recognize the clinical presentation and treatment of radial head subluxation?
● Recognize a "toddler fracture"?

CASE 8

You are evaluating a newborn male following a normal spontaneous vaginal delivery. You note the following on exam: significant plantar flexion of both feet, right slightly greater than left; calcaneus seems to be drawn inward and upward bilaterally; moderate forefoot adduction bilaterally; and neither foot can be placed in a neutral position by passive manipulation (Figure 12–2).

Which of the following is the most likely diagnosis?

A) Talipes equinovarus.
B) Calcaneovalgus.

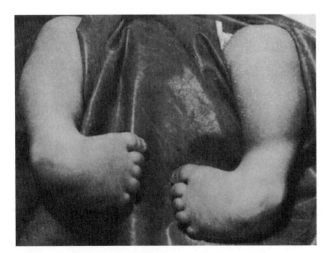

Figure 12–2 **From Brunicardi FC et al.** *Schwartz's Principles of Surgery,* **8th ed. Copyright The McGraw-Hill Companies, Inc.**

C) Flexible flatfeet.
D) Metatarsus valgus.
E) None of the above.

Discussion

The correct answer is A. This is also known as "clubfoot." The other answer choices are incorrect and are discussed separately.

Which of the following is true about talipes equinovarus?

A) It is most often a component of another congenital syndrome.
B) It is associated with lower extremity paralysis.
C) It is bilateral in the great majority of cases.
D) It is more common in females.
E) None of the above.

Discussion

The correct answer is E. None of the above statements is true. Answer A is incorrect because clubfoot is usually found as an isolated deformity **not** associated with another deformity although it can be found as part of a congenital syndrome. Answer B is incorrect. There is no relationship to paralysis. Answer C is incorrect because clubfoot is bilateral in only 30%–50% of patients. Answer D is incorrect because males are affected more commonly than females (approximately 2:1 ratio).

The most appropriate form of treatment for this patient would be:

A) Reassurance and watchful waiting.
B) Surgical reconstruction.
C) Serial casting and manipulation (Ponseti method).
D) Physical therapy referral for stretching and exercise.
E) Corrective shoes.

Discussion

The correct answer is C. A patient with clubfoot requires specialty referral. Treatment is most effective when initiated early.

* *

You refer this patient to an orthopedic surgeon who appropriately manipulates and casts the patient. The treatment is considered a success.

What is the most likely long-term outcome in patients with unilateral clubfoot?

A) Chronic foot pain.
B) Severe disability.
C) Difficulty finding a pair of shoes at a mainstream shoe store.
D) No further problems.

Discussion

The correct answer is C. For patients who are left untreated, severe disability is the usual result. For those who are appropriately treated, the repaired clubfoot will be smaller than the normal foot, resulting in the need for specialty shoe fitting for most patients.

Objectives: Did you learn to . . .

- Diagnose talipes equinovarus and recognize syndromes that may be associated with it?
- Recognize the need for early referral for patients with talipes equinovarus?
- Describe the prognosis of talipes equinovarus?

CASE 9

A concerned father presents to your clinic with his 1-month-old daughter. He is worried that his daughter appears to be pigeon-toed, and his mother-in-law is sure that the child will need immediate surgery for correction. Your exam reveals a pleasant, well-developed 1-month-old female with moderate medial deviation of the forefoot bilaterally. A line bisecting the heel passes through the fourth toe on each foot. The lateral borders of the feet are convex; the heels are in a normal neutral position. The feet are flexible.

The above description is best characterized as?

A) Clubfoot.
B) Internal tibial torsion.
C) Flexible flatfoot.
D) Excessive femoral anteversion.
E) Metatarsus adductus.

Discussion

The correct answer is E. This is a classic description of the foot shape of metatarsus adductus. In the normal foot, a line bisecting the heel would pass between the second and third toes. In those with metatarsus adductus

it passes through the fourth toe. In addition to the heels remaining in a neutral position—indicating that the problem is isolated to the shape of the foot and **not** to an internal rotation of the tibia—the forefoot is flexible and easily straightened into normal position. This is in contrast to metatarsus varus in which the forefoot is rigid.

The most appropriate treatment for this patient would be?

A) Surgical reconstruction.
B) Serial casting.
C) Physical therapy referral for stretching and exercise.
D) Watchful waiting and reassurance.
E) Orthopedic outflare shoes.

Discussion

The correct answer is D. Spontaneous correction occurs in most children. Parents can begin a regimen of gentle foot stretching. It gives them something to do but **does not change the outcome.** Care should be avoided to keep the child from the prone position with the feet in an inward position.

If the **deformity is severe and inflexible, serial casting and/or surgical intervention may be indicated. A rigid** metatarsus adductus in a child >3 months or a residual problem in a child >6 months with a flexible metatarsus adductus is an indication for pediatric orthopedic referral.

Objectives: Did you learn to . . .

- Identify a patient with metatarsus adductus?
- Discuss treatment approaches to metatarsus adductus?

CASE 10

A 28-year-old male presents to your clinic for evaluation of lower back pain (LBP). Yesterday morning he first noticed the discomfort, manifesting as stiffness and soreness in the lower back. He had spent the day before running a floor polisher. He describes his pain as sharp in nature and 8/10 in intensity. He denies radiation of the pain, sensory changes, and constitutional symptoms. He is concerned this may be an injury to a disk and that he may be permanently disabled due to his extreme pain.

Which of the following signs or symptoms are "red flags" that indicate the need for early imaging and/or referral?

A) Pain radiating down one or both legs into the posterior thigh.

B) Severe pain, prompting the patient to request narcotics.

C) Pain greater with active lumbar extension than with forward flexion.

D) New-onset erectile dysfunction with back pain.

E) None of the above.

Discussion

The correct answer is D. The onset of erectile dysfunction is suggestive of neurologic involvement and warrants further investigation. None of the other answers are suggestive of significant disease requiring immediate intervention. Answer A could represent disk disease; however, this does not require immediate intervention.

Early imaging should be obtained in all of the following situations EXCEPT:

A) Neurologic symptoms such as bowel or bladder disfunction and impotence.

B) History of fever, night sweats, weight loss.

C) History of cancer.

D) Trauma.

E) Age >30 years.

Discussion

The correct answer is E. Patients >50 years should have early imaging. Table 12–1 lists indicators for early imaging.

Table 12–1 INDICATIONS FOR EARLY IMAGING FOR BACK PAIN

Bowel or bladder dysfunction
New onset of impotence
Fevers or night sweats
Unplanned weight loss
Night pain
Personal history of cancer
Saddle anesthesia
History of recent trauma (eg, fall or direct blow ..... **not** twisting or lifting)
Age >50 or <18 years
Patient with current or recent use of steroids
Suspicion of an infectious or neoplastic cause for low back pain
Pain for >6 weeks

 HELPFUL TIP: Several of the indicators listed in Table 12–2 are associated with cauda equina syndrome. Cauda equina syndrome is the result of an acute reduction in the volume of the spinal canal resulting in compression and paralysis of multiple nerve roots distal to the conus medullaris. It is often caused by central disk herniations, epidural abscesses and hematomas, fractures, and other trauma. Cauda equina syndrome is an orthopedic emergency, and MRI and surgical consultation should be sought without delay.

 HELPFUL TIP: Patients who do **not** have films done initially have better outcomes than those who do. When we order imaging studies, we "medicalize" the illness, and cause the patient to expect a longer recovery and the need for intervention in order to get better.

* *

Upon physical examination, you note the vital signs are normal. Straight leg raise (SLR) testing on the right leg at 55 degrees reproduces the patient's pain in the lower back and a painful "tightness" in the posterior thigh. He complains of the same discomfort on the left at 30 degrees.

Based on these findings, which of the following statements is true?

A) This is a positive SLR test bilaterally and is specific for disk herniation.

B) This is a positive SLR test on the left and is specific for disk herniation.

C) This is a positive SLR test on the right and is specific for disk herniation.

D) This is a negative SLR test bilaterally.

Discussion

The correct answer is D. The SLR test can be preformed in several ways, as listed:

Seated active: With the patient seated on the exam table, ask that he dorsiflex the foot and extend the knee.

Seated passive: With the patient seated on the exam table, the examiner passively extends the knee, and radicular symptoms will be exacerbated with passive ankle dorsiflexion.

Lying passive: With the patient in a supine position, the examiner holds the knee in full extension and passively flexes the hip, and radicular symptoms will be exacerbated with passive ankle dorsiflexion.

In all cases, **the test is positive when radicular symptoms occur (eg, pain, paresthesias down the leg below the level of the knee—not back or thigh pain from muscle stretching)** between 25 and 75 degrees of hip flexion while lying or with knee extension while seated. The symptoms will be exacerbated with active or passive ankle dorsiflexion. **Straight leg raise is neither sensitive nor specific for disk disease. "Crossover" pain with radicular symptoms in the leg not lifted is specific for disk disease.**

* *

Even though SLR is negative, you continue your neurologic exam. You note symmetric patellar reflexes, diminished Achilles reflex on the right, and symmetric strength in the legs except for decreased strength with ankle eversion on the right. You also note decrease in gross sensation to light touch over the right lateral malleolus.

Which of the following nerve roots is most likely compromised?

A) L3
B) L4
C) L5
D) S1
E) S2-3-4

Discussion
The correct answer is D. A summary of nerve root innervation is given in Table 12–2.

Appropriate initial treatment for this patient's acute back pain should include which of the following?

A) Strict bed rest.
B) NSAIDs.
C) Corset or lumbar belt.
D) Referral for epidural steroid injection or endoscopic disk resection.
E) A and B.

Discussion
The correct answer is B. In acute mechanical back pain (no longer than 6 weeks), regardless of the method of treatment, 40% of patients are better within 1 week, 60% to 85% in 3 weeks, and 90% in 2 months. Negative prognostic factors include more than 3 episodes of back pain, gradual onset of symptoms, and prolonged absence from work. **Bedrest does not contribute to a return of function and may worsen outcomes.** Early mobilization of the patient is best to allow him to continue activities as tolerated.

HELPFUL TIP: If you have a choice between acetaminophen and an NSAID for an acute injury, acetaminophen will always be the right choice. Most acute injuries are not inflammatory and acetaminophen is a lot safer without gastropathy or platelet inhibition.

HELPFUL TIP: For low back pain, early mobilization and walking is important. Epidural steroid injections, while intuitively appealing, have demonstrated no long-term benefit. Chiropractic care and acupuncture may be useful.

Table 12–2   EXAM FINDINGS OF LUMBAR AND SACRAL SPINAL NERVE ROOTS

Nerve Root	Reflex	Motor	Sensory
L2–3	None	Quadriceps	Anterior thigh
L4	Patella	Tibialis anterior (foot dorsiflexion, inversion)	Medial lower leg and foot
L5	Medial hamstring (difficult to assess)	Extensor hallucis longus (dorsiflexion of big toe)	Dorsal foot
S1	Achilles	Peroneus longus and brevis (ankle eversion) and plantar flexion of foot	Lateral foot
S2–4	Anal wink	Intrinsic foot muscles, anal sphincter tone	Perianal

* *

You prescribe your NSAID of choice and recommend rehabilitation exercises.

Which of the following has been shown to be effective at reducing the recurrence of back injury in the workplace?

A) Back support belts.
B) "Back School" which teaches proper lifting techniques, stretches, etc.
C) Increasing physical fitness and muscle tone.
D) A and C.
E) B and C.

Discussion

The correct answer is C. The only thing that has been unequivocally shown to reduce further back injuries is improving the overall fitness of the patient and his muscle tone. **Back support belts, long worn in industry, have equivocal data with most studies being negative.** "Back School" (answer B) does not seem to help.

 HELPFUL TIP: Physical therapy modalities such as application of heat, cold, and ultrasound, and muscle stimulation may have short-term benefit. Rehabilitation exercises focusing on trunk extensors, abdominal muscles, and aerobic conditioning promote early mobilization, which is critical in treating acute back pain. **The specific exercise does not matter as much as the mobilization.** Sham therapy works as well as specific exercises as long as the patient is mobile.

Objectives: Did you learn to . . .

- Generate a differential diagnosis and understand the etiology of lumbar spine pain?
- Evaluate and treat acute low back pain?
- Recognize warning signs of low back pain?

 QUICK QUIZ: BACK PAIN

Spondylolysis commonly occurs in which part of the spine?

A) Cervical spine lateral processes.
B) Thoracic spine pars interarticularis.
C) Thoracic spine lateral processes.
D) Lumbar spine pars interarticularis.

Discussion

The correct answer is D. Spondylolysis is characterized by bilateral pars interarticularis fractures and most commonly occurs in the lumbar region.

 QUICK QUIZ: SPONDYLOLYSIS

Spondylolysis generally presents with pain:

A) When the slippage is 10%–15% and the patient is early teenaged (12–14 years).
B) When the slippage is 25% and the patient is early teenaged (12–14 years).
C) When slippage is 25% and the patient is late teenaged to early 20s.
D) When slippage is 10%–15% and the patient is >60 years.
E) When slippage is 25% and the patient is >60 years.

Discussion

The correct answer is C. Spondylolysis is a problem in late teenaged and early 20s patients. Patients become symptomatic when there is ≥25% slippage. Predisposing factors include recurrent lumbar hyperextension (gymnasts, football players, etc) although many patients do not have an identifiable cause. Patients present with back pain that is made worse by hyperextension. Treatment is usually conservative but may require surgical intervention if cord-compromise occurs.

 QUICK QUIZ: BACK PAIN

Anterior slippage of one vertebra on another is called:

A) Spondylolysis.
B) Spondylolisthesis.
C) Spondylitis.
D) Spondyloarthropathy.
E) Scheuermann disease.

Discussion

The correct answer is B. Slippage of one vertebra on another is called spondylolisthesis. Spondylolysis (answer A) is discussed above. Spondyloarthropathy (answer D) is a nonspecific term referring to inflammation of the spine and encompasses such diseases as ankylosing spondylitis, Reiter disease, enteropathic arthritis, etc. Spondylitis (answer C) is a more specific term for the same thing (eg, ankylosing spondylitis). Scheuermann disease (answer E) is a process causing a kyphosis. The cause is unknown but it tends to present in adolescence.

QUICK QUIZ: BACK PAIN IN CHILDREN

A 4-year-old child presents to your office accompanied by his mother who says he has a limp and lower back pain. This has been getting progressively worse over the past 2 weeks. When the patient sits, he sits in a "tripod" position supporting his weight on his hands. Vitals are normal without a fever and a CBC is normal.

This history is most consistent with:

A) Discitis.
B) Occult fracture.
C) Growing pains.
D) Juvenile rheumatoid arthritis.

Discussion

The correct answer is A. This history is most consistent with discitis. Discitis is an inflammatory process of the disk usually found in children aged infancy to 3 years but may occur at any age. The etiology is usually staphylococcus (low-grade infection) but there may be sterile inflammation. Fever is usually absent in discitis (seen in only 25%), and blood cultures are sterile. The white count is usually normal although the erythrocyte sedimentation rate is elevated in 90% of patients. Treatment is not standardized, but most experts would include anti-staphylococcal antibiotics.

Occult fracture (answer B) is unlikely in a child this age. Growing pains (answer C) does not present with back pain (see Case 6 for a discussion of growing pains). Juvenile rheumatoid arthritis (answer D) presents with small joint involvement as opposed to back pain.

CASE 11

A 24-year-old male presents to clinic two days after a collision during a softball game in which he fell on his outstretched right hand. He reports he could not continue playing and that his pain has not improved. He has some general edema around the right wrist, poor grip strength secondary to pain, point tenderness over the radial aspect of the wrist ("snuff box tenderness"), and decreased ROM. There is no obvious deformity, and he is neurovascularly intact.

Of the following, what would be the most likely diagnosis for this patient?

A) Colles fracture.
B) Scaphoid fracture.
C) Smith fracture.
D) Extensor carpiradialis strain.
E) Scapholunate sprain.

Discussion

The correct answer is B. Although all of the answer choices could be in the differential diagnosis, scaphoid fracture is the most likely based on mechanism of injury and clinical findings. The scaphoid spans both the proximal and distal carpal row. In this position it is quite vulnerable to high-impact injuries, such as a fall on an outstretched hand, and is the most commonly fractured carpal bone.

* *

Plain film radiographs, including AP and lateral of the hand and wrist as well as scaphoid views, are negative for fracture.

What is the most appropriate next step for this patient?

A) Short arm thumb spica cast with follow-up in 10–14 days.
B) NSAIDs, ice, compression, and elevation followed by physical therapy.
C) Bone scan or CT to rule out an occult fracture.
D) Orthopedic referral.
E) None of the above.

Discussion

The correct answer is A. Scaphoid fractures are often occult acutely and usually will be evident on plain films after 10–14 days due to bony resorption along the fracture line. If repeat films are negative but suspicion remains high, an MRI or bone scan should be considered.

* *

Repeat wrist radiographs including scaphoid views 2 weeks postinjury indicate a nondisplaced fracture of the **proximal** pole of the scaphoid.

You recommend which of the following treatment plans?

A) Wrist and thumb spica splint and physical therapy, because good blood supply at the proximal pole allows fast healing.
B) Thumb spica cast for 6 weeks, then repeat x-rays.
C) Short-arm cast excluding the thumb for 4–6 weeks.
D) Orthopedics referral for open reduction/internal fixation.
E) B or D.

Discussion

The correct answer is E. A spica cast with the thumb included is important; whether a short (answer C) or long arm cast is optimal is still a matter of debate. Open fixation is another option. Treatment of scaphoid fractures should be overseen by an orthopedic surgeon because there is a high rate of complications. A proximal pole fracture has high risk for nonunion and avascular necrosis. **The blood supply to the scaphoid is through the distal pole, putting the proximal pole at high risk for complications.** Evidence of healing may not be well visualized on plain films, and a CT or MRI may be needed to confirm the degree of healing. The closer the fracture line is to the proximal pole, the lower the threshold for orthopedic referral.

 HELPFUL TIP: Healing time for a distal pole fracture is 6–8 weeks, for middle third or waist fractures, 8–12 weeks, and for proximal pole fractures, 12–24 weeks.

Objectives: Did you learn to . . .

- Generate a differential diagnosis for radial wrist pain?
- Recognize a patient at risk for scaphoid fracture?
- Manage a patient with a scaphoid fracture?

 QUICK QUIZ: FRACTURES

A Colles fracture consists of:

A) A fracture of the midshaft of the radius and ulna.
B) A fracture of the head of radius and ulna that is displaced dorsally and is angulated.
C) A fracture of the head of the radius and ulna that is displaced ventrally and is angulated.
D) None of the above.

Discussion

The correct answer is D, none of the above. You may have chosen answer B. However, the **head of the radius** is at the elbow and **not at the wrist**. Therefore, none of the answers is correct. A Colles fracture is a fracture of the distal radius at the metaphysis, which is displaced dorsally and often angulated. It is the most common wrist fracture in adults. The ulnar styloid is often involved, and there may be intraarticular involvement as well.

 QUICK QUIZ: DE QUERVAIN TENOSYNOVITIS

Which of the following physical exam findings would be associated with the diagnosis of de Quervain tenosynovitis?

A) Positive Finkelstein test.
B) Positive Phalen test.
C) Positive Tinel sign.
D) Sensory loss over the C7 dermatome.
E) Weakness of the intrinsic muscles of the hand.

Discussion

The correct answer is A. De Quervain tendonitis is a tendonitis of the abductor pollicis longus, the extensor pollicis brevis, and occasionally the extensor pollicis longus. Full flexion of the thumb into the palm and ulnar deviation of the wrist produces exquisite tenderness over the radial aspect of the wrist (positive Finklestein test). Other findings may include soft tissue swelling and pain over the abductor pollicis longus and extensor pollicis brevis tendons near the radial styloid. Crepitus may also be palpable or audible with ROM.

 QUICK QUIZ: DE QUERVAIN TENOSYNOVITIS

The appropriate treatment of de Quervain tendonitis includes which of the following?

A) Thumb spica splint.
B) NSAIDs.
C) Steroid injection.
D) Surgical release of the tendon.
E) All of the above.

Discussion

The correct answer is E. All of the above treatments have been used successfully for the treatment of de Quervain tendonitis. Some prefer steroid injection as the first-line therapy rather than NSAIDs. Surgery is obviously a last choice.

CASE 12

A patient presents to your office after a gentlemen's disagreement. Another man's face accidentally hit his fist, and he suffered a laceration over dorsum of the left fifth MCP joint. Exam reveals a painful erythematous and edematous fifth MCP joint with ROM limited secondary to pain. The patient states, "You should see the other guy. I knocked out 2 of his teeth and broke 2 others." He brightens at this memory, confirming your suspicion that he was involved in something like a bar brawl.

Which of the following are concerns about this injury?

A) A septic joint.
B) Fracture.
C) Extensor tendon injury.
D) Foreign body.
E) All of the above.

Discussion

The correct answer is E. This is a so-called "clenched fist injury" that occurred when the patient's hand struck the opponent in the mouth. It is associated with a high risk of infection in the joint (generally in the second MCP joint). Even a small laceration may produce a devastating infection involving the deep palmar space, osteomyelitis, and joint sepsis. A boxer fracture (a fracture of the neck of the fourth or fifth metacarpal), tendon laceration, and foreign body (tooth fragments) are common with this mechanism of injury.

Appropriate treatment for the laceration described above would include all of the following EXCEPT:

A) Tetanus prophylaxis, antibiotics, and admission if clinical evidence of infection is already present.
B) Radiographs to rule out fracture and radiopaque foreign body.
C) Anesthetize wound edges followed by wound exploration, debridement, and irrigation.
D) Primary closure of deep and superficial layers after exploration, debridement, and irrigation.

Discussion

The correct answer is D. Primary closure may lead to a significant infection. A wound suspected of being caused by human bite should be allowed to close by secondary intention. The wound edges should be anesthetized and the wound explored for foreign body, debridement of necrotic tissue, and assessment for damage to tendons or joint capsule. Evaluate the tendons with the fingers flexed, as the injured area of the tendon may retract with extension. Irrigation with at least 1,000 mL of normal saline followed by application of a sterile dressing is indicated. Referral is appropriate if there is tendon, bone, nerve, or joint capsule damage, or if deep infection is suspected.

 HELPFUL TIP: Inserting a needle in the joint capsule and trying to inject methylene blue or saline can help to determine if the joint capsule is intact. If the fluid rushes out easily, there is likely a breech in the joint capsule.

* *

Radiographs demonstrate a fifth metacarpal fracture with some angulation.

What is the maximal acceptable angulation and rotation for a boxer fracture, fourth or fifth metacarpal, to maintain full hand function?

A) 10 degrees of dorsal angulation and 5 degrees of rotation.
B) 30 degrees of dorsal angulation and 5 degrees of rotation.
C) 40 degrees of dorsal angulation and 5 degrees of rotation.
D) 60 degrees of dorsal angulation and 0 degrees of rotation.
E) None of the above.

Discussion

The correct answer is E. **Any degree of rotation**, or **>40 degrees of dorsal angulation**, may result in significant functional deficits. Reduction should be attempted if angulation is >10 degrees. Patients should be advised that with angulations >10–15 degrees there will likely be a loss of MCP prominence although there should be no loss of function. If this is unacceptable to the patient, referral is recommended.

HELPFUL TIP: Boxer fracture is **not** caused by a fall on an outstretched hand regardless of what patients may claim.

Objectives: Did you learn to . . .

- Manage a patient at risk for a human bite infection?
- Manage a patient with a boxer fracture?

* *

The next patient in the ED was trying to break up the bar fight when he was tripped and fell onto his side, landing on the tip of his right shoulder. He states that he can actively move his arm but is limited by pain on the top of his shoulder. He has also noticed a small painful bump on top of the right shoulder and is concerned that he "broke his collarbone."

Based on the mechanism of injury and patient history, the MOST likely injury is:

A) Acromioclavicular (AC) sprain.
B) Biceps tendon rupture.
C) Glenohumeral dislocation.
D) Rotator cuff tear.
E) Scapula fracture.

Discussion

The correct answer is A. Although any of these injuries may be present, an AC sprain is the most likely based on the history and the way the patient fell. A thorough exam should be able to further distinguish between these injuries. "B" is not likely, given the mechanism of injury. The deformity associated with biceps tendon rupture (a defect in tendon with pain and deformity in the muscle belly representing the contracted, detached muscle) would be on the upper arm or at the elbow, not on the "top" of the shoulder. "C" is incorrect. The deformity and loss of ROM of a glenohumeral dislocation (shoulder dislocation) is usually obvious. The mechanism of injury is typically a forced abduction and external rotation. "D" is less likely. A rotator cuff tear will present with pain more laterally over the subacromial space and should not have an associated deformity. The range of motion is generally markedly limited by pain. "E" is unlikely. Scapula fractures are uncommon and are usually the result of high velocity blunt trauma such as a blow from a baseball bat or motorcycle accident. Plain film

radiographs should be obtained to rule out a clavicle fracture, especially when any suspected deformity is present.

* *

Your patient is worried that he broke his "collarbone."

If he did sustain a clavicle fracture, which of the following would be appropriate treatment?

A) External fixation with molded plaster to maintain alignment.
B) A sling for comfort only.
C) A figure 8 splint.
D) B and C.
E) Any of the above choices is appropriate.

Discussion

The correct answer is D. Although the traditional teaching has been that a figure 8 splint is required, it adds nothing to the treatment of a clavicle fracture. Pain control and using a sling work as well. Figure 8 splints often increase a patient's pain and can cause a brachial plexus injury. Thus, a sling is preferable although a figure 8 splint can be used.

The proper treatment for a clavicle fracture that is displaced is:

A) Closed reduction and then a sling.
B) Open reduction and immobilization.
C) Open reduction and early mobilization.
D) A sling.
E) None of the above.

Discussion

The correct answer is D. The ends of a displaced clavicle fracture need not be approximated for healing to occur and for function to return. Therefore, any reduction is generally not necessary.

* *

You send the patient for x-rays. AP radiographs show slight widening of the AC joint on the injured side with symmetric distance between the clavicles and coracoid processes. The exam and radiograph confirm your suspicion of an AC injury.

For this patient with an acromioclavicular sprain, you offer:

A) Sling for comfort, ice, and NSAIDS or analgesics for pain control.
B) Referral for open fixation.
C) Figure 8 strap for 4–6 weeks.
D) Corticosteroid injection followed by physical therapy.
E) Manual reduction then sling immobilization for 6–8 weeks.

Discussion

The correct answer is A. Surgical fixation is rarely needed for AC injuries unless an anterior or posterior displacement of the clavicle is present or in injuries in which the coracoclavicular interspace distance is increased >100% more than the distance seen on the uninjured side without weights. Answers C, D, and E are incorrect because they are not appropriate for this type of injury.

Objectives: Did you learn to . . .

- Differentiate between causes of shoulder injuries?
- Treat a clavicular fracture?
- Manage acromioclavicular injuries?

CASE 13

A 65-year-old male presents with left shoulder pain and weakness that began after he put a new roof on his house. The pain came on gradually and is made worse with abduction and flexion of the shoulder joint. He describes himself as active and healthy, and he takes only acetaminophen when needed for shoulder pain. You suspect that he may have a rotator cuff injury.

If this is the case, what do you expect to find on exam?

A) Tenderness to palpation of the greater tuberosity of the humerus.
B) Limited active range of motion.
C) Normal passive range of motion.
D) Shoulder shrug with attempted abduction.
E) Any of the above.

Discussion

The correct answer is E. This might fit under the category of "trick question," but the shoulder exam can be normal in a patient with rotator cuff tear, or it can include any of the elements in answers A through D.

Which of the following muscles is NOT a part of the rotator cuff?

A) Supraspinatus.
B) Infraspinatus.
C) Subscapularis.
D) Teres major.
E) Teres minor.

Discussion

The correct answer is D. The rotator cuff consists of the other four muscles listed, and it functions to rotate the arm and stabilize the humeral head.

Which of the following muscles is the most commonly torn in the rotator cuff?

A) Supraspinatus.
B) Infraspinatus.
C) Subscapularis.
D) Teres minor.

Discussion

The correct answer is A. The supraspinatus is the point of origin for most tears.

 HELPFUL TIP: Full thickness tears are uncommon in individuals <40 years, unless associated with trauma.

* *

Based on your history and physical exam, you diagnose a rotator cuff tendonosis.

Appropriate initial management of this 65-year-old male should be:

A) Acetaminophen and physical therapy.
B) Oral corticosteroids and physical therapy.
C) Subacromial injection with corticosteroid and physical therapy.
D) Surgical repair and physical therapy.
E) None of the above.

Discussion

The correct answer is A. For initial management in an individual >60 years, acetaminophen and physical therapy for 6 weeks is the best answer. If they have no improvement or inadequate response, a corticosteroid injection may be used judiciously. Injection will likely cause at least short-term pain relief but is thought to weaken the tendon and may accelerate extension of the tear. Oral steroid administration may provide relief, but it is associated with a higher incidence of systemic side effects. Patients with significant symptoms or failed therapy should be considered for MRI, orthopedic referral, and surgical management. Patients <60 years with acute traumatic tears should be considered for surgery, with best results within 6 weeks of injury.

> **HELPFUL TIP:** The old adage about corticosteroids causing weakening of the tendon has recently been questioned. It is now thought that the steroid injection provides enough relief of the pain that the patient will start using the extremity in ways he or she had not done before. This leads to tendon rupture from the additional load. However, the issue remains that steroid injections may be associated with, but not causative of, tendon rupture.

* *

Your patient is successful in rehabilitating his left shoulder, but he returns 2 years later with right shoulder problems. The right shoulder has become progressively stiff and painful, and his ROM is now significantly limited in all directions. Your examination is consistent with "frozen shoulder" or adhesive capsulitis.

Adhesive capsulitis is most commonly associated with which of the following?

A) Diabetes mellitus type 1.
B) Hyperthyroidism.
C) Spondyloarthitis.
D) Nondominant arm.
E) Male gender.

Discussion

The correct answer is A. Adhesive capsulitis shows no preference for gender, race, arm dominance, or occupation. It is characterized by loss of ROM of the shoulder in all directions, with loss of both passive and active motion. It has a high incidence in patients with type 1 diabetes and tends to be more recalcitrant in those patients, of whom up to 50% will have bilateral involvement—although not necessarily concomitantly. Adhesive capsulitis is not typically related to trauma, but it can be associated with disuse due to pain, osteoarthritis, sling use, etc. Other conditions that are associated with adhesive capsulitis include **hypo**thyroidism, cervical disc disease, and Parkinson disease.

> **HELPFUL TIP:** Adhesive capsulitis is considered to be idiopathic and separate from posttraumatic or postoperative joint stiffness or adhesions.

What initial treatment do you recommend for this patient?

A) Arthroscopic debridement.
B) Oral corticosteroids.
C) NSAIDs and a sling for comfort.
D) Extended progressive physical therapy.
E) Mobilization under anesthesia.

Discussion

The correct answer is D. A progressive stretching program with heat and NSAIDs to improve comfort is the most appropriate early treatment. A corticosteroid injection may be beneficial, but should be used cautiously in diabetic patients. Oral steroids (answer B) have no greater benefit than NSAIDs. Answer C is incorrect because a sling will contribute to further immobilization and worsening of the problem. Mobilization under anesthesia (answer E) may be a last resort in true adhesive capsulitis, but is more commonly used for posttraumatic or postoperative joint stiffness or adhesions that do not respond to conservative treatment.

> **HELPFUL TIP:** The typical clinical course for adhesive capsulitis evolves over 1–2 years with an initial "freezing" phase characterized by progressing pain and stiffness followed by a slow "thawing" phase with decreasing pain and increasing ROM.

Objectives: Did you learn to . . .

- Define the muscles of the rotator cuff?
- Identify, evaluate, and treat a rotator cuff injury?
- Recognize the presentation, associations, and treatment of adhesive capsulitis?

CASE 14

A 58-year-old male presents after sudden onset of right upper arm pain. He was working in the yard, cutting and pulling out some bushes, when he heard a "snap" and felt the pain. He has a history of rotator cuff tendonosis and osteoarthritis.

You look for all of the following on physical examination EXCEPT:

A) A positive elevated arm stress test ("Roos" test).
B) A palpable biceps muscle defect.
C) Normal grip strength.
D) An asymmetric bulge in the affected arm.

Discussion

The correct answer is A. The elevated arm stress test is used to evaluate a patient for thoracic outlet syndrome and is positive if neurologic or vascular symptoms are reproduced when the arm is elevated for a prolonged period. This patient's presentation is not consistent with thoracic outlet syndrome. However, the history is consistent with biceps tendon rupture. Answers B through D would be expected in a patient with biceps tendon rupture.

HELPFUL TIP: Provocative maneuvers for thoracic outlet syndrome (Roos test, etc) have poor sensitivity and specificity (<60%). They are most helpful if test results are positive and the patient's symptoms are reproduced.

Which portion of the biceps is most commonly involved in ruptures?

A) Distal tendon.
B) Proximal short head tendon.
C) Proximal long head tendon.
D) Mid-muscle belly.
E) Proximal short-head belly.

Discussion

The correct answer is C. The long head is most commonly affected due to its position and risk for weakening secondary to rotator cuff tendonosis and shoulder impingement.

* *

You decide this patient has a rupture of the long head of the biceps tendon.

How is this injury treated initially?

A) Immediate surgical repair.
B) Delayed surgical repair.
C) Immobilization for 4–6 weeks with sling.
D) NSAIDs and physical therapy.

Discussion

The correct answer is D. For most isolated proximal long- or short-head tears (with the exception of some young athletes and heavy laborers who would not tolerate the slight decrease in strength), treatment is conservative. Analgesics and physical therapy typically suffice. Surgical repair may be indicated if conservative therapy fails. You should discuss with patients the cosmetic deformity that will be permanent when these injuries are unrepaired vs. scarring associated with surgery. There is approximately a 10% loss of elbow flexion and supination strength with an isolated proximal tear.

HELPFUL TIP: Although proximal biceps tendon ruptures are treated conservatively, distal ruptures should be referred for early surgical repair, as the continuity of the entire muscle is lost and function at the elbow joint is significantly impaired with a 30%–40% loss of strength across the elbow joint.

Objectives: Did you learn to . . .

- Identify the clinical presentation of biceps tendon rupture?
- Manage a patient with biceps tendon rupture?

CASE 15

A 25-year-old male presents to you with a history of a soccer injury. Another player fell on his right foot while trying to steal the ball. The patient rapidly and forcefully

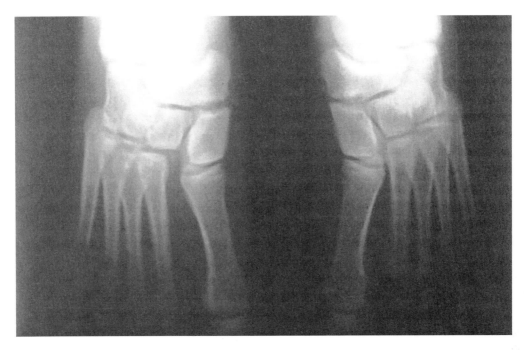

Figure 12–3

twisted around the fixed foot. Since then he has had significant pain and swelling of the foot. His x-ray is shown in Figure 12–3.

This radiographic abnormality is notable for:

A) Often being difficult to identify on radiograph.
B) Marked instability.
C) Association with significant pain.
D) All of the above.
E) None of the above.

Discussion

The correct answer is D, all of the above. This is a Lisfranc fracture, which occurs between the metatarsals and the tarsal bones (the space between the metatarsals and the tarsal bones is known as the Lisfranc joint). Look for a widened space between the first and second and/or second and third metatarsals. There may also be a stepoff between the second metatarsal and middle cuneiform. These fractures may be difficult to identify unless you are looking for them. Significant foot pain should be a tip off. See Figure 12–4 for further explanation.

HELPFUL TIP: Weight bearing "stress" films may be required in order to identify a Lisfranc fracture.

Appropriate treatment for this type of injury should include:

A) Weight bearing as tolerated in a postop or hard-soled shoe.
B) Rest, ice, compression, elevation, NSAIDs, and activity as tolerated. Will heal well and can be treated like a mid-foot sprain.
C) Orthopedic referral for open reduction/internal fixation (ORIF).
D) Walking boot that can be removed for several weight-bearing hours a day.

Discussion

The correct answer is C. This fracture and dislocation will lead to significant long-term pain if not recognized and treated appropriately. Any significant displacement (>2 mm) should be referred for surgical consideration. These are generally complex injuries prone to poor outcomes and should be managed by an orthopedic consultant.

Objectives: Did you learn to . . .

• Identify a Lisfranc fracture?
• Manage a patient with a Lisfranc fracture?

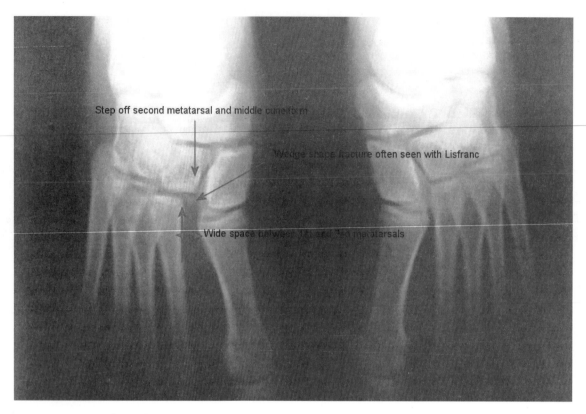

Figure 12–4   Lisfranc fracture.

CASE 16

An 18-year-old female gymnast lands her dismount from the balance beam awkwardly. She reports the knee buckling, hearing a pop and experiencing immediate right knee pain. She presents to your office 45 minutes after the injury. She is able to bear some weight on the leg but reports it is already swollen and feels loose. On exam there is a knee effusion present.

The MOST likely isolated injury experienced by this athlete is:

A) Medial meniscus tear.
B) Medial collateral ligament (MCL) sprain.
C) Distal quadriceps/patellar tendon rupture.
D) Anterior cruciate ligament (ACL) rupture.
E) None of the above.

Discussion

The correct answer is D. Did the patient or someone else hear a pop? If yes, suspect ACL tear (80%), meniscal injury (15%), and rarely a fracture. When did you notice swelling? If 0–12 hours after the injury, suspect

ACL tear or patellar dislocation/subluxation; if 12–24 hours, suspect meniscal injury. If there is hemarthrosis on aspiration, suspect ACL injury (>75%), patellar subluxation, or intraarticular fracture. A history of "My knee gives way; buckles; feels loose; or comes apart" may be secondary to patellar subluxation/dislocation, ACL deficiency, or arthritis. Collateral ligament injuries, MCL, or lateral collateral ligament (LCL) do not typically present with significant effusion and typically feel stable with forward ambulation but are painful with side-to-side movements. Muscle or tendon rupture may cause buckling, but will not typically cause effusion and will generally have an obvious deformity and inability to bear weight.

The best test to confirm the diagnosis of the above injury would be:

A) Plain film radiographs.
B) McMurray test.
C) Lachman test.
D) Anterior drawer test.
E) None of the above can confirm this diagnosis independently.

Discussion

The correct answer is C. **In the hands of an experienced clinician**, the Lachman test is the most sensitive test for ACL insufficiency (80%–95%). The anterior drawer sign is negative in about 50% of acute ACL tears, and often is negative subacutely. McMurray test is used to evaluate for a meniscal tear. Plain films should be obtained for all patients with acute knee injury with effusion or suspected ACL tear. However, x-rays are rarely positive for more than effusion or Segond fracture (avulsion of the lateral joint capsule from the tibia). Although an MRI may be considered a gold standard test, its sensitivity has been reported as 97% when compared with arthroscopy findings, and is positive in only 82% in cases of complete rupture. An orthopedic consult is generally indicated if ACL injury is suspected, and obtaining one is less expensive than MRI.

 HELPFUL TIP: The Lachman test is performed with the knee flexed at 20–30 degrees with the patient in a supine position. The examiner then attempts to anteriorly displace the tibia on the femur while stabilizing the femur. Always remember to check the contralateral side. Some patients have naturally lax joints.

* *

You feel that this patient is appropriate for radiographic evaluation, and you obtain x-rays of the knee.

Which of the following is NOT one of the criteria of the Ottawa knee rules predicting the need for knee radiographs?

A) Age <18.
B) Pain isolated to the patella.
C) Tenderness at the head of the fibula.
D) Inability to flex the knee 90 degrees.
E) Inability to bear weight for 4 steps.

Discussion

The correct answer is A. The age criterion for the Ottawa knee rules is age >55 years. All of the other answer choices are correct. If **any** of these criteria are present (including a patient >55 years), a radiograph should be obtained. These rules have been validated and are 97% sensitive for fracture. The Pittsburgh rules, which are reportedly 99% sensitive, have only

two criteria: (1) age <12 years or >50 years and (2) inability to bear weight in the clinic or ED. Of the two, the Ottawa rules are the more commonly accepted.

* *

The x-ray shows no fracture. You prescribe a knee immobilizer, rest, ice, NSAIDs, and refer the patient to an orthopedic surgeon. The patient returns 2 days later with marked effusion and pain. To help relieve the pain you perform an arthrocentesis and 90 mL of bloody aspirate is obtained. As per your clinic's standard protocol, the joint fluid is sent for analysis. The analysis returns with the only abnormalities being blood and **a small amount of fat droplets**.

Based on the effusion, you suspect what diagnosis?

A) Complete ACL rupture.
B) Meniscal tear.
C) ACL and PCL tear.
D) Intraarticular fracture.
E) Patellar subluxation.

Discussion

The correct answer is D. **Fat from bone marrow** may be seen even with a small intraarticular fracture. Consider CT or MRI if fracture is not noted on plain film.

Objectives: Did you learn to . . .

- Generate a differential diagnosis for knee pain in an athlete?
- Diagnose anterior cruciate ligament injury?
- Determine when knee radiographs are appropriate?

 QUICK QUIZ: KNEE PAIN

The best clinical test(s) for determining the presence of a meniscal injury is (are):

A) Posterior sag test.
B) Apley test.
C) McMurray test.
D) Pivot shift test.
E) B and C.

Discussion

The correct answer is E. The McMurray test is the best test for determining meniscal injury. This is done by flexing the knee and then extending the knee while performing internal and external rotation of the tibia/fibula. Keep one hand on the knee. The test is positive when the examiner feels a pop during the maneuver or when there is significant pain during internal or external rotation. The Apley test is done with the patient in a prone position. Move the knee to 90 degrees of flexion. Put downward pressure on the tibia/fibula while internally and externally rotating the lower leg. Pain suggests a meniscal tear. Pain should be relieved by distracting the joint.

CASE 17

A 24-year-old female presents to clinic 24 hours after slipping on a patch of ice outside her home. She reports feeling a "pop" and immediate pain on the lateral aspect of the ankle. She reports significant swelling in the first few hours with pain and inability to bear weight initially, but now she is able to walk with a significant limp. She reports no significant past injuries to the foot or ankle. On exam, you note edema/effusion over the lateral ankle, some ecchymosis, tenderness, but no laxity on anterior drawer and inversion stress. There is no bony tenderness on palpation of the foot and ankle, but there is tenderness anterolaterally in the soft tissue.

The most likely injury this patient has suffered is:

A) Fracture of the distal tibia.
B) Fracture of the distal fibula.
C) Sprain of the lateral ligament complex.
D) Sprain of the medial ligament complex.
E) Syndesmosis sprain.

Discussion

The correct answer is C. A sprain is most likely because there is no bony tenderness. And, since she is tender laterally, the lateral ligament complex is most likely sprained.

In this case, the most likely structure injured would be the:

A) Anterior talofibular ligament.
B) Distal fibula.
C) Distal tibia.
D) Deltoid ligament.
E) Achilles tendon.

Discussion

The correct answer is A. This is a sprain of the anterior talofibular ligament. This is the first ligament injured

with an inversion ankle sprain. It is followed by the calcaneofibular ligament if enough force is involved. Answer E, Achilles tendon injury (specifically rupture), is of special note. First, this injury presents as pain in the Achilles tendon area. With a complete Achilles tendon tear, the patient will have marked weakness of plantar flexion. A diagnostic test (Thompson test) is to squeeze the posterior calf. In response, the foot should plantar flex. If this does not occur, consider Achilles rupture. Operative and nonoperative treatments have been used. Operative treatment carries a lower risk of re-rupture.

 HELPFUL TIP: The Ottawa criteria reliably predict who needs an ankle radiograph and who does not. The criteria are listed in Figure 12–5.

Which of the following is the most appropriate management of this patient's injury?

A) Cast for 4 weeks followed by physical therapy.
B) Crutches, non-weight-bearing for 2 weeks, and then progressive physical therapy.
C) Rest, ice, elevation, and early mobilization using external support, crutches or cane if needed. Progress to activity as tolerated.
D) Refer for orthopedic consultation.
E) Immobilization with short leg walking cast, heat for comfort, analgesics or NSAIDs, and progress to activities as tolerated.

Discussion

The correct answer is C. Treatment for most grade I and II sprains includes external support, such as an air or gel splint, ice application, and elevation; early mobilization is critical and will hasten recovery. NSAIDs or acetaminophen should be used for pain control. The patient should be allowed partial weight bearing as tolerated with crutches or a cane. Patients with recurrent problems of instability or an acute grade III sprain should be referred to an orthopedist for evaluation.

 HELPFUL TIP: Early mobilization and weight bearing reduces the time of disability for ankle sprains. Rest and non-weight-bearing should be minimized. Allow the patient to advance activities as tolerated.

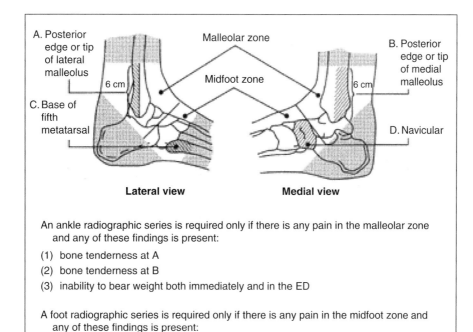

A. Posterior edge or tip of lateral malleolus

Malleolar zone

B. Posterior edge or tip of medial malleolus

6 cm

Midfoot zone

6 cm

C. Base of fifth metatarsal

D. Navicular

Lateral view   **Medial view**

An ankle radiographic series is required only if there is any pain in the malleolar zone and any of these findings is present:

(1) bone tenderness at A

(2) bone tenderness at B

(3) inability to bear weight both immediately and in the ED

A foot radiographic series is required only if there is any pain in the midfoot zone and any of these findings is present:

(1) bone tenderness at C

(2) bone tenderness at D

(3) inability to bear weight both immediately and in the ED

Figure 12–5   Ottawa criteria.

Objectives: Did you learn to . . .

- Identify a patient with an ankle sprain?
- Differentiate ankle sprain from fracture based on history and exam?
- Use the Ottawa ankle rules to determine when to obtain an ankle radiograph?
- Manage a patient with an ankle sprain?

CASE 18

A 27-year-old male presents to your clinic following an inversion type injury to the foot and ankle. He cannot bear weight on the foot. He complains of pain and swelling laterally on the foot and ankle. There is some soft tissue swelling but no obvious deformity. There is tenderness over the lateral ankle ligaments as well as over the base of the fifth metatarsal. AP and lateral films of the foot and ankle are obtained and reveal a nondisplaced transverse fracture through the proximal base/tuberosity of the fifth metatarsal. The radiograph is shown in Figure 12–6.

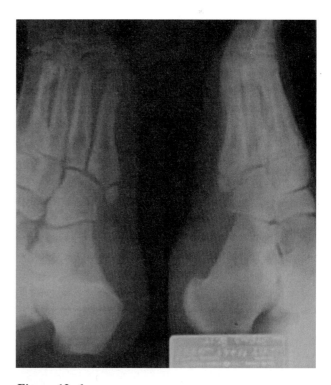

Figure 12–6

What is this injury called?

A) Jones fracture.
B) Lisfranc fracture.
C) Maisonneuve fracture.
D) Kirschner's fracture.
E) Avulsion fracture of tuberosity, base 5th metatarsal.

 HELPFUL TIP: An unfused apophysis in children and adolescents may be confused with a 5th metatarsal avulsion injury. Tuberosity avulsion fractures are transverse, while the unfused apophysis is oriented vertically along the long axis of the metatarsal. Table 12–3 lists fracture terminology.

Discussion

The correct answer is E. This is an avulsion fracture of the base of the fifth metatarsal which commonly results from an inversion ankle injury. Attempts at dynamic stabilization by the peroneus brevis cause an **avulsion of the proximal portion of the metatarsal base**. This type of fracture generally heals well. If it does not, it is generally asymptomatic. A **Jones fracture** is a transverse fracture through the proximal fifth metatarsal shaft (Figure 12–7). Jones fractures have a high incidence of nonunion because they occur in a watershed area of blood supply.

Appropriate treatment for the avulsion fracture described would be:

A) A wooden postoperative shoe or walking boot, with weight bearing as tolerated for 2–4 weeks.
B) Non-weight-bearing short-leg cast for 6–8 weeks.
C) Operative internal fixation.
D) Rest, ice, compression, elevation, and NSAIDs as needed.
E) None of the above.

Discussion

The correct answer is A. Nondisplaced tuberosity fractures can be managed with a wooden postoperative shoe or cast fracture boot, with weight bearing as tolerated for 2–4 weeks. For a fracture with a displaced fragment >3 mm, orthopedic referral should be considered. Fractures to the metaphyseal-diaphyseal junction (**Jones fractures**) result from a vertical load placed on the lateral foot, such as an inversion injury or a stress injury. Jones fractures can be managed with 6–8 weeks in a non-weight-bearing short-leg cast if nondisplaced **but are best referred due to high incidence of nonunion.** All displaced Jones fractures and intraarticular tuberosity fractures should be referred for orthopedic management.

Table 12–3 FRACTURE TERMINOLOGY

Closed fracture. Fracture that does not communicate with the outside.
Open fracture. Fracture that communicates with the external environment.
Comminuted fracture. Consisting of three or more fragments.
Avulsion fracture. Fragment of bone pulled from its normal position by a muscular contraction or resistance of a ligament.
Greenstick fracture. Incomplete, angulated fracture of a long bone, particularly in children.
Torus fracture. Described as a buckle fracture or compression of the bone without cortical disruption. Seen especially in the distal forearms of children.

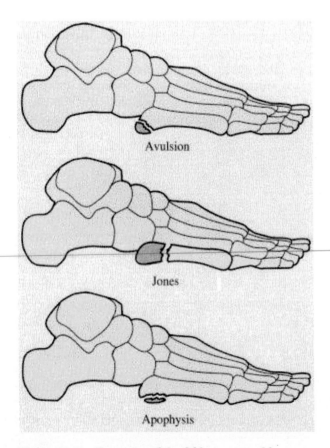

Figure 12–7 Fractures of the fifth metatarsal bone.

HELPFUL TIP: Stress fractures of the forefoot are common in competitive and recreational athletes, especially after a sudden increase in activity, intensity, duration, frequency, or a change in surface type. They may be occult on plain films acutely, but some subtle periosteal change may be evident on close exam in the area of maximal tenderness. If plain films are negative but suspicion remains high, consider an MRI or bone scan (less specific). The same treatment considerations apply to metatarsal stress fractures as to any other nondisplaced forefoot fracture.

Objectives: Did you learn to . . .

- Evaluate foot injuries?
- Describe metatarsal fractures?
- Manage straightforward metatarsal fractures and identify which fractures should be referred?

CASE 19

A 40-year-old female factory worker presents with progressively worsening heel pain. She has pain when she first gets out of bed in the morning. The pain tends to subside after 20–45 minutes but is worsened by standing on the concrete floor of the factory where she works. She has a history of diabetes and hyperlipidemia. On examination, you find an obese female with a normal stance and gait. She has exquisite tenderness to palpation just distal to the heel on the underside of the foot. Pain is exacerbated by dorsiflexion of the toes.

Which of the following is the most likely diagnosis?

A) Tarsal tunnel syndrome.
B) Achilles tendon tear.
C) Charcot foot.
D) Plantar fasciitis.
E) Plantar fascia rupture.

Discussion

The correct answer is D. Plantar fasciitis, the most common cause of heel pain in adults, is a degenerative condition of the origin of the plantar fascia. Answer A is incorrect. Tarsal tunnel syndrome is caused by posterior tibial nerve entrapment and presents with diffuse pain at the medial ankle and arch of the foot. Paresthesias and dysesthesias often occur as well. Achilles tendon rupture (answer B) is incorrect because the pain is sudden, stabbing, and is located in the calf (not the plantar aspect of the heel). Answer C is incorrect. Charcot foot does occur in diabetics, but it is the result of neuropathy and so generally does not present with pain. Instead, Charcot foot presents as an inflammatory condition (eg, warmth, erythema, edema) and progresses to joint instability and severe foot deformities. Answer E is incorrect because plantar fascia rupture should have a sudden onset and is related to trauma.

Which of the following is true of plantar fasciitis?

A) It more commonly occurs in individuals with pes cavus.
B) It is more common in women.
C) It is commonly an acute injury.
D) Radiographic identification of a "heel spur" or osteophyte is pathognomonic.
E) None of the above.

Discussion

The correct answer is B. Plantar fasciitis is not associated with any particular foot type. It is nearly twice as common in women as men. It is more common in overweight individuals. Although a tear of the plantar fascia may occur acutely, more typically a degenerative or repetitive trauma causes tendonosis. Radiographs are not recommended. Spurring may be seen in up to 50% of patients with plantar fasciitis, but is present in 20% of age-matched asymptomatic adults. **Therefore, the finding of a spur does not mandate surgical intervention and radiographs are not mandatory.**

Appropriate initial treatment for this patient's plantar fasciitis should include:

A) A heel cup or silicon pad.
B) Achilles stretching.
C) Ice or heat.
D) NSAIDs.
E) All of the above.

Discussion

The correct answer is E, all of the above. Other initial treatments to consider include night splints to maintain ankle dorsiflexion and stretch the Achilles tendon and plantar fascia. Physical therapy modalities such as ultrasound may be helpful as well.

HELPFUL TIP: Not all heel pain is plantar fasciitis. Remember tarsal tunnel syndrome (described above), painful heel pad syndrome (pain located over the heel secondary to breakdown of fibrous septae from overuse and which may take up to 6 months to heal), and piezogenic papules (pain over medial/inferior aspect of heel, tender papules noted when patient standing).

Objectives: Did you learn to . . .

● Diagnose plantar fasciitis and consider other causes of heel and foot pain?
● Describe the natural history of and treatments for plantar fascitis?

QUICK QUIZ: HAND INJURIES

A "gamekeeper's thumb" would likely be seen as the result of which of the following injuries?

A) Fall on an outstretched hand.
B) Crush injury, for example, between two pieces of machinery.
C) Fall by a skier using a ski pole.
D) Excessive electronic gaming (eg, Nintendo, XBOX).
E) Fall from a mountain bike.

Discussion

The correct answer is "C." A gamekeeper's thumb is defined as an injury (partial or complete tear) of the ulnar collateral ligament of the first metacarpophalangeal joint. This injury can occur with hyperextension of the thumb, as happens when falling with a ski pole. These injuries do well with casting or surgery in the event of a very unstable joint. The term "gamekeeper's thumb" comes from the injury occurring more often in gamekeepers when twisting the neck of fowl after hunting.

QUICK QUIZ: FRACTURES

The most specific finding on radiograph for a radial head fracture is:

A) Anterior fat pad sign.
B) Posterior fat pad sign.
C) Trousseau sign.
D) Medial fat pad sign.

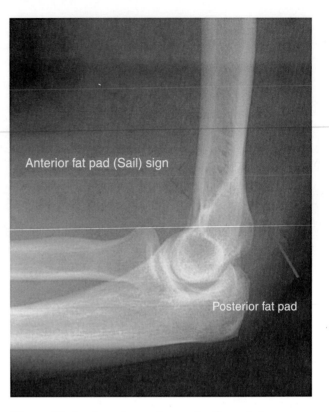

Figure 12–8   Anterior and posterior fat pads in a radial head fracture.

Discussion

The correct answer is B. The posterior fat pad sign, which indicates an effusion in the joint, is the most **specific** of the findings for a radial head fracture. An **anterior** fat pad sign is the most sensitive. Figure 12–8 demonstrates both the anterior and posterior fat pad signs. There is no medial fat pad sign, and Trousseau sign is related to hypocalcemia and is carpal spasm with arterial occlusion (as with a blood pressure cuff).

QUICK QUIZ: RADIAL HEAD FRACTURE

The proper treatment of a nondisplaced, fractured radial head is:

A) Internal fixation.
B) Sling with early mobilization.
C) Short arm cast.
D) Long arm cast.

Discussion

The correct answer is B. For a nondisplaced radial head fracture, the treatment is a sling for comfort and early mobilization. Mobilization is especially important to avoid a stiff elbow.

CASE 20

A 45-year-old female hospital clerk presents with bilateral aching pain in the forearms and thenar eminences. The pain is made worse with driving and typing. She also has intermittent numbness over the same areas. She tried to ignore the symptoms, but today she dropped her coffee mug on her computer keyboard and became alarmed at her loss of strength. She has hypothyroidism and is obese, but she reports that her health is otherwise good.

Based on the history alone, which of the following is the most likely diagnosis?

A) Carpal tunnel syndrome.
B) Osteoarthritis.
C) Ulnar neuropathy.
D) Diabetic neuropathy.

Discussion

The correct answer is A. Carpal tunnel syndrome results from median nerve entrapment in the carpal tunnel of the wrist. Typical symptoms include numbness, paresthesias, and pain at the palmar/radial aspect of the hand, quintessentially the thenar eminence. In more severe or long-lasting cases, you may see atrophy of the thenar eminence. Patients may also develop weakness of thumb opposition. Ostoearthritis of the wrists (answer B) does not usually cause nerve symptoms but can cause spondylosis and nerve root impingement on occasion. Ulnar neuropathy (answer C) involves the ulnar aspect of the arm, rather than the radial aspect, which is involved with carpal tunnel syndrome. Diabetic neuropathy (answer D) typically presents in the feet since they are innervated by the longest nerves in the body. **This could represent cervical disc disease as well, especially given that it is bilateral.**

* *

Phalen sign is positive (placing the wrists in a flexed position causes aching and numbness in the median nerve distribution).

What is the best next step in the continuing evaluation and management of this patient?

A) Nerve conduction studies.
B) Radiograph of the wrist.
C) MRI of the cervical spine.
D) Orthopedic referral.
E) Initiation of treatment.

Discussion

The correct answer is E. In a clear-cut case of carpal tunnel syndrome, there is no need for further studies. If the diagnosis is in doubt, EMG/nerve conduction studies may be of benefit. If the ROM in the wrist is limited, x-rays may be helpful. MRI and orthopedic referral now are not likely to add much.

Which of the following is NOT associated with carpal tunnel syndrome?

A) Hypothyroidism.
B) Diabetes mellitus.
C) Amyloidosis.
D) Polycythemia vera.
E) RA.

Discussion

The correct answer is D. All of the above are associated with carpal tunnel syndrome except for polycythemia vera. Polycythemia vera can cause a painful condition of the hands called erythromelalgia which is a burning pain of the hands and feet associated with erythema, pallor or cyanosis. It responds to aspirin. Other conditions associated with carpal tunnel syndrome include pregnancy, menopause, obesity, acromegaly, and end-stage renal disease. A patient with carpal tunnel syndrome should have a systemic cause ruled out either clinically or with labs.

What is the most appropriate initial treatment?

A) Thumb spica splint.
B) Steroid injection.
C) NSAIDs and neutral position wrist splints.
D) Short arm casts.

Discussion

The correct answer is C. Conservative therapy should be initiated first, unless there is a compelling reason for more aggressive therapy (eg, severe weakness of the hands and loss of function). Most patients respond well to NSAIDs and the use of neutral position splints. The traditional cock-up splints are not as effective as neutral position splints. The splints should be worn at night. The patient may wear the splints during the day, too, but should take them off for several hours per day to avoid disuse muscle atrophy. Answer A is incorrect because a thumb spica is not needed. Answer B, steroid injection, might be tried if initial conservative measures fail. If you choose to perform a steroid injection, **avoid injecting steroids directly into the median nerve.** Answer D is incorrect—do not cast patients with carpal tunnel syndrome!

 HELPFUL TIP: Oral steroids have been used for carpal tunnel with limited success. Most modalities (NSAIDs, splints, steroids, etc) are no better than placebo in randomized trials.

 HELPFUL TIP: Phalen and Tinel signs are crude tools at best. Tinel sign, which is a painful sensation of the fingers induced by percussion of the median nerve at the level of the palmar wrist, may be positive, but is only 50% sensitive and 54% specific. Phalen sign, keeping both wrists in a palmar-flexed position, may reproduce symptoms. Sensitivity ranges from 10% to 88% depending on study; its specificity is 80%.

Objectives: Did you learn to . . .

- Diagnose carpal tunnel syndrome and consider other causes of wrist pain?
- Manage a patient with carpal tunnel syndrome?

 QUICK QUIZ: CASTING

A few days ago, your partner placed a cast on the arm of a 20-year-old male for a distal radial fracture. The patient calls your office today, when your partner has gone fishing. The patient has complaint of increasing pain and numbness of his fingers in the casted arm.

Which course of action is most appropriate?

A) Have the patient follow up tomorrow, when your partner is back in the office.

B) Send the patient to the ED for compressive Doppler exam of the arm to rule out venous thrombosis.

C) Ask the patient to come to clinic to have the cast replaced.

D) Tell the patient that these are expected symptoms and advise him to take some aspirin.

Discussion

The correct answer is C. This patient has symptoms that are most likely due to an improperly fitted cast. The problem could be vascular compromise, nerve compression, or a compartment syndrome. He should be seen without delay, and the cast should be adjusted or replaced. The cast can be bivalved or have a window cut into it.

BIBLIOGRAPHY

Adkin SB. Hip pain in athletes. *Am Fam Physician.* 2000;61(7):2109.

DeLee JC, Drez D, et al, eds. *Orthopaedic Sports Medicine Principles and Practice.* 2nd ed. St. Louis: W.B. Saunders; 2003.

Griffin LY, et al, eds. *Essentials of Musculoskeletal Care.* 3rd ed. Rosemont, IL: American Academy of Orthopaedic Surgeons; 2005.

Kindale S. Evaluation and treatment of acute low back pain. *Am Fam Physician.* 2007;75(8):1181.

Leet AI. Evaluation of the acutely limping child. *Am Fam Physician.* 2000;61(4):1011.

Margaretten ME, Kohlwes J, Moore D, Bent S. Does this adult patient have septic arthritis? *JAMA.* 2007 Apr 4; 297(13):1478.

McGillicuddy DC, Shah KH, Friedberg RP, Nathanson LA, Edlow JA. How sensitive is the synovial fluid white blood cell count in diagnosing septic arthritis? *Am J Emerg Med.* 2007 Sep;25(7):749.

Phillips TG, Reibach AM, Slomiany WP. Diagnosis and management of scaphoid fractures. *Am Fam Physician.* 2004;70(5):879.

Steill IG, Greenberg GH, Wells GA, et al: Prospective validation of a decision rule for the use of radiography in acute knee injuries. *JAMA.* 1996;275:611.

Wilson JJ, Best TM. Common overuse tendon problems: a review and recommendations for treatment. *Am Fam Physician.* 2005;72(5):811.

Wolfe MW, Uhl TL, McCluskey LC. Management of ankle sprains. *Am Fam Physician.* 2001;63:93.

Woodward TW. The painful shoulder: part II. Acute and chronic disorders. *Am Fam Physician.* 2000;61(1):3291.

13

Pediatrics

Jason K. Wilbur

CASE 1

You have just delivered a term male infant born via normal spontaneous vaginal delivery to a 28-year-old G2 P2 married female. There was spontaneous rupture of membrane 2 hours prior to delivery. Thick particulate meconium was noted. The infant is brought under the radiant warmer where he appears peripherally cyanotic. He is crying and moving vigorously, and his heart rate is 160 beats per minute.

Which one of the following is the most appropriate next step in the resuscitation of this infant?

A) Perform bulb suction of the oropharynx and nasopharynx.
B) Proceed with routine neonatal evaluation and observe since the infant is vigorous.
C) Proceed with routine neonatal evaluation and observe since the infant should have been suctioned at the perineum before delivery of the shoulders.
D) Provide positive pressure ventilation via bag-valve mask.
E) Under direct visualization, suction the trachea via an endotracheal tube to remove any meconium below the vocal cords.

Discussion

The correct answer is B. The recommendations have changed with the publication of the 2005 AHA/AAP Neonatal Resuscitation Program guidelines. Although the presence of meconium in the amniotic fluid should alert the caregiver to the possibility of neonatal distress,

a vigorous infant is a good sign and further intervention is not warranted. Answers A and C are of special note. **Routine suctioning of the nose and mouth as the head is delivered is no longer recommended because it does not reduce the risk of meconium aspiration syndrome.** In the presence of meconium-stained fluid, suctioning is recommended if the infant has a low heart rate (<100 bpm), depressed respirations, or poor muscle tone. In an infant with one or more of these signs of distress, suctioning should be performed. Prior to drying, the infant should have visible, residual meconium removed from the nose and mouth by bulb suction. Then, under direct visualization, the trachea should be suctioned with an appropriately sized endotracheal tube. The infant in this case is clearly vigorous and should receive routine care (standard positioning, warming, etc).

 HELPFUL TIP: Overvigorous suctioning can lead to a vagally mediated bradycardia in neonates.

* *

At 1 minute his heart rate is 160 beats per minute. The infant continues to have some peripheral cyanosis. He appears to be breathing easily and demonstrates good tone. He grimaces and pulls away with stimulation.

What is the infant's 1-minute Apgar score?

A) 10
B) 9

435

C) 8
D) 7
E) 6

Discussion

The correct answer is B. The Apgar score is an objective measure of the newborn's condition. It is routinely determined at 1 and 5 minutes after birth. An Apgar of 8 or higher is normal; if the Apgar is 7 or lower, further evaluation is warranted. However, the Apgar score is not used to determine the need for resuscitation. The initiation and course of resuscitation are primarily determined by respiration, heart rate, tone, and color, assessed individually rather than as an overall score. The Apgar score is assigned as shown in Table 13–1.

CASE 2

You are having a busy day on labor and delivery. In the next room, a male infant born at 35 weeks' gestation is brought to the radiant warmer bed. The amniotic fluid was clear and labor was uncomplicated. Despite drying and stimulation, he appears cyanotic. He is noted to have gasping respirations and a heart rate of 110 beats per minute.

What is the most appropriate next step in the resuscitation of this neonate?

A) Begin positive pressure ventilation with a bag-valve mask.
B) Continue tactile stimulation and drying only.
C) Open the airway via positioning and bulb suctioning.
D) Perform endotracheal intubation to ensure adequate ventilation.
E) Provide free-flow oxygen via an oxygen mask.

Discussion

The correct answer is C. After the infant is brought to the radiant warmer, drying and stimulation are performed immediately. This is followed by clearing of the airway via positioning the infant with the neck in a neutral position ("sniffing position"). The oropharynx and nasopharynx are then suctioned. In the majority of newborns who require resuscitation, proper attention to these steps will lead to the establishment of spontaneous respirations and improvement in heart rate and color.

* *

Despite proper opening of the airway and tactile stimulation, the infant continues to have poor respiratory effort and central cyanosis. His heart rate has dropped to 90 beats per minute.

What is the next appropriate step in the resuscitation of this neonate?

A) Begin chest compressions.
B) Begin positive pressure ventilation with a bag-valve mask.
C) Continue tactile stimulation and drying only.
D) Perform endotracheal intubation to ensure adequate ventilation.
E) Provide free-flow oxygen via an oxygen mask.

Discussion

The correct answer is B. Despite establishing an open airway, the neonate continues to require further resuscitation. This is based on the absence of strong, spontaneous respirations and a drop in the heart rate <100 beats per minute. Both are indications for initiation of positive pressure ventilation with a bag-and-mask. If this infant had a heart rate >100 beats per minute but persistent central cyanosis, supplemental oxygen would have been the next step.

Table 13–1   APGAR SCORE

	0	1	2
Heart rate	Absent	<100 bpm	>100 bpm
Color	Cyanotic	Peripheral cyanosis	Pink
Tone	Limp	Some flexion	Active motion
Reflex irritability	None	Grimace	Cough/sneeze/retracts
Respirations	Absent	Weak cry	Strong cry

What is the appropriate rate (breaths per minute) to begin ventilating the infant?

A) 10–20
B) 20–40
C) 40–60
D) 60–80
E) 80–90

Discussion

The correct answer is C. When a seal between the mask and the infant is ensured, ventilation should start with an initial breath of >30 cm H_2O followed by normal breaths of 15–20 cm H_2O; check to see chest wall rise with each breath. Ventilation should occur at a rate of 40–60 breaths per minute. An orogastric tube should be inserted after several minutes of bag-and-mask ventilation.

 HELPFUL TIP: Most "pop off" valves used for positive pressure ventilation are set to release at 30–40 mm Hg. Since the initial breaths may require a pressure >30 mm Hg, it may be necessary to occlude the valve for the first few breaths. Once the lungs are inflated, the pop-off valve may be allowed to function normally to prevent barotrauma.

* *

After 30 seconds of ventilation, the infant develops a strong respiratory effort. Heart rate has increased to 130 beats per minute. He continues to appear cyanotic.

What is the most appropriate next step in the resuscitation of this neonate?

A) Begin chest compressions.
B) Continue positive pressure ventilation with a bag-valve mask.
C) Discontinue positive pressure ventilation and provide free-flow oxygen via an oxygen mask.
D) Perform endotracheal intubation to ensure adequate ventilation.
E) Stop positive pressure ventilation and observe.

Discussion

The correct answer is C. If the heart rate has increased to >100 beats per minute and the infant is breathing spontaneously, positive pressure ventilation may be stopped. Due to the persistent central cyanosis, free-flow oxygen should be continued. Once the infant becomes pink, oxygen may gradually be withdrawn. The infant must be reassessed frequently to ensure that respirations, heart rate, and color are appropriate.

* *

The infant becomes more vigorous with a strong respiratory effort, and his cyanosis resolves.

Indications for initiating chest compressions during neonatal resuscitation, include(s):

A) Heart rate <60 bpm despite adequate ventilation.
B) Heart rate <80 bpm that does not increase despite adequate ventilation.
C) Heart rate of 90 bpm that appears to be increasing with ventilation.
D) All of the above.
E) None of the above.

Discussion

The correct answer is A. Chest compressions should be started on the infant with a heart rate <60 beats per minute despite adequate positive pressure ventilation (assessed via chest wall movement and adequate breath sounds) for 30 seconds. The compression site is between the xiphoid and nipple level at the lower third of the sternum. Each compression should depress the sternum one-third of the anterior-posterior diameter of the chest. Two hands should be used in either of the following manners: (1) two fingers used to compress the sternum while one hand supports the back, or (2) two thumbs used to compress the sternum with the fingers wrapped around the infant's torso. The rate is 3:1 compression:ventilation (90 chest compressions to 30 respirations per minute). If the heart rate is between 60–100 bpm, positive pressure ventilation should be continued while the heart rate is reassessed every 30 seconds. Continue positive pressure ventilation until the heart rate is >100 and spontaneous respirations have been established.

Indication(s) for administering epinephrine during neonatal resuscitation include which of the following?

A) Heart rate of zero.
B) Heart rate <60 beats per minute after 30 seconds of positive pressure ventilation and chest compressions.
C) Heart rate of 100 beats per minute despite administering epinephrine 5 minutes earlier.

D) A and B.

E) All of the above.

Discussion

The correct answer is D. Epinephrine should be administered to an infant with a heart rate of zero and if the heart rate remains <60 beats per minute despite performing chest compressions for 30 seconds. In both instances, ventilation must be assured (with 100% oxygen) as determined by chest wall movement and auscultation demonstrating good air entry. In the severely depressed infant, endotracheal intubation should be performed and the stomach decompressed via nasogastric tube placement. Epinephrine may then be given via endotracheal route until vascular access is obtained. The correct epinephrine dose is 0.1–0.3 mL/kg of 1:10,000 concentration, either IV or via ET tube (can also give 0.3–1 mL/kg for ET tube). It may be diluted in 1–2 mL of normal saline if giving via the ETT. If the heart rate remains <60 beats per minute, epinephrine may be readministered every 3 to 5 minutes. If the heart rate is not improving, consider volume expansion (10 mL/kg of 0.9% saline) if there is evidence or suspicion of acute blood loss with signs of hypovolemia.

 HELPFUL TIP: Administration of drugs via ET tube is second-line. An umbilical vein catheter or peripheral line is preferred if possible.

Objectives: Did you learn to . . .

- Describe indications for endotracheal suction for infants exposed to meconium-stained amniotic fluid?
- Describe the indications for providing free-flow oxygen?
- Describe the indications for initiating and stopping positive pressure ventilation?
- Describe the indications for initiating chest compressions?
- Describe the indications for administering epinephrine and fluids?

CASE 3

Amy, a 4-day-old female, comes to clinic because "she is yellow." She was born at term to a 25-year-old married woman. Maternal labs are as follows: blood type A +, RPR nonreactive, rubella immune, Group B Strep negative. Amy has been breast-feeding every 3 to 5 hours. She has had 1 stool and 3 urine diapers a day. Stools are transitional. On your exam you notice jaundice from the head to the thighs. Her total bilirubin level is 25.2 mg/dL. The conjugated (direct) fraction is 0.4 mg/dL.

Which of the following statements is true?

A) She has breast-feeding failure jaundice.

B) She has physiologic jaundice.

C) She has biliary atresia; you must consult pediatric gastroenterology.

D) There is an ABO incompatibility between the mother and child.

Discussion

The correct answer is A. Amy most likely has **breast-feeding failure jaundice.** This occurs within the first several days of birth before the mother's milk supply is adequate. This must be distinguished from **breast milk jaundice** which can occur in the same time frame. One sign that Amy is not receiving adequate breast milk feedings—and this is breast-feeding failure jaundice **not** breast milk jaundice—is that she is having fewer than 6 wet diapers per day and fewer than 2 to 5 stools a day. You should try to evaluate the mother's milk supply by asking about the mother's feeling of engorgement, if she feels her breasts empty with feeding, and if she hears the baby swallow with feedings. Checking the patient's weight is an important part of the evaluation; watch for an increase in the baby's weight.

Answer B is incorrect. Even though physiologic jaundice peaks at this age, the level of 25.2 mg/dL is higher than would be expected with physiologic jaundice (not higher than 13 mg/dL in a term infant). Answer C is incorrect because biliary atresia presents with conjugated hyperbilirubinemia and thus would not be considered in Amy's case. Answer D is incorrect because ABO incompatibility is unlikely in a mother whose blood type is other than O. Additionally, Rh incompatibility is impossible because the mother is Rh +.

All of the following are risk factors for severe neonatal hyperbilirubinemia EXCEPT:

A) Exclusive breast feeding.

B) Gestational age ≥41 weeks.

C) Significant birth trauma.

D) Visible jaundice in first 24 hours of life.

Discussion

The correct answer is B. A major risk factor for severe hyperbilirubinemia in term and near-term infants is lesser gestational age, not greater gestational age. The other answer choices are true statements. Answer A is true because infants who are exclusively formula-fed are less likely to have severe hyperbilirubinemia (but this is not a reason to recommend bottle feeding). Answer C is true because cephalohematoma and large bruises result in increased bilirubin production from heme breakdown. The earlier jaundice occurs, the higher the peak is likely to be, so answer D is true. Other major risk factors for severe hyperbilirubinemia include a sibling who required phototherapy, East Asian race, and blood group incompatibility.

 HELPFUL TIP: Infants with total serum bilirubin levels >5 mg/dL typically have visible jaundice. The jaundice usually starts at the head and progresses distally to the feet. It resolves in the opposite pattern with the distal extremities resolving first.

* *

Amy's CBC is unremarkable and blood type is A +.

Which of the following is the most appropriate initial treatment for this patient?

A) Admission for exchange transfusion.
B) Admission for IV fluids.
C) Admission for phototherapy.
D) Discharge to home with recommendations for formula feeding, light exposure, and follow-up bilirubin tomorrow.

Discussion

The correct answer is C. Amy should be treated with intensive phototherapy with her level of hyperbilirubinemia. Answer A is incorrect because phototherapy should be employed first and an exchange transfusion would follow if phototherapy failed to lower the bilirubin level. Exchange transfusion is recommended for term infants >72 hours old who have total bilirubin levels >30 mg/dL. Answer B is incorrect because this patient does not show signs of dehydration requiring IV fluids, and IV fluids will not do much for the hyperbilirubinemia. Answer D is incorrect because this patient needs intensive phototherapy.

Decisions regarding treatment vary depending on the infant's risk, age (in hours after delivery), gestational age, and total bilirubin level. Graphs, tables, and nomograms are available to assist with decision making. Decision-making software is available at: http://www.babydoc.co.il/article-364.htm.

* *

You admit Amy for further management, and you formulate a plan. On admission, you check Amy's weight, which is down about 200 g from birth (about 5%). Children often lose about 10% of their weight after birth.

When is it considered problematic if the patient has not returned to his or her birth weight?

A) 5 days.
B) 7 days.
C) 10 days.
D) 14 days.
E) None of the above. Don't worry, be happy.

Discussion

The correct answer is D. Children should regain their birth weight by 2 weeks. Anything beyond this is reason for concern.

* *

Amy does well and is discharged after 2 days of phototherapy. She is back to breast-feeding when she returns for her 2-month well-child exam. The mother reports discharge, clear or white, from Amy's right eye. Amy has otherwise been healthy without ill symptoms or fever. Her conjunctivae are clear.

What is the diagnosis and treatment of choice for Amy's eye?

A) Conjunctivitis: Culture before treatment.
B) Conjunctivitis: Treat with antibiotic eye drops.
C) Lacrimal duct obstruction: Refer to ophthalmology for probing to prevent problems with conjunctivitis in the future.
D) Lacrimal duct obstruction: Teach the parents duct massage and refer to ophthalmology if the duct has not opened >1 year.
E) Normal eye: No treatment necessary.

Discussion

The correct answer is D. Congenital lacrimal duct obstruction occurs in estimated 5% of newborns. Patients often present with tearing, crusting, and mucoid discharge of the eyes. These patients are at increased risk of developing conjunctivitis and cellulitis. Usual treatment is conservative with duct massage and referral to an ophthalmologist if the obstruction lasts longer than one year. Whether or not massage adds anything to the treatment is a matter of debate. However, it gives the parents something to do while nature effects a cure. Antibiotic drops should be given when conjunctivitis occurs (conjunctival injection and mucopurulent discharge). Culture of the discharge is not generally necessary.

 HELPFUL TIP: Congenital glaucoma can also cause excessive tearing but it is much less common than lacrimal duct obstruction and presents with corneal enlargement and corneal clouding.

* *

You teach Amy's mother duct massage and plan to check in on the symptoms when Amy is 4–6 months old. Mom questions the need for immunizations during the well-child exam "since we never see these archaic diseases anymore." She has read information on the Internet and has concerns about immunization safety. And there was a TV drama about a kid who suffered autism because of thimerosal in a vaccine. Amy's mother's concerns are not unusual. Parents often bring up misconceptions about vaccinations.

What common side effect might Amy have after her immunizations at THIS visit?

A) Fever to 104°F.
B) Autism.
C) Diabetes.
D) Erythema at the site of immunization.
E) Shedding of virus in her stool.

Discussion

The correct answer is D. Vaccine side effects, such as **low-grade fevers** (not to 104°F as in answer A), induration and redness at the site, and fussiness are common. However, they are self-limited. Answers B and C are incorrect. Autism and diabetes have not been linked to vaccines in large, well-designed studies. Answer E is incorrect because the DTaP, HIB, and IPV vaccines are inactivated. Thus, the virus or bacteria is killed and purified for a specific component. The hepatitis B vaccine is constructed with genetic engineering in a yeast cell. Thus one would not shed virus in the stool. The MMR, oral polio, and varicella vaccines are

live attenuated vaccines. With these immunizations, the virus has been weakened but can still replicate and be shed in stool. Answer E is incorrect because this is a 2-month checkup and the patient will not receive these immunizations.

* *

Amy's mother accepts that advice but still has concerns.

What other true information can you share with her about vaccines?

A) Giving a child multiple vaccines at the same time weakens her immune system.
B) The fever and rash side effects of the MMR caused by the measles component usually occurs 1 week after the vaccine is given.
C) If Amy receives her MMR at a 9-month visit (before she travels to visit Aunt Tilley who lives in Outer Mongolia), her MMR immunization would be considered complete after this dose and another one at 5 years of age.
D) If Amy had an acute otitis media and fever of 100.4°F, we should delay her immunizations until she is afebrile.
E) Immunizations are not important because these diseases are rare in the United States.

Discussion

The correct answer is B. The measles component can cause a fever and rash 5–10 days after the immunization. This occurs in 5%–15% of infants. Up to 25% of adult women may have arthralgias after the vaccine. The MMR dosing schedule includes 2 doses of MMR. Answer C is incorrect. The first must be **after** 1 year of age. It may be given sooner if the child is at risk (such as with travel or with a measles outbreak) but must be repeated after the first birthday. Answer A is incorrect; there is no evidence that multiple vaccines given at the same time weaken the immune system. Answer D is incorrect. Minor illnesses should not prevent vaccination. True contraindications include anaphylactic reactions to a vaccine or vaccine constituent, moderate to severe febrile illness, and encephalopathy within 7 days of DTP. Answer E is incorrect as we do have outbreaks of many vaccine preventable diseases in the US every year.

* *

Amy's mother consents to vaccines after a lengthy discussion about the common misconceptions regarding vaccines and ways to evaluate information on the Internet. Amy continues her scheduled well-child exams. At one of those visits she was babbling and crawling around the office. She poked her fingers at the outlet covers and could use a pincer grasp to pick up a raisin.

These behaviors are developmentally appropriate for a child at age:

A) 6 months.
B) 9 months.
C) 15 months.
D) 24 months.

Discussion

The correct answer is B. Nine-month-old children can respond to their own name, babble with possible non-specific "mama" and "dada," crawl, creep, sit unsupported, poke with fingers, bang objects, and throw objects. They enjoy peekaboo and may have some stranger anxiety. Six-month-olds can sit with support, grasp and mouth objects, and transfer objects. They can rake small objects, squeal, and blow raspberries. Twelve-month-olds can pull to stand, cruise, and take a few steps alone. They enjoy pat-a-cake and waving "bye-bye." They can say 1–5 words with meaning. Fifteen-month-olds can say 3–6 words and point to body parts. They can walk well and stoop to pick up an object. They can stack two blocks and feed self with fingers.

* *

Amy is 9 months old and 25 pounds. Part of your anticipatory guidance is about child restraint systems to keep Amy safe.

Which of the following is a true statement about childhood injuries and car seats you can discuss with the parents?

A) Unintentional injury is the largest cause of death of children under 14 years.
B) Nine out of 10 car seats are used properly.
C) Amy may use a forward-facing convertible car seat now.
D) A rear infant seat may be placed in front of an airbag as long as it is rear-facing.
E) Nine-year-olds may ride in the front seat.

Discussion

The correct answer is A. Educating about car seats and childhood injury is an important part of anticipatory guidance. Unintentional injury is the largest cause of death in children with motor vehicle crashes being the leading cause of unintentional injury. Car seats are a very cost-effective way to prevent injury and death in children. Answer B is incorrect. Nine out of 10 car seats are used **incorrectly**. Answer C is incorrect. A child <1 year **and** <20 pounds needs to be in a rear-facing car seat. After the child is 1 year old **and** 20 pounds, she may switch to a forward-facing car seat. A child >40 pounds may switch to a booster seat but remain in a booster seat until an adult seat belt fits appropriately (at 60–80 pounds). Answer D is incorrect. A child should **not** sit in front of an airbag; especially not an infant seat that is rear-facing. Answer E is incorrect. A child <12 years should sit in the back seat.

* *

Amy continues her scheduled well-child exams. However, at 14 months old, her mother brings Amy for a sick visit because she turned blue. You appropriately diagnose breath-holding spells after taking a complete history and physical exam.

Which of the following statements about breath-holding spells is true?

A) The incidence of breath-holding spells for children between 6 months old and 6 years old is 50%.
B) If a color change occurs, it occurs after loss of consciousness.
C) Seizure-like activity may occur with breath-holding spells.
D) A child typically takes 60–90 minutes to return to her baseline after a breath-holding spell.
E) The evaluation should include an echocardiogram and electroencephalogram (EEG).

Discussion

The correct answer is C. A typical breath-holding spell begins with an inciting event (like Santa did not bring the right toy). The child begins to cry, holds his or her breath, turns blue, and loses consciousness. After loss of consciousness some rhythmic jerking of the extremities may occur. The loss of consciousness is brief and the child returns quickly to normal activity. The differential diagnosis includes cardiac arrhythmias, seizures, and apnea. If the history is classic for breath-holding spells, no further evaluation is necessary. The treatment is parental reassurance. Parents should be encouraged to ignore the episodes and not to give in to the child's requests in an attempt to avoid the spells.

HELPFUL TIP: An ALTE (Apparent Life-Threatening Event). ALTE is nonspecific and is defined by what the parents observe: apnea, cyanosis, decreased responsiveness, etc. By the time they get to you the spell has generally resolved. There is no relationship between an ALTE and SIDS. Common causes of ALTEs include: GERD with choking (sputtering and cyanosis), seizures or breath-holding spells, CNS problems (bleeds, etc). Other etiologies to consider (which are far less common) include cardiac abnormalities/dysrhythmia, true airway obstruction, among others. Always consider child abuse in your differential. These spells should be taken seriously and evaluation should include laboratory testing (electrolytes, glucose, etc) and EKG. Home oxygen/bradycardia monitoring may be indicated depending on the history.

Between 12 and 15 months of age, Amy should receive all of the following vaccines, as per CDC recommendations, EXCEPT:

A) MMR.
B) Varicella.
C) Hepatitis A.
D) Rotavirus.
E) Influenza.

Discussion
The correct answer is D. Vaccination schedules and recommendations represent quickly moving targets, so a regular review is required to keep up to date. The Centers for Disease Control and Prevention (CDC) recommends initial MMR, varicella, and hepatitis A vaccinations for all U.S. children 12–15 months. Influenza recommendations are updated annually and have become progressively more inclusive. At the writing of this book, the CDC recommends that children 6 months to 18 years receive the influenza vaccine during the appropriate season. Of note, rotavirus vaccine should not be administered to children >32 weeks, and the first dose should not be given after 12 weeks.

**

Amy's breath-holding spells resolve by the time she is 3 years old, and she continues to grow and develop

normally. Amy's next issue comes when she is 5 years old and in your office for her prekindergarten physical. You notice a new murmur.

Which of the following suggests that this is a benign murmur?

A) Murmur is grade II/VI.
B) Murmur has a thrill.
C) Murmur radiates to the apex.
D) Murmur is diastolic.
E) Murmur is holosystolic.

Discussion
The correct answer is A. Not all murmurs need to be referred to a cardiologist. There are features that can help differentiate pathologic from benign murmurs. A murmur that is diastolic, grades IV–VI, pansystolic, or associated with cardiac symptoms is likely pathologic and requires further investigation. A benign murmur is systolic, soft (grades I–II, occasionally III), nonradiating, and short. A "benign" murmur is not a diagnosis of exclusion. You should try to make a decision about which innocent murmur it is. See Table 13–2.

**

On Amy's exam you hear a Grade III/VI **holosystolic** murmur in the pulmonic area with fixed splitting of the second heart sound. She is otherwise healthy without any cardiac symptoms.

Table 13–2 "BENIGN" CARDIAC MURMURS OF CHILDHOOD*

Still murmur: A grade I–III murmur heard best in the 2nd to 5th left intercostal interspace. It is a "musical," vibratory, or buzzing systolic ejection murmur which gets worse when the patient is supine and better when upright. A still murmur may get louder as blood flow increases with fever, exercise, or excitement.

Venous hum: A grade I–VI murmur heard best in the supraclavicular area. It should get better when the patient is recumbent or with pressure over the jugular vein.

Pulmonic murmur: Heard as a grade I–III systolic ejection murmur in the first half of systole. It is generally best heard in the 2nd left intercostal space.

*Murmurs that change with respiration are generally, but not always, benign.

What is the appropriate next step in management of this issue?

A) Family reassurance.
B) Endocarditis prophylaxis at the dental visit next week.
C) ECG and chest radiograph (CXR).
D) Limit physical activity.
E) Refer for immediate operative repair.

Discussion

The correct answer is C. Most likely, Amy has an ASD or atrial septal defect. The murmur is a holosystolic murmur heard best at the upper left sternal border. The murmur is caused by increased flow across the pulmonic valve creating a relative stenosis (more volume needs to get through a relatively fixed outlet) and **not** from flow across the ASD. The increased flow across the pulmonic valve causes a wide, fixed split S2. There may be a diastolic murmur at the lower left sternal border from flow across the tricuspid valve if the ASD is very large. The chest x-ray may demonstrate cardiomegaly with increased pulmonary vascular markings. The ECG might show mild right ventricular hypertrophy. Children with an ASD do **not** need endocarditis prophylaxis (except for the first 6 months after their surgical repair) and rarely need to limit their physical activity. If the ASD does not spontaneously close, and most small ASDs will do so by 5 years, then it is electively repaired by one of a variety of methods.

Consistent with the CDC recommendations, which of the following immunizations will you recommend for Amy at this visit (5 years old), assuming she has had all of her routine vaccines and no immunizations since she turned 2 years old?

A) MMR.
B) Varicella.
C) Td.
D) A and B.
E) A and C.

Discussion

The correct answer is D. Td should not be given at this age. Rather DTaP is recommended for children aged 4–6 years. The other recommended vaccines for this age group include boosters of varicella, MMR, and polio. Hepatitis A vaccine should be considered if not given between 12–23 months. Influenza vaccine should be administered according to age, risk, season, and potential for exposure.

Objectives: Did you learn to . . .

- Describe the causes of neonatal hyperbilirubinemia?
- Manage an infant with breastfeeding failure jaundice?
- Identify risk factors for severe hyperbilirubinemia?
- Discuss the differential diagnosis and treatment of lacrimal duct obstruction?
- Identify vaccine misconceptions, list MMR side effects, and identify contraindications to immunization?
- Recognize stages of infant development?
- Recognize the importance of child passenger safety?
- Describe and manage ALTEs?
- Differentiate benign from pathologic cardiac murmurs in childhood?
- Recommend vaccines for children in accordance with CDC guidelines?

 QUICK QUIZ: NEONATAL POLYCYTHEMIA

Causes of polycythemia (hematocrit of >65%–70%) in the immediate postpartum period include all of the following EXCEPT:

A) "Milking" the cord.
B) Twin-twin transfusion.
C) Congenital adrenal hyperplasia.
D) Diabetic mother.
E) Congenital hyperthyroidism.

Discussion

The correct answer is E. Neonatal polycythemia can be caused by all of the above except for congenital hyperthyroidism. Congenital **hypothyroidism** can cause neonatal polycythemia. Other causes of neonatal polycythemia include chronic intrauterine hypoxia (eg, mother is a heavy smoker), intrauterine growth restriction, and chromosomal abnormalities (eg, trisomy 21 and others).

 QUICK QUIZ: NEONATAL POLYCYTHEMIA

Patients with neonatal polycythemia are at risk for hyperviscosity syndrome including venous stasis and thrombosis, hypoxia, cyanosis, etc. Heart failure, stroke, and necrotizing enterocolitis may occur.

The best treatment for these patients is:

A) Phlebotomy.
B) Exchange transfusion with normal RBCs.
C) Exchange transfusion using D5W.
D) Exchange transfusion using normal saline.
E) Aspirin.

Discussion

The correct answer is D. Exchange transfusion using either normal saline, fresh frozen plasma, or albumin is the treatment of choice. Answer A is incorrect because phlebotomy will do nothing to reduce the hematocrit and can exacerbate the problem. Answer B is incorrect. If you chose this, back home for you! What is the point of taking out cells and then putting more in? Answer C is incorrect because large amounts of D5W can cause fluid shifts, electrolyte abnormalities, and hemolysis. Answer E is incorrect because aspirin will not do anything to reduce blood viscosity, which is the main problem. Of note, patients with a hematocrit of 65%–70% can be observed if they are asymptomatic. There is no direct relationship between hematocrit and blood viscosity.

 QUICK QUIZ: JAUNDICE

The current recommendation for the treatment of breast milk jaundice (not breast-feeding failure jaundice) is:

A) Continue to breast-feed.
B) Stop breast-feeding and change to a cow's milk formula.
C) Stop breast-feeding and change to soy milk formula.
D) Stop breast-feeding and treat with rehydration solution (eg, Pedialyte).

Discussion

The correct answer is A. Patients with hyperbilirubinemia resulting from breast milk jaundice should continue to breast-feed. Supplementation with a rehydration solution or small amounts of glucose water may be helpful.

CASE 4

A family has moved into the area and bring their 1-year-old girl in for a well child check. They bring her medical records with them. Her parents have no concerns, and she has been healthy. Her growth chart concerns you, however. Her length tracks along the 25th percentile. But her weight has gone gradually from the 25th to 50th percentile at 0–6 months, to the 10th percentile at 9 months, and is now at the 5th percentile at 1 year.

Which of the following most likely explains her pattern of growth?

A) It is normal. Her parents are petite. She is finding her destined genetic pattern of growth.
B) Familial short stature or constitutional delay.
C) IUGR or prenatal insult such as exposure to drugs or infection.
D) Hypothyroidism, growth hormone deficiency, or Cushing syndrome.
E) Feeding behaviors, lack of parental knowledge of infant feeding, or poverty.

Discussion

The correct answer is E. This patient's pattern of growth is most consistent with failure to thrive. The criteria for diagnosis include: weight below the 3rd to 5th percentile (depending on the source) **or** a fall of weight of >2 major percentile lines in 6 months, **or** weight <80% of ideal weight for age, **and/or** weight for height below the 5th percentile.

Answer A is incorrect because the patient meets more than one of these criteria. Answer B is incorrect because both height and weight would be affected. In this child, only the weight (and not the height) is affected. Answer C is incorrect because a child with a prenatal insult tends to be smaller globally in both height and weight, and the weight percentile would not be expected to drop so dramatically from birth. Answer D is incorrect because the endocrinologic causes listed create a child who stops gaining height but continues to gain weight. Therefore, answer E is the most likely cause of this patient's failure to thrive.

* *

Taking more history, you learn that the patient eats mostly rice and fruit. She does not like meat. She is picky. She drinks about 12 ounces of whole milk and 12 ounces of apple juice each day. She is active and developmentally appropriate. Her review of systems is negative as well as her past medical history.

What is the LEAST appropriate way to proceed with evaluation and management of this patient?

A) Allow the child to feed herself whenever she is hungry or thirsty. Parents should offer food and drink frequently throughout the day.

B) Obtain CBC, iron studies, and urinalysis.

C) Limit the amount of juice the child can have and limit it to meal times. Add extra calories to foods using butter, salad dressings, cheese, etc.

D) Consult with a nutritionist.

E) Prescribe a multivitamin.

Discussion

The correct answer (and least appropriate approach) is A. The goals of management of failure to thrive are to increase caloric intake, identify treatable causes of failure to thrive, and look for effects of her malnutrition. Thus, a CBC, iron studies, electrolytes, bicarbonate, glucose and urinalysis (answer B) may be helpful to investigate possible iron deficiency, anemia, or renal tubular acidosis. Juice should be limited, meals scheduled, and caloric intake boosted. Although children should feed themselves, they take in more calories when given a set schedule for meals and snacks instead of being allowed to graze on food or drink throughout the day (answer C). A nutritionist (answer D) can help educate the family on appropriate food choices for an infant and ways to boost calories. A child with a restrictive eating pattern, especially poor in iron containing foods, may benefit from a multivitamin with iron (answer E).

* *

Your patient presents to the ED at 15 months old. Her mother states that she has had several episodes of emesis over the last 48 hours and today began to have watery, foul-smelling diarrhea. Mother has lost track of number of episodes of emesis and diarrhea. She cannot tell if the child has had urine output because of the watery diarrhea.

On your exam the temperature is 102.5°F, heart rate 180, respiratory rate 50, blood pressure 80/50. Her weight is 8 kg. She has dry, cracked lips and dry skin. She lies in her mother's arms and is not very interested in your exam. Her capillary refill is about 4 seconds.

What is the most appropriate next step in the management of this patient's condition?

A) Evaluate for underlying bacterial source with blood, urine, and stool cultures.

B) Admit to an inpatient unit and begin maintenance IV fluids.

C) Infuse 20 cc/kg normal saline IV over 20 minutes.

D) Begin oral rehydration.

E) Infuse 10 cc/kg D5 1/2 normal saline over 2 hours.

Discussion

The correct answer is C. This patient is severely dehydrated (estimated 15%), and she should have fluid resuscitation quickly with a 20 cc/kg normal saline bolus. Although she might need admission, she should be stabilized in the ED before transfer to the inpatient unit. Answer B is incorrect because starting with maintenance fluids is inappropriate. Answer D is incorrect. Oral rehydration is cost-effective in less severe dehydration. However, because of the severity of dehydration, history of emesis, and likely acidosis, oral hydration would quickly fail and the attempt would delay her rehydration. There are several tables published listing the clinical exam with various degrees of dehydration. See Table 13–3 for symptoms of dehydration.

 HELPFUL TIP: Laboratory findings are variable in childhood dehydration. It is a clinical diagnosis, and the BUN/Cr ratio used in adults is not reliable in children. Signs and symptoms of dehydration are only 75% sensitive, so you need to have a high clinical suspicion in the proper patient.

* *

After completing the initial management, the patient is more interested in her surroundings. Her vital signs are now pulse 160, respiratory rate 36, and blood pressure 80/50. Her lips are still dry and she is still irritable. The capillary refill is 2–3 seconds. She is more interactive with her mother.

Table 13–3   SIGNS AND SYMPTOMS OF DEHYDRATION

Mild (<5%): Normal skin turgor, moist lips, tears present, normal vital signs, consolable

Moderate (10%): Dry skin and lips, slightly increased pulse, decreased urine output, normal capillary refill

Severe (15%): Parched lips, sunken eyes, decreased or no urine output, elevated pulse, prolonged capillary refill, lethargic or obtunded

What further treatment is indicated for her dehydration?

A) 80 cc/hour × 2 hours of D5 1/4 NS.

B) 33 cc/hour × 24 hours of D5 1/2 NS with 20 mEq KCl.

C) 50 cc/hour × 24 hours of D5 1/4 NS.

D) 20 cc/kg NS over 20 minutes.

E) 10 cc/kg D5 1/2 NS over 2 hours.

Discussion

The correct answer is D. After an initial bolus, the patient should be reassessed. This patient is still quite dehydrated. Although she has responded to her initial bolus of normal saline, she still has abnormal vital signs as well as signs of dehydration on exam. Therefore, the normal saline bolus should be repeated. Hyponatremic solutions (eg, 1/2 NS) or those containing glucose and/or potassium should never be used as a bolus. Also, potassium should be withheld until the patient urinates and has better hydration status.

 HELPFUL TIP: Maintenance fluids can be calculated using the Holiday-Segar method: Daily water needs for the first 10 kg of body weight is 100 mL/kg/day; water needs for 11–20 kg is 50 mL/kg/day; each additional kg over 20 kg is 20 mL/kg/day. Remember to account for dehydration, which will require additional fluids (usual weight – current weight in kg = water replacement in L over 24 hours). Also, replace ongoing losses from diarrhea, emesis, etc.

* *

The patient recovers well from her GI illness, but she returns a few months later to your clinic with a new illness. She has had temperatures of 103°F at home for 2–3 days. She has had no upper respiratory symptoms. Her oral intake has decreased, but she is maintaining good urine output. She has had no vomiting or diarrhea. Your exam reveals a febrile child who is slightly irritable. She is nontoxic and not dehydrated. Her oral cavity shows increased tonsil size with ulcers on her tongue and lips but not on the tonsillar pillars. Her anterior cervical lymph nodes are enlarged. The rest of her exam is noncontributory.

What is the most likely diagnosis?

A) Streptococcal pharyngitis.

B) Hand, foot, and mouth disease (Coxsackie virus).

C) Herpetic gingivostomatitis.

D) Varicella.

E) Infectious mononucleosis.

Discussion

The correct answer is C. Primary oral herpes (herpetic gingivostomatitis) is associated with a relatively high fever and anteriorly placed ulcerations (gums, tongue, and lips). Symptoms tend to start relatively abruptly with pain, salivation, refusal to eat, and fever. Herpes gingivostomatitis may recur during life in the form of "cold sores." Answer B is incorrect because the patient does not have hand and foot lesions. Varicella (answer D) can occur in the oral pharynx but would have lesions elsewhere in various stages and respiratory symptoms as well. Infectious mononucleosis (answer E) and streptococcal pharyngitis (answer A) are not associated with vesicular lesions or mucosal ulcerations.

 HELPFUL TIP: Herpangina (also known as aphthous stomatitis) is another consideration here. Herpangina tends to cause lower fevers (<102°F) than herpetic gingivostomatitis, is associated with fewer ulcers, and those that do occur are found on the posterior soft palate and tonsillar pillars and fossa. There are often other viral symptoms involved, such as headache, vomiting, or rhinorrhea. There may be additional lesions on the hands, feet, and buttocks.

CASE 5

Next, you see the patient's sister, aged 10 years, who presents for a school physical. Her mother is concerned because this patient has pubic hair, which her mother thinks is premature. On your exam she has enlarged areola and a small amount of breast tissue. She also has sparse, dark, but mostly straight pubic hair.

This patient is Tanner stage:

A) 1

B) 2

C) 3

D) 4

E) 5

Table 13–4 TANNER STAGES

Stage 1: Prepubertal
Stage 2: Sparse growth of hair at base of penis or along labia
- Girls: Breast bud development
- Boys: Enlargement of scrotum and testes with reddening and thickening of scrotal skin

Stage 3: Darkening, coarser hair sparsely in pubic area
- Girls: Enlargement of breasts
- Boys: Elongation of penis and increased size of testes

Stage 4: Adult pubic hair distribution but smaller area covered with no extension to medial thighs
- Girls: Areola and papilla begin to mound above the level of the breast
- Boys: Increase in breadth and development of penis, darkening of scrotal skin, enlargement of tests

Stage 5: Adult breasts, genitals, and hair distribution

Discussion

The correct answer is B. Breast buds and sparse pubic hair put the patient in Tanner stage 2. Tanner stage 1 is prepubertal. Any sign of puberty moves a child from Tanner 1 to Tanner 2. Tanner stage 5 is adult or fully matured secondary sexual characteristics. Table 13–4 lists Tanner stages.

* *

The mother has several questions about puberty. She is nervous about discussing sexual development with her daughter.

Which one is a developmental fact that you can provide mother?

A) Typically, in females, the first sign of puberty is pubic hair.
B) At 10 years, the patient is experiencing premature puberty.
C) The height spurt occurs early during puberty and is almost complete at menarche.
D) Menarche occurs approximately 1 year after breast budding.
E) Schools discuss puberty and relieve mother of that duty.

Discussion

The correct answer is C. In girls, the growth spurt occurs early and is almost complete at menarche. Female secondary sexual characteristics appear estimated 1–2 years before male characteristics. Answer A is incorrect because approximately 80%–85% of females begin puberty with breast development while only 10% have pubic hair development first. Answer B is incorrect. The average age of breast budding is 10.9 years. Thus, Sara is appropriate in her pubertal timing. Precocious puberty is diagnosed in a female with development of secondary sexual characteristics <8 years. Answer D is incorrect. Menarche typically begins 2 years after breast budding. Answer E is incorrect. Although schools may discuss puberty they are often limited in the time and content. It is important for the child to get information from mother about puberty and sex.

Objectives: Did you learn to . . .

- Define failure to thrive in a child?
- Evaluate a child with failure to thrive?
- Evaluate a dehydrated child and determine severity of dehydration?
- Manage dehydration in the ED?
- Calculate rehydration fluids for a dehydrated child?
- Generate a differential diagnosis for pharyngitis with blisters?
- Describe changes of puberty and Tanner staging in a female?

CASE 6

A 2-year-old male presents to your office with his father with complaint that the patient has had intermittent crying followed by episodes of profound lethargy during which he is difficult to arouse. The father relates that his son will sometimes clutch at his abdomen and roll into the fetal position during episodes. These episodes have been going on for about 4 hours. He has had no fever, no vomiting, and no diarrhea. Nobody else at home has been sick. The child is developmentally normal and has no significant past medical history. His exam reveals that he is afebrile and lethargic but can be aroused. His abdominal exam is benign. The rest of the exam is unremarkable.

Given his normal abdominal exam and lack of diarrhea, your working diagnosis is:

A) Meningitis.
B) Renal colic.
C) Intussusception.
D) Gastric outlet obstruction.
E) Appendicitis.

Discussion

The correct answer is C. The patient may have intussusception. The combination of abdominal colic **plus** mental status changes should suggest intussusception. The etiology of the mental status changes is not clear, but mental status changes are one of the classical findings of intussusception. Meningitis (answer A) should be a consideration in a patient with mental status changes, but abdominal pain is not usually part of the presentation. Additionally, the patient is afebrile and his symptoms are intermittent, making meningitis less likely. Renal colic (answer B) is not associated with mental status changes. Gastric outlet obstruction (answer D) and appendicitis (answer E) usually present with some abnormal findings on abdominal exam.

Which laboratory finding will help you confirm the diagnosis of intussusception?

A) CBC.
B) Urinalysis.
C) Glucose.
D) Serum lactate.
E) None of the above.

Discussion

"The correct answer is E". None of the above findings will help to make the diagnosis of intussusception. Early in the course, the CBC may be normal. Only 70% of patients will have heme positive stools early in the course.

 HELPFUL TIP: "Currant jelly stools" are a late finding in intussusception and are a reflection of mucosal ischemia. You want to make the diagnosis before you see "currant jelly" per rectum.

* *

Based on your history and physical, you decide that this patient has intussusception.

The next step in diagnosing and treating this patient is:

A) Upper GI with barium.
B) A plain film of the abdomen.
C) An air enema.
D) An abdominal ultrasound.
E) C or D.

Discussion

The correct answer is E. An air enema can be used to reduce the intussusception obviating the need for surgery. An ultrasound may show a typical "bull's eye" lesion. Answer A is incorrect. An upper GI will be of no use because intussusception is a distal process. Answer B is incorrect. A plain film of the abdomen will most likely be nondiagnostic as is the case in most abdominal processes (except perhaps bowel obstruction).

 HELPFUL TIP: For intussusception, an air enema is preferred over traditional barium enema. It can reduce the intussusception and has less risk of perforation with barium leaking into the peritoneum.

* *

The patient's intussusception reduces with an air enema.

Which of the following is the next step in the treatment of this patient?

A) Discharge to home since the process has been resolved.
B) Admission for IV antibiotics to treat any microperforation that may have occurred with the enema.
C) Discharge to home, planning for elective surgery to fix the area of intussusception to the posterior peritoneal cavity to prevent recurrence.
D) Admission to the hospital for observation.
E) Admission to the hospital with surgery within the next 24 hours to fix the area of intussusception to the posterior peritoneal cavity to prevent recurrence.

Discussion

The correct answer is D. No further treatment needs to be undertaken now or in the future if the patient does well. However, the patient should be admitted for observation for 24 hours. An estimated 25% of cases that are successfully reduced will recur within the first 24 hours, so observation is prudent.

 HELPFUL TIP: Although classic teaching is that majority of patients with intussusception will have a "lead point" (eg, a polyp, a patch from HSP, etc) that initiates the process of intussusception, only <10% of patients have a lead point. The old rotavirus vaccine was removed from the U.S. market because of intussusception, presumably resulting from the vaccine. The new vaccines (RotaTeq and Rotarix) do not appear to be associated with an increased risk of intussusception, but cautious use is recommended in patients with a history of intussusception.

Objectives: Did you learn to . . .

- Recognize the clinical presentation of intussusception?
- Evaluate and treat a child with intussusception?

 QUICK QUIZ: INFECTIOUS DIARRHEA

Which of the following organisms may be associated with diarrhea and mental status changes, including seizures (in the absence of severe dehydration or other metabolic cause for seizures)?

A) *Salmonella.*
B) *Cryptosporidium.*
C) *Giardia.*
D) *Campylobacter.*
E) *Shigella.*

Discussion
The correct answer is E. Through a toxin-mediated process, *Shigella* can cause fever, mental status changes, and seizures.

CASE 7

Benjamin, a 4-month-old male, presents to your office for a well-baby check. Parents have no concerns. Development and feeding are progressing as expected. On your exam his head is >95th percentile, but his weight and height are still at the 50th percentile. His previous head circumferences have been at the 50th percentile. He is a social infant but is having difficulty supporting his large head.

Which imaging study is LEAST likely to assist in the diagnosis of the macrocephaly?

A) X-ray.
B) CT scan.

C) MRI scan.
D) Ultrasound.

Discussion
The correct answer is A. Because the change of head size is so dramatic, an imaging study is needed, but skull radiographs are not likely to assist you in arriving at a diagnosis. The other modalities are used in this setting, and each has its benefits and detractions. Ultrasound or CT scan is frequently obtained first. Ultrasound offers the advantage of no radiation exposure, but it is limited in its application. Ultrasound is primarily used to assess fluid filled spaces (ventricles in hydrocephalus, subdural hematoma, etc). CT scan is a rapid and readily available test that can detect bleeds, intracranial calcifications, skull fractures, Chiari malformations, and more. CT is limited in its ability to delineate soft tissue problems, which is where MRI becomes important.

The differential diagnosis of macrocephaly is long and includes a premature infant showing catch-up growth, hydrocephalus, brain tumor, benign familial macrocephaly, neurocutaneous disorder (eg, neurofibromatosis, tuberous sclerosis), trauma, and metabolic disorders (eg, Tay-Sachs disease, mucopolysaccharidoses).

 HELPFUL TIP: Unfortunately, the amount of radiation in a single head CT scan in an infant of this age may affect cognitive development later. There are no controlled studies but radiation exposures at this level from other sources have been shown to adversely affect development.

* *

Benjamin had his CT scan, which shows subdural hematomas.

What is your next step in management of Benjamin?

A) Admit to the hospital.
B) Ophthalmological exam of eyes in an ophthalmologist's office.
C) "Babygram" to view entire skeleton of infant for fractures.
D) Alert the Department of Human Services within the next week.
E) Send the patient to a neurosurgeon's office for the next available appointment.

Discussion

The correct answer is A. Subdural hematomas in an infant are highly suspicious of abusive head trauma. Your first priority is to protect the child by admission to the hospital. A retinal exam and skeletal survey are important in the evaluation but are secondary to protection of the child.

Answer C is incorrect. A "babygram" should never be done to evaluate for skeletal trauma. There is a specific procedure for performing a skeletal survey for abuse. "Babygrams" miss more fractures than they find. More honed views are necessary to discern small fractures, especially at distal long bones. Answer D is incorrect. Your state agency responsible for investigating child abuse must be notified within **24 hours** (although clinicians are encouraged to know their legal responsibilities in the state in which they practice). Protection of the child is most important; if the family flees, calling the police or the appropriate state agency would be the first step. Answer E is incorrect. Suspicion of abuse, especially abusive head trauma, is an emergency, and it should not wait for a neurosurgeon's next available appointment.

 HELPFUL TIP: Retinal hemorrhages are **not** caused by seizures, falls, etc, and are essentially diagnostic of abuse. The exception is major motor vehicle trauma. Here, retinal hemorrhages can be seen but only in association with significant head trauma.

* *

As you have done in this case, radiologic studies should always be obtained in the evaluation of suspected child abuse. However, the cause of fractures has a broader differential than abuse.

Which patient's injuries and/or radiologic studies would be diagnostic of abuse?

A) A 9-month-old male with widened distal radius and ulna with fraying and cupping evident on radiograph.
B) A 21-month-old female with multiple fractures at different ages on radiograph. She has delayed tooth eruption and sparse hair.
C) A colicky 1-month-old male with callus on the left clavicle.

D) A 2-year-old female with a spiral fracture of the distal right tibia.
E) None of the above.

Discussion

The correct answer is E. None of these injuries is diagnostic of abuse. Although each of these children would make you think of possible abuse, none of them has been abused. Answer A is a child with rickets. Answer B is a child with osteogenesis imperfecta. Answer C is a child who sustained a clavicle fracture at birth. Answer D is a child with a "toddler fracture." A toddler fracture is a spiral tibial fracture found in children age 9–36 months (see Chapter 12, Orthopedics and Sports Medicine). These fractures are found in the distal one-third of the tibia. **Fractures in the mid-tibia are more likely to be from abuse.**

 HELPFUL TIP: Suspicious fractures include posterior rib fractures; fractures through the growth plate; spinal, scapular, or multiple fractures; fractures of different ages; fractures inconsistent with the developmental capabilities of the child; and corner fractures.

* *

Benjamin's evaluation shows bilateral subdural hemorrhages and retinal hemorrhages. His skeletal survey is negative. The state agency removes him from the home and places him in foster care. Benjamin then returns for his 6-month well-child exam. He has been in foster care since you last saw him. His vision is being followed by an ophthalmologist. He smiles and squeals. His foster mother says, "Looks like he's right-handed. Does that mean that he's advanced for his age?" He rolls both ways. He has started on rice cereal and bananas. He sleeps well.

On your exam he continues to have macrocephaly but a soft fontanelle. His left hand is fisted. The rest of the exam is unremarkable.

What is your assessment and plan for Benjamin?

A) Normal 6-month-old. Routine anticipatory guidance and immunizations.
B) Infant with history of head trauma. Delay pertussis vaccination.

C) Infant with history of head trauma. Perform Denver Developmental Screening Test (DDST) and document findings. Repeat in 3 months.

D) Hypertonic left upper extremity. Monitor progress at next well-child check.

E) Hypertonic left upper extremity. Refer for further evaluation and treatment of his delay.

Discussion

The correct answer is E. Benjamin has a risk of developmental delays as a result of his abusive head injury. He should be monitored closely for delays. One way to monitor for delays is by performing a screening test, such as the DDST. However, Benjamin has concerns that go beyond screening. The concerns are the tightly fisted left hand with corresponding favoring of his right hand. Early hand preference is a worrisome sign. Typically hand preference is not definite before 18–24 months. Hand preference should prompt the physician to examine the other extremity. In this patient there is hypertonicity resulting from his trauma. Any child with evidence of developmental delay should be referred for further evaluation. Some local and state agencies offer a free service to families to evaluate development and offer therapy. Do **not** watch and wait with a suspected delay. The earlier intervention begins, the better the outcome.

Objectives: Did you learn to . . .

- Recognize and evaluate macrocephaly in an infant?
- Generate a differential diagnosis of macrocephaly in an infant?
- Identify a child who is probably being abused?
- Determine when child abuse should be included in the differential diagnosis?
- Describe some aspects of developmental delay and its management?

CASE 8

A 5-year-old male presents to your clinic with his mother with a complaint of enuresis. Evidently, this child has **never** been completely continent at night, wetting his bed several times per week. This has become somewhat of a problem for him now that his friends are having sleep-over birthday parties. His mother confides that she is tired of paying for pull-ups

and cleaning sheets. His incontinence is monosymptomatic (ie, he is dry during the day and has only nocturnal symptoms).

What percent of 5-year-old males continue to have enuresis?

A) 5%
B) 10%
C) 15%
D) 20%
E) 25%

Discussion

The correct answer is C. An estimated 15% of males continue to have enuresis at 5 years. Even though this would suggest that it is a variant of normal, there is extreme social pressure on children this age to remain dry at night. Parental expectations are affected by their experience with other children. For example, if an older sibling was dry at night at 3 years or if a younger sibling is dry while an older child has enuresis, parents may not accept the bed-wetting as normal.

 HELPFUL TIP: Note that the child in this case is male. Enuresis affects twice as many males as females.

* *

Because he has had no period of nocturnal dryness, this patient has primary enuresis.

Which of the following is likely to be part of this child's history?

A) A family history of enuresis.
B) A stressful event in the family such as the birth of a new child or parental divorce.
C) Increased fluid intake over the past 2 months.
D) History of urinary tract infections.

Discussion

The correct answer is A. Enuresis is divided into primary and secondary enuresis. Primary enuresis exists when there is **never** a period of dryness at night. Secondary enuresis exists when there is a period of dryness (by convention, 6 months) but the patient then develops enuresis. Answers B, C, and D are more likely seen in children with **secondary** enuresis. Primary enuresis tends to be a familial trait.

 HELPFUL TIP: Approximately 15% of patients with enuresis become dry each year. The longer enuresis persists, the less likely it is to resolve; 1%–2% of patients >15 years continue to have primary enuresis.

* *

This patient's exam is essentially normal including neurologic evaluation.

Further evaluation of this patient should include all of the following EXCEPT:

A) Asking about a history of bowel problems.
B) Assessment of growth and development.
C) Investigation into family history of nocturnal enuresis.
D) Spine MRI to rule out pathologic lesion.
E) Urinalysis.

Discussion

The correct answer is D. Patients with enuresis who have an otherwise normal neurologic exam need not have an MRI done. If on exam this child had neurologic findings, an MRI would be indicated. All of the other answer choices are part of a thorough evaluation of nocturnal enuresis. Of special note is the assessment of growth and development (is this child neurologically delayed leading to enuresis?). Attention to bowel problems is also important. Fecal impaction can lead to incontinence.

* *

You find no indication of an underlying cause, and you decide that this is primary enuresis. The parents are desperate for some sort of intervention to fix the problem since it is becoming a major source of anxiety in the home and of teasing at school.

Which of the following has been shown to be effective in the treatment of primary enuresis?

A) Motivational training (eg, rewards for staying dry).
B) Bladder retention training (holding in urine in an attempt to stretch the bladder and increase capacity).

C) Enuresis alarms.
D) Pharmacologic therapy (eg, desmopressin and tricyclic antidepressants).
E) All of the above.

Discussion

The correct answer is E. All of the above are effective in the treatment of enuresis. Most of these modalities have about a 60%–80% success rate in reducing enuresis. Relapse is more common when pharmacologic therapy (answer D) is discontinued than with the other modalities. The treatment with the best long-term result is the enuresis alarm (answer C), but it relies on conditioning and therefore must be used regularly for an extended period of time until the child is reconditioned to wake when he needs to urinate. Another option for treatment is the use of a traditional alarm clock (or several alarm clocks), which prompts the child to awake and void.

Of particular note is answer B. Most children with enuresis have a small bladder capacity. Bladder retention training will improve enuresis in about 60% of patients and leads to complete nocturnal dryness in 35%. It is inexpensive and without significant side affects and is thus worth a try.

 HELPFUL TIP: Another option for the treatment of enuresis is fluid management. Have the child discontinue fluids after 5:00 p.m. or so. However, it is important that the child be able to meet all of his or her fluid needs. Thus, **increase** fluids during the rest of the day to compensate.

 HELPFUL TIP: Nasal DDAVP (desmopressin) is no longer approved for nocturnal enuresis due to problems with hyponatremia. Oral DDAVP still carries the enuresis indication, but it can cause hyponatremia—it just occurs less often.

Objectives: Did you learn to . . .

• Define primary and secondary enuresis?
• Describe the epidemiologic characteristics of enuresis?

- Evaluate a patient with enuresis?
- Develop a management strategy for enuresis?

 QUICK QUIZ: MECONIUM

Delayed meconium passage occurs in which of the following conditions?

A) Encopresis.
B) Hirschsprung disease.
C) Cystic fibrosis.
D) Hyperthyroidism.
E) B and C.

Discussion

The correct answer is E. Seventy percent of newborns will pass meconium within the first 12 hours of life. In those with delayed passage of meconium (generally >24 hours of life), consider Hirschsprung disease, cystic fibrosis, hypothyroidism, sepsis, intrauterine narcotic exposure, or imperforate anus.

CASE 9

An 8-year-old boy presents to the ED while you are on call. Within the last hour he had an unwitnessed fall off his scooter. He was not wearing a helmet or pads. His memory of the event is poor, and he is unsure if he lost consciousness. He has been confused, continually asking his mother about what happened and where he is. On your exam, vital signs are stable. His exam is remarkable for fracture of his secondary central incisors and abrasion of the upper lip. He has no other obvious trauma to his head. His elbows and forearms have abrasions. He is not oriented to place or time. He is definitely confused and cannot recall 3 objects. His neurologic exam is otherwise negative.

Which of the following is the most appropriate first step in his evaluation?

A) Skull films.
B) Observation of his mental status.
C) Head CT.
D) Dental evaluation.
E) Neuropsychology testing.

Discussion

The correct answer is C. All of the answer choices are part of his evaluation. However, a head CT should be first. Because of his level of confusion (and the presumption that he lost consciousness since he is amnestic and the injury was not witnessed), brain contusions and intracranial bleeding should be ruled out. Skull films are not necessary because the CT scan can detect fractures. Plus, one can have an intracranial injury with a normal CT scan. Likewise, a linear skull fracture does not mean that there is any intracranial injury. A dental exam is important but secondary to his head injury. Neuropsychology testing could be used after he has recovered from his initial trauma.

* *

There are no skull fractures, brain contusions, or intracranial hemorrhages on CT scan. He continues to be significantly confused and disoriented for about 5 hours after the event. He was amnestic for the time right before the event until after he arrived at the hospital. Using one of the various grading scales for concussion, this patient would be on the severe end of the scale because of his prolonged amnesia and altered mental status. Thankfully, the morning after the event his neurologic exam is normal.

When can this patient return to normal activity, sports, or using his scooter?

A) Today, since his symptoms are resolved.
B) In 1–2 weeks after a follow-up examination by his physician.
C) In 4 weeks after a follow-up examination by his physician.
D) He should be out of sports and activities for this season.
E) Whenever he learns to be more responsible and wear a helmet.

Discussion

The correct answer is B. Because grading scales of concussion differ, the guidelines differ about when to allow return to normal activities. It is reassuring that your patient's headache is gone and his mental status has normalized. However, he sustained a severe concussion and is at risk for "second impact syndrome." **Second impact syndrome** occurs when a child who has had a concussion suffers another blow to the head. The second blow may be trivial, such as occurs routinely during sports like football or soccer. Following this second—seemingly minor—injury, the patient rapidly loses consciousness and may suffer from brainstem herniation. The exact mechanism is not clear, but it may be related to hyperemia from a loss of autoregulation. Thus, he should be kept out of activities for 2 weeks to allow his brain to recover. His physician should perform a complete exam at rest and after exertion; if normal, he may return to normal activities. Of course, he should always wear a helmet and other safety gear. Parents and teachers should monitor him for signs of postconcussive syndrome, which includes moodiness, fatigue, difficulty concentrating, and headaches. Neuropsychology testing would be indicated if symptoms of postconcussive syndrome are observed.

Objectives: Did you learn to . . .

- Diagnose concussion?
- Manage head trauma and concussion in a child?
- Describe appropriate follow-up of concussion and when to return to activity?

QUICK QUIZ: OVERDOSE

Next in the ED, an irritable 16-year-old female presents with her tearful mother. The mother states she found an empty bottle of acetaminophen in her daughter's bedroom. The 16-year-old admits to taking a "handful" of the medication about 2 hours ago. Activated charcoal is administered. You order laboratory tests, including an acetaminophen level.

When should blood levels of acetaminophen be obtained in order to determine if treatment is required?

A) 4 hours.
B) 8 hours.
C) 30 hours.
D) A and B.
E) A and C.

Discussion

The correct answer is D. This reflects a change in thinking. Classically, 4-hour levels were considered sufficient. With the advent of sustained-release acetaminophen,

this is no longer the case. Additionally, medications such as Tylenol PM, which contain an anticholinergic, may delay acetaminophen absorption. If a 4-hour level is >10 micrograms/mL, checking an 8–12-hour acetaminophen level is prudent. If the time-zero (time of ingestion) is unknown, any acetaminophen level >10 micrograms/mL or any abnormal liver enzymes warrant treatment. Answer C is incorrect. Levels obtained after 24 hours are not useful to determine if treatment is indicated (see Chapter 1, Emergency Medicine for a more complete discussion of overdoses).

QUICK QUIZ: RASH

Your next patient in the ED is a 3-year-old female with a rash. After playing outside, her father found spots on her legs, and she did not want to walk because her knees hurt. On exam she is afebrile with normal vitals and slightly irritable but otherwise interactive. She has slight nasal drainage which her father says is a residual from a cold last week. Her legs and buttocks have palpable purpura. Her knees are mildly swollen and are painful with range of motion. Her CBC and coagulation studies are normal, and her urinalysis is significant for 2 + hematuria.

The most likely diagnosis in this patient is:

A) Acute exposure to lawn chemicals.
B) Henoch-Schönlein Purpura.
C) Juvenile rheumatoid arthritis.
D) Meningococcemia.
E) Rocky Mountain spotted fever.

Discussion

The correct answer is B. This is classic Henoch-Schönlein Purpura (HSP), an IgA-mediated, self-limited vasculitis. The symptoms and signs of HSP are a rash (typically nonthrombocytopenic purpura), abdominal pain (from bowel ischemia secondary to localized vasculitis), arthritis/arthralgia, and nephritis. Typically the vasculitis follows an upper respiratory infection or streptococcal pharyngitis, such as in this case. Treatment for HSP is supportive.

Answer A is incorrect because, although there may be long-term health problems from lawn chemicals, these problems are not acute. Answer C is incorrect.

Juvenile rheumatoid arthritis (JRA) is not likely because the rash of JRA is evanescent salmon-pink rash on the trunk and axilla that classically occurs when the patient spikes a fever. Answer D is incorrect. Meningococcemia is not likely because the patient is afebrile, alert and nontoxic-appearing. Answer E is incorrect. Rocky Mountain spotted fever presents with headache, high fever, and the patient appears toxic. Additionally, patients with Rocky Mountain spotted fever have thrombocytopenia when their petechiae appear.

 HELPFUL TIP: The rash of HSP is frequently initially urticaria with surrounding edema. The rash tends to be dependent, developing first on the legs.

CASE 10

The next patient in your ED is Howard, a 17-year-old male with a sore throat. He is sitting up on the examination table, leaning forward, and drooling. He has a muffled, "hot potato" voice when speaking and prefers not to speak due to pain. Therefore, his father gives the history. He states that Howard has had subjective fevers, chills, and sore throat for 4 days. He has not eaten anything solid for the past 2 days because of difficulty swallowing. Howard has refused all liquids today due to pain with swallowing.

Which one of the following is the most likely diagnosis?

A) Streptococcal pharyngitis.
B) Peritonsillar abscess.
C) Epiglottitis.
D) Adenovirus infection.
E) Herpangina.

Discussion

The correct answer is B. Because of Howard's severe sore throat and drooling, a serious infection such as a peritonsillar abscess or retropharyngeal abscess should be considered. His distress is more severe than would be explained by a streptococcal pharyngitis or viral

pharyngitis. Epiglottitis (caused by *Haemophilus influenza* type b) might be considered in an under- or unimmunized child. However, the presence of sore throat for several days argues against epiglottitis, which tends to have a rapid onset in a previously healthy patient. Epiglottitis **does** occur in adults and presents with a severe sore throat but without drooling. However, it is rare since the widespread use of the Hib vaccine.

* *

Howard's temperature is 40°C with heart rate 150, respiratory rate 18, and blood pressure 120/60. His exam is significant for enlarged tonsils (4 +) bilaterally with airway obstruction and a swollen, enlarged uvula. There is erythema and exudate. He has dry cracked lips. His cervical lymph nodes, including posterior nodes, are very enlarged (2–3 + cm) and tender. Axillary and inguinal adenopathy is also present. He has mild hepatomegaly and no splenomegaly. His extremities are well perfused. A normal saline bolus is started. A CBC shows increased atypical lymphocytes.

What is your treatment of choice?

A) Acyclovir.
B) Clindamycin.
C) Corticosteroids.
D) Amoxicillin.
E) Supportive care.

Discussion

The correct answer is C. Howard has infectious mononucleosis. His infection is accompanied with severe tonsillar swelling, putting his airway at risk. Therefore, corticosteroids are indicated. Steroids should be avoided in cases of mononucleosis unless there is potential airway compromise. If impending airway obstruction is a concern, an otolaryngologist should be consulted immediately.

Acyclovir (answer A) has not demonstrated benefit in mononucleosis. Antibiotics are not necessary in this patient's disease process. Ampicillin or amoxicillin (answer D) can cause a maculopapular rash when given during infectious mononucleosis. Supportive care (answer E) is the treatment of choice unless the symptoms are severe enough to warrant steroids.

HELPFUL TIP: The muffled, "hot potato" voice is also found with peritonsillar abscess. In this patient, one of the tonsils will be asymmetrical with one tonsil protruding towards the midline and the uvula pointing **away** from the infected side. The treatment is antibiotics and drainage, which can be either surgical or by needle drainage in the office or ED. The preferred antibiotics are clindamycin and ampicillin-sulbactam.

Objectives: Did you learn to . . .

- Generate a differential diagnosis for pharyngitis?
- Diagnose and manage mononucleosis?

CASE 11

A 7-month-old female presents to the ED with fever. Her mother reports her child has "not been herself" and felt "a bit warm on the forehead." Vitals reveal a temperature of 39.2°C. Physical exam reveals a slightly fussy and sleepy infant. You perform a complete history and physical but are unable to identify a source of the fever.

What is the first step in your approach to this child?

A) Obtain WBC count and urinalysis before proceeding with further evaluation.
B) Admit for observation and perform blood, urine, and CSF for culture.
C) Give an intramuscular dose of ceftriaxone.
D) Order acetaminophen 30 mg/kg and discharge the patient if the temperature comes down.
E) Admit for IV fluids overnight.

Discussion

The correct answer is A. At this age, occult serious bacterial infection is less likely than during the neonatal period. Because the patient's temperature is >39°C, a WBC count and urinalysis are indicated. The other answer choices are incorrect. Answer B is overly aggressive, and answer C is not indicated. Answer D might be appropriate; the dose of acetaminophen is incorrect (it should be 15mg/kg Q 4–6 hours) and whether the patient becomes afebrile is not relevant here. What is relevant is how the patient looks. An afebrile child who is listless and lethargic is still a child

to worry about. Since you are not seeing signs of dehydration, answer E is incorrect. See Chapter 1, Emergency Medicine for guidelines for the evaluation of pediatric fever.

HELPFUL TIP: The **rectal loading** dose for acetaminophen is between 25 and 30mg/kg. Subsequent rectal doses are 10–20 mg/kg every 4–6 hours.

* *

The WBC count is 17,500/mm³ with 2,000 bands. You determine further investigation is warranted.

What is the most appropriate manner in which to obtain a urine specimen in this child?

A) Midstream "clean-catch."
B) Bag specimen from sterile plastic bag taped to the perineal region.
C) Bladder catheterization.
D) Suprapubic aspiration.
E) C or D.

Discussion

The correct answer is E. The American Academy of Pediatrics (AAP) has published practice guidelines to aid clinicians in diagnosing and managing urinary tract infection (UTI) in febrile infants and children (aged 2 months to 2 years). The standard test for the diagnosis of UTI is a quantitative urine culture. While the urinalysis and microscopy may suggest UTI, no single or combination of components is as sensitive or specific as culture. Therefore, if a child is likely to require antimicrobial therapy, one should attempt to obtain urine for culture in a manner not likely to cause contamination. The midstream "clean-catch" may be obtained in older children who are toilet trained, and the perineum should be cleansed first. Bag specimens are prone to contamination, and are most useful to **rule out** UTI if the urinalysis and microscopy are negative. However, if the results of a bag specimen suggest a UTI, a second specimen collected via transurethral catheterization or suprapubic aspiration is necessary for culture. According to AAP Practice Guidelines, if an infant or young child with unexplained fever is assessed as being sufficiently ill to need antimicrobial therapy, a urine specimen should be obtained by suprapubic aspiration or transurethral bladder catheterization.

* *

The patient has 20 WBC/hpf on UA.

Before you have the culture and susceptibility results, which antibiotic would be the LEAST appropriate choice for the treatment of a UTI in this child?

A) Trimethoprim/sulfamethoxazole.
B) Amoxicillin.
C) Cephalexin.
D) Cefixime.

Discussion

The correct answer is B. The resistance rate to amoxicillin is high. Thus, amoxicillin is not a good choice for treating a UTI in children (or anyone with a UTI who is not pregnant). The usual choice for oral antibiotic treatment of UTI includes amoxicillin/clavulanate, sulfonamides, or cephalosporins. The duration of treatment should be 7–10 days for uncomplicated UTI. If the child appears clinically ill suggesting pyelonephritis, initial parenteral treatment with ceftriaxone would be an appropriate first-line agent. A 14-day course is recommended for those with pyelonephritis.

* *

Her urine culture reveals *E. coli* susceptible to trimethoprim/sulfamethoxazole, and you treat her appropriately.

Following her initial treatment, what diagnostic study should be performed next?

A) Abdominal supine and upright radiographs.
B) Renal ultrasound and voiding cystourethrogram.
C) Spiral CT of abdomen and pelvis.
D) Urology consultation for urodynamic studies.

Discussion

The correct answer is B. A UTI in a young child often serves as a marker for anatomic abnormalities of the urinary tract. Imaging is recommended following a first UTI to identify those at risk for recurrence and subsequent damage to renal parenchyma. Urinary tract ultrasonography should be performed at the earliest convenient time. Ultrasound is useful in the evaluation for kidney size and hydronephrosis, but it is limited in the evaluation of vesicoureteral reflux

(VUR), a common abnormality associated with recurrent UTI. VUR is evaluated with a voiding cystourethrogram (VCUG) or radionuclide cystogram (RNC). **The VCUG or RNC should be done after the child has been treated for the current UTI** (typically several weeks after antibiotic treatment) as reflux is often present during the acute infection. The child should remain on prophylactic antibiotics, such as trimethoprim/sulfa or nitrofurantoin, until these studies have been performed. If an abnormality is detected, urology consultation should be obtained for further management.

 HELPFUL TIP: There is controversy over optimal management of pediatric UTI vis-à-vis radiologic evaluation. Many clinicians will do an evaluation on a female with a second UTI and a male with a first UTI. Others feel that these evaluations are not helpful and should be performed only on individuals with several UTIs. The AAP practice parameter recommends radiologic evaluation after the first UTI diagnosed in any child aged 2–24 months. You are in good company with just about any decision you make here.

* *

The patient is found to have grade 2 reflux (Table 13–5).

Which of the following would be the most appropriate initial management of her reflux?

A) Prescribe prophylactic antibiotics.
B) Refer for surgical intervention.
C) Perform GFR to assess renal scarring.

Table 13–5 INTERNATIONAL REFLUX STUDY COMMITTEE GRADING OF VESICOURETERAL REFLUX

Grade 1: Involves the ureter only.
Grade 2: Involves the ureter, pelvis, and calyces without dilatation.
Grade 3: Involves the ureter, pelvis, and calyces with moderate ureter and pelvis dilatation.
Grade 4: Involves the ureter, pelvis, and calyces with significant dilatation and blunting of the calyceal fornices.
Grade 5: Demonstrates dilatation and tortuosity of the ureter as well as loss of the calyceal fornices.

D) Obtain monthly urine cultures to assure sterility.

E) Observe for now with repeat VCUG in 6 months.

Discussion

The correct answer is A. There is no evidence to support surgical management over medical management or vice versa. Children with mild forms of reflux (grades 1–3) are placed on daily prophylactic antibiotics to minimize renal injury secondary to reflux of infected urine. Mild reflux tends to resolve with maturity, and the antibiotics are discontinued after negative repeat cystogram or when the child reaches 5–7 years. **There are questions about the effectiveness of antibiotic prophylaxis: it may do nothing to prevent recurrence of UTI, breeds resistant organisms, and may not prevent renal scarring. Prophylactic antibiotic treatment (or surgery for that matter) has no benefit** (see *Pediatrics* 2006;117:626). To quote the Cochrane Collaboration, "It is unclear whether the identification and treatment of children with vesicoureteric reflux has any clinically important benefit. Surgery reduced febrile UTIs but not overall UTIs or renal damage." However, for purposes of your board exam, antibiotics are still indicated as prophylaxis. Surgical intervention (answer B) is reserved for those with severe reflux (grades 4–5) or recurrent UTI despite prophylactic antibiotics.

 HELPFUL TIP: Renal scarring is best detected by radioisotope scanning with 99m-technetium dimercaptosuccinate. Assessing renal function with a GFR may be indicated in children who demonstrate significant scarring.

Objectives: Did you learn to . . .

- Approach an older infant with fever?
- Diagnose and treat a child with an initial urinary tract infection (UTI)?
- Recognize that UTI is often a marker for urinary tract abnormalities in children?
- Manage a patient with vesicoureteral reflux?

CASE 12

Steven is a 14-year-old male who presents to your clinic for evaluation of fever. His parents report he has had high (39° to 40°C) intermittent fevers for the past 3–4 weeks. They were trying to wait it out, but the fever apparently won. The fevers are most noticeable in the evening when he often has shaking chills. His mother has noticed a blotchy rash on his chest that appears during these febrile episodes. Upon further questioning, he also complains of aching in his knees and hands that has been present since the onset of fevers. He reports occasional chest pain but denies significant cough or shortness of breath. On physical exam you note diffuse lymphadenopathy. He has mild warmth and swelling in both knees.

Which of the following is true regarding fever of unknown origin (FUO) in the pediatric population?

A) The majority of FUO are due to significant illness such as malignancy or collagen-vascular disorders.

B) Extensive laboratory investigation including cultures of blood, urine, and CSF should be obtained on all children with FUO.

C) The final diagnosis is often suggested by history or physical findings.

D) FUO is best treated empirically with broad-spectrum antibiotics.

E) Mortality is approximately 50%.

Discussion

The correct answer is C. FUO in children is characterized as fever lasting **>2 weeks** (compared to 3 weeks in adults) without a diagnosis despite careful history and physical exam. An estimated 50% of pediatric FUO are due either to localized or systemic infection. Multisystem collagen inflammatory disorders and life-threatening malignancies are the next most common etiologies. Approximately 20% of FUO resolve spontaneously and are presumed to be viral infections. However, a higher percentage will have a disorder requiring specific intervention. A complete history and physical exam (often performed repeatedly) are critical in the making the final diagnosis and avoiding unnecessary testing.

Answer B is incorrect. Specific tests, including cultures and imaging, should be undertaken as suggested by the history and physical findings. Answer D is incorrect. There is no indication for treating FUO empirically with antibiotics unless a specific infectious process is suspected. Answer E is incorrect. Mortality in pediatric FUO has been reported between 6% and 17%.

Which one of the following is the most likely etiology of fever in this patient?

A) Kawasaki disease.

B) Henoch-Schöenlein Purpura.

C) Juvenile idiopathic (rheumatoid) arthritis.

D) Rheumatic fever.

E) Cat-scratch disease.

Discussion

The correct answer is C. The combination of high intermittent fever associated with an evanescent rash and arthritis is most characteristic juvenile idiopathic arthritis (JIA) (formally known as juvenile rheumatoid arthritis [JRA]), a condition of chronic synovitis in children. There are three disease subgroups: systemic-onset, polyarticular, and pauciarticular. **Systemic-onset disease** presents with fever and large and small joint arthritis as well as multiple extraarticular manifestations including rash, hepatosplenomegaly, lymphadenopathy, serositis (pleural or pericardial), leukocytosis, anemia, and rarely DIC. **Polyarticular JIA** is characterized by symmetric arthritis of small and large joints and a female preponderance. A subset of these individuals will be rheumatoid factor (RF) positive, with 50% continuing to experience severe arthritis into adulthood. **Pauciarticular JIA** may be grouped into early-onset or late-onset. Early-onset disease demonstrates fairly mild, asymmetric large joint arthritis. It is characterized by chronic iridocyclitis in 30% of individuals affected. Late-onset disease is characterized by a male preponderance and sacroiliac involvement. HLA-B27 is positive in 75% of individuals and some will continue to have spondyloarthropathy as adults.

Kawasaki disease (aka mucocutaneous lymph node syndrome) (answer A) is a vasculitic syndrome with a predilection for the coronary arteries. Criteria for diagnosis include fever lasting at least 5 days and four of the following: conjunctivitis, lymphadenopathy, mucosal changes such as cracked lips or strawberry tongue, a polymorphous exanthem, and extremity involvement causing hand/foot edema and desquamation. Answer B is incorrect because HSP presents with purpura, which is not described here. HSP is discussed in more detail earlier in this chapter.

Rheumatic fever (answer D) is suggested in a child who has recently had a streptococcal infection. The Jones criteria are often used to establish a diagnosis. Major Jones criteria (acronym PECCS) include **p**olyarthritis that is often migratory, a serpiginous rash termed **e**rythema marginatum, **c**arditis often manifested as a new murmur, Sydenham **c**horea, and **s**ubcutaneous nodules. Minor criteria include fever, arthralgias, elevated acute phase reactants, and prolonged PR interval.

Cat-scratch disease (answer E) is caused by inoculation with *Bartonella henselae*, a small pleomorphic Gram-negative bacillus. It is commonly transmitted following a scratch from a cat and typically presents with fever and local lymphadenopathy.

Which of the following is the most appropriate initial therapy for this patient?

A) Naproxen.

B) IVIG.

C) Penicillamine.

D) Systemic corticosteroids.

E) Azithromycin.

Discussion

The correct answer is A. NSAIDs, such as ibuprofen and naproxen, remain the front-line therapy for JIA. In controlled studies, traditional antirheumatic agents such as penicillamine have not been shown to have an effect over placebo in the control of symptoms. Corticosteroids are sometimes used in severe cases and may be useful in short-term management of recalcitrant symptoms as well as iridocyclitis. IVIG would be useful in Kawasaki disease. Azithromycin is used in treating cat-scratch disease.

Objectives: Did you learn to . . .

- Define fever of unknown origin (FUO)?
- Develop a differential diagnosis of FUO?
- Recognize the clinical manifestations of juvenile idiopathic arthritis (JIA)?

CASE 13

Anthony is a 2,300-gram male born at 35 weeks' gestation to a 23-year-old G2P2 single female. The mother did not seek prenatal care and routine screening labs were not available. She presented to the ED in active labor shortly following spontaneous rupture of membranes at home. Upon transfer to the obstetric ward, she was noted to be febrile (38.3°C) and received intravenous antibiotics. Five hours later, the infant was delivered via spontaneous vaginal delivery.

Management of this newborn infant whose mother probably has chorioamnionitis (not simply GBS screen positive) should include which of the following?

A) Empiric therapy with gentamicin.
B) Empiric therapy with ampicillin.
C) Empiric therapy with vancomycin.
D) A and B.
E) All of the above.

Discussion

The correct answer is D. The organism that is most responsible for chorioamnionitis is group B streptococcus. Adequate treatment requires at least two antibiotics, and ampicillin and gentamicin represent one recommended regimen.

The following tests are routinely recommended in all children of mothers with known or suspected chorioamnionitis EXCEPT:

A) CBC with differential.
B) Blood culture.
C) Urinalysis and urine culture.
D) Chest radiograph.

Discussion

The correct answer is D. Not all neonates need a chest radiograph. However, all children born to mothers with chorioamnionitis should have the other testing done, and any child with respiratory symptoms should have a chest radiograph done. Additionally, any child that appears septic or is febrile should have a lumbar puncture performed.

* *

Anthony is started on appropriate antibiotics. Subsequently, your exam of this neonate reveals hepatosplenomegaly, lymphadenopathy, petechia, and white mucocutaneous patches in the infant's mouth. His CBC reveals a hemoglobin of 12 g/dL and a platelet count of 85,000/mm³ with evidence of hemolysis on the peripheral smear.

The most likely pathogen infecting this infant is:

A) Rubella.
B) Cytomegalovirus.
C) *Toxoplasma gondii.*
D) *Treponema pallidum.*
E) *Candida albicans.*

Discussion

The correct answer is D. Congenital syphilis is caused by transplacental transmission of the spirochete *Treponema pallidum*. Intrauterine infection can result in stillbirth, hydrops fetalis, or prematurity. Neonatal manifestations of syphilis include hepatosplenomegaly, lymphadenopathy, jaundice, rash, hemolytic anemia, and thrombocytopenia. Abnormalities specific to congenital syphilis include white, patchy mucocutaneous lesions, edema, rhinitis (snuffles), osteochondritis, and pseudoparalysis. These findings overlap with other congenital TORCH (**T**oxoplasmosis, **O**ther [congenital syphilis and viruses], **R**ubella, **C**MV, **H**erpes) infections.

 HELPFUL TIP: Late sequelae of congenital syphilis involve the bones and joints, teeth, eyes, and CNS, and include bowed shins, frontal bossing, saddle nose, pegged central incisors, interstitial keratitis, and sensorineural deafness. The Hutchinson triad includes interstitial keratitis, deafness, and notched, peg-shaped teeth.

* *

In addition to the laboratory data obtained above, you order an ultrasound of the patient's head, which appears normal.

Intracerebral calcifications are MOST associated with which congenital infection(s)?

A) Cytomegalovirus.
B) Toxoplasmosis.
C) *Treponema pallidum.*
D) Rubella.
E) A and B.

Discussion

The correct answer is E. The clinical manifestations of congenital cytomegalovirus and toxoplasmosis are often similar. Infants are typically asymptomatic at birth, but a significant number develop visual impairment, learning disabilities, and mental retardation months to years later. Those infants who are symptomatic at birth may demonstrate intrauterine growth retardation, hepatosplenomegaly, jaundice, hemolytic anemia, and thrombocytopenia. Intracerebral calcifications also occur in both infections. The calcifications tend to be periventricular in CMV (mnemonic to help remember this: **C**alcifications in **C**MV are **C**-shaped and around the ventricles) and more dispersed throughout the cortex in toxoplasmosis. Additional central nervous system abnormalities include microcephaly, chorioretinitis, and sensorineural hearing loss.

Objectives: Did you learn to . . .

- Appropriately manage the neonate born to a mother who has evidence of chorioamnionitis?
- Recognize that congenital TORCH (**T**oxoplasmosis, **O**ther, **R**ubella, **C**MV, **HSV**) infections have overlapping signs and symptoms?
- Recognize that many infants with congenital TORCH infections are asymptomatic at birth?

 QUICK QUIZ: CONGENITAL INFECTIONS

A small-for-gestational-age newborn infant is found to have hepatosplenomegaly, jaundice, and thrombocytopenia. Cardiac examination reveals a grade 2/6 continuous murmur heard best at the left upper sternal border. An ophthalmologic examination demonstrates micro-ophthalmia and cataracts.

The result of which maternal prenatal screening lab is likely to have been abnormal in the above case?

A) VDRL.
B) Rubella immunity status.
C) HIV status.
D) Varicella zoster immunity status.
E) GBS cultures.

Discussion

The correct answer is B. Cardiac, ophthalmologic, auditory, and neurologic findings predominate in the symptomatic infant with congenital rubella. Up to 85% of infants infected during the first 4 weeks of gestation will have some form of congenital defect. This decreases to 5% when the primary infection occurs after the third to fourth month of gestation. Ophthalmologic findings include microphthalmia, cataracts, glaucoma, and retinopathy. Infants are often microcephalic and develop sensorineural hearing deficits, meningoen-

cephalitis, and mental retardation. Additional findings of hepatosplenomegaly, thrombocytopenia, and osteitis may be present. A characteristic "blueberry muffin" appearance may be present due to the combination of jaundice and extramedullary (skin) hematopoiesis.

Answers A and E are incorrect. Syphilis and GBS infections are described elsewhere, and they do not typically cause the ophthalmologic findings described in this case. Answer C is incorrect because congenital HIV infection is commonly asymptomatic. Evidence of immune deficiency may present later in the child's life with failure to thrive, generalized lymphadenopathy, hepatosplenomegaly, and recurrent infections. Answer D is incorrect because congenital herpes infections do not cause cardiac abnormalities.

 QUICK QUIZ: CONGENITAL INFECTIONS

Which of the following cardiac lesions is likely to be found in an infant with congenital rubella?

A) Patent ductus arteriosus.
B) Tetralogy of Fallot.
C) Transposition of great vessels.
D) Coarctation of aorta.
E) Bicuspid aortic valve.

Discussion

The correct answer is A. The most common cardiac lesions associated with congenital rubella are patent ductus arteriosus (PDA) and peripheral pulmonary artery stenosis. PDA is characterized by a continuous "washing machine" murmur heard best over the left upper sternal border.

Answers B and C are incorrect. **Tetralogy of Fallot and transposition of great vessels are classically cyanotic heart defects that have no known association with congenital infections.** Both coarctation of the aorta (answer D) and bicuspid aortic valve (answer E) cause harsh systolic murmurs. The murmur of coarctation radiates to the back. Both coarctation and bicuspid aortic valve are commonly found in females with Turner syndrome.

CASE 14

A term newborn infant is noted to have a solitary, tense bulla located on the dorsum of his wrist. The underlying skin is nonerythematous. Pregnancy was uncomplicated; however, the infant was delivered via cesarean section for failure to progress. The infant appears to be a vigorous feeder and is noted to frequently suck on his hands and wrists while in the nursery. He is otherwise asymptomatic.

Which of the following is MOST appropriate at this time?

A) Start acyclovir.
B) Perform lumbar puncture and send a sample of the CSF for HSV PCR.
C) Perform a Tzanck smear of the bulla fluid.
D) All of the above.
E) Observation with no intervention at this time.

Discussion

The correct answer is E. Nothing needs be done at this time. The appearance and location of the bulla is consistent with a sucking blister. A solitary bulla or blister on normal appearing skin may be present at birth from in utero sucking. Often when presented with the affected extremity, the infant will demonstrate the sucking behavior in that location. Such blisters are often mistaken for herpes simplex, but the solitary nature and location help to establish the correct diagnosis—although there may be multiple blisters at times. Additional history of cesarean section makes HSV less likely in this scenario. Nonetheless, a sucking blister is a diagnosis of exclusion, and other more serious diagnoses should be ruled out by history and exam and further testing as indicated.

Of course, herpes should have been included in the differential diagnosis of this patient, but the infant did not have any other signs or symptoms of herpes infection.

Which statement is FALSE regarding neonatal herpes simplex virus infection?

A) The majority of infants with neonatal HSV are born to mothers with symptomatic herpetic lesions.
B) The incidence of neonatal transmission is higher when the pregnant woman experiences primary infection versus secondary reactivation.
C) Most neonatal HSV infections are caused by HSV-2.
D) Intrauterine exposure accounts for the minority of perinatal HSV infection.
E) Typical skin lesions are present in <50% of infants with HSV infection.

Discussion

The correct answer is A. Fewer than one-third of infants with neonatal HSV are born to mothers with active genital lesions. Most cases of neonatal HSV are found in the infants of asymptomatic mothers who are shedding the virus. Neonatal herpes simplex virus often results in serious morbidity and mortality. Clinical manifestations are variable and HSV may present as localized disease (typically to skin, eyes, or mouth), CNS disease, or disseminated infection. Encephalitis may occur without skin involvement; therefore, HSV infection should be suspected in an infant from birth to approximately 4 weeks of age who presents with fever or mental status abnormalities such as lethargy, irritability, or poor feeding.

The other answer choices are correct. A woman who contracts a primary infection during pregnancy has a 33% chance of transmitting the virus to her infant. There is <5% transmission if she experiences a secondary reactivation intrapartu. Between 70% and 85% of neonatal HSV is caused by infection with HSV-2. Only 5% of congenital infections occur in utero, as the majority occurs via exposure to infected cervical secretions during birth, and <50% of infants with encephalitis or disseminated disease demonstrate the typical vesicular lesions.

 HELPFUL TIP: Most neonates with HSV infection do not present with skin findings at birth. It is more typical for neonates to develop HSV skin lesions 1–2 weeks after delivery.

 HELPFUL TIP: Empiric therapy with acyclovir (after obtaining blood and CSF for culture) is indicated if vaginal delivery occurs over an active HSV lesion or if membranes are ruptured for >4 hours in a mother with genital HSV lesions.

Objectives: Did you learn to . . .

• Differentiate between a herpes lesion and a sucking blister?
• Recognize rates and modes of transmission of herpes in neonates?
• Identify some of the clinical manifestations of neonatal herpes?

CASE 15

Several parents in your neighborhood decide to have a "chickenpox" party. They want to synchronize their kids' chickenpox outbreaks with their busy schedules. One of the mothers, who has never had chickenpox, finds out that she is pregnant the day after being exposed to chickenpox. She is not yet symptomatic (from the pregnancy or the chickenpox).

The best advice for this potential parent about her pregnancy is:

A) Consider termination since it is likely that the child will have congenital varicella.
B) Get treated within 48 hours of exposure with varicella immune globulin.
C) Get treated within 48 hours of exposure with varicella immune globulin plus varicella vaccine.
D) Get treated within 48 hours of exposure with IVIG plus varicella vaccine.

Discussion

The correct answer is B. Women who are varicella-susceptible, are pregnant, and are exposed to chickenpox should be treated with varicella immune globulin. Answer C and D are incorrect. **The vaccine should be avoided during pregnancy. It is a live, attenuated, virus and carries some risk to the fetus (although the degree of risk is unknown).**

You can let the mother know that:

A) Varicella immune globulin has been shown to reduce the risk of congenital varicella.
B) Varicella immune globulin is aimed mostly at attenuating the case in the mother should she be infected.
C) Varicella immune globulin has not been shown to prevent congenital varicella.
D) Both A and B are true.
E) Both B and C are true.

Discussion

The correct answer is B. Varicella immune globulin is aimed at reducing the symptoms in the mother and attenuating her case of varicella. Answers A and C are incorrect. There is no firm data either way about how varicella immune globulin will affect the child's outcome vis-à-vis congenital varicella. The old varicella immune globulin is not readily available everywhere and is being replaced by VariZIG (a newer immune globulin). If VariZIG or traditional varicella immune globulin is not available, IVIG can be used or the patient can be observed to see if chickenpox symptoms occur and then be treated with acyclovir.

Manifestations of intrauterine infection with varicella zoster include all of the following defects EXCEPT:

A) Microphthalmia.
B) Congenital cataracts.
C) Cardiac abnormalities.
D) CNS abnormalities.
E) Limb hypoplasia.

Discussion

The correct answer is C. Cardiac abnormalities are not seen with varicella zoster exposure in utero. In addition to the findings above, patients with congenital varicella zoster will have cutaneous scarring called cicatrix.

* *

Now that all of these children have been infected with varicella zoster, the question arises about how long they should be kept out of school.

These children are considered infectious until:

A) 5 days after the first lesion appears.
B) 10–14 days after the first lesion appears.
C) New lesions are no longer forming.
D) All lesions are crusted over.
E) They are no longer febrile.

Discussion

The correct answer is D. Patients are considered infectious until all lesions are crusted over. Lesions need not have healed entirely, only crusted over.

Objectives: Did you learn to . . .

- Offer treatment for varicella exposure to a pregnant nonimmune female?
- Recognize the uses of varicella immune globulin?
- Identify symptoms of congenital varicella infection?

CASE 16

A 3-year-old child presents to you office with a history of bright red cheeks. Over the past several days, she has had mild fever with mild muscle aches. Except for the rash, the child is now asymptomatic.

The most likely cause of this patient's illness is:

A) Parvovirus B19.
B) Herpes virus 6.
C) Rubeola.
D) Rubella.
E) Influenza virus.

Discussion

The correct answer is A. A mild systemic illness followed by red, "slapped cheeks" is typical of erythema infectiosum (fifth disease). The red, slapped cheeks are generally followed by a lacy, reticular rash on the extremities and trunk. This is generally a self-limited illness in children.

Complications of parvovirus B19 infection—either congenital or acquired—include all of the following EXCEPT:

A) Aplastic anemia.
B) Birth defects, including CNS and limb disease.
C) Hydrops fetalis.
D) Inflammatory arthritis.
E) Intrauterine fetal death.

Discussion

The correct answer is B. Parvovirus B19 causes all of the above except for birth defects. Fetal death, anemia, and nonimmune-mediated hydrops fetalis are potential outcomes of intrauterine exposure (33% of infected women will transmit the virus to their fetus). If the child survives, a good outcome is the usual result without any limb abnormalities or other birth defects. Aplastic anemia can occur and is especially common in those with sickle-cell anemia. Inflammatory arthritis is common in adults.

* *

The question is raised about whether or not to exclude this child from preschool. There are two pregnant teachers at the school.

You can tell the child's mother that:

A) This child is infectious and should be excluded from school until the rash resolves.
B) Since almost all adult women are already immune, there is no need to worry about transmission to the teachers.

C) Since this virus is an enterovirus, careful hygiene in the school will prevent spread.
D) This child is no longer infectious and can be allowed back into school.

Discussion

The correct answer is D. Once the rash is present, this child is no longer infectious and can be allowed back into school. Answer B is incorrect because only about 50% of adult women are immune. Answer C is incorrect. First, this is not an enterovirus. Second, it is spread via droplets.

 HELPFUL TIP: Just try getting this child with a rash back in school and past the school nurse—it is impossible. On the other hand, schools are well aware that there is a magical effect of topical antibiotics to prevent the spread of viral conjunctivitis.

Objectives: Did you learn to . . .

• Recognize the clinical manifestations of parvovirus B19 infection (fifth disease) and describe how the disease is transmitted?
• Identify complications of parvovirus B19 infection?

 QUICK QUIZ: CHILDHOOD INFECTIONS

Which of the following is characterized by a high fever, possibly >40°C, a bulging fontanelle, a maculopapular rash which begins after the fever abates, conjunctivitis, and upper respiratory symptoms?

A) Roseola infantum (erythema subitum).
B) Rubeola (measles).
C) Rubella (German measles).
D) Erythema infectiosum (fifth disease).
E) Meningococcal meningitis.

Discussion

The correct answer is A. This clinical presentation is typical of roseola infantum. Roseola infantum, caused by the herpes 6 (and rarely herpes 7) virus, is characterized by a high fever for 3–5 days (often >40°C), generalized malaise, a bulging fontanelle in up to 26% of infants, conjunctivitis, perhaps oral mucosal ulcers, and a rash that appears as the fever begins to defervesce.

 QUICK QUIZ: TAKING A TEMPERATURE

Which of the following correctly describes the relationship between rectal, axillary, and tympanic temperature?

A) Rectal equals axillary plus 2°, tympanic plus 1°.
B) Rectal equals axillary plus 1°, tympanic plus 2°.
C) Rectal and tympanic temperatures are equivalent.
D) Rectal equals axillary minus 1°, tympanic minus 2°.
E) None of the above.

Discussion

The correct answer is E. **There is no consistent relationship between rectal, axillary, and tympanic temperatures.** If you need to know the temperature and are going to base evaluation and therapy on it (such as in the neonate) **you must do a rectal temperature.** Axillary and tympanic temperatures are notoriously unreliable.

 QUICK QUIZ: GASTROINTESTINAL SYMPTOMS

A young couple brings in their 18-month-old daughter because of a 12-hour history of vomiting and diarrhea. The patient has felt warm, and her oral intake has been depressed. However, she continues to make tears with crying and has wet diapers. Her medical history is unremarkable. On exam, you find a lethargic-looking female who perks up slightly when you open a bag of toys. Her temperature is 38.5°C, and her capillary refill is <3 seconds. The remainder of the exam is nonfocal. You think that she has a viral gastroenteritis, and give the parents some advice regarding rehydration.

Which of the following is the most appropriate advice for this patient?

A) Avoid all solid food for the next 24–48 hours.
B) Use milk as the primary rehydration solution.
C) Use only watered-down tea for rehydration.
D) Use a commercially prepared oral rehydration solution and reintroduce foods as tolerated.
E) Use cola beverages (eg, Coca-Cola or Pepsi) because they contain more sodium than commercially available oral rehydration solutions.

Discussion

The correct answer is D. Effective oral rehydration can be accomplished with any one of the rehydration solutions on the market (eg, Pedialyte). Answer A is incorrect. There is no need to limit the food intake of patients with vomiting or infectious diarrhea. They can have whatever they can tolerate. The concept of "gut rest" is obsolete and leads to increased bowel permeability and prolonged diarrhea. So, early feeding is optimal. **There is no need to avoid lactose-containing products.** The diet should be dictated only by what the child can tolerate orally **unless the child is <3 months** or malnourished (*Pediatrics.* 2006;118:1279). **In children <3 months or in those who are malnourished, avoid lactose containing products.**

Answers C and E are incorrect. There is no role for weak tea, flat soda, "Jello water," etc, in the treatment of the vomiting child. The most common cause of hyponatremic seizures in the child is improper rehydration during gastroenteritis. Answer E is incorrect. Commercial drinks, like cola beverages and sports drinks, are not specifically designed for oral rehydration, and the sodium concentration is typically much lower, risking hyponatremia. Additionally, these drinks usually have a high sugar content.

 HELPFUL TIP: In the exclusively breast-fed infant with vomiting and/or diarrhea, breast-feeding should be encouraged and not replaced with oral rehydration solutions.

 HELPFUL TIP: Avoid nonabsorbable sugars, like those found in apple or grape juice. These can promote an osmotic diarrhea.

CASE 17

A new mother and father bring their 2-month-old infant to your office with a complaint of inconsolable crying. This started at about 3 weeks of age and occurs about the same time every day. The crying will last for hours and is becoming quite disruptive. The infant will draw up his knees and appears to be in quite a bit of pain. They have tried pretty much everything that they can think up including car rides, swings, swaddling, various types of music, etc, but to no avail. Shivers run up and down your spine as you recall your own early parenting experiences.

The most likely diagnosis is:

A) Colic.
B) Intussusception.
C) Hair around the penis or toes or corneal abrasion.
D) Constipation.
E) Cluster headache.

Discussion

The correct answer is A. Colic generally begins at 3 weeks of age, peaks at about 6 weeks of age, and abates by 3 months of age. The cause is unknown. Answer B is incorrect. While intussusception can present with colicky abdominal pain, it is not likely to be recurrent for several days or weeks without a more significant problem (eg, bloody stools) developing. Answer C is incorrect. A hair or thread around a child's toes or penis, or corneal abrasion, need to be considered in any child with inconsolable crying. However, they are not likely to result in crying that is daily and episodic. Answer D is incorrect because this history is not consistent with constipation. Answer E, a cluster headache, is not likely to occur in this age group.

You can advise the parents that:

A) Phenobarbital is safe and effective for controlling infant colic (when given to the parents to help them chill out).
B) Infants who breast-feed are less likely to develop colic.
C) Elimination of cruciferous vegetables from the diet of breast-feeding mothers has been shown to reduce infant colic.
D) Simethicone has been shown to be effective in infant colic.
E) Anticholinergic drugs are effective in treating infant colic but the risks are unacceptable.

Discussion

The correct answer is E. Anticholinergic drugs have been shown to be effective in the treatment of colic. However, the risks associated with the use of these drugs are considered unacceptable. The rest of the answers are incorrect. It does not seem as though breast-fed infants are any less likely to develop colic than are bottle-fed infants. The evidence for elimination of cruciferous vegetables is inconclusive. Simethicone is **not** effective in treating infantile colic, but it gives the parents something to do.

 HELPFUL TIP: Most studies of infantile colic are flawed. Whey hydrolysate milk is probably effective. Sucrose solution (12%) has shown modest, very short-term benefit. **It is important to identify alternative caregivers because infant colic can be a major stress on parents and can possibly lead to abuse.**

* *

You next see the same child when he is 2 years old. His parents bring him to your ED with a history of "barky" cough. He has had an antecedent upper respiratory infection for a couple of days with a runny nose and a temperature of 38.2°C. On arrival in the ED, he has retractions, a "barky" cough, and stridor but does not look toxic. He also has vomiting after episodes of coughing.

The MOST LIKELY diagnosis in this child is:

A) Epiglottitis.
B) Laryngotracheobronchitis.
C) Bacterial tracheitis.
D) Retropharyngeal abscess.
E) Gastroenteritis.

Discussion

The correct answer is B. This represents laryngotracheobronchitis (aka croup). Typically, patients have an antecedent URI with a low-grade fever, a barky cough, and stridor, which are usually worse at night. Answer A is incorrect because patients with epiglottitis generally do **not** have an antecedent URI, but they do have a much higher temperature with sudden onset of symptoms and a toxic appearance. Answer C is incorrect. Patients with bacterial tracheitis do have an antecedent URI but then develop a second stage of the illness (eg, a biphasic illness) with sudden onset of high fever, purulent sputum production, and stridor. These patients look toxic. Answer D is incorrect. A retropharyngeal abscess occurs in conjunction with high fever, drooling, refusal to swallow, and toxic appearance. Answer E is incorrect. This child has posttussive emesis. Gastroenteritis does not include the other features found in this child with croup.

* *

You decide to treat this patient in the ED.

All of the following are appropriate treatments EXCEPT:

A) Racemic epinephrine.
B) Antibiotics.
C) L-epinephrine 5 cc of 1:1,000.
D) Dexamethasone 0.6 mg/kg IM.
E) Humidified oxygen.

Discussion

The correct answer is B. One would not want to use antibiotics in this patient. This is a viral illness, usually parainfluenza virus. All the other answers are appropriate treatments. Of particular note is answer C. Although classically we have used racemic epinephrine, the "d" isomer is inactive. Additionally, racemic epinephrine is more expensive and must be kept refrigerated if a multidose vial is used. L-epinephrine, 5 cc of 1:1,000, delivered by nebulizer is as effective—if not more—than racemic epinephrine, is cheaper, and is the same dose for everyone.

* *

You give the patient nebulized epinephrine, and his stridor resolves. You now need to decide what to do with this patient.

You tell the parents that since the child had nebulized epinephrine:

A) He needs to be admitted because of the "rebound" effect seen with epinephrine in croup.
B) He needs to be observed in the ED for 6 hours to make sure his symptoms do not recur.
C) He must be observed for 2 hours in the ED to make sure his symptoms do not recur.
D) He must be observed in the ED for 1 hour to make sure that his symptoms do not recur.
E) He can be discharged immediately with follow-up tomorrow.

Discussion

The correct answer is C. The patient should be observed for 2 hours. The thinking about this has changed. Admission after nebulized epinephrine was the rule. Now, 2-hour observation is considered sufficient. There is no "rebound effect." The patient may return to his pretreatment state but will not get worse as the result of the epinephrine treatment.

* *

You decide to do a radiograph of this child's neck to aid in the diagnosis (although this is not necessary nor advocated in most cases—but this is a board review book, not real life).

You are most likely to see which of the following on cervical radiograph?

A) Thumb sign.
B) Sign of Lesser-Trélat.
C) Spine sign.
D) Retropharyngeal space swelling.
E) Steeple sign.

Discussion

The correct answer is E. Radiographs in croup show the "steeple sign" which is a subglottic narrowing of the trachea from edema, giving it a steeple-like appearance. The thumb sign (answer A), is seen in epiglottitis. The sign of Lesser-Trélat (answer B) is the sudden development of numerous seborrheic keratoses in a patient with internal malignancy—it is rare, not seen in children, and nearly useless knowledge. The spine sign (answer C) is loss of progressive radiolucency of the spine on lateral chest radiograph. This is seen when something is overlaying the lower thoracic spine making it appear more dense, classically an infiltrate indicative of pneumonia. Retropharyngeal space swelling (answer D) is seen in retropharyngeal abscess.

* *

The patient is breathing a little easier after the nebulized epinephrine and has received acetaminophen for his fever. He is drinking a little and does not appear significantly dehydrated.

Which of the following is the MOST appropriate treatment for this patient?

A) Prednisone 1 mg/kg PO once.
B) Prednisone 2 mg/kg PO followed by a taper.
C) Dexamethasone 0.2 mg/kg IV once.
D) Dexamethasone 0.6 mg/kg PO once.
E) Dexamethasone 5 mg/kg IM once.

Discussion

The correct answer is D. The most appropriate treatment is dexamethasone 0.6 mg/kg with a maximum dose of 10 mg. Dexamethasone is chosen because of its relatively long half-life that allows it to remain active during the duration of the illness (about 3 days). The least invasive route is recommended, and oral dexamethasone is appropriate in patients tolerating PO intake. The other answer choices are not appropriate for treating croup.

HELPFUL TIP: 0.3 mg/kg and 0.15 mg/kg of dexamethasone are as effective as 0.6 mg/kg. For some reason, the authors cannot make the leap to 0.15 mg/kg, so we use 0.3 mg/kg.

* *

You treat the child as noted above with epinephrine and dexamethasone. His oxygen saturation improves to 92% on room air. His stridor and retractions are much milder now.

Your next step is to:

A) Admit the patient to the hospital for further treatment.
B) Discharge the patient for follow-up in your office the next day.
C) Discharge the patient with instructions to use a cool-mist humidifier.
D) Discharge the patient with a course of azithromycin in case it is bacterial.
E) Observe the patient for an additional 2 hours in the ED.

Discussion

The correct answer is A. An oxygen saturation of 92% is distinctly abnormal in a child of this age. He or she should be running 95% or better. In addition, he still has stridor and retractions, signifying some potential respiratory compromise. He may require further neb-ulized epinephrine treatments. Sending this child home would not be a great idea.

Objectives: Did you learn to . . .

- Evaluate a patient with colic and offer management strategies to the parents?
- Diagnose laryngotracheobronchitis (croup)?
- Manage a patient with laryngotracheobronchitis?
- Identify radiographic abnormalities seen with soft-tissue neck infections?

 QUICK QUIZ: EPIGLOTTITIS

You have a child in the ED who is toxic appearing with the sudden onset of high fever, drooling, and stridor. You suspect epiglottitis.

What is the FIRST step in the treatment of this patient?

A) Draw blood work including a CBC.
B) Place an IV for access and fluids.
C) Give a dose of IM steroids (eg, dexamethasone 0.6 mg/kg) to help shrink the epiglottis.
D) Put a face mask on the child and administer albuterol via face mask.
E) Leave the child on the mother's lap and do not upset the child (you don't want a temper tantrum in the ED).

Discussion

The correct answer is E. Anything that upsets the child can lead to increased airway obstruction. Leave the child in the parent's lap and do not upset him. Answers A and B are incorrect because they may upset the child, leading to increased work of breathing and increased obstruc-tion. Answer C, dexamethasone, is indicated for croup and not for epiglottitis. Answer D is incorrect. However, it would **not** be wrong to give blow-by oxygen or blow-by nebulized epinephrine **if it did not agitate the child.**

 QUICK QUIZ: EPIGLOTTITIS

Which of the following is NOT needed in the optimal diagnosis and treatment of epiglottitis?

A) "Thumb sign" on radiograph.
B) Antibiotics to cover *Haemophilus influenza.*
C) Antibiotics to cover *Streptococcus pneumonia.*
D) An operating room.
E) Personnel able to emergently manage the airway.

Discussion

The correct answer is A. The use of radiographs in sus-pected epiglottitis is fraught with problems and delays life-saving therapy. **Do not do it.** Epiglottitis is a clin-ical diagnosis that requires visualization of the epiglot-tis. This is preferably done in the operating room (answer D) with a setup for both intubation and tra-cheostomy should that become necessary. If the child is mildly ill, looking at the epiglottis in the ED is per-missible. However, be prepared to manage the airway (answer E). Answers B and C are both used in the treat-ment of epiglottitis. Since the advent of *H. influenza* vaccine, there is no longer a single organism causing most cases of epiglottitis. Bacteria that can cause epiglottitis include *H. influenza, S. pneumoniae, S. aureus,* and groups A, B, and C beta-hemolytic streptococci. Epiglottitis may also be of viral origin.

 QUICK QUIZ: NEONATAL INFECTIONS

What is the most likely etiologic agent in a 2-week-old male with conjunctivitis, cough, rales, nasal congestion, and infiltrate on radiograph, but no fever or wheezes?

A) Influenza.
B) Chlamydia.
C) RSV.
D) Parainfluenza.
E) Gonorrhea.

Discussion

The correct answer is B. This is a classic description of *Chlamydia* infection in the newborn. Patients usually present between 5–14 days with conjunctivitis and pneumonia. These patients should have cultures done via swab under the upper eyelid and should be treated with systemic antibiotics **even if conjunctivitis is the only symptom present.** Erythromycin is the drug of choice. Sulfisoxazole is the second-line drug. **Currently, azithromycin is not considered adequate treatment.** Topical treatment is not indicated (if you want to give the parents something to do, a little topical erythromycin ointment won't hurt).

CASE 18

A 12-month-old presents to your office in January with a 2-day history of runny nose and cough. The child now has wheezing with nasal flaring and retractions, and his oxygen saturation is 89%. There has been no fever, and several of the other children and adults in the family have had "a cold" over the past several weeks. On exam you hear scattered wheezes and rales. You diagnose bronchiolitis.

The MOST LIKELY organism involved in this child's illness is:

A) Rhinovirus.
B) Adenovirus.
C) Respiratory syncytial virus.
D) Parainfluenza.
E) Human metapneumovirus.

Discussion

The correct answer is C. The **most common** cause of bronchiolitis in children is respiratory syncytial virus (RSV). All of the other organisms can cause bronchiolitis, as can influenza virus, but less commonly than RSV.

Which of the following treatments have been unequivocally shown to be effective in bronchiolitis?

A) Nebulized albuterol.
B) Nebulized epinephrine.
C) Corticosteroids such as prednisone or dexamethasone.
D) All of the above are unequivocally effective.
E) None of the above are unequivocally effective.

Discussion

The correct answer is E. None of the above has been shown to be effective in bronchiolitis. Does this mean we don't use albuterol, epinephrine, and steroids? No, even though they are of no use, these are still prescribed for bronchiolitis. Just don't expect to see any benefit. One argument for the use of steroids—and bronchodilators—is that it may be difficult to determine which patients have reactive airway disease in addition to (or instead of) bronchiolitis at the initial presentation. However, in **bronchiolitis,** these medications have demonstrated no benefit.

 HELPFUL TIP: Nebulized 3% saline has demonstrated benefit in patients who are admitted for bronchiolitis. Several studies support this practice. (*J Pediatr* 2007;151(3):266).

RSV is usually diagnosed by:

A) Nasal wash using immunofluorescence or antigen detection.
B) Baseline and convalescent antibody titers.
C) Blood culture for RSV.
D) Sputum Gram stain.
E) Induced sputum culture.

Discussion

The correct answer is A. A nasal wash for RSV immunofluorescence or antigen detection is used to diagnose RSV. The others answer choices are incorrect.

* *

Your patient stabilizes after nebulized albuterol and blow-by oxygen. But you were ready with ribavirin just in case.

Consideration of ribavirin is indicated for which of these patients with RSV?

A) Patients with congenital heart disease.
B) Patients with chronic lung disease, such as bronchopulmonary dysplasia.
C) Infants <6 weeks of age.
D) Immunosuppressed infants.
E) All of the above.

Discussion

The correct answer is E. Additionally, patients with decreasing oxygen saturations and increasing pCO_2 should be considered for ribavirin therapy.

Which of the following most accurately describes the role of ribavirin therapy?

A) It has been shown unequivocally to be beneficial in high-risk patients (eg, those with immunosuppression, chronic lung disease, etc).
B) It can be administered orally for RSV, as is done with other illnesses such as hepatitis.
C) It is safe and effective without any adverse effects on the fetus.
D) It is of marginal benefit, if any.
E) A and B.

Discussion

The correct answer is D. Ribavirin can be **considered** for use in the most ill patients. However, randomized studies show that it **may increase the length of stay and requirement for artificial ventilation in an ICU.** Additionally, it can have adverse effects on the fetus in pregnancy. Thus, pregnant women should not be caring for patients receiving nebulized ribavirin. Answer B is incorrect because ribavirin must be administered via inhalation for patients with RSV bronchiolitis.

Which of the following is indicated for the prevention of RSV in high-risk infants?

A) Vaccination against RSV.
B) Prophylactic oral ribavirin.
C) Rimantadine or oseltamivir.
D) RSV-IVIG IV (RespiGam) q 30 days or palivizumab (Synagis) IV q 30 days.
E) None of the above.

Discussion

The correct answer is D. High-risk patients can be treated with either RSV-IVIG or palivizumab IV every 30 days to prevent infection with RSV. All the other answers are incorrect.

Objectives: Did you learn to . . .

● Recognize the clinical presentation of a patient with RSV bronchiolitis?
● Diagnose and treat RSV bronchiolitis?
● Describe what patients may possibly benefit from ribivarin and RSV prophylaxis?

CASE 19

A 4-week-old infant presents to your office with his parents. The parents note that he has had vomiting every time he eats. His vomitus is mostly formula and nonbilious. He seems to be hungry and is demanding to be fed often. Except for the vomiting, he seems to be well, without diarrhea. Exam reveals an afebrile infant in no distress with normal cardiac and pulmonary exams and a relatively benign abdomen. There is no "olive" palpable.

Your working diagnosis is:

A) Midgut volvulus.
B) Gastroenteritis.
C) Pyloric stenosis.
D) CNS injury with increased intracranial pressure.

Discussion

The correct answer is C. This most likely represents pyloric stenosis. The classic presentation of pyloric stenosis is the sudden development of nonbilious, often projectile, vomiting shortly after feeding, followed by a demand to feed again soon after. Classically, pyloric stenosis occurs in infants aged 2 weeks to 2 months. Midgut volvulus (answer A) is incorrect because these patients have bilious vomiting. Our patient has nonbilious vomiting. Gastroenteritis (answer B) is incorrect because there is no diarrhea, fever, or appetite loss. Answer D is incorrect. Although CNS injury with increased intracranial pressure and vomiting is a possibility, you would expect to see other evidence of CNS injury such as lethargy, possibly signs of head injury, etc.

The metabolic abnormality most likely to be seen in this patient is:

A) Hyperchloremic metabolic acidosis.
B) Hypochloremic metabolic alkalosis.
C) Hyperglycemia.
D) Elevated CPK reflecting muscle hypertrophy.
E) None. This patient will have normal electrolytes.

Discussion

The correct answer is B. This answer proceeds from knowing that the stomach produces hydrochloric acid (HCL). Patients with pyloric stenosis are losing acid and chloride and present with a hypochloremic metabolic alkalosis.

Which of the following patients is most likely to present with pyloric stenosis?

A) A first-born male.
B) A first-born female.
C) A second-born male.
D) A second-born female.
E) The rate of pyloric stenosis is equal in all of these groups.

Discussion

The correct answer is A. There is a 4:1 male:female preponderance, and estimated 30% of all cases occur in a first-born child. Thus, first-born males are at risk for pyloric stenosis.

 HELPFUL TIP: Infants receiving erythromycin, especially those <2 weeks old, appear to be at increased risk of developing pyloric stenosis. This association may extend to other macrolides as well.

* *

You give the patient a bolus of IV normal saline and decide to confirm the diagnosis with a Gastrografin test.

What are you most likely to see on radiograph if this patient has pyloric stenosis?

A) "Bullseye" or "target" lesion.
B) Corkscrew pattern of small bowel.
C) Ulcerations of the gastric mucosa.

D) String sign.
E) Rapid filling of the bowel distal to the pylorus.

Discussion

The correct answer is D. The string sign is formed when contrast material trickles through the hypertrophied pyloric sphincter (and thus looks like a thin string on x-ray). "Bullseye" or "target" lesions (answer A) are seen on ultrasound with intussusception. A corkscrew pattern (answer B) is seen with midgut volvulus. Ulcerations of the gastric mucosa are seen, of course, with gastric ulcers. Answer E is incorrect. The problem with pyloric stenosis is that little of anything can get from the stomach to the small bowel. Ultrasound can be used to make the diagnosis of pyloric stenosis; the ultrasonographer will note a hypertrophied pylorus. However, this is more operator-dependent than is a Gastrografin swallow, so choose ultrasound only if you can count on your ultrasonographer.

 HELPFUL TIP: Checking for gastric volume after 2–3 hours is another way to diagnose pyloric stenosis. Gastric volumes of >10 cc 2–3 hours after feeding are sensitive (92%) and specific for pyloric stenosis. However, you do not want to miss this diagnosis, and 92% may not be good enough.

 HELPFUL TIP: The definitive treatment for pyloric stenosis is surgical although a number of other treatments have been used, including nitrous oxide and nutritional support with watchful waiting.

* *

You have a surgical consultant see the patient, surgery is done, and everybody is happy.

Objectives: Did you learn to . . .

- Identify clinical manifestations of pyloric stenosis?
- Diagnose and manage pyloric stenosis?

QUICK QUIZ: PEDIATRIC BELLY PAIN

The treatment for midgut volvulus is:

A) Watchful waiting.
B) Maneuver of Leopold.
C) Emergent surgery.
D) Air enema.
E) Nasogastric suction and bowel rest.

Discussion

The correct answer is C. Midgut volvulus is a surgical emergency. None of the other answers is correct. Watchful waiting is dangerous and risks ischemic bowel with perforation, so answers A and E are incorrect. Leopold's maneuvers (answer B) are used to move a breech pregnancy to vertex and have nothing to do with the bowel. Answer D is incorrect. because air enema can be used to reduce an intussusception but has no role in the treatment of midgut volvulus.

CASE 20

A 5-year-old presents to your office with his mother. The mother complains that the child has been soiling himself frequently. He states that he does not notice that he has to have a bowel movement until he soils himself. This tends to be problematic in his kindergarten class because he is being called "smelly belly" and other, even less pleasant, names. In other words, he is having some social problems.

What percent of patients children with fecal incontinence (encopresis) have a primary form (eg, never have had a period of stool continence)?

A) 10%
B) 20%
C) 30%
D) 40%
E) 50%

Discussion

The correct answer is D. Sixty-percent of patients with this problem will have secondary fecal incontinence (this term is preferred to encopresis) and 40% have primary fecal incontinence. Many children will have been continent for a time prior to experiencing significant fecal incontinence. Contrast this with enuresis, which is more often primary than secondary.

* *

Your patient was doing well, per his mother, with rare episodes of soiling prior to starting kindergarten. His mother reports that his habit was to defecate after lunch every day. Now, 3 months into school, he refuses to defecate in the school bathroom and has only about 2 bowel movements per week at home. At least once or twice per week he has fecal incontinence at school, so his mother has been sending spare clothes with him daily.

What is the LEAST likely cause of his fecal incontinence?

A) Primary variceal encopresis.
B) Overflow fecal incontinence.
C) Dysfunction of anal sphincter.
D) Psychological fecal incontinence.

Discussion

The correct answer is A. Primary variceal encopresis does not exist. All of the other answer choices are types of fecal incontinence. Overflow encopresis (answer B) occurs when patients become constipated (usually with voluntary withholding of stool as the inciting factor). Patients then become obstipated with overflow stool incontinence. Anal sphincter dysfunction (answer C) is a rare cause of fecal incontinence. Psychological fecal incontinence (answer D) is usually the result of oppositional disorder or another significant psychiatric or developmental disorder.

Which of the following may result in constipation (and thus fecal incontinence)?

A) Hypothyroidism.
B) Hypercalcemia.
C) Laxative use.
D) Lead poisoning.
E) All of the above.

Discussion

The correct answer is E. All of the above can cause constipation and fecal incontinence. Other metabolic causes, including diabetes, hypokalemia, etc, can cause constipation. Of particular note is laxative use (answer C). Parents may use laxatives in a misguided effort to have a child stool every day. Thus, the patient becomes laxative-dependent.

All of the following are useful in the treatment of overflow fecal incontinence EXCEPT:

A) Polyethylene glycol (PEG).
B) Cascara.
C) Mineral oil.
D) Psyllium.
E) Milk of magnesia.

Discussion

The correct answer is B. Bowel stimulants (eg, cascara, phenolphthalein, senna) are contraindicated in the treatment of overflow fecal incontinence—and in chronic constipation in general. They are addictive with the bowel becoming dependent on stimulant laxatives. This can lead to worsening fecal incontinence. All the other answer choices may be helpful in treating constipation and overflow incontinence.

 HELPFUL TIP: The treatment of overflow fecal incontinence begins with disimpaction, which may be accomplished in a variety of ways. Some authors promote the use of enemas to clear out the rectal ampulla. Others recommend polyethylene glycol or mineral oil orally (especially in the case of children who have had perirectal trauma or who cannot tolerate enemas). Still others recommend a combination of oral and rectal treatments. After disimpaction, the patient should be put on a regimen containing a nonstimulative laxative such as milk of magnesia, mineral oil, or polyethylene glycol. These should be incrementally increased until the patient is having regular, soft, formed bowel movements. Relapse is common (20%–30% over 3 years). Mineral oil should never be used in a child who is at risk of aspiration. It can cause a chemical pneumonitis.

Objectives: Did you learn to . . .

- Recognize a patient with constipation causing fecal incontinence?
- Identify types and causes of constipation and fecal incontinence?
- Manage fecal incontinence and constipation?

CASE 21

A 5-year-old male who was recently diagnosed with influenza presents to your ED with complaints (via the parents) of intractable vomiting and mental status changes. On exam, the child is febrile and is vomiting but has neither meningeal signs nor focal neurologic findings. His liver is palpable.

Influenza is associated with which of the following complications?

A) Bacterial pneumonia.
B) Rhabdomyolysis.
C) Myocarditis.
D) Viral pneumonia.
E) All of the above.

Discussion

The correct answer is E. All of the above can be a result of influenza. In addition to these, influenza may cause CNS problems such as encephalitis, transverse myelitis, etc.

* *

You get labs on this patient. He is noted to be hypoglycemic and to have markedly elevated liver enzymes. His bilirubin is normal. The patient's white blood cell count and differential suggest a viral illness.

The MOST LIKELY diagnosis based on this patient's history, physical, and laboratory findings is:

A) Reye syndrome.
B) Bacterial meningitis.
C) Transverse myelitis.
D) Hepatic encephalopathy secondary to hepatitis.
E) Diabetes mellitus in the "honeymoon" period with Somogyi phenomenon.

Discussion

The correct answer is A. This patient most likely has Reye syndrome. Reye syndrome presents with intractable vomiting, elevated liver enzymes, hypoglycemia, and mental status changes (excitability, delirium, coma). It is generally associated with a viral illness such as influenza or chickenpox. This patient is not likely to have meningitis (answer B) given the absence of an elevated white blood cell count and lack of meningeal signs. He clearly does not have transverse myelitis (answer C), an autoimmune condition producing rapidly progressive weakness and sensory disturbance. Answer D is possible but less likely than Reye syndrome given the history. Answer E is incorrect because the Somogyi phenomenon refers to stress hormone-induced morning hyperglycemia in a patient on insulin who is having unrecognized hypoglycemia at night.

The medication MOST associated with Reye syndrome is:

A) Ibuprofen.
B) Celecoxib (Celebrex).
C) Aspirin.
D) Acetaminophen.
E) Naproxen.

Discussion

The correct answer is C. The use of aspirin in a child with a viral illness, classically influenza or chickenpox, has been associated with the development of Reye syndrome. The incidence of Reye syndrome has been steadily declining now that parents are aware that they should avoid aspirin use in children. Reye syndrome is now a very rare disease.

HELPFUL TIP: The treatment of Reye syndrome is supportive and includes controlling hypoglycemia and treating cerebral edema. There is no specific treatment for this illness. Mortality rate is estimated 10%, which is much lower than in the past.

* *

For some reason, you found heme-positive stool in this patient. You must have been thinking that every patient in the ED deserves at least one rectal exam.

All of the following are common causes of heme-positive stools in children aged 1–5 years EXCEPT:

A) Colon polyps.
B) Ulcers.
C) Esophageal varices.
D) Gangrenous bowel.
E) Intussusception.

Discussion

The correct answer is D. Gangrenous bowel is found in neonates and younger infants resulting from necrotizing enterocolitis, midgut volvulus, etc. See Table 13–6.

Table 13–6 CAUSES OF HEME POSITIVE STOOLS IN CHILDREN

<1 year: swallowed maternal blood, anal fissure, intussusception, duodenal or gastric ulcers, gangrenous bowel, Meckel diverticulum.
>1 year: Colon polyps (up to 50% of rectal bleeding in this age), ulcers, anal fissure, esophageal varices, intussusception, hemorrhoids.

Objectives: Did you learn to . . .

- Recognize sequelae of influenza infection?
- Describe Reye syndrome and how it occurs?
- Manage a patient with Reye syndrome?
- Identify some causes of heme-positive stools in children?

CASE 22

A mother comes to you with concerns about sudden infant death syndrome (SIDS) in her infant. Her sister had a child who died of SIDS, and she is concerned that her child is now at elevated risk.

You can tell her:

A) Twin concordance studies suggest that SIDS is a genetic disorder.
B) Since her child is now 5 months old there is no risk of SIDS, which generally occurs <3 months.
C) Siblings of an infant with SIDS have a 5-fold increase in the risk of SIDS.
D) If one twin died of SIDS, the other has a 5%–10% chance of dying of SIDS.
E) Young maternal age (<20 years) is associated with reduced risk of SIDS.

Discussion

The correct answer is C. A sibling of child who died with SIDS has a 5-fold increased risk of dying of SIDS (although the absolute risk is still <1%). Answer A is incorrect. SIDS does not appear to be a genetic disorder. Answer B is incorrect. SIDS generally occurs between 2–4 months (median age 11 weeks). However, 90% of cases occur <6 months, so a 5-month-old infant is still at risk. Answer D is incorrect because the risk of a twin dying of SIDS is greater than another sibling dying of SIDS but is <1%. Answer E is incorrect. The opposite is true: maternal age <20 years is a risk factor, as is maternal smoking.

All of the following have been associated with an increased incidence of SIDS EXCEPT:

A) Side-sleep positioning.
B) Prone-sleep positioning.
C) Early introduction of solid foods.
D) Premature birth.
E) Intrauterine exposure to drugs.

Discussion

The correct answer is C. The introduction of solid foods is not related to the development of SIDS. All of the other factors increase the rate of SIDS. Of note: nonsupine positioning (answer B) is associated with an increased incidence of SIDS.

The most important advice you can give to prevent SIDS is:

A) Avoid feeding close to bedtime to reduce aspiration risk.
B) Place the child in the prone position (stomach and face down) when sleeping.
C) Use a child alarm in the room to alert the parent(s) if something is wrong.
D) Place the child in the recumbent position (stomach and face up).
E) Use sheepskin or polystyrene bedding to prevent suffocation.

Discussion

The correct answer is D. Putting the child in the recumbent position ("**back** to sleep") reduce the risk of SIDS by an estimated 50%. Answer B (prone sleeping position) and answer E (polystyrene or sheepskin bedding) **increase the risk** of SIDS. Additional advice is to quit smoking during the pregnancy. Smoking during pregnancy increases the risk of SIDS 3-fold.

HELPFUL TIP: The use of pacifiers in bed decreases the risk of SIDS as well. Give it to the child when he or she is put down for sleep. Do not reinsert it once the child is asleep if he/she spits it out.

HELPFUL TIP: Recumbent sleeping has increased the rate of plagiocephaly (flattening of the head, in this case in the occipital region). This has been associated with developmental delay although it is not known if these children will catch up later. The child should be placed in a **prone** position **while awake** (referred to as "tummy time"). Hopefully this will mitigate the plagiocephaly.

Objectives: Did you learn to . . .

● Identify risks of sudden infant death syndrome (SIDS)?
● Give advice on how to reduce the risk of SIDS?

CASE 23

The parents of a 1-month-old female are in your office for a routine check-up. They are first-time parents and are concerned about feeding. One of the grandmothers is "from the old country." Back in her day, they would start children on solid foods at 2 months of age—usually starting with strained liver (lots of vitamins and stuff plus it is disgusting and the adults wouldn't eat it). The grandmother also cannot figure out why the couple is wasting their money on formula when cow's milk (sometimes goat's milk when available) "worked just fine for me." They would like your advice about feeding.

You let them know that:

A) Solid foods should be introduced at 3 months for all children. Two months of age is too soon.
B) Cow's milk is considered adequate only after 6 months of age.
C) Early introduction of cow's milk has been irrefutably linked to type 1 diabetes mellitus.
D) The first foods introduced should be strained meats.
E) Children should have good head control before solid foods are introduced.

Discussion

The correct answer is E. Children should have good head control before starting solid foods. Answer A is incorrect for two reasons. First, solid foods are generally not recommended until 4 months of age. Second, note that the answer says "all children." Some children do not want solid foods until 6 months of age. Answer B is incorrect. Cow's milk should be avoided for the first year of life. Breast-feeding is optimal. This failing, infant formula contains additional nutrients not found in cow's milk. Additionally, the use of cow's milk has been linked to an increase in gastrointestinal blood loss and anemia. Answer C is incorrect. There has been some observational evidence to suggest a connection between diabetes type 1 and cow's milk, but the data is quite suspect. Answer D is incorrect. Cereals are usually the first food introduced, followed by fruits and vegetables, and foods should be introduced one at a time.

 HELPFUL TIP: New AAP guidelines recommend 200 IU/day of vitamin D from birth through the teenage years, no exceptions. This can come either from supplements or foods. Breast milk does not contain enough vitamin D and these children should be supplemented as well.

* *

The parents manage to fend off the grandmother. The child continues on formula feedings. However, the child gets somewhat fussy on occasion and has occasional bouts of diarrhea. The family wants to know what to do.

Your advice is to:

A) Change formulas because this represents an allergy to the cow's milk formula.
B) Do not change formulas.
C) Change formulas because this likely represents lactase deficiency.
D) Switch to a formula based on short-chain fatty acids since this likely represents an inability to absorb and metabolize fats.

Discussion

The correct answer is B. Children will occasionally be fussy and have occasional diarrhea. This does not indicate a formula allergy or intolerance. Reflux and vomiting are common in infants. Again, this does not indicate a formula allergy. The parents should be reassured that as long as the child is growing and is not having significant difficulties, continuing the current formula is acceptable.

 HELPFUL TIP: Reflux or spitting up does not mean formula intolerance. **Do not make multiple formula changes.** This medicalizes a normal pattern in children. The majority of reflux will resolve by 1 year. If the child looks well and is growing, there is no need to change the formula.

* *

The parents decide that you are correct and continue to feed the child the cow's milk formula. As you predicted, the child does well on this formula. However, the child is now becoming "constipated" and the grandmother would like to give this child a laxative. She is only having 1 bowel movement per day rather than the 3 or 4 per day that occurred during the first several months of life.

You let the parents know that:

A) One stool a day is likely normal for this infant.
B) An infant having fewer than 2–3 bowel movements per day is likely constipated since bowel transit time is only 8.5 hours or so.
C) Infants fed soy-based formula tend to have softer stools than those fed cow's milk formula.
D) Breast-fed infants may normally have up to 10 stools per day.
E) A and D.

Discussion

The correct answer is E. The number of bowel movements in a normal infant can vary widely from up to 10 a day in a breast-fed infant to 1 a day in a formula-fed infant. What is more important is whether the child has to strain to pass stool, how hard the stool is, etc. The number of stools per day is less important. Of particular note is answer C. Infants on soy-based formulas tend to have **harder** stools than those on cow's milk formula.

* *

On further questioning, it becomes clear that the grandmother may be correct. This child is having a hard time passing stool and passes only small amounts of hard stool with great effort (red-purple face, lots of crying, etc). The parents would like some advice.

All of the following are reasonable suggestions EXCEPT:

A) Change to a formula with a preponderance of whey protein such as Carnation Good Start.

B) Add corn syrup to the formula (15–20 cc/8-oz bottle).

C) Add fruit juices if the child is >2 months.

D) Add lactulose to the child's formula.

E) Use a glycerin suppository for occasional constipation.

Discussion

The correct answer is C. Fruit juices should not be used <4 months. Of particular note is answer B. There was concern a number of years ago that corn syrup caused infant botulism. This has since been shown to be unfounded. All of the other answer choices are viable options.

* *

The child does well after the parents implement your plan, but she continues to have significant reflux symptoms. This is getting to be quite a problem because the child sputters and coughs frequently and then vomits feedings.

Which of the following is NOT recommended as standard therapy in treating this child?

A) Elevating the head of the bed.

B) Metoclopramide.

C) Use of a proton pump inhibitor.

D) Cisapride.

E) Thickening the formula with rice cereal.

Discussion

The correct answer is D. Cisapride has been associated with torsade de pointes and is no longer recommended. Its use has been restricted by the FDA; it can only be obtained directly from the manufacturer after providing documentation of the child's disease and the failure of other methods of treatment. In addition to the advice above, H_2-blockers have also been used with some success. In infants with gastroesophageal reflux **disease** (not just physiologic reflux), a trial of milk-free diet for 1–2 weeks is reasonable.

Objectives: Did you learn to . . .

- Give appropriate advice for nutrition and feeding during infancy?
- Diagnose and manage constipation in infancy?
- Treat an infant with significant gastroesophageal reflux?

CASE 24

A 23-year-old G2 P1 female at 31 weeks' gestation presents to the ED and delivers precipitously. Her pregnancy was uncomplicated. The neonate is a 1.25-kg male. The helicopter is on its way to transport this premature infant to your regional pediatric hospital.

The BEST treatment for this newborn now is:

A) Antibiotics.

B) Corticosteroids.

C) High pressure 100% oxygen.

D) Routine care (warmth, stimulation, etc.).

E) Surfactant.

Discussion

The correct answer is E. Without further information, you must assume that this patient is at significant risk for neonatal respiratory distress syndrome (RDS). The appropriate treatment is surfactant. The dose of surfactant depends on the preparation, and the timing of administration varies by source (some sources favor immediate administration while others recommend "early" treatment—usually within 2 hours of delivery). Surfactant therapy has good evidence for decreasing morbidity and mortality and should be used in all premature infants who are at risk for RDS (see next question). Some sources recommend combination therapy with **antenatal** corticosteroids for the mother and surfactant for the premature infant.

Answer A is incorrect because you have no reason to believe that the mother—or the infant—has an infection. Answer B is incorrect as corticosteroids for the premature infant at risk for RDS probably cause harm without any evidence of benefit. Answer C is incorrect because you have no information on the patient's respiratory status and do not need to be so aggressive without an indication. Answer D is incorrect. It might be the second-best option if surfactant were unavailable.

All of the following are risk factors for neonatal RDS EXCEPT:

A) Cesarean section.

B) Gestational diabetes.

C) Male sex of infant.

D) Prolonged rupture of membranes.

Discussion

The correct answer is D. Prolonged rupture of membranes is associated with a **decreased** risk of neonatal RDS. All of the other answer choices are associated with an increased risk. Increasing prematurity is associated with increasing risk of RDS as is multifetal pregnancy, especially in the second fetus delivered in a twin pregnancy.

> **HELPFUL TIP:** The lecithin/sphingomyelin (L/S) ratio is the traditional method for assessing fetal lung maturity. If the L/S ratio is >2, the risk of RDS is low. Other options include phosphatidylglycerol level and direct surfactant measures. It is important to realize that these tests have fairly low positive predictive values.

> **HELPFUL TIP:** As premature infants grow into adults, pay attention to their blood pressures and glucose levels. Infants who were born prematurely and at very low weight (<1.5 kg) have more problems with hypertension and glucose intolerance.

CASE 25

This family returns to see you many times over the ensuing years. You now turn your attention to the newest addition to the family, a 4-day-old male infant you delivered—this time in the labor and delivery unit. He is the product of a full-term, uncomplicated pregnancy. He is breast-fed and was doing well until this morning. His mother noticed today that he is breathing harder, eating poorly, and looking more yellow. You note a respiratory rate of 72 and crackles on lung exam, so you order a chest x-ray.

Which of the following diagnoses is most likely?

A) Neonatal respiratory distress syndrome.
B) Persistent pulmonary hypertension.
C) Pneumonia.
D) Pneumothorax.
E) Transient tachypnea of the newborn.

Discussion

The correct answer is C. Pneumonia is more likely than the other answer choices because of the timing of the symptoms. Neonatal pneumonia may occur early (shortly after birth) or late (days or weeks later). The pathogenic organisms involved are different for early and late disease. Patients presenting with early pneumonia are more likely to have acquired the infection in utero or during delivery; group B streptococcus is the most common pathogen in these cases. Patients presenting with late pneumonia may have acquired the disease during delivery, during hospitalization, or while in the community; Gram-positives, Gram-negatives, and *Chlamydia* may all cause pneumonia in these patients.

Answer A is incorrect because RDS should not occur in a full-term infant. Answer B is incorrect because persistent pulmonary hypertension should present shortly after birth with hypoxemia and cyanosis. Answer D is incorrect because pneumothorax is a common result of the trauma of birth, and up to 2% of infants may sustain a pneumothorax during delivery. However, very few infants with a pneumothorax are symptomatic, and you would expect the symptoms to occur shortly after delivery. Answer E is incorrect because transient tachypnea of the newborn (TTN) occurs within 1–2 hours of birth and resolves on its own.

* *

You found your thermometer, and your patient is febrile. The chest x-ray shows a left lower lobe infiltrate.

Which of the following antibiotics is LEAST appropriate in this setting?

A) Ampicillin.
B) Ceftriaxone.
C) Gentamicin.
D) Vancomycin.

Discussion

The correct answer is B. There are a few potential problems with ceftriaxone in this case: it should not be given to neonates with hyperbilirubinemia (this infant is jaundiced); it may induce resistance in Gram-negative organisms (which are more likely to be the cause of pneumonia in the neonate); and it may cause fatal precipitates in the lung and kidney when coadministered with calcium (not an immediate concern for this patient). Because of the patient's age, it is difficult to say if this is "early" or "late" pneumonia. It would be prudent to provide empiric antibiotic coverage for all likely pathogens. The combination of ampicillin and gentamicin is preferred for coverage of group B strep-tococcus and also covers *Listeria*. Because of the potential for MRSA to cause pneumonia in the neonatal period, vancomycin is reasonable but should not be used alone.

 HELPFUL TIP: Remember the possibility of sustained PSVT with CHF in this patient who is tachypneic, has rales, and is feeding poorly. Not all rales in infants are from an infectious cause.

Objectives: Did you learn to . . .

- Provide appropriate treatment to an infant at risk for neonatal respiratory distress syndrome?
- Identify risk factors for neonatal respiratory distress syndrome?
- Describe causes of respiratory distress in the neonatal period?

BIBLIOGRAPHY

Alper BS, Curry SH. Urinary tract infection in children. *Am Fam Physician.* 2005;72(12):2483.

American Academy of Neurology. The Management of Concussion in sports [practice parameter]. *Neurology.* 1997;48:581.

American Academy of Pediatrics. Practice Parameter: Management of Hyperbilirubinemia in the Newborn Infant 35 Weeks or More of Gestation. *Pediatrics.* 2004;114(1):297.

American Academy of Pediatrics. *2006 Red Book: Report of the Committee on Infectious Diseases.* 27th ed. Elk Grove, IL: Author, 2006.

American Academy of Pediatrics. *Car Safety Seats: A Guide for Families.* Elk Grove, IL: Author, 2002.

American Academy of Pediatrics. Practice parameter: The diagnosis, treatment and evaluation of the initial urinary tract infection in febrile infants and young children. American Academy of Pediatrics. Committee on Quality Improvement. Subcommittee on Urinary Tract Infection. *Pediatrics.* 1999;103:843.

Bithoney W, Dubowitz H, Egan H. Failure to thrive/growth deficiency. *Pediatrics* Rev 1992;13(12):453.

Cooper WO, Griffen MR, Arbogast P, et al. Very early exposure to erythromycin and infantile hypertrophic pyloric stenosis. *Arch Pediatr Adolesc Med.* 2002;156:647.

Corneli HM, Zorc JJ, Majahan P, et al. A multicenter, randomized, controlled trial of dexamethasone for bronchiolitis. *N Engl J Med.* 2007;357:331.

Dennery P, Seidman D, Stevenson, D. Neonatal hyperbilirubinemia. *N Engl J Med.* 2001;344(8):581.

Gartner LM, Greer FR. Prevention of rickets and vitamin D deficiency: new guidelines for vitamin D intake. *Pediatrics.* 2003;111:908.

Glazener CM, Evans JH, Peto RE. Alarm interventions for nocturnal enuresis in children. *Cochrane Database Syst Rev.* 2005;CD002911.

Immunization Action Coalition. Summary of Childhood and Adolescent Immunization Recommendations. Accessed February 2, 2008, at http://www.immunize.org/catg.d/p2010.pdf.

Kattwinkel J, et al. *Neonatal Resuscitation Textbook.* 5th ed. American Academy of Pediatrics/American Heart Association, 2006. Chicago, IL.

Kliegman RM, et al. *Nelson Textbook of Pediatrics.* 18th ed. Philadelphia: Saunders, 2007.

Mitchell EA, Hutchison L, Stewart AW. The continuing decline in SIDS mortality. *Arch Dis Child.* 2007;92:625.

Offit P, et al. Addressing parents' concerns: do multiple vaccines overwhelm or weaken the infant's immune system? *Pediatrics.* 2002;109(1):124.

Patel H, Platt R, Lozano J, Wang E. Glucocorticoids for acute viral bronchiolitis in infants and young children. *Cochrane Database Syst Rev.* 2004;3:CD004878.

Pichichero M. Group A beta-hemolytic streptococcal infections. *Pediatr Rev.* 1998;19(9):291.

Rosenthal A. How to distinguish between innocent and pathologic murmurs in childhood. *Pediatr Clin North Am.* 1984;31(6):1229. (Yes, it's old but it's the best!)

Woolf A. Poisoning in children and adolescents. *Pediatr Rev.* 1993;14(11):44.

14

Adolescent Medicine

Anne Sullivan

CASE 1

A 14-year-old male presents to your clinic with his mother for a routine well-child examination. The patient's mother has some questions about puberty. Her son enjoys playing sports and she is concerned that he may be too small to play football. The past medical history is unremarkable.

Which of the following can you tell the mother will likely be the first sign of puberty in this boy?

A) Increase in penile length.
B) Enlargement of the testes.
C) Deepening of the voice.
D) Rapid increase in linear growth.
E) Coarsening of pubic hair.

Discussion

The correct answer is B. Increase in the volume of the testes is the first sign of pubertal development in boys, with average age of onset 12 years (range 10–14 years). Answer E is of special note. While pubic hair appears shortly after the onset of puberty, it is initially long and straight and not in a mature distribution. Coarsening of the pubic hair is a more advanced pubertal stage, occurring approximately 1.5 years after the onset of puberty. An increase in penile length occurs simultaneously. The maximal growth spurt occurs on average at 14 years, approximately 2 years after onset of puberty. Changing of the voice is a secondary hormonal effect that is quite variable in nature.

* *

The mother tells you that the patient's father began going through puberty during high school, and he did not reach his adult height until he was in college at about 20 years. The patient's father is 5'10" tall (approximately 178 cm). The mother is 5'3" tall (approximately 160 cm). Physical examination reveals that your patient is Tanner stage I for genitalia and pubic hair. His height and weight continue to track along their previously established curves on the growth chart, both at approximately the 5th percentile. The remainder of the examination is unremarkable.

What is your next step in evaluation this patient's short stature?

A) Obtain hand radiographs to assess bone age.
B) Draw blood to test for growth hormone and testosterone levels.
C) Obtain an endocrinology consult.
D) Order computed tomography (CT) imaging of the brain to rule out hypothalamic tumors.
E) Order magnetic resonance imaging (MRI) of the brain to rule out hypothalamic tumors.

Discussion

The correct answer is A. In the face of a normal physical examination and appropriate linear growth velocity, the likelihood of an intracranial process in very low. An assessment of bone age can be obtained easily (and relatively inexpensively) and would be useful prior to performing other tests.

* *

You decide to obtain a bone age, and the radiologist reports bone age as 12 years, 3 months (remember that the patient is 14 years old).

What is the most likely diagnosis for your patient?

A) Growth hormone deficiency.
B) Sella turcica tumor.
C) Constitutional delay.
D) Idiopathic testicular atrophy.
E) Testosterone receptor abnormality.

Discussion

The correct answer is C. The bone age of 12 years, 3 months is reassuring. His bones are immature and still have the ability to grow; there is no fusion of the growth plates. If the bone age were 14 years, his adult height would likely be short: the bones would no longer have the inherent ability to grow. Bone age assessment is an accurate tool for determination of expected growth. Constitutional delay is the most common diagnosis for short stature, and it is often associated with a delayed onset of puberty. Constitutional delay is a diagnosis of exclusion; a complete history and physical often rules out other diagnoses. Family history often reveals a parent who was a late bloomer but eventually had normal pubertal development. This adolescent's history of normal linear growth velocity (albeit along the 5th percentile) is reassuring for the absence of growth hormone deficiency or intracranial abnormalities. The combination of appropriate linear growth velocity, appropriate adjustment for bone age, and paternal history of late pubertal development is classic for constitutional delay.

* *

When your patient's height is plotted on a growth curve, and adjusted for bone age rather than chronological age, the height now plots just below the 50th percentile. Your patient now has a question of his own. His main concern is that some of his classmates are starting to get taller, and he is afraid he will be too short to continue competing in sports. The mother's height is 5′3″ and the father's is 5′10″.

Based on what you know today, what is your best estimate of this patient's adult height?

A) 5′3″ ± 2″ (160 ± 5 cm)
B) 5′5″ ± 2″ (165 ± 5 cm)
C) 5′7″ ± 2″ (170 ± 5 cm)
D) 5′9″ ± 2″ (175 ± 5 cm)
E) 5′11″ ± 2″ (180 ± 5 cm)

Discussion

The correct answer is D. You can provide a rough estimate of the patient's adult height using the calculation for midparental height (MPH). The parent of the opposite gender—the mother in this case—must have the height adjusted for this calculation. For a boy, add 5 inches to the mother's height (12.5 cm); then average the corrected maternal height and the paternal height to determine the MPH. For a girl, subtract 5 inches from the paternal height; then average this corrected paternal height and the maternal height to calculate the MPH. In our patient's case, his mother's corrected height is 68 inches, averaged with his father's height of 70 inches to get an MPH of 69 inches. A margin of error of ±2 inches (5 cm) is often given with MPH estimates.

Objectives: Did you learn to . . .

- Evaluate a patient with growth concerns?
- Identify the clinical presentation of constitutional delay?
- Calculate midparental height (MPH)?

CASE 2

Your next patient is a 16-year-old female cross-country runner who you are seeing in follow-up for right shin pain. She was diagnosed in the local ED 1 week ago with "shin splints" and told to limit her activities. In your office, she tells you that the pain has been worsening over the last 3 months, and she has progressively decreased the distance and time of her runs. Her pain has now reached the point where effectively she cannot run. She denies fever, swollen joints, or other systemic symptoms. She normally has regular menses but notes on review of symptoms that she has irregular menses every cross-country season. The patient's past medical history is significant for a stress fracture in her left foot 18 months ago. Your exam reveals tenderness at the middle one-third of the right tibia. Also, she has pain on a single-leg hop. You review her x-rays from the ED, which do not reveal any fractures or other abnormalities.

What is the appropriate next step to diagnose your patient's leg pain?

A) Ultrasound of the lower extremity.
B) MRI of the lower extremity.
C) Dual-energy x-ray absorptiometry (DEXA) scan.
D) Thyroid-stimulating hormone (TSH) level.
E) Urine pregnancy test.

Discussion

The correct answer is B. MRI is sensitive and specific for stress fractures and has become the preferred study. The patient's history and examination are of concern for the presence of a tibial stress fracture. Stress fractures often present insidiously and cause gradual progression in symptoms over time until a critical point is reached regarding sports participation. Fifty percent of stress fractures are not visible on plain radiographs.

Answer A is incorrect. Ultrasound can help evaluate soft tissue masses, but it does not play a role in evaluating stress fractures. Answer C is incorrect. DEXA scan can provide whole-body and site-specific measurement of bone mineral density, which may be related to the pathophysiology of stress fractures, but does not help diagnose a site of injury. Radionuclide bone scans are often less expensive than CT or MRI, and they demonstrate sites of injury based on increased uptake of the radionuclide material. However, bone scans are not specific for stress fractures and are often false positive. Given the patient's other complaints, TSH (answer D) and urine pregnancy test (answer E) may be warranted but will not assist in the diagnosis of her leg pain.

* *

An MRI is obtained and confirms the presence of a stress fracture in the middle one-third of the right tibia. Because of your patient's history, especially that of multiple stress fractures, you are concerned she may be suffering from the female athlete triad.

What are the components of the female athlete triad?

A) Disordered eating, menstrual dysfunction, altered bone mineral density.
B) Depression, weight loss, sports-related injury.
C) Poor sports performance, low self-esteem, injury.
D) Weight gain, bony injury, mood changes.
E) Sports participation, emotional disturbance, chronic injury.

Discussion

The correct answer is A. The female athlete triad was identified in the early 1990s and characterized as anorexia, amenorrhea, and osteoporosis. As more has been learned about the triad, it is likely that there is a broader spectrum of disorders within each category. Many young women with the triad will exhibit disordered eating behaviors, such as caloric restriction or use of diuretics and diet pills, but would not meet the criteria for anorexia or bulimia nervosa. Menstrual dysfunction may include oligomenorrhea (irregular, intermittent menses), as well as amenorrhea (absence of menses). These young women may also have abnormal bone mineral density, with predisposition to bony injury, without meeting the criteria of osteoporosis.

* *

The patient comes back to the office to receive her test results, and you take the opportunity to obtain more history. The patient admits that she is very concerned about her diet during her cross-country season, and she is very careful to choose foods that have very little fat but are often high in protein. She will occasionally "go overboard" and eat a lot, for which she compensates by taking part in extra workouts. She has also used laxatives in the past "to not gain weight when I eat too much."

Which of the following findings is NOT consistent with bulimia nervosa?

A) Loss of dental enamel.
B) Enlarged parotid glands.
C) Metabolic acidosis.
D) Skin changes over the dorsum of the hands.
E) Weight <85% of ideal.

Discussion

The correct answer is E. Anorexia nervosa has diagnostic criteria requiring maintenance of body weight at <85% of ideal body weight. **Individuals with bulimia nervosa often maintain a normal weight.** Loss of dental enamel, skin changes over the dorsum of the hands, and enlarged parotid glands are a result of repetitive self-induced vomiting. Although self-induced vomiting causes a metabolic alkalosis through loss of stomach acid, repetitive use of laxatives can cause gastrointestinal losses of bicarbonate, resulting in a metabolic acidosis.

* *

Your patient also relates that she began having her periods about 12 years of age. While they were initially irregular, they seemed to become more regular before starting high school. As she became involved in high school sports, her periods became more irregular. During her off-season, her menses are "more regular," though she cannot predict when they will occur. She recalls that her last period was about 7 weeks ago.

In order to evaluate your patient's menstrual dysfunction, what is your next course of action?

A) Obtain serum luteinizing hormone (LH), FSH, and estradiol levels.
B) Order an abdominal and pelvic ultrasound.
C) Perform a speculum-assisted pelvic exam with Papanicolaou smear.
D) Confirm urine β-hCG levels.
E) Prescribe an oral progestin-only pill (progestin challenge).

Discussion

The correct answer is D. The most common cause of secondary amenorrhea in women of childbearing age is pregnancy. If pregnancy is excluded, and the history and physical are reassuring, a progestin challenge is helpful to determine if adequate estrogen is present; the progestin challenge should induce menses if adequate estrogen exists. Imaging studies and hormonal levels may help to exclude other diagnoses or if warranted by exam. "Pap and pelvic" exams are recommended for sexually active women, but may not be necessary in the initial evaluation of menstrual dysfunction in this setting.

* *

Your patient's pregnancy test is negative, and a progestin challenge induced menses. A comprehensive plan was developed that included psychological counseling, dietary modification, physical therapy, consultation with a nutritionist, and frequent follow-up. Over the next several months, the patient recovers from her injury, and has been able to run again on a modified schedule. However, she now complains of heavy, painful menses and wants to go on the "shot" to stop them.

In your counseling about birth control options, which of the following statements is FALSE?

A) The birth control pill can be used to treat irregular menses of the female athlete triad and will also increase bone deposition.
B) The effect of Depo-Provera (medroxyprogesterone) is to suppress the hypothalamic-pituitary-ovarian axis, creating a low-estrogen state similar to perimenopause.
C) The FDA issued a "black box" warning that prolonged use of Depo-Provera may result in loss of bone density which may not be completely reversible after discontinuation of the drug.
D) The risk of future fracture using Depo-Provera is unknown, as bone density is an incomplete measure of bone strength and remodeling and recovery are significant.

Discussion

The correct answer is A. A combined estrogen/progesterone contraceptive pill will restart a menstrual cycle but may not increase bone density. IGF-1 (insulin-like growth factor 1) **can** increase bone density and **endogenous** IGF-1 levels increase when caloric intake increases (Grinspoon, et al, 2002). The other statements are all true.

* *

In your routine anticipatory guidance, you learn that she avoids most dairy products because of prior concerns about fat content and lactose intolerance.

What do you recommend for her daily intake of calcium?

A) 900 mg.
B) 1,100 mg.
C) 1,500 mg.
D) 1,700 mg.
E) 2,100 mg.

Discussion

The correct answer is C. Although the optimum intake of calcium for individuals is unknown, studies show positive calcium balance for adolescents with an intake of 1,200–1,500 mg daily. The National Academy of Sciences has set 1,300 mg/day as the "adequate" dietary intake for boys and girls, aged 9–18 years. This guideline was set to meet the needs of 95% of healthy children, with the upper limit of calcium intake set at 2,500 mg/day.

For most individuals, 1,300 mg/day of calcium intake can be accomplished with 4 servings of dairy products (8 oz of milk = 8 oz of yogurt or cottage cheese = 1-inch cube of cheese) plus a varied diet that includes calcium-rich foods (eg, broccoli, collard greens, turnip greens). Despite numerous non- and lowfat dairy options and supplements, concern over fat intake has resulted in an average adolescent intake of only 700–800 mg/day for girls and about 1,000 mg/day for boys.

On average, what percentage of total body mineral content has a young woman deposited by 12 years of age?

A) 20%–30%
B) 40%-50%
C) 70%–75%
D) 80%–85%
E) 95%–100%

Discussion

The correct answer is D. Research suggests that by 12 years, a young woman has reached approximately 83% of her peak bone mineral content. Fifty percent deposition takes place from "peak height velocity," which is premenarchal, through 1 year postmenarche. The ability to absorb calcium from the diet is also enhanced during this period. Rates of deposition begin to decline approximately 2 years postmenarche, and no significant gains are seen after 17 years. These statistics emphasize that osteoporosis, although a manifestation of older adults, is an issue of adolescent preventive medicine.

* *

Your patient returns from a high-powered sports medicine clinic. She brings her DEXA results consistent with osteopenia.

You scour the literature and recommend:

A) Alendronate.
B) Calcium and vitamin D.
C) Vigorous weight-bearing exercise.
D) DHEA (dihydroepiandrosterone).
E) All of the above.

Discussion

The correct answer is B. Stick with the standard of care: calcium in the daily doses recommended above and vitamin D 400 IU daily. Alendronate (answer A) has no demonstrated benefit in adolescent osteopenic females. Weight-bearing exercise (answer B) is the usual course for older patients with osteopenia, but you need to be careful in the adolescent with weight concerns who may exercise excessively at baseline. DHEA (answer C) is investigational and has not been shown to increase bone mineral density.

Objectives: Did you learn to . . .

• Evaluate leg pain in a runner?
• Identify the female athlete triad?
• Recognize the importance of calcium intake and osteoporosis prevention in adolescence?

QUICK QUIZ: ADOLESCENT ATHLETES

For adolescent athletes, what is the leading cause of sudden cardiac death (SCD)?

A) Marfan syndrome.
B) Coronary artery disease.
C) Congenital malformation of coronary arteries.
D) Hypertrophic cardiomyopathy.
E) Long QT syndrome.

Discussion

The correct answer is D. Hypertrophic cardiomyopathy is an autosomal dominant trait with highly variable penetrance that results in asymmetric septal wall hypertrophy. This may cause functional aortic outflow tract obstruction as well as predispose the athlete to arrhythmias. This condition is often asymptomatic prior to the terminal event and screening tests such as electrocardiographs and echocardiograms have not been shown to be effective for early detection of this condition. Aberrant coronary arteries (answers B and C) are the second leading cause of SCD in young athletes. Marfan syndrome (answer A) and long QT syndrome (answer E) are less common causes of death.

CASE 3

You are participating in a sports physical screening. One of the students is noted to be hypertensive with a blood pressure of 143/95. There is no family history of sudden death or early heart attack. He has never experienced any symptoms with exercise. His parents indicated on the form that they did not recall any history of previous heart murmur or high blood pressure. The athlete passes through the remaining stations, and an I/VI systolic murmur is heard. The examiner asks the athlete to perform a Valsalva maneuver by holding his breath and bearing down while auscultation is repeated.

Which of the following correctly describes the role of Valsalva maneuver in the relationship between murmur intensity and the type of murmur?

A) Valsalva maneuver increases flow murmur, decreases outflow tract obstruction murmur.
B) Valsalva maneuver increases both flow murmur and outflow tract obstruction murmur.
C) Valsalva maneuver decreases both flow murmur and outflow tract obstruction murmur.
D) Valsalva maneuver decreases flow murmur, increases outflow tract obstruction murmur.

Discussion

The correct answer is D. The Valsalva maneuver decreases venous return to the heart, resulting in decreased diastolic filling. You would expect this to cause decreased flow through the outflow tract and thus a softer flow murmur. However, the decreased flow exacerbates the **functional** outflow tract obstruction of hypertrophic cardiomyopathy (there is less volume to push the septum out of the way, resulting in a tighter functional stenosis), resulting in a louder murmur. In summary, **benign flow murmurs will decrease in intensity with Valsalva maneuver while the murmur of hypertrophic cardiomyopathy will increase with a Valsalva maneuver.**

 HELPFUL TIP: The systolic crescendo-decrescendo murmur of hypertrophic cardiomyopathy increases in intensity when the patient moves from a supine to an upright position. S_4 may be heard as well.

* *

Reassured by a murmur that disappears with Valsalva maneuver and an otherwise unremarkable exam, you are now faced with an adolescent athlete with an elevated blood pressure confirmed by manual retesting.

What is the best recommendation for this athlete regarding sports participation and follow-up of his elevated blood pressure?

A) Qualified participation pending serial blood pressure checks over the next three weeks.
B) Complete disqualification for 2 months, followed by return if normal ECG and echocardiogram.
C) Disqualification from competition only for 1 month, but allowed to practice after being seen by a nephrologists.
D) Full participation with no required follow-up, based on reassuring history and examination.
E) Full participation with blood pressure recheck prior to the next competitive sport season.

Discussion

The correct answer is A. It is important to remember that the diagnosis of hypertension cannot be made at a single screening visit. The screening test may be affected by patient anxiety (white coat hypertension), recent caffeine ingestion, drugs, or other factors (including a common occurrence of scheduling PPEs for right after practice). Most recommendations include 3 separate recordings of blood pressure on different occasions after several minutes at rest, sitting comfortably.

Because exercise is beneficial for blood pressure control, continued aerobic activity is encouraged while the serial blood pressure readings are obtained. Debate exists over recommendations regarding static exercises, such as weightlifting. While lifting of heavy weights can exacerbate high blood pressure, there is some evidence to suggest that use of light to moderate weights with repetition is beneficial. Certainly, the presence of additional symptoms with exercise, such as headache or lightheadedness, would require more significant limitations in activity.

Objectives: Did you learn to . . .

- Identify important issues to address at the preparticipation physical exam?
- Evaluate an adolescent athlete with elevated blood pressure?
- Evaluate a cardiac murmur revealed on preparticipation physical exam?

CASE 4

A 15-year-old female presents to your office for a well-adolescent examination. She is a healthy teenager with no complaints. You have incorporated into your routine a screening tool, the Guideline for Adolescent Preventive Services (GAPS), one of many such tools available. The questions cover all areas of adolescent development and are designed so that areas of concern are easily identified.

What are the three leading causes of mortality for adolescents?

A) Leukemia, suicide, accidental drowning.
B) Childhood cancers, perinatally acquired HIV, suicide.
C) Congenital malformations, childhood cancers, suicide.
D) Accidental injury, homicide, suicide.
E) Childhood cancers, sudden cardiac death, suicide.

Discussion

The correct answer is D. Accidental injury, homicide, and suicide are the three leading causes of death for adolescents and should be addressed during preventive health visits. Accidental injuries often involve the use of alcohol or other substances in combination with motor vehicle operation or other risk-taking behaviors. Ask not only about personal use of alcohol, but also if they are ever passengers of another teenager (or adult) who drives while impaired or intoxicated.

* *

You noticed that your patient checked "yes" for a history of use of alcohol and marijuana.

What is the approximate frequency of lifetime use of these substances among 9th–12th-grade students according to the Center for Disease Control and Prevention (CDC) 2005 Youth Risk Behavioral Survey?

A) Alcohol 30%–40%; marijuana <5%
B) Alcohol 40%–50%; marijuana 5%–10%
C) Alcohol 50%–60%; marijuana 10%–20%
D) Alcohol 60%–70%; marijuana 20%–30%
E) Alcohol 70%–80%; marijuana 30%–40%

Discussion
The correct answer is E. The survey found 74.3% of adolescents reporting lifetime use of alcohol, and 38.4 % lifetime use of marijuana, and incidentally, 54.3% have tried cigarettes.

HELPFUL TIP: Screening tools for adolescent substance use include the CRAFFT questions, developed by the Center for Adolescent Substance Abuse Research (CeASAR), Children's Hospital Boston. It is a tool similar to the CAGE tool for adult alcohol assessment. The acronym CRAFFT stands for:
Cars (Have you ever gotten into a car under the influence, or with a driver who is?)
Relax (Do you use a substance to help you relax?)
Alone (Do you use a substance alone?)
Forget (Have you ever had spells of forgetfulness/ black-outs when using?)
Friends (Are your friends concerned about your use?)
Trouble (Have you gotten into trouble from your use?)

* *

After eliciting a positive response to questions about drug use, you ask the patient about depression, and she states that she has been feeling "down" for several months now.

What will your next step be?

A) Call the police and report the illegal use of substances by a minor.
B) Reassure the patient about her confidentiality rights, counsel her to quit using drugs, and see her back annually.
C) Begin the patient on a SSRI and see her back in a month.
D) Negotiate next steps to guarantee the patient's safety and consider counseling referral.
E) Obtain a nonconsented urine drug screen to document recent use.

Discussion
The correct answer is D. Most states and HIPAA guarantee teenagers confidentiality, to be broken only when there is an issue of personal danger to self or others or physical/sexual abuse. It is recommended that the patient be involved and consent to who and how the information is shared. Rarely is there a need to involve police, unless there is an issue of abuse requiring a report or concern over safety releasing the patient to the home environment.

Answer C is incorrect. If an SSRI is started, close supervision is required for adolescents. For depression, studies reporting increased suicidality in teenagers treated with antidepressants caused the FDA to issue a black-box warning in 2004. The American Academy of Child and Adolescent Psychiatry Web site has resources outlining patient and parent information about the risks and benefits of pharmacologic treatments. CBT (cognitive behavioral therapy), along with talk therapy, has been shown to be the best first-line treatment for adolescents with mood disorders. Close follow-up of a depressed adolescent (weekly visits or phone calls) is recommended.

HELPFUL TIP: SSRIs are not that effective for pediatric/adolescent depression. The NNT to benefit one patient is ten. Fluoxetine has the most favorable benefit/risk profile in adolescents and is recommended as first-line therapy by most published guidelines.

HELPFUL TIP: The American Academy of Pediatrics has a position statement against the use of nonconsented urine drug screens as a screening tool because of its lack of accuracy and violation of patient trust.

Objectives: Did you learn to . . .

- Identify and employ useful screening tools for routine adolescent exams?
- Recognize the importance of depression in adolescents?
- Describe causes of death in adolescents?
- Understand the common lifetime experience use of alcohol, tobacco, and marijuana?
- Describe screening and treatment options for mood disorders and substance abuse?

CASE 5

Your afternoon continues with a number of patients with sports-related complaints. A 14-year-old wrestler has arrived in the office with complaint of a rash on his left shoulder. The rash appears to consist of several small lesions with a vesicular appearance but no purulence and minimal erythema. There is no tenderness to palpation, and there is no tactile warmth in the affected area.

What is the best test to confirm your diagnosis of these lesions?

A) Microscopic evaluation with potassium hydroxide (KOH) preparation of the contents of one of the lesions.
B) Gram stain of the contents of one of the lesions.
C) Culture of the contents of one of the lesions.
D) Tzanck smear of the contents of one of the lesions.

Discussion

The correct answer is D. A Tzanck prep will give you immediate information about whether this is herpes simplex. This is important information to determine whether or not this patient can return to wrestling.

* *

The lesions have appeared within the past day, and your laboratory testing confirms the diagnosis of herpes simplex. Your patient does not recall any previous lesions like these. He denies any systemic symptoms.

What is the best course of treatment for this patient?

A) Cover the involved area to allow return to wrestling.
B) Treat with topical acyclovir and return to wrestling when lesions have crusted over.
C) Treat with oral acyclovir and return to wrestling when lesions have crusted over.

D) Treat with oral steroids to suppress the response and promote quicker return to wrestling.
E) Treat with topical antifungal medication and allow return to wrestling.

Discussion

The correct answer is C. Cutaneous herpes, also referred to in wrestling as herpes gladiatorum, is a highly contagious illness. With herpes simplex, all lesions must be fully crusted over **and** the athlete must have had at least 3 days of oral antiviral therapy before returning to competition. Most high school athletic associations have rules regarding the treatment of cutaneous disorders in wrestling, including herpes, tinea corporis, and impetigo. Answer B is incorrect because topical acyclovir is **not** effective in treating herpes simplex. Answer D is incorrect because oral steroids suppress the athlete's immune response, which allows further spread of the lesions.

Objectives: Did you learn to . . .

- Identify cutaneous herpes (herpes gladiatorum) and describe its treatment?

CASE 6

A 15-year-old male presents to your clinic for a sports physical. You review your patient's chart and scan his immunizations. The patient's mother recalls that her son received his "kindergarten shots," but he has had no immunizations since. His records reveal the following vaccines: 5 doses of diphtheria-tetanus-acellular pertussis (DTaP); 2 doses of oral polio vaccine (OPV); 2 doses of injectable polio vaccine (IPV); 4 doses of *Hemophilus influenzae* type B (HiB); 2 doses of measles-mumps-rubella (MMR); a clinical history of chickenpox.

Which, if any, immunizations would you offer today?

A) None; the patient is up-to-date for all immunizations.
B) Conjugate pneumococcal vaccine.
C) Hepatitis A/B vaccine; conjugate meningococcal vaccine; oral polio vaccine.
D) Hepatitis A/B vaccine; tetanus, diphtheria and pertussis (Tdap) vaccine; conjugate meningococcal vaccine.
E) Human papillomavirus (HPV) vaccine; Tdap; varicella vaccine.

Discussion

The correct answer is D. Universal vaccination for hepatitis B is now the standard recommendation, and the vaccine is included in most primary immunization series for infants. Because adolescence is a time when experimentation with drugs and sexual activity becomes more prevalent, vaccination for hepatitis B becomes even more relevant. Hepatitis A vaccine is now being required in many states before entry to school and is universally recommended for all children aged 12 months to 2 years. A catch-up vaccination schedule is now recommended for those aged 2–18 years. For those not vaccinated against hepatitis B, a combined hepatitis A and B vaccine exists.

Most children receive their last DTaP prior to entering preschool or kindergarten (4–5 years). Beginning in 2005, the ACIP has recommended giving the tetanus booster **with pertussis** at entry to middle school/ junior high (11–12 years). A Tdap "catch-up" vaccination is recommended for those who missed the prejunior high school booster, and the Tdap can be given within 5 years of the last Td vaccine for those who want pertussis protection (and has been safely administered within 18 months of Td). For protection against some serotypes of *Neisseria meningitidis*, the ACIP recommends universal vaccination with the new conjugate vaccine (Menactra) for teens. Answer E is incorrect, because the patient here is a male and HPV vaccine is indicated for females only (as of the writing of this book).

Which statement does NOT accurately describe how the conjugated vaccine (Menactra) differs from the older polysaccharide meningitis vaccine, Menomune?

A) Menactra elicits a T-cell immune response that gives long-term immunity and allows for herd immunity.

B) Menactra protects against all the types of *N. meningitidis*: A, B, C, Y, W-135.

C) Menomune does not elicit a booster effect, may be given only once, and is recommended only at the onset of high-risk activity, such as living in dorms or being a military recruit.

D) Menactra should be offered at entry to middle school/ junior high (11–12 years), as the highest incidence of mortality for *N. meningitidis* is for individuals aged 15–25 years, and may be given again at entry to college.

Discussion

The correct answer is B. Unfortunately neither the Menomune nor the Menactra vaccine protects against serogroup type B. *N. meningitidis* type B is endemic in North America. The CDC estimates 75% prevention of *N. meningitidis* using the Menactra vaccine.

For an unvaccinated teen, what is the recommended schedule for the hepatitis B series?

A) 1 vaccination only.

B) 2 vaccinations: day 0, 1 month later.

C) 2 vaccinations: day 0, 12 months later.

D) 3 vaccinations: day 0, 1 month later, 6 months later.

E) 3 vaccinations: day 0, 2 weeks later, 1 month later.

Discussion

The correct answer is D. The schedule of three vaccinations, administered on day 0, 1 month later, and 6 months later, is the standard schedule recommended by the CDC. Accelerated dosing with shorter intervals may be appropriate for some patients but there must be 4 weeks between dose #1 and #2, and 8 weeks between doses #2 and #3.

* *

If your patient returned 1 year late for the second hepatitis B vaccine, how would this change the series schedule?

A) Restart the series schedule.

B) Give today and complete in 4 weeks.

C) Check hepatitis titers and adjust schedule accordingly.

D) Give today and complete series in 2 to 6 months.

Discussion

The correct answer is D. It is not required to restart a series of vaccines if there is a departure from the administration schedule. In the scenario described, this patient would receive vaccine at day 0, 12 months later (due to being late), and 2 months after the second dose, which is an acceptable schedule by recommended guidelines. It is important to ascertain that 2 months separate the second and third doses of hepatitis B vaccine. The practice of checking titers for vaccine efficacy is not routinely recommended, and it is often reserved for persons in high-risk occupations.

CASE 7

Upon return for his final hepatitis B vaccination, your patient's mother asks about the human papillomavirus

(HPV) vaccine. The mother has a daughter almost 12 years old who will come in for her annual exam soon, so she wants to know if her daughter should get the HPV vaccine.

All of the following statements about the quadrivalent HPV vaccine are true EXCEPT:

A) The vaccine will prevent about 70% of cervical cancer.

B) The vaccine will prevent >90% of anal/genital warts.

C) The vaccine requires 3 injections, at 0, 2, and 6 months.

D) The vaccine does not work on males, and so they are not eligible to receive it.

E) After completion of the vaccine series, routine gynecologic preventive care (Pap and pelvic) is still recommended.

Discussion

The correct answer is D. It is not a true statement because the vaccine **can** be given to males and is given to males in other countries to decrease the disease burden. However, as of the writing of this book, no major vaccine organization is recommending HPV vaccine to U.S. males.

The currently approved quadrivalent HPV vaccine (Gardasil) is active against HPV types 16 and 18, which cause an estimated 70% of cervical cancer worldwide (answer A). It is active against types 6 and 11, which cause over 90% of anal and genital warts (answer B). It has a 3-injection schedule and is recommended by the ACIP to be given to all girls aged 11–12 years (answer C), with catch-up vaccination through 26 years of age. The vaccine is approved for girls as young as 9 years in high-risk groups, and can be given even if a woman has an abnormal Pap smear. It is not approved during pregnancy, but it is approved during nursing.

 HELPFUL TIP: Up to 30% of patients with only one varicella vaccine get chicken pox, although it is usually mild. A booster varicella vaccine, which may be combined with the booster MMR at 4–6 years, is recommended. Adolescents who have had only one varicella vaccine should get the booster. The combination varicella-MMR is **not** recommended for children >12 years.

Objectives: Did you learn to . . .

• Identify immunizations important for adolescents?

BIBLIOGRAPHY

American Psychiatric Association. *Diagnostic and Statistical Manual of Mental Disorders*, 4th ed. Washington, DC: APA, 1994.

Elster AB, Kuznets NJ, eds. *AMA Guidelines for Adolescent Preventive Services (GAPS):Recommendations and Rationale.* Baltimore: Williams & Wilkins, 1994.

Gomez JE, Lantry BR, Saathoff KN. Current use of adequate preparticipation history forms for heart disease screening of high school athletes. *Arch Pediatr Adolesc Med.* 1999;153(7):723.

Grinspoon S, Thomas L, Miller K, et al. Effects of recombinant human IGF-1 and OCP administration on BMD in AN. *J Clin Endocrinol Metab.* 2002;87(6):2883.

Hoyert DL, Arias E, Smith BL, Murphy SL, Kochanek KD. Deaths: final data for 1999. *National Vital Statistics Reports.*, 2001;49(8).

Immunization Action Coalition. 2006 Immunization Schedule. Adapted from the Advisory Committee on Immunization Practices. Accessed September 6, 2007, at http://immunize.org/catg.d/rules1.pdf.

Kliegman RM, Behrman RE, Jenson HB, eds. *Nelson Textbook of Pediatrics*, 17th ed. Philadelphia: W.B. Saunders, 2007.

Lloyd T, Rollings N, Andon MB, Demers LM, Eggli DF, et al. Determinants of bone density in young women. I. Relationships among pubertal development, total body bone mass, and total body bone density in premenarchal females. *J Clin Endocrinol Metab.* 1992;75(2):383.

NIH Consensus Conference. Optimal calcium intake. NIH Consensus Development Panel on Optimal Calcium Intake. *JAMA.* 1994;272:1942.

Otis CL, Drinkwater B, Johnson M, Loucks A, Wilmore J. ACSM position stand on the female athlete triad. *Med Sci Sports Exer.* 1997;29(5):i.

Patel DR, Gordon RC. Contagious diseases in athletes. *Contemp Pediatr.* 1999;16(9):139.

Sallis RE, Massimino F, eds. *American College of Sports Medicine's Essentials of Sports Medicine.* St Louis: Mosby-Year Book, 1997.

Samuels RC, Cohen LE. Understanding growth patterns in short stature. *Contemp Pediatr.* 2001;18:94.

Tanner, JM, Goldstein, H, Whitehouse, RH. Standards for children's heights at ages 2 to 9 years allowing for height of parents. *Arch Dis Child.* 1970;45:755.

Theintz G, Buchs B, Rizzoli R, Slosman D, Clavien H, et al. Longitudinal monitoring of bone mass accumulation in healthy adolescents: evidence for a marked reduction after 16 years of age at the levels of lumbar spine and femoral neck in female subjects. *J Clin Endocrinol Metab.* 1992;75(4):1060.

United States Food and Drug Administration, Center for Food Safety and Applied Nutrition. Accessed November 4, 2007, at http://www.cfsan.fda.gov.

15

Obstetrics and Women's Health

David A. Bedell, Lori J. Day and Colleen M. Kennedy

CASE 1

A 24-year-old nulligravida female presents for her annual exam. Her gynecologic history is remarkable for irregular menses, occurring every 4 weeks to 8 weeks. She would like a more reliable form of contraception (currently uses condoms) and would like to have predictable menses, but is very concerned regarding weight gain with various contraception methods.

How would you counsel her regarding weight changes and oral contraceptive pills (OCPs)?

A) Weight gain of 10 pounds during the first year of use with any type of OCPs is expected.
B) Studies show there is no significant difference in weight gain of women initiating OCPs versus placebo.
C) Weight gain of 10 pounds during the first year of use with monophasic pills is expected, but not with triphasic formulations.
D) Weight loss of 10 pounds during the first year of use with Depo-Provera (medroxyprogesterone acetate) is expected.

Discussion

The correct answer is B. Studies have shown no significant weight gain with OCP use when compared to placebo. Trials have been conducted evaluating estrogen components of 20–50 micrograms, both monophasic and triphasic. Answers C and D are incorrect. **There is no evidence to support the premise that triphasic formulations offer improvement in weight changes.** Depo-Provera has variable effects on weight gain. Several studies have shown a weight gain of 3–6 kg in the first year of use; however, other studies have shown no difference in weight gain between Depo-Provera and placebo.

* *

After reassuring her regarding the concerns of weight gain, you tell her about the additional potential benefit(s) of OCPs, which include:

A) Improvement in acne.
B) Decreased dysmenorrhea.
C) Decreased menstrual flow.
D) Decreased risk of ovarian cancer.
E) All of the above.

Discussion

The correct answer is E. Besides these, additional benefits of OCP use include regulation and predictability of menses, decreased anemia, decreased hirsutism, and decreased risk of endometrial cancer.

* *

After further discussion, she reports that she occasionally takes over-the-counter medications for headaches that occur every 1 to 2 months. She has never been evaluated for migraines, but reports that her headaches are bilateral, posterior, throbbing, and relieved with sleep and over-the-counter medication. She denies associated aura, nausea, or focal neurologic changes.

How would you counsel her regarding OCPs and headaches?

A) Headaches are an uncommon reason for discontinuation of OCPs.

B) She should not use OCPs, because they are contraindicated in anyone with headaches.

C) She should use progestin-only pills.

D) She should use OCPs, as it is hard to predict whether her headaches will be affected.

Discussion

The correct answer is D. Although headache is a frequently cited reason for women to discontinue OCPs, there is not a strong correlation between headache frequency or intensity for most women. There is no evidence that the type of progestin or amount of estrogen will alter the headaches, except in women with menstrual migraines. Among women with migraines, headaches can improve, worsen, or remain unchanged after initiation of OCPs. This patient describes characteristics of a tension headache rather than a migraine. **There is an increased risk of cerebral thromboembolism in women with a history of pseudotumor cerebri or migraines with aura or focal neurologic changes; therefore, OCPs are contraindicated in this group of women.**

* *

Three years later the patient returns again for her "annual exam" (see Helpful Tip below). She has used OCPs and is satisfied with her regular menses and no worsening in her headaches. However, she and her partner are interested in starting a family. She has no new medical problems and her partner is healthy.

What should NOT be addressed during her prepregnancy counseling session?

A) Implications of advanced maternal age.

B) Tobacco and alcohol use.

C) Initiation of a prenatal vitamin.

D) Vaccination status.

Discussion

The correct answer is A. This patient is 27 years old now, and advanced maternal age is considered to be 35 years at the time of delivery. Tobacco and alcohol cessation programs should be offered to patients who need this assistance. Folic acid 400 micrograms daily should be taken prior to conception and should be recommended to all women of child-bearing age. Rubella and varicella susceptibility should be assessed as well. It is recommended that women delay conception for 1 month after receiving a live rubella or varicella vaccination. Other items that should also be included are family history of genetic diseases, mental health and social support, occupational or environmental exposures, and common over-the-counter medications to avoid. Although this patient does not have any other medical conditions or pregnancy history, these items are important to review with those patients who may have them.

 HELPFUL TIP: Note that this patient followed up for a repeat PAP smear 3 years after starting OCPs; this is appropriate for a low-risk patient with a normal PAP. **However, the patient should be followed up for blood pressure checks, etc after starting OCPs.**

* *

In 8 months, the patient calls to speak with your nurse regarding nausea and vomiting. Her last menstrual period was 10 weeks ago, and she had a positive home pregnancy test 5 weeks ago. She has stopped taking her prenatal vitamins, since these were making the nausea worse. Over the last week, she has been vomiting once every day, at various times, but is nauseated throughout most of the day. She wants to know if there is anything else that is safe that she can do to decrease the nausea.

What is your most appropriate response?

A) This level of nausea and vomiting is abnormal and needs an immediate workup to rule out other pathology.

B) This level of nausea and vomiting is very common, and there are several modifications and over-the-counter medications that are safe.

C) This level of nausea and vomiting is very common; however, there are no medications that can be initiated in the first trimester.

D) This level of nausea and vomiting is very common. Metoclopramide, promethazine, and ondansetron are first-line therapies.

Discussion

The correct answer is B. Mild-to-moderate nausea and vomiting are very common in the first trimester of pregnancy, often improving by 16 weeks' gestation. Several modifications can improve symptoms, including small, frequent meals, avoiding fatty foods, and avoiding environmental triggers (perfumes, smoking, position changes, or certain movements). Over-the-counter remedies include ginger ale, vitamin B_6 (10–25 mg 3–4 times daily), and doxylamine (12.5 mg 3 to 4 times daily). These remedies resolve symptoms for many patients. For those who do not respond, antiemetics including metoclopramide or promethazine should be considered. Answer D is incorrect because it represents a next step, not a first step. Rarely is ondansetron necessary. Up to 2% of the time, nausea and vomiting represent characteristics of hyperemesis gravidarum, which involves weight loss of more than 5% of prepregnancy weight or dehydration and ketonuria.

If the patient had presented with 6–8 episodes of emesis daily, an 8-pound weight loss since her LMP, and a urine specific gravity of >1.030 and ketonuria, your workup should have included:

A) Quantitative β-HCG.
B) Serum electrolytes, BUN and creatinine.
C) Thyroid-stimulating hormone (TSH).
D) Pelvic ultrasound.
E) All of the above.

Discussion

The correct answer is E. As with any other severely nauseated and vomiting patient, it is reasonable to check for electrolyte imbalances. Severity of nausea and vomiting correlates with higher levels of β-HCG, as would be seen with a molar or twin pregnancy. Gestational trophoblastic disease, although rare, should be evaluated for with β-HCG level. The ultrasound would confirm a twin pregnancy and could provide evidence of a molar pregnancy. TSH can exclude hyperthyroidism.

* *

Fortunately, the patient did not have severe nausea and vomiting and her symptoms improved with the conservative dietary changes, vitamin B_6, and doxylamine. She presents for her initial prenatal visit at 12 weeks' gestation.

You offer her the routine prenatal tests at this visit, which include all of the following EXCEPT:

A) Syphilis testing.
B) HIV testing.

C) One-hour postcarbohydrate load serum glucose level.
D) Blood type and antibody screen.
E) Fetal nuchal lucency with maternal HCG and PAPP-A.

Discussion

The correct answer is C. Diabetes screening (50 g carbohydrate load with blood glucose obtained at 1 hour) is typically not completed until 24–28 weeks' gestation. Patients with a history of gestational diabetes or those who are suspected to have diabetes may be candidates for earlier screening. Syphilis and HIV testing are completed to decrease the risk of perinatal transmission. The blood type and antibody screen is used to identify mothers with blood antibodies that could cause hemolytic disease of the fetus. Mothers who are Rh negative will subsequently receive RhoGAM as well.

Additional first trimester screening should be offered to mothers of all ages with a gestation of between 11 weeks 0 days and 13 weeks and 6 days. This represents a change in the ACOG guidelines (ACOG Practice Bulletin 2007). Two maternal serum markers, HCG (human chorionic gonadotropin) and PAPP-A (plasma-associated pregnancy protein A), and one fetal marker, nuchal thickness, are used for early screening for Down syndrome and trisomy 18. This method offers a Down syndrome detection rate of approximately 85% with a 5% false-positive rate.

 HELPFUL TIP: Since it does not screen for neural tube defects, first-trimester screening does not negate the need for a second-trimester maternal serum triple or quad screen, including AFP (alpha-fetoprotein), HCG, uE3 (unconjugated estriol), and inhibin A, which is done between 15 weeks 0 days and 19 weeks 6 days gestation.

* *

The patient has passed all of her screening tests with flying colors so far. She returns at 36 weeks' gestation.

What additional screening test(s) is (are) obtained near 36 weeks' gestation?

A) Amniocentesis.

B) 3-hour glucose tolerance test.

C) Fetal fibronectin.

D) Group B streptococcus (GBS) culture.

E) All of the above are appropriate at 36 weeks' gestation.

Discussion

The correct answer is D. The CDC recommends maternal screening for GBS between 35 and 37 weeks' gestation. The only persons who should be excluded are women who had bacteruria with GBS during the current pregnancy or those who had an infant previously infected with GBS. These mothers are treated empirically with antibiotics in labor and do not need screening. Mothers whose culture status is unknown should receive antibiotic prophylaxis only if one of the following exists: (1) intrapartum fever (>38°C), (2) preterm labor (<37 weeks' gestation), or (3) prolonged rupture of membranes (>18 hours). Amniocentesis is not a routine screening test at 36 weeks, but is recommended to patients for various indications including genetic diagnosis, isoimmunization, and fetal lung maturity. A 3-hour glucose tolerance test is used to diagnose gestational diabetes, and is completed after a patient has failed a 1-hour glucose challenge screening test. Fetal fibronectin is not recommended as a routine screening test, but you will see more on this later.

Objectives: Did you learn to . . .

- Describe contraception options?
- Provide appropriate routine prenatal care?
- Recognize nausea and vomiting of pregnancy and the appropriate management?

CASE 2

You are taking obstetric calls for your group this weekend. Labor and delivery calls you to notify you regarding a patient coming in. She is a 27-year-old G1 P0 at 38 weeks' gestation who awoke this morning complaining of wetness. However, when she went to the bathroom she discovered significant vaginal bleeding that had soaked her bed. She denies any cramping or abdominal pain. She is on her way to the hospital.

You tell the nurses to initiate all of the following interventions immediately upon the patient's arrival EXCEPT:

A) Obtain IV access.

B) Draw blood for type and screen.

C) Perform a digital vaginal exam.

D) Initiate fetal monitoring.

E) Draw blood for complete blood count.

Discussion

The correct answer is C. A small-to-moderate amount of bleeding is not unexpected during labor; however, the profuse bleeding described by the patient is an obstetric emergency. The first priorities are to obtain IV access and ensure that the mother is hemodynamically stable. Baseline laboratory evaluation will give some indication of the amount of blood loss and establish that blood is available for transfusion if necessary. Monitoring of the fetal heart rate will establish viability. Also, an ultrasound should be done to evaluate for placenta previa. A digital vaginal examination should **not** be performed until the diagnosis of placenta previa has been excluded. An obstetrical consultation should be obtained if the initial evaluation suggests that immediate fetal delivery is necessary.

 HELPFUL TIP: Classically, placenta previa presents as painless third-trimester bleeding, whereas, placental abruption classically presents as painful third-trimester bleeding.

* *

When the patient arrives at the hospital, she alters her recollection of events to say that the fluid soaking the bed sheets was blood-tinged and pink in color and first occurred 2 hours ago. She continues to have vaginal leakage but denies any bright-red bleeding or contractions. Ultrasound reveals a fundal placenta without any evidence of abruption. Fetal heart tones are in the 140s and reactive. Sterile speculum examination reveals fluid which is nitrazine and ferning positive. Her GBS culture performed 3 weeks ago is negative.

What is the most appropriate next step in the management of this patient?

A) Begin an induction of labor.

B) Send her home after 4 hours of reassuring fetal monitoring.

C) Treat her with IV penicillin for GBS prophylaxis.

D) Repeat her GBS culture.

Discussion

The correct answer is A. Even if labor does not ensue, the patient should not be sent home after rupture of membranes has been diagnosed. She is at risk for intrauterine infection. Induction of labor, even with an unfavorable cervix, is not associated with an increase in cesarean or operative vaginal delivery, but it is associated with fewer maternal infections and fewer neonatal intensive care unit admissions. Her GBS culture was negative 3 weeks ago. Although GBS colonization can be transient, since the culture was completed within 5 weeks, it should be reliable. Even if her membranes were ruptured for more than 18 hours, she would not require treatment with antibiotics unless she developed a fever.

* *

Sterile vaginal exam reveals a cervix that is 1 cm dilated, 3 cm long (effacement), and vertex at −1 station. The patient agrees to an induction of labor.

The best method for this patient is to:

A) Insert intracervical Laminaria.
B) Begin IV oxytocin at 2 milliunits per minute.
C) Begin IV oxytocin at 2 units per minute.
D) Insert intravaginal dinoprostone.

Discussion

The correct answer is B. The use of intravaginal and intracervical methods for cervical ripening may increase the risk of infection after membranes have ruptured. Oxytocin should be closely titrated via IV route for labor induction or augmentation. There is a wide variance in administration protocols at hospitals. However, the general starting doses are 0.5 to 6 milliunits per minute, increased by 1–6 milliunits every 20–40 minutes, to a maximum dose rarely exceeding 40 milliunits per minute. If you chose answer C, you were off by only a factor of 10^3—at least it's not heparin.

* *

The patient is currently in labor (success!), and now her cervical exam is: 6 cm dilation, 1 cm effaced, and −1 station. The amniotic fluid is still clear, having ruptured approximately 22 hours ago. She has an epidural for analgesia. The fetal heart rate baseline has increased to 165 beats per minute with decreased variability. Contractions occur every 3 minutes. Maternal temperature is now 38.6°C, and her pulse is 110. The patient denies any complaints.

What is the most likely diagnosis?

A) Normal labor.
B) Epidural fever.
C) Nosocomial infection.
D) Chorioamnionitis.

Discussion

The correct answer is D. Chorioamnionitis is the most likely diagnosis, given the prolonged rupture of membranes, maternal fever, and fetal tachycardia. Treatment should be initiated immediately. There is an association between the use of epidural analgesia and a rise in maternal temperature. Etiologies proposed for this temperature increase include lack of pain-induced hyperventilation and decreased perspiration due to sympathetic blockade. However, until we prove otherwise, one must assume this is chorioamnionitis.

What is the next step in the care of this patient?

A) Stop the oxytocin.
B) Remove the epidural.
C) Initiate broad-spectrum antibiotics.
D) Call the obstetrician/surgeon for cesarean section.

Discussion

The correct answer is C. Initiation of antibiotics is associated with a decrease in both maternal and neonatal morbidity. Multiple organisms are isolated in more than 66% of test cases; therefore, antibiotics should be broad. Approved regimens include ampicillin and gentamicin, ticarcillin/clavulanate, or piperacillin. The patient's labor is progressing, and the ultimate treatment for the chorioamnionitis is delivery. However, there is no need to stop the oxytocin and proceed with a cesarean delivery immediately, unless there is another indication. Although epidural anesthesia is associated with increased maternal temperature, it should only be removed if it is felt to be contributing to maternal pathology (eg, meningitis, epidural abscess, or epidural bleed).

* *

The patient's labor is progressing. Her cervix is 9 cm dilated, completely effaced, and station is +3. Her temperature is 39.0°C. The fetal heart rate pattern is shown in Figure 15–1.

What is the FHR interpretation?

A) Baseline 165 beats per minute, reactive.
B) Baseline 165 beats per minute, with periods of bradycardia.

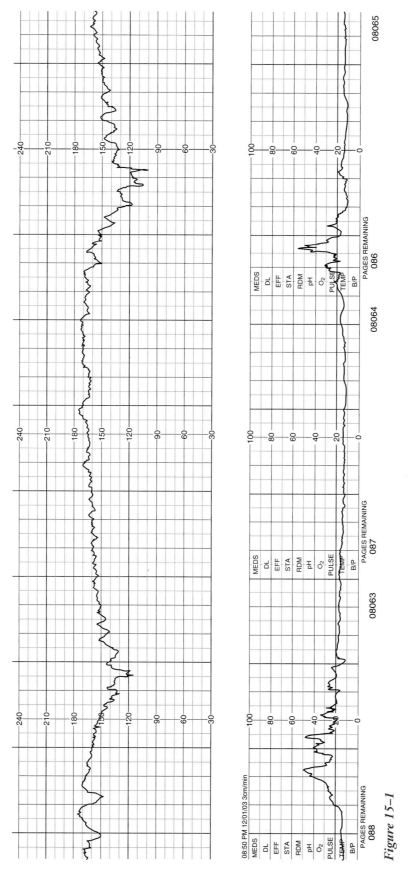

495

Figure 15-1

C) Baseline 165 beats per minute, with late decelerations.

D) Baseline 165 beats per minute, with variable deceleration.

Discussion

The correct answer is C. The fetal heart rate shown in Figure 15–1 is about 165 beats per minute. There is good long-term and short-term (beat-to-beat) variability present. Following each contraction, there are late decelerations to the 110s. Answer A is incorrect because "reactive" refers to a nonstress test. Reactive is defined as 2 accelerations, of at least 15 beats above baseline and lasting at least 15 seconds, within a 20-minute interval. Fetal bradycardia is defined as a fetal heart rate of <90 beats per minute. Variable decelerations vary with respect to timing, duration, and depth.

What is the likely etiology of the fetal heart rate tracing in Figure 15–1?

A) Head compression.

B) Placental insufficiency.

C) Cord compression.

D) All of the above.

Discussion

The correct answer is B. Late decelerations are believed to be secondary to transient fetal hypoxia in response to decreased placental perfusion. Prompt evaluation and intervention are warranted. Early decelerations are generally reassuring and attributed to fetal head compression. Variable decelerations are the most common decelerations seen in labor and indicate cord compression. Variable decelerations can sometimes be relieved by maternal repositioning or amnioinfusion.

What is the LEAST appropriate course of action now?

A) Administer maternal oxygen.

B) Stop oxytocin.

C) Forceps- or vacuum-assisted vaginal delivery.

D) Consider cesarean delivery.

E) Reposition mother (roll to one side or knee-chest).

Discussion

The correct answer is C. The arterial pO_2 in the fetus is normally approximately 25% of the arterial pO_2 in the mother. Increasing maternal O_2 may improve fetal oxygenation. Oxytocin can decrease placental blood flow via uterine stimulation, and hence should be decreased or stopped if non-reassuring fetal **heart rate** changes are present. If there is evidence of maternal hypotension, maternal hydration may be indicated. Another option is position changes (left lateral) to improve placental perfusion. Maternal position can affect uterine blood flow and placental perfusion. The gravid uterus may compress the vena cava while supine. Because the patient is 9 cm dilated, forceps- or vacuum-assisted vaginal delivery (also known as "operative vaginal delivery") is **not** indicated. Prior to operative vaginal delivery, several criteria must be evaluated, including: complete dilation and effacement; appropriate fetal position and station; adequate maternal pelvis; appropriately sized fetus; and adequate analgesia.

* *

The fetal heart rate changes resolve with your appropriate interventions. The patient progresses to complete dilation and delivers vaginally one hour later. No antibiotics are continued following delivery, and the maternal temperature 2 hours after delivery is 37.0°C. On postpartum day 1, your patient complains of sore breasts from breast-feeding, and her abdomen is sore "all over." She is having a moderate amount of lochia, and her temperature is 38.4°C.

The most likely diagnosis at this time is:

A) Endometritis.

B) Mastitis.

C) Deep vein thrombosis.

D) Septic pelvic thrombophlebitis.

Discussion

The correct answer is A. Postpartum endometritis is most likely in this patient who had chorioamnionitis. Prolonged rupture of membranes and prolonged labor with multiple cervical examinations increase the risk of postpartum endometritis to 6%. The presence of intraamniotic infection increases the risk of postpartum endometritis to 13%. Antibiotics are not routinely continued for chorioamnionitis after a vaginal delivery because the "source" of the infection (the placenta) has been removed. Whenever fever occurs in the immediate postpartum period, endometritis should be suspected. Mastitis is characterized by a swollen, firm, tender breast with systemic symptoms including fevers, chills, and flu-like symptoms. *Staphylococcus aureus* is the typical pathogen. However, in the immediate postpartum period, breast engorgement without infection is the most likely reason for the patient's sore breasts. Pregnancy and the postpartum period increase a woman's risk of thrombogenesis. However, DVT is not a likely source of the fever. Septic pelvic thrombophlebitis is a diagnosis of exclusion and is usually entertained when fever spikes continue following treatment for endometritis.

What is the best course of action?

A) Monitor closely and avoid antibiotics since she is breast-feeding.
B) Obtain uterine cultures.
C) Begin oral antibiotics.
D) Begin IV antibiotics.
E) Begin IV heparin.

Discussion

The correct answer is D. Broad-spectrum antibiotics should be administered promptly by the parenteral route. Similar to chorioamnionitis, multiple bacterial organisms (usually normal vaginal and perineal flora) are likely to be responsible for this infection. Therefore, uterine cultures are unlikely to be helpful for guiding antibiotic therapy. Parenteral therapy should be continued until the patient has been afebrile for at least 24 hours. Oral antibiotics would be appropriate for the treatment of mastitis; however, this is not the most likely diagnosis. Heparin therapy should not be considered at this time, as there is a low clinical suspicion for thrombosis. However, should the patient not respond to antibiotics, septic pelvic thrombophlebitis should be reconsidered and heparin therapy reconsidered.

HELPFUL TIP: One of the greatest concerns with prolonged membrane rupture is the risk of maternal or fetal infection. If chorioamnionitis is diagnosed, prompt efforts to affect delivery, preferably vaginally, are initiated. Unfortunately, fever is the only reliable indicator for making this diagnosis; a temperature of ≥38°C accompanying ruptured membranes implies infection. Infants born to women with chorioamnionitis have a four-fold increase in neonatal mortality and a three-fold increase in the incidence of respiratory distress, neonatal sepsis, and intraventricular hemorrhage.

Objectives: Did you learn to . . .

- Triage and manage third-trimester bleeding?
- Recognize and treat a patient with premature rupture of membranes?
- Evaluate and manage intrapartum fever?
- Interpret fetal heart rate patterns and manage abnormal patterns?
- Appreciate the risk factors, evaluation, and management of postpartum infection?

CASE 3

You are seeing a 31-year-old G2P1 at 41 weeks' gestation by definite last menstrual period and 16-week ultrasound. You have been following her for prenatal care, and her pregnancy has been uncomplicated. At her visit today she has no complaints; she denies vaginal bleeding or loss of fluid. She continues to note fetal movement. Her examination is normal: BP 120/68, urine dipstick negative for protein and glucose, fundal height 42 cm, vertex, fetal heart rate 156. Her cervix is soft, anterior, 2–3 cm dilated, 50% effaced, and +1 station. You have discussed induction with your patient given her postdates, multiparity, and favorable cervix. However, she was induced with her first pregnancy, and this time she wants to have a "natural labor."

* *

Bishop score is a measure to assess success with induction.

Which of the following is NOT included in the Bishop score?

A) Cervical dilation.
B) Cervical effacement.
C) Station.
D) Cervical consistency.
E) Number of previous vaginal births.

Discussion

The correct answer is E. The Bishop pelvic scoring system evaluates cervical dilation, effacement, consistency, and position as well as fetal station. If the total score is more than 8, the probability of vaginal delivery for labor induction is similar to that of spontaneous labor. Table 15–1 describes the scoring.

* *

The Bishop score for the patient is 9 to 10 (dilation 2 cm is 1 less point than 3 cm).

Table 15–1 BISHOP SCORE

Points	0	1	2	3
Cervical dilation (cm)	0	1–2	3–4	5+
Cervical effacement (%)	0–30	40–50	60–70	80+
Fetal station	–3	–2	–1	≥+1
Cervical position	Posterior	Midposition	Anterior	—
Cervical consistency	Firm	Medium	Soft	—

Which of the following are the most appropriate recommendations now?

A) She should be induced at once; there is a high chance of fetal mortality after 41 weeks' gestation.

B) Since her antepartum course has been uncomplicated to date, it is safe for her to await spontaneous labor until 43 weeks' gestation.

C) She should undergo a nonstress test and ultrasound for amniotic fluid index.

D) She should plan for a cesarean section.

Discussion

The correct answer is C. A term gestation is one completed in 38 to 42 weeks' gestation. There is no significant increase in fetal mortality in an uncomplicated pregnancy at term. Virtually all reports suggest an increase in perinatal morbidity and mortality when pregnancy goes beyond 42 weeks' gestation. Antenatal surveillance of postterm pregnancies should be initiated at 41 weeks' gestation.

 HELPFUL TIP: Accurate determination of conception is important in reducing the false diagnosis of postterm pregnancy. The estimated date of delivery is most reliably and accurately determined early in pregnancy.

Which of the following nonpharmacologic methods of augmenting or inducing labor is LEAST likely to be effective?

A) Stripping the amniotic membranes.

B) Prolonged walking.

C) Amniotomy.

D) Nipple stimulation.

Discussion

The correct answer is B. Stripping membranes appears to be associated with a greater frequency of spontaneous labor and was demonstrated to be effective in initiating spontaneous labor within 72 hours in a randomized trial of postterm pregnancies. Amniotomy may be used for labor induction, especially if the Bishop score is favorable; however, early addition of oxytocin is associated with a shorter induction-to-delivery interval. Nipple stimulation causes release of oxytocin and may be utilized for labor induction, but its marginal benefit is only seen in patients with a favorable Bishop score. Walking does not result in labor induction or augmentation, but it is not harmful either.

 HELPFUL TIP: Sexual intercourse is sometimes recommended to induce labor. Studies are of low quality and use various endpoints. One of the better quality studies (Tan PC, et al, *Obstet Gynecol.* 2006;108(1):134) did find that coitus was associated with reduced need for labor induction at 41 weeks.

Which of the following pharmacologic methods would be the best approach to your patient, assuming the cervical exam above and no other interventions yet?

A) IV oxytocin.

B) Intracervical PGE$_2$ (dinoprostone).

C) Intravaginal PGE$_2$ (dinoprostone).

D) Intravaginal PGE$_1$ (misoprostol).

E) None of the above.

Discussion

The correct answer is A. This patient does not need further cervical ripening but instead is a candidate for induction of labor. The physiology of oxytocin-stimulated labor is similar to spontaneous labor. Uterine response begins after 3–5 minutes of infusion. It would be reasonable and appropriate to start induction with IV oxytocin. PGE_2 gel (dinoprostone, Cervidil or Prepidil) is administered vaginally—not intracervically—and is used for cervical ripening when induction is indicated but the status of the cervix is unfavorable. PGE_2 gel is not indicated for induction of labor. PGE_1 (answer D) can be administered intravaginally or orally and has been found to be effective for both cervical ripening and labor induction in studies. However, the FDA has not approved it for use in pregnancy. Because the cervix is favorable, proceeding with oxytocin is the best option.

**

Your patient's husband is called up for active duty in Iraq (or Afghanistan . . . or insert appropriate country at the time you are reading this) and is due to report in the next few days. She is now 41 2/7 weeks' gestation and desires induction so he can be with her for the delivery. You admit her to labor and delivery the following morning. The initial fetal heart rate monitoring **before any induction** is shown in Figure 15–2.

What is the correct interpretation?

A) Baseline = 150 beats per minute; not reactive.
B) Baseline = 150 beats per minute; reactive.
C) Baseline = 180 beats per minute; decelerations to 150s.
D) Baseline = 150 – 180 beats per minute; good variability, reassuring.

Discussion

The correct answer is B. The baseline is 150 beats per minute. There are 2 accelerations >15 beats and lasting longer than 15 seconds, which meets the criteria for a reactive nonstress test. There is one contraction and evidence of uterine irritability noted as well. There are no decelerations. The long-term and short-term (beat-to-beat) variability is excellent.

**

You perform amniotomy with return of particulate meconium-stained fluid. Her cervix is now 5 cm dilated, 80% effaced, with vertex at +1 station. You elect to continue monitoring progress.

Which of the following choices of labor analgesia is MOST appropriate now?

A) Epidural analgesia.
B) Local perineal anesthetic infiltration.
C) Bilateral pudendal nerve block.
D) All of the above.

Discussion

The correct answer is A. Epidural analgesia offers the most effective form of pain relief and generally may be utilized once the patient is determined to be in active labor. Various local anesthetic agents are available for local infiltration of the perineum and vagina to provide analgesia for **episiotomy or laceration repair following delivery but not for labor.** Bilateral pudendal nerve blocks are useful during the **second** stage of labor, as a supplement to epidural analgesia for anesthesia of the sacral nerves, or as an option for operative vaginal delivery anesthesia (forceps, vacuum), especially if the patient does not have an epidural. Opioid agonists and agonist-antagonists are also available and commonly employed. However, recent reports suggest that the analgesic effect in labor is limited.

**

The nurse notices some changes on the fetal heart monitor. The current fetal heart rate is shown in Figure 15–3.

What is the correct interpretation of this fetal monitor?

A) Baseline 160 beats per minute; reactive.
B) Baseline 160 beats per minutes; variable decelerations to the 90s.
C) Baseline 160 beats per minute; late decelerations to the 90s.
D) Baseline 160 beats per minute; early decelerations to the 90s.

Discussion

The correct answer is B. The baseline fetal heart rate is 160 beats per minute. There is good long-term and short-term variability noted. Variable decelerations to the 90s occur with the first and last contractions on this strip. Variable decelerations vary with respect to timing, duration, and depth—thus, the name "variable." They are not uniform. Variable decelerations represent

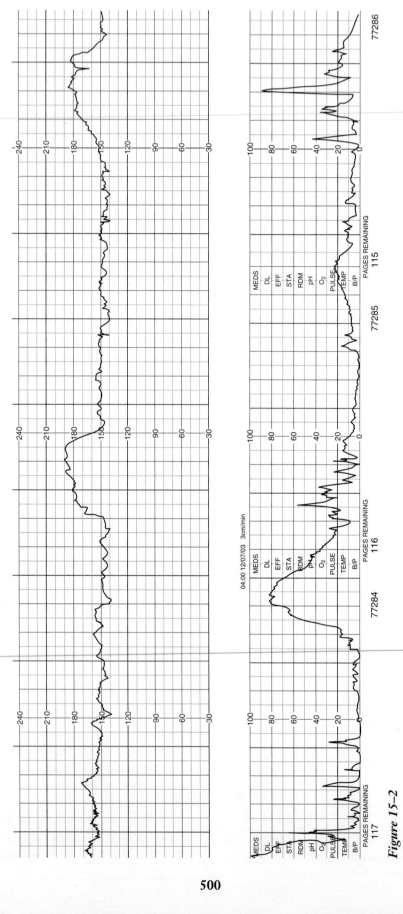

Figure 15–2

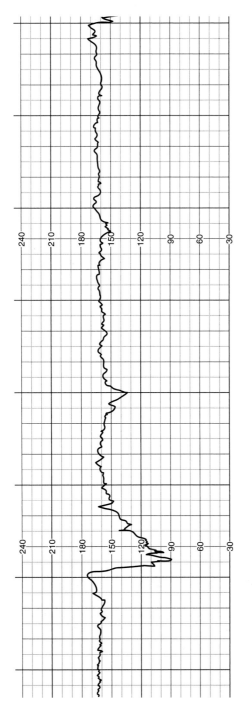
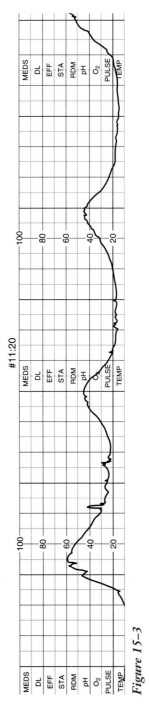

Figure 15–3

changes in the fetal heart rate in response to cord compression. Early decelerations are typically more repetitive and uniform and begin with the onset of the contraction and nadir with the contraction peak (mirroring the contraction). Early decelerations represent fetal head compression. Late decelerations are also repetitive and uniform. They begin after the contraction peak and represent placental insufficiency. Late decelerations are more concerning and should be investigated and treated aggressively.

Given the findings in Figure 15–3, which of the following should be performed next?

A) Check the patient's cervix.
B) Place a fetal scalp electrode.
C) Begin IV oxytocin infusion.
D) Place an intrauterine pressure catheter and begin an amnioinfusion.

Discussion

The correct answer is A. Variable decelerations are common in labor, and brief variable decelerations are benign. When variable decelerations become persistent, progressively deeper, longer lasting, and with delayed return to baseline, they are nonreassuring and may reflect hypoxia. In this situation, the variable decelerations are not ominous in nature. There is still good variability in the fetal baseline. A pelvic examination should be performed to determine if the umbilical cord is prolapsed or if there has been rapid descent of the fetal head or rapid progression of labor. The fetal heart rate is tracing being picked up well on the external monitor, and a fetal scalp electrode would add nothing. Oxytocin should not be considered until one learns more regarding the progression—or lack thereof—of labor. Replacement of the amniotic fluid with normal saline infused through a trans-cervical catheter has been reported to decrease both the frequency and severity of repetitive variable decelerations. However, it would first be helpful to assess the cervical status. **Amnioinfusion is no longer recommended as a prophylactic intervention for moderate or severe meconium.**

* *

Labor progresses without incident. Your patient is now completely dilated and effaced, with vertex at +3 station. She is comfortable with her epidural and able to push with good effort. The fetal heart rate tracing is reassuring. Contractions are every 3 minutes.

Appropriate management now is:

A) Continue pushing.
B) Vacuum-assisted delivery.
C) Forceps-assisted delivery.
D) Midline episiotomy.
E) Augment with oxytocin.

Discussion

The correct answer is A. Labor is progressing now and maternal-fetal status is reassuring. You should continue expectant management. No intervention is indicated.

 HELPFUL TIP: No indication for operative vaginal delivery (forceps, vacuum extraction) is absolute. Operative vaginal delivery is considered for prolonged second stage, potential fetal compromise, and shortening of the second stage for maternal benefit, among others.

 HELPFUL TIP: Episiotomies should not be performed routinely. Indications for episiotomy are typically related to nonreassuring fetal status and dystocia. **There is no evidence that episiotomies reduce tears, etc.**

* *

She pushes for 3 hours. She is now exhausted. The fetal head now separates the labia with contractions, and then recedes slightly. You consider offering assistance with delivery.

In counseling your patient and her husband about the maternal risks of operative vaginal delivery, which of the following should you discuss?

A) Vaginal trauma.
B) Shoulder dystocia.
C) Fetal injury.
D) Perineal and rectal trauma.
E) All of the above.

Discussion

The correct answer is E. Maternal risks of operative vaginal delivery include injury to the lower genital tract and rectal sphincter involvement in the case of a third- or fourth-degree laceration. Prolonged second-stage of labor is associated with an increased risk of shoulder dystocia. Fetal complications need to be discussed as well.

Each of the following is a fetal risk of operative vaginal delivery EXCEPT:

A) Cephalohematoma.
B) Skull fracture.
C) Brachial plexus injury.
D) Respiratory distress syndrome.
E) Facial nerve palsy.

Discussion

The correct answer is D. Neonatal cephalohematoma, retinal hemorrhage, and jaundice (secondary to breakdown and reabsorption of the cephalohematoma) are more common with vacuum-assisted delivery than with forceps-assisted delivery. Skull fracture and facial nerve injury are more common with forceps-assisted delivery than with vacuum-assisted delivery. Shoulder dystocia with resultant brachial plexus injury is more common with vacuum-assisted delivery, prolonged time required for delivery, and birth weight. Note that injury can occur before operative delivery as a result of abnormal labor forces. Operative vaginal delivery has not been associated with an increased incidence of respiratory distress syndrome.

* *

Delivery of an 8-pound baby is accomplished without operative vaginal assistance. The mere presence of the vacuum on the table was enough to entice the uterus to perform one last massive contraction. Following spontaneous delivery of the placenta 15 minutes later, you note a large gush of blood.

Which of the following is the most likely source of the bleeding?

A) Uterine atony.
B) Vaginal laceration.
C) Cervical laceration.
D) Retained placenta.

Discussion

The correct answer is A. Postpartum hemorrhage is most commonly associated with uterine atony. Risk factors for uterine atony include: overdistended uterus (such as from twins), prolonged labor, very rapid labor, high parity, chorioamnionitis, retained placental tissue, poorly perfused myometrium, halogenated hydrocarbon anesthesia, and previous atony. Maternal trauma to the genital tract may result in postpartum hemorrhage, is more likely following operative vaginal delivery than spontaneous vaginal delivery, and should be routinely investigated following assisted delivery. A retained placenta cotyledon is another common source for postpartum hemorrhage. The placenta should be inspected, and if there is any question of retained products of conception, the uterus should be manually explored.

Which of the following should be undertaken next?

A) Obtain IV access and initiate hydration.
B) Begin bimanual uterine compression.
C) Inspect vagina and cervix for lacerations.
D) Obtain blood for type and screen for possible blood transfusion.
E) All of the above.

Discussion

The correct answer is E. Postpartum hemorrhage is an obstetrical emergency and must be addressed immediately. The gravid uterus receives 500 mL of blood per minute, which can lead to massive hemorrhage if not addressed quickly. Additional personnel should be notified to help with obtaining IV access and blood draws, while you quickly try to identify the source of bleeding.

* *

After thorough exploration of the vagina and uterus, you suspect uterine atony is the cause of bleeding.

While continuing uterine massage, you instruct the nurse to prepare to administer which of the following?

A) Dilute IV oxytocin.
B) Methergine IM.
C) Hemabate IM.
D) Misoprostol PR.
E) All of the above.

Discussion

The correct answer is E. Oxytocin can be given as a dilute IV solution or IM. It should never be administered as an undiluted IV bolus, due to the risk of hypotension and cardiac arrhythmia. Methergine (methylergonovine) may be administered orally or intramuscularly. Caution should be used in women with hypertension, as Methergine can cause hypertension. Hemabate (carboprost tromethamine) is an F-2α prostaglandin analog that is administered IM or directly into the uterine myometrium. Caution should be used in women with asthma, as Hemabate can cause bronchoconstriction. Misoprostol is a prostoglandin E_1 analog that can be administered to women with asthma or hypertension. Rectal or oral administration can be used, but rectal administration is preferred in a patient with potential hemodynamic instability.

> **HELPFUL TIP:** Methergine (an ergot alkaloid), oxytocin, Hemabate, and misoprostol all cause smooth-muscle contraction in the uterus.

* *

She requires a large amount of IV crystalloid and 4 units of packed red cells for symptomatic anemia following delivery, but your patient and her baby are ultimately discharged home on postpartum day 2. You schedule a follow-up appointment in 2 days. You are concerned about Sheehan syndrome because of the severe postpartum hemorrhage.

All of the following are characteristic of Sheehan syndrome EXCEPT:

A) Failure in lactation.
B) Amenorrhea.
C) Hyperthyroidism.
D) Decreased LH/FSH.
E) Adrenal cortical insufficiency.

Discussion
The correct answer is C. Severe intrapartum or postpartum hemorrhage may result in pituitary necrosis due to hypovolemia and hypoperfusion. This leads to a global hypopituitarism known as Sheehan syndrome. Initial symptoms may be vague (lethargy, anorexia, weight loss, difficulty with lactation), and the syndrome can go unrecognized. It is characterized clinically by endocrine deficiency syndromes as a result of loss of anterior pituitary function. Characteristic manifestations include failure of lactation, amenorrhea, breast atrophy, loss of pubic and axillary hair, **hypo**thyroidism, and adrenal cortical insufficiency.

Objectives: Did you learn to . . .

- Recognize the risks of prolonged pregnancy and identify appropriate timing of intervention?
- Describe the indications and risks associated with induction of labor?
- Interpret intrapartum fetal heart rate patterns and choose appropriate management options?
- Evaluate analgesia options, contraindications, and risks during labor and delivery?
- Recognize the indications for and management of operative vaginal and abdominal delivery?
- Evaluate and manage postpartum hemorrhage?

CASE 4

While you are on call for your small community hospital, a nurse on the labor and delivery ward calls you about a patient with preterm contractions. You come in to see the patient and find a 33-year-old G1 at 26 weeks' gestation by in vitro fertilization. She is in the area to attend her aunt's funeral but is usually followed at an academic hospital 400 miles away. She looks worried and says, "I'm going to have twins. But not now!" She has a copy of her prenatal record (you nearly fall over backward at her foresight and planning), and her prenatal labs are unremarkable. Her most recent ultrasound was 1 week ago, confirming a dichorionic, diamniotic gestation with concordant growth.

All of the following risks are increased with a multifetal gestation EXCEPT:

A) Preterm labor.
B) D-isoimmunization (Rh isoimmunization).
C) Preterm rupture of membranes.
D) Intrauterine growth restriction.
E) Twin-twin transfusion syndrome.

Discussion
The correct answer is B. The most significant complication of multiple gestations is preterm labor resulting in preterm delivery. Preterm rupture of membranes and intrauterine growth restriction also occur more frequently in multiple gestations than in singleton pregnancies. The

risk of all these complications is directly proportional to the number of fetuses. Twin-twin transfusion syndrome rarely occurs and is associated with monochorionic gestations. D-isoimmunization is not associated with multifetal gestation. D-isoimmunization occurs when a nonimmunized D-negative (Rh negative) woman receives blood or blood fractions (including fetal to maternal bleed) from a D-positive infant and becomes immunized.

＊＊

The nurse asks if you want to check fetal fibronectin.

A negative fetal fibronectin is associated with:

A) Fetal lung immaturity.
B) Ruptured fetal membranes.
C) A decreased risk of preterm birth.
D) An increased risk of preterm birth.

Discussion

The correct answer is C. Fetal fibronectin (FFN) is a basement membrane protein produced by the fetal membranes. A negative test is useful in assessing the risk of preterm delivery during the following 2-week period. A negative test is reassuring. A positive test is not useful as the test has low positive predictive value. The test is performed on a sample from the posterior vaginal fornix or the external cervical os. In performing FFN testing, the following criteria must be met: intact amniotic membranes, minimal cervical dilation (<3 cm), and sampling between 24 0/7 weeks and 34 6/7 weeks. FFN does not assess fetal lung maturity. Ruptured membranes would cause a positive FFN.

 HELPFUL TIP: The main use for fetal fibronectin lies in its high negative predictive value. With a properly performed test in a symptomatic patient, up to 99.5% of patients with a negative FFN will not deliver in the subsequent 7 days.

＊＊

You are wondering if this patient is a good candidate for corticosteroid therapy.

Regarding the risks and benefits of corticosteroid therapy for fetal lung maturation, which of the following is NOT true?

A) Corticosteroid therapy is recommended for all pregnant women between 24 and 34 weeks' gestation who are at risk of preterm delivery within 7 days.
B) Corticosteroid therapy has been associated with an increased risk of neonatal infection.
C) Multiple courses of corticosteroids have been associated with fetal adrenal suppression.
D) Corticosteroids accelerate the appearance of pulmonary surfactant in the fetal lungs.

Discussion

The correct answer is B. There is no evidence that antenatal corticosteroid therapy increases the risk of neonatal infection. However, maternal infection is a **relative** contraindication to corticosteroid therapy. Corticosteroids are recommended for all pregnant women between 24 and 34 weeks' gestation who are at risk of preterm delivery within 7 days. Corticosteroids may be given after 34 weeks if there is documented fetal lung immaturity and delivery will likely occur before lung maturation. Multiple courses have been associated with fetal adrenal suppression and are no longer recommended because they offer no additional clinical benefit.

 HELPFUL TIP: Antenatal corticosteroids reduce not only the incidence of neonatal respiratory distress in preterm infants but also the rates of intraventricular hemorrhage, necrotizing enterocolitis, and overall mortality. **It is imperative that mothers who fall into the 24- to 34-week gestation window and who are at risk of imminent delivery receive steroids.**

Which of the following agents has been approved by the FDA for tocolysis?

A) Calcium channel blocker.
B) Magnesium sulfate.
C) Prostaglandin inhibitors.
D) Ritodrine.
E) Terbutaline.

Discussion

The correct answer is D. The use of tocolytics is controversial. The only FDA-approved agent for use as a tocolytic is ritodrine, a β-adrenergic receptor agonist.

The side effects of ritodrine are significant. Thus, other agents have been investigated not only to identify a more reliable tocolytic but also to minimize the side effects. Terbutaline, magnesium sulfate, prostaglandin inhibitors, and calcium channel blockers have all been studied and may be utilized in select cases for tocolysis—but realize that these drugs are not approved by the FDA for this indication.

 HELPFUL TIP: Tocolysis only delays labor by 48 hours at best, so the real goal should be to prolong the pregnancy until steroids have time to be effective.

 HELPFUL TIP: Contraindications to tocolysis include evidence of fetal distress, fetal anomalies, abruptio placentae, placenta previa with heavy bleeding, and severe maternal disease.

* *

You ponder the risks of tocolytic medications.

Which of the following is a TRUE statement?

A) Hyperglycemia is a potential complication of magnesium sulfate.
B) Seizures have been associated with the use of calcium channel blockers during pregnancy.
C) Transient hypotension is a potential complication of prostaglandin inhibitors.
D) Pulmonary edema is a potential complication of several tocolytic agents.
E) All of the above.

Discussion

The correct answer is D. Pulmonary edema is a specific complication of β-adrenergic agents and magnesium sulfate. Hyperglycemia (answer A) is a potential complication of terbutaline, not of magnesium. Gastrointestinal bleeding has been associated with prostaglandin inhibitors (answer C). Transient hypotension is a potential complication of calcium channel blockers (answer B). The combination of calcium channel blockers and magnesium sulfate for tocolysis has the potential to cause cardiorespiratory collapse.

* *

You examine the patient after collecting a fetal fibronectin. Her cervix is 1 cm dilated at the external os

and closed at the internal os, long, and posterior. The first infant is vertex. The monitor shows fetal heart rate baselines of 140 and 145. Contractions are irregular, occurring every 4–9 minutes. Urine dipstick shows a specific gravity of 1.030.

The LEAST appropriate intervention is:

A) Continuation of monitoring.
B) Oral hydration.
C) Obstetrical consult for cerclage placement.
D) Cultures for group B streptococci, gonorrhea, and chlamydia.
E) Administration of corticosteroids.

Discussion

The correct answer is C. Cerclage (stitch to hold the cervix closed) is indicated for incompetent cervix, not preterm labor. The other answers are appropriate interventions. The patient should be evaluated carefully and the frequency of uterine contractions should be assessed during the initial management. Oral or intravenous hydration may be administered for the patient who is volume depleted (in this situation, the patient is relatively dehydrated as established by a high urine specific gravity). Because dehydration may result in uterine irritability, rehydration may eliminate irritability if present; however, there is no proven benefit of hydration in the patient who is euvolemic. The practice of obtaining cultures is based on the need to prevent perinatal transmission even though treatment of positive cultures has not been established to aid in the prevention of preterm birth. Corticosteroids should be considered for the induction of fetal lung maturity for all women between 24 and 34 weeks' gestation who are at risk for preterm delivery.

A cerclage is typically placed in the first part of the second trimester after fetal viability has been established. A rescue cerclage may be placed later for the finding of cervical dilation in the absence of preterm labor. It is usually not placed after 23–24 weeks' gestation.

Objectives: Did you learn to . . .

- Identify risks and evaluate a multifetal pregnancy?
- Recognize preterm labor and manage it appropriately?

● Understand the indications, contraindications, risks, and benefits of tocolytics and corticosteroids?

 HELPFUL TIP: Delivery rates in Israel go up around Jewish holiday fast days likely because of the relative dehydration.

* *

A 33-year-old G1 at 35 2/7 weeks presents to labor and delivery while you are on call. Her pregnancy has been complicated by preterm labor. She was in last week with contractions and has been on pelvic rest (no tampons, no intercourse, etc) ever since. On admission she is uncomfortable with regular contractions every 3–4 minutes. The fetal heart rate baseline is 135 with good long-term variability. Her cervix is 6 cm dilated, completely effaced, with a bulging bag of water, and fetus in vertex presentation.

Which of the following is your best course of management?

A) Administer corticosteroids.
B) Administer tocolytics.
C) Initiate GBS prophylaxis.
D) Discharge her to home until she is in active labor.
E) A, B, and C.

Discussion

The correct answer is C. GBS prophylaxis is indicated for preterm delivery, and appropriate antibiotics include penicillin or ampicillin, or alternative intravenous agent if the patient has a penicillin allergy. The patient likely received corticosteroids during her recent admission. If not, she is now 35 2/7 weeks' gestation and thus beyond the window for corticosteroid administration (24–34 weeks). Given the gestational age (>34 weeks), advanced cervical dilation, and high likelihood of imminent delivery, tocolysis should be avoided.

 HELPFUL TIP: Indications for GBS prophylaxis are (1) GBS screen positive during current pregnancy; (2) GBS bacteriuria anytime during this pregnancy; (3) prior history of giving birth to a neonate with GBS disease; (4) unknown GBS status **plus** fever, preterm labor, or prolonged rupture of membranes. No GBS prophylaxis is indicated in women who are **culture-negative** with fever, preterm labor, or prolonged rupture of membranes.

* *

Her labor progresses and she is now 9 cm dilated. She is very uncomfortable with contractions and requests analgesia.

Which of the following will provide the best pain relief while maintaining patient safety?

A) Spinal anesthesia.
B) Pudendal block.
C) Opioid agonist-antagonist.
D) All of the above choices are equally good.

Discussion

The correct answer is A. Single-shot spinal analgesia provides excellent pain relief for procedures of limited duration, such as the second stage of labor and rapidly progressing labor. A pudendal block may provide adequate pain relief and would be a reasonable second choice. An opioid agonist-antagonist given at this late time will likely suppress the infant's respiratory drive. The infant may then require naloxone therapy in addition to close monitoring. The other choices would be better.

* *

The anesthesiologist likely will not get here in time, so you place a pudendal block. Shortly after placement, she has the urge to push. You confirm that she is completely dilated, and she delivers vaginally without incident. The baby is vigorous. Before discharge she asks about her risk of recurrent preterm delivery.

Which is the most appropriate response?

A) Her risk is not increased above the background risk.
B) Her risk is increased to about 15%.
C) Her risk is increased to about 50%.
D) Her risk is unquantifiable.

Discussion

The correct answer is B. A history of preterm delivery strongly correlates with subsequent preterm labor. After one preterm delivery, the risk for a subsequent preterm birth is approximately 15%. Progesterone therapy can be used prophylactically in women with a prior preterm delivery. Starting at 16–20 weeks, weekly injections of 17 α-hydroxyprogesterone caproate significantly reduced the incidence of preterm birth.

Smoking cessation and appropriate nutrition are other interventions to potentially decrease the risk of recurrent preterm delivery.

Objectives: Did you learn to . . .

- Recognize preterm labor and manage it appropriately?
- Identify appropriate analgesia options for labor?
- Identify risk of recurrent preterm birth and potential prevention options?

 QUICK QUIZ: PRETERM BIRTH

Risk factors for preterm birth include each of the following EXCEPT:

A) Multiple gestation.
B) Maternal history of preterm birth.
C) Maternal history of preterm contractions, with term birth.
D) Maternal smoking.
E) Maternal hypertension.

Discussion

The correct answer is C. Although preterm contractions are concerning in the evaluation of preterm labor, a maternal history of preterm contractions with term birth does not increase the risk of preterm delivery in a subsequent pregnancy. Multiple gestations, history of preterm birth, smoking, cocaine use, asymptomatic bacteriuria, and hypertension are all risk factors for preterm birth.

CASE 5

A 37-year-old G3 P0111 (full term, preterm, abortions, living children) presents for routine obstetric care at 10 weeks' gestation. Her OB history is remarkable for an induced abortion at 8 weeks' gestation with her first pregnancy, in addition to a second pregnancy complicated by severe preeclampsia which required induction of labor and magnesium sulfate therapy at 35 weeks' gestation. Her past medical history is uncomplicated. She is feeling well, other than mild nausea. She has not started her prenatal vitamins. Her blood pressure is 132/86, urine protein is negative, physical exam is unremarkable. Uterine size is consistent with dates and fetal heart tones are auscultated. The patient wonders if she will develop pre-eclampsia and need that "magnesium medicine" again.

You counsel her that her risk of recurrent severe preeclampsia is in the range of:

A) <5%
B) 20%–50%
C) 60%–75%
D) >90%

Discussion

The correct answer is C. The risk of recurrence of preeclampsia is affected by both gestational age at diagnosis and the severity of preeclampsia. Earlier gestation at diagnosis and more severe forms of preeclampsia increase the risk of recurrence. The overall recurrence risks are estimated at <10% for mild preeclampsia and >20% for severe preeclampsia. Because her preeclampsia was severe and mildly preterm, her risk of recurrence is at least 20% but <50%. Other risk factors for preeclampsia include young maternal age, advanced maternal age, and chronic hypertension.

* *

The patient would do anything reasonable to prevent the preeclampsia again.

In addition to obtaining baseline laboratory evaluation (CBC, AST, ALT, Creatinine, 24-hour urine for protein) to aid in early diagnosis, you recommend the following therapy:

A) Low-sodium diet.
B) Diuretic for hypertension and edema.
C) Aspirin 81 mg daily.
D) Subcutaneous heparin therapy at prophylactic doses.
E) None of the above.

Discussion

The correct answer is E. There is currently no approved therapy to reduce the risk of preeclampsia in a subsequent pregnancy. Management includes early identification of patients with preeclampsia so that therapy and monitoring of the pregnancy can be instituted. The diagnosis of preeclampsia can often be challenging, so the additional knowledge of liver, renal and platelet function at the beginning of pregnancy can help clarify the diagnosis, especially in an individual with chronic hypertension.

* *

Because of her age (37 years), the patient inquires about her risk for delivering a baby with Down syndrome.

What is her estimated risk of a Down syndrome baby with this pregnancy?

A) 1/9,000
B) 1/1,200
C) 1/150
D) 1/12

Discussion

The correct answer is C. Meiotic nondisjunction, which increases the risk of Down syndrome and other trisomies, increases with maternal age. The risk begins to rise more rapidly at 35 years, with an estimated risk of 1/250 at 35 years, 1/150 at 37 years, and 1/70 at 40 years.

* *

After hearing her age-related risk for Down syndrome, the patient asks about what tests she should have to screen for Down syndrome.

You counsel her regarding various tests and offer:

A) First-trimester PAPP-A, HCG, and nuchal lucency.
B) Chorionic villus sampling.
C) Amniocentesis.
D) Quadruple screening (HCG, MSAFP, estriol, inhibin-A).
E) All of the above.

Discussion

The correct answer is E. All patients should be offered first-trimester screening, and if declined, they should be offered second-trimester quadruple screening. Because of her advanced age (>35 years at the time of delivery), the patient should be offered chorionic villus sampling (CVS) and amniocentesis as well. Patients should understand that the first-and second-trimester screening tests are just that—**screening methods**. However, both CVS and amniocentesis can diagnose Down syndrome, in addition to other chromosomal abnormalities. CVS is typically completed between 10 and 13 weeks' gestation, whereas amniocentesis is performed after 15 weeks. Both are invasive procedures that carry risks, including pregnancy loss, rupture of membranes, and fetal injury.

* *

The patient undergoes first-trimester screening which decreases her Down syndrome risk to 1/800. She declines an amniocentesis. You draw her maternal serum alpha fetal protein (MSAFP) only at 17 weeks, because you know that the first-trimester screening does not evaluate for neural tube defects. The AFP is normal. She subsequently undergoes diabetes screening with a 1-hour post-50 g glucose test, which shows a glucose level of 170 mg/dL.

The next step is:

A) Order a 3-hour glucose tolerance test.
B) Set up diabetes teaching and a consult with a nutritionist/dietician.
C) Start glyburide.
D) Start insulin.
E) All of the above.

Discussion

The correct answer is A. The 1-hour, 50-gram glucose load (Glucola) test is a screening test for gestational diabetes. The next step is to perform a more specific test, which is the 3-hour glucose tolerance test, which utilizes a 100-gram glucose load. It is not appropriate to diagnose and treat for diabetes based on the screening test alone.

* *

The patient completes her glucose tolerance test with values of:

Fasting: 92 mg/dL

1-hour: 194 mg/dL

2-hour: 169 mg/dL

3-hour: 148 mg/dL

The next step in management is:

A) Nothing.
B) Set up diabetes teaching and a consult with a nutritionist/dietician.
C) Start glyburide.
D) Start insulin.

Discussion

The correct answer is B. The recommended upper limit of normal serum glucose levels for the 3-hour glucose tolerance test are:

Fasting: 95 mg/dL

1-hour: 180 mg/dL

2-hour: 155 mg/dL

3-hour: 140 mg/dL

If a patient has glucose levels which are above these at 2 or more times, she is considered to have gestational diabetes. Your patient fails 3 of the 4 tests. The recommendation is to initiate dietary modifications including carbohydrate restriction with frequent blood sugar monitoring. Medication such as glyburide or insulin should be started only if the patient fails to control her diabetes with dietary changes.

* *

The patient is seen for her 32-week visit and her fundal height is only 28 cm (which surprises you, given her diagnosis of gestational diabetes!). She has been compliant with the dietary changes and her blood sugars are usually 80s fasting and 120s 2 hours postprandial. She has gained 20 pounds so far in the pregnancy. You send her for an ultrasound, which reveals an infant measuring only 28 3/7 weeks' gestation, weighing 1168 g (<10th percentile). Amniotic fluid volume and umbilical artery Dopplers are normal.

Appropriate follow-up includes:

A) Changing the estimated due date.
B) Scheduling an induction.
C) Repeating the ultrasound for growth in 1 week.
D) Repeating the ultrasound for growth in 3–4 weeks.

Discussion

The correct answer is D. This infant demonstrates intrauterine growth restriction. The patient had a first-trimester ultrasound with her first-trimester screening, which establishes her due date. It is inappropriate to change her due date based on this ultrasound. Initiating an induction would be inappropriate without further investigation, given the early gestational age. Current ultrasound techniques are not sensitive enough to assess growth at weekly intervals, and therefore waiting at least 3 weeks would give a better assessment of growth rate. Completing an ultrasound for amniotic fluid volume and Doppler assessment in 1 to 2 weeks could be considered in this growth-restricted infant. A nonstress test would also be indicated at this point.

* *

The patient continues with weekly nonstress tests and her ultrasound at 35 weeks reveals appropriate interval growth, but remains growth restricted at a weight of 1846 g (<10th percentile). The patient is otherwise well. However, today her blood pressure is 146/88 and urine protein on dipstick is +1.

Appropriate intervention now includes:

A) Administering corticosteroids.
B) Obtaining a 24-hour urine for protein.
C) Follow up with a routine appointment in 1 week.

D) Start labetalol.
E) All of the above.

Discussion

The correct answer is B. Given the patient's elevated blood pressure and proteinuria, you need to be concerned about recurrent preeclampsia. Urinary excretion of protein is transient, and a 24-hour urine protein level is a more accurate reflection of proteinuria and the preferred method for diagnosis of preeclampsia. The patient is at 35 weeks' gestation (although measuring smaller), which is beyond the recommended gestation at which corticosteroids are administered. Arranging follow-up for the patient in 1 week would potentially miss the diagnosis of preeclampsia. Although antihypertensives such as labetalol can be utilized in pregnancy, they are not routinely initiated for mild elevations in blood pressure at later gestations.

* *

Serial blood pressure measurements in the clinic reveal no blood pressures >146/88. Her nonstress test is reactive. The patient is sent home to collect her 24-hour urine and returns in 2 days. Her blood pressure is now 148/90 and she has trace protein on urine dipstick. The 24-hour urine returns at 180 mg (her baseline 24-hour urine protein at the beginning of the pregnancy was 116 mg). She denies any headache, visual changes, nausea, or abdominal pain.

Your diagnosis is:

A) Gestational hypertension.
B) Mild preeclampsia.
C) Severe preeclampsia.
D) Acute renal failure.

Discussion

The correct answer is A. She now has 2 blood pressure readings >140/90 and >6 hour apart, which satisfies the criteria for hypertension. Given that this elevation in blood pressure started after 20 weeks' gestation, it is likely pregnancy related. However, her blood pressure at her initial visit was 132/86. Although this is not technically hypertensive, it is in the higher range of normal. The patient may be predisposed to having chronic hypertension. She does not have protein >300 mg in a 24-hour urine collection, so she does not meet that diagnostic criterion for mild preeclampsia. Nor does she qualify for severe preeclampsia. Criteria for mild and severe preeclampsia are outlined in Table 15–2.

Table 15–2 PREECLAMPSIA CRITERIA

Criteria for preeclampsia
- Proteinuria ≥300 mg in a 24-hour specimen **and**
- Systolic blood pressure of ≥140 mm Hg **or**
- Diastolic blood pressure of ≥90 mm Hg **that**
- Occurs after 20 weeks' gestation in a woman with previously normal blood pressure

Criteria for severe preeclampsia (1 or more of the following)
- Systolic blood pressure of ≥160 mm Hg **or**
- Diastolic blood pressure of ≥110 mm Hg
- BP must be obtained on 2 occasions at least 6 hours apart while the patient is on bed rest
- Proteinuria of ≥5 g in a 24-hour urine specimen
- Oliguria
- Cerebral or visual disturbances, including headache
- Pulmonary edema
- Epigastric pain or right upper quadrant pain
- Impaired liver function
- Thrombocytopenia
- Fetal growth restriction

She returns to the office for her appointment 5 days later, after having felt well over the weekend. However, today she developed a headache. Her blood pressure is 166/112 and her urine dipstick reveals 3 + protein.

Your next step is to:

A) Start oral labetalol and see the patient back in 2 days for a blood pressure check.
B) Repeat the 24-hour urine for protein.
C) Admit to labor and delivery for blood work and monitoring, with plans to move toward delivery.
D) Administer corticosteroids.

Discussion

The correct answer is C. The clinical picture is now developing into severe preeclampsia (headache, systolic BP >160, diastolic BP >110, and 3 + proteinuria). The patient needs to be admitted for further monitoring of blood pressure and symptoms. In addition, blood work should be obtained for CBC and liver and renal function. Starting oral labetalol would treat the patient's hypertension, but this step alone is not prudent for a patient who probably has severe preeclampsia. The 24-hour urine protein collection may be helpful in meeting the technical criteria to diagnose preeclampsia and can be done during admission; however, the results would not change the immediate

management of the patient. The patient is at 36 weeks' gestation, and corticosteroids are not indicated.

* *

You admit her to the hospital. Repeat blood pressure is 164/98 and urine dipstick shows 3+ protein. Her cervix is soft, 2 cm dilated, 50% effaced, with fetus vertex at –2 station.

What is the most appropriate intervention at this point?

A) Begin induction for vaginal delivery.
B) Start magnesium sulfate.
C) Prepare for a cesarean delivery in case it is needed.
D) All of the above.

Discussion

The correct answer is D. All of these options are important to consider at this time. Induction with oxytocin and treatment of preeclampsia with magnesium are appropriate at this point. Obstetrical backup should be involved earlier rather than later unless you plan to do the cesarean section yourself.

 HELPFUL TIP: Delivery of the baby (baby and placenta, really) is the ultimate treatment for preeclampsia and should be affected as soon as feasible when the mother's condition demands it.

* *

You begin magnesium sulfate and oxytocin. The induction proceeds without incident, and she delivers a viable male infant.

How long will you continue the magnesium sulfate?

A) Until delivery.
B) For 12 hours after delivery.
C) For 24 hours after delivery.
D) Until the urine protein dipstick is negative.
E) Until discharge.

Discussion

The correct answer is C. All women with preeclampsia should receive intravenous magnesium sulfate to prevent eclamptic convulsions. Magnesium sulfate is administered by controlled intravenous infusion with a loading dose of 6 grams in 100 mL over 15–20 minutes, followed by maintenance at 2 grams per hour. Treatment should be continued for 24 hours following delivery.

 HELPFUL TIP: Monitor deep tendon reflexes, level of consciousness, and urine output for all patients on magnesium. Turn off the magnesium infusion if signs of toxicity emerge (eg, decreased mental status, hyporeflexia) or if the patient is at risk for impending toxicity (eg, from renal failure).

Objectives: Did you learn to . . .

- Evaluate, diagnose, and manage hypertension in pregnancy?
- Define and manage preeclampsia?
- Recognize and manage complications that can arise with advanced maternal age?
- Identify fetal intrauterine growth restriction?

CASE 6

A 37-year-old G3 P1112 (full-term, preterm, abortions, living children) presents for an annual gynecologic exam. She has questions regarding contraception. She may be done with child-bearing but does not like the permanence of a tubal ligation. She is 6 months postpartum and is currently breast-feeding and using condoms for supplemental contraception. She has used oral contraceptives in the past but is concerned about the potential side effect of hypertension. Although her past medical history is not notable for hypertension, she had preeclampsia with both of her prior deliveries and has a family history of hypertension. She is wondering if she is a candidate for an intrauterine device (IUD).

All of the following are contraindications to IUD placement EXCEPT:

A) Pregnancy.
B) Acute pelvic infection.
C) Undiagnosed vaginal bleeding.
D) History of chlamydia infection.

Discussion

The correct answer is D. Although active cervicitis and acute pelvic inflammatory disease are contraindications to placement of an IUD, a prior positive chlamydia culture does not exclude a patient from obtaining an IUD. Verification of no acute infection can be obtained through cervical cultures prior to the insertion date. Undiagnosed vaginal bleeding can be a sign of either endometritis or structural abnormalities of the uterine cavity, which would require treatment prior to considering the IUD as an option for contraception.

* *

Your patient has none of these contraindications, and she would like to proceed with the IUD. Her friends have told her that all IUDs cause abortions, and she is unsettled by this idea.

The mechanism of action of IUDs (copper or progesterone) is:

A) Abortifacient.
B) Causes a sterile inflammatory reaction to a foreign body.
C) Impairs sperm transport from the cervix to the fallopian tube.
D) B and C.
E) All of the above.

Discussion

The correct answer is D. Studies detecting levels of human chorionic gonadotropin reveal that this hormone is not present in IUD users during the luteal phase. Thus, the IUD is **not** an abortifacient. Studies suggest the mechanism of action of IUDs include: interference with sperm transport from the cervix to the fallopian tube, inhibition of sperm capacitation or survival, and endometrial inflammatory changes which inhibit implantation. The newest IUD product on the market is Mirena, which offers the benefit of immediate resumption of menses and fertility following discontinuation of the progesterone-releasing IUD.

The risk of infection with IUD use is HIGHEST with:

A) Insertion.
B) Removal.
C) First 3 years of use.
D) Patient >30 years.

Discussion

The correct answer is A. The risk of infection is most strongly associated with insertion, estimated at 1/1,000 to 1/100. It does not increase with prolonged use. However, because the risk of infection is so low, routine prophylaxis with antibiotics is **not** recommended. For women with complicated valvular heart disease, prophylactic antibiotics prior to insertion should be considered to prevent infective endocarditis.

* *

After extensive counseling regarding the IUD and other contraceptive methods, your patient discusses her options with her husband. They decide that based on her last pregnancy complications, they would be best served by permanent sterilization. Her husband undergoes a vasectomy. She returns in 2 years for another annual exam. She now complains of worsening menorrhagia. Currently she uses 20 pads or tampons on her heaviest days of bleeding, with the total duration of menses 7 days. She denies any intermenstrual spotting. She has not noticed any lightheadedness or dizziness, but does complain of generalized fatigue. On physical exam, you find a normal-sized thyroid and an enlarged, irregular uterus measuring 10–12 weeks in size. There are no distinct adnexal masses, but this is somewhat difficult to discern due to the irregular uterus.

Your initial workup in this 39-year-old female should include all of the following EXCEPT:

A) CBC.
B) TSH.
C) CA-125.
D) Pelvic ultrasound.

Discussion

The correct answer is C. CA-125 is not a test to include in the initial workup. A CBC (answer A) will provide information regarding the hematocrit (and therefore the level of anemia) and platelet count—important information for someone bleeding so heavily. TSH (answer B) will screen for hypothyroidism, which is a common cause of menorrhagia in a 39-year-old female. Correction of the hypothyroidism may be the only treatment necessary for her menorrhagia. A pelvic ultrasound (answer D) will aid in the evaluation of the mass palpated on examination and characterize the location and size of any uterine fibroids that may contribute to the bleeding; it also will evaluate for any adnexal masses.

CA-125 is a nonspecific tumor marker that has a high false positive rate in premenopausal women. Thus, CA-125 is not recommended as a screening test for ovarian cancer. It can be used as an adjunct to pelvic ultrasound when a complex adnexal mass is identified.

* *

The patient returns in 2 weeks following her ultrasound. Her hematocrit was 31% (indices are consistent with iron-deficiency anemia), platelets 195,000, and TSH 2.8 mU/L. The ultrasound reveals a uterus measuring $12 \times 8 \times 6$ cm, with multiple small intramural fibroids measuring <2 cm in diameter. There is one subserosal, pedunculated fibroid measuring 3.5 cm at the fundus.

What is the best initial management?

A) Expectant management and reassurance.
B) Nonsteroidal antiinflammatory drugs (NSAIDs).
C) Gonadotropin-releasing hormone (GnRH) agonists.
D) Blood transfusion.
E) Hysterectomy.

Discussion

The correct answer is B. Most fibroids are asymptomatic, although the most common symptom associated with leiomyomata (fibroids) is abnormal bleeding. This patient's fibroids are not impinging on the uterine cavity but may be contributing minimally to the patient's menorrhagia. Given the presence of anemia, the menorrhagia should be treated in this case. Initial treatment of menorrhagia may include NSAIDs that inhibit prostaglandin synthesis in appropriate doses. Antiprostaglandins have been shown to reduce menstrual blood loss by 30%–50% in women with menorrhagia. If the patient's anemia was more severe or she had symptoms associated with it, she would be a candidate for a blood transfusion. This decrease in blood count has likely been chronic, and the patient should be started on iron therapy. GnRH agonists may be utilized to produce a medical menopause. However, they are expensive, and long-term usage is associated with significant side effects. Generally, use of GnRH agonists is recommended only in selected cases. Hysterectomy is the definitive treatment for leiomyomata in symptomatic women who have completed childbearing. The mortality associated with hysterectomy is approximately 1/1,000 procedures. It is generally reserved for women who have failed medical management for abnormal bleeding or have symptoms or signs related to fibroid size.

What is the prevalence of fibroids in reproductive-age women?

A) <5%
B) 20%–30%
C) 50%–60%
D) >90%

Discussion

The correct answer is B. Uterine leiomyomata are the most common benign neoplasm of the female pelvis, estimated to occur in 20%–30% of reproductive-age women. They are more common with increasing age, African-American race, and a familial history of fibroids.

**

The patient returns in 4 months for follow-up. Her bleeding is improved with ibuprofen, and she continues to deny any symptoms of pelvic pressure or pain. On repeat pelvic exam, the uterus is still palpable at 10–12-week size, without any tenderness. You discuss a trial of oral contraceptives in addition to NSAIDs.

Contraindications to the use of combination oral contraception include all of the following EXCEPT:

A) Active liver disease.
B) History of pulmonary embolism.
C) Pregnancy.
D) Tobacco use in patients >35 years.
E) Polycystic ovary syndrome.

Discussion

The correct answer is E. Polycystic ovary syndrome is an indication for oral contraception use. Combination oral contraceptive use is contraindicated in women with all of the other conditions listed.

**

The patient continues to be pleased with NSAID and OCP therapy for control of her menorrhagia. This patient's fibroids are asymptomatic and she responded well to medical therapy for her menorrhagia. However, if the patient had not responded to medical therapy, she would have been referred to a gynecologist for potential surgical therapy.

What other characteristic(s) would have prompted evaluation for surgery?

A) Prolapsing fibroid through the cervix.
B) 5 cm submucosal myoma protruding 50% into the uterine cavity.
C) Rapidly enlarging uterus.
D) 20-week-sized uterus and pelvic pressure.
E) All of the above.

Discussion

The correct answer is E. A fibroid prolapsing through the cervix has a potential for necrosis and infection; therefore, it may require surgical removal. A submucosal myoma, especially one that distorts the uterine cavity, would be more likely to contribute to menorrhagia. A rapidly enlarging uterus would be more concerning for a uterine malignancy and would require further investigation. Larger uterine fibroids are more likely to contribute to symptoms of pelvic pressure and pain, which may only respond to surgical correction.

**

The patient returns in 1 year for her annual exam, and her pelvic exam is unchanged. However, she expresses concern that these fibroids could become cancerous.

What is the risk of malignancy (leiomyosarcoma) in a patient with fibroids?

A) <1%
B) 5%–10%
C) 40%–50%
D) 90%–95%

Discussion

The correct answer is A. A leiomyosarcoma is a malignant tumor that does **not** arise from preexisting benign leiomyomata. Leiomyosarcomas typically arise in the fifth or sixth decade of life and are usually associated with abnormal bleeding or a rapidly enlarging uterus. The estimated incidence of leiomyosarcoma discovered at the time of surgery for fibroids is <1%.

Objectives: Did you learn to . . .

• Treat menorrhagia?
• Describe management principles for uterine leiomyomas?
• Recognized contraindications to OCP and IUD use?

C) Cytological follow-up.
D) LEEP or laser ablation.
E) 5-fluorouracil intravaginally.

Discussion

The correct answer is D. Although some patients with severe dysplasia (CIN III) may be candidates for a hysterectomy, it would be an overly aggressive approach in this 31-year-old female who has never been pregnant and may wish to conceive in the future. Additionally, women who had high-grade CIN before hysterectomy can develop recurrent vaginal dysplasia (VaIN) or cancer at the vaginal cuff. Likewise, trachelectomy (removal of the entire cervix) would be overly aggressive with no added benefit over a simple cone excision or destructive procedure. Cytological follow-up or "expectant management" is **not** recommended for high-grade dysplasia. The likelihood of regression is low, while the likelihood of persistence or progression to cancer is unacceptably high. A conization or destructive procedure would be the best recommendation in this patient. The advantage of a cone procedure is that it provides further tissue for evaluation. The use of 5-fluorouracil intravaginally is typically not recommended for initial treatment of **cervical dysplasia.** It is used instead for **vaginal dysplasia**, when the extent of disease precludes complete excision or destruction.

LEEP or conization is indicated in which of the following?

A) Inability to see the extent of the lesion.
B) Cervical biopsy demonstrating microinvasion.
C) Positive endocervical curettage.
D) Inadequate colposcopy.
E) All of the above.

Discussion

The correct answer is E. A LEEP or cone procedure is indicated for diagnosis (exclusion of cervical cancer) and in some cases treatment of cervical dysplasia. There are 5 classic indications for performing a cone procedure, of which 4 are listed above. The fifth indication is a discrepancy between Pap smear and biopsy (eg, high-grade Pap smear and normal biopsy or biopsy with minimal atypia), in which case you have not explained the Pap smear findings and need to continue the evaluation. This patient does not have any of the classic indications. Thus, the goal is treatment of her CIN III. Either a

destructive mechanism (such as laser) or an excisional mechanism may be utilized in this case. A cone procedure has the additional advantage of removing further tissue to exclude micro-invasive or invasive disease.

* *

Your patient wants to know the likelihood of regression to "normal" without treatment.

What will you counsel?

A) This will almost certainly become invasive cancer without aggressive treatment.
B) The natural history of untreated CIN III is characterized by high rates of spontaneous regression.
C) Approximately 33% of CIN III lesions spontaneously regress.
D) Approximately 66% of CIN III lesions spontaneously regress.

Discussion

The correct answer is C. 32% of untreated CIN III lesions will spontaneously regress, approximately 56% will persist, and 14% will progress to invasive carcinoma.

* *

She is concerned about future childbearing if she undergoes a LEEP.

All of the following are possible complications of LEEP EXCEPT:

A) Cervical incompetence.
B) Cervical stenosis.
C) Cervical ectopy.
D) Decreased fertility.
E) Premature rupture of membranes.

Discussion

The correct answer is C. Cervical incompetence, stenosis, decreased fertility, and premature rupture of the membranes have been identified following all types of cone procedures, including LEEP, and are estimated to occur following <1% of procedures. Each of these complications seems to be related to the volume of tissue removed with the procedure rather than the procedure itself, though studies are ongoing to evaluate the effect of cone procedures on the function of the cervix. Cervical ectopy or ectopic cervical pregnancy is also quite rare and has **not** been associated with cone or LEEP procedures.

* *

She undergoes treatment as recommended. The pathology reveals CIN III with negative margins.

What do you counsel her about follow-up?

A) She should return for a Pap smear and pelvic exam in 1 year.
B) She should return for a Pap smear in 4–6 months.
C) She should return for a Pap smear in 2–3 months.
D) She should return for a colposcopy and Pap smear in 2–3 months.
E) No follow-up is indicated.

Discussion

The correct answer is B. The current recommendations for follow-up include Pap smears every 4–6 months until 3 sequential Pap smears return as normal following treatment. Then, the patient may resume yearly cytological follow-up. If any of the Pap smears reveal cells of higher grade than ASC (atypical squamous cells), the patient should undergo repeat colposcopy.

* *

At the follow-up evaluation her cervix appears normal, without lesions or discharge. The Pap smear returns as normal, limited by absence of endocervical cells.

What is the best recommendation for management of this patient now?

A) Repeat the endocervical portion of the Pap smear at her convenience in the next month.
B) Cervical dilation and endocervical curettage.
C) Cervical dilation and endocervical Pap smear.
D) Repeat LEEP.
E) Repeat the Pap smear in 1 year.

Discussion

The answer is A. Since the Pap smear was limited by the absence of endocervical cells, the patient should have a repeat Pap smear at her convenience (within the next month) to exclude abnormality. The additional Pap smear would not count as one of the required follow-up evaluations (the Pap and repeat Pap count as one).

Objectives: Did you learn to . . .

- Manage an abnormal Pap test?
- Recognize the indications for colposcopy?

- Interpret colposcopic findings?
- Evaluate and manage cervical dysplasia?
- Recognize the risks and potential complications of loop electrosurgical excision procedure?
- Manage the absence of endocervical cells on a Pap test?

CASE 10

You are called to the ED to evaluate a patient with a 2-day history of abdominal pain. She is a 24-year-old G1 P1 female whose LMP was 1 week ago. On a scale of 1 to 10, her pain is "12." She is on oral contraceptives for birth control. She has "never missed a pill" and "could not possibly be pregnant." Her pain is across her lower abdomen and a little more on the right side than the left. She has felt feverish. She has had some nausea but no vomiting, and her appetite has remained fairly normal. She denies bowel or bladder problems. Her pain improves with acetaminophen and worsens with activity.

On examination, she appears uncomfortable but not toxic. Her temperature is 38°C, but the rest of her vitals are normal. Her abdominal examination reveals decreased bowel sounds, with tenderness to palpation primarily across the lower quadrants. She has minimal guarding and no rebound tenderness. Her pelvic examination is remarkable for cervical motion tenderness. The uterus is of normal size and consistency with no masses.

Which of the following diagnoses can be excluded from your differential now?

A) Ectopic pregnancy.
B) Appendicitis.
C) Pelvic inflammatory disease.
D) Pyelonephritis.
E) None of the above should be excluded.

Discussion

The correct answer is E. The differential for lower abdominal pain in a young female includes all of the above and more. Even though your patient seems unlikely to be pregnant due to her consistent use of contraceptives and recent menses, you should not exclude pregnancy without a negative urine HCG.

All the following are appropriate INITIAL diagnostic tests EXCEPT:

A) Urine HCG.
B) CBC with differential.
C) Pelvic ultrasound to rule out ectopic pregnancy.
D) Urinalysis.

Discussion

The correct answer is C. Although pregnancy seems unlikely based on history, the urine HCG is absolutely necessary. A CBC with differential is needed to look for evidence of systemic infection in a febrile patient, while a urinalysis will help evaluate for a urinary tract infection. An ultrasound to rule out an ectopic pregnancy is not indicated now. It may be indicated if the urine HCG comes back positive or exam findings warrant it.

* *

The urine pregnancy test is negative, the urinalysis is negative for nitrites and leukocytes, and the WBC is 15,600/mm^3 with an increase in bands. You feel the patient's history, examination, and diagnostic tests are most consistent with a diagnosis of pelvic inflammatory disease (PID).

What is the most appropriate next step?

A) Consult surgery and gynecology to confirm your findings.
B) Admit for IV antibiotics and IV hydration.
C) Treat as an outpatient with antibiotics and schedule follow-up for 36–48 hours.
D) Treat with IV antibiotics on an outpatient basis utilizing visiting nurse care.
E) Obtain cultures, discharge the patient, and treat based on culture results.

Discussion

The correct answer is C. PID is a clinical syndrome caused by the ascent of microorganisms from the lower genital tract (eg, vagina) to the upper genital tract (eg, endometrium). Most patients with PID can be managed in the outpatient setting. Indications for hospitalization are listed in Table 15–3. Appropriate treatment for PID rests on prompt antibiotic administration. Surgical consultation (answer A) is not necessary, and awaiting culture results (answer E) in order to initiate treatment is not appropriate—although patients should be tested for gonorrhea and chlamydia.

Table 15–3 CRITERIA FOR ADMISSION FOR TREATMENT OF PID

- Uncertain diagnosis
- Surgical emergencies (eg, appendicitis) cannot be excluded
- Suspected pelvic abscesses
- Concurrent pregnancy (due to high risk of maternal mortality, fetal wastage, and preterm delivery)
- Adolescent patient with uncertain compliance with therapy
- Severe illness
- Patient cannot tolerate outpatient regimen (eg, severe vomiting)
- Lack of response to 72 hours of treatment
- Concurrent HIV infection
- Clinical follow-up cannot be arranged within 72 hours

 HELPFUL TIP: The diagnosis of PID is a **clinical** one and not laboratory-based! Because untreated PID has significant morbidity and mortality, empiric treatment is recommended if the patient meets the following minimal diagnostic criteria:

Uterine/adnexal tenderness, **or**
Cervical motion tenderness, **and**
No other cause for illness identified.

Other helpful (but not necessary) criteria include:

Temperature ≥38°C
WBC ≥10,500/mm^3
Adnexal mass
Laboratory evidence of gonorrhea or chlamydia infection
Elevated C-reactive protein and/or ESR

 HELPFUL TIP: Empiric therapy is unlikely to impair diagnosis and management of other important causes of lower abdominal pain, so do not delay treatment while pursuing additional laboratory studies if the history and physical are suggestive of PID.

* *

You review the most recent antibiotic recommendations for treatment of PID and administer ceftriaxone (Rocephin) 250 mg IM now, and doxycycline 100 mg

PO BID for 14 days after ensuring the cultures you obtained for gonorrhea and chlamydia are sent to the laboratory. **Single-dose azithromycin is not indicated for the treatment of PID—only for cervicitis.** The patient calls your office the next morning with worsening nausea and vomiting. She is unable to keep fluids or the antibiotic down.

What do you advise her to do now?

A) Come to your office for repeat evaluation now.
B) Go to the pharmacy; you will call in an antiemetic.
C) Go to the pharmacy; you will call in stronger antibiotics.
D) Rest. The ceftriaxone injection needs more time to work.

Discussion

The correct answer is A. Inability to tolerate the outpatient regimen may be an indication for hospitalization, so the patient should be seen for evaluation and possible admission.

* *

She returns for evaluation. She appears ill now. Otherwise, her examination is essentially unchanged.

What is the most appropriate action?

A) Repeat the CBC with differential.
B) Consider a pelvic ultrasound to assess for tubo-ovarian abscess or appendicitis.
C) Admit for IV antibiotics and serial examinations.
D) All are appropriate actions now.

Discussion

The correct answer is D. All the above options are acceptable, and all might be done in such a circumstance. As the patient's illness seems to be getting worse and she is not tolerating her oral antibiotics, she should be admitted for IV treatment and further diagnostic workup.

* *

Again, you feel the history, examination, and diagnostic tests are most consistent with PID. You admit her for failed outpatient management and initiate IV antibiotics. She does well and is discharged when she is tolerating oral intake and has been afebrile for 48 hours. You instruct her to finish a 14-day course of doxycycline. She presents for follow-up a week later, when her symptoms have completely resolved and she is feeling well.

Which of the following is a potential consequence of PID?

A) Infertility.
B) Chronic pelvic pain.
C) Increased risk for ectopic pregnancy.
D) Recurrent PID.
E) All of the above.

Discussion

The correct answer is E. All the answer choices are potential sequelae of PID. Additionally, tubal ovarian abscess may develop.

> **HELPFUL TIP:** The etiology of PID is polymicrobial, although sexually transmitted infections, predominantly gonorrhea and/or chlamydia, are implicated in up to 66% of cases. Antibiotic regimens are chosen for broad coverage. The CDC no longer recommends the use of fluoroquinolones for treatment of PID/gonorrhea due to increasing resistance.

* *

You see her next for her annual examination. She quit taking her oral contraceptive 5 months ago after she separated from her husband (the jerk gave her chlamydia, after all). Subsequently, her periods have been irregular. With further investigation you note that she was started on oral contraception for cycle regulation following her delivery 4 years previously. Her height and weight are appropriate (BMI = 23 kg/m²). She has minimal acne and no hirsutism or galactorrhea. Her physical examination is essentially normal.

What is the most appropriate diagnostic test?

A) Urine pregnancy test.
B) FSH.
C) TSH.
D) Hysterosalpingogram.
E) Each of the above tests should be obtained now.

Discussion

The correct answer is A. If the patient is complaining of irregular or missed menses and she is of reproductive age, you cannot go wrong getting a urine pregnancy test. Other tests can follow once pregnancy has been ruled out.

**

Urine HCG is negative, and a serum TSH is normal.

What is the most likely etiology of the irregular cycles?

A) Anovulation.
B) Pituitary tumor.
C) Polycystic ovarian syndrome.
D) Premature ovarian failure.
E) Androgen-secreting tumor.

Discussion

The correct answer is A. OCPs work by suppressing ovulation. Resumption of ovulation after pill cessation can take several months. In the absence of abnormal history, physical exam, or laboratory findings, the other choices are unlikely to be the etiology of the irregular cycles in this patient.

Each of the following is appropriate initial management EXCEPT:

A) Expectant management.
B) Reestablishment of cycle regulation with OCPs.
C) Progestin-induced withdrawal cycles.
D) Colposcopy with cervical and endometrial biopsies.

Discussion

The correct answer is D. Anovulation is expected following OCP cessation, thus expectant management is a reasonable option, as most women will resume regular cycling within 6 months. She could also opt to resume OCPs for cycle regulation. Withdrawal bleeds could be induced by cyclical progestin challenges. Colposcopy is not indicated in this patient as she has no cytologic abnormalities noted that would require follow-up with colposcopy and biopsy.

**

The patient is reluctant to resume "hormone therapy." She decides to monitor her cycles for another 3–6 months. You next evaluate her 8 months later. She notes that her periods have remained irregular, typically occurring every 3–6 weeks. Her last period was 7 weeks earlier. A urine pregnancy test is positive. Given her history of PID, you request a quantitative serum β-HCG and are considering a pelvic ultrasound to confirm intrauterine pregnancy.

What is the minimum expected increase in quantitative HCG in early gestation in a normal pregnancy?

A) 20% increase in 24 hours.
B) 66% increase in 48 hours.
C) 200% increase in 24 hours.
D) 10% increase in 48 hours.
E) 75% increase in 72 hours.

Discussion

The correct answer is B. Human chorionic gonadotrophin typically doubles every 48 hours in normal gestation. The minimum increase typically compatible with a viable pregnancy is 66%.

**

If the quantitative serum β-HCG is 8,000 ng/mL and the pelvic ultrasound reveals no intrauterine pregnancy but a probable right tubal pregnancy (no fetal heart rate), what would be the most appropriate management choice?

A) Medical management with methotrexate.
B) Laparoscopic surgery with evacuation of the products of conception.
C) Gynecological consultation.
D) Dilation and curettage.
E) Hysterectomy.

Discussion

The correct answer is C. An ectopic pregnancy may rupture and become a life-threatening event at any point before complete resolution. If the patient becomes hemodynamically unstable, she will need emergent surgery. Thus, an early referral for management is warranted.

If the quantitative serum β-HCG had come back at 1,000 ng/mL and no ultrasound were available, how would you have counseled the patient?

A) Given the history of PID this is most likely an ectopic pregnancy. She should abort the pregnancy at once.
B) Given the history of PID, she should remain on bed rest until a definitive diagnosis is made.
C) She should be given ectopic pregnancy and miscarriage precautions.
D) She does not need counseling until a diagnosis is made.

Discussion

The correct answer is C. This β-HCG level is consistent with an early gestation given her history of irregular cycles. However, with her history of PID she is at risk for ectopic pregnancy. Thus she should be given ectopic pregnancy and miscarriage precautions. Although a history of PID increases the risk of ectopic pregnancy by 7- to 10-fold, only 8% of these patients will ever have an ectopic. So, it is still highly probable that the patient has a normal intrauterine pregnancy. Bed rest is not indicated in pregnancy for a history of PID.

* *

Her quantitative serum β-HCG is 6,000 ng/mL. A pelvic ultrasound confirms a viable intrauterine pregnancy at 8 4/7 weeks' gestation.

How do you counsel her now?

A) Routine first-trimester counseling.
B) Ectopic pregnancy counseling. This may be a heterotopic pregnancy.
C) Miscarriage counseling. She will almost certainly miscarry, given her history.
D) Chromosomal defect counseling. She is at an increased risk for fetal malformation.

Discussion

The correct answer is A. She has a reassuring ultrasound, which confirms an intrauterine pregnancy. Spontaneous heterotopic pregnancies (simultaneous uterine and ectopic pregnancies) are extremely rare. There is no reason to believe the patient is at higher risk of having a miscarriage or a fetal malformation based on her history.

 HELPFUL TIP: Fertility treatment substantially increases the risk of a heterotopic pregnancy (≤3%).

Objectives: Did you learn to . . .

- Evaluate a patient with pelvic pain?
- Diagnose and treat pelvic inflammatory disease?
- Evaluate and treat irregular menses?
- Diagnose and manage ectopic pregnancies?

⧗ QUICK QUIZ: ECTOPIC PREGNANCY

A 25-year-old married female presents to your office for preconception care. She had an ectopic pregnancy 2 years ago. She wants to know her risk of an ectopic pregnancy if she conceives again.

In comparison with average women her age, her risk for ectopic pregnancy is:

A) Increased.
B) The same as the background risk (1%–2%).
C) Decreased.
D) Unable to discern given her history.
E) 100%.

Discussion

The correct answer is A. An ectopic pregnancy has significant implications for future pregnancies. The overall conception rate after an ectopic is only 60%. In subsequent pregnancies following the ectopic, recurrent ectopics are frequent and spontaneous abortions occur in 1/6. Only 33% of women with a history of ectopic pregnancy deliver a live-born infant.

CASE 11

A 52-year-old female patient presents for an annual exam and Pap smear. Her last menstrual period was 3 months ago. She has intermittent hot flashes and night sweats. Her examination is remarkable for mild vaginal atrophy. She wonders about "estrogen testing" to determine if she needs hormone replacement therapy.

How will you counsel her about the role of estrogen testing?

A) Recommend **AGAINST** estrogen testing.
B) Recommend buccal swab testing as it is the most accurate.
C) Recommend fasting morning serum estradiol testing.
D) Recommend estrogen testing with FSH to ensure menopause status.
E) Recommend initiating annual estrogen testing >55 years.

Discussion

The correct answer is A. In a person of the right age with symptoms consistent with menopause, no testing is recommended. Testing is recommended only if the diagnosis is unclear (eg, patient <35 years). It can also be useful when a patient on OCPs presents with a symptoms suggestive of menopause. In this case, an FSH could be done after the patient has discontinued hormonal contraception for 1 week.

**

She jokes that you're probably getting kickbacks from the insurance company for ordering fewer tests, and then she asks, "How will you know if I'm going through menopause without an estrogen level?"

How will you counsel her about menopause and its diagnosis?

A) FSH is the definitive test.
B) There is no definitive test of menopause.
C) Six months amenorrhea, elevated FSH, and decreased estradiol confirm the diagnosis.
D) Twelve months amenorrhea, elevated FSH, and decreased estradiol is the definitive test.

Discussion

The correct answer is B. Menopause is a clinical syndrome characterized by the cessation of spontaneous menstrual periods along with associated symptoms of estrogen deficiency such as hot flashes, vaginal atrophy, and psychological symptoms. There is no definitive test.

**

She is concerned about menopause and wonders if she needs hormone replacement therapy.

All of the following are benefits of estrogen-containing hormone therapy (HT) EXCEPT:

A) Osteoporosis prevention.
B) Decrease in colon cancer.
C) Decrease in hot flashes and vasomotor symptoms.
D) Decrease in risk of stroke.

Discussion

The correct answer is D. The role of hormone therapy in menopause has been controversial for years. Until recently, observational data had suggested wide-ranging benefits for HT. However, recent well-conducted randomized controlled trials, the largest of which was the Women's Health Initiative (WHI) study, suggest that these benefits may be overstated. Proven benefits of HT are limited to the following:

- Reduced risk of osteoporosis and related fractures.
- Decreased colon cancer risk.
- Improvement of vasomotor symptoms such as hot flashes.

HT may increase the risk of the following (variable findings):

- Breast cancer (WHI estrogen-only arm showed no increased risk).
- Myocardial infarction (WHI estrogen-only arm showed no increased risk).
- Venous thromboembolic events.
- Stroke.

Only women with vasomotor symptoms appear to have improved overall quality of life scores with HT. Given the significant excess risks with HT usage, many practitioners now recommend short-term HT use only for vasomotor symptoms and not for osteoporosis or other purported benefits.

An absolute contraindication to use of hormone therapy is:

A) Heart disease.
B) Breast cancer.
C) Endometrial cancer.
D) Previous thromboembolic event.
E) All of the above.

Discussion

The correct answer is D. Previous thromboembolic disease is the only **absolute** contraindication to HT. The others are **relative** contraindications. Although HT is not routinely recommended for women who have heart disease or a history of breast or endometrial cancer, it may be useful in women who have significant impairment in their quality of life from vasomotor symptoms refractory to other management methods.

You discuss menopause and the potential risks and benefits of HT with your patient. She decides against HT for the time being.

**

Your patient returns in 6 months. She notes continued amenorrhea and hot flashes, as well as vaginal dryness. She remains reluctant to initiate HT.

Options to treat the vaginal dryness include which of the following?

A) HT.
B) Vaginal estrogen.
C) Lubrication.
D) All of the above.
E) None of the above.

Discussion

The correct answer is D. Systemic and local estrogen administration are both effective for treating vaginal dryness. Lubrication with vegetable oil and specifically manufactured lubricants can be effective.

How is vaginal atrophy most rapidly and accurately diagnosed?

A) Biopsy.
B) Culture.
C) Wet mount evaluation.
D) Direct visualization.
E) All of the above.

Discussion

The correct answer is C. Vaginal atrophy is most easily diagnosed with microscopy. The wet mount will reveal an abundance of basal and parabasal cells and a paucity of mature squamous epithelium. A biopsy may reveal atrophic changes. However, it is not necessary for diagnosis and is invasive and would not be cost effective. Culture is utilized for identification of infectious pathogens. Direct visualization will aid in the diagnosis but is not as reliable as microscopy.

* *

She decides to try HT to reduce hot flashes.

Assuming the initial hormone replacement fails to resolve her symptoms, further options to treat symptomatic hot flashes include which of the following?

A) Increase the estrogen component.
B) Increase the progestin component.
C) Trial of an SSRI.
D) All of the above.

Discussion

The correct answer is D. HT is the most efficacious treatment for vasomotor symptoms with almost 90% of women responding. Other options include progestins like medroxyprogesterone (Provera) or megestrol (Megace), SSRIs, clonazepam, gabapentin (Neurontin), venlafaxine (Effexor), clonidine, and exercise. Although there is conflicting evidence for the efficacy of vitamin E and black cohosh, there is no good data to suggest that propranolol or phytoestrogens, such as soy, are effective in treating vasomotor symptoms.

Objectives: Did you learn to . . .

- Evaluate menopausal symptoms?
- Describe hormone replacement therapy; including risks, benefits, and contraindications for its use?
- Diagnose and manage atrophic vaginitis?
- Treat menopausal symptoms?

CASE 12

A 57-year-old postmenopausal patient presents for her annual examination. Since you last saw her, she stopped hormone replacement because of vaginal spotting. She is now experiencing hot flashes and night sweats, as well as continued vaginal bleeding. Her medical history is otherwise unremarkable. She wants your opinion about resuming hormone replacement.

Her pelvic examination is remarkable for atrophic vaginal mucosal changes, a stenotic cervix without lesions, normal size uterus, no adnexal masses, and no masses palpable on rectovaginal examination. The remainder of her exam is normal.

All of the following are possible causes of her vaginal bleeding EXCEPT:

A) Cervical cancer.
B) Uterine polyp.
C) Polycystic ovarian disease.
D) Atrophic vaginitis.
E) Uterine/endometrial cancer.

Discussion

The correct answer is C. Polycystic ovarian disease does not cause vaginal bleeding in postmenopausal women. All the other choices are diagnostic considerations in a postmenopausal female with vaginal bleeding/spotting.

Which of the following studies should you consider obtaining?

A) Urinalysis.
B) Pap smear.

C) Endometrial biopsy.

D) Stool guaiac.

E) All of the above.

Discussion

The correct answer is E. The patient could easily mistake the source of the bleeding; thus, it is prudent to rule out a rectal or urinary source. Cervical and endometrial evaluations are necessary to rule out gynecological pathology, such as endometrial polyp, hyperplasia, or cancer.

All of the following are risk factors for endometrial cancer EXCEPT:

A) Smoking.

B) Obesity.

C) Unopposed estrogen.

D) Diabetes.

E) Hypertension.

Discussion

The correct answer is A. Endometrial cancer is believed to be caused by overexposure to unopposed estrogen stimulation of the endometrium. States that increase estrogen exposure (exogenous or endogenous) increase risk, while those that decrease estrogen exposure decrease risk. Smoking decreases luteal phase estrogen and is epidemiologically linked to a **decrease** in the risk for endometrial carcinoma (this risk is offset by the other adverse health affects of smoking). Risk and protective factors are listed in Table 15–4.

* *

You review your patient's test results: normal Pap smear and urinalysis, stool guaiac negative for blood, and endometrial biopsy with fragments of benign polyp. As you discuss these test results, the patient asks if taking all of that extra estrogen she bought over the Internet might make a difference. Why didn't she tell you this before? Well, it's called "Natural Female Hormone," so she figured it was safe and not worth mentioning.

What treatment will you recommend?

A) Consult gynecology for a hysterectomy.

B) Discontinue the unopposed exogenous estrogen.

C) Start high-dose progestin.

D) Start tamoxifen.

E) Take more "Natural Female Hormone."

Table 15–4 RISK AND PROTECTIVE FACTORS FOR ENDOMETRIAL CANCER

Risk factors

Advancing age
Obesity*
Nulliparity
Early menarche
Late menopause
Chronic anovulation (eg, PCOS)
Unopposed exogenous estrogen use
Tamoxifen
Hypertension
Diabetes

Protective factors[†]

Progesterone
OCPs
Cigarette smoking
Multiparity

* Obesity leads to increased estrogen levels from peripheral conversion of androstenedione. The presence of DM and HTN as risk factors may simply reflect the high incidence of obesity in patients with these disorders.

[†] All reduce exposure to unopposed estrogens.

Discussion

The correct answer is B. You have ruled out worrisome pathology with the workup that you have performed thus far. Her use of unopposed estrogen puts her at risk of endometrial carcinoma. Thus, she should discontinue the exogenous estrogen supplements she has been taking.

* *

She follows your recommendations. Over the next 3 years she continues to have rare occurrences of vaginal spotting. She has declined further evaluation given the infrequency of the episodes. However, over the last several months, she has experienced an increase in the amount and frequency of the bleeding. Other than an interval weight gain of 27 pounds, there has been no change in her examination. Repeat endometrial biopsy reveals complex hyperplasia with atypia, and the pathologist cannot rule out endometrial cancer.

Which is the most appropriate intervention?

A) Repeating the endometrial biopsy.

B) Performing a transvaginal ultrasound to assess endometrial thickness.

C) Starting high dose progestin therapy.

D) Starting high dose SERM therapy.

E) Arrange for definitive management (hysterectomy if carcinoma found on further evaluation).

Discussion

The correct answer is E. Her biopsy findings are highly abnormal and may indicate already existing carcinoma that was not contained in the sample examined. Referral to a gynecologist for definitive management is warranted now.

 HELPFUL TIP: In postmenopausal women, an endometrial stripe of >5 mm on ultrasound is suggestive of endometrial cancer. In the editor's opinion, this is too insensitive a test and an in-office endometrial biopsy should be done in cases of postmenopausal bleeding.

Objectives: Did you learn to . . .

● Evaluate postmenopausal bleeding?

● Manage a patient with postmenopausal bleeding?

● Assess a patient for risk of endometrial cancer?

● Evaluate, diagnose, and manage endometrial hyperplasia?

CASE 13

A 15-year-old nulligravida female presents with her mother for evaluation of painful periods. Menarche was at age 14. Her periods are typically every 4–8 weeks and are very painful. She has missed 1–2 days of school with each menses because of the severe pain and has been suspended from the volleyball team because of missed practices. She denies intercourse. She has never had a pelvic examination. Her review of systems is otherwise negative.

What is the MOST likely etiology of her irregular cycles?

A) Pregnancy.

B) Endometriosis.

C) Anovulation.

D) Hyperthyroidism.

E) Imperforate hymen.

Discussion

The correct answer is C. Dysfunctional uterine bleeding is common in adolescent girls who have reached menarche. The first few years of menstruation are often characterized by irregular cycles as a result of anovulation. This is as a result of immaturity of the still-developing hypothalamic-pituitary-ovarian axis. It can take a few years after menarche before regular ovulatory cycles begin. Pregnancy and imperforate hymen lead to absence of menses, not irregular menses. Although hyperthyroidism may lead to irregular cycles, it does not typically cause dysmenorrhea, is usually associated with other systemic complaints, and would be unusual in a patient of this age. Endometriosis may cause dysmenorrhea, but is unlikely to occur in a patient this young; most cases of endometriosis present in patients in their twenties and thirties.

What is the etiology of her dysmenorrhea?

A) Prostaglandin release.

B) Streptococcal endotoxin release.

C) Estrogen release.

D) Excessive testosterone production.

Discussion

The correct answer is A. The pathogenesis of dysmenorrhea involves excess prostaglandin release which causes prolonged, painful uterine contractions. Dysmenorrhea (excessive pain in association with menstruation) is the most common gynecologic complaint, affects about half of all adolescent females, and is the leading cause of periodic school absenteeism. It can be divided in two main subtypes: primary and secondary. Primary dysmenorrhea usually starts <20 years and tends to occur with menarche. It is caused by prostaglandin stimulation of the myometrium. Secondary dysmenorrhea typically arises >20 years and is associated with pelvic pathology or other organic disease.

* *

You perform a physical examination, revealing normal vital signs, normal weight, a benign abdomen, Tanner stage V, and no signs of androgen excess.

What is the best first-line treatment for this patient?

A) Expectant management.

B) Hormonal combined contraception.

C) GnRH agonist.

D) Narcotic analgesic.

E) She should **not** be treated without a complete evaluation including diagnostic laparoscopy.

Discussion

The correct answer is B. OCPs offer cycle regulation and reduction in dysmenorrhea. Expectant management is inappropriate given the severity of symptoms and availability of safe and effective treatment. A further workup is not needed now, as her history is straightforward and her physical exam is reassuring. Narcotic analgesics do not help reduce prostaglandin levels and are not appropriate for pain control in this patient. GnRH agonists will not regulate the patient's irregular cycles, are expensive, and require add-back estrogen when utilized >6 months. **Although not listed in the answers, NSAIDs are also effective at treating dysmenorrhea and should be considered as a first-line drug. Anecdotal evidence suggests that mefenamic acid (Ponstel) may be more effective for dysmenorrhea than other NSAIDs.**

* *

The patient's mother inquires about "normal menarche." She is concerned that the irregular and painful cycles indicate abnormal maturation, especially because her own cycles have always been "regular—every 28 days." She also expresses concern about her daughter's "late" menstrual onset.

What is the MOST LIKELY etiology of her menarche timing?

A) Chromosomal abnormality.

B) Hypothyroidism.

C) Prolactinoma.

D) Normal menarche.

E) Obesity.

Discussion

The correct answer is D. The average age of menarche is 12.8 years in the United States, with the range from 10 to 15 years. Therefore, menarche at 14 years is within the normal range.

 HELPFUL TIP: Primary amenorrhea is defined as (1) the absence of menses with no secondary sexual characteristics by 14 years or (2) the absence of menses by 16 years regardless of the development of secondary sexual characteristics (or lack thereof).

* *

Your patient and her mother opt to try hormonal regulation with birth control pills. She returns for follow-up in 4 months and is doing well. She has appropriate withdrawal cycles with minimal dysmenorrhea. She asks if the pills she is taking are good for birth control. She confides that she had intercourse with her boyfriend of 2 months and is concerned that she may be pregnant. She has continued on the oral contraceptive as prescribed at your last visit. Her last menstrual period was 3 weeks ago, and her first intercourse was 4 days ago.

When is the best time to administer a pregnancy test?

A) Today.

B) After she misses a withdrawal period.

C) Before starting her next pill pack.

D) A pregnancy test is never indicated when oral contraception is taken as directed.

Discussion

The correct answer is B. Currently available pregnancy tests have very good sensitivity and specificity and are able to pick up most pregnancies (approximately 90%) **by the first day of the missed period.** Testing before a period is missed will result in many false negatives. Compliance with OCPs is rarely perfect, and there is up to a 5% failure (pregnancy) rate with OCPs with "normal" (eg, imperfect) use. With perfect use, OCPs have a success rate of up to 99%. Remember that the failure rate is higher in teenagers, so a pregnancy test would be appropriate if her period does not occur as expected.

In addition to reviewing the use of birth control pills, she should be questioned or counseled about which of the following?

A) Knowledge of sexually transmitted diseases and use of condoms.

B) Age of her boyfriend.

C) Consensual nature of her relationship.

D) HPV vaccination.

E) All of the above.

Discussion

The correct answer is E. Visits for contraception are great opportunities for you to discuss safe sexual practices with the patient. The interview should include evaluation for sexual assault, coercion, or abuse. The quadrivalent human papillomavirus (HPV) vaccination was approved by the FDA for use in females aged 9 to 26 years. This vaccination prevents infection by HPV types 6, 11 (responsible for 90% of genital warts), and types 16 and 18 (responsible for 70% of cervical cancer) and is administered in a series of 3 injections at 0, 2, and 6 months.

 HELPFUL TIP: HPV is the most common viral sexually transmitted infection in the United States.

* *

The patient's dysmenorrhea and irregular cycles are well controlled with the oral contraceptives through high school and college. However, she is concerned about the risk of cancer with long-term use and wonders if the benefits offset the risks.

All of the following are benefits of currently available combined hormonal oral contraceptives EXCEPT:

A) Decreased incidence of ovarian cancer.
B) Decreased incidence of endometrial cancer.
C) Decreased amount of menstrual flow with cycles.
D) Decreased prostaglandin release and dysmenorrhea with cycles.
E) Decreased incidence of venothromboembolism.

Discussion

The correct answer is E. OCPs increase the risk of venothromboembolism. All of the other responses are noncontraceptive benefits of combined OCPs. Additional benefits include decreased incidence of PID, decreased risk of benign breast disease, lower incidence of ectopic pregnancy, improvement in acne, decreased risk of osteoporosis, and prevention and treatment of endometriosis.

 HELPFUL TIP: Smoking may add to the risk of venothromboembolism for women on OCPs, but it does **not** act in a synergistic way (as has been suggested in the past).

All of the following are risks or complications associated with OCP use EXCEPT:

A) Increased rate of breast cancer.
B) Increased rate of cervical adenocarcinoma.
C) Slight vaginal bleeding ("spotting") with initiation of OCP.
D) Amenorrhea after discontinuing OCP use.
E) Increased blood pressure.

Discussion

The correct answer is A. No blanket statement can be made regarding the association of OCPs and breast cancer. There is considerable conflict among epidemiologic studies that have tried to examine the relationship between OCP use and breast cancer rates—some have shown decreased rates in certain populations, others have shown increased rates, and others have shown no association. Answer B is true. Although the most common type of cervical cancer (squamous cell) is not associated with OCP use, increased rates of cervical adenocarcinoma have been observed in OCP users. Answer C is true. Spotting may occur with initiation of OCPs or with intermittent use. Amenorrhea may persist for months after stopping OCPs, so answer D is true. Answer E is true. OCPs cause small degrees of blood pressure elevation and may cause overt hypertension in some women.

Which of the following is a contraindication to the use of combined oral contraceptives?

A) <2 weeks postpartum.
B) History of thromboembolic disease.
C) Diabetes with vascular disease.
D) >35 years and cigarette use.
E) All of the above.

Discussion

The correct answer is E. Each of the above conditions places women at risk for adverse event related to the use of combined oral contraceptives. Safer methods of birth control may include: barrier methods, progestin-only contraceptives, implants, and sterilization.

* *

You lose touch with the patient, and she discontinues her OCP. Years later when she returns for a physical examination, she complains of increasing irritability along with intermittent bloating and swelling during the week before her period each month. Although she is annoyed by these symptoms, they are not severe enough to interfere with her usual activities. You review activity and dietary changes over the last year (none), as well as changes in her health status (none). Her menstrual cycles are now occurring monthly, without intermenstrual spotting or missed periods.

What is her most likely diagnosis?

A) Major depression.
B) Premenstrual dysphoric disorder.
C) Premenstrual syndrome.
D) Polycystic ovarian syndrome.
E) Hypothyroidism.

Discussion

The correct answer is C. PMS is a constellation of physical, emotional, and behavioral symptoms. It is cyclical in nature, occurs during the second half of the menstrual cycle (luteal phase, 7–10 days before menses), and resolves soon after menses. A symptom-free interval occurs during the first half of the cycle (follicular phase). Premenstrual dysphoric disorder (PMDD) is more severe but occurs during the same time frame as PMS. Symptoms of PMDD include labile mood, depressed mood, irritability, feelings of hopelessness, hypersomnia or insomnia, and decreased interest in usual activities. PMDD is diagnosed by DSM-IV criteria and some functional impairment must be present. The cyclic nature of the symptoms present in this patient makes diagnoses of depression, hypothyroidism, and PCOS less likely. However, a patient may experience a perimenstrual exacerbation of an underlying psychiatric disorder, so it is important to determine whether the patient suffers symptoms at other times during her cycle as well.

 HELPFUL TIP: Perimenstrual symptoms exist on a continuum with up to 90% of women affected by minimal PMS symptoms while 10% are affected severely. The group with more severe symptoms can be categorized as having PMDD.

Each of the following is a key element of the diagnosis of PMS EXCEPT:

A) Physical symptoms of bloating, swelling, and/or fatigue.
B) Elevated luteinizing hormone to follicle stimulation hormone (LH:FSH) ratio.
C) Restriction of symptoms to the luteal phase of the menstrual cycle.
D) Exclusion of other diagnoses that may better explain the symptoms.

Discussion

The correct answer is B. PMS is a clinical entity and no laboratory data exist to aid in diagnosis. The other answer choices are key elements. An elevated LH: FSH ratio of 3:1 in the face of appropriate symptoms is suggestive of PCOS.

Each of the following is a possible treatment option for PMS and PMDD EXCEPT:

A) Supportive therapy/counseling.
B) Aerobic exercise.
C) Selective serotonin reuptake inhibitors.
D) Thiazide diuretics.
E) Calcium.

Discussion

The correct answer is D. Thiazide diuretics are not helpful in premenstrual syndrome or PMDD. The other answer choices are potentially useful. Treatment options for PMS are listed in Table 15–5.

Table 15–5   TREATMENT OPTIONS FOR PREMENSTRUAL SYNDROME

- Aerobic exercise
- Supportive therapy
- Calcium, magnesium
- Vitamin B_6 (pyridoxine), Vitamin E
- NSAIDs
- Serotonergic antidepressants such as SSRIs and venlafaxine
- Anxiolytics such as buspirone and benzodiazepines
- Spironolactone (*not* thiazide diuretics)
- Reduction of sodium, caffeine, and alcohol intake
- Danazol
- Hormonal (OCPs, GnRH agonists, progesterones)
- Increased intake of complex carbohydrates and fiber
- Bromocriptine

Objectives: Did you learn to . . .

- Evaluate concerns about menarche?
- Evaluate and manage dysmenorrhea?
- Counsel a patient regarding contraception and sexually transmitted disease prevention?
- Diagnose and treat premenstrual syndrome?

CASE 14

A frantic patient calls you. She and her boyfriend were having intercourse about 16 hours ago and the condom broke at the time of ejaculation. She does not use any other form of contraception. Her last menstrual period was about 2 weeks ago.

What is her risk of pregnancy (assuming she and her partner are fertile)?

A) <1%
B) ~8%
C) ~52%
D) ~94%

Discussion

The correct answer is B. Approximately 8% of women will get pregnant after a single act of coitus.

Appropriate methods of "emergency contraception" include which of the following?

A) Plan B.
B) Yuzpe (combined estrogen and progesterone).
C) Preven (ethinyl estradiol and levonorgestrel).
D) A and B only.
E) A, B, and C.

Discussion

The correct answer is D. While all of the above are effective methods for postcoital pregnancy prevention, Preven is no longer manufactured (it remains "FDA approved," and appears to be available on the Internet). Many OCPs are also effective if used at the right doses and within 72 hours (the Yuzpe method). Plan B and Preven are the only FDA-approved drugs for postcoital contraception. Plan B is levornegestrel and is more effective than the combined OCPs for postcoital contraception.

 HELPFUL TIP: Prescribe an antiemetic with postcoital OCPs, as nausea and vomiting are common side effects. Plan B has fewer GI side effects.

Contraindications for the use of emergency contraception include which of the following?

A) Positive urine pregnancy test.
B) Diabetes mellitus
C) Hypertension.
D) All of the above.

Discussion

The correct answer is A. Emergency contraception is not effective once a pregnancy is established. Therefore, if the patient has a positive urine pregnancy test, it is pointless to use emergency contraception. The patient should be referred for appropriate counseling to discuss other options (eg, continuing pregnancy versus abortion). Emergency contraception may be offered to women with contraindications to the use of conventional oral contraceptives, such as in the case in a smoker >35 years. The progestin-only regimen is preferred in women with a history of thrombosis.

* *

You decide to prescribe Plan B. Several months later, she schedules an appointment with you for evaluation of abdominal and pelvic pain. The same pain occurred 2 years ago, and appendicitis was ruled out at that time. She was advised to try acetaminophen for the discomfort, which she has not found useful. Her pain has gradually worsened over the last 2 years and is almost omnipresent. She complains of severe abdominal cramping and stabbing in the right lower quadrant. The pain radiates to the left lower quadrant at times and is worse during her menstrual periods. Her periods have become heavier and occasionally irregular. She has no bowel or bladder symptoms. She has been missing work 1–2 days each month and is now concerned about her job.

Your examination reveals a well-developed woman who looks depressed and uncomfortable. Her abdomen is soft, nondistended, and diffusely tender to palpation in the lower quadrants. There is no evidence of guarding, rebound tenderness, or palpable masses. She has no back tenderness. The external genital and vaginal examinations show no lesions or erythema. There is a creamy discharge noted at the cervix. Bimanual reveals a retroverted uterus with uterosacral nodularity palpable. Both adnexal areas are tender to examination, but without masses.

Each of the following is an appropriate test to order now EXCEPT:

A) Urine pregnancy test.
B) Cervical culture for chlamydia.
C) Cervical culture for gonorrhea.
D) Erythrocyte sedimentation rate (ESR).
E) CT scan of the abdomen and pelvis.

Discussion

The correct answer is E. Imaging technologies have a limited place in the evaluation of chronic pelvic pain. Ultrasound is often the better choice for imaging as it gives better definition of pelvic gynecologic structures. Other laboratory studies should be dependent on the history and physical exam. Each of the other laboratory studies may be appropriate at this time.

 HELPFUL TIP: Chronic pelvic pain is a symptom, not a specific disease, and is often accompanied by various other symptoms that may seem unrelated. Chronic pelvic pain is defined as pain that has been present >6 months and for which a thorough investigation has been negative. To go by the textbook, the "diagnosis" of chronic pelvic pain requires a negative diagnostic laparoscopy. However, laparoscopy may be excluded in some cases.

What is the most likely etiology of the patient's chronic pelvic pain?

A) Irritable bowel syndrome.
B) Myofascial pain disorder.
C) Endometriosis.
D) Dysplasia.
E) Interstitial cystitis.

Discussion

The correct answer is C. There were no bowel symptoms elicited on the history to suggest irritable bowel syndrome. There were no signs elicited on the examination to suggest a myofascial pain disorder. The patient's history and physical examination (including uterosacral nodularity) are consistent with a diagnosis of endometriosis. Dysplasia is typically asymptomatic. There were no bladder symptoms elicited on the history to suggest interstitial cystitis.

* *

CBC, urine pregnancy test, and cervical cultures are all negative or normal.

What is the most appropriate next step at this time?

A) Consult for diagnostic laparoscopy.
B) Have the patient complete pain calendar for 3 months.
C) Offer her a trial of depot-Lupron for suppression.
D) All of the above.

Discussion

The correct answer is D. Treatment of chronic pelvic pain is aimed at the underlying etiology. The history and physical exam are consistent with endometriosis. Therefore a trial of cycle suppression or diagnostic laparoscopy to confirm your impression would be appropriate. A pain calendar is often useful to further identify aggravating factors and follow treatment outcomes.

* *

In your discussion with the patient on how to proceed, she says that she wants a "definitive diagnosis."

Which of the following will allow for a definitive diagnose of endometriosis?

A) Transvaginal ultrasound.
B) Transabdominal ultrasound.
C) Diagnostic laparoscopy with biopsy.
D) CA 125 level.
E) Hysterosalpingogram.

Discussion

The correct answer is C. The diagnosis of endometriosis continues to rely upon direct visualization confirmed by histologic examination. The presence of 2 or more of the following features is required for pathologic diagnosis: endometrial epithelium, endometrial glands, endometrial stroma, and hemosiderin-laden macrophages. However, empiric therapy may be used when the signs and symptoms support the diagnosis of endometriosis and the consequences of an inaccurate diagnosis are likely to be minimal.

* *

When she hears the word "surgery," she nearly has a panic attack and says, "Nobody's cutting me open!" You offer alternatives, and she elects to undergo cycle suppression with a 3-month trial of leuprolide (Lupron) and to complete a pain calendar. You see her in follow-up at the conclusion of the trial. She is feeling much better. The pain has been almost completely suppressed, and she has missed only 1 day of work since you last saw her. She has noted hot flashes, but they are minor.

What is the most appropriate management now?

A) Continue the Lupron for another 3 months (total 6 months).
B) Stop the Lupron and monitor.
C) Switch to a trial of cycle suppression using Depo-Provera (medroxyprogesterone acetate) or continuous low-dose OCPs.
D) Switch to a trial of Premarin (conjugated estrogens).
E) A or C.

The correct answer is E. For pain relief, treatment with a GnRH agonist for 3–6 months is effective in most patients. Oral contraceptives and oral or depot progestins are more effective than placebo. Given the marked treatment success with the depot-Lupron, discontinuing treatment would likely result in recurrence of the patients pain symptoms. Since endometriosis is estrogen-dependent, use of estrogen (Premarin) would be inappropriate. Another option is treatment with danazol. However, danazol is less well tolerated than GnRH agonists, Provera, or OCPs.

> **HELPFUL TIP:** NSAIDs are useful monotherapy in patients with mild endometriosis and are useful in combination with hormonal therapy for patients with more severe symptoms.

* *

The patient is concerned about how endometriosis may affect her future fertility. You recall that she is 25 years old and has never attempted pregnancy. She has regular menstrual cycles.

What will you tell her?

A) She is surely infertile.
B) It is impossible to know if she will have problems achieving pregnancy until she has tried to conceive.
C) There is no association between endometriosis and infertility.
D) Her risk of infertility is ~50%.
E) Her risk of infertility is ~70%.

Discussion

The correct answer is B. Early-stage endometriosis is more likely to be associated with pain symptoms without associated alterations in fecundity. Thus it is impossible to predict fertility and infertility based on the available information. Diagnostic laparoscopy may aid in visualization of anatomic pathology and allow one to render a guess as to tubal disease. The better approach would be continued medical management until attempts for pregnancy are desired.

Objectives: Did you learn to . . .

- Manage patients who desire emergency oral contraception?
- Define and evaluate chronic pelvic pain?
- Describe the ramifications, evaluation, diagnosis, and management of endometriosis?

 QUICK QUIZ: SEXUALLY TRANSMITTED INFECTIONS

A 19-year-old female presents to your urgent care center with a foul-smelling vaginal discharge. She has noted the discharge for about 3 days. She is sexually active and sporadically uses condoms for birth control. On examination she is in no acute distress, and her vital signs are normal. Her pelvic examination is remarkable for mild vaginal erythema and a frothy gray discharge. You note a "fishy odor" and suspect *Trichomonas*. A wet prep confirms your diagnosis.

You recommend now that she also be tested for:

A) *Chlamydia* and gonorrhea.
B) Herpes simplex.
C) Hepatitis A.
D) All of the above.
E) None of the above.

Discussion

The correct answer is A. Routine screening for chlamydia and gonorrhea infection is recommended for all sexually active adolescents. Given the presence of one STD, it is appropriate to offer testing for other STDs at this visit. Currently, HSV is not routinely tested for in asymptomatic persons, and the USPSTF recommends against serologic screening for HSV. Hepatitis A is not a sexually transmitted disease. It may be appropriate to offer testing for hepatitis B, HIV, syphilis, etc, as individual cases dictate.

QUICK QUIZ: PROLAPSE

An 80-year-old woman presents for evaluation of a "bulge" she noted after gardening over the weekend. She has no discomfort and no difficulty with bowel or bladder elimination. On examination you note her cervix extends 1 cm beyond the vestibule (vaginal opening) with straining. There are no lesions or excoriations noted.

What is the best initial treatment option?

A) Hysterectomy.
B) Trachelectomy.
C) Pessary trial.
D) Bed rest.
E) Hormone therapy.

Discussion

The correct answer is C. Pelvic floor prolapse will not resolve with bed rest or hormone therapy. Hysterectomy and trachelectomy (removal of the cervix) are both unnecessarily invasive for this 80-year-old patient. Although advanced age alone is not a contraindication for surgery, less invasive therapies should be tried initially. Seventy percent of women who are fitted with a pessary are satisfied at 5-year follow-up.

QUICK QUIZ: OVARIAN MASS

What is the best way to manage an ASYMPTO-MATIC 4-cm ovarian mass found on routine pelvic exam in a 22-year-old female who is otherwise healthy?

A) Referral to a gynecologist.
B) Start hormonal therapy to reduce ovulation.
C) Expectant management with repeat examination in 2 months.
D) Serum CA-125 level.

Discussion

The correct answer is C. A 4-cm ovarian mass likely represents a functional cyst in a woman who is cycling (reproductive age). Since it is asymptomatic and easily palpable, expectant management is the best option. No

further evaluation is warranted at this time. **If you are not sure of your exam, ultrasound is a good option.** CA-125 is a tumor marker for epithelial ovarian cancer, but it is not useful as a screening test.

QUICK QUIZ: OVARIAN MASS

What is the best first step in managing an asymptomatic 4-cm ovarian mass in a 76-year-old postmenopausal woman?

A) Referral to a gynecologist.
B) Pelvic ultrasound.
C) Expectant management with repeat exam in 2 months.
D) Serum CA-125 level.

Discussion

The correct answer is B. Unlike a relatively small palpable ovarian mass in a reproductive-age woman, a palpable ovarian mass in a postmenopausal woman represents ovarian malignancy until proven otherwise. The best initial imaging study for evaluation of a pelvic mass is ultrasound. Ultrasound will not only identify the location of the mass but will also identify its internal consistency. Characteristics suggestive of cancer include: bilaterality, solid and cystic components, thick septations, and the presence of ascites. CA-125 is a marker for epithelial ovarian cancer and may assist in evaluation, but it cannot be relied upon to rule in or to rule out cancer as a diagnosis. CA-125 levels >65 U/mL in postmenopausal women with pelvic masses are predictive of malignancy in 75% of patients.

QUICK QUIZ: GYNECOLOGIC CANCERS

What is the leading cause of death from a gynecologic malignancy in American women?

A) Ovarian cancer.
B) Uterine cancer.
C) Cervical cancer.
D) Fallopian tube cancer.
E) Vaginal cancer.

Discussion

The correct answer is A. Ovarian cancer is the leading cause of death from gynecologic malignancy, is the second most common gynecologic malignancy, and is the fourth leading cause of cancer death in women. Endometrial cancer is the most common gynecologic malignancy. Cervical cancer is the third most common gynecologic malignancy. Both fallopian tube and vaginal malignancy are relatively uncommon.

 QUICK QUIZ: OVARIAN CANCER

How does ovarian cancer typically present?

A) Early satiety.
B) Abdominal fullness and pain.
C) Urinary obstruction.
D) Asymptomatic mass noted on routine exam.
E) A and B.

Discussion

The correct answer is E. There are no specific early symptoms of ovarian cancer. Thus, most patients present with symptoms associated with increasing tumor mass: early satiety, abdominal fullness, and abdominal pain. Unfortunately, ovarian cancer is rarely identified on routine annual exam.

CASE 15

While covering the ED on the graveyard shift (so called because of the time of day, not because of the number of patients who die), a 21-year-old college student presents sobbing with a friend. Her friend says, "She's been raped."

Relevant history includes all of the following EXCEPT:

A) Whether force was used and what type.
B) Physical characteristics of the assailant.
C) Details regarding penetration (vaginal, anal, oral).
D) Number of sexual partners the victim has had in her lifetime.
E) Condom use.

Discussion

The correct answer is D. The patient's past sexual history is not immediately relevant in the evaluation of sexual assault, and asking directly about the number of sexual partners she has had may make the interview sound accusatory in nature. The other issues are pertinent to the case. Although it may be difficult for the patient to relive the experience, you should try to

obtain a detailed history of the assault. In order to assess her risk for pregnancy and infection, you need to ask about the area penetrated (eg, vaginal, oral, or anal penetration), whether the assailant ejaculated, and if a condom was used. In a sexual assault case, your job is also to collect evidence, including pertinent historical elements (eg, number of assailants, names, physical appearance, whether force was used and what type—threat, restraints, weapons, etc).

 HELPFUL TIP: Sexual assault includes genital, anal, or oral penetration by a part of the accused's body or by an object. By definition, it occurs without the victim's consent and need not involve direct force or violence.

Which of the following are important physical elements to collect for the forensic evaluation in this case?

A) Combed specimens from the scalp and pubic hair.
B) Swabs of the oral, vaginal, and rectal mucosa.
C) The patient's clothing.
D) Fingernail scrapings.
E) All of the above.

Discussion

The correct answer is E. All of the items listed will be important to the investigation. Evidence collection kits for sexual assault cases (rape kits) should be available in your ED.

* *

Although apparently inebriated, the patient is able to give a coherent history. When you broach the subject of physical examination, her friend says, "Look, she was raped an hour ago. Can't you let her recover a bit before you violate her all over again?"

Which of the following is the most appropriate response?

A) "Of course. Come back tomorrow come back tomorrow when you feel better."
B) "An examination is important for your health and in the event that this becomes a criminal case. The yield of the exam declines with time. Even if you don't feel like prosecuting now, you may decide to do so in the future, and the best evidence is gathered early."

C) "The exam has a fairly high yield even a week after the assault, so take your time on this."
D) "Under federal law I am required to perform this exam."

Discussion

The correct answer is B. The yield of a forensic exam declines with time. Even if a patient states that she does not want to prosecute the assailant, she should be encouraged to have the exam done in case she changes her mind. Also, you are concerned about her health, and she may be at risk for sexually transmitted diseases, pregnancy, and traumatic injury, so it is important to try to complete an exam. Although yield does decline with time, reliable evidence may still be gathered up to 5 days after the assault. However, you should not encourage patients to postpone the exam. There is no federal law in this matter, so practitioners are encouraged to know and observe their state laws.

HELPFUL TIP: "Rape Trauma Syndrome" generally occurs in 3 stages. The first includes anger, anxiety, guilt, shame, sleep disturbance, etc. The second stage includes somatic complaints (pelvic pain, other pain) and psychiatric complaints (depression, phobias, etc). Some patients will go on to resolve these issues while others will develop posttraumatic stress syndrome. A further discussion of this is beyond the scope of this book but practitioners should familiarize themselves with this disorder.

Which of the following is the LEAST appropriate to offer this patient now?

A) HIV antibody testing.
B) HSV antibody testing.
C) Prophylactic treatment for gonorrhea and chlamydia.
D) Mental health services referral.
E) Emergency contraception (eg, Plan B).

Discussion

The correct answer is B. Herpes virus antibody testing will only tell you if she has been exposed to HSV in the past. Testing on the day of presentation will not reveal anything about transmission from the assailant, and since HSV is only treated when symptomatic, this information will not lead to any useful changes in her management. HIV antibody testing carries more significance. This patient should be counseled on HIV testing and offered a baseline test on the day of presentation. You should consider HIV prophylaxis and encourage the patient to return for follow-up testing in 6 weeks. You should also consider testing and/or treating for gonorrhea and chlamydia. The patient should be offered mental health services, a crisis center number to call, emergency contraception, and a follow-up appointment within a week or 2. Further recommendations include syphilis testing, hepatitis B antibody testing, performing a wet prep of a vaginal sample, and checking a urine pregnancy test.

* *

The patient consents to a physical examination. You use the sexual assault kit to collect samples. You note what appear to be new ecchymoses on her arms. There is no sign of vulvar or vaginal trauma. Upon palpation, you find a discrete mass measuring about 8 cm in the left adnexal area.

Which of the following is the most appropriate next step in the management of this new issue?

A) Follow-up pelvic examination in 6 months.
B) Pelvic ultrasound.
C) Chest/abdomen/pelvis MRI.
D) Serum FSH and LH levels.
E) Determine BRCA gene status.

Discussion

The correct answer is B. An ovarian mass of ≥6 cm is more likely to be cancerous than a mass <6 cm. Ultrasound will allow you to better characterize the mass, determine the risk of malignancy, and provide a more accurate measurement. If findings on ultrasound are reassuring, even a 6-cm mass may be followed over time provided the patient is otherwise at low risk. Typically, patients are asked to return in 2 months for repeat pelvic exam and ultrasound. In this case, an MRI is overkill and unlikely to yield any more useful information than the ultrasound. Serum LH and FSH are not indicated here. If a patient has a BRCA gene, she is at higher risk of developing ovarian cancer. However, BRCA would not be the first step in evaluation of this patient.

HELPFUL TIP: The following characteristics place a patient at higher risk of having a malignant ovarian mass: premenarcheal, postmenopausal, mass >10 cm in diameter, and solid mass on ultrasound.

HELPFUL TIP: When you find an adnexal mass in a woman of child-bearing years, rule out pregnancy.

Objectives: Did you learn to . . .

- Evaluate a patient for sexual assault?
- Manage a patient who has been the victim of sexual assault?
- Evaluate an adnexal mass?

CASE 16

A 21-year-old woman presents to your office with complaint of pelvic pain with intercourse. The pain seems worse over the last 2 weeks. She also complains of not getting pregnant, even though she's had several partners over her last 3 years of sexual activity and has been trying to get pregnant with the same partner for the past 6 months. She states she never has used birth control of any type—not even once. She started her periods around 14 years but has only had a couple of periods since then. Apparently, this pattern of menstruation is normal for her family, as her mother was the same way. Finally, she wants something to treat facial hair and acne, both of which have been worse lately.

On physical exam, you note the patient is a centrally obese young woman, afebrile, with (culturally defined) excess hair noted down the side of her face and under her chin. She also has some erythematous pustules on her cheeks.

Which of the following lab results would be most consistent with the history and exam findings?

A) Positive urine pregnancy test.
B) Low TSH level.
C) Elevated CA-125 level.
D) LH: FSH ratio >3:1.
E) Prolactin level >3 times normal.

Discussion

The correct answer is D. While there are several issues to address with this patient, she certainly gives a history and has an appearance consistent with polycystic ovarian syndrome (PCOS). The clinical features of PCOS include oligomenorrhea (90%), hirsutism (80%), obesity (50%), amenorrhea (40%), and infertility (40%). Early symptoms in an adolescent may consist only of irregular periods, acne, and central obesity. An LH: FSH ratio >3:1 adds further support to the diagnosis. A positive pregnancy test is the most common cause of amenorrhea in reproductive age women, but pregnancy would not account for the other symptoms. Nonetheless, a urine HCG test should be one of the first things ordered for this patient, and with the above clinical history and physical appearance, would most likely be negative. A low TSH would be indicative of hyperthyroidism, which may cause more frequent, heavy menses, would usually cause weight loss, and does not cause hirsutism. CA-125 is used to follow ovarian cancer, and sometimes severe endometriosis, but is not a good screening test because it lacks sensitivity. A normal to mildly elevated prolactin level can be found with PCOS. However, a level 3 times normal would not only cause amenorrhea, but would probably cause galactorrhea and, again, does not explain her hirsutism.

**

On closer inspection, you see slightly hyperpigmented areas of roughened skin in her axilla, which she states appeared in the last 6 months.

Which of the following lab values would correlate with this finding?

A) Elevated testosterone level.
B) Elevated dehydroepiandrosterone sulfate (DHEAS) level.
C) Elevated serum 17-hydroxyprogesterone (17-OHP) level.
D) Prolactin level 3 times normal.
E) Elevated fasting insulin level.

Discussion

The correct answer is E. The hyperpigmented, almost dusty-appearing areas in the skin folds are known as acanthosis nigricans, which suggests significant insulin resistance. The most recent evidence points to insulin resistance as the underlying cause of PCOS. Insulin resistance can be quantified by calculating the ratio of fasting glucose to insulin. A ratio of <4.5 indicates decreased insulin sensitivity. Insulin resistance stimulates ovarian androgen production, which leads to anovulation. Prolonged anovulation can lead to the development of enlarged ovaries with multiple cysts that were first seen on ultrasound and thus gave the name to the syndrome. Hyperinsulinemia and hyperandrogenemia interfere with the secretion of gonadotropins from the pituitary gland, resulting in changes, in the mid-cycle LH surge and its diurnal variation.

An elevated testosterone level would certainly correlate with the findings of hirsutism and acne but does not contribute to the development of acanthosis nigricans. DHEAS elevation may represent a virilizing tumor, while serum 17-OHP is associated with adult-onset congenital adrenal hyperplasia, but neither will cause acanthosis nigricans. Finally, an elevated prolactin level sometimes is seen in PCOS or is consistent with a pituitary adenoma, but not acanthosis nigricans.

* *

You proceed with the pelvic portion of the exam, noting the patient also has a large diamond-shaped, rather than triangular-shaped, pubic hair pattern. You find no lesions on the vulva or in the vagina. However, the cervix appears reddened, with an almost strawberry texture. And, although there is a generous amount of yellowish, malodorous leukorrhea in the vaginal vault, there is no notable pus at the cervical os. On bimanual exam, there is questionable cervical tenderness and fullness in both adnexa, but the exam is somewhat limited because of the patient's obesity.

Of the following, which is the most likely diagnosis?

A) Herpes simplex virus (HSV) infection.
B) *Trichomonas vaginalis* infection.
C) *Candida albicans* infection.
D) Pelvic inflammatory disease (PID).
E) Bacterial vaginosis.

Discussion

The correct answer is B. Trichomonas is a protozoan that is sexually transmitted and can cause urethritis in both sexes. However, in women, it most commonly causes ulceration of the cervical mucosa with punctuate hemorrhages known as a "strawberry cervix." Signs and symptoms also include a malodorous discharge and

occasional vulvar and vaginal irritation. The cervix can be somewhat tender to touch, either during exam or intercourse, and patients often complain of a nonspecific pelvic pain. Males are often asymptomatic.

HSV is a DNA virus that causes a recurrent lifetime infection and is characterized by painful vesicles that ulcerate. There is not usually a significant discharge or cervicitis. *Candida albicans* is a yeast infection, perhaps the most common vaginal infection, and usually is best described as very itchy with thick, white discharge. PID is a clinical diagnosis (see discussion earlier in this chapter). Bacterial vaginosis is due to an overgrowth of *Haemophilus* bacteria, which causes a malodorous discharge and vulvar itching but no cervicitis or pelvic pain.

* *

You proceed to send a wet mount that does indeed demonstrate the one-celled protozoan with a flagellum, and there is no evidence of yeast or clue cells. You send samples for chlamydia and gonorrhea tests as well as a Pap smear. You recommend testing for HIV, syphilis, and hepatitis, and she agrees.

For her trichomonas vaginal infection you prescribe:

A) Flagyl (metronidazole) 2 g orally in a single dose.
B) MetroGel-Vaginal (topical vaginal metronidazole) 5 g applied nightly for 5 days.
C) Diflucan (fluconazole) 150 mg orally in a single dose.
D) Zithromax (azithromycin) 1 g orally in a single dose.
E) Levaquin (levofloxacin) 250 mg orally in a single dose.

Discussion

The correct answer is A. The best choice is oral metronidazole. Topical antibiotic gels, creams, or ovules—either metronidazole or clindamycin (Cleocin)—treat only bacterial vaginosis, as the concentration is insufficient to reach the protozoa in the glands and urethral areas. Diflucan is an antifungal that best treats *Candida*. Azithromycin, dosed once, will treat chlamydia cervicitis, in both pregnant and nonpregnant patients. However, doxycycline 100 mg BID for 1 week is a less expensive alternative. Levaquin and other fluoroquinolones should be avoided for gonorrhea due to resistance.

HELPFUL TIP: As with other STDs, a patient with trichomonas should have her partner tested and treated (or treated only).

 HELPFUL TIP: Although it makes sense that single dose azithromycin would work better in treating chlamydia because of compliance issues, the cure rate is the same whether azithromycin or the doxycycline is used.

* *

You have her return in a week. She states that she took metronidazole and that her boyfriend was treated also. You review her lab results: HIV and RPR negative; chlamydia negative; gonorrhea positive.

Which of the following is the best strategy regarding her positive gonorrhea test?

A) Repeat the test in 2 weeks.
B) Don't worry about it since she has been treated with metronidazole and has no symptoms.
C) Prescribe erythromycin 500 mg 4 times a day for 7 days.
D) Administer ceftriaxone 250 mg IM in the office and prescribe doxycycline 100 mg twice daily for 7 days.
E) Any of the above strategies is equally acceptable.

Discussion
The correct answer is D. Uncomplicated—including asymptomatic—gonococcal infection must be treated with antibiotics. Due to the fact that there is frequently coinfection with *Chlamydia trachomatis* (perhaps even with a negative chlamydia culture), concomitant treatment for chlamydia is recommended by the CDC. Treatment regimens for gonorrhea include single doses of cefixime, ceftriaxone, and azithromycin. Increased resistance has been noted with the fluoroquinolones, which are no longer recommended by the CDC for treatment of gonorrhea. Treatment of the partner(s) is imperative, and patients should practice abstinence during treatment.

* *

After prescribing appropriate therapy for her GC, you turn your attention to her abnormal Pap smear. The pathology report reads "atypical squamous cells of undetermined significance—cannot rule out high grade squamous intraepithelial lesion (ASC-H)."

According to the 2006 Consensus Guidelines for the Management of Women with Abnormal Cervical Cancer Screening Tests by the ASCCP (American Society of Cervical and Cytological Pathology), which of the following statements is correct?

A) ASC can be safely followed up with a repeat Pap smear in 1 year if the Pap is performed using a liquid-based media and the reflex test for HPV is negative.
B) ASC-H can be safely followed up with a repeat Pap smear in 1 year regardless of HPV test result.
C) Atypical glandular cells (AGC) can be safely followed up with a repeat Pap smear in 1 year if the Pap is performed using a liquid-based media and the reflex test for HPV is negative.
D) Low-grade squamous intraepithelial lesion (LSIL) can be safely followed up with a repeat Pap smear in 1 year if the Pap is performed using a liquid-based media and the reflex test for HPV is negative.
E) All of the above.

Discussion
The correct answer is A. The finding of ASC can be safely followed up with a repeat Pap smear in 1 year, provided that the Pap is performed using a liquid-based media and the reflex test for HPV is negative. This is the only use for testing the residual liquid in a liquid-based Pap for HPV. A negative test on the liquid for HPV puts an ASC at no greater risk than a normal Pap, and so patients in this category can return to routine follow-up. If the liquid-based Pap shows ASC **positive** for high-risk strains of HPV, the patient should proceed directly to colposcopy.

 HELPFUL TIP: The new guidelines for PAP smears are hopelessly complex and include differences based on patient age, pregnancy status, etc. If you want to review the documents, they are available at http://www.asccp.org/consensus.shtml. See following quick guide discussion of abnormal PAP smears.

ASCUS (atypical squamous cells of undetermined significance) does not indicate dysplasia or a precancerous lesion. It may be secondary to infection or reparative changes (eg, after pregnancy). ASCUS is categorized further as:

ASC-US: Do HPV testing only if >20 years old (see note below). If negative, repeat PAP in 12 months. If positive, proceed to colposcopy. If cannot do HPV testing, repeat the PAP in 6 and 12 months. If both negative, resume normal screening intervals.

ASC-H (favor high-grade): Proceed directly to colposcopy. If no CIN 2 or CIN 3, do repeat PAP at 6 and 12 months **or** HPV testing at 12 months. If either abnormal, repeat colposcopy. If negative, resume routine screening.

LGSIL/LSIL (low-grade squamous intraepithelial lesion which encompasses HPV & CIN I): Proceed to colposcopy and endocervical Pap smear (although recommendations vary depending on patient age, pregnancy, etc). If no CIN 2 or CIN 3, repeat PAP at 6 and 12 months **or** HPV testing at 12 months. If either abnormal, repeat colposcopy. If negative, resume routine screening.

Pap reads HGSIL/HSIL (high-grade squamous intraepithelial lesion which encompasses CIN II, CIN III, CIS (carcinoma in situ): Options include: immediate loop electrosurgical excision procedure (LEEP) **or** colposcopy and endocervical assessment (preferred). If no CIN 2 or CIN 3 is found in your biopsy specimens (from colposcopy or excision) you have the option of PAP + colposcopy Q 6 months for a year or diagnostic excision of lesions. If you choose PAP + colposcopy and both the 6- and 12-month exams are normal, resume routine screening intervals.

AGUS (atypical glandular cells of undetermined significance): Do endometrial sampling (eg, Pipelle) + colposcopy + HPV testing. Another option is to do endometrial **and** endocervical sampling and if this is negative to proceed to colposcopy.

> **HELPFUL TIP:** The ASCCP Guidelines 2006 are a major change in the way adolescents are approached. A woman ≥20 years (here considered an adolescent) who has ASC or LSIL on Pap should **not** have colposcopy right away. Rather, repeat cytology in 12 months is recommended. Also, adolescents with ASC should

> **not** have reflex HPV testing done. These recommendations recognize the high prevalence of HPV in this population and the high likelihood of cervical changes being transient and regressing to normal. Colposcopy should be performed in adolescent women with high-grade squamous intraepithelial lesion (HSIL) or higher **and** in adolescent women with ASC persisting >24 months.

* *

You proceed with the colposcopy, and after the application of 5% acetic acid, you note a thickened, white area along the posterior border of the transformation zone with an internal white border and coarse mosaic changes of the blood vessels.

This appearance on colposcopy is most consistent with which of the following pathology reports on your biopsy?

A) Normal metaplasia of the cervix.
B) Low-grade squamous intraepithelial lesion (LSIL).
C) High-grade squamous intraepithelial lesion (HSIL).
D) Cervical cancer.

Discussion

The correct answer is C. This appearance is most consistent with HSIL. Colposcopic exam of HSIL will show internal borders with vascular changes on white epithelium. LSIL shows only the white epithelium, with normal, fine vasculature. Normal metaplasia has translucent, white changes, with indistinct borders and gland formation. In addition to changes seen in HSIL, cervical cancer will appear with heaping up and peeling of the white epithelium and abnormally branching blood vessels with hemorrhage into the lesion.

* *

Your interpretation on colposcopy was correct, and pathology of the biopsy is indeed HSIL. You refer the patient to your partner for a loop electrosurgical-excision procedure (LEEP). The entire transformation zone, with the area of HSIL around the external cervical os, is excised, and the margins are reported as clear. Six months later, your patient's follow-up Pap smear is normal.

* *

You now return your attention to her PCOS (remember, way back then?). Her labs demonstrated a LH:FSH ratio >3; normal TSH and prolactin; slightly elevated testosterone, but still well below the normal male range; fasting glucose:insulin <4.5; slightly elevated total cholesterol and triglycerides. Her LH:FSH ratio was consistent with the diagnosis of PCOS. She has not menstruated for 12 months, and she denies sexual activity. A urine HCG is negative, and a repeat fasting glucose is 120 mg/dL.

Which of the following recommendations should you make now?

A) Initiate metformin.
B) Attempt weight loss through a nutritious diet and increased exercise.
C) Initiate oral contraceptives to regulate menses.
D) A and C
E) All of the above.

Discussion

The correct answer is E. This patient has glucose intolerance (elevated fasting glucose and ratio of glucose:insulin <4.5), and it is reasonable to initiate dietary and medical therapy now. Another option is to start with lifestyle modifications and check fasting glucose again 3–6 months later. Due to increased risk of endometrial carcinoma in patients who have rare menses, it is important to regulate her cycles. OCPs (answer C) can accomplish menstrual regulation. For hirsutism, spironolactone is usually first-line therapy, unless the patient has a contraindication; traditional hair removal techniques will still be required for the existing hair growth. Since spironolactone can result in feminization of a male fetus, patients taking spironolactone must be using reliable birth control (eg, oral contraceptives).

 HELPFUL TIP: Not all women with PCOS are obese and hirsute. Many patients may be thin with sparse body hair, and present with menstrual irregularities and fertility concerns.

Objectives: Did you learn to . . .

• Identify the clinical presentation of polycystic ovarian syndrome?
• Diagnose and treat trichomonas infection?

• Treat gonorrhea?
• Manage abnormal Pap smear results?
• Diagnose and manage polycystic ovarian syndrome?

 HELPFUL TIP: When an older woman sustains a wrist fracture, it doubles risk for a hip fracture, and the mortality rate of hip fractures approaches 20% within 1 year. This mortality rate exceeds that of breast cancer, and the cost of osteoporotic fractures in the U.S. approaches $14 billion per year.

* *

You next see her for a health maintenance examination, including pelvic examination. She complains of a vulvar "itching" due to recurrent yeast infections, and her symptoms have worsened over the last few months. She is sexually active with her new husband and has experienced dyspareunia with penetration lately. She always uses a water-based lubricant with intercourse. On examination, you find complete loss of the borders of the labia minora, constriction of the vaginal outlet, and several thin white plaques (like parchment paper) on the vulva. There is no other skin or mucosal involvement.

What is the most likely diagnosis?

A) Lichen planus.
B) Lichen simplex.
C) Lichen sclerosus.
D) Vulvovaginal candidiasis.
E) Squamous carcinoma.

Discussion

The correct answer is C. The clinical description above is characteristic of lichen sclerosus, which occurs more commonly in older women but also has a second peak of incidence in young girls. Almost all lichen sclerosus is intensely pruritic. As lichen sclerosus progresses, there may be loss of labial architecture, stenosis of the introitus, and obliteration of the clitoris. The lesions are usually multiple and appear as thin, shiny, white, wrinkled patches or plaques. Initial treatment for lichen sclerosus involves local steroid ointment application. Typically, high-potency steroids are initiated and then tapered to the lowest potency and frequency that maintain symptom control. Testosterone creams, which have been used in the past, are now generally **avoided** due to lesser efficacy and secondary virilization.

Lichen planus (answer A), is an autoimmune disease that is often difficult to treat. Lesions may be papular or ulcerated. If you suspect lichen planus of the genitalia, look elsewhere, as it can be diffuse. Lichen simplex (answer B), although also pruritic, does not result in the loss of labial architecture as with lichen sclerosus. However, the patient should be carefully evaluated for the presence of a "mixed dystrophy" or the combination of both lichen sclerosus and lichen simplex, as the two often coexist. Candida (answer D) is not likely to cause the discrete lesions and vulvar changes described in this case. Squamous carcinoma (answer E) occasionally can be confused for lichen sclerosus. However, the examination is more likely to reveal a lesion with ulceration and induration, and squamous carcinoma is less common (though if you are suspicious of cancer, a biopsy is indicated).

* *

You initiate topical treatment with clobetasol 0.05% ointment daily and have the patient follow up in 1 month to assess the response. On follow-up 2 months later, she notes marked improvement of the vulvar pruritus. However, she continues to have pain with vaginal penetration which she describes as a "tearing sensation." On examination, you again note complete loss of the borders of the labia minora, and mild constriction of the vaginal outlet. The white plaques have resolved.

Given the clinical response, the next step in treatment should be:

A) Reduce the frequency and potency of the steroid ointment.
B) Discontinue the clobetasol ointment.
C) Begin vaginal dilator therapy.
D) Perform a random biopsy.
E) A and C.

Discussion

The correct answer is E. The patient has responded well to the initial topical steroid as demonstrated by the reduction in symptoms and resolution the white plaques. Thus, the steroid ointment should be tapered to avoid steroid atrophy while maintaining symptom control. Additionally, the patient continues to have dyspareunia, which is likely due to the mild vaginal constriction. Treatment options include graded vaginal

dilators (to gently "stretch" the vaginal vestibule) or perineoplasty. Dilator therapy is preferred as it avoids the risks of surgery.

Answer B is incorrect. Discontinuation of the steroid would likely result in rebound of symptoms. Lichen sclerosus is a chronic disorder and requires long-term maintenance therapy to prevent further loss of anatomy. Answer D is incorrect. The patient responded well to therapy and had resolution of the white plaques.

* *

The patient asks you about her risk of developing vulvar squamous cell cancer given the lichen sclerosus. She notes vulvar diseases were featured on a recent TV talk show and cancer was mentioned.

You counsel the patient that her risk of developing vulvar squamous cell cancer with her history of lichen sclerosus is about:

A) 5%
B) 20%
C) 50%
D) Almost certain, and she will need yearly biopsies.

Discussion

The correct answer is A. The risk of subsequent vulvar squamous cell cancer is 3%–7% in women with lichen sclerosus. For this reason, patients with lichen sclerosus require vulvar examinations every 6–12 months, more often if symptoms are not well controlled. If a lesion occurs and does not respond to treatment, a biopsy should be performed.

Objectives: Did you learn to . . .

• Recognize various vulvar pathologies?

 QUICK QUIZ: VULVOVAGINAL CANDIDIASIS

A 48-year-old perimenopausal female presents with a 3-day history of vulvar pruritus. Her history is significant for mitral valve replacement, on warfarin with INR 2–3. A limited vulvar and vaginal exam reveals significant erythema with satellite lesions on the labia majora. Wet prep microscopy reveals abundant pseudohyphae and inflammatory cells. You diagnose yeast vulvovaginitis. She inquires about use of oral therapy as vaginal creams are "messy."

How will you counsel this patient regarding use of oral fluconazole (Diflucan)?

A) "You have no contraindications to oral fluconazole."

B) "Given use of warfarin, you should not use oral fluconazole."

C) "You will need to adjust your warfarin dose when using oral fluconazole."

D) "You should take extra warfarin if you take oral fluconazole."

Discussion

The correct answer is B. There are numerous drug interactions with oral fluconazole, including warfarin (both inhibit CYP 3A4). The INR will increase following oral fluconazole therapy, increasing the patient's risk of hemorrhage. Similarly, the ubiquitous statins are affected by oral fluconazole with several case reports of rhabdomyolysis in the literature. A thorough drug history should be ascertained before prescribing oral fluconazole for a simple yeast vulvovaginitis. Even a single dose of fluconazole can through off the INR. In cases such as this, topical azoles are the better choice.

CASE 17

A 27-year-old female presents with her husband seeking advice regarding pregnancy loss. She recently had a miscarriage. Because this is your first meeting, you take a detailed history.

Of the following historical elements, which is the MOST important when exploring the patients history of pregnancy loss?

A) History of pelvic infections.

B) Woman's age.

C) Partner's (male's) age.

D) Number and outcomes of prior pregnancies.

E) Menstrual history.

Discussion

The correct answer is D. It is important to determine if this patient is experiencing recurrent (>2) pregnancy loss and whether she has carried a pregnancy to term. The other historical elements, while important in prenatal screening and fertility counseling, are not relevant in establishing whether or not this couple has recurrent pregnancy loss.

* *

Your patient states that this was her second miscarriage in the last year. Her menarche was at age 12 and her menses have been regular since midadolescence. She had been using oral contraceptives until they married 2 years ago. Since this time she has become pregnant twice (missed period and positive home pregnancy test) with miscarriage before establishing OB care (about 9 weeks' gestation each time). Her Pap smears have always been normal, and she has never had any sexually transmitted diseases.

Possible explanations for recurrent pregnancy loss in this patient include all of the following EXCEPT:

A) Parental structural chromosome abnormalities.

B) Uterine anatomic abnormalities.

C) History of appendicitis at 6 years.

D) Unexplained etiology.

Discussion

The correct answer is C. History of appendicitis would not cause pregnancy loss. Parental structural chromosome abnormalities (balanced structural chromosome rearrangement in one partner) are responsible for pregnancy loss in 2%–4% of couples. Answer B is true. Uterine anatomic abnormalities have been associated with 10%–15% of pregnancy loss (septum, bicornuate, didelphic. Answer D is true. The majority of couples with recurrent pregnancy loss will have an uncertain etiology despite extensive evaluation (>50%).

 HELPFUL TIP: Recurrent pregnancy loss is defined as 3 consecutive spontaneous abortions. However, the risk of another miscarriage after 2 successive spontaneous abortions is clinically similar to the risk of recurrence among women with 3 or more spontaneous abortions.

* *

The couple desires testing for possible causes of the pregnancy losses.

Of the following, which test(s) should be included in the evaluation?

A) Cultures for bacteria.

B) Test for glucose intolerance.

C) Maternal antipaternal antibodies.

D) Lupus anticoagulant and anticardiolipin antibody.

E) All of the above.

Discussion

The correct answer is D. Antiphospholipid syndrome is associated with pregnancy loss in 3%–15% of women with recurrent pregnancy loss. Each of the other choices is not beneficial in the evaluation of otherwise normal women with recurrent pregnancy loss. However, you should also evaluate parental chromosomes to identify if one parent has a balanced chromosome abnormality.

 HELPFUL TIP: The most commonly recognized cause of early pregnancy loss is abnormality of chromosome structure or number.

* *

Evaluation of the recurrent pregnancy loss fails to identify a cause. Thus, like most couples with recurrent pregnancy loss, the etiology remains unexplained.

What is the likelihood that this couple will have a successful pregnancy outcome in the next pregnancy?

A) Highly unlikely; they should consider adoption.

B) Less than 1 in 4 chance of successful pregnancy.

C) 60%–70% chance of successful next pregnancy.

D) You cannot hazard a guess. This has not been studied.

Discussion

The correct answer is C. Studies suggest that 60%–70% of couples with unexplained recurrent pregnancy loss will have a successful next pregnancy.

* *

You advise the couple and recommend prenatal vitamins with 0.4 mg folic acid given the desire to attempt pregnancy in the near future. The patient calls 4 months later, 5 days following her missed period. She desires an ultrasound to confirm pregnancy and to make sure "everything is all right." You correctly inform her that her best course of action is to check a urine pregnancy test to confirm pregnancy.

When should this patient be seen to establish OB care?

A) As soon as the pregnancy is confirmed.

B) She should have an amniocentesis to determine chromosomes prior to a new OB visit.

C) At 8 to 11 weeks' gestation.

D) At 14 to 20 weeks' gestation.

E) All early testing has been done, she does not need to be seen until the fetus is viable.

Discussion

The correct answer is C. Despite this patient's obvious anxiety related to her history of two prior losses, there is no benefit to establishing "earlier than normal OB care" (answer A). All the other incorrect answers would delay the initiation of OB care and potentially miss the window for first-trimester and early second-trimester screening.

* *

She presents for her new OB at 10 weeks' gestation. The fetal heart is auscultated with Doppler at 140 beats per minute. Her uterus is consistent with gestation, and the remainder of the exam is unremarkable. You obtain a Pap smear along with the routine initial OB labs. The Pap smear reveals atypical glandular cells.

How will you proceed?

A) Repeat the Pap smear postpartum.

B) Repeat the Pap smear in 4–6 months.

C) Luckily you use liquid-base Pap testing and can test for high risk HPV types.

D) Perform colposcopy with directed biopsy.

E) Perform colposcopy with directed biopsy, endocervical curettage, and endometrial biopsy.

Discussion

The correct answer is D. Atypical glandular cells (AGC) are associated with underlying high-grade dysplasia in up to 41% and cervical adenocarcinoma in 1% of women. Thus the evaluation of AGC includes colposcopy with directed biopsy. Because the patient is pregnant, endocervical sampling should not be performed now (likewise endometrial biopsy). Endometrial sampling is indicated in women with atypical endometrial cells and women with AGC who are ≥35 years. Repeat Pap screening is not appropriate (answers A and B). Reflex HPV testing is reserved for management of atypical squamous cells of undetermined significance and will avoid the necessity of colposcopy in approximately 40% (negative high-risk HPV). HPV testing has not been found to be useful in the evaluation of AGC.

* *

You perform the colposcopy, but the cervix appears normal and biopsy is unnecessary.

Which of the following is the best follow-up approach?

A) Repeat the Pap smear postpartum.
B) Repeat the Pap smear in 4–6 months.
C) Repeat the colposcopy in 3 months.
D) Repeat the colposcopy with directed biopsy and endocervical Pap smear postpartum.
E) The patient should have an immediate cone procedure to exclude cancer.

Discussion

The correct answer is C. Colposcopy should be repeated in 3 months because of concern for high-grade dysplasia. During pregnancy the squamocolumnar junction will evert, aiding in the colposcopic evaluation. Repeating the Pap smear is inappropriate given the initial Pap smear and concern for a high-grade lesion. Delay of follow-up colposcopy until the postpartum period may result in a delay of diagnosis. Excisions should be considered for pregnant women only if a lesion detected at colposcopy is suggestive of invasive cancer.

* *

You repeat the colposcopy at 5 months' gestation (the pregnancy is otherwise going well) and note punctuation and atypical vessels at the 6 o'clock squamocolumnar junction.

What is the MOST appropriate action now?

A) Repeat the Pap smear postpartum.
B) Routine Pap smear in 1 year (all evaluation has been normal thus far).
C) Repeat the colposcopy postpartum.
D) Refer the patient for a cone procedure.
E) Biopsy the lesion.

Discussion

The correct answer is E, biopsy the lesion. Given the initial AGC Pap smear and findings including atypical vessels, you are concerned about high-grade dysplasia,

presence of microinvasion, or adenocarcinoma *in situ* (ACIS). Follow-up postpartum in 1 year would delay diagnosis and may impact optimal treatment. The benefit of biopsy during pregnancy outweighs the risks if colposcopy is suspicious of high-grade dysplasia or worse.

* *

The biopsy returns demonstrating ACIS.

What do you recommend?

A) Repeat the Pap smear postpartum.
B) Repeat the colposcopy postpartum.
C) Refer the patient for a cone procedure postpartum.
D) Refer the patient to a gynecologic oncologist for evaluation prior to delivery.

Discussion

The correct answer is D, refer the patient to a specialist in gynecology-oncology for evaluation prior to delivery. Delaying treatment to postpartum may affect her prognosis.

Objectives: Did you learn to . . .

- Define recurrent pregnancy loss and discuss some of its epidemiologic aspects?
- Enumerate potential causes of recurrent pregnancy loss?
- Identify etiologies and the work-up of recurrent pregnancy loss?
- Evaluate abnormal Pap smear findings during pregnancy?
- Manage the patient with atypical glandular cells (AGC) on Pap smear?

QUICK QUIZ: WEIGHT GAIN IN PREGNANCY

A 28-year-old primigravida female presents for an initial obstetric visit. Her last menstrual period was about 2 months before this visit. You find that she is in good health and is taking no medications. On physical examination, her blood pressure is 112/68, heart rate 76, temperature 36.7°C, weight 140 pounds, and height 5 feet 4 inches. Pelvic examination is consistent with a 6–8-week gestation uterus, and the remainder of the exam is unremarkable. As this is her first pregnancy, she has a number of questions. She wants to know how much weight gain is expected and whether she should "watch her weight."

You calculate her body mass index (BMI) as 24 kg/m² and recommend the following:

A) "Eat anything you want. You cannot gain too much weight."
B) "Your BMI is normal. Your goal is to gain no more than 20 pounds."
C) "Your BMI is low. Your goal is to gain 40 pounds."
D) "Your BMI is high. Your goal is to gain no more than 15 pounds."
E) "Your BMI is normal. Your goal is to gain 30 pounds."

Discussion

The correct answer is E. The Institute of Medicine recommends weight gain in pregnancy based on pregravid BMI. .In this patient, her BMI is in the normal range, so her goal for weight gain in pregnancy is 25–35 pounds. Women with a normal prepregnancy BMI should gain about 1 pound per week during their second and third trimesters. Those with a BMI of <19.8 should gain 28–40 pounds while those with a BMI of >26–29 should gain 15–25 pounds.

BIBLIOGRAPHY

ACOG Practice Bulletin No. 77: Screening for fetal chromosomal abnormalities. Clin *Obstet Gynecol.* 2007;109:217.

Allen RH, Goldberg AB. Emergency contraception: A clinical review. *Clin Obstet Gynecol.* 2007;50(4):927.

Briscoe D, Nguyen H, Mencer M. Management of pregnancy beyond 40 weeks' gestation. *Am Fam Physician.* 2005;71:1935.

Creasy RK, Resnik R, Iams J. *Maternal-Fetal Medicine.* 5th ed. Philadelphia: Saunders 2004.

Crossman SH. The challenge of pelvic inflammatory disease. *Am Fam Physician.* 2006;73:859.

Cunningham G, Leveno KJ, Bloom SL, et al. *Williams Obstetrics.* 21st ed. New York: McGraw-Hill, 2005.

Frey KA, Patel KS. Initial evaluation and management of infertility by the primary care physician. *Mayo Clin Proc.* 2004;79(11):1439.

Johnson BE, Johnson CA, Murray JL, Apgar BS. *Women's Health Care Handbook.* 2nd ed. Philadelphia: Hanley & Belfus, 2000.

Kirkham C, Harris S, Grzybowski S. Evidence-based prenatal care: Part I. General prenatal care and counseling issues. *Am Fam Physician.* 2005;71:1307.

Kirkham C, Harris S, Grzybowski S. Evidence-based prenatal care: Part I. Third-trimester care and prevention of infectious diseases. *Am Fam Physician.* 2005;71:1555.

Hatcher RA, Nelson AL, Zieman M, et al. *A Pocket Guide to Managing Contraception.* 6th ed. Ardent Media; 2005.

Magnotti M, Futterweit W. Obesity and the polycystic ovary syndrome. *Med Clin North Am.* 2007;91(6):1151.

Raina R, Pahlajani G, Khan S, et al. Female sexual dysfunction: classification, pathophysiology, and management. *Fertil Steril.* 2007;88(5):1273.

Scott A, Glasier A. Evidence based contraceptive choices. *Best Pract Res Clin Obstet Gynecol.* 2006;20(5):665.

Centers for Disease Control and Prevention. Sexually transmitted diseases treatment guidelines, 2006. *MMWR.* 2006;55(RR-11):1.

Wright TC, Massad S, Dunton CJ, et al. 2006 consensus guidelines for the management of women with abnormal cervical cancer screening tests. *Am J Obstet Gynecol.* 2007;197(4):346.

16

Men's Health

Victoria Sharp and Jason K. Wilbur

CASE 1

A 58-year-old black male presents to your clinic complaining of hesitancy, frequency, and nocturia 3–4 times per night, which has been steadily worsening over the past few years. His urinary stream is weaker than it was a few years ago. He is not sure if he empties his bladder completely, but he denies a history of urinary tract infections, dysuria, or any pain. He is otherwise well with no significant past medical or surgical history. Currently he takes no medications and has no allergies. On reviewing his family history, you find that his father and older brother died of prostate cancer in their fifties. General physical exam is normal. Genital exam reveals a circumcised penis with no lesions or discharge. There is no inguinal adenopathy. Testicles are descended bilaterally with no lesions or masses. Rectal exam reveals a smooth prostate with no nodules or tenderness.

Based on this patient's history and physical exam, all of the following would be appropriate at this stage EXCEPT:

A) Screening prostate specific antigen (PSA) blood test.
B) AUA symptom score.
C) Postvoid residual urine volume.
D) Transrectal ultrasound with prostate biopsies.
E) Urinalysis.

Discussion

The correct answer is D. Although your patient has an increased risk of prostate cancer, transrectal ultrasound with prostate biopsies is not indicated at this stage. This

diagnostic test should be reserved for suspicion of prostate cancer. Based on this patient's family history and because he is black (blacks have a 50% higher incidence of and mortality from prostate cancer in comparison with whites), PSA screening is appropriate. A rectal exam, while classically taught to be important, adds no additional information in most cases and is not recommended by the U.S. Preventive Services Task Force. Since your patient may not empty his bladder well, a post-void residual urine volume and urinalysis will help determine if he is likely to get a urinary tract infection from urine retention and if he already has an infection. The AUA (American Urological Association) symptom score is a 7-item questionnaire about symptoms of urinary outlet obstruction. The AUA symptom score can assist in the initial diagnosis as well as in following a patient over time to assess status of obstruction.

When considering benign prostatic hyperplasia (BPH), you reflect on the common symptoms of this syndrome, which include all of the following EXCEPT:

A) Urinary retention.
B) Post-void dribbling.
C) Frequency.
D) Nocturia.
E) Hematuria.

Discussion

The correct answer is E. Hematuria is not usually associated with BPH. However, it can occur if a man's prostatic urethra is very enlarged and friable. Enlargement of the prostate often results in obstructive flow symptoms (eg, hesitancy and slow, weak stream), which in turn can lead to irritative symptoms (eg, frequency, urgency, and nocturia). Obstruction from an enlarged prostate alone can cause hypertrophy of the detrusor, or it can lead to an infection that results in detrusor instability—the cause of irritative symptoms. **If irritative symptoms are present without obstructive symptoms, other diagnoses should be considered, including bladder cancer, urolithiasis, infection, or neurogenic bladder.**

* *

Your patient's urinalysis and PSA are normal. After emptying 250 mL of urine, the post-void residual urine volume is 50 mL.

With this information, you recommend which of the following strategies?

A) Urodynamic studies.
B) Medical therapy.
C) Surgical therapy.
D) Scheduled bladder catheterization.
E) Biofeedback.

Discussion

The correct answer is B. You have enough information to diagnose symptomatic BPH, and further studies are not necessary. Depending on the patient's preferences, the next step is to begin treatment, and in most cases medical therapy is initiated first. If medical therapy fails or if a patient has severe BPH with ongoing obstruction, retention of large volumes of urine, or recurrent urinary tract infections, surgical therapy should be considered. The most commonly performed surgery is transurethral resection of the prostate, but other techniques are employed as well, including transurethral incision of the prostate, minimally invasive procedures, and open surgery for extremely enlarged glands.

Scheduled bladder catheterization is unlikely to benefit your patient since his post-void residual is not very large. A post-void residual >200 mL is associated with an increased risk of urinary tract infections, and such patients may benefit from scheduled catheterizations if medical or surgical interventions do not correct the problem or are contraindicated. Biofeedback may be used to treat urge incontinence but is not used in BPH.

* *

You are satisfied that the patient's urinary symptoms are due to BPH. Your patient desires treatment.

You prescribe which of the following?

A) Finasteride.
B) Oxybutynin.
C) Terazosin.
D) Imipramine.
E) Furosemide.

Discussion

The correct answer is C. Timing and type of intervention should depend on how much the patient is bothered by his symptoms and whether complications of BPH are present. If the symptoms do not significantly interfere with your patient's life, he may choose to wait and take no treatment once he is reassured that he does not have a life-threatening illness. Generally, medical management begins with a selective α_1-receptor blocker, such as doxazosin or terazosin. A medication specific for the α_{1A}-receptor subtype (eg, tamsulosin) may be used in patients who cannot tolerate traditional α_1-receptor blockers. If the patient does not receive sufficient relief from maximum doses of an α_1-blocker (terazosin 10 mg daily, doxazosin 8 mg daily or tamsulosin 0.8 mg daily), a 5α-reductase inhibitor (eg, finasteride 5 mg daily or dutasteride 0.5 mg daily) may be added if symptoms are not well controlled. However, it may take up to 6 months for a 5α-reductase inhibitor to result in a noticeable difference in symptoms (thus, answer A should not be the first treatment), whereas, the full benefit of an α-blocker will be apparent within 4–6 weeks. Answers B and D are incorrect because these anticholinergic drugs are used for incontinence due to detrusor instability and may make urinary retention worse in this patient. Answer E, furosemide, is a potent diuretic and would be a cruel joke to play on this patient.

* *

As you write the prescription for terazosin, you review the side effects.

Potential side effects of α-blockers include all the following EXCEPT:

A) Retrograde ejaculation.
B) Hypotension.
C) Intraoperative floppy iris syndrome.
D) Priapism.

Discussion

The correct answer is D. α-Blockers do not help with erectile dysfunction and do not cause priapism. The most commonly encountered problem is hypotension (answer B). In elderly males, the hypotension can be particularly problematic as the propensity for falling may increase. Additionally, α-blockers in combination with phosphodiesterase inhibitors (eg, sildenafil) can cause dangerously low blood pressures; terazosin and doxazosin should be used with caution with this class of medication. Retrograde ejaculation (answer A) is not common but can occur. Here is more evidence for a direct link between the male ocular and genital systems: intraoperative floppy iris syndrome (answer C) has been observed in men taking α-blockers and undergoing cataract surgery; causality has not been proven. You may have thought we made this up but we didn't.

* *

You start terazosin, slowly increasing the dose and administering the medication at night. Unfortunately, the patient is unable to tolerate the medication due to dizziness. His symptoms are bothersome enough that he wishes to try something else, and you prescribe tamsulosin. He tolerates this medication well, but his symptoms are not relieved to his satisfaction. You consider finasteride.

Which of the following is true of finasteride?

A) It permanently reduces prostate volume, even after the drug is stopped.
B) It is approved by the FDA for abnormal hair growth in women.
C) It may reduce the overall risk of developing prostate cancer but increase the risk of developing high-grade prostate cancers.
D) It improves symptoms within 1 week of starting the drug.
E) None of the above.

Discussion
The correct answer is C. Finasteride (and dutasteride) work by inhibiting 5α reductase, which is the enzyme that converts testosterone to dihydrotestosterone. Dihydrotestosterone stimulates hyperplasia of the prostate gland, and removing this stimulus results in decreased prostate volume. However, removal of finasteride allows hyperplasia to continue, and thus answer A is incorrect. Answer B is incorrect because finasteride for hirsutism in women is not approved by the FDA. Additionally, finasteride is category X in pregnancy, with potential teratogenic effects on the fetus. Answer D is incorrect because finasteride takes time to work—a

lot of time. As previously mentioned, its peak effectiveness is not seen for 3–6 months after starting the medication.

 HELPFUL TIP: In comparison trials with α-blockers, 5α-reductase inhibitors have shown variable results. The addition of a 5α-reductase inhibitor to an α-blocker does not seem to have additional benefit over α-blocker therapy alone in the **near term,** but combination therapy has shown reduced incidence of clinical progression of BPH in longer trials.

* *

You decide to add finasteride. You see the patient again 2 months later when he presents with a febrile illness. He thinks that he might have the flu, but his BPH symptoms worsened at the same time. For the last 2 days he has felt feverish with back pain, perineal pain, and generalized malaise. He complains of dysuria and worsening urinary frequency and urgency.

During your exam you make sure NOT to:

A) Perform a rectal exam.
B) Massage the prostate.
C) Swab the urethra for chlamydia.
D) Perform urinalysis and microscopic exam of the urinary sediment.

Discussion
The correct answer is B. There is a risk of seeding bacteria into the bloodstream when an infected prostate is massaged. This patient has symptoms of prostatitis; thus, you should **avoid prostatic massage.** Nonetheless, you should perform a prostate exam. The following physical findings are associated with prostatitis: tenderness, warmth, enlargement, and bogginess.

* *

You suspect prostatitis and obtain urine for analysis.

All of the following laboratory abnormalities are consistent with the diagnosis of acute prostatitis EXCEPT:

A) Leukocytosis.
B) Hematuria.
C) Bacteriuria
D) Elevated creatinine.
E) Elevated PSA.

Discussion

The correct answer is D. Tests of renal function should not be abnormal in simple, acute prostatitis. Chronic partial or complete urinary outlet obstruction may cause abnormal renal function but not acute prostatitis. Abnormal serum BUN and/or creatinine in the setting of prostatitis should prompt further investigation. During the evaluation, urine should be analyzed, and bacteriuria, pyuria, and hematuria are often found. Urine should also be sent for culture and sensitivity to identify the pathogen and direct further treatment. Answer E is true because the PSA is often elevated in prostatitis. However, it is not necessary nor is it recommended to obtain a PSA in order to diagnose prostatitis. When the PSA is elevated due to acute prostatitis, it may not return to normal levels for 1 month or longer after the resolution of inflammation.

> **HELPFUL TIP:** It is important to obtain urine in the diagnosis of prostatitis, but you should avoid bladder catheterization due to the potential to spread infection with this procedure. Besides, you want urine that has been in contact with the prostate.

* *

On exam, you find an uncomfortable-appearing male in no distress. His temperature is 38.4°C, and the rest of his vital signs are normal. The prostate is tender, enlarged, warm, and boggy. The remainder of the exam is unremarkable. Urinalysis is consistent with an infection. He has a **sulfa allergy**.

Which of the following is the most appropriate treatment plan for this patient?

A) Amoxicillin 500 mg TID for 10 days.
B) Ciprofloxacin 500 mg BID for 28 days.
C) Admit for IV levofloxacin 500 mg daily for 14 days.
D) Admit for IV levofloxacin 500 mg daily, followed by completion of therapy with oral levofloxacin 500 mg daily for 14 days when the patient is stable.
E) Unable to determine at this time because a transrectal ultrasound must be performed to rule out prostatic abscess.

Discussion

The correct answer is B. The most appropriate treatment for this patient is a fluoroquinolone, such as ciprofloxacin, for at least 28 days. Some authorities recommend longer treatment (up to 6 weeks) to reduce the risk of chronic prostatitis. In patients who are not allergic, a sulfa antibiotic could be considered as an alternative to a fluoroquinolone. In this case, answers C and D are overkill. Admission is appropriate for patients who appear septic, have not responded to oral antibiotics, or who have significant comorbidities. However, fluoroquinolones have 100% bioavailability PO. Therefore, there is no indication for giving these drugs IV unless the oral route is unavailable (eg, vomiting). Answer E is incorrect because abscesses are rare and imaging for an abscess is only undertaken if the patient does not respond to appropriate antibiotics.

> **HELPFUL TIP:** The most common cause of acute prostatitis is *E. coli.*

* *

When you see this patient again, his symptoms of prostatitis have cleared, but he does not think that finasteride is really helping. His AUA symptoms score is 21 (severe). He is wondering if a transurethral resection of the prostate (TURP) might help him, and he wants to discuss the downsides of the operation.

Compared with watchful waiting, all of the following are observed at greater rates in men who undergo TURP EXCEPT:

A) Erectile dysfunction.
B) Urinary incontinence.
C) Urethral stenosis.
D) Increased urine flow.
E) Decreased post-void residual urine volume.

Discussion

The correct answer is A. TURP is a commonly performed procedure for BPH. Indications for TURP include failure of medical therapy, recurrent infections, bladder calculi, renal insufficiency, and patient preference. Patients who undergo TURP typically experience decreased AUA symptom scores, increased urine flow rates, and decreased post-void residual volumes. There are downsides to TURP, including urinary incontinence, urethral stenosis, and the need to repeat the surgery. Strange as it may seem, several studies have shown that erectile dysfunction does **not** occur at increased rates in patients undergoing TURP compared with watchful waiting.

Objectives: Did you learn to . . .

- Recognize the pattern of voiding dysfunction seen in benign prostatic hyperplasia (BPH)?
- Manage a patient with BPH and understand the potential adverse effects of medications used to treat BPH?
- Diagnose and treat acute prostatitis?
- Describe indications for and complications of transurethral resection of the prostate?

QUICK QUIZ: SEXUALLY TRANSMITTED INFECTIONS

A 21-year-old college student, self-described as a "ladies' man," presents because of a concerning spot that developed on his penis. He complains of pain at the spot but denies itching. He reports no fever. When asked further about his sexual practices, he reports no condom use because his partners are all "on the pill." He had chlamydia in high school but is otherwise healthy. His review of systems is negative. On examination of the penis, you find a tender, erythematous papule with a deep central ulceration. There is some mild, tender lymphadenopathy in the inguinal area. The rest of the exam is unremarkable.

This lesion most likely is caused by:

A) *Haemophilus ducreyi.*
B) *Neisseria gonorrhoeae.*
C) *Staphylococcus aureus.*
D) *Treponema pallidum.*
E) None of the above.

Discussion

The correct answer is A. This is the lesion of *Haemophilus ducreyi* (aka chancroid). It can be confused with the chancre of primary syphilis, caused by *Treponema pallidum*, but the syphilis chancre is painless. Gram stain (Gram-negative rods in chains), culture, or biopsy may confirm the diagnosis. Chancroid is rarely diagnosed in the United States and is likely underdiagnosed; it frequently coinfects with syphilis and tends to occur in clusters. A number of treatments are available, including ceftriaxone (250 mg IM once), azithromycin

(1 g PO once), ciprofloxacin (500 mg PO BID for 3 days), and others.

CASE 2

A 22-year-old male presents with complaint of a painless lump on his left testicle. He denies penile discharge, dysuria, or other urinary complaints. He underwent a left orchidopexy for an undescended testicle at 6 years of age. Otherwise, his past medical history is unremarkable. On exam, the penis is circumcised with no lesion or discharge. There is adenopathy in the left inguinal area. His testicles are descended bilaterally with a 1-cm palpable, irregular mass on the midlateral portion of the left testicle. His exam is otherwise unremarkable. Your patient is worried about testicular cancer and wants to know if he is at risk.

All of the following are associated with an increased risk of testicular cancer EXCEPT:

A) Vasectomy.
B) HIV infection.
C) Cryptorchidism.
D) Klinefelter syndrome.
E) Family history.

Discussion

The correct answer is A. Epidemiologic data do not support an association between testicular cancer and vasectomy. As is true of some other malignancies, males with HIV infection have an increased risk of testicular cancer. Also, males with cryptorchidism (failure of one or both testicles to descend into the scrotum) and Klinefelter syndrome are at increased risk of testicular cancer. Approximately 25% of testicular cancers occurring in patients with cryptorchidism arise in the contralateral (normally descended) testicle. Although testicular cancer does not have as strong of a hereditary component, a positive family history is a risk factor for testicular cancer. Of note, black males have a much **lower** incidence of testicular cancer than do white males.

If your patient had not had an orchidopexy to repair the undescended testicle, he would be at risk for developing all of the following problems EXCEPT:

A) Infertility.
B) Inguinal hernia.

C) Testicular torsion.
D) Testicular malignancy.
E) Impotence.

Discussion

The correct answer is E. Organic impotence is not a consequence of cryptorchidism. All of the other problems listed occur at an increased frequency in males with an undescended testicle. The best time to begin treatment for an undescended testicle to minimize future sequelae is between 6 and 18 months of age. The consequence of not treating an undescended testicle is a 20%–40% increase in risk of developing a testicular malignancy, which often presents as a painless mass. Therefore, the reasons to treat cryptorchidism are: (1) to better palpate the testicle to assess for potential malignant transformation; (2) to decrease the risk of malignant transformation; (3) to improve chances of fertility; (4) to decrease risk of testicular torsion; (5) to decrease psychological effects from having an empty scrotum; (6) to repair an inguinal hernia at the same time, if it is present.

After an appropriate history and physical examination, which of the following tests is the initial diagnostic study of choice?

A) CT scan.
B) Ultrasound.
C) CBC.
D) α-Fetoprotein (AFP).
E) Pelvic x-ray.

Discussion

The correct answer is B. The best initial diagnostic test would be a scrotal ultrasound to determine if this mass is cystic or solid. If it is determined to be a solid mass suspicious for malignancy, other diagnostic studies would be warranted, such as β-HCG and AFP. Answer A is incorrect, as ultrasound is considered the test of choice. In conjunction with a radical inguinal orchiectomy for testicular cancer, a CT scan would be indicated to evaluate for metastatic disease. CBC (answer C) would have a role in suspected infection. X-ray (answer E) has no role in the evaluation of this patient.

> **HELPFUL TIP:** If the ultrasound is equivocal, MRI or urological referral should be considered next.

In taking this patient's history, if he had described a *painful* lump in his scrotum, the LEAST likely cause would be:

A) Chlamydia.
B) Inguinal hernia.
C) Hyrdrocele.
D) Testicular torsion.

Discussion

The correct answer is C. Spermatoceles and hydroceles are usually not painful. In a young, sexually active male, epididymitis from chlamydia or gonorrhea should be considered. Testicular torsion often has a very abrupt onset of pain and is a surgical emergency. Inguinal hernias can be intermittently painful if moving freely in the inguinal canal. However, if one becomes incarcerated, intense pain occurs. Of note, varicoceles are usually an incidental finding; however, large varicoceles may occasionally be painful. Likewise, testicular cancers are usually not painful but can become so if tumor growth is rapid.

* *

Your patient's ultrasound is concerning for testicular cancer, and you refer him to a urologist.

CASE 3

The next day, the patient's younger brother, a 15-year-old, presents with scrotal pain. His pain is on the right and he can localize it well to the front of the testicle. It has been present for 3 days and seemed to occur gradually over a few hours. There is no radiation of the pain. Running makes it worse, and cool packs seem to help. Yesterday, he noticed a slight swelling of the scrotum on the same side. He denies trauma to the area, any history of sexual activity, other genitourinary complaints, fever, nausea, or vomiting. On exam you find normal vitals. He has a well-localized tender spot at the anterior superior right scrotum with a bluish discoloration under the skin.

Which of the following is the most likely diagnosis?

A) Torsion of the appendix testis.
B) Torsion of the testicle.
C) Varicocele.
D) Abscess.
E) Spermatocele.

Discussion

The correct answer is A. This is the classic presentation of torsed appendix testis. The appendix testis is a pedunculated, vestigial structure at the anterior superior testicle. Torsion of it is one of the most common causes of scrotal pain in children. The pain is usually well localized. There may be a reactive hydrocele. Diagnosis is confirmed by ultrasound. Unlike a torsed testicle, a torsed appendix testis is not an emergency. It may be treated by conservative therapy (rest, NSAIDs, ice) or surgical excision.

Objectives: Did you learn to . . .

- Recognize potential causes of a painless scrotal mass?
- Evaluate a testicular mass?
- Identify different types of testicular cancer and recognize the age groups in which they occur?
- Recognize the significance of cryptorchidism?
- Identify torsion of the appendix testis?

QUICK QUIZ: HEMATOSPERMIA

A 28-year-old male presents to your office looking quite concerned. Several days ago after sexual intercourse with his girlfriend, he noticed bloody ejaculate in the condom. Since then he has avoided sex and masturbation. He denies pain, hematuria, dysuria, fevers, night sweats, and weight loss. He reports that he is otherwise healthy. His examination, including genitourinary and rectal exam, is normal, and a urinalysis shows 1–2 RBCs/hpf.

What is your next step in the evaluation and management of this patient?

A) Reassurance and follow-up.
B) Scrotal ultrasound.
C) Pelvic CT scan.
D) Transrectal ultrasound.
E) PSA.

Discussion

The correct answer is A. Hematospermia, the name given to bloody penile ejaculate, is fairly uncommon. It can occur in men of any age and is perhaps most common after prostate biopsy or prostate surgery. In otherwise healthy young men, the cause is most often idiopathic and is almost always benign. History should focus on traumatic causes, symptoms of prostate disease, and symptoms of infection. A genital and prostate examination should be performed. Urinalysis is helpful to exclude infection. Consider gonorrhea and chlamydia cultures in the appropriate patients. In this patient, reassurance is adequate. In an older male (>40 years) with the same complaint, PSA and transrectal ultrasound may be indicated. Other studies (eg, MRI, cystoscopy, etc) may be indicated depending on the findings on history, physical exam, and initial lab studies. Of note, in other parts of the world, schistosomiasis is a frequent cause of hematospermia and hematuria. In most cases of hematospermia, semen analysis is not warranted, but it can be diagnostic in patients with schistosomiasis. Finally, otherwise healthy patients with **persistent hematospermia** (>1 month) should be treated with a month trial of antibiotics (although there is no evidence for benefit) to treat possible prostatitis, and then be referred to a urologist if hematospermia persists.

CASE 4

A couple you have known for a few years come to your office to announce that they are expecting and that they want you to be the baby's doctor (strange that they didn't ask you to be the mother's doctor, but you let it slide). According to an ultrasound, the fetus is male. The couple is ambivalent about neonatal circumcision and wants your advice.

You start the conversation by saying:

A) "Circumcision is a relic of history and should be illegal."
B) "All major medical organizations (eg, AAFP, AAP, AMA) recommend routine neonatal circumcision."
C) "The decision to perform circumcision is a personal one, influenced by a number of factors—but primarily influenced by cultural, religious, and familial issues."
D) "Do whatever you want. I don't really care what you do with a tiny piece of skin."

Discussion

The correct answer is C. One of the strongest predictors of whether a newborn in the United States will be circumcised is the circumcision status of the father. There are other reasons cited by parents as well (discussed later in the case). Answer A is incorrect because the statement is effused with emotion and lacks logic. Answer B is incorrect. The AAFP has no policy statement on circumcision. The 1999 AAP (American Academy of Pediatrics) statement reads, "Existing scientific evidence demonstrates potential medical benefits of newborn male circumcision; however, these data are not sufficient to recommend routine neonatal circumcision." The AMA endorses this statement as well. As of the writing of this book, the AAP is reviewing this recommendation. If you chose answer D, you need to work on your bedside manner!

Potential benefits of circumcision include which of the following?

A) Overall reduction in mortality of circumcised infants in comparison with uncircumcised infants.
B) Reduction in urinary tract infections in the first year of life.
C) Reduction in the number of sexual partners.
D) All of the above.

Discussion

The correct answer is B. The rate of urinary tract infections (UTIs) in uncircumcised males in the first year of life is about 10 times greater than the rate for circumcised males. In order to prevent one UTI in the first year of life, about 100 circumcisions need to be performed. The effect of circumcision on rates of UTI later in life is not well studied. The rate of UTI may be higher shortly after circumcision (within the first 2 weeks). Answer A is incorrect because there are no data showing any difference in mortality between circumcised and uncircumcised infants. Answer C is incorrect. Some surveys have shown increased frequency and variety of sexual practices in circumcised males in comparison with uncircumcised (note that this is an association, not a causal relationship).

 HELPFUL TIP: Circumcision reduces the rate of cervical cancer in female partners of men who engage in high risk sex (eg, have had more than 6 sexual partners).

 HELPFUL TIP: It is clear that circumcision reduces the transmission of HIV. This has led to a call for circumcision in high-risk populations (eg, some parts of sub-Saharan Africa, etc).

Neonatal circumcision is associated with all of the following EXCEPT:

A) Risk of hemorrhage with the procedure.
B) Psychological trauma and decreased sexual satisfaction later in life.
C) Reduced risk of infection with HPV.
D) Reduced risk of penile cancer.

Discussion

The correct answer is B. Despite what some anticircumcision Web sites maintain, circumcision does not appear to result in any significant psychological trauma or decreased sexual satisfaction for most men later in life. Answer A is true. There is a small but real risk of hemorrhage with the procedure, and this occurs mostly in patients who have an unknown or unrealized coagulopathy. Abnormal bleeding after circumcision is a common way in which sporadic cases of hemophilia are discovered (including one case discovered this way by one of the editors—and he still feels bad!). Answer D is true. Several studies have demonstrated that circumcised men are less likely to have HPV infection. The data for the risk of other sexually transmitted infections are somewhat contradictory, but generally favor a reduced risk of STIs in circumcised males. Answer D appears to be true—at least in the United States. Retrospective studies have shown that the rate of squamous cell carcinoma of the penis is about 3-fold higher in uncircumcised men. However, other risk factors are associated with penile cancer, including smoking, risky sexual behavior, poor hygiene, and genital warts. The American Cancer Society does **not** recommend routine neonatal circumcision for the prevention of penile cancer but does recommend that all risk factors be addressed.

 HELPFUL TIP: Some insurers do not consider neonatal circumcision a necessary procedure, but rather a cosmetic one, and therefore do not cover it. Parents should check with their insurance company to determine if the procedure is covered.

* *

You have a nice, long conversation with the couple, discussing the potential benefits and risks, and they decide to have their son circumcised. After the birth, you are performing a thorough examination when you find something slightly abnormal with the penis.

Routine circumcision is absolutely or relatively contraindicated in all of the following situations EXCEPT:

A) Congenital phimosis.
B) Micropenis.
C) Hypospadias.
D) Ambiguous genitalia.
E) Religious beliefs of the parents that circumcision is wrong.

Discussion

The correct answer is A. Significant congenital phimosis rarely occurs and is an **indication** for circumcision. Phimosis is defined as the inability to retract the foreskin (prepuce) over the glans. This is a **normal** finding in uncircumcised infants. However, **significant** congenital phimosis may completely cover the urethra and not allow the normal passage of urine. Answers B, C, and D are reasons to avoid routine circumcision and to enlist the aid of a urologist. Answer E should be obvious. If the parents have a religious or cultural objection to circumcision, it should be avoided.

> **HELPFUL TIP:** When performing circumcision, local anesthetic is recommended, and either dorsal penile nerve block or subcutaneous ring block is preferred. Other pain control modalities may be used as well, including preprocedure acetaminophen, sucrose-coated pacifier, etc.

* *

You identify hypospadias in this patient. You also note that the left scrotum is empty and the testis is not palpable. You request a urology consultation.

You tell the parents that:

A) Definitive treatment of an undescended testis should occur before 5 years of age.
B) Definitive treatment of an undescended testis should occur before 1 year of age.
C) Orchidopexy will eliminate the risk of malignancy but not the risk of infertility.
D) This patient is **not** at increased risk of chromosomal anomalies.
E) None of the above.

Discussion

The correct answer is B. Currently, the trend is for early referral and orchidopexy for the newborn with an undescended testis. If the testis remains undescended for longer than 1 year, a significant amount of reproductive function is lost. Answer C is incorrect. Orchidopexy will reduce the risk of infertility and reduce, but not eliminate, the risk of malignancy. You cannot be certain now that this patient has an undescended testis; you can only be sure that he has an empty scrotum. The left testis may be undescended or it may not even be present. In patients with hypospadias and unilateral or bilateral empty scrotum, there is a higher rate of chromosomal anomalies.

Objectives: Did you learn to . . .

- Discuss the benefits and risks of circumcision with parents?
- Identify indications and contraindications for routine neonatal circumcision?
- Recognize trends in circumcision?
- Employ pain control measures for the procedure of circumcision?
- Manage a patient with an undescended testis?

CASE 5

A 32-year-old male presents to discuss permanent sterilization. He clearly states that he wants a vasectomy, and sooner is better than later. He is married and has 3 children at home. His wife just gave birth to twins. He is healthy and takes no medications. He looks tired and anxious. You examine him and find no abnormalities. The vas deferens is easily isolated bilaterally.

What is your next step?

A) Refer him for psychological counseling as he is clearly under a great deal of stress.
B) Provide him with detailed counseling on vasectomy, give him written material on the procedure, and ask him to discuss it with his wife.
C) Schedule the procedure as soon as possible.
D) Tell him that he is not an appropriate candidate for vasectomy.

Discussion

The correct answer is B. Patient education, counseling, and selection are very important aspects of vasectomy. When you counsel him on vasectomy, you should explore his reasons for wanting the procedure. You should not schedule a vasectomy without providing counseling and ensuring that he understands the procedure in detail. This patient appears to be fatigued—an issue that should be explored further. However, immediate referral for psychological counseling without investigating the underlying cause is not appropriate.

While counseling this patient, you discuss which of the following issues?

A) Partner's desire for permanent sterility.
B) Effect of the procedure on sexual function.
C) Reversibility of the procedure.
D) Complications.
E) All of the above.

Discussion

The correct answer is E. All of these issues are important to discuss prior to scheduling the procedure. It is important that the couple agree on this procedure because it is the couple—not just your patient—who will be sterile. Aside from psychological effects of vasectomy, the procedure should not directly affect sexual function, orgasm, or ejaculation. Patients should be aware that vasectomy results in permanent sterility and that reversal procedures are successful approximately only 50% of the time. Potential complications include failure and unwanted pregnancy, infection, pain, bleeding, hematoma, etc.

* *

After discussing the situation with his wife, the patient calls to ask your opinion on another option that they are considering. Although he is ready to have the vasectomy, his wife recently thought that maybe she should have a tubal ligation instead.

All of the following are advantages of vasectomy compared to tubal ligation EXCEPT:

A) Effectiveness of the procedure.
B) Risks of anesthesia.
C) Risks of complications due to the procedure.
D) Cost.
E) Verification of sterility.

Discussion

The correct answer is A. The failure rates of vasectomy and tubal ligation are similar and are generally <1%.

All the other statements are true. Generally, local anesthesia is used for vasectomy, compared to spinal or epidural anesthesia for tubal ligation. Vasectomy is safer and less expensive. Men usually leave the office shortly after the vasectomy is completed, whereas, tubal ligation is typically performed in a surgical suite and requires 2 or 3 hours of postoperative observation. Abdominal organs can be injured during tubal ligation (eg, bowel perforation). If you injure abdominal organs during a vasectomy, you need to go to remedial anatomy class. Another advantage of vasectomy is the ability to verify sterility with a semen analysis after the vasectomy.

* *

Your patient decides to "get snipped" as he puts it. You perform the vasectomy using a no-scalpel technique. The procedure was fairly easy, and the patient tolerated it well. One month after the procedure, the patient calls to complain about a painful swelling that has developed superior and slightly posterior to the left testis. He has no other symptoms.

Which of the following is the most likely diagnosis?

A) Hematoma.
B) Variococoele.
C) Congestive epididymitis.
D) Abscess.

Discussion

The correct answer is C. Without any further information, congestive epididymitis is the most likely cause of this patient's current complaint. Congestive epididymitis occurs in approximately 3% of patients postvasectomy, and the onset is usually within weeks to months after the procedure. Answer A, hematoma, can be avoided in most cases if hemostasis is achieved during the procedure and the patient does not overdo it immediately postop. A hematoma is more likely to develop early rather than a month later. An infection (answer D) would be unlikely so far out from the procedure. Answer B is incorrect because varicoceles do not develop after vasectomy (unless you are operating far away from where you are supposed to be). Overall, the most common scrotal pathology after vasectomy is sperm granuloma, which occurs in up to 40% of patients but is generally asymptomatic.

HELPFUL TIP: The treatment of congestive epididymitis can be frustrating. Most men who have a vasectomy will have some element of congestive epididymitis, but most will have minor swelling without pain. For patients with painful congestive epididymitis, a trial of NSAIDs and sitz baths for several months is indicated. Failing conservative therapy, steroid injection or surgery may be indicated.

* *

Two months after the vasectomy, your patient returns with a semen sample, showing no sperm. His surgery was successful, but failures occasionally do occur.

Vasectomy failure is usually due to:

A) Failure to identify and transect the vas at time of surgery.
B) Recanalization.
C) Left-handed doctors.
D) Infection.
E) Immaculate Conception.

Discussion

The correct answer is B. Although "redundant systems" (removing a segment of the vas deferens, clipping or suturing the free ends, cauterizing the transected vas, suturing fascia around one free end while leaving the other outside the fascia) are employed to avoid this complication, recanalization can occur. A new pathway can form between the free ends of the transected vas deferens, allowing sperm into the ejaculated semen. Therefore, all patients should return postvasectomy for semen analysis. Answers A and D are potential, but infrequent, causes of failure. Answer C is incorrect. What have you got against lefties? As to answer E, only God knows.

* *

Your patient is ultimately pleased with his vasectomy results. He returns to see you several years later because of concerns that he is balding. On exam, you find nonscarring hair loss at the vertex. The scalp appears normal otherwise.

You should entertain all of the following diagnoses EXCEPT:

A) Androgenetic alopecia.
B) Telogen effluvium.
C) Alopecia areata.
D) Hypothyroidism.
E) Tinea capitis.

Discussion

The correct answer is E. Hair loss is common in males, affecting up to 66% of all men. Alopecia is often divided in scarring and nonscarring forms. Most infectious causes of hair loss (eg, tinea capitis, folliculitis, etc) are scarring if not treated, whereas the other causes listed (Answers A through D) are nonscarring. Without any signs of inflammation or hyperkeratosis, tinea capitis is unlikely. Androgenetic alopecia (answer A) is quite common in adult males. Telogen effluvium (answer B) presents with diffuse hair loss, as the rate of shedding of hairs in the resting (telogen) phase increases. Alopecia areata (answer C) results in patchy hair loss in round or oval shapes. Metabolic conditions should also be in the differential diagnosis of hair loss, and these might include hypothyroidism (answer D), hyperthyroidism, and iron deficiency.

 HELPFUL TIP: Secondary syphilis causes a noninflammatory, nonscarring hair loss that may be patchy or diffuse. Consider testing for syphilis in appropriate patients.

* *

The patient reports a strong family history of baldness. On your exam, the patient has thin hair at the vertex and recession of the hairline in an "M" shape at the frontotemporal area. Based on the history and exam, you diagnose androgenetic alopecia. He would like to do something about his hair loss.

Which of the following is a true statement concerning androgenetic alopecia?

A) Minoxidil must be used for at least 2 years to achieve permanent hair regrowth.
B) Lower doses of 5α-reductase inhibitors (eg, finasteride) are used in treating androgenetic alopecia compared to BPH.
C) Hair transplant should be avoided unless all other therapeutic attempts have failed.
D) Topical steroids are an effective therapy for androgenetic alopecia.
E) A toupee looks great on anyone.

Discussion

The correct answer is B. Finasteride (Propecia) is FDA approved for androgenetic alopecia, and the dose is 1 mg per day rather than the 5 mg per day dose used to treat BPH symptoms. Minoxidil applied to the scalp is also an effective therapy for androgenetic alopecia. Both minoxidil and finasteride must be continued indefinitely, or hair loss will continue. Answer C is incorrect. Hair transplant is a viable option for men and women with androgenetic alopecia, and it is sometimes used as a first-line therapy. Answer D is incorrect. Topical steroids are not effective for this type of hair loss. Answer E is clearly incorrect—there are a lot of bad toupees out there.

Objectives: Did you learn to . . .

- Provide prevasectomy counseling?
- Recognize complications of vasectomy?
- Identify causes of hair loss in men?
- Describe current treatment options for androgenentic alopecia?

QUICK QUIZ: DEATH RATES IN MEN

For all of the following causes of death, the age-adjusted death rate is higher for males than females EXCEPT:

A) Liver disease.
B) Alzheimer disease.
C) Coronary artery disease.
D) Suicide.
E) Cancer.

Discussion

The correct answer is B. When it comes to Alzheimer disease, men get a break; the death rate is higher for females. All of the other causes of death listed have greater death rates in males. For example, compared to women with liver disease, same-age men with liver disease are twice as likely to die of liver disease.

QUICK QUIZ: DEATH RATES IN MEN

The relative risk of death for males is greater throughout the life span.

Compared to same-age females, at what age range is the relative risk of death greatest for males?

A) <1 year.
B) 5–14 years.
C) 15–24 years.
D) 25–34 years.
E) >85 years.

Discussion

The correct answer is C. Males aged 15–24 years have a relative risk of death >2.5 compared to same-aged females. Mother nature has a way of making up for boys and young men dying: more males fetuses are conceived than female. However, the miscarriage rate is also greater for male fetuses. Nonetheless, 105 males are born for every 100 females in the United States. By 35 years, enough males have died off that the number of males and females that age is nearly equal, and thereafter the number of females exceeds the number of males.

CASE 6

A 14-year-old male presents with his mother, who is worried that he is growing breasts. Over the last 2 or 3 months, the patient has developed swellings beneath both nipples. He denies discharge or pain, but the nipples are tender at times.

You can tell this patient that physiologic gynecomastia (subareolar breast tissue) is a disease that effects:

A) Newborns.
B) Adolescents.
C) Elderly males.
D) All of the above.

Discussion

The correct answer is D. The incidence of physiologic gynecomastia is trimodal, with peaks in the neonatal period, adolescence, and old age. Data can be contradictory, but clinically palpable breast tissue (either fat or true breast tissue) may be present in >50% of males in each of these three age groups.

Which of the following hormones is responsible for the proliferation of breast tissue?

A) Testosterone.
B) Estrogen.
C) Androstenedione.
D) Growth hormone.
E) Progesterone.

Discussion

The correct answer is B. Estrogens induce ductal hyperplasia and growth of glandular tissue. Testosterone and androstenedione inhibit the actions of estrogens on the breast tissue. Some men with gynecomastia have increased sensitivity of breast tissue to circulating estrogens, others may have an increased proportion of estrogens compared to androgens, yet others may have a mixture of both processes or another process altogether.

Potential causes of gynecomastia include all of the following EXCEPT:

A) Renal failure.
B) Marijuana use.
C) Testicular cancer.
D) Hypothyroidism.
E) Phenothiazines.

Discussion

The correct answer is D. **Hyper**thyroidism, not **hypo**thyroidism, can cause gynecomastia through increased production of androstenedione. A number of drugs are associated with gynecomastia, including marijuana, alcohol, 5α-reductase inhibitors, phenothiazines, tricyclic antidepressants, androgens, estrogens, growth hormone, calcium channel blockers, and spironolactone. Some testicular tumors secrete estrogens, causing gynecomastia. Renal and liver diseases (cirrhosis) are other causes of gynecomastia.

* *

A thorough drug history is negative. On physical examination, you find palpable, nontender tissue beneath the nipples, with slightly more prominent tissue mass on the right. The tissue is about 2–3 cm in diameter, and no discrete masses are palpable. There is no nipple discharge. An adult male hair growth pattern is evident in the axillary and inguinal areas. The testicles are normal size without masses.

You recommend which of the following now?

A) Observation.
B) Referral to a surgeon.

C) Limited laboratory studies, including TSH, testosterone, and liver enzymes.
D) Biopsy of the tissue.
E) Mammogram and/or ultrasound.

Discussion

The correct answer is A. As discussed, physiologic gynecomastia is quite common in adolescent males. The findings on exam are reassuring. This patient does not display any other signs of testosterone deficiency, and further workup is not indicated now. If there are no discrete masses on exam, a mammogram, ultrasound, or biopsy is not likely to be helpful. Referral to a surgeon is premature, as 90% of these patients experience spontaneous involution of the breast tissue over 3 years.

HELPFUL TIP: In adolescent males with gynecomastia, further evaluation with laboratory studies and imaging is indicated if the breast tissue is rapidly enlarging or is >5 cm in diameter, a mass is palpable, or other signs of under-androgenization are present.

* *

You provide the patient and his mother with reassurance and have them follow up in a year. When they return, there is no palpable tissue. When you see the patient again, he is 17 years old and presents alone but with a signed letter from his mother giving permission for him to be diagnosed and treated. He told his mother that he was having abdominal pain, but really he is worried that he may have contracted a sexually transmitted infection (STI). He has become fairly promiscuous and does not use condoms. In the last week, he has developed dysuria and a yellowish urethral discharge. He has no other symptoms.

Which of the following is the most likely diagnosis?

A) HPV.
B) Syphilis.
C) Gonorrhea.
D) Trichomonas.
E) Herpes simplex.

Discussion

The correct answer is C. This patient's symptoms are typical of gonococcal urethritis. However, *Neisseria gonorrhoeae* **may be present in the urethra without any symptoms and** *Chlamydia trachomatis* **can present with similar symptoms**, so that gonorrhea and chlamydia cannot be reliably distinguished on clinical grounds. Answer A is incorrect because HPV causes genital warts, not urethritis. Answer B, syphilis, may present as a painless ulcer (primary syphilis). Answer D is incorrect because most men infected with *Trichomonas vaginalis* are asymptomatic, although some will have mild urethritis. Answer E, herpes simplex, presents with painful vesicles at the area of inoculation.

* *

You take urethral samples for gonorrhea and chlamydia. You discuss other STIs and decide to perform some other tests (eg, HIV, hepatitis B, RPR/VDRL).

You are compelled to do all of the following now EXCEPT:

A) Recommend safe sexual practices.
B) Inform the public health services if he tests positive.
C) Treat him with antibiotics.
D) Encourage him to contact his partners and tell them to get tested.
E) Inform his mother of your findings.

Discussion

The correct answer is E. In general, adolescents can seek care for STIs and be treated without parental consent. However, clinicians should refer to the laws of the state in which they practice for ultimate legal authority in this matter. Of course, the time of diagnosis and treatment should be used as an opportunity to educate the patient regarding safe sexual practices (answer A). Answer B is true. Gonorrhea and chlamydia are reportable diseases in every state. Clinicians should refer to the laws of their state and the reporting protocols of the clinic in which they practice. Empiric treatment is the rule here, so answer C is true. Answer D is true because all of this patient's partners should be contacted, tested, and treated. There are several ways to contact the partners, and allowing the patient to do so is only one way. The clinician or the public health authorities could contact the partners as well.

Which of the following methods maintains a high degree of sensitivity and is also the quickest and least expensive way to diagnose gonococcal urethritis in a symptomatic male?

A) Culture.
B) Gram stain.
C) Serologic antibody assay.
D) PCR.
E) DNA probe.

Discussion

The correct answer is B. In **symptomatic** males, Gram stain of a urethral sample can identify Gram-negative diplococci (*N. gonorrhoeae*) with a sensitivity of near 90%–95%. The sensitivity drops to about 70% in asymptomatic males. If the materials and expertise are readily available, a Gram stain is quick and inexpensive. Culture of a urethral specimen on Thayer-Martin agar takes longer and false-negative tests can occur with high frequency (due to the need to have a CO_2-rich environment and to keep the culture in a narrow temperature range). However, culture is still the gold standard. PCR and DNA probe techniques are entering into more widespread use, and the sensitivity and specificity of these tests appear to be excellent. PCR is particularly attractive as a screening test, as it can be performed on urine specimens instead of urethral swab specimens. Serologic assays for gonorrhea would not be helpful in diagnosing urethritis.

* *

Your clinical suspicion of gonorrhea is high.

What is your next step?

A) Single doses of ceftriaxone 125 mg IM and azithromycin 1 g PO.
B) A single dose of penicillin G 1.2 million units IM and erythromycin 500 mg PO QID for 7 days.
C) Tetracycline 500 mg PO QID for 10 days.
D) Single doses of ciprofloxacin 500 mg PO and cefixime 400 mg PO.
E) Await laboratory results to determine which antibiotics to use.

Discussion

The correct answer is A. If there is any concern for compliance, it is best to treat the patient in the office if you have access to the appropriate antibiotics. When you are treating for gonorrhea either empirically or on the basis of a positive test result, **you should also treat for chlamydia**. Therefore, of the answer choices listed, A is most appropriate. Ceftriaxone 125 mg IM as a single dose is indicated for uncomplicated gonococcal urethritis, and azithromycin 1 g PO as a single dose is indicated for chlamydia urethritis. The first-line treatments for gonorrhea are third-generation cephalosporins. **Fluoroquinolones are no longer recommended for gonorrhea due to high rates of resistance in some communities.**

Answer B is incorrect because penicillin should never be used to treat gonorrhea (due to the prevalence of penicillinase-producing strains of the bacteria). Answer C is incorrect. Tetracycline antibiotics provide adequate coverage for chlamydia and some strains of *N. gonorrhoeae*, but other strains of *N. gonorrhoeae* are resistant to tetracyclines, so these drugs are not used as first-line agents in treating gonorrhea. Answer D is incorrect because it gives two medications that are used for the treatment of gonorrhea and none for the treatment of chlamydia. Answer E is incorrect because this patient should be treated as soon as possible, and empiric therapy is recommended in such instances.

 HELPFUL TIP: Another equally effective regimen for chlamydia is doxycycline 100 mg BID for 7 days. Doxycycline is equal in efficacy to azithromycin even if some doses may be missed.

* *

You treat this patient with ceftriaxone and azithromycin and tell him to contact his partners so that they can get tested. When your patient returns to discuss his lab tests, he is feeling much better. You tell him that he was infected with both gonorrhea and chlamydia but that the rest of his tests were negative. He is relieved that he does not have HIV, but he wonders which problems chlamydia can cause.

Chlamydia trachomatis has been implicated in which of the following?

A) Reiter syndrome.
B) Lymphogranuloma venereum.
C) Proctitis.
D) Epididymitis.
E) All of the above.

Discussion

The correct answer is E. A small percentage of men with chlamydia urethritis develop reactive arthritis, and a subset of these will go on to have the triad of Reiter

syndrome (urethritis, arthritis, uveitis) (answer A). Lymphogranuloma venereum (answer B) is also due to a particularly virulent strain of Chlamydia, but it produces genital ulcers and lymphangitis and is generally seen in tropical areas. Lymphoganuloma venereum is treated with extended courses of doxycycline (100 mg PO BID for 21 days) or azithromycin (1 g PO weekly for 3 weeks). Chlamydia proctitis (answer C) occurs almost exclusively in homosexual men and presents with rectal pain, bleeding, and discharge. Diagnosis is confirmed by rectal swab, and the treatment is the same as for chlamydia urethritis. Epididymitis (answer D) occurring in young men is most often the result of infection with *C. trachomatis* or *N. gonorrhoeae*. CDC guidelines recommend treatment with a single injection of ceftriaxone 250 mg IM and doxycycline 100 mg PO BID for 10 days.

 HELPFUL TIP: The majority of males (and females) who are infected with chlamydia and/or gonorrhea **do not have symptoms.** Therefore, a good argument is made for screening asymptomatic individuals in high-risk populations (eg, adolescents, young adults, those with multiple sexual partners, etc)

Objectives: Did you learn to . . .

- Define gynecomastia and understand its causes?
- Identify when to initiate further evaluation in a patient with gynecomastia?
- Recognize symptoms of gonorrhea and chlamydia?
- Initiate treatment in a male with urethritis?
- Recognize manifestations of chlamydia infection in men?

 QUICK QUIZ: AN INFLAMED GLANS

A 36-year-old male diabetic presents with a 3-day history of irritation, itching, dysuria, and redness at the tip of his penis. He is monogamous with his wife, and he denies any history of high-risk sexual behavior or STIs. On exam, you find an afebrile patient in no acute distress. The penis is circumcised, and the glans penis is red, tender, and edematous. There are numerous small, white papules on the glans.

Which of the following is the most appropriate treatment?

A) Sitz baths and improved hygiene.
B) Oral doxycycline.
C) Topical bacitracin.
D) Topical miconazole.
E) Topical steroids.

Discussion

The correct answer is D. This patient has balanitis, defined as an inflammatory condition of the glans penis (balanoposthitis is inflammation of the glans and foreskin). Some authors believe that balanitis is a noninfectious, inflammatory condition. Others implicate infectious causes. Of infectious causes, the most common is *Candida albicans*, especially in diabetics. This patient has classic findings of candidal balanitis and he is diabetic. Therefore, the most appropriate therapy is a topical antifungal agent, such as miconazole. Topical and oral antibiotics will not help, and topical steroids should be avoided. Sitz baths and improved hygiene should be encouraged, but they should not be employed without an antifungal agent.

CASE 7

While you are covering the ED, a 40-year-old male presents with a painful erection that began 4 hours ago "out of the blue." You quickly identify priapism.

Which of the following is true regarding priapism and normal erections?

A) Duration of erection cannot be used to differentiate the two because normal erections can last up to 12 hours.
B) Abnormally prolonged sexual desire can "convert" a normal erection into priapism.
C) The corpus spongiosum and glans penis are not involved in priapism.
D) Acute urinary retention may lead to priapism and vice versa.
E) All of the above are true statements.

Discussion

The correct answer is C. Priapism is defined as the prolonged engorgement of the penis (in females, the clitoris), unrelated to sexual desire or stimulation. The word priapism comes from the Greek god Priapus, well known for his lasciviousness and generous genital endowment. In most cases of priapism, the corpus spongiosum and glans penis are not involved. Only the corpora cavernosa are engorged and rigid.

Answer A is incorrect. Priapism typically lasts longer than 6 hours, whereas normal erections last minutes to hours. With normal erections, detumescence occurs after ejaculation or after the stimulus is removed. This is not the case with priapism, and sexual desire does not play a role in the development of priapism; thus, answer B is incorrect. Answer D is incorrect. Urinary retention is not thought to cause priapism, and priapism does not lead to urinary retention.

Priapism may be secondary to all of the following EXCEPT:

A) Sickle-cell disease.
B) Penile trauma.
C) Leukemia.
D) Iron deficiency anemia.
E) Trazodone use.

Discussion

The correct answer is D. A number of different disease states and drugs have been implicated in the etiology of priapism. In one way or another, these diseases and drugs affect the balance of blood flow into the penis, leading to increased arterial blood flow and/or decreased venous outflow. Local malignancies, such as bladder and prostate cancers, can cause obstruction. Likewise, any condition that increases blood viscosity (eg, sickle-cell disease, polycythemia, leukemia) or results in thromboembolic phenomena (eg, vasculitis) can cause priapism. Penile trauma that results in laceration of penile arteries can cause priapism. Numerous drugs have also been implicated, but in most cases the cause is not identified (Table 16–1).

What is your next step in management of this patient?

A) Reassurance.
B) Call for emergent urologic consultation.
C) Give oral α-blockers.
D) Engage patient in guided imagery to lead his thoughts away from sex.

Discussion

The correct answer is B. Priapism is a urologic emergency and needs to be treated ASAP.

Table 16–1 DRUGS ASSOCIATED WITH PRIAPISM

Psychotropics
- Trazodone
- Chlorpromazine

Agents Used to Treat Erectile Dysfunction
- Intracavernosal injections (eg, papaverine)
- Phosphodiesterase (PDE) inhibitors (eg, sildenafil)

Antihypertensives
- Hydralazine
- Prazosin

Anticoagulants
- Heparin

Drugs of Abuse
- Alcohol
- Cocaine
- Marijuana

 HELPFUL TIP: After recovery, approximately 50% of men with priapism suffer erectile dysfunction. Also, a disproportionate percentage of cases of priapism lead to litigation. From a medicolegal perspective, you want to have a urologist involved.

* *

The urologist will be in the ED in 30 minutes.

What should you do while you wait?

A) Administer intracavernosal metoprolol.
B) Administer supplemental oxygen, IV hydration, and analgesics.
C) Insert a needle into the glans penis and withdraw blood.
D) "Take 5" and get a cup of coffee.

Discussion

The correct answer is B. Until the urologist arrives, conservative measures are probably best, and you should try to make the patient comfortable using analgesics, oxygen, and hydration. Check a CBC since leukemia can rarely present with priapism. Some patients will respond to analgesics and ice packs. Oral or subcutaneous terbutaline may be helpful. Some authors recommend sedatives, such as benzodiazepines. Answer A is incorrect because giving metoprolol is the opposite of what you should be doing. Answer C is incorrect because any attempt to withdraw blood from the penis should be directed at the corpora cavernosa, not the glans. Answer E may be tempting, but you can get your coffee after you do B.

 HELPFUL TIP: If a urologist is not available and/or you are comfortable performing the procedure (and you have a good lawyer), you can attempt detumescence. A needle is inserted into the corpora cavernosa and blood is withdrawn. Then a vasoactive agent (eg, phenylephrine) is injected. This procedure is repeated every 5 minutes until detumescence occurs. It should go without saying that the patient's vital signs must be closely monitored during this intervention.

Objectives: Did you learn to . . .
- Recognize priapism and its causes?
- Manage a patient with priapism?

 QUICK QUIZ: DEPRESSION AND SUICIDE

Which of the following groups makes up the majority of completed suicides (death by suicide)?

A) Black males.
B) White males.
C) Black females.
D) White females.
E) Hispanic males.

Discussion

The correct answer is B. White males make up 73% of deaths by suicide. Although females account for more suicide attempts, males are at greater risk of death by suicide. Men tend to use deadlier means, such as guns, hanging, and car collisions. In other words, men are very efficient at suicide. White males >85 years have one of the highest rates of death by suicide: 59/100,000 (the rate in the general public is 10.6/100,000). Black males have the second highest rate of suicide. Of the groups listed, black females have the lowest risk of death by suicide.

CASE 8

A 78-year-old male presents to your office after sustaining a backward fall last night. He went to the bathroom and slipped on a throw rug. He complains of mid-back pain. He smokes cigarettes, considers himself healthy, and takes no medication. On examination, you find a pleasant male in some discomfort. His vital signs are normal. Radiographs of the thoracic spine show an acute wedge compression fracture of the T11 vertebral body.

Which of the following is the most appropriate next step in the evaluation of this patient?

A) Bone scan.
B) DEXA scan.
C) Chest x-ray.
D) PSA.

Discussion

The correct answer is B. Normal, healthy vertebral bodies should not break from low-impact trauma, such as falling from a standing height. This patient almost certainly has diseased bone, most likely osteoporosis. The next step is to confirm your suspicion by obtaining a bone mineral density test, and DEXA (dual energy x-ray absorptiometry) is the most standardized test currently available. The other radiologic studies are less likely to be useful. Fracture due to metastatic prostate cancer is a reasonable concern, and a PSA and rectal exam can help rule out or rule in prostate disease. However, prostate cancer metastatic to bone typically causes lytic lesions, which should be seen on x-ray. Therefore, a PSA would be expected to have lower yield than a DEXA scan.

 HELPFUL TIP: Regarding bone mineral density, the numbers to watch do not change for men. Use T-scores. If the T-score is between −1 and −2.5, the diagnosis is osteopenia. If the T-score is ≤−2.5, the diagnosis is osteoporosis.

* *

The DEXA scan results show that this patient has osteoporosis.

What further tests are indicated in this patient at this point in time?

A) TSH.
B) Calcium.
C) Skeletal survey.
D) A and B.
E) All of the above.

Discussion

The correct answer is D. Secondary causes of osteoporosis are found more commonly in men compared to women. You should not assume that this patient's osteoporosis is idiopathic, because ≥50% of males with symptomatic vertebral fractures resulting from osteoporosis have a secondary cause of osteoporosis. Common causes of osteoporosis in males include long-term corticosteroid use, thyroid and parathyroid disorders, gastrointestinal disease (adversely effecting calcium and vitamin D absorption), testosterone deficiency, alcoholism, and renal disease. Although multiple myeloma may result in decreased bone mineral density, it is less common, and a skeletal survey (answer C) is not the preferred screening test. Instead, you would want to order serum and urine protein electrophoresis, looking for a monoclonal band.

* *

Your patient's laboratory tests are normal. In addition to calcium and vitamin D, you want to start him on a medication for osteoporosis.

Which of the following medications has the best evidence for use in men with primary osteoporosis?

A) Alendronate.
B) Estrogen.
C) Testosterone.
D) Calcitonin.
E) Fluoride.

Discussion

The correct answer is A. Amino bisphosphonates, such as alendronate, have the best evidence for treatment of primary osteoporosis in men. In addition to stabilizing bone density, alendronate and risedronate have been shown to decrease the incidence of osteoporotic fractures in men. If you choose to treat with bisphosphonates, the doses are the same for men and women. The other medications listed simply do not have the efficacy data published for bisphosphonates If a patient cannot tolerate oral bisphosphonates, calcitonin nasal spray (answer D) and intravenous bisphosphonate preparations should be considered. Estrogen (answer B) may be effective, but the side effect profile would prohibit its use and bisphosphonates are preferred. Fluoride (answer E) does not appear to be effective.

* *

> **HELPFUL TIP:** If a male patient with osteoporosis has testosterone deficiency, testosterone supplementation may be a reasonable treatment option but the efficacy of testosterone in this scenario is **not** well studied. Although testosterone contributes to peak bone mass in young men and low testosterone is associated with an increased fracture risk in older men, testosterone for the treatment of osteoporosis has been disappointing.

> **HELPFUL TIP:** Teriparatide (recombinant parathyroid hormone (PTH) 1-34) is FDA approved for treatment of men at high risk for osteoporotic fractures (severe osteoporosis, failed other therapies, previous osteoporotic fractures). However, its use is limited by cost, need for daily injection, and the finding of increased osteosarcoma incidence in lab rats.

* *

To be on the safe side, you order several laboratory tests, all of which are normal except for serum testosterone. His testosterone level is low. You are considering starting testosterone supplementation.

Which of the following testosterone supplementation products would you AVOID?

A) Transdermal testosterone.
B) Buccal testosterone.
C) Oral testosterone.
D) Intramuscular testosterone.
E) None of the above.

Discussion
The correct answer is C. Oral testosterone should be avoided due to significant first-pass metabolism and potential liver toxicity. The other choices listed are viable options for testosterone replacement. See Table 16–2.

Which of the following is true regarding testosterone supplementation in older men with testosterone deficiency?

A) Testosterone supplementation has markedly beneficial effects on depression.

Table 16–2   TESTOSTERONE SUPPLEMENTATION PRODUCTS

Agents	Dosages	Comments
Striant (buccal tablet)	Dosed 30 mg BID and must be kept beside buccal mucosa	The product does not dissolve completely.
Androgel, Testim (transdermal gels)	Dosed daily	Cover the application area to reduce risk of spreading by contact with others.
Androderm (transdermal patch)	Applied daily	Rotate sites to reduce skin irritation.
Scrotal patches (Testoderm)		Now rarely used due to scrotal irritation and more acceptable alternatives.
Intramuscular injections (Depo-testosterone, Delatestryl)	Dosed every 2 to 4 weeks	Serum testosterone levels fluctuate significantly between doses.
Subcutaneous pellets (Testopel)		These are implanted (like Norplant) and are rarely used for supplementation.
Oral agents (methyltestosterone)		AVOID due to significant first-pass metabolism, fluctuating serum levels, and risk of liver toxicity.

B) The effects of testosterone supplementation in young hypogonadal males and older testosterone deficient males are the same.

C) In testosterone-deficient older males with erectile dysfunction, testosterone supplementation dramatically improves erections.

D) In testosterone-deficient older males with poor libido, testosterone supplementation improves libido.

E) Testosterone supplementation has no effect on lean muscle mass or grip strength.

Discussion

The correct answer is D. In testosterone-deficient older males, testosterone supplementation does improve libido. Answer C is incorrect: The effects of testerone on erectile dysfunction are not impressive. Even in testosterone-deficient men with erectile dysfunction, a phosphodiesterase inhibitor (eg, sildenafil) is more likely to be successful. Answer A is incorrect. Many questions are as yet unanswered about the neuropsychiatric effects of testosterone. Testosterone supplementation does not appear to significantly improve depression. Answer E is incorrect because testosterone has been shown to consistently improve lean muscle mass and grip strength. Answer B is incorrect. Young hypogonadal males who are treated with testosterone have increased peak bone mass and virilization. The effects on older males are different: older males have improved strength, libido, and sense of well-being without some of the effects seen in the young hypogonadal males.

 HELPFUL TIP: Hypogonadal males should **not** take testosterone replacement while trying to impregnate their partners because it will further decrease their sperm counts (due to the effect of exogenous testosterone feeding back on the hypothalamic-pituitary-gonadal axis). To improve fertility in these patients, unproven empiric therapy is often used, including clomiphene, human chorionic gonadotropin, and gonadotropin-releasing hormone.

---

* *

You have a conversation with your patient about starting testosterone therapy. He would like to try it.

You tell him about adverse effects and monitoring and tell him it's important to periodically check:

A) Hematocrit.

B) Potassium.

C) Alanine aminotransferase.

D) A and B.

E) A and C.

Discussion

The correct answer is E. There are good reasons behind the recommendation for periodic monitoring with certain serum tests. Testosterone increases erythropoietin production and can cause erythrocytosis. Testosterone should not be started in a patient with a hematocrit >50% (or severe heart failure or untreated sleep apnea). Testosterone can cause elevated liver enzymes, increased cholesterol, and growth of prostate and breast tissue, including prostate and breast cancers. Prostate exam and PSA is recommended prior to starting therapy and periodically while on testosterone. Periodically monitor serum testosterone levels to ensure that the patient is in the normal range and not sub- or supratherapeutic. Potassium (answer B) is not directly affected and no monitoring is recommended.

Objectives: Did you learn to . . .

- Recognize osteoporosis in older males?
- Evaluate a patient with an osteoporotic fracture?
- Discuss management strategies for osteoporosis in males?
- Identify testosterone replacement products and discuss how older males might benefit from them?
- Recognize some of the risks associated with testosterone supplementation?

CASE 9

A 50-year-old male presents for a get acquainted visit. He has a history of hyperlipidemia treated with lovastatin. He takes no other medications and states that he is otherwise healthy. He has no particular complaints today but wants your opinion regarding various screening measures. After watching a television feature on prostate cancer, he thought he should be screened. As he puts it, he wants "the works" and is willing to pay for any tests not covered by his insurer.

In order to assess his risk for prostate cancer, you should take into account all of the following factors EXCEPT:

A) Age.
B) Race.
C) Family history.
D) Diet.
E) Ultraviolet light exposure.

Discussion

The correct answer is E. Ultraviolet light exposure increases the risk of skin cancer but not prostate cancer. Advancing age is strongly and directly associated with the development of prostate cancer. Between 50 and 70 years, the incidence of prostate cancer more than quadruples, and it continues to increase thereafter. Black race and positive family history are associated with an increased risk. Dietary factors may have a role in the development of prostate cancer. A diet rich in fish and vegetables (especially lycopene in tomatoes) and low in red meat may reduce the risk of prostate cancer. Selenium in the diet seems beneficial.

* *

Your patient is white and denies any family history of prostate cancer. He has no urinary symptoms and denies sexual dysfunction.

If he did have urinary symptoms, which of the following could be used to reliably distinguish BPH from prostate cancer?

A) Urgency.
B) Nocturia.
C) Frequency.
D) Hesitancy.
E) None of the above.

Discussion

The correct answer is E. A male who presents with urinary symptoms of urgency, nocturia, frequency, and/or hesitancy most likely has BPH and not prostate cancer. However, prostate cancer can present with these symptoms and must be considered as well. The point is: we cannot always attribute urinary symptoms in an older male to BPH. Similar symptoms are found in high rates in older *women* and are often attributable to bladder problems rather than prostate problems.

* *

You discuss prostate cancer screening with him, and he chooses to undergo digital rectal exam and PSA testing. The exam is remarkable for a slightly enlarged, smooth, nontender prostate with no nodules. The PSA level is 16 ng/mL (normal 0–4 ng/mL).

The most appropriate next step is to:

A) Repeat the PSA in 3–6 months.
B) Order a transrectal ultrasound of the prostate.
C) Refer to urology for further evaluation and prostate biopsy.
D) Repeat the rectal exam and try to find that nodule that you missed.
E) Order a free PSA.

Discussion

The correct answer is C. This patient is at relatively high risk of having prostate cancer based on his PSA level and age at presentation. Sending him to a urologist for prostate biopsy is the most prudent step. Follow-up for PSA alone (answer A) would be defensible if the PSA level were <10 ng/mL and/or the patient were much older. Transrectal ultrasound (answer B) is likely to miss more than it would find in this case. With this patient's PSA and current life expectancy, ultrasound should only be used as part of a larger urologic evaluation, including biopsy. To repeat the rectal exam (answer D) is just nuts. There is no need for this. Did you miss a nodule? Maybe. If so, you will eventually get over it. More likely, there was no palpable nodule. This patient could have stage T1 prostate cancer in which, by definition, no nodules are palpable. He could have a nodule located anteriorly in the prostate—a location you cannot palpate. He also may have a PSA elevation for reasons other than prostate cancer. Finally, answer E is incorrect. The free PSA is most helpful when the total PSA is in the intermediate risk zone (4.1–10 ng/mL). When the PSA is higher (>10 ng/mL), the risk of cancer is too great to make the free PSA useful. The fraction of PSA that is free (not bound to plasma proteins) is inversely proportional to the risk of prostate cancer: the lower the free PSA compared to total PSA, the greater the risk of prostate cancer (cutoff percentages vary from 10%–25%).

 HELPFUL TIP: The determination of when to send a patient for prostate biopsy is made on clinical grounds and must take into account the patient's risk, comorbidities, exam findings, PSA level, possibility of false-positive or false-negative tests, patient's preference, etc. **This decision cannot be made based on an arbitrary PSA value.**

Which of the following is true of the PSA test for screening purposes?

A) The positive predictive value approaches 100%.

B) Since PSA testing has become widespread, prostate cancer incidence and mortality have increased.

C) The false-negative rate is 20%–25%.

D) Age-specific cutoff values for PSA have proven to increase positive predictive value and specificity.

E) Race-specific cutoff values for PSA have proven to increase positive predictive value and specificity.

Discussion

The correct answer is C. There is a substantial false-negative rate—from 20% to 25%—limiting the use of PSA for screening purposes. Answer A is incorrect by a long shot. The positive predictive value (likelihood of a positive test indicating true prostate cancer) ranges from about 20%–60%, depending on the PSA level. The positive predictive value increases with increasing PSA level. Answer B is incorrect. Since the PSA test has come into widespread use, the incidence of prostate cancer has increased but mortality due to the disease has decreased. The reason for these trends has not been completely explained, and the role of the PSA test in these trends is not known. Answers D and E are incorrect. Because older males seem to have higher PSA values in the absence of prostate cancer and black males tend to have prostate cancer found at lower PSA levels, age-specific and race-specific cutoff values have been proposed and investigated. However, the use of age-specific and race-specific PSA cutoff values is of questionable value.

 HELPFUL TIP: It is important to realize that there is great controversy over the role of digital rectal exam and PSA in screening for prostate cancer. Neither is considered a "good" screening test (high rate of false-positives and false-negatives), but there is nothing else to offer at this time. The AUA and American Cancer Society recommend routine prostate cancer screening with DRE and PSA, but the U.S. Preventive Services Task Force and the AAFP do not. However you approach this issue, you're not alone, and the company you keep is just as confused.

 HELPFUL TIP: Decisions on the treatment for prostate cancer are complicated. There are many different treatment options and combinations. The expertise of urology and oncology is necessary to arrive at a treatment plan. Other than surgery and radiation, antiandrogen hormonal therapy, chemotherapy, and finasteride are often employed in more advanced disease.

Objectives: Did you learn to . . .

● Identify risk factors for prostate cancer?

● Discuss prostate cancer screening with a patient?

● Interpret an elevated PSA?

● Recognize the limitations of prostate cancer screening?

CASE 10

A 32-year-old male accompanied by his wife presents for evaluation of infertility. They have been married for 5 years and have been attempting conception for 3 years without success. The patient's wife has a 7-year-old daughter from a previous marriage. The patient has no significant past medical or surgical history. He does not smoke but drinks a 6-pack of beer and 1 cup of coffee daily. He relaxes after work and on weekends by sitting in their hot tub. The patient is 5'8" tall and weighs 220 pounds. On physical exam, he has normal facial and body hair and his testicles are descended bilaterally. You estimate the testicular volume to be 13 cc on the left and 18 cc on the right. You note a moderate-sized varicocele on the left.

Which of the following is NOT a modifiable risk factor for male subfertility?

A) Alcohol intake.

B) Hot tub usage.

C) Varicocele.

D) Tobacco use.

E) Obesity.

Discussion

The correct answer is D. We should note that the study of infertility risk factors and treatments is complicated by inconsistent outcome measures (eg, sperm count, sperm motility, conception, pregnancy resulting in live birth). However, there are no conclusive studies correlating tobacco use with male subfertility. The other answers are modifiable risk factors and have been directly linked to subfertility, either in decreased sperm count or decreased sperm motility. It is important to ask about alcohol use (answer A). Other drug use, such as marijuana, should be investigated as well. Answer B is true. Hot tub usage, febrile illnesses, and the presence of a varicocele raise the temperature of the testicles, thereby decreasing the optimal environment for the maturation of sperm. Boxers or briefs? Type of underwear does not seem to affect scrotal temperature significantly, and more to the point, tight underwear is not associated with decreased fertility. The presence of a varicocele (answer C) is an interesting issue. It certainly is modifiable in that the patient could undergo a varicocelectomy which might help if the varicocele is moderate to large in size. However, the degree to which a varicocele contributes to infertility is not well known. Varicoceles are noted to occur more commonly in infertile men, but they also occur in 10%–15% of the normal, fertile male population. Obesity (answer E) contributes to the increased peripheral aromatization of testosterone into estradiol in fatty tissue.

Other factors which contribute to subfertility/infertility include a history of cryptorchidism, hypospadias, viral orchitis after puberty, prior chemotherapy or radiation, intake of calcium channel blockers, and retrograde ejaculation associated with diabetes and multiple sclerosis. It has been noted that roughly 33% of men with a history of unilateral cryptorchidism and 66% of men with bilateral cryptorchidism are infertile.

 HELPFUL TIP: Infertility in a couple is defined as inability to conceive despite 1 year of frequent (how frequent is not defined), unprotected sexual intercourse. In the developed world, the 1-year prevalence of infertility is approximately 15%.

Which of the following laboratory tests would you order first?

A) Seminal fluid analysis (SFA) including sperm count.
B) Testosterone.
C) Karyotype.
D) FSH.
E) Y chromosome analysis for microdeletion.

Discussion

The correct answer is A. If the main concern is infertility, the initial step in evaluation beyond the history and physical exam is the SFA. Depending on the results of the SFA, additional laboratory studies may need to be ordered. If the count is abnormal, then hormonal studies (eg, testosterone, FSH, Luteinizing Hormone [LH]) should be ordered. If the patient is obese, an estradiol level may also be appropriate since obesity contributes to the increased peripheral aromatization of testosterone into estradiol in fatty tissue. Karyotype and Y chromosome analysis are important tools in the right patient population but should not be employed in the early stages of the evaluation unless a chromosomal disorder is strongly suspected.

* *

This patient's sperm density is 12 million/mL with a motility of 35%. You repeat the SFA 2 weeks later, and again it is abnormal. His testosterone level is low for his age, and his FSH and LH are high.

Which of the following is most likely to be the cause of his decreased fertility?

A) Congenital absence of the prostate gland.
B) Primary hypogonadism.
C) Bilateral complete vas deferens obstruction.
D) Androgen resistance.
E) None of the above.

Discussion

The correct answer is B. A low testosterone level accompanied by elevated LH and FSH could indicate testicular failure, or primary hypogonadism. Answer A is not a known cause of infertility, and in fact is not a known disorder as far as the editors can determine. Additionally, the prostate gland does not seem to play a role in male fertility. Answer C, an obstruction of the vas deferens, would most likely result in azoospermia with normal or high testosterone levels. Answer D is incorrect. You would expect to see elevated testosterone levels in patients with androgen resistance. Table 16–3 lists causes of infertility in males.

How can you now best help this patient achieve fertility, assuming that there are no problems with his partner?

A) Empiric treatment for gonorrhea and chlamydia.
B) Empiric treatment with testosterone injections.

Table 16–3 CAUSES OF MALE INFERTILITY

Mechanism	Examples
Hypothalamic-pituitary disorders	Congenital disorders (Kallmann syndrome), pituitary tumors, pituitary infarction, hormonal or psychotropic drug use
Primary hypogonadism	Klinefelter syndrome, cryptorchidism, alcohol use, chemotherapeutic agents, testicular torsion, hyperthermia
Disorders of sperm transport	Congenital absence of the vas deferens, epididymal dysfunction, spinal cord injury
Idiopathic infertility	Unexplained satisfactorily by history, exam, and laboratory evaluation

C) Empiric treatment with gonadotropin-releasing hormone (GnRH).

D) Referral to an infertility treatment center.

Discussion

The correct answer is D. You have now performed a reasonably complete evaluation and even arrived at a potential cause of infertility. However, treatments for male infertility are the subject of much debate, and the patient is probably best served by referral to an infertility treatment specialist. Answer A is incorrect. Genital infections are not thought to play a major role in male subfertility/infertility, so without clear evidence of gonorrhea and/or chlamydia, treating for these diseases is not recommended. Answer C is incorrect because this patient does not appear to have a hypothalamic source for his infertility. Testosterone injection (answer B), can actually make the problem worse. The most effective therapy for patients with infertility and primary hypogonadism (ie, this patient) may be sperm retrieval for intracytoplasmic sperm injection (not typically thought of as an office procedure for the family physician).

CASE 11

You refer this patient to an infertility treatment center in your neck of the woods. He is so pleased with your attention to detail and well-reasoned approach that he refers his best friend to you for the same problem—infertility. This new patient reports never fathering a child, although his wife has had one child from a previous marriage. On physical exam, you note thin frame, mild symmetric gynecomastia, and small testicles. He has complete azoospermia on two semen analyses.

His most likely diagnosis is:

A) Cystic fibrosis.

B) History of vasectomy.

C) Klinefelter syndrome.

D) Testicular cancer.

E) Turner syndrome

Discussion

The correct answer is C. The triad of small firm testicles, gynecomastia, and azoospermia are classic findings in patients with Klinefelter syndrome (KS). Klinefelter syndrome occurs in 1 in 500 live male births and is responsible for 14% of cases of azoospermia. The most common (90%) chromosomal abnormality in KS is 47, XXY. In a patient who has had a vasectomy, azoospermia should be present; however, the consequences of the vasectomy, if performed properly, should not result in gynecomastia or small testicles (of course if the knife slips . . .). Male patients with cystic fibrosis can have congenital absence of the vas deferens. While this would be associated with azoospermia, these patients usually have normal-sized testicles and no gynecomastia. Turner syndrome (45, X) is associated with unambiguously female genitalia with no breast development. Patients with testicular cancer usually have an enlarged testicle with a mass on the surface or inside the testicle. Although the treatments for testicular cancer may result in infertility, patients with testicular cancer do not typically present with infertility.

Objectives: Did you learn to . . .

- Define modifiable risk factors for male subfertility/infertility?
- Recognize the significance (or lack of significance) of a varicocele?
- Identify the appropriate indications for obtaining laboratory studies in male patients with infertility concerns?
- Recognize some important causes of infertility?

CASE 12

A 63-year-old male with a history of insulin-dependent diabetes complains of decreased libido and difficulty maintaining an erection. He has noticed increasing difficulty over the last several years. He had a similar problem years ago when he was experiencing a deep depression. He does have occasional erections sufficient for penetration and awakens with an erection at times. His medical history is also significant for hypertension and an appendectomy. His medications include insulin, lisinopril, and hydrochlorothiazide. He has been married for 30 years and has 2 grown children, aged 24 and 26.

Which of the following historical elements is NOT likely to contribute to this patient's erectile dysfunction?

A) Diabetes.
B) Depression.
C) Hypertension.
D) History of appendectomy.
E) Antihypertensive medications.

Discussion

The correct answer is D. All the other options could cause some degree of erectile dysfunction (ED). Any disease process that affects the nervous, vascular, endocrine, or smooth-muscle systems can result in ED. A partial list of other risk factors for ED includes: advancing age, prostate disease or surgery, pelvic fracture, alcohol or other substance abuse, medications (eg, antihypertensives, antidepressants), spinal radiculopathy or spinal cord injury, multiple sclerosis, endocrine disorders (eg, hypothyroidism, hyperthyroidism), smoking, cardiovascular disease, chronic renal failure, and Peyronie disease.

 HELPFUL TIP: There are two types of ED—psychogenic and organic. In men <35 years, psychogenic ED is more common. Men >50 years are more likely to have an organic cause for their ED.

What further historical element(s) is/are useful in the evaluation of ED?

A) Rapidity of onset of sexual dysfunction.
B) Presence of nocturnal erections.

C) Status of relationship with the sexual partner.
D) Partner's interest in sex.
E) All of the above.

Discussion

The correct answer is E. Further history should involve all of the elements listed. Patients with a sudden onset of ED often have a primary psychogenic ED. The presence of nocturnal erections establishes that the patient's neurologic and vascular mechanisms work to produce an erection. An organic disorder may still be playing a role, but the circuit is working. The status of the relationship with the patient's partner, his attraction to that partner, and the partner's interest in sex are important. If the patient and his partner are having relationship problems outside of the sexual arena, counseling may be the best first step in trying to address the ED.

All of the following drugs or classes of drugs can adversely affect male sexual function EXCEPT:

A) Cimetidine.
B) Chlorthalidone.
C) Prednisone.
D) Clonidine.

Discussion

The correct answer is C. Prednisone is not known to cause significant ED. There are many drugs, prescription and recreational, that affect sexual function, and some of these include: antihypertensives, antidepressants, antipsychotics, anxiolytics, hormonal agents (eg, antiandrogens, estrogens, progestational agents, and anabolic steroids), and the H_2-blocker cimetidine (apparently not ranitidine or famotidine). The effects range from decreased libido to impotence and/or ejaculatory dysfunction. Various recreational drugs such as alcohol, marijuana, heroin, and cocaine may initially cause a state of disinhibition and enhanced libido. However, excessive or chronic use leads to ED (both acutely with excessive use and chronically with prolonged use).

* *

On physical examination, you find normal genitalia, normal femoral and dorsalis pedis pulses, appropriate virilization, and slightly diminished sensation at the plantar aspects of the feet with an otherwise intact neurologic exam.

Which of the following will be most useful in evaluating a cause for his ED and directing further therapy?

A) BUN and creatinine.
B) TSH and free thyroxine.
C) PSA.
D) Nocturnal penile tumescence study.
E) Arterial and venous Doppler studies.

Discussion

The correct answer is B. With the advent of safe and efficacious therapy for ED, many clinicians proceed directly to a medication trial without laboratory studies. In many patients, this approach is acceptable. Other patients may benefit from a limited laboratory evaluation—especially those men with other symptoms and/or comorbidities. Initial labs might include TSH and free thyroxine, testosterone, and prolactin. If not done already, screening for diabetes and vascular risk (eg, lipids) is appropriate. The role of nocturnal penile tumescence is debated, but it is not necessary prior to a therapeutic trial and this patient reported having nocturnal erections. BUN, creatinine, and PSA are not likely to be helpful. Doppler flow studies of femoral vessels are unlikely to change therapy as long as the physical exam demonstrates normal distal blood flow. In this patient, you know that he has vascular disease (diabetes, hypertension, and now ED), so his treatment should already involve lowering his vascular risk factors.

Concurrent use of which of the following drugs is an absolute contraindication to taking a PDE-5 inhibitor (eg, Viagra, Levitra, Cialis)?

A) Hydrochlorothiazide.
B) Isosorbide dinitrate.
C) Testosterone.
D) Finasteride.
E) Saw palmetto.

Discussion

The correct answer is B. In patients who take nitrates for coronary heart disease, PDE inhibitors are contraindicated. The combination has been shown to cause hypotension, in rare cases severe enough to result in stroke. While concurrent use of finasteride is safe, the α-blockers used to treat BPH are another story (see below). Drugs that inhibit cytochrome P-450 isoenzyme, such as cimetidine, erythromycin, clarithromycin, itraconazole, ketoconazole, and HIV protease inhibitors, may warrant dosage reductions. Caution with phosphodiesterase inhibitors is advised in patients with uncontrolled hypertension, recent stroke or myocardial infarction, life-threatening arrhythmias, unstable angina, or heart failure. Other potential medical therapies for ED include testosterone supplementation and yohimbine. There are more treatment modalities: sex therapy, vacuum erection devices, intracavernosal injection therapy, intraurethral pharmacotherapy, arterial revascularization, penile prosthesis implantation, and combined therapy.

An important difference between the phosphodiesterase inhibitors is:

A) Tadalafil and vardenafil have a shorter half-life than sildenafil.
B) Tadalafil and vardenafil are contraindicated with α-blockers, but sildenafil is safe.
C) Tadalafil and vardenafil must be taken at least 6 hours before intercourse, whereas sildenafil acts much faster.
D) Tadalafil and vardenafil affect color vision changes, whereas sildenafil does not.
E) None of the above.

Discussion

The correct answer is E. Tadalafil and vardenafil both have a longer half-life than sildenafil, and tadalafil has a duration of action of 24–36 hours, thus earning it the title "the weekender." Tadalafil, vardenafil, and sildenafil all have precaution warnings for use with α-blockers (α-blocker + phosphodiesterase inhibitors = hypotension). Sildenafil can cause some changes in color vision (everything looks a little blue) because it affects phosphodiesterase in the retina. All of the phosphodiesterase inhibitors have about the same time to onset of action and should be taken 30–60 minutes before sexual activity. Tadalafil and vardenafil are supposed to be more specific for phosphodiesterase in the penis, but this claim has yet to be proven in clinical practice.

* *

You start the patient on sildenafil. He discovers love again, but his wife finds out. Now you're in trouble!

Objectives: Did you learn to . . .

- Evaluate a patient with ED?
- Describe various etiologies of ED?

- Identify medications that affect erectile function?
- Recognize indications, contraindications, and side effects of therapeutic modalities for ED?

BIBLIOGRAPHY

Nseyo U; Weinman E, Lamm D. *Urology for Primary Care Physicians.* Philadelphia: W.B. Saunders, 1999.

Lipshultz LI, Kleinman I. *Urology and the Primary Care Practitioner.* St Louis: Mosby-Wolfe, 2000.

Lipshultz LL, Howards SS. *Infertility in the Male. 3rd ed.* St Louis: Mosby, 1996.

Mulcahy JJ. *Male Sexual Function: A Guide to Clinical Management.* Totowa, NJ: Humana Press, 2001.

Resnick MI, Novick AC. *Urology Secrets.* 3rd ed. Philadelphia: Hanley & Belfus, 2003.

Teichman JMH. *Urology: 20 Common Problems.* New York: McGraw-Hill, 2001.

17

Dermatology

Jason K. Wilbur

Since dermatology is a visual science, take a look at pictures at http://www.dermnet.org.nz/sitemap.html or www.dermnet.com.

CASE 1

A 37-year-old white female presents to clinic for her annual well-adult physical exam. After a complete skin examination you find a suspicious lesion on her back (Figure 17–1; see also color section). It measures 16 mm × 8 mm. She has approximately 20 nevi that appear normal. The patient reports never performing skin self-exams and does not know if the lesion in question is new. She denies any symptomatic lesions. Her family history is remarkable for "skin cancer" on her father's side. Many family members have "tons of moles." She frequented a tanning parlor in college and occasionally still does so before social events.

How do you evaluate the lesion?

A) Take a photograph and see her back in 3 months.
B) Take a shave biopsy of the lesion.
C) Excise the entire lesion with 1- to 2-mm margins.
D) Excise the entire lesion with 3-cm margins.

Discussion

The correct answer is C. This lesion is worrisome for malignant melanoma. Any time you suspect melanoma, you are obligated to perform at minimum a punch biopsy or preferably complete excision of the lesion and send it for pathology. Do not throw away the specimen; do not perform a pathologic exam yourself. These cases end badly in court.

Answer A is incorrect. If you suspect melanoma, the sooner you make the diagnosis the better. A shave biopsy (answer B) is not recommended because the biopsy is often too shallow and the deep margins are not visible. The depth of the lesion is necessary to stage the melanoma. An excisional or punch biopsy has the greatest likelihood of obtaining a diagnosis and giving you information on the depth. Since a punch biopsy will only get a portion of the lesion, sampling error is a possibility, which is why excisional biopsy with narrow (eg, 2 mm) margins is preferred. Answer D is preferable to answers A and B; however, it would be unnecessary to remove the lesion with such large margins when the histopathology is not yet known.

* *

You excise the lesion with a small border. The pathology report reveals a malignant melanoma.

Which of the following lesion characteristics will determine your patient's prognosis?

A) The depth and ulceration.
B) The histologic level of invasion (Clark level).
C) The number of colors in the lesion.
D) Whether or not it arose in a preexisting mole.
E) Number of mitoses per high power field on microscopy.

Discussion

The correct answer is A. As discussed, the depth of the melanoma is the most important prognostic indicator. Breslow tumor thickness is most commonly used to arrive at a prognosis. Breslow tumor thickness measures

Table 17–1 DERMATOLOGY TERMS

Macule/Patch: A circumscribed area of change without elevation or depression; definitions vary, but generally "macule" if <0.5–1 cm and "patch" if >1 cm.

Papule/Plaque: A palpable, superficial, elevated, solid lesion; definitions vary, but generally "papule" if <0.5–1 cm and "plaque" if >1 cm.

Ulcer: A crater-like lesion with loss of epidermis.

Wheal: A round or irregular, light-red patch that is typically evanescent.

Crust: Dried exudate on the skin surface (eg, impetigo).

Desquamation: Heaped-up scales and flakes, representing malformed stratum corneum (eg, psoriasis).

Nodule: A solid, firm, round lesion of varying depths.

Pustule: A well-circumscribed cavity in the skin filled with purulent exudate.

Vesicle/Bulla: A well-circumscribed cavity in the skin filled with fluid; definitions vary, but generally "vesicle" if <0.5–1 cm and "bulla" if >1 cm.

the depth of the melanoma from the granular layer in the epidermis to the base of the melanoma in millimeters. The best prognosis is achieved with a Breslow depth ≤0.75 mm. Ulceration is associated with more aggressive cancers and a poorer prognosis. Clark level of invasion (answer B) is still reported by many pathologists, but it has less bearing on prognosis than the Breslow depth. The diameter of the lesion has not been associated with prognosis. A very large, clinically atypical pigmented lesion can often be benign. Melanomas can also be one color, many colors, or non-

pigmented; color does not correlate with prognosis. Up to 66% of melanomas arise in normal skin. They can be just as aggressive as those arising from moles. The number of mitoses in a lesion can be a clue of more aggressive melanomas in some instances but does not possess the same prognostic value as the Breslow depth.

 HELPFUL TIP: For a patient with no metastasis and a melanoma completely excised, Breslow depth is the most important prognostic factor. However, the worst prognostic factor overall is regional or distant spread of disease, with the overall survival dropping to <50% for regional metastases and <10% for distant metastases.

In the United States the current lifetime risk of developing a melanoma in the white population is approximately:

A) 1/10
B) 1/75
C) 1/200
D) 1/1,000

Discussion

The correct answer is B. The lifetime incidence of melanoma in the year 2004 was approximately 1 in 76. The closest answer is B.

* *

Your biopsy reveals a malignant melanoma in situ. You excise the entire lesion with 0.5-cm margins. **There is no penetration of the epidermis.**

What additional evaluation is necessary?

A) Chest x-ray.
B) CT scan of the chest.
C) Serum lactic acid dehydrogenase (LDH).
D) All of the above.
E) None of the above.

Discussion

The correct answer is E. If the melanoma has not penetrated the epidermis, it is referred to as a melanoma in situ. If excised with 0.5-cm to 1-cm margins, the long-term survival at 5 and 10 years approaches 100%. Therefore, any additional workup is not usually necessary

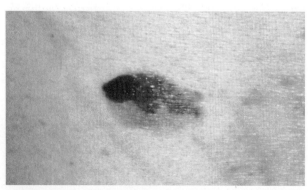

Figure 17–1

according to the most recent data collected from The American Joint Commission on Cancer. When the melanoma depth is >1 mm, there is wide variation in clinical practice regarding imaging and serologic evaluation. Generally, chest radiography and an LDH serum level are recommended for malignant melanomas >1 mm in depth. Serum LDH levels are usually positive in very advanced cases that have metastasized to bone or the liver. A CT scan of the chest and pelvis and MRI of the brain can be ordered if metastatic disease is suspected, but these studies are not recommended routinely. Metastatic disease has not been reported with malignant melanoma in situ.

> **HELPFUL TIP:** Sentinel lymph node biopsy is often undertaken in patients at risk for metastatic melanoma (based on ulceration and tumor thickness) who have no clinically evident lymphadenopathy. However, there is no proven survival benefit to this approach.

Which of the following has NOT been associated with an increased risk of the development of melanoma?

A) Blistering sunburns in childhood.
B) Sister with melanoma.
C) Fair hair color.
D) >50 moles on a person's body.
E) Smoking.

Discussion

The correct answer is E. Smoking has not been linked to malignant melanoma—unlike many other malignancies. A history of blistering sunburns, melanoma in first-degree relatives, fair hair, and >50 moles are all associated with an increased risk of developing melanoma. Also, high socioeconomic class and immunosuppression appear to be risk factors.

The most common subtype of melanoma in people of African descent is:

A) Superficial spreading melanoma.
B) Lentigo maligna melanoma.
C) Nodular melanoma.
D) Acral lentiginous melanoma.
E) Amelanotic melanoma.

Discussion

The correct answer is D. There are 4 classical subtypes of malignant melanoma. They do not predict prognosis independently. **Superficial spreading melanoma** is the most common type in fair skin populations. It can occur at any site and clinically presents as a brown macule with irregular, notched borders. It grows radially (outward) initially. **Nodular melanoma** is the second most common type in fair-skinned individuals, and as the name suggests, is an exophytic nodule. **Lentigo maligna melanoma** is usually a brown macule with hue variations that spread outward slowly. It occurs in the elderly on sun-exposed areas, such as the face and hands. When there is dermal invasion, lentigo maligna is referred to as lentigo maligna melanoma. **Acral lentiginous melanoma** (ALM) is the least common type in white populations but is the most common type in non-whites, such as people of African descent. ALM occurs on the palms, soles, or near the nails. **Amelanotic melanoma** is a subtype of nodular melanoma.

Objectives: Did you learn to . . .

- Evaluate a patient with suspected melanoma?
- Describe how the prognosis of melanoma is determined?
- Recognize the lifetime risk of malignant melanoma in the U.S.?
- Identify risk factors for the development of melanoma?
- Recognize the 4 classic subtypes of melanoma and which are the most common in African and white populations?

CASE 2

A 7-month-old male is brought to clinic for a "rash all over." Six weeks ago his parents noticed him rubbing his legs against his crib and scratching his head frequently. They are concerned because they find blood on his sheets in the morning, and he has become increasingly irritable. He is eating and drinking normally. His past medical history is unremarkable. His father has sensitive skin and hay fever, but no one else in the family currently has a rash. On skin exam you find lichenified and erythematous patches of skin with fissures and bleeding on the ventral heels, dorsal feet, and hands. His cheeks are bright red with scale. His diaper area is uninvolved and there are no lesions in the web spaces of the hands and feet.

Based on the description, which of the following is the MOST LIKELY diagnosis?

A) Seborrheic dermatitis.
B) Atopic dermatitis.
C) Scabies.
D) Tinea corpora.
E) Tinea versicolor.

Discussion

The correct answer is B. The most likely diagnosis is atopic dermatitis (AD) or eczema. AD is characterized by dryness of the skin that is intensely pruritic. A red rash subsequently develops. AD is often referred to as the "itch that rashes." It occurs in characteristic locations. In younger infants, the cheeks and neck are involved. As they begin to crawl, their extensor surfaces are involved. The diaper area, because it is moist, is not usually involved. In older children, the flexural areas, like the antecubital and popliteal fossae, are involved. AD tends to worsen in the dry winter months.

Seborrheic dermatitis (answer A) is common in infants and usually is seen on the scalp and face, although it can involve the whole body. Seborrheic dermatitis is typically not hyperkeratotic and is less erythematous than AD. Scabies (answer C) rarely involves the scalp, but it can do so in infants and the immunocompromised. However, other more typical locations (web spaces, wrists, waist, etc) should be involved in scabies. Tinea corpora (answer D) is not usually widespread or brightly erythematous. Often, tinea corpora presents with a ring of advancing erythema and a central clearing ("ringworm"). Tinea versicolor (answer E) typically involves the trunk and extremities, not the scalp, and is not very pruritic.

* *

You diagnose the patient with atopic dermatitis (AD).

Which of the following is NOT true about AD?

A) The prevalence of AD appears to be increasing worldwide.
B) AD tends to worsen in the winter months.
C) In some patients, food allergies can exacerbate AD.
D) Positive skin prick tests and RAST testing correlate highly with food challenges (eg, those with positive tests will have worsening of their rash when given a food challenge).
E) In most infants AD will significantly improve or resolve by school age.

Discussion

The correct answer is D. It is an incorrect statement. AD does tend to improve as the affected child ages. Sixty percent of atopic dermatitis appears in the first year of life, usually >2 months. The cause of AD is not yet known. The role of specific allergens is controversial. In some patients, a food allergy can worsen the disease but is not thought to be the cause. However, in severe, unresponsive AD, food allergens should be evaluated. Most patients who have positive allergy testing to foods do not have improvement in their skin with removal of the allergen.

The hallmark of AD is:

A) Lichenification of the skin.
B) Pruritus and relapsing nature.
C) Associated asthma or allergic rhinitis.
D) Associated food allergy.
E) Redness of the skin with honey crusting.

Discussion

The correct answer is B. Although all of the above can be associated with atopic dermatitis, waxing and waning pruritus defines this common skin condition. Chronic scratching often leads to thickened skin with accentuation of skin lines (lichenification). Early lesions will not have lichenification. Asthma and allergic rhinitis can be associated with atopic dermatitis. This common hypersensitivity triad is referred to as atopy. As discussed, food allergy can exacerbate some patients with AD, but it is not common. Erythema of the skin is a nonspecific sign of inflammation and is seen in many skin disorders. Honey crusting implies a secondary bacterial infection which is common in AD but does not define the disease.

Your initial recommendation should include the mainstay of long-term management of AD, which is:

A) Daily use of thick emollients such as white petrolatum.
B) Decrease of bathing frequency to twice per week.
C) Topical corticosteroids or topical immunomodulators.
D) Oral antihistamines.
E) Oral antibiotics.

Discussion

The correct answer is A. The protective barrier of skin is broken down in patients with AD. By adding a protective barrier such as petrolatum frequently, the skin becomes less pruritic resulting in less itching-induced skin trauma and rash, thus decreasing the "itch-scratch cycle." This is the most important long-term management. Topical steroids and immunomodulators work well to decrease the inflammation in the skin and are first-line antiinflammatory treatment; however, the goal is to protect the skin with thick emollients so that the skin does not dry out and cause itch that leads to scratching and subsequent inflammation. Daily bathing with mild cleansers and cool water is recommended. Patients with AD have a higher bacterial count of *Staphylococcus aureus* on their skin. By bathing for short periods daily, the bacterial count is decreased, thus decreasing the risk of secondary infection. Oral antihistamines cause some level of sedation which is often helpful at night when the child is awake and itching. Oral antibiotics are necessary in more extensive impetigo, especially if lymphadenopathy is appreciated.

 HELPFUL TIP: Mid-potency steroid (eg, triamcinolone) ointments are the mainstay of pharmacotherapy for AD. For the face, low-potency steroid (eg, hydrocortisone) creams can be used for a maximum of 2–3 weeks at a time. For severe, acute flares, systemic steroids can be employed for 10–14 days.

 HELPFUL TIP: Topical calcineurin inhibitors (tacrolimus and pimecrolimus) should be considered second-line therapies in the treatment of AD. Although they are generally safe and well tolerated, they are expensive and carry a "black box warning" related to possible cancer risk. There are a few reported cases of lymphoma and cutaneous cancers that develop in humans who use topical calcineurin inhibitors. Animal studies support this association.

* *

A recent ear infection has caused your patient's skin to worsen. He returns to clinic and your physical exam reveals the skin lesion shown in Figure 17–2 (see also color section). He has appreciably enlarged cervical lymph nodes. The patient has no known drug allergies.

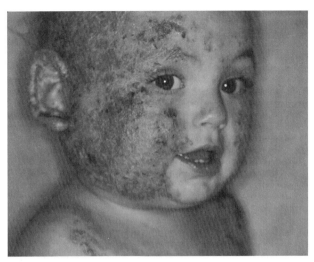

Figure 17–2

Which of the following oral antibiotics would be the best initial choice while you wait for culture and antimicrobial sensitivities?

A) Ciprofloxacin.
B) Trimethoprim/sulfamethoxazole.
C) Amoxicillin/clavulanic acid.
D) Tetracycline.
E) Metronidazole.

Discussion

The correct answer is B. Patients with AD are prone to certain skin infections that may exacerbate their disease. Ninety percent of patients with AD will grow *S. aureus* on swab cultures of their crusted lesions. By decreasing the bacterial count, inflamed lesions often heal faster. With the rapid spread of community-acquired methicillin-resistant *S. aureus* (CA-MRSA), it is safe to assume that many, or in some communities most, skin infections are caused by CA-MRSA; therefore, trimethoprim/sulfamethoxazole (Bactrim or Septra) is the most appropriate initial choice. Tetracycline (answer D) is another option. However, this should be avoided in young children < 8 years of age for doxycycline, 18 for ciprofloxacin as should fluoroquinolones (except in rare cases such as cystic fibrosis). Although not an option, cephalexin (answer A), a first-generation cephalosporin, would also be a reasonable initial choice as it has good skin penetration with good coverage of Gram-positive cocci. However, neither cephalexin nor amoxicillin/clavulanate (answer C) will cover CA-MRSA. E, metronidazole, is for anaerobes and will not cover *S. aureus*.

Which of the following vaccinations is contraindicated in patients with AD?

A) Smallpox (Vaccinia).
B) Varicella.
C) Measles/Mumps/ Rubella.
D) Hepatitis B.
E) Pneumococcus.

Discussion

The correct answer is A. Vaccination against smallpox (vaccinia), a live virus vaccine, is contraindicated in people with AD even when the condition is in remission. Vaccination may result in eczema vaccinatum, a severe and potentially fatal reaction. Vaccinia vaccine is also contraindicated in all household contacts (eg, parents of children with AD). A family history of AD is not a contraindication.

* *

As the patient grows, he improves significantly. However, his skin continues to be sensitive to many products. As a teenager he presents with a recurring rash near his wrist that is intensely pruritic. He has recently started wearing a metal bracelet (Figure 17–3; see also color section).

The test most likely to confirm your presumptive diagnosis is:

A) Potassium hydroxide of a skin scraping.
B) Tzanck preparation.
C) Patch testing.
D) Serum thyroid-stimulating hormone (TSH) level.
E) Serum IgE levels.

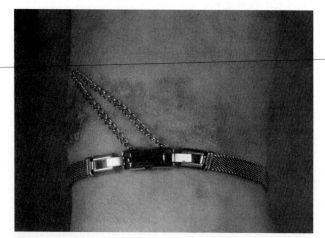

Figure 17–3

Discussion

The correct answer is C. The patient most likely has an allergic contact dermatitis to the nickel in the metal bracelet on his wrist. Patients with a history of AD are more likely to have contact hypersensitivities. Nickel is the most common contact allergen and can also be seen with contact to earrings, optical glasses, and buttons on jeans. Patch testing identifies many of the common contact allergens in the skin. KOH (potassium hydroxide) application to a skin scraping is used to identify fungal elements. KOH dissolves keratin, the protein in skin, to better identify the fungal elements. Tzanck preparations stain blister scrapings to evaluate lesions suspicious for herpes or varicella viruses. Thyroid disease can cause many skin conditions but is not a known cause of allergic contact dermatitis. An abnormality in the TSH level is the least likely to yield a diagnosis in this case. Serum IgE levels may be elevated in atopic patients, but this is not diagnostic as IgE can be elevated in many states.

Objectives: Did you learn to . . .

- Recognize atopic dermatitis by its classic presentations?
- Identify the hallmarks of atopic dermatitis?
- Manage a patient with atopic dermatitis and its complications?
- Recognize that smallpox vaccination is contraindicated in atopic dermatitis?

CASE 3

A 49-year-old obese white male with poorly controlled diabetes mellitus, hypertension, and hyperlipidemia presents to clinic for a regularly scheduled visit. He complains that his left leg is red. He denies constitutional symptoms or pain. His vital signs are within normal limits. He has a warm leg with circumferential erythema extending from the ankle to the mid-calf. He has 2 + pitting edema bilaterally with hemosiderin staining (brownish macular lesions) of the ankles. There are no open sores or minor trauma noted (Figure 17–4; see also color section). His complete blood count with differential is within normal limits. You send him for Doppler studies that fail to reveal venous thromboses. You prescribe 7 days of oral antibiotics and send him home.

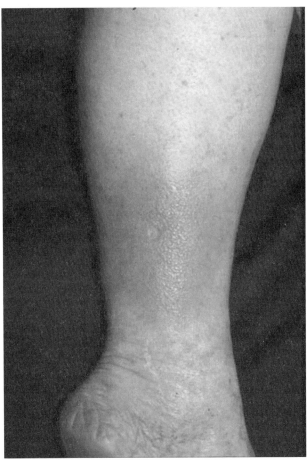

Figure 17–4

* *

He returns 3 days later with modest improvement in the redness. After completing the antibiotic course, he presents to clinic 3 weeks later complaining of return of the redness.

The most effective treatment or study at this time would be:

A) Another course of oral antibiotics for 14 days.
B) Admit the patient to the hospital for intravenous antibiotics.
C) Send a punch biopsy of skin for bacterial culture.
D) Recommend daily leg elevation and compression hose use.
E) Prescribe diuretics (eg, furosemide).

Discussion

The correct answer is D. This patient has a classic history of stasis dermatitis, a condition that is often misdiagnosed as recurrent or chronic cellulitis. Stasis dermatitis is a chronic dermatitis of the lower extremities that results from chronic edema. It can start relatively abruptly and be unilateral or bilateral. The pitting edema with hemosiderin staining is a clue that there is chronic fluid extravasation from the vessels of the lower extremities. Ectatic veins may also be present. The goal of therapy is directed at resolution of the edema. Patients must lose weight and employ a strict routine of compression hose and leg elevation. In the short term, topical corticosteroids can improve the inflammation. In general, diuretics should not be used simply to treat edema as these drugs have a number of systemic effects, some of which may be untoward. Paradoxically, diuretics can make edema worse in the long term by causing low circulating volume and renal retention of sodium and water to make up for the diuretic-induced hypovolemia. Chronic lower extremity edema can lead to local tissue necrosis, resulting in ulceration.

* *

As a result of years of diabetic nephropathy, the patient's kidneys eventually fail, leading to transplantation. After 5 years of stable renal function and improved control of his diabetes, he develops a new nonhealing lesion on the left forearm.

What cutaneous malignancy is he at the highest risk of developing?

A) Basal cell carcinoma.
B) Malignant melanoma.
C) Squamous cell carcinoma.
D) Metastases from an undiagnosed internal malignancy.

Discussion

The correct answer is C. All primary cutaneous malignancies are increased in immunosuppressed patients. However, squamous cell carcinoma is the most common in transplanted, immunosuppressed patients. In an immunocompetent population, basal cell carcinoma (answer A) is the most common malignancy. Any non-healing lesion should be investigated further with a biopsy.

* *

The patient develops a shallow ulcer superior to the medial malleolus.

The most common cause of an ulceration at this location is?

A) Arterial insufficiency.
B) Diabetic neuropathy.
C) Chronic venous stasis.
D) Pyoderma gangrenosum.
E) Prolonged pressure (eg, decubitus ulcer).

Discussion

The correct answer is C. Your patient is at risk for many of the above diagnoses; however, venous ulcerations classically occur over the medial lower leg. In contrast to this patient's venous ulceration, arterial insufficiency ulcers classically have a punched-out appearance and occur over bony prominences (eg, malleoli) or distal aspects (eg, tips of toes) and are extremely painful. Poor peripheral pulses, cool extremities, and hairlessness are clues to arterial insufficiency. Abnormal ankle-brachial indices help to confirm peripheral artery disease.

Neuropathic ulcers, such as those associated with diabetic neuropathy, also occur over pressure points on the plantar surface of the foot. The patient may complain of burning or tingling of the foot, but the ulcer is asymptomatic (because of lack of pain sensation from diabetic neuropathy). Pyoderma gangrenosum is a rare cause of ulceration associated with systemic problems such as Crohn and ulcerative colitis. Pressure ulceration is common and results from tissue ischemia from prolonged pressure, usually over bony prominences, such as the sacrum, coccyx, and heels.

* *

As you start to exit the exam room the patient states, "Oh, by the way, Doc, can you do anything for my toenails?" Your exam reveals 3, yellow heaped-up nails on the left foot. You suspect a dermatophyte infection.

What do you do next?

A) Perform a KOH exam of toenail scrapings.
B) Send toenail clippings for culture.
C) Empirically treat with an oral antifungal.
D) Empirically treat with a topical antifungal.
E) Tell the patient that his nails are the least of his worries.

Discussion

The correct answer is A. Because of the high cost of antifungals, the potential toxicity of therapy, and that many dystrophic nails are not a result of fungal infection, a test is warranted to determine if there is an organism.

Potassium hydroxide (KOH) is an inexpensive and easy test to perform in the clinic setting. If it is negative, a toenail clipping could be sent for fungal culture.

* *

The KOH is negative, so you send a toenail clipping for culture. It grows a *Candida* species.

Which of the following would be the LEAST efficacious medication?

A) Fluconazole.
B) Amphotericin.
C) Terbinafine.
D) Voriconazole.
E) Nystatin.

Discussion

The correct answer is C. All the above medications have some *Candida* species coverage, but terbinafine (Lamisil) has the least yeast coverage. Of note, amphotericin (answer B) would be the most toxic (but still would work well) and should be avoided.

 HELPFUL TIP: Terbinafine (Lamisil) **is** effective against most dermatophyte infections of the nails. Most cases of onychomycosis are caused by various *Tinea* species, which are sensitive to terbinafine.

* *

The patient wants to know why he has this problem with his toenails.

You tell him that it is related to:

A) Occlusive footwear.
B) Cotton socks.
C) Poor peripheral arterial circulation.
D) Being called "stinky-stinky-fat-feet" in kindergarten.
E) A and C.

Discussion

The correct answer is E. Patients with peripheral artery disease are more likely to develop onychomycosis. Likewise, occlusive footwear is thought to play a role. Cotton socks are more breathable than nylon or other materials and do not increase the risk of onychomycosis as much as other materials.

 HELPFUL TIP: "Cold," nontender nodules and abscesses at injection sites are often caused by *Mycobacterium chelonei*. These are found most commonly in immunocompromised patients, such as those with diabetes, organ transplantation, etc.

Objectives: Did you learn to . . .

- Recognize the presentation of stasis dermatitis and describe its etiology?
- Treat stasis dermatitis?
- Recognize the cutaneous malignancies seen in transplanted, immunosuppressed patients?
- Differentiate between common causes and sites of lower-extremity ulcerations?
- Diagnose and treat onychomycosis?
- Identify injection site reactions can be caused by atypical *Mycobacteria*?

CASE 4

You are working in the student health clinic at the local university when a previously healthy 19-year-old female presents with malaise for 3 weeks and a severe sore throat for 3 days. She has enlarged tonsils with exudates and large cervical lymph nodes, including prominent posterior nodes. She takes an oral contraception pill and a multivitamin daily and denies medicine allergies. You suspect a group A streptococcal pharyngitis. You are all out of the rapid strep assay reagents, so you swab the patient's throat and send it for culture. You give her a prescription for amoxicillin and tell her not to fill it until you call her the next day with the culture results. She is miserable and fills her prescription anyway.

Within 24 hours of her starting the medication, she develops a macular, red skin eruption that starts on her chest and soon spreads to involve her extremities. Her mucous membranes, palms, and soles are free of lesions. In the meantime the culture is negative. The patient, worried about prematurely starting the amoxicillin, does not call until the rash involves nearly her entire body.

You suspect:

A) A common drug reaction to the amoxicillin.
B) An Epstein-Barr virus infection (mononucleosis).
C) An enterovirus infection.
D) A gonococcal infection.
E) Scarlet fever.

Discussion

The correct answer is B. All of the above infections except for enterovirus can present with an exudative pharyngitis; enterovirus presents with gastrointestinal or meningeal symptoms. The clinical scenario describes the usual course of infectious mononucleosis: a college-age student, a few weeks prodrome of malaise, and posterior cervical lymphadenopathy. Amoxicillin or ampicillin given to patients with infectious mononucleosis can result in a macular, diffuse rash. Note that this rash does not occur with penicillin which is the drug of choice for streptococcal phayngitis anyway. This is not an allergy but can be confused for one. Scarlet fever, which this patient does not have, is a complication of group A streptococcal infection which presents with an erythematous, coarse ("sandpaper") rash, strawberry tongue, and skin desquamation.

CASE 5

Later that day, a 20-year-old male presents with a mildly pruritic rash on his trunk. He had a cold a few weeks earlier but is otherwise healthy. He denies high-risk sexual behavior or intravenous drug use. Your exam reveals the findings as shown in Figures 17–5 and 17–6 (for both figures see also color section).

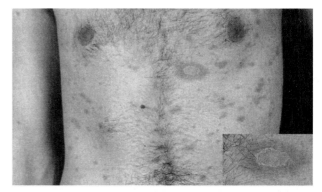

Figure 17–5 **Wolff K, Johnson RA, Suurmond D.** *Fitzpatrick's Color Atlas and Synopsis of Clinical Dermatology,* **5th ed. New York, NY: McGraw-Hill; 2005:119. Copyright The McGraw-Hill Companies, Inc.**

Figure 17–6

without treatment and does not usually recur. Topical steroids are not necessary for healing but may be helpful in the minority of patients that experience itching. Answer E is incorrect. This rash is not that serious.

> **HELPFUL TIP:** Pityriasis rosea starts with a "herald patch," a salmon-colored 2–5 cm oval-shaped lesion on the back, neck, or chest (see inset Figure 17–5). The herald patch may clear a bit and scale and is followed by numerous smaller lesions that crop up mostly on the trunk. These lesions tend to be oval in shape and are oriented along skin lines, giving a "Christmas tree" appearance.

CASE 6

Your next patient is a 20-year-old female complaining of "a rash down below." You confirm that she is talking about a vulvar rash and ask about her sexual history. She says that she had not been sexually active with anyone for about 1 year until a recent spring break liaison in Florida. On exam, you find a rash over the pubic region and extending into the inguinal areas and medial thighs. There is no pain or pruritus. See Figure 17–7; see also color section.

You tell the patient:

A) This skin condition is usually chronic and relapsing.
B) That although you trust his history, you suspect a sexually transmitted disease is the cause.
C) Topical corticosteroids are needed to speed up the healing.
D) The rash usually resolves within 6–8 weeks without treatment.
E) The rash is likely to be fatal.

Which of the following statements is FALSE?

A) These lesions are transmitted in adults only by sexual contact.
B) If not treated, the lesions may resolve on their own.

Discussion

The correct answer is D. The rash is consistent with pityriasis rosea (PR) which is an acute, often asymptomatic eruption on the trunk and proximal extremities. The etiology is unknown. Secondary syphilis, which is on the rise in some areas of the United States, can mimic PR. A sexual history is necessary, and appropriate laboratory studies should be undertaken if high-risk behaviors have occurred or if local syphilis rates are high. PR, unlike syphilis, often resolves within 8 weeks

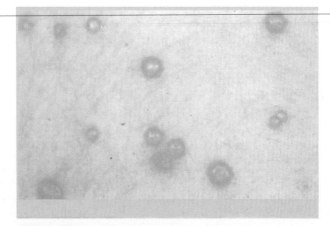

Figure 17–7

C) Topical corticosteroids do not improve this skin condition.

D) The lesions are contagious and can spread readily and rapidly.

E) The skin lesions are a result of a viral infection.

Discussion

The correct answer is A. These lesions, referred to as molluscum contagiosum, result from a pox virus. Molluscum is commonly spread via sexual contact in adults; however, **any** physical human contact (not necessarily sexual) can spread it. Molluscum is extremely common in children in day-care settings. The lesions generally resolve in time without treatment. Because they can be autoinoculated, the molluscum lesions rapidly increase, and for this reason treatment is recommended. Treatment consists of destructive methods, such as cryotherapy or curetting. Newer immune modulators (eg, Imiquimod) are being used but are not yet approved by the FDA for this purpose; topical steroids are not indicated. In immunocompromised patients, molluscum lesions can be widespread and persist much longer.

CASE 7

A healthy 18-year-old male presents for treatment of plantar warts. He has tried topical salicylic acid 17% at home. He used it for a few weeks without significant improvement.

Which of the following is FALSE about the treatment of plantar warts?

A) Duct tape occlusion at night has been shown to be as effective as a destructive method (cryotherapy).

B) Regardless of the therapeutic modality used such as burning, freezing, cantharidin (blistering), and CO_2 laser, there is a high recurrence rate.

C) If left alone, most warts will resolve in time.

D) Systemic antiviral therapy is successful in treating recurrent or widespread warts.

Discussion

The correct answer is D. There is currently no specific antiviral therapy available to cure human papilloma viral infections such as plantar warts (verruca plantaris). As we all know, duct tape (answer A) can be used for anything and it has been shown to be as effective as cryotherapy for the treatment of warts. However, the

trial that showed success with duct tape has not been successfully reproduced. Destructive methods are all approximately 70% effective at eradicating warts. It is important to remind patients that one method is no more likely to work than another. In immunocompetent patients, most warts resolve in time without treatment. For young children, this is an important issue since they cannot understand the pain associated with most treatment modalities.

 HELPFUL TIP: To use duct tape for warts, the patient should put a piece of duct tape on the wart and leave it on for 6 days. On day 7, remove the duct tape, soak and abrade the wart with a "pumice stone." Reapply the duct tape the next day and continue until the warts have resolved.

Objectives: Did you learn to . . .

● Recognize that ampicillin/amoxicillin given to patients with mononucleosis will often result in a macular rash?

● Diagnose pityriasis rosea and recognize secondary syphilis as a mimic?

● Recognize and treat molluscum contagiosum?

● Describe the treatment modalities for verruca plantaris?

 QUICK QUIZ: ID REACTIONS

Which of the following represents an id reaction?

A) Granuloma annulare.

B) Dyshidrotic eczema.

C) Sézary syndrome.

D) Tinea versicolor.

E) Acanthosis nigricans.

Discussion

The correct answer is B. Dyshidrotic eczema does not have a well-characterized etiology and several causes have been implicated. Some cases are "id" reactions which occur as a result of a dermatophyte infection. Dyshidrotic eczema is characterized by pruritic, small, fluid filled blisters (tapioca-like) generally on the sides of the fingers and toes. You should look for a dermatophyte infection and treat it if present. Otherwise, if no dermatophyte is found, topical steroids of medium to high potency are useful.

CASE 8

Within the first 24 hours of life, you notice yellow, 1- to 2-mm inflamed pustules the trunk and buttocks of this term infant (Figure 17–8; see also color section). The palms and soles are not affected. The neonate is feeding well, has normal vital signs, and does not seem to be bothered by this rash.

The most likely diagnosis now is:

A) Neonatal acne.
B) Miliaria crystalline.
C) Scabies.
D) Erythema toxicum neonatorum.
E) Herpes simplex.

Discussion

The correct answer is D. See below for further discussion.

* *

To help confirm your suspected diagnosis you perform a Wright stain on a scraping of a pustule. Numerous eosinophils are present. The parents are worried about the rash and mention that they have an 18-month-old son at home.

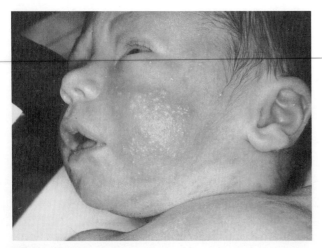

Figure 17–8

You recommend:

A) Keeping the neonate in the hospital until the rash resolves as it could be spread from skin-to-skin contact.
B) Keeping the neonate in the hospital and starting intravenous antibiotics immediately.
C) Discharging the patient home because this is a noncontagious, self-limited condition.
D) Discharging the patient home and recommending daily benzoyl peroxide to the lesions.
E) Discharging the patient home and recommending strict contact precautions for the 18-month-old sibling.

Discussion

The correct answer is C. Erythema toxicum neonatorum is a common condition of full-term infants. It is rarely seen in premature infants or those <2,500 grams. It presents during the first and second day of life. The rash is characterized by inflammatory macules and pustules and often begins on the face and involves the torso, buttocks, and proximal extremities. It is never seen on the palms and soles. The rash can come and go but resolves without treatment in several days. The diagnosis is usually made by a typical clinical presentation in a healthy infant. The etiology is unknown. If the diagnosis is in question, a Wright stain of a pustule scraping can be performed, revealing numerous eosinophils.

In contrast, neonatal acne presents as a pustular, facial eruption with a mean onset at 2 to 3 weeks. It is asymptomatic and diagnosed clinically. Fungal organisms have been found in some pustules. Treatment for acne is not necessary as most lesions resolve in several weeks. Some physicians have tried topical low-potency corticosteroids. Miliaria, or prickly heat rash, present as inflammatory vesicles on the face and upper trunk and are associated with excessive warming of the infant. Miliaria result from a blockage of sweat ducts, and no treatment is necessary. Neonatal scabies does not present on the first day of life. Most scabies cases result in an extremely irritable infant with a nonspecific rash; flexural areas and palm and sole involvement are the most frequent locations. Neonatal herpes presents with blisters or erosions and a sick-appearing child. Diagnosis is made via a Tzanck preparation demonstrating multinucleated giant cells, viral culture, or direct fluorescent antibody for HSV 1 or 2.

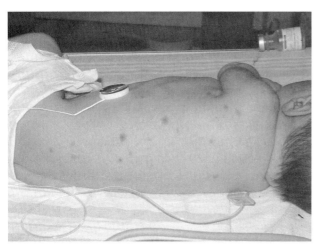

Figure 17–9

CASE 9

As you are taking care of the neonate in the newborn nursery, you notice a child in isolation. His skin catches your eye (Figure 17–9; see also color section).

The most common cause of this rash in newborns in the United States is:

A) Cytomegalovirus.
B) Rubella.
C) Langerhan cell histiocytosis.
D) Rh incompatibility.
E) Parvovirus B19.

Discussion

The correct answer is A. All the above can present as a "Blueberry muffin" baby. However, Cytomegalovirus (CMV) is the most common cause in the United States. CMV is the most common congenital viral infection, affecting approximately 1%–2% of all newborns. Rubella was the most common cause in the prevaccination era. In most cases, the purple plaques represent extramedullary hematopoiesis.

CASE 10

At 3 weeks of age, a previously healthy neonate presents to your clinic with peeling of the skin and a fever (Figure 17–10; see also color section). She had been feeding well until 2 days ago when she became more irritable. Her mother noted a decrease in her urine output. The child was born vaginally without complications and has no known medical conditions. On physical exam

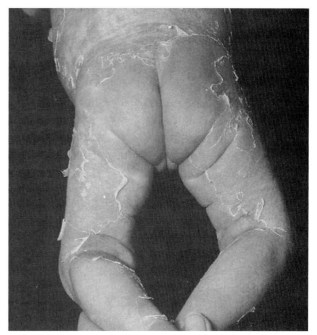

Figure 17–10 **Wolff K, Johnson RA, Suurmond D.** *Fitzpatrick's Color Atlas and Synopsis of Clinical Dermatology,* **5th ed. New York, NY: McGraw-Hill; 2005:623. Copyright The McGraw-Hill Companies, Inc.**

you note a well-nourished, crying infant with large sheets of desquamating skin on her extremities. Her mucous membranes appear normal. You order complete blood count and urine analysis.

The most likely diagnosis is:

A) Toxic epidermal necrolysis.
B) Bullous impetigo.
C) Staphylococcal scalded skin syndrome.
D) Diffuse cutaneous mastocytosis.

Discussion

The correct answer is C. See Discussion below.

In this patient with staphylococcal scalded skin syndrome, peeling of the skin is a result of:

A) Necrosis of the entire epidermis from lymphocyte attack.
B) A widespread bacterial skin infection.
C) Histamine released in the skin with edema and blistering.
D) Toxin-mediated skin blistering from a nonskin source of infection.

Discussion

The correct answer is D. This clinical scenario describes staphylococcal scalded skin syndrome (SSSS), which is an epidermolytic toxin-driven disease. Extreme tenderness of the skin precedes superficial, widespread desquamation. The skin is usually bright red with areas of flakiness. Radial wrinkling of the mouth, giving an "old man" appearance, is common. The source of infection is not the skin but rather an occult site such as nasopharynx or urinary tract; therefore, investigation for a causative infection should be undertaken (eg, blood and urine cultures, etc) Bullous impetigo is a result of *Staphylococcus aureus* skin infection in 85% of the cases. The erosions and blisters result from the local production of epidermolytic toxins. Toxic epidermal necrolysis (TEN) presents with shedding of sheets of skin and often has mucosal involvement which separates it clinically from SSSS. Usually, TEN is a result of drug hypersensitivity or bacterial sepsis in the case of the neonate. These children are quite ill in comparison with SSSS. In TEN, a biopsy would show full thickness necrosis of the epidermis versus an intraepidermal split in SSSS. Diffuse cutaneous mastocytosis can present with hemorrhagic blisters and erosions, but these are usually focal areas, not sheets of skin loss.

Objectives: Did you learn to . . .

- Recognize neonatal benign cutaneous eruptions?
- Identify a "blueberry muffin" neonate and know the common causes?
- Recognize staphylococcal scalded skin syndrome (SSS) and consider its differential diagnosis?

 QUICK QUIZ: NAILS

Which of the following pairs of nail findings—systemic disease are matched incorrectly?

A) Muehrcke nails—nephrotic syndrome.
B) Plummer nail—hyperthyroidism.
C) Periungual fibroma—tuberous sclerosis.
D) Splinter hemorrhages—infective endocarditis.
E) Koilonychia—systemic lupus erythematosus.

Discussion

The correct answer is E. Koilonychia (aka "spoon nail"), is a result of softening and thinning of the nail plate and is found in patients with long-standing iron-deficiency anemia, Plumer-Vinson syndrome, Raynaud, hemachromatosis, and trauma. It can also be inherited as an autosomal dominant trait. Connective tissues diseases, such as lupus, are more commonly characterized by nail-fold abnormalities, such as nail-fold telangiectasias, rather than koilonychia.

The other answer choices are paired correctly. Muehrcke nails (answer A) have paired narrow horizontal white bands, separated by normal color, that remain static as the nail grows. They are most often seen in patients with nephrotic syndrome, and their presence reflects the degree of hypoalbuminemia. When you see onycholysis (separation of the nail plate from the nail bed that appears opaque) consider trauma, onychomycosis, psoriasis, and other systemic disease. When onycholysis is present in hyperthyroidism, it is called Plummer nail (answer B) and often affects the ring finger only for unclear reasons. A periungual fibroma (answer C) should prompt evaluation for tuberous sclerosis with brain imaging for tuberous lesions. Splinter hemorrhages (answer D) are usually a result of trauma but can be a sign of infectious endocarditis.

 HELPFUL TIP: Paronychia, inflammation around the nail, may be acute or chronic. Acute paronychia is often a result of bacterial infection and is treated with oral antibiotics, warm compresses, and soaks. Chronic paronychia is related to eczema and may have secondary *Candida* infection. Treatment is with topical steroids, topical antifungals, and oral antifungals.

 QUICK QUIZ: DERM PHOTO

A 52-year-old white male presents to clinic with a non-healing, asymptomatic "pimple" on the cheek. It has been present for 6 months and has recently started to bleed when he shaves. On exam you note his fair skin, blue eyes, and ruddy complexion. The lesion is shown in Figure 17–11 (see also color section).

Your preliminary diagnosis is:

A) Sebaceous hyperplasia.
B) Squamous cell carcinoma.

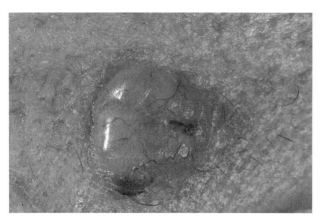

Figure 17–11

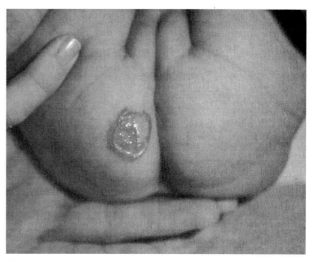

Figure 17–12

C) Basal cell carcinoma.
D) Metastases from internal malignancy.
E) Merkel cell carcinoma.

Discussion

The correct answer is C. The photograph is a classic picture of a basal cell carcinoma with its rolled, pearly pink borders and telangiectasias. It is found commonly on the head and neck. People with fair skin and light hair and eyes are at particular risk. Sebaceous hyperplasia can look similar but is ivory or yellow in appearance and has a central pore. Squamous cell carcinoma is usually a hyperkeratotic or ulcerated papule or plaque. Metastases from solid organ malignancies are subcutaneous, firm nodules although they may ulcerate. Merkel cell carcinoma is a rare tumor on the head and neck that usually appears as an ill-defined, violaceous nodule or plaque.

CASE 11

While you are working in the ED, a 6-month-old healthy female infant is brought in by her grandmother. She is bleeding from a birthmark on her buttocks (Figure 17–12; see also color section). Her grandmother watches her during the day when her mother is at work and has noticed the lesion getting larger recently. After holding pressure on the lesion for about 20 minutes, the bleeding stops. You educate the grandmother about the natural history of the "birthmark."

Which of the following is NOT a true statement about this type of birthmark?

A) This is the most common type of soft tissue tumor of infancy.
B) Most of these birthmarks undergo complete or partial resolution.
C) Treatment is indicated in all lesions.
D) Pulse dye laser therapy is used primarily for ulcerated lesions.
E) Many are not present at birth but develop shortly thereafter.

Discussion

The correct answer is C. The child has an ulcerated hemangioma of infancy. Infantile hemangiomas are benign proliferations of endothelial cell lineage that are usually present at birth or soon thereafter. They are characterized by rapid growth in the first several months of life and then stop growing about 1 year of age. They spontaneously involute over years. Treatment options must be individually tailored. Most are treated if they ulcerate or if they are impairing a normal function, such as vision. Pulse dye laser therapy can heal ulcerated hemangiomas but does not significantly change the size of lesions. Most ulcerated lesions are successfully treated with topical antibacterial agents and nonadhesive dressings. Hemangiomas on the head and neck or multiple hemangiomas should be further evaluated with imaging studies.

* *

The patient, now 5 years, returns, this time with her mother. The hemangioma has healed. About 2 months ago the mother noticed a spot on the patient's left index

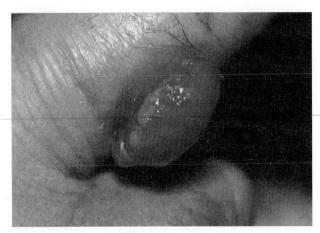

Figure 17–13

finger, and now she is concerned that it is not resolving. The patient is not bothered by the lesion, except that it occasionally bleeds when she bumps it on something. On exam, you find a 3-mm dome-shaped, bright red nodule on the palmar aspect of the left index finger. It is nontender and smooth (Figure 17–13; see also color section).

The most likely diagnosis is:

A) Basal cell carcinoma.
B) Squamous cell carcinoma.
C) Acne.
D) Pyogenic granuloma.
E) Nodular melanoma.

Discussion

The correct answer is D. This patient most likely has a pyogenic granuloma, which is essentially a nodular hemangioma arising at sites of trauma, especially the fingers and toes. Although pyogenic granuloma is not cancerous, it can be confused with basal (answer A) and squamous cell carcinomas (answer B) as well as melanoma (answer E). For this reason, it is prudent to perform excision and histologic examination. After excision, the base of the lesion should be ablated (electrocautery or laser), or the pyogenic granuloma may return. Acne (answer C) should not be a consideration because sebaceous glands are not found on the palms.

Objectives: Did you learn to . . .

- Describe the natural history of infantile hemangiomas?
- Identify options for treating ulcerated hemangiomas?
- Describe the features and management of pyogenic granuloma?

CASE 12

A 78-year-old female presents with a rash on her legs. It started 1 week ago and was preceded by itching of the legs without any visible changes. Then red blotches developed which quickly became blisters. She denies pain or drainage. She also has some sores in her mouth. Her medical history is otherwise remarkable in that she has been very healthy and takes no medications.

On exam, you find an afebrile, comfortable-looking female. There are several small ulcers on her hard palate. She has 1 + pitting edema at her ankles. You note round, tense bullae erupting on erythematous patches on the lower extremities bilaterally. The bullae break open with slight pressure applied to the edge, and several are draining clear fluid. There is no purulence or bleeding (Figure 17–14; see also color section).

Which of the following is the most likely diagnosis?

A) Pemphigus vulgaris.
B) Bullous pemphigoid.
C) Varicella zoster.
D) Dermatitis herpetiformis.
E) Stevens-Johnson syndrome.

Discussion

The correct answer is B. Bullous pemphigoid is an autoimmune disorder and is primarily a disease of the elderly. Often patients will have some sort of prodrome prior to the eruption of typical bullous lesions. Prodromal symptoms can include pruritus, erythema, and urticaria.

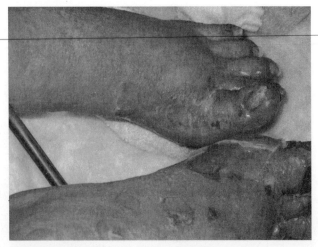

Figure 17–14

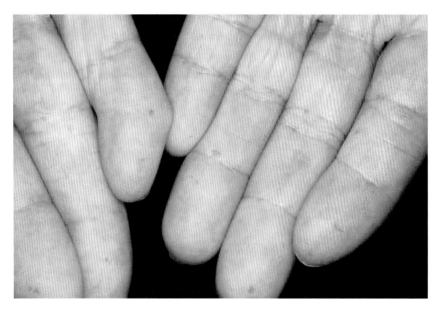

Figure 7–1

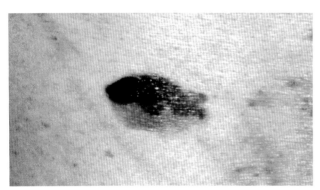

Figure 17–1

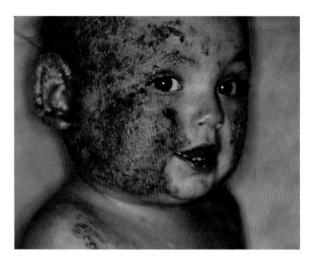

Figure 17–2

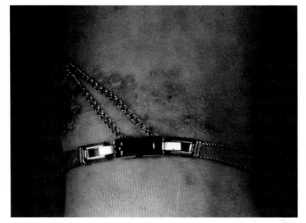

Figure 17–3

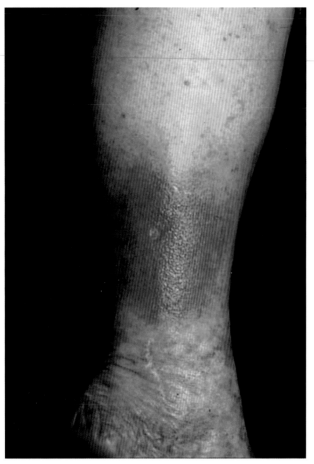

Figure 17–4

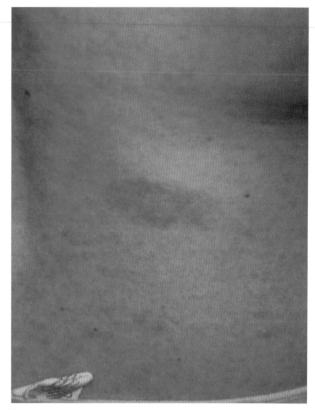

Figure 17–6

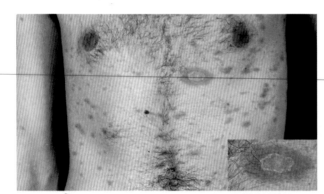

Figure 17–5   Wolff K, Johnson RA, Suurmond D.
*Fitzpatrick's Color Atlas and Synopsis of Clinical
Dermatology*, 5th ed. New York, NY: McGraw-Hill;
2005:119. Copyright The McGraw-Hill Companies,
Inc.

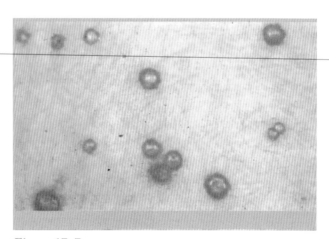

Figure 17–7

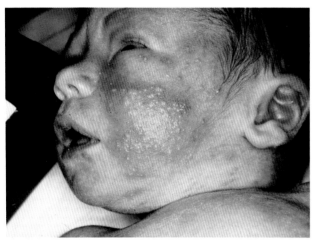

Figure 17-8

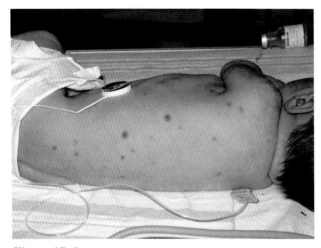

Figure 17-9

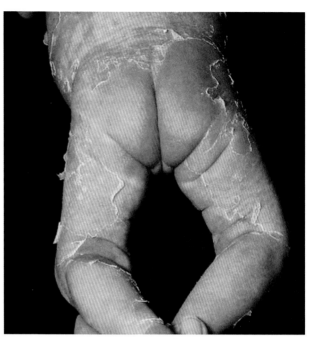

Figure 17-10 Wolff K, Johnson RA, Suurmond D. *Fitzpatrick's Color Atlas and Synopsis of Clinical Dermatology*, 5th ed. New York, NY: McGraw-Hill; 2005:623. Copyright The McGraw-Hill Companies, Inc.

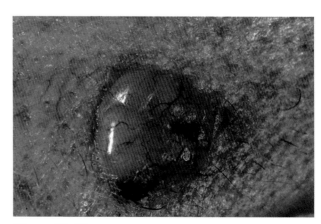

Figure 17-11

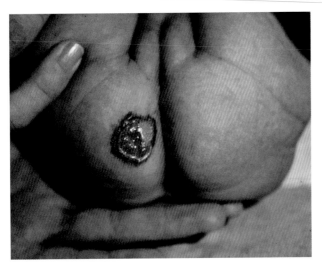

Figure 17–12

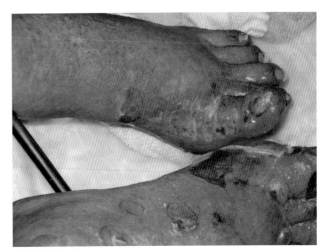

Figure 17–14

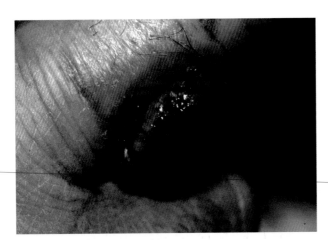

Figure 17–13

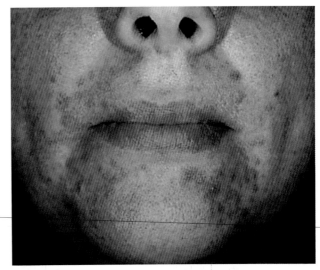

Figure 17–15

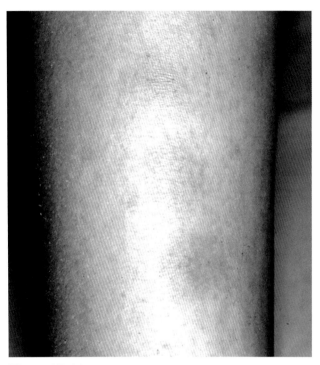

Figure 17–16

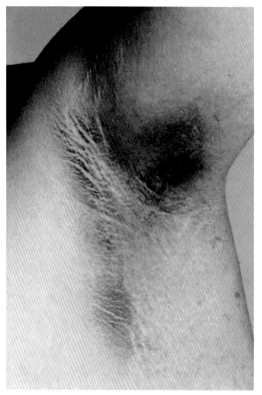

Figure 17–18   Wolff K, Johnson RA, Suurmond D.
Fitzpatrick's Color Atlas and Synopsis of Clinical
Dermatology, 5th ed. New York, NY: McGraw-Hill;
2005:87. Copyright The McGraw-Hill Companies,
Inc.

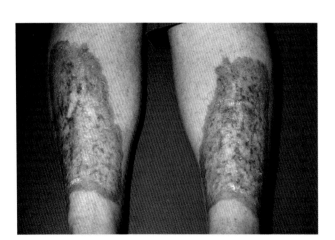

Figure 17–17   from www.dermnet.com

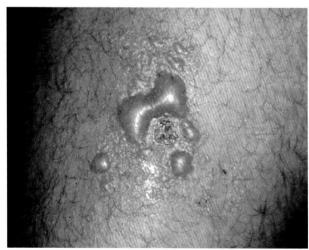

Figure 17–19

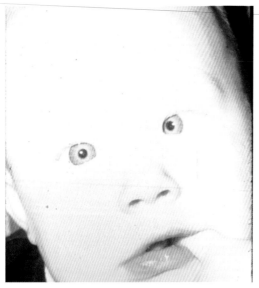

Figure 19–1   *Congenital esotropia. Note the large deviation with abnormal corneal light reflexes. The corneal light reflex of the left eye appears more temporal than that of the right eye. Therefore, the eye is deviated inwards.*

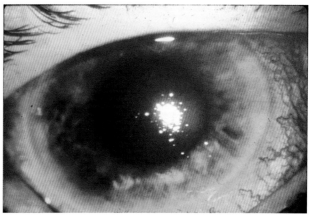

Figure 19–3   *Acute Angle Closure Glaucoma. Note the injection, hazy corneal reflex, and mid-dilated pupil.*

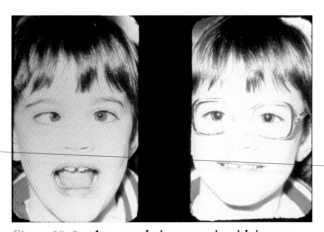

Figure 19–2   *Accommodative esotropia with improvement when vision is corrected.*

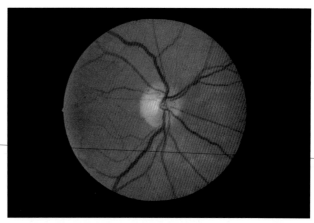

Figure19–4   *Normal optic nerve.*

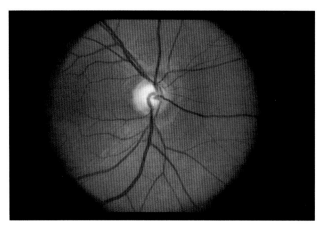

Figure 19–5 *Glaucomatous optic nerve. Observe the cupping of the optic nerve head.*

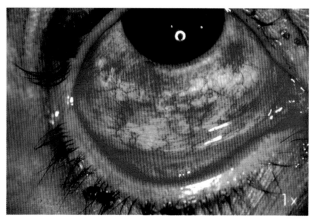

Figure 19–8 *Viral conjunctivitis. Note the follicles which are round collection of lymphocytes in the inferior fornix.*

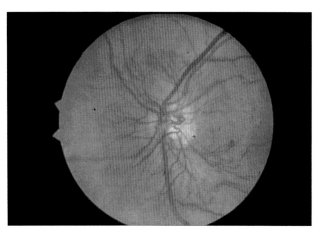

Figure 19–6 *Proliferative diabetic retinopathy. Neovascularization of the optic nerve.*

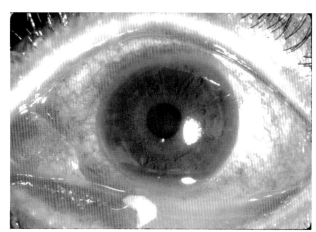

Figure 19–9 *Bacterial conjunctivitis. Note the mucopurulent discharge.*

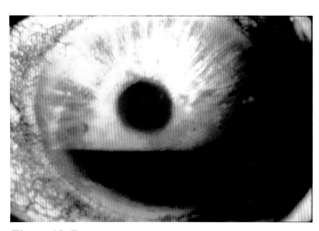

Figure 19–7

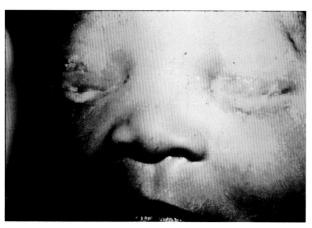

Figure 19–10 *Ophthalmia neonatorum. Note the severe mucopurulent discharge.*

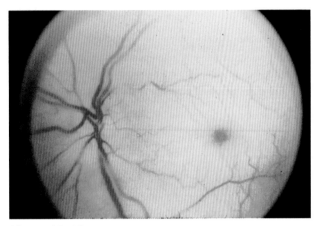

Figure 19–11

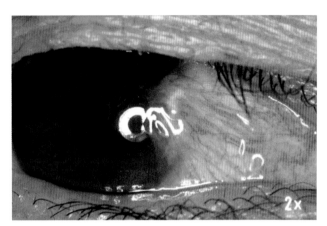

Figure 19–13

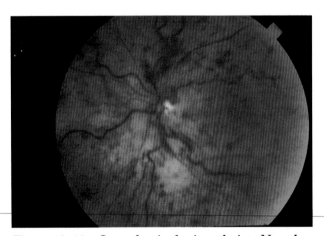

Figure 19–12 *Central retinal vein occlusion. Note the dilated tortuous veins, optic disc edema, and retinal hemorrhage/edema.*

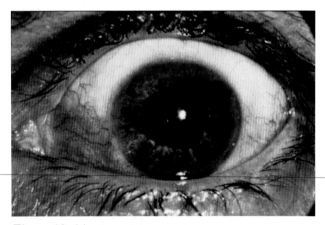

Figure 19–14

When the bullae form, they are frequently asymptomatic but can be intensely pruritic and mildly tender. In contradistinction to pemphigus vulgaris (answer A) and Stevens-Johnson syndrome (SJS) (answer E), systemic symptoms are not part of bullous pemphigoid. Additionally, pemphigus vulgaris lesions are painful, and classically the bullae are flaccid rather than tense. SJS generally occurs in response to medications, and this patient is taking none. Varicella zoster (answer C) should follow a dermatomal pattern rather than appear bilaterally; zoster is usually associated with pain and paresthesia. Dermatitis herpetiformis (answer D) presents with crops of vesicles and excoriations rather than bullae.

* *

Although she feels well, the lesions are dramatic, and the patient is very concerned that she might have cancer. To confirm your diagnosis, you decide to biopsy the skin.

The most appropriate way to perform a biopsy in this situation is:

A) 4-mm punch biopsy of the margin of an intact bulla for light microscopy.

B) 4-mm punch biopsy of normal skin for light microscopy.

C) 4-mm punch biopsy of normal skin for immunofluorescence.

D) A and B.

E) A and C.

Discussion

The correct answer is E. For a definitive diagnosis, both A and C should be done. Bullous pemphigoid is diagnosed definitively by demonstration of autoantibodies deposited along the basement membrane of **normal** skin. Immunofluorescent exam of normal-appearing skin can demonstrate IgG and complement deposits. A biopsy of the edge of an intact bulla will show the characteristic pathology of separation at the basement membrane and subepidermal blister.

* *

You assure her that the lesions are not cancerous.

What else can you tell her about the prognosis of bullous pemphigoid?

A) It is a chronic condition which increases the risk of melanoma.

B) It is associated with a high mortality rate.

C) It often resolves, never to occur again.

D) A and B.

Discussion

The correct answer is C. Bullous pemphigoid may undergo complete resolution and never recur. Alternatively, the disease may have resolutions and exacerbations over time. It is not associated with an increased risk of cancer or a high mortality rate. Very extensive involvement may lead to skin infections and bacteremia.

* *

She seems miserable. You want to offer her the safest, most effective therapy to treat this condition.

What intervention do you offer her now?

A) Oral azathioprine.

B) Oral cephalexin.

C) Oral prednisone.

D) Topical antimicrobials.

E) Topical clobetasol.

Discussion

The correct answer is E. Bullous pemphigoid is an autoimmune disease, so antiinflammatory medications and immunosuppressive agents are used to treat it. There is some concern about increased mortality in elderly patients treated with systemic steroids, and there is good evidence that even moderate to severe cases will respond to topical steroids. Therefore, potent topical steroids (eg, clobetasol) are currently the preferred therapy. However, topical clobetasol may be impractical and is much more expensive than oral prednisone. Thus, many cases are still treated with oral steroids, sometimes in combination with another immunosuppressive agent such as azathioprine or methotrexate. Dapsone may be used as well. When using oral steroids, it is prudent to taper the medication to achieve the lowest effective dose. Topical antimicrobials are used when treating infected, open bullae but are not effective for the treatment of the disease itself.

Objectives: Did you learn to . . .

- Distinguish bullous diseases from one another?
- Diagnose and treat bullous pemphigoid?

QUICK QUIZ: PAPULAR ERUPTION

A 30-year-old female presents with a several-month history of bumps on her chin and around her mouth. Although she has never had problems with acne, she thought that she was developing some and tried treating it with benzoyl peroxide. A month ago she stopped the benzoyl peroxide because it did not seem to work, and she switched to hydrocortisone cream, which has worsened the outbreak if it has done anything. The rash is neither itchy nor painful. She works in an office and cannot recall any contact irritants. On exam you find erythematous papules with small pustules on the chin and laterally around her mouth (Figure 17–15; see also color section). The neck and the remainder of the face are not involved.

Which of the following treatments do you recommend?

A) Oral tetracycline.
B) Oral isotretinoin (Accutane).
C) Topical high-potency steroids.
D) Topical triple-antibiotic ointment.
E) Topical retinoic acid.

Discussion

The correct answer is A. This patient appears to have perioral dermatitis. Appropriate treatments for perioral dermatitis include topical metronidazole or erythromycin or oral tetracycline antibiotics (tetracycline, minocycline, or doxycycline). The etiology of perioral dermatitis is unknown. Answers B and E are incorrect because they are treatments of acne vulgaris. Answer C is incorrect because high-potency topical steroids can make the condition worse, with more severe erythema. Topical triple-antibiotic ointment (answer D) is not likely to be effective.

CASE 13

A 15-year-old male presents to your office complaining of "zits" on his face and back. He has several scattered comedones on his face and several deep nodules on his back. He also has some papulopustular lesions on his chin. You diagnose him with acne vulgaris.

Which of the following is NOT true about acne?

A) Acne is an inflammatory process.
B) It commonly presents first in adolescence.
C) It may first appear in adulthood.
D) It is more severe in females than in males.
E) The incidence is lower in Asians and Africans than in whites.

Discussion

The correct answer is D. Acne is more severe in **males than females.** Acne is an inflammatory process that involves the pilosebaceous units of the face and trunk. It can be comedonal, papulopustular, or nodulocystic in presentation. It typically presents first in adolescence with girls aged 10 to 17 years and boys aged 14 to 19 years. However, it may not appear until early adulthood. It is less prevalent in Asians and Africans.

> **HELPFUL TIP:** Open comedones (blackheads) and closed comedones (whiteheads), are considered noninflammatory lesions while papular and cystic lesions are considered inflammatory.

* *

Your patient has heard many things about acne and wonders if they are true.

Which of the following is TRUE?

A) Acne is not caused by medications.
B) Acne is improved in the winter months.

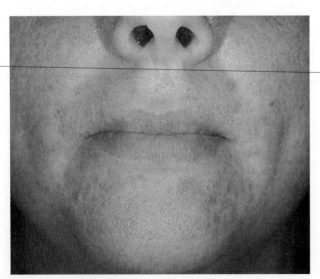

Figure 17–15

C) Certain foods (eg, chocolate) can worsen acne.

D) Emotional stress does not affect the course of acne.

E) Birth control pills can sometimes worsen acne.

Discussion

The correct answer is E. Medications such as lithium, steroids, and oral contraceptives can lead to acneiform outbreaks or exacerbation of acne. Acne is improved in the summer months and worse in the fall and winter. Despite popular myths, acne is not caused, or exacerbated by any foods or a "dirty face." Emotional stresses have been shown to lead to acne exacerbations. Many women tend to flare up right before menses.

For acne, which of the following treatment principles is (are) correct?

A) Treatment can often lead to initial worsening of lesions.

B) Therapeutic response often takes several months.

C) Mild acne can be treated with over-the-counter preparations (OCPs).

D) Often, 2 or more therapeutic agents must be combined for effective treatment.

E) All of the above are correct.

Discussion

The correct answer is E. Topical retinoids, topical antibiotics, and benzoyl peroxide are the first-line agents and can be titrated as needed. Retinoids should be applied at bedtime. The main oral antibiotic agents are tetracyclines and should be used as **add-on therapy** to topical agents for moderate to severe acne. OCPs with low androgenic progesterone can also be helpful.

* *

Isotretinoin (Accutane) is indicated for severe, recalcitrant, nodular acne.

Which of the following is FALSE regarding the use of Isotretinoin?

A) Two methods of contraception are required in all reproductive-age women along with frequent pregnancy tests.

B) It should not be used with tetracycline.

C) Hypertriglyceridemia is a possible side effect.

D) Severe depression is a contraindication to its use.

E) A patient can receive only one course of isotretinoin.

Discussion

The correct answer is E. Isotretinoin is category X in pregnancy and the FDA requires two contraceptive methods in all reproductive-age females who use it. They must also have frequent pregnancy tests. As both tetracycline and isotretinoin can lead to pseudotumor cerebri, they should not be used together. Hypertriglyceridemia, dry skin, and decreased night vision are common side effects. There have been reports in the popular press and the scientific literature of suicide in patients on isotretinoin though there is no good controlled data to suggest that the drug is responsible. The drug should not be used in patients at high risk for suicide, however, and this includes patients with severe depression. After 2 months off, patients who failed to respond completely may be treated again. Informed consent is needed before isotretinoin can be prescribed.

 HELPFUL TIP: Retinoids (isotretinoin and topicals) are related to Vitamin A, so vitamin A supplements should be avoided as the combination may lead to vitamin A toxicity.

 HELPFUL TIP: Women should have a pregnancy test monthly while on isotretinoin (Accutane) and should avoid becoming pregnant for 1 month after discontinuing treatment.

Objectives: Did you learn to . . .

• Diagnose and treat acne?

• Identify side effects of isotretinoin?

• Describe the natural history of acne?

CASE 14

A 26-year-old female patient presents to your office with a painful, nonpruritic pink rash that started last week on her shins. You find the firm lesions easier to palpate that visualize (Figure 17–16; see also color section).

What is the most likely diagnosis in this patient?

A) Erythema multiforme.

B) Urticaria.

C) Erythema nodosum.

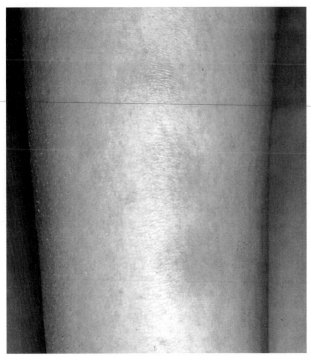

Figure 17–16

D) Erythema migrans.
E) Big lumps on the shins.

Discussion

The correct answer is C. This is erythema nodosum. Typically, these firm nodules occur first on shins and are often more easily palpated than seen. They may then spread to the thighs, trunk, and extensor surfaces of the arms. Erythema multiforme (answer A) presents as erythematous, targetoid lesions usually affecting the distal extremities including palms and soles. Urticaria (answer B) is not tender but would be intensely pruritic. Erythema migrans (answer D) is the quintessential lesion of Lyme disease: a nontender, nonpruritic red plaque with a central clearing. Although answer E is technically correct, you're not likely to ever find this sort of answer on the board exam.

Which of the following can cause erythema nodosum?

A) Oral contraceptives.
B) Streptococcal pharyngitis.
C) Sarcoid.
D) Viral upper respiratory infection (URI).
E) All of the above.

Discussion

The correct answer is E. All of these entities may cause erythema nodosum, but viral URI and streptococcal pharyngitis are most common. Multiple medications can also be responsible.

* *

This patient does relate a history of URI symptoms about 1 week prior to the onset of her symptoms.

What advice are you going to give this patient?

A) The rash will be present for 3–6 weeks and will heal **with** scarring.
B) The rash will be present for 3–6 weeks and will heal **without** scarring.
C) This is an inflammation primarily of blood vessels and requires oral steroids.
D) This is an inflammation primarily of fat and requires oral steroids.

Discussion

The correct answer is B. Generally erythema nodosum heals spontaneously in 3–6 weeks without scarring. The other answer choices are incorrect. Of special note is answer D. Erythema nodosum **is** an inflammation of the fat. However, **oral steroids are contraindicated** although intralesional or topical steroids under occlusion can be useful. Oral steroids may worsen the underlying problem (eg, TB, etc).

Objectives: Did you learn to . . .

● Recognize erythema nodosum?
● Describe some of the causes and natural history of erythema nodosum?

> **HELPFUL TIP:** Erythema migrans is often thought of as a single "bull's eye" lesion in the area of the tick attachment. However, the bull's eye is present in a minority of patients, and erythema migrans can have multiple widespread lesions in some patients with Lyme disease.

 QUICK QUIZ: ERYTHEMA MULTIFORME

Which of the following cause(s) erythema multiforme?

A) Viral URIs.
B) Cimetidine.
C) Herpes simplex outbreak.
D) Nifedipine.
E) All of the above.

Discussion

The correct answer is E. All of the above are causes of erythema multiforme as are many other medications, etc. **The most common precipitator of erythema multiforme is herpes simplex.** Look for this association in your patients.

 HELPFUL TIP: Sunlight is a frequent precipitator of an outbreak of herpes labialis.

CASE 15

A patient presents to your office with a 1-week history of a pruritic rash that is evanescent but involves his entire body except for his face. He cannot remember any new products with which he has been in contact (eg, soaps, detergents, etc). He is quite concerned. You correctly diagnose urticaria.

Your next step is:

A) Skin testing for various commercial products.
B) Viral titers for CMV, EBV, etc.
C) RAST test for common allergens.
D) Recommend no further evaluation.

Discussion

The correct answer is D. No workup is needed at this time. Beyond a good history, an extensive workup is pretty much futile. It is almost impossible to identify a cause of urticaria by laboratory testing.

Urticaria is categorized as which of the following?

A) Type I hypersensitivity reaction.
B) Type II hypersensitivity reaction.
C) Type III hypersensitivity reaction.
D) Type IV hypersensitivity reaction.

Discussion

The correct answer is A. Urticaria is a clinical feature of a type I reaction. Other clinical presentations of type I reactions include anaphylaxis and angioedema. Type II reactions are antibody dependent and present as nephritis or hemolytic anemia. Type III reactions present as serum sickness. Type IV reactions present as contact dermatitis.

* *

You decide to provide symptomatic care for this patient.

Appropriate medications include which of the following?

A) Cimetidine.
B) Doxepin.
C) Diphenhydramine.
D) Cetirizine (Zyrtec).
E) All of the above.

Discussion

The correct answer is E. All of the above can be useful in the symptomatic treatment of urticaria. Of the choices, cimetidine and other H_2-blockers are effective in the 10%–15% of patients who do not respond to H_1-blockers. This is as opposed to anaphylaxis where H_2-blockers are very useful. Finally, doxepin is a particularly effective H_1- and H_2-blocker that can be helpful when other drugs are ineffective.

* *

The patient returns to see you 4 weeks later and is still having symptoms. You are wondering a bit more about potential causes of this unfortunate individual's urticaria.

Which of the following are causes of urticaria?

A) Sweating.
B) Cold (OK, move to Hawaii and quit whining!).
C) Water.
D) Pressure (OK, use an antigravity unit and quit whining!).
E) All of the above.

Discussion

The correct answer is E. All of the above can cause urticaria. These are not uncommon causes and can be identified by history. Patients may develop urticaria with exercise and sweating (cholinergic urticaria), cold

Table 17–2   CAUSES OF URTICARIA

Physical
- Pressure
- Water
- Vibration
- Cold
- Sunlight
- Dermatographism

Allergic
- Foods (nuts, fish)
- Insect stings
- Drugs

Systemic
- Malignancy
- SLE
- RA
- Chronic hepatitis B and C
- EBV

(during the winter), and pressure (eg, from walking). Of particular note is water urticaria, which occurs with bathing and showering. Table 17–2 lists causes of urticaria.

 HELPFUL TIP: Cold urticaria often starts with lesions appearing on exposed skin, but then is worsened with rewarming.

* *

You decide that this patient probably has cold urticaria (the fact that it is summer does not dissuade you).

The next drug you might want to try on this patient is:

A) Cyproheptadine (Periactin).
B) Prednisone.
C) Montelukast.
D) Nifedipine.
E) Aspirin.

Discussion

The correct answer is A. The physical urticaria (cold and pressure especially) may respond better to cyproheptadine than other modalities. If this patient had a "typical" urticaria you might want to try prednisone, one of the leukotriene inhibitors, or nifedipine (which interferes with mast cell degranulation). **Leukotriene inhibitors, steroids, etc, are second-line drugs and should be used only when first-line drugs have failed or are not tolerated** (cyproheptadine for physical urticaria; doxepin, H_2-blockers, etc, for typical urticaria). There are no good studies on the effectiveness of leukotriene inhibitors but they might be worth trying when all else fails.

 HELPFUL TIP: Any number of drugs can cause urticaria. Always think about prescribed medications first.

Objectives: Did you learn to . . .
- Recognize urticaria?
- Identify potential causes of urticaria?
- Develop a treatment strategy for patients with urticaria?

 QUICK QUIZ: DERMATOLOGY

Actinic keratoses are precursors of:

A) Nothing.
B) Melanoma.
C) Basal cell carcinoma.
D) Squamous cell carcinoma.
E) Granuloma annulare.

Discussion

The correct answer is D. Actinic keratoses are precursors to squamous cell carcinomas. As such, they should be treated. Options include cryotherapy, laser therapy, or 5-fluorouracil topically.

 QUICK QUIZ: DERMATOLOGY

Seborrheic keratoses are precursors of:

A) Nothing.
B) Melanoma.
C) Basal cell carcinoma.
D) Squamous cell carcinoma.
E) Granuloma annulare.

Discussion

The correct answer is A. Seborrheic keratoses are precursors of nothing. They are the greasy-looking, stuck-on growths that occur with age. They can be treated, if necessary, with freezing and curetting.

CASE 16

A 50-year-old female with type 2 diabetes controlled with insulin complains of a rash that has developed on her legs over the past year. It started as a small patch on her left leg and then "spread" to her right leg. It is neither painful nor pruritic. You are impressed by the rash shown in Figure 17–17 (see also color section).

The most appropriate next step in the management of these lesions is:

A) A topical mid-potency steroid under occlusion or intralesional steroids.
A) Discontinue insulin.
B) Increase her insulin dose.
C) Liberal use of emollients (eg, petrolatum).
D) Leg elevation and application of compressive stockings.

Discussion

The correct answer is A. This patient has developed necrobiosis lipoidica, a benign condition of the skin that affects a low percentage of diabetics, usually those on insulin. Look for brownish red patches or plaques with yellowish areas through the center. The center is often shiny with telangiectasias. The legs are most often involved and the lesions may be painful. The name describes the pathology: necrobiosis refers to the inflammation around destroyed collagen, and lipoidica refers to the yellowish color associated with lipid deposits.

Answers B and C are incorrect because necrobiosis lipoidica does not seem to be caused by insulin or affected by glucose control. The lesions can be confused with eczema, and they may respond to topical steroids; however, emollients are not useful. Necrobiosis lipoidica might be confused for skin changes associated with venous stasis and chronic edema, which would be treated as in answer D. Patients should know that necrobiosis lipoidica is often chronic and difficult to treat but benign. The diagnosis is clinical but can be confirmed by biopsy, and treatment is not always necessary.

* *

Your patient also complains of thick, dark, velvety patches under her arms (Figure 17–18; see also color section). She is unsure of the duration, but states, "They've been with me a while. I just wonder if my medication might cause these." You have to admit, she takes a few medicines related to her diabetes.

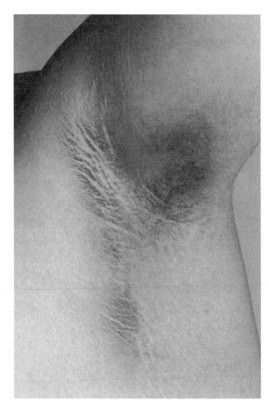

Figure 17–18 Wolff K, Johnson RA, Suurmond D. *Fitzpatrick's Color Atlas and Synopsis of Clinical Dermatology*, 5th ed. New York, NY: McGraw-Hill; 2005:87. Copyright The McGraw-Hill Companies, Inc.

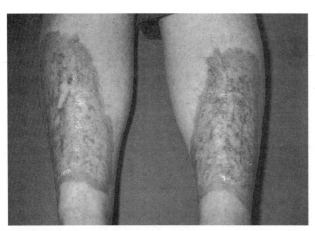

Figure 17–17 from www.dermnet.com

The most likely cause is:

A) Aspirin.
B) Lisinopril.
C) Insulin.
D) Simvastatin.

Discussion

The correct answer is C. The lesions are typical of acanthosis nigricans, a hyperkeratotic, hyperpigmented condition affecting skin folds (neck, inguinal area, axilla, etc.). The common causes of acanthosis nigricans are obesity, insulin resistance, and diabetes. Some drugs have been known to cause it, including insulin, corticosteroids, and nicotinic acid. We remember from med school that acanthosis nigricans is a cutaneous manifestation of internal malignancy. But such a presentation is rare. Cancer is more likely in patients with extensive and quickly progressing lesions, and as you might expect, it is a bad sign.

 HELPFUL TIP: Another cutaneous manifestation of internal malignancy is the Leser-Trélat sign: a large crop of seborrheic keratoses (SKs) that erupt quickly. Note that SKs are benign, and that knowing about Leser-Trélat is mostly good for looking smart.

* *

Your patient returns a year later and the lesions on her legs have disappeared. Now she has a new concern. She reports a sore on the bottom of her great toe. She's uncertain how it occurred and thinks it has only been present for a few days. You find a 1-cm circular ulcer at the plantar aspect of her great toe.

The most important next step is to:

A) Culture the wound.
B) Assess for adequate vascular supply to the foot.
C) Perform MRI of the foot.
D) Perform monofilament testing to check sensation in the foot.
E) Debride the wound.

Discussion

The correct answer is B. The described wound is most likely a diabetic foot ulcer, but the location and the patient's history of diabetes elicit concern for an ulcer related to vascular disease. Additionally, good vascular supply to the foot is necessary for wound healing. Therefore, we need to know the status of blood flow to the foot. This may be accomplished by physical exam. For patients at high risk for peripheral vascular disease or without strong pulses, ankle-brachial indices would be the next step. With regard to the other answers: culture of an open foot ulcer is pretty much worthless; x-ray may be warranted to evaluate for osteomyelitis, but MRI is jumping the gun; sensation is important, but not as urgent to wound healing as vascular supply; wound debridement may be needed, but you would want to know that the debrided area will have good blood flow first.

* *

Her pulses are good, her feet are warm, and the rest of her skin is in good condition. Through her diligent care and control of her diabetes, the ulcer heals. She returns 3 months later with a new skin concern. Between her fingers, she has developed clear fluid-filled blisters measuring 5–10 mm that are irregularly shaped. There is no erythema, no pruritus, and no pain. She denies trauma and new environmental contacts.

Which of the following is the most likely diagnosis?

A) Dyshidrotic eczema.
B) Contact dermatitis.
C) Staphylococcal scalded skin syndrome.
D) Bullosis diabeticorum.
E) Drug eruption.

Discussion

The correct answer is D. Bullosis diabeticorum, or bullous disease of diabetes, is not common. However, patients may be alarmed by it and seek treatment. The cause is unknown, but it typically follows a benign course and resolves spontaneously over several weeks or months. Because it requires no intervention, it is useful to distinguish bullosis diabeticorum from dyshidrotic eczema and contact dermatitis, both of which may mimic the disease except for pruritus and inflammation.

Objectives: Did you learn to . . .

- Identify necrobiosis lipoidica, acanthosis nigricans, and bullosis diabeticorum?
- Treat these conditions (if necessary)?
- Evaluate a diabetic foot ulcer?

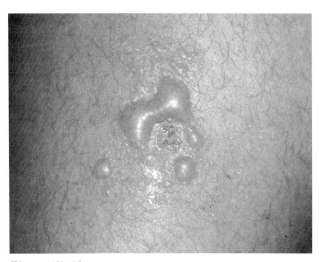

Figure 17–19

 QUICK QUIZ: DERMATOLOGY

The pruritic lesion in Figure 17–19 (see also color section) is most likely:

A) Grover disease.
B) Lichen planus.
C) Contact dermatitis.
D) Atopic dermatitis.
E) Pyoderma gangrenosum.

Discussion
The correct answer is C. This is contact dermatitis, which may be acute, subacute, or chronic. It is an erythematous, pruritic eruption that usually blisters and leaves a crust. More chronic forms of contact dermatitis present with lichenification and scaling. The rash shown in Figure 17–19 does not look like any of the other answer choices.

Again, since we cannot print pictures of all diseases mentioned, please look at one of the Web sites included at the beginning of this chapter.

 QUICK QUIZ: SKIN CONDITION

A 76-year-old male comes to your clinic with a 1-year history of pruritic, eczematous rash on his chest and back. He has no atopic history or eczema as a child. He has no other active medical issues. He has tried moisturizers and OTC hydrocortisone cream, which have provided minimal relief.

Which of the following is the most appropriate next step in his management?

A) Tacrolimus ointment.
B) Skin scraping for KOH preparation.
C) High-dose topical steroids.
D) Skin biopsy.
E) Oral antihistamines.

Discussion
The correct answer is D. The development of a new, eczematous rash in an adult patient should raise the concern for a more serious condition. It is rare for an elderly person to develop atopic dermatitis de novo. This may be indicative of an underlying lymphoproliferative malignancy such as cutaneous T-cell lymphoma. Bowen disease (squamous cell carcinoma *in situ*) is another possibility. The most appropriate next step in this patient's management would be skin biopsy.

 QUICK QUIZ: ALLERGY

A 4-year-old girl comes to clinic accompanied by her mother for her yearly checkup. Her mother requests that you examine her daughter's skin because of a rash. Upon examination, you identify scattered reddish-brown macules on the back and chest. When stroked, the lesions urticate. There are no other complaints or abnormalities on physical examination.

What is the most likely diagnosis?

A) Atopic dermatitis.
B) Contact dermatitis.
C) Congenital nevi.
D) Cutaneous lupus.
E) Urticaria pigmentosa.

Discussion
The correct answer is E. This child's rash is most likely secondary to urticaria pigmentosa which is a cutaneous form of mastocytosis. Clinical findings include reddish-brown macules or slightly raised papules, which represent cutaneous accumulations of mast cells. These occur most commonly on extensor surfaces, thorax, and abdomen. When stroked, these lesions can urticate (Darier sign). Urticaria pigmentosa is the most common skin manifestation of mastocytosis in children and adults. Eighty percent of cases appear during the first

year of life. Lesions resolve by adolescence in >50% of patients. The diagnosis is confirmed by skin biopsy. In children, urticaria pigmentosa is rarely associated with systemic disease.

BIBLIOGRAPHY

Balch CM, et al. Final version of the American Joint Committee on Cancer staging system for cutaneous melanoma. *J Clin Oncol.* 2001;19:3635.

Bruckner AL, Frieden IJ. Hemangiomas of infancy. *J Am Acad Derm.* 2003;48;477.

Chartier MB, Hoss DM, Grant-Kels JM. Approach to the adult female patient with diffuse nonscarring alopecia. *J of Am Acad Derm.* 2002;47:809.

Edwards BK, Brown ML, Wingo PA, et al. Annual report to the nation on the status of cancer. *Natl Cancer Inst.* 2005;97(19):1407.

Eichenfield LF, Frieden IJ, Esterly NB. *Textbook of Neonatal Dermatology.* Philadelphia: Saunders, 2001.

Fitzpatrick TB, Johnson RA, Wolff K, Polano MK, Suurmond D. *Color Atlas and Synopsis of Clinical Dermatology.* 5th ed. New York: McGraw-Hill, 2005.

Gilbert DN, Moellering Jr. RC, Ellopoulos GM, eds. *The Sanford Guide to Antimicrobial Therapy.* 37th ed. Sperryville, VA: Antimicrobial Therapy, Inc., 2007.

Graham-Brown R, Bourke J. *Mosby's Color Atlas and Text of Dermatology.* 2nd ed. New York: Mosby, 2005.

Hurwitz S,. Eczemetous Eruptions in Childhood. In: *Clinical Pediatric Dermatology.* 3rd ed. Philadelphia: Saunders, 2005.

Khumalo N, Kirtschig G, Middleton P, et al. Interventions for bullous pemphigoid. *Cochrane Database Syst Rev.* 2003;(3):CD002292.

Ramsey HM, Fryer AA, Hawley CM, et al. Factors associated with nonmelanoma skin cancer following renal transplantation. *J Am Acad Dermatol.* 2003;49(3):397.

Smallpox vaccination: contraindications. Retrieved August 13, 2003, from http://www.CDC.gov.

Sober AJ, Chuang TY, Duvic M, et al. Guidelines of care for primary cutaneous melanoma. *J Am Acad Dermatol.* 2001;45:579.

18

Neurology

Mark A. Graber

CASE 1

A 75-year-old right-handed male presents with dizziness that started 1 hour ago. His dizziness consists of a spinning sensation and he feels off balance as he walks. He reports coughing when trying to drink water earlier, but otherwise notes no symptoms. He has an unremarkable past medical history and is taking no medications. On exam, he is found to have left-sided ptosis and left facial numbness to pinprick. Gag reflex is absent. Motor examination is otherwise unremarkable. Sensory examination revealed decreased pinprick sensation of the right arm and leg. He is unsteady while walking, tending to lean leftward.

What is the most likely diagnosis in this patient?

A) Acute vestibulitis/labyrinthitis.
B) Benign paroxysmal positional vertigo (BPPV).
C) Cerebellar stroke.
D) Brainstem stroke.
E) Ménière attack.

Discussion

The correct answer is D. Although dizziness can be associated with all of the above disorders, a brainstem stroke is the most likely answer. The associated symptoms of ptosis (suggestive of Horner syndrome), absent gag with patient report of possible dysphagia, and crossed sensory findings (left side face, right side body) are most consistent with brainstem localization. In peripheral etiologies of vertigo (answers A, B, E), one would not expect sensory phenomena, ptosis, or swallowing difficulties. In BPPV, one would expect brief

attacks, lasting seconds to minutes, and not a prolonged attack. In Meniere disease, one would generally have a history of tinnitus and/or hearing loss (low-frequency initially). A pure cerebellar stroke would not be expected to have sensory findings.

 HELPFUL TIP: When a patient complains of dizziness, ask what the patient means by "dizziness." Dizziness is defined differently by different patients. The report of "dizziness" may represent vertigo, light-headedness, presyncope, disequilibrium when walking (eg, falling to one side), anxiety, etc.

* *

In considering the management of this patient, TPA (tissue plasminogen activator) was discussed.

Which one of the following is NOT a contraindication to intravenous TPA?

A) Age >75.
B) INR >1.7.
C) Platelets <100,000.
D) Stroke within last 3 months.
E) Glucose <50.

Discussion

The correct answer is A. Acute stroke treatment with thrombolytics **may be** of benefit if administered to carefully selected patients within **3 hours** of symptom onset. When administered properly, the number needed to treat for improvement at 3 months is **6**. However, there is no survival benefit. The risk of hemorrhage is 6% (1 in 16). Of those with symptomatic hemorrhagic transformation, 60% are fatal. There is no age cutoff range for administration of TPA. Strong contraindications include minor or rapidly improving symptoms. In selected patients, there is a role for neurointerventional procedures including intra-arterial TPA. Unlike intravenous TPA, there are no clearly defined criteria for inclusion/exclusion. Generally, patients should be within 6 hours of onset of symptoms and have well-localized symptoms for treatment with intra-arterial, intracranial TPA. See Table 18–1 for contraindications.

> **HELPFUL TIP:** Unfortunately, the experience in the community with TPA for stroke is much worse than in the NINDS study; in real world, community studies there is no benefit and probably harm. Make sure you are **compulsive about inclusion and exclusion criteria!!** Otherwise, your outcomes will be poor.

* *

The patient is outside of the 3-hour window for thrombolysis and has a blood pressure of 200/100.

Table 18–1 CONTRAINDICATIONS TO THE USE OF INTRAVENOUS TPA IN STROKE

Absolute Contraindications
- >3 hours since onset of stroke
- Stroke or serious head trauma within 3 months
- Major surgery within 14 days
- Known history of intracranial hemorrhage
- Symptoms suggestive of subarachnoid hemorrhage (headache, vomiting, stiff neck)
- Sustained blood pressure of >185/110
- GI or urinary hemorrhage within 7 days
- Platelet count of <100,000
- Heparin within last 48 hours that reached therapeutic level or anticoagulation with an INR of >1.7

Relative Contraindications
- Seizure
- Glucose <50mg/dL or >400mg/dL
- Hemorrhagic eye disorder
- Myocardial infarction in last 6 weeks
- Suspected septic embolism
- Infective endocarditis

The best next step in treatment now is to:

A) Administer IV labetalol with a blood pressure goal of 140/90.

B) Administer IV labetalol with a blood pressure goal of 130/85.

C) Administer IV nitroglycerin with a blood pressure goal of 150/90.

D) Administer sublingual nifedipine with a blood pressure goal of 160/95.

E) Monitor the patient's blood pressure and avoid antihypertensives.

Discussion

The correct answer is E. Do not treat this patient's blood pressure unless the blood pressure is >220 mm Hg systolic or 120 mm Hg diastolic. Treating the blood pressure reduces CNS perfusion and puts ischemic brain at risk. Obviously, this does not apply if the patient has a hypertensive urgency or hypertensive crisis (CHF or other end-organ dysfunction—renal, CNS, optic, etc). **Note that this is for ischemic stroke and not hemorrhagic stroke. Lowering the blood pressure to a MAP of 130 mm Hg or so is indicated in hemorrhagic stroke.** Sublingual nifedipine should **never** be used to lower blood pressure in the ED. Absorption is erratic and the effect on blood pressure is unpredictable.

* *

After admission to a monitored bed, which of the following diagnostic evaluations is LEAST likely to be of further benefit in this patient?

A) Fasting lipid profile.

B) Magnetic resonance angiography of the head and neck.

C) Fasting glucose.

D) Carotid duplex examination.

Discussion

The correct answer is D. Carotid duplex can be extremely helpful in determining the degree of stenosis **in the anterior circulation** and is an essential part of the workup for **anterior circulation strokes.** However, in the case of isolated posterior circulation stroke, as in this patient, carotid duplex would be of low yield although it should be done to be complete. In addition to monitoring the patient for signs of neurologic decline or complications, evaluation of potential risk factors for recurrent stroke is an integral part of stroke care. Hypertension, hyperlipidemia, and diabetes mellitus are risk factors for recurrent stroke and should be evaluated. Magnetic resonance angiography (MRA) allows noninvasive evaluation of intracranial and cervical blood vessels in both the anterior and posterior circulation. Echocardiography (not listed above) is also an important part in the evaluation of stroke, especially in the setting of dysrhythmia (eg, atrial fibrillation) or structural heart disease; transesophageal echocardiography is more sensitive for identifying thrombotic sources for stroke etiology when compared to transthoracic echo.

What would be the optimal medical management in this patient for prevention of recurrent stroke?

A) Coumadin (warfarin).
B) Aspirin.
C) Plavix (clopidogrel).
D) Aggrenox (aspirin/dipyridamole).
E) Pletal (cilostazol).

Discussion
The correct answer is B. In patients with a noncardiogenic source for their stroke, there are no data to support the use of anticoagulation (warfarin) in stroke prevention. Similarly, there are no prospective data to support a role for cilostazol or pentoxifylline in the prevention of stroke.

With regard to antiplatelet agents, aspirin is the first-line choice. There is no benefit to dual therapy (ie, clopidogrel (Plavix) and aspirin). If a patient fails aspirin, change to clopidogrel. Finally, the combination of aspirin and dipyridamole (50 mg ASA, 400 mg dipyridamole) is a bit more effective than aspirin alone. Because of cost, most authors recommend aspirin as a primary preventive agent in those who have had a transient ischemic attack (TIA).

 HELPFUL TIP: Patients on a "stroke service" have better outcomes than those taken care of by other services (eg, family medicine). **This is because stroke services are compulsive about evaluation and treatment (swallow studies, early physical therapy, etc).** There is nothing a stroke unit can do that you can't. It just takes being compulsive.

CASE 2

You have a 60-year-old patient who has a simple TIA with left-sided focal weakness. The TIA lasted <10 minutes and the patient has a normal blood pressure and is nondiabetic.

His risk of a having a stroke in the 48 hours after a simple TIA is:

A) 1%
B) 5%
C) 10%
D) 20%
E) 30%

Discussion
The correct answer is A. The overall risk of stroke ranges from 4% to 20% in the 90 days after a TIA. This is a pretty wide range. To narrow the range a bit, the $ABCD^2$ has been developed that takes into account age, duration of symptoms, blood pressure, and diabetes. This can be used to predict the 48-hour risk of stroke.

The acronym $ABCD^2$ stands for:

Age: 1 point for ≥60 years

Blood pressure: 1 point for systolic >140 or diastolic >90

Clinical features: Focal weakness (2 points) or speech difficulty only (1 point)

Duration of symptoms: >60 minutes (2 points), ≤59 minutes (1 point)

Diabetes (1 point).

The 2-day risk of stroke is **0–3 points**: 1%, **4–5 points**: 4.1%, **6–7 points**: 8.1%

Rapid evaluation of the at-risk patient is warranted although it is unclear if earlier interventions make a difference (beyond starting antiplatelet agents, etc).

Which of the following referrals for carotid endarterectomy is most likely to result in a benefit to the patient?

A) A symptomatic **woman** with ≥70% or stenosis to a surgeon who has a 5% complication rate.
B) An asymptomatic **man** with 60% stenosis to a surgeon who has a 7% complication rate.
C) A symptomatic **woman** with a 50%–69% stenosis and a life expectancy of >5 years to a surgeon who has a 5% complication rate.
D) None of the above.

Discussion

The correct answer is A. All sources agree that a symptomatic patient who has ≥70% stenosis will benefit from surgery. Men, but not women, seem to have a benefit with symptomatic stenosis of 50%–69% if there is >5 years life expectancy **and** the surgeon's complication rate is <6% (NNT 22). In asymptomatic patients, those with >60% stenosis will benefit from carotid endarterectomy but NNT is 33 and the benefit is less than those with symptomatic disease.

Objectives: Did you learn to . . .

- Identify signs/symptoms suggestive of acute ischemic stroke (cerebral infarction)?
- Initiate a diagnostic evaluation for a patient with a possible stroke?
- Describe the role of intravenous and/or intra-arterial tissue plasminogen activator in the treatment of acute ischemic stroke?
- Evaluate options for secondary prevention of stroke?

CASE 3

A 24-year-old right-handed woman presents to you in the ED after her second episode of loss of consciousness. The first spell occurred 6 months ago and was associated with a 60-second loss of consciousness and jerking movements of her arms and legs. Following the spell, she was confused for about 15 minutes. At that time, her initial ED evaluation was unremarkable. She presents today following a spell that occurred about 45 minutes ago. Her friends observed her to fall to the ground and shake her arms and legs for about 2 minutes. They could not get her to respond during this time. Afterwards, she was confused and they chose to bring her to the ED. Upon arrival in the ED, she is mildly drowsy but otherwise oriented. She has no memory of the earlier events. Her general medical examination and neurologic examination are unremarkable.

Which of these tests would be LEAST helpful in determining the etiology of this spell?

A) Urine toxicology screen.
B) Electrolytes.
C) Neuroimaging (head CT or MRI).
D) Electrocardiogram (ECG).

Discussion

The correct answer is D. In this patient, ECG would be the lowest yield, as this spell is most suggestive of seizure. Syncopal episodes, which can be caused by cardiac disease, are generally of shorter duration without postictal confusion. Although a few tonic-clonic movements can be seen with syncope (convulsive syncope), it would be atypical for those movements to continue throughout the entire period of loss of consciousness.

All of the other tests would be useful. Evaluation of a first-time seizure should include assessment for alcohol or other drug withdrawal (especially benzodiazepines and barbiturates) as well as drug intoxication (cocaine, methamphetamine, and other sympathomimetics) or withdrawal. Infection, including meningitis and encephalitis, can provoke a seizure. Hyponatremia, hypernatremia, hypocalcemia, hypoglycemia, hyperglycemia, hypomagnesemia, hypophosphatemia, and uremia are all associated with seizures. To rule out structural lesions (eg, tumor, AV malformation, etc) and hemorrhage, neuroimaging should be performed. Although MRI has greater sensitivity, it is often not available in a timely manner, and thus, CT is the modality of choice.

 HELPFUL TIP: All patients with syncope (not seizure), including children, deserve at least one ECG in order to rule out prolonged QT interval, Brugada syndrome, etc. If the spell is not clearly a seizure and could be syncope, get an ECG.

 HELPFUL TIP: One of the most common causes of breakthrough seizures in those with a known seizure disorder is sleep deprivation. Another common cause is poor compliance with medications.

* *

Evaluation in the ED, including electrolytes, CBC, brain CT scan and urine toxicology, is unremarkable. An emergent electroencephalogram (EEG) is obtained in the ED and read as normal. The patient is feeling well and does not wish to remain in the hospital. Her friends assure you that they will be with her over the next 24 hours. She returns to your clinic in 2 days.

After reviewing her test results with her, what do you recommend for further management?

A) Continued follow-up with no further workup or treatment.
B) Video/EEG monitoring.
C) Initiate treatment with antiepileptic drug(s).
D) Tilt table testing.

Discussion

The correct answer is C. This is the patient's second seizure. In adults with a first seizure, between 30% and 60% will go on to have a second seizure. In patients who have a second seizure, the likelihood of going on to have a third is 80%–90%; therefore, after a second unprovoked seizure, treatment is recommended. Video/EEG monitoring is appropriate for classifying spells of unclear etiology. In order for video/EEG to be an effective tool, the patient should have spells frequently enough to capture them during a reasonable inpatient stay (3–7 days average). Tilt table testing would not be of value as syncope is unlikely to be the cause of these spells of loss of consciousness.

* *

You discuss her case with the neurologist who recommends that she start an antiepileptic drug because this is her second unprovoked seizure. "What?" you say. "Start her on an antiepileptic drug? Didn't she have a negative EEG?"

What is the sensitivity of a singe interictal EEG for seizure focus?

A) 20%
B) 30%
C) 50%
D) 60%
E) 90%

Discussion

The correct answer is D. A single interictal EEG has only a 60% sensitivity for picking up a seizure focus. The sensitivity increases to 90% after 3 interictal EEGs. However, this still means that an EEG will be negative in 10% of those with seizures after 3 EEGs.

* *

She has many questions about antiepileptic drugs.

Which of the following drugs is NOT typically associated with weight gain?

A) Depakote (valproic acid).
B) Lamictal (lamotrigine).
C) Tegretol (carbamazepine).
D) Neurontin (gabapentin).

Discussion

The correct answer is B. Depakote, Tegretol, and Neurontin are all associated with weight gain. Gabitril (tiagabine) is also associated with weight gain. Lamictal is typically weight neutral. Felbatol (felbamate) and Topamax (topiramate) are associated with weight loss.

Which of the following adverse effects is NOT typically associated with phenytoin (Dilantin)?

A) Cerebellar atrophy.
B) Hirsutism.
C) Gingival hyperplasia.
D) Stevens-Johnson syndrome.
E) Hypertension.

Discussion

The correct answer is E. Phenytoin (Dilantin) is associated with a number of idiosyncratic effects including cerebellar atrophy, hirsutism, Stevens-Johnson syndrome, and gingival hyperplasia. Diplopia and nystagmus can be prominent side effects, particularly with supratherapeutic doses. Dizziness, drowsiness, fatigue, headache, nausea, vomiting, weight loss, and urine discoloration (pink, red, or reddish-brown) are among the side effects seen with phenytoin. Phenytoin is associated with hypotension and cardiac dysrhythmia (particularly with IV administration) and should **not** be administered through a central line.

Which of the following drugs is NOT Class D for pregnancy?

A) Valproic acid (depakote).
B) Dilantin (phenytoin).
C) Topamax (topiramate).
D) Phenobarbital.
E) Primidone.

Discussion

The correct answer is C. Valproic acid, phenytoin, phenobarbital, primidone, and carbamazepine are all Class D drugs in pregnancy. The newer antiepileptics drugs (AEDs), including Neurontin (gabapentin), Lamictal (lamotrigine), Keppra (levetiracetam), Trileptal (oxcarbazepine), Gabitril (tiagabine), Topamax, and Zonegran (zonisamide) are currently Class C in pregnancy. In particular, valproic acid has a known association with neural tube defects. As a result, it is recommended that **all** women of childbearing age be on folate and a prenatal vitamin while on AEDs. It is **not** recommended that women discontinue AEDs when pregnant, but simplifying to monotherapy is recommended if possible.

 HELPFUL TIP: In the third trimester, vitamin K, 10 mg PO daily, should be administered due to depression of clotting factor levels with many antiepileptics.

Which of the following drugs does NOT have potential interactions with oral contraceptives?

A) Depakote (valproic acid).
B) Tegretol (carbamazepine).
C) Trileptal (oxcarbazepine).
D) Dilantin (phenytoin).
E) Topamax (topiramate).

Discussion

The correct answer is A. Interactions with oral contraceptives (decreasing efficacy of the OCP, **not** the anticonvulsant) have been reported with oxcarbazepine, phenobarbital, phenytoin, lamotrigine, and topiramate. Zonisamide (Zonegran), valproic acid (Depakote), tiagabine (Gabitril), levetiracetam (Keppra), gabapentin (Neurontin), and felbamate (Felbatol) do not interfere with oral contraceptives. A barrier method of contraception, in addition to oral contraceptives, is recommended in women on AEDs, particularly those with known interactions with oral contraceptives.

Which of the following is NOT part of routine counseling with epilepsy and *initiation of therapy with an antiepileptic drug?*

A) Work safety.
B) Calcium and vitamin D supplementation.
C) Driving.
D) Alcohol consumption.
E) Epilepsy surgery.

Discussion

The correct answer is E. Epilepsy surgery is reserved for patients that are intractable to medical management and have failed at least 2 AEDs. Exceptions would include patients with focal pathology (eg, malignancy or vascular malformation). Answer B, calcium and vitamin D supplementation, should be initiated in patients on AEDs due to increased risk of osteoporosis. Answers A and C, work and driving safety issues, should be discussed. Most states have specific laws regarding driving and seizures and the time before resumption of driving privileges varies greatly; check the laws in your state(s) of practice. Epileptic patients should be warned of potentially dangerous activities at work and home (eg, working on ladders, with heavy equipment, bathing, swimming, etc). Answer D, alcohol use, should be discussed with patients. Patients should also be warned of potential factors that could lower their seizure threshold, including alcohol consumption, herbal ephedra supplements, sleep deprivation, infection, and medication non-compliance.

Objectives: Did you learn to . . .

• Evaluate a patient with a potential new diagnosis of epilepsy?
• Identify some areas of specific concern regarding women's issues in epilepsy?
• Recognize commonly encountered or serious side effects with antiepileptic drugs (AEDs)?
• Counsel patients with epilepsy for daily activities and regarding medication management?

 QUICK QUIZ: SEIZURE DISORDERS

All of the following are indicated in the treatment of petit mal seizures (aka absence seizures, aka generalized nonconvulsive epilepsy) EXCEPT:

A) Ethosuximide.
B) Acetazolamide.
C) Valproic acid.
D) Clonazepam.
E) Phenytoin.

Discussion

The correct answer is E. Phenytoin is not indicated in the treatment of petit mal seizures. The other options are indicated. Other drugs known to be useful in petit mal seizures include lamotrigine, phenobarbital, and topiramate. Generally, ethosuximide is considered the first-line drug.

 HELPFUL TIP: For grand mal seizures, valproic acid seems to be the drug that is most effective and thus the best drug to start with. For partial seizures (eg, temporal lobe epilepsy), lamotrigine seems to be the best drug to start with.

CASE 4

A 60-year-old left-handed man presents with complaint of numbness and tingling in his lower extremities for about 10 months. He notes no weakness. He has had diabetes mellitus type 2 for 6 years and has a 30-pack per year smoking history. Examination reveals decreased sensation to light touch, pin prick, and vibratory sensation in the feet extending to 7 centimeters below the knees symmetrically. Chest, abdomen, and upper extremities have normal sensation. His reflexes are 1 + /4 in the upper extremities and quadriceps with absent Achilles bilaterally. The remainder of his neurologic and general medical examination is unremarkable. He says his diet is good but always brings you a dozen donuts when he visits with one or two missing.

This history is most consistent with:

A) Stroke.
B) Early mononeuritis multiplex.
C) Guillain-Barré syndrome.
D) Brown-Sequard syndrome.
E) Peripheral neuropathy.

Discussion

The correct answer is E, peripheral neuropathy. Answer A is incorrect because of the distribution. Bilateral distal lower extremity sensory changes are not likely from a stroke. Answer B, mononeuritis multiplex, is—at least initially—not in a stocking-glove distribution. Patients with mononeuritis multiplex will notice a stepwise loss of feeling/motor ability in discrete nerve distributions. Eventually, these may become confluent and resemble a stocking-glove neuropathy. However, this is found late in the disease. Additionally, there is usually motor involvement. Answer C is incorrect

because Guillain-Barré syndrome has a relatively rapid onset and is associated with motor findings. Answer D, Brown-Sequard syndrome, is the result of a lesion in one side of the spinal cord. Patients have diminished proprioception, vibration sense, and strength on the side of the lesion and decreased sharp sensation and loss of temperature sense on the other side. Because your patient's findings are symmetrical in both distribution and manifestation, it is not likely Brown-Sequard syndrome.

Which of the following lab tests would NOT be useful in helping to determine a *particular cause* of this patient's neuropathy?

A) Serum immunofluorescence electrophoresis.
B) TSH/free T4.
C) Hemoglobin A1C.
D) Electrolytes (Na, K, Cl, CO2).
E) Vitamin B_{12}.

Discussion

The correct answer is D. Electrolytes are not likely to give us a diagnosis in this patient. The initial evaluation of a patient with "stocking-glove" sensory loss should focus on finding potentially treatable causes of neuropathy. These would include hypothyroidism and vitamin B_{12} deficiency. In addition, serum immunofluorescence electrophoresis can help to identify monoclonal gammopathy, which is associated with neuropathy. Hemoglobin A1C is a marker of glycemic control in diabetes and would be associated with diabetic polyneuropathy.

 HELPFUL TIP: A history of alcohol use is important as chronic alcohol abuse is commonly associated with polyneuropathy, even in the absence of vitamin B_{12} or other nutritional deficiencies.

Your patient is on a number of medications. Which of the following medications does NOT cause a peripheral neuropathy?

A) Metronidazole.
B) HMG-CoA reductase inhibitors.
C) Amiodarone.
D) Disulfiram.
E) All of the above can cause a peripheral neuropathy.

Table 18–2 PARTIAL LIST OF CAUSES OF PERIPHERAL SENSORY NEUROPATHY

Infectious
- Syphilis
- Lyme disease
- Mycoplasma
- West Nile virus
- Leprosy

Nutritional
- Vitamin B_{12} deficiency
- Thiamine (vitamin B_1) deficiency
- Folic acid deficiency
- Vitamin B_6 toxicity
- Celiac disease

Drugs
- Metronidazole
- Isoniazid
- Phenytoin
- Thalidomide

Metabolic
- Diabetes
- Hypothyroidism

Toxic
- Mercury
- Thallium
- Other heavy metals
- Alcohol

Miscellaneous
- Amyloid
- Paraneoplastic syndromes
- Mitochondrial disease
- Chronic inflammatory demyelinating polyneuropathy (motor >sensory)

Discussion

The correct answer is E. All of the above can cause a peripheral neuropathy. Some of the other drugs that can cause neuropathy include phenytoin, gabapentin, gold, isoniazid, several chemotherapeutic agents, nitrofurantoin, ddC, and D4T. See Table 18–2 for causes of peripheral neuropathy.

Electrophysiological testing (electromyography and nerve conduction studies, EMG/NCV) can be helpful for all of the following EXCEPT:

A) Confirming the presence of sensory deficits.
B) Identifying subclinical motor deficits.
C) Identifying a specific etiology of the neuropathy (eg, diabetes versus B_{12} deficiency).
D) Determining axonal damage versus demyelination as the primary pathologic process.
E) Differentiating between primarily myopathic versus neuropathic processes.

Discussion

The correct answer is C. EMG and NCV are not capable of yielding results specific to the etiology of neuropathy (eg, identifying diabetic neuropathy versus B_{12} versus syphilis); however, they can yield a pattern suggestive of a particular etiology. For example, increasing motor reaction to repeated stimulation is classic Eaton-Lambert syndrome (a paraneoplastic syndrome), while a decreasing motor response with repeated stimulation is suggestive of myasthenia gravis. These tests can be helpful in confirming the presence of a radiculopathy in the proper clinical setting. They can also determine if the process is primarily axonal (damage directly to the axons/reduction in the number of axons) versus demyelinating (damage to the myelin sheath). NCV can confirm the presence of sensory deficits (although NCV is looking at large fibers and may not identify small-fiber, painful neuropathies) as well as identify subclinical motor involvement. EMG and NCV can be used to differentiate between myopathic and neuropathic processes.

 HELPFUL TIP: If electrophysiological testing shows a primary demyelinating neuropathy, a neurologic consult is recommended. These may respond to IVIG, steroids or other immunosuppressives, and plasma exchange, among others.

* *

After being followed in clinic for several years, the patient begins to complain of a painful, burning sensation developing in his feet and ankles. This pain developed gradually over the last few years in the areas that were numb previously. He has a friend who was started on gabapentin (Neurontin) for a similar problem and is wondering if this would be a good drug for him.

Which of the following is NOT an adverse reaction or contraindication to gabapentin?

A) Dizziness.
B) Peripheral edema.
C) Fatigue and drowsiness.
D) Hepatic failure.
E) Paresthesias.

Discussion

The correct answer is D. Gabapentin (Neurontin) is not hepatically metabolized or cleared. In the setting of renal dysfunction, reduced dosing is necessary. Although gabapentin is generally well tolerated, numerous side effects have been reported. Among the most prominent complaints are those of dizziness, vertigo, and ataxia. Fatigue and drowsiness are also relatively common adverse effects; paresthesias, myalgias, and weakness have also been reported. Peripheral edema (particularly lower extremities) and facial edema are also seen as a result of therapy with gabapentin. Titrating slowly to the target dose over several weeks can improve tolerance.

* *

Your patient is concerned about swelling in his legs, as he has had problems with this in the past and does not want to try gabapentin now.

Which of the following medications would NOT be a reasonable FIRST choice for treatment of painful neuropathy (not specifically in this patient but in general)?

A) Amitriptyline.
B) Topical Lidoderm patch.
C) Oxycodone.
D) Capsaicin cream.
E) Valproic acid.

Discussion

The correct answer is C. Narcotics are not the treatment of choice for peripheral neuropathy and tend not to be as effective in this setting as in other types of pain. **Tricyclic antidepressants are commonly used in the setting of neuropathic pain and remain the first-line therapy.** The evidence for TCAs suggests they are superior to other classes of drugs. If pain is confined to a small area, a topical treatment such as capsaicin cream or a Lidoderm patch may be effective. The use of Lidoderm patches outside the setting of postherpetic neuralgia is an off-label use.

 HELPFUL TIP: Other treatments for neuropathic pain once the patient has failed a TCA include valproic acid and carbamazepine. Newer antiepileptics such as gabapentin (Neurontin), and topiramate (Topamax) should be third-line treatments. Finally, methadone is more effective than other opiates for neuropathic pain.

What is the most common INFECTIOUS cause of peripheral neuropathy in the world (not just in the U.S.)?

A) HIV.
B) Lyme.
C) Leprosy.
D) Hepatitis C.

Discussion

The correct answer is C. The most common infectious cause of peripheral neuropathy in the world is leprosy. Leprosy (Hansen disease) is caused by *Mycobacterium leprae*, an acid-fast bacillus. It usually presents with a hypopigmented anesthetic patch. The sensory deficits start with loss of temperature sensation followed by loss of pain and then tactile sensations. Modalities carried by the posterior columns (proprioception and vibration) are spared. Sensation in the palms, soles, mid-chest, and mid-back is preserved until late in the disease.

Lyme disease is caused by *Borrelia burgdorferi* and is transferred by the *Ixodes* tick. Early neurologic manifestations of Lyme disease include lymphocytic meningitis, cranial neuropathy (a Bell's palsy-like picture) or painful radiculoneuritis. Guillain-Barré syndrome and mononeuritis multiplex can be seen early in the course of Lyme disease. Advanced (late) neurologic complications of Lyme disease include peripheral neuropathy and encephalomyelitis.

Human Immunodeficiency Virus type 1 (HIV-1) can cause a peripheral neuropathy. The most common neuropathy is a symmetric, distal polyneuropathy. Autonomic dysfunction and mild weakness accompany distal paresthesias and burning sensations with sensory loss. Keep in mind that many of the medications used in HIV-1 therapy are also associated with peripheral neuropathies.

Hepatitis C and hepatitis B can cause peripheral nerve manifestations. Hepatitis B has been associated with Guillain-Barré syndrome (demyelinating) and mononeuritis multiplex. Hepatitis C is also associated with multiple mononeuropathies.

 HELPFUL TIP: In the United States, diabetes and alcohol use disorders are the most common causes of peripheral neuropathy.

Objectives: Did you learn to . . .

- Recognize common etiologies of peripheral neuropathy?
- Identify appropriate uses of electrophysiological testing?
- Identify types of neuropathy that are potentially treatable?
- Prescribe medical therapy for painful peripheral neuropathy?

 QUICK QUIZ: WRIST DROP

Which of the following is most likely to cause an isolated wrist drop?

A) C-3 disk lesion.
B) Ulnar nerve compression.
C) Radial nerve compression.
D) C-4 disk lesion.
E) Median nerve compression.

Discussion

The correct answer is C. Compression of the radial nerve (such as sleeping with someone's head on your arm) can cause an isolated wrist drop (aka "Saturday night palsy"). Suspect alcohol or other drug abuse in patients with this lesion. It is pretty hard to get this type of compressive lesion if you are not passed out or very sedated. Answer B, ulnar nerve compression (cubital tunnel syndrome), presents with pain and numbness in the elbow and fourth and fifth fingers and weakness of the intraosseous muscles (weakness with spreading fingers). Answer E, median nerve compression (including carpal tunnel syndrome), leads to numbness on the palmar surface of the thumb and fingers 2, 3 and the radial 1/2 of 4. There is weakness and perhaps atrophy of the thenar muscles (unable to maintain opposition of thumb to fifth finger against resistance).

CASE 5

A 25-year-old female presents to your clinic with complaint of a bifrontal headache that started this morning. She describes the pain as throbbing and 8/10 in severity. She is complaining of photophobia and nausea. She has had similar headaches in the past, lasting hours to 1 day. She is unable to work during these headaches and prefers a dark, quiet, room. The physical examination, including neurologic exam, is unremarkable.

Which of the following statements is most accurate?

A) She likely does not have migraine headaches because her headache is bilateral.
B) She likely dose not have migraine headaches because they most commonly present between 40 and 50 years.
C) She likely does not have migraine headaches because they rarely occur in the morning.
D) She likely has migraine headaches.

Discussion

The correct answer is D. She likely has migraine headaches. Migraine headaches may vary considerably in severity, time of day, and characteristics. The International Headache Society (IHS) has a useful classification system with criteria for the diagnosis of migraine headaches (Table 18–3).

Answer B is incorrect because migraine headaches typically present in the first 3 decades of life. Attacks

Table 18–3 CRITERIA FOR THE DIAGNOSIS OF MIGRAINE WITHOUT AURA

At least five attacks fulfilling the following criteria:
Headache lasting 4–72 hours (untreated or unsuccessfully treated)
Headache has at least 2 of the following characteristics: • Unilateral location • Pulsating quality • Moderate or severe intensity (inhibits or prohibits daily activities) • Aggravation by walking stairs or similar routine physical activity
During headache at least 1 of the following: • Nausea and/or vomiting • Photophobia **and** phonophobia
No evidence of organic disease

typically last <1 day although they may occasionally last longer. Migraine headaches are typically moderate to severe in intensity, may occur at any time during the day, and occur with or without aura. Most migraine headaches are unilateral, preceded by aura, and accompanied by nausea and vomiting. They are more prevalent among women, with a 1-year prevalence rate of approximately 18% in women, 6% in men, and 4% in children. Family history is important as 80% of patients with migraine headache have a first-degree relative with migraines.

Migraine headaches were formerly classified as classic type (migraine with aura) and common type (migraine without aura.) Typical auras develop over several minutes and last for <60 minutes. Auras may involve visual, language, sensory, or motor deficits. The visual auras are the most common and may appear as photopsias (flashes of light), scotomas (blind spots), or complex shapes that build or move across the visual field. The IHS criteria for migraine with aura are listed in Table 18–4.

 HELPFUL TIP: The IHS criteria are meant as research criteria rather than strict clinical criteria. Although patients with a certain type of migraine headache will ideally meet all criteria, it is not necessary to meet all criteria to make a clinical diagnosis of migraine headache.

* *

You have decided to treat this woman's migraine headache.

Table 18–4 CRITERIA FOR THE DIAGNOSIS OF MIGRAINE WITH AURA

At least 2 migraines fulfilling at least 3 of the following characteristics:
- One or more fully reversible aura* symptoms indicating brain dysfunction.
- At least 1 aura symptom develops gradually ≥5 minutes, or 2 or more symptoms occur in succession.
- No single aura symptom lasts >60 minutes.
- Headache begins during aura or within 60 minutes of the end of the aura.

History, physical, and appropriate diagnostic tests exclude a secondary cause.

*An aura should have symptoms from 2 neurologic domains—visual and/or sensory and/or speech. The symptoms may be positive (eg, flickering lights, pins/needles sensation) or negative (eg, scotoma, numbness).

Which medication would be LEAST appropriate for acute management of her headache?

A) Oral ibuprofen.
B) Intranasal sumatriptan.
C) IV meperidine (Demerol).
D) Intranasal DHE.

Discussion

The correct answer is C. The least appropriate treatment from the above list would be meperidine (Demerol). The long-term use of opiates for rescue therapy has not been found to improve the quality of life in patients with migraines.

Oral noninflammatory antiinflammatory agents (NSAIDs) (answer A), including aspirin and combination analgesics containing caffeine, are a first-line choice for mild to moderate migraine attacks or severe attacks that have been NSAID-responsive in the past. Answer B, the "migraine specific" treatments, commonly called the "triptans" (eg, sumatriptan, zolmitriptan, naratriptan, rizatriptan, almotriptan, eletriptan, and frovatriptan), are effective and relatively safe for the acute treatment of migraine headaches. Triptans are an appropriate initial treatment choice in patients with moderate to severe migraines who have no contraindications to their use. Recall, however, that the patient populations studied by pharmaceutical companies all meet the research definition of "migraine." Thus, the "triptans" may not be as effective in an unselected, primary care population. Alternative vasoconstrictive agents, including DHE nasal spray (dihydroergotamine) (answer D), can provide a safe and effective treatment of acute migraine attacks. DHE can be administered IV as well. Vasoconstrictive side effects, including the risk of coronary artery spasm, should specifically be discussed with patients prior to initiation of therapy.

 HELPFUL TIP: Adding oral metoclopramide to aspirin or NSAIDs will improve their rate of success. Part of the nausea and vomiting from migraines (and the reason that oral medications often do not work) is from gastric paresis. Metoclopramide overcomes this problem and treats nausea as well.

Which of the following statements is true?

A) If a patient doesn't respond to sumatriptan, there is no point in trying another triptan since the patient will not respond.

B) DHE and sumatriptan may be safely used within the same 24-hour time period.

C) Sumatriptan use is contraindicated in patients with known coronary artery disease, regardless of age.

D) Flushing, sweating, and paresthesias after a dose of sumatriptan is an indication of a severe reaction and continued use of this medication is contraindicated.

Discussion

The correct answer is C. The triptans should not be used in patients with known coronary disease. Patients that do not respond to one triptan may respond to other triptans, and a trial of other triptans is appropriate. Also, a patient may respond initially to a triptan but not respond on other occasions. Each triptan has a maximum recommended dose and a good rule of thumb is that the initial dose may be repeated once in a 24-hour period. However, avoid the use of DHE within 24 hours after a triptan has been given due to increased vasoconstriction and the possibility of vasospasm.

Contraindications to the use of triptans include all of the following EXCEPT:

A) Lung cancer.

B) Coronary artery disease.

C) Uncontrolled hypertension.

D) Use of an MAO inhibitor within the last 2 weeks.

E) Use of an ergot preparation within the last 24 hours.

Discussion

The correct answer is A. Lung cancer is not a contraindication to the use of triptans. In addition to answers B–D, caution should be used in patients with history of stroke, known cardiac risk factors, and impaired liver function.

HELPFUL TIP: Common reactions to triptans include jaw tightness, flushing, anxiety, dizziness, and sweating. These are uncomfortable but not dangerous. Serious reactions to triptans include coronary vasospasm, anaphylaxis, or hypertensive crisis in patients with known CAD, hypersensitivity to triptans, or uncontrolled hypertension.

HELPFUL TIP: Consider dexamethasone as an adjunct therapy in severe headache. A single dose of dexamethasone 10 mg PO, IV or IM after abortive therapy (eg, triptan, antiemetic, etc) in the ED **may** prevent headache recurrence in patients who have had a headache for >24 hours. However, there is conflicting evidence for this approach.

* *

Your patient has decided to take ibuprofen for her headaches. This medication seemed to be effective at first, but she notes for the last several weeks that she is taking 2–3 doses of ibuprofen per day without significant headache relief. She has had a dull bilateral headache that is moderate in severity for the last 2 weeks. She has no personal or family history of coronary artery disease.

Which of the following statements is true?

A) She likely has a tension headache and should increase her frequency of ibuprofen and continue to take it on a daily basis.

B) She likely has a medication-overuse headache in addition to chronic migraine headache (status migrainous) and should taper and then discontinue ibuprofen.

C) A medication such as sumatriptan used on a daily basis does not increase the risk of rebound headache.

D) She likely does not have medication-overuse headache because opiates are the only medications that increase the risk of these headaches.

Discussion

The correct answer is B. See Discussion below.

Which of the following medications taken on a frequent basis is LEAST likely to cause medication-overuse or rebound headache?

A) Sumatriptan.

B) Morphine.

C) Ibuprofen.

D) Amitriptyline.

E) All of the above are equally likely to cause rebound headache.

Discussion

The correct answer is D. Frequent use of opiates, ergotamine, triptans, and any other analgesics may put a patient at risk for medication-overuse or rebound headache. Although analgesic rebound headache characteristics can vary significantly, the patient typically reports a pattern of headache that decreases modestly in severity with the use of their analgesic of choice, and then in 2–4 hours (depending on the medication) the headache returns to its previous severity or worsens further. Failure to repeat analgesic use results in a withdrawal headache (similar to the caffeine withdrawal headaches physicians often experience when they miss their morning coffee). In the case of triptans, the headache may not worsen for many hours or even until the next day, but a cycle of regular use of the medication is still established. At this time, no clear consensus on the duration of therapy necessary to produce analgesic rebound is reported. As a general rule, it is best to limit the use of these types of medications to no more than 2–3 headache days per week. In addition, limit the patient's analgesic use to no more than 2–3 weeks per month. Patient education is the most important part of therapy in treating analgesic rebound or medication-overuse headaches.

 HELPFUL TIP: Treatment of rebound headaches consists of discontinuing the medication. Several approaches have been tried to reduce headaches after the analgesic has been withdrawn. These include IV or oral steroids, long-acting NSAIDs (naproxen) and elective admission and therapy with IV DHE (dihydroergotamine). These should be combined with amitriptyline (or other tricyclic) used on a daily basis as preventive therapy. Patients can also take hydroxyzine and promethazine when they have a breakthrough headache; these medications do not cause rebound headaches.

Which of the following medications would be the LEAST appropriate for the preventative treatment of your patient's migraine headaches?

A) Verapamil.
B) Propranolol.
C) Amitriptyline.
D) Clonazepam.

Discussion
The correct answer is D. Clonazepam is not commonly used as a preventive treatment for migraine headaches.

Keep in mind the common side effects of these medications and the appropriateness in your specific patient. For example, valproate would be a bad choice for many patients secondary to weight gain. Propranolol may cause hypotension. Amitriptyline may cause cognitive difficulties, constipation, and urinary retention—especially in elderly patients. Topiramate (Topamax) may cause weight loss, and impaired cognition is common.

 HELPFUL TIP: A number of medications are useful in the prevention of migraine headaches.
Medications that have been found to have medium to high efficacy, good strength of evidence, and mild to moderate side effects include amitriptyline (and likely other tricyclics), divalproex sodium, and propranolol/timolol.
Medications of lower efficacy include atenolol/metoprolol/nadolol, nimodipine/verapamil, aspirin/naproxen/ketoprofen, fluoxetine, ACE inhibitors, gabapentin, feverfew, magnesium, and vitamin B_2.
Antidepressants such as fluvoxamine, paroxetine, nortriptyline, sertraline, trazodone, and venlafaxine have also been found to be clinically efficacious based on consensus and clinical experience, but no scientific evidence of efficacy has been established. Efficacy has also been demonstrated for the antiepileptic drugs valproic acid (Depakote) and topiramate (Topamax); other antiepileptic drugs have been tried as well, although there is little to no evidence to support their use at this time.

 HELPFUL TIP: Combination products like butalbital/caffeine/acetaminophen/codeine (eg, Fiorinal with codeine) have a limited, if any, role in the treatment of migraine or other headaches. They have no role in treatment or prophylaxis of chronic daily headaches. Addiction, abuse, and diversion are potential issues with these drugs.

Which one of the following medications is rated Class B or better in pregnancy?

A) Phenergan (promethazine).
B) Imitrex (sumatriptan).
C) Codeine.
D) Amitriptyline.
E) None of the above.

Discussion

The correct answer is E. Headache treatment in pregnancy remains a difficult problem. Although numerous medications are available for headache treatment, their safety in pregnancy has not been established. Amitriptyline and valproic acid are class D in pregnancy. Other commonly used tricyclics include imipramine (class C) and nortriptyline (class D); venlafaxine is Class C. Promethazine, prochlorperazine, codeine, hydrocodone, and meperidine are all class C. Ergotamine (DHE 45) is class X. The triptan class of medications, including sumatriptan, remains class C.

In which of the following patients is neuroimaging LEAST likely to be useful?

A) A 30-year-old woman with a headache typical of a migraine.
B) A 23-year-old woman with a history of migraine headaches who is very concerned because her current headache of 1-week duration is more severe than her typical migraine headaches.
C) A 60-year-old man with new headache, worse in the morning and of 6-weeks duration.
D) A 40-year-old man with a headache and right arm weakness.

Discussion

The correct answer is A. According to the U.S. Headache Consortium, neuroimaging is not typically recommended in **migraine** patients with a normal neurologic examination. Imaging may be considered in patients who are disabled by their fear of serious pathology or if the provider is suspicious about underlying pathology. Factors that may lead one to consider neuroimaging include a nonacute, atypical headache or unexplained abnormal neurologic examination. There is not enough evidence to support or refute neuroimaging in patients with headaches that are not migrainous in nature.

Objectives: Did you learn to . . .

- Recognize and diagnose migraine headaches?
- Initiate appropriate acute therapy for migraine headaches?
- Identify contraindications and adverse reactions of the triptan medications?
- Recognize and treat analgesic-related headaches?
- Identify appropriate preventive therapy for chronic headaches?

CASE 6

A 30-year-old woman presents to your office with a 2-day history of progressive, **unilateral** arm (proximal and distal) numbness without weakness. She has been diagnosed with fibromyalgia in the past. She is taking fluoxetine for depression and has a history of previous hospitalizations for depression.

Which of the following is the most appropriate next step?

A) Monitor her symptoms and reassure her that her numbness is likely related to her fibromyalgia.
B) Order nerve conduction (NCV) studies.
C) Order a head CT.
D) Get additional history; ask about previous similar episodes or other neurological concerns.
E) Order a chest radiograph and complete blood count.

Discussion

The correct answer is D. With the history of a progressive neurological deficit, the first step in the workup is to further explore the history. Frequently, patients will not mention previous neurologic symptoms because they—the symptoms, not the patients—are vague.

* *

When she is asked about previous spells, she notes that she had an episode of left leg numbness that lasted about 1 week several years ago, but she thought nothing of it as it was mild. Six months ago she had a 3-day visual disturbance in her right eye, during which she found it difficult to read and focus on objects; no blind spot was noticed. However, she had pain in the eye, especially when moving it.

What is the most likely diagnosis based upon the history given?

A) Multiple sclerosis.
B) Fibromyalgia.
C) Conversion disorder.
D) Migraine.

Discussion

The correct answer is A. Multiple sclerosis (MS) would be the most likely diagnosis based upon the history related above. MS most commonly presents in women aged 20–35 years and men aged 35–45 years. It is almost 5 times more prevalent among women than men and is more common in the white population. MS is a central nervous system demyelinating disease that is thought to occur by an immune-mediated process. The demyelinating lesions of MS can occur anywhere in the CNS including the brainstem and spinal cord. The presenting symptoms of MS vary, but common symptoms are visual complaints, weakness, and sensory deficits. Although migraine can be associated with neurologic symptoms, one would expect more stereotypic events and a history of previous headaches. Fibromyalgia is associated with numerous somatic complaints, but is not typically associated with sensory deficits or visual problems. Conversion disorder can produce all of the symptoms described above but is a diagnosis of exclusion.

HELPFUL TIP: MS has a geographic predilection. The incidence of MS increases with increasing distance from the equator. Various theories have suggested an association with sunlight exposure, vitamin D, or ethnicity.

If your patient indeed does have multiple sclerosis, which type is most likely?

A) Devic disease.
B) Relapsing-remitting.
C) Primary progressive.
D) None of the above.

Discussion

The correct answer is B. The two common forms of MS are primary progressive and relapsing-remitting. The diagnosis of relapsing-remitting MS is based on clinical grounds and laboratory data. Clinically, symptoms of CNS dysfunction develop over hours to days, stabilize, and then improve. It is important to identify clinical events disseminated in space and time. In this case, your patient had a prior history of optic neuritis and lower extremity numbness and now has arm numbness. Answer A, Devic disease (neuromyelitis optica), is a central nervous system demyelinating illness that is characterized by **bilateral** optic neuritis, which may be simultaneous or may occur at different times, and spinal cord demyelination.

Which of the following tests would NOT be helpful in further diagnosing MS?

A) MRI brain.
B) Lumbar puncture.
C) Nerve conduction studies.
D) Visual evoked potentials.

Discussion

The correct answer is C. Multiple sclerosis is a central demyelinating process and does not produce abnormalities that would be seen on nerve conduction studies. Answer A, an MRI, would be helpful. Brain MRI is 85%–97% sensitive in detecting MS plaques. Multiple areas of increased signal in the periventricular area are suggestive but not specific for MS. Gadolinium enhancing lesions suggest active disease. Answer B, an LP, can also be useful. CSF abnormalities suggestive of MS include oligoclonal bands and increased synthesis of IgG. A spinal fluid examination may be considered if the clinical diagnosis of MS is suspected but is not definite; however, the positive and negative predictive value of CSF oligoclonal bands is inadequate to do more than support the clinical diagnosis. Recent evidence for serum antibody testing to other myelin components has yielded promising initial results as a supportive diagnostic tool. Answer D, visual evoked potentials may be helpful. Evoked potential may be used to aid in the diagnosis MS by indicating prior demyelination of the optic tract (optic neuritis) if the clinical history is vague (eg, eye pain without vision loss or no recollection of symptoms). This will aid in proving the occurrence of different events separated by space and time.

Which of the following is NOT a recognized therapy for MS?

A) Corticosteroids.
B) Interferon-beta.

C) Glatiramer acetate.
D) Sulfasalazine.
E) Amantadine.

Discussion

The correct answer is D. Sulfasalazine is not useful in the treatment of MS. Immune modulating therapy reduces the number of exacerbations and active lesions on MRI. These include interferon beta 1a (Avonex and Rebif) and interferon beta 1b (Betaseron) as well as glatiramer acetate (Copaxone). These medications are more efficacious if started early in the course of the disease. Common adverse affects of interferon include fatigue, depression, and myalgias. Amantadine is given commonly as monotherapy and in combination with immunomodulatory therapy to treat fatigue associated with multiple sclerosis. Corticosteroids have a role in treating severe acute exacerbations (eg, optic neuritis, severe neurological impairments limiting activities of daily living) in the form of a short burst and taper (typically methylprednisolone 1 g per day, which may be in divided doses, for 3 days followed by oral prednisone taper). Oral steroid use does not appear to offer long-term functional benefit, excluding the possible exception of IV pulsed steroid dosing. Currently, oral immunosuppressive therapies (mycophenolate mofetil, azathioprine, and cyclosporin) are being considered in treating refractory multiple sclerosis, but their long-term efficacy and safety are not known. Similarly, the value of IVIG and plasma exchange has not been conclusively demonstrated and use of these treatment modalities is reserved for refractory patients.

Which of the following treatments would you most likely choose for this patient, given her history of depression?

A) Avonex (interferon beta 1a).
B) Amantadine.
C) Copaxone (glatiramer acetate).
D) Betaseron (interferon beta 1b).

Discussion

The correct answer is C. The interferon agents (Avonex, Rebif, and Betaseron) and amantadine are associated with worsening of depression. Given this patient's history of severe depression requiring hospitalization, one would favor Copaxone as an initial therapy, although treatment with interferon is not absolutely contraindicated.

* *

The patient is wondering what she can do to prevent exacerbations.

Which of the following is associated with exacerbation of MS symptoms?

A) Cold temperatures (you could recommend she move to Florida).
B) Urinary tract infection.
C) Influenza vaccination.
D) Trauma.

Discussion

The correct answer is B. Urinary tract infections can exacerbate multiple sclerosis. Unfortunately, urinary tract infections are particularly common in those with MS because of the frequent occurrence of neurogenic bladder. Systemic infection has also been reported to provoke multiple sclerosis exacerbations. Answer A is of special note. Cold is not associated with exacerbations, **but heat is** notorious, and this phenomenon actually has a name—Uhthoff phenomenon. Patients with MS should be instructed to avoid hot tubs, saunas, steam rooms, etc. Answer C, vaccinations, including influenza vaccine, had been posited as a cause of exacerbations. However, a review of multiple clinical trials showed no increased risk of exacerbations in patients with multiple sclerosis receiving the influenza, hepatitis B, or tetanus vaccinations. **Note that we do not have experience with nasal influenza vaccine and multiple sclerosis. Since the nasal vaccine contains live virus, it should probably be avoided in patients with multiple sclerosis.** Answer D, trauma, has been suggested as a possible exacerbation trigger, but the American Academy of Neurology clinical practice guidelines state that the majority of class II evidence available on this issue supports no connection.

Objectives: Did you learn to . . .

- Identify demographic characteristics of multiple sclerosis (MS)?
- Identify appropriate workup for patients with possible MS?
- Diagnose MS?
- Discuss potential treatment options available for long-term disease modification as well as acute exacerbations?
- Recognize factors that might result in exacerbations of MS?

CASE 7

A 43-year-old woman with a history of myasthenia gravis presents to the ED while on vacation. She reports she is feeling tired and run-down and endorses flu-like symptoms in addition to some worsening of her proximal lower extremity weakness. On examination, she is afebrile with a respiratory rate of 18. She has mild diplopia with lateral gaze. Her strength is 4/5 proximally and 4 + /5 distally bilaterally. Her sensory examination is normal. Plantar responses are downgoing bilaterally.

In determining this patient's further disposition, what is the most important test?

A) Arterial blood gas (ABG).
B) Chest radiograph (CXR).
C) Head CT.
D) Forced vital capacity (FVC).
E) Complete blood count (CBC).

Discussion

The correct answer is D. This patient is experiencing an exacerbation of her myasthenia gravis. This could be occurring for any number of reasons including concurrent illness or possibly noncompliance with her regimen. The greatest morbidity and mortality for this patient lie in the potential for respiratory failure and arrest. In primary neuromuscular respiratory failure (eg, myasthenia gravis, acute inflammatory demyelinating polyradiculoneuropathy, or Guillain-Barré syndrome), the arterial blood gas may remain normal despite impending respiratory collapse. The best way to evaluate respiratory status is with the forced vital capacity (FVC). If the FVC is <15 mL/kg, elective intubation is recommended, although some centers will choose to monitor these patients closely in an intensive care setting without initial intubation. Monitoring the FVC should be done regularly throughout the hospital course until the patient is clinically improved and stable.

* *

You decide to give this patient a dose of edrophonium to try to reverse her symptoms. When you do this she becomes increasingly weak, requiring intubation.

The BEST explanation of this is:

A) Because she has missed multiple doses of her pyridostigmine, she has become desensitized and will have an overwhelming response to small doses of IV edrophonium.
B) Influenza has made her particularly susceptible to edrophonium.
C) The patient has taken too much pyridostigmine by accident.
D) The alcohol which she has had on vacation has changed her pyridostigmine requirement.

Discussion

The correct answer is C. Myasthenic crisis can be due to two causes. First, the patient may have not taken enough medication or may have missed doses. In this case, edrophonium will improve symptoms. The second cause is **too much** pyridostigmine. This will also cause weakness. In this case, the edrophonium will worsen the patient's symptoms.

 HELPFUL TIP: Pyridostigmine and edrophonium are both cholinesterase inhibitors similar to organophosphates. They act by binding to acetylcholinesterase and preventing the breakdown of acetylcholine. Thus, too much of either drug (or a combination of the drugs) will cause weakness and an organophosphate toxicity-like syndrome (salivation, lacrimation, defecation, urination, weakness, etc).

Which of the following is NOT likely to contribute to the diagnosis of myasthenia gravis?

A) Tensilon (edrophonium) test.
B) Nerve conduction studies.
C) Anti-thymocyte antibodies.
D) Anti-acetylcholine receptor antibodies.

Discussion

The correct answer is C. Antithymocyte antibodies are used to treat renal rejection and have also been used in aplastic anemia, red cell aplasia, and other disorders. They have no relationship at all to myasthenia gravis. All of the others can be used in the diagnosis of myasthenia gravis. The edrophonium test is a functional test. One must be ready to intubate the patient when performing an edrophonium test. Nerve conduction studies show a reduction in the amplitude of the response to repeated stimulation (thus, patients get weaker with repeated muscle use). Antiacetylcholine receptor antibodies are found in the majority (80%–90%) of patients with myasthenia gravis. When an ultrasensitive test is done, it is found in 70% of "antibody negative" cases of myasthenia gravis.

 HELPFUL TIP: Myasthenia gravis can be systemic or limited to the ocular muscles. It is often associated with a thymoma (or thymus hyperplasia), and patients with myasthenia gravis should have a chest CT scan to rule out thymoma or thymus hyperplasia. If present, removal of the thymoma will often "cure" the patient's disease.

Which of the following is LEAST likely to be confused with myasthenia gravis on the basis of its neurologic symptoms?

A) Eaton-Lambert syndrome.
B) Guillain-Barré syndrome.
C) Amyotrophic lateral sclerosis.
D) Botulism toxicity.
E) Penicillamine-induced myasthenia gravis.

Discussion
The correct answer is B. Guillain-Barré syndrome includes sensory findings of pain, paresthesias, numbness, etc, that are generally absent in the other syndromes. Answer A, Eaton-Lambert syndrome, is a paraneoplastic process which consists of weakness **that gets better with repetitive movement.** This is the opposite of what is seen with myasthenia gravis where repetitive tasks lead to increased weakness. Thus, Eaton-Lambert syndrome is often worse in the morning and better towards the afternoon—the reverse of what is seen with myasthenia gravis. Patients with ALS, botulism, and penicillamine-induced myasthenia gravis do not have sensory symptoms. Thus, these can be confused with myasthenia gravis.

* *

The patient and her husband have some questions about myasthenia gravis and are wondering if there are any medications that might exacerbate this patient's weakness.

Which of the following can worsen myasthenia gravis?

A) Fluoroquinolones.
B) Verapamil.
C) β-Blockers.
D) Oral contraceptives.
E) All of the above can exacerbate myasthenia gravis.

Discussion
The correct answer is E. All of the above can worsen myasthenia gravis. Other drugs of note include aminoglycosides, anesthetic and paralytic agents, diuretics, tetracyclines, and magnesium among many others.

Objectives: Did you learn to . . .

• Manage a patient with an exacerbation of myasthenia gravis?
• Understand the use of diagnostic tests in myasthenia gravis?
• Recognize diagnoses that can be confused with myasthenia gravis?

CASE 8

A 29-year-old female presents to the ED with sudden onset of a severe headache involving **bilateral occipital** pain associated with nausea. The headache has not responded to her sumatriptan (Imitrex) injection. She has a history of migraine headaches consisting of **right-sided throbbing** pain that typically respond to sumatriptan but occasionally require IM hydroxyzine and morphine. She appears to be in moderate pain but otherwise has a normal general and neurological examination. This is the worst headache of her life.

What is the next step in the management of this patient?

A) Ketorolac (Toradol) IM or IV.
B) Aspirin plus metoclopramide.
C) IV Dihydroergotamine (DHE).
D) Head CT.
E) Lumbar puncture.

Discussion
The correct answer is D. Although this patient has a history of migraines, she is reporting a sudden onset

headache that is markedly changed from her typical pattern of headache. In this setting—especially with the "worst headache of her life"—the diagnosis of sub-arachnoid hemorrhage (SAH) must be ruled out. Requiring a CT before LP is dogma which is unsupported in the literature. None of the other answers is correct. While pain management can be given before CT (eg, IV morphine or fentanyl), ketorolac, aspirin, and DHE are inappropriate if there is a question of SAH. Ketorolac and aspirin have antiplatelet effects which can increase bleeding. DHE can cause vasospasm and worsen brain ischemia. Finally, if you recall, this patient tried her sumatriptan. One should not use DHE within 24 hours of a triptan.

 HELPFUL TIP: Did you notice that the patient usually gets hydroxyzine and morphine IM? IM hydroxyzine has been known to cause severe muscle necrosis and should be avoided.

The patient's head CT is negative. What do you do next?

A) Lumbar puncture.
B) IV hydroxyzine and meperidine and discharge when the patient is comfortable.
C) IV hydroxyzine and promethazine (Phenergan) and discharge when the patient is comfortable.
D) Discharge home with prescription for acetaminophen and oxycodone (Percocet).
E) Discharge home with prescription for rizatriptan (Maxalt).

Discussion

The correct answer is A. In the setting of a worst headache of life, a CT scan to rule out subarachnoid hemorrhage (SAH) is required. The sensitivity of CT scan of the brain for hemorrhage in the setting of SAH is 90%–95% within 24 hours of the event (decreases to 80% at 72 hours). As a result, **a negative head CT does not adequately rule out SAH** and should be followed with a lumbar puncture. The cerebrospinal fluid from the lumbar puncture must be spun down immediately to examine for xanthochromia; delay in examining the CSF may result in false-positive results. Xanthochromia is a yellow discoloration of the normally clear CSF resulting from degradation of hemoglobin.

In addition to xanthochromia, markedly elevated RBC counts are indicative of SAH. If either the CT or LP are positive for SAH, an emergent 4-vessel cerebral angiogram (or MR-angiogram or CT-angiogram) is indicated.

 HELPFUL TIP: 39% of patients with SAH have no neurologic signs or symptoms. Only 10% of patients with SAH have an initially focal exam. Patients with SAH may have a fever and leukocytosis. Although looking at the patient's fundi is important, the absence of papilledema does not rule out SAH. SAH can present as back pain. Since each bleed carries 50% mortality, this is one diagnosis you do not want to miss. Use LP liberally in appropriate patients.

Objectives: Did you learn to . . .
* Identify a patient presenting with symptoms of sub-arachnoid hemorrhage?

CASE 9

A 40-year-old male with diabetes presents with a complaint of low back pain that is dull in nature, which started 2 days ago. This morning he woke up with a feeling of numbness in his feet, which gradually seemed to worsen. By noon, he noted difficulty walking and decided to come to the ED. He denies bowel or bladder incontinence. On exam, he is in no acute distress and has a respiratory rate of 12. He has strength 5/5 in his upper extremities, and in his lower extremities strength is 4/5 proximally and 3/5 distally. Sensory examination reveals a mild decrease in pinprick and light touch in a stocking distribution to the mid-calf. Reflexes in the upper extremities are 2 + /4 and in the lower extremities are trace at the knees and absent at the Achilles. Plantar response is down going bilaterally.

What is the most likely diagnosis?

A) Diabetic polyneuropathy.
B) Guillain-Barré syndrome.
C) Diabetic amyotrophy.
D) Stroke.

Discussion

The correct answer is B. Of the choices given above, the most likely diagnosis is acute inflammatory demyelinating polyradiculoneuropathy (Guillain-Barré syndrome). With an acute onset of bilateral lower extremity weakness and sensory deficits, the diagnosis of an acute cord-compressing lesion (eg, tumor, epidural abscess) should also be considered and ruled out, especially with back pain. The time course described above is not consistent with diabetic polyneuropathy nor would one expect to see weakness as a prominent symptom. Diabetic amyotrophy is characterized by painful **proximal** muscle weakness with minor sensory loss. The onset of diabetic amyotrophy can be subacute or acute. The time course described above of gradually progressing deficits is not consistent with stroke. Additionally, the findings of a stroke should not be bilateral.

Which of the following is/are associated with Guillain-Barré syndrome?

A) *Campylobacter jejuni* infection.
B) Lyme disease.
C) Epstein-Barr virus.
D) CMV virus.
E) All of the above.

Discussion

The correct answer is E. All of the above are associated with Guillain-Barré syndrome. Other associations include URIs, HIV, immunizations (rare), mycoplasma, epidural anesthesia, sarcoid, lupus, etc. The point here is that one should look for an underlying illness in patients with Guillain-Barré disease.

 HELPFUL TIP: Antibodies to *Campylobacter* have recently been shown to cross-react with nerve tissue. Thus, the association of *Campylobacter* with Guillain-Barré syndrome.

Which of the following actions would NOT be appropriate for additional diagnosis and/or management?

A) Cardiac monitoring.
B) Forced vital capacity (FVC).

C) Discharge to home on steroids with a follow-up in the morning.
D) Electromyography/nerve conduction velocity (EMG/NCV).

Discussion

The correct answer is C. This patient should not be sent home. This is especially true since his disease has worsened rapidly over the last 12 hours. As with other potential causes of neuromuscular respiratory failure, a forced vital capacity (FVC) is necessary to determine adequate respiratory reserve (15 ml/kg is the cutoff for elective intubation). The FVC should be monitored closely during the acute illness. Guillain-Barré syndrome can have a rapid and catastrophic worsening that necessitates monitoring during the acute phase of illness. Typically, patients reach the peak of severity about 2 weeks into the illness. Autonomic dysfunction is associated with GBS, and close cardiovascular monitoring, including telemetry, is important. EMG/NCV can be of value in diagnosing Guillain-Barré syndrome—although early on in the course of the disease these tests may be normal.

* *

A diagnosis of Guillain–Barré syndrome is made.

Which of the follow is NOT an appropriate treatment modality?

A) Intravenous immunoglobulin (IVIG).
B) Plasma exchange (PLEX).
C) Elective intubation if FVC <15 cc/kg.
D) Corticosteroids.

Discussion

The correct answer is D. Treatment options for GBS include careful monitoring of disease with no intervention, IVIG, or PLEX. Corticosteroids are not used in the treatment of GBS. Multiple studies have shown no benefit to corticosteroids in this disease. If a patient requires ventilatory support or has weakness that precludes ambulation, treatment should be started immediately. Elective intubation is appropriate if the FVC is <15 cc/kg. As discussed in regard to neuromuscular respiratory failure with myasthenia gravis, arterial blood gases are not reliable markers of impending failure, and the FVC must be closely monitored. Cardiac monitoring is appropriate given the prominent autonomic fluctuations that are seen in many patients with the syndrome.

* *

The family would like to know what the outcome in this patient with Guillain-Barré syndrome will be.

You let them know that FULL RECOVERY can be expected in the following percentage of patients:

A) 15%
B) 50%
C) 80%
D) >95%

Discussion

The correct answer is A. Fifteen percent of all patients with GBS will have **complete** resolution of their symptoms. Sixty-five percent will be left with minor deficits, and approximately 10% will become disabled. Despite excellent care, some patients still die.

 HELPFUL TIP: West Nile virus infection can present either as a Guillain-Barré syndrome (symmetrical neurological symptoms with loss of reflexes) or a poliomyelitis syndrome (generally asymmetrical weakness with worse weakness proximally, loss of reflexes, fasciculations).

 HELPFUL TIP: In addition to the FVC, another helpful measurement in those with neurologic disease is the negative inspiratory force (NIF). If the NIF is ≤25 mm H₂O (eg, with myasthenia gravis or GBS), elective intubation should be considered.

Objectives: Did you learn to . . .

- Recognize the clinical presentation of Guillain-Barré syndrome?
- Identify underlying illnesses that are associated with GBS?
- Manage a patient with GBS?

CASE 10

A 38-year-old female is brought to the ED by her husband who expresses concerns over changes in her mental status over the past 2 days. She has become confused, forgetting the names of persons well known to her, and forgetting what she is doing. Her conversations have become increasingly more difficult to follow, and over the past 12 hours she has gradually become sleepier. On examination, she has a temperature of 38°C. She is drowsy but can be aroused. She has no meningismus. She is oriented only to person. She responds to questions slowly and incorrectly and follows only simple commands (stick out your tongue). The remainder of her neurological examination is essentially normal, given her limited ability to cooperate. Complete blood count, coagulation studies, and electrolytes (including calcium, magnesium, and phosphorous) are normal.

What is the best next step in evaluating this patient?

A) Lumbar puncture.
B) Head CT.
C) EEG.
D) Chest radiograph.

Discussion

The correct answer is B. Although performing all of the above tests will be helpful in evaluating this patient, the most important test to do at this time is a head CT to rule out any mass lesion or hemorrhage. You could argue that answer A, an LP, could be done first and you would technically be correct. However, the standard in the United States is to do the CT scan first if there is any possibility of a mass lesion. There is a possibility that nonconvulsive status epilepticus is causing these mental status changes. However, even if the EEG showed nonconvulsive status epilepticus, a head CT and lumbar puncture would be necessary. Although pneumonia could cause confusion, a chest radiograph is unlikely to be of high yield in this setting.

* *

Her head CT is normal. Lumbar puncture revealed 18 WBCs (all lymphocytes), 12 RBCs, CSF protein 67 mg/dL (elevated), and CSF glucose 70 mg/dL (normal). An EEG is normal.

What is the next step in managing this patient?

A) Admit for viral encephalitis with close monitoring.
B) Admit for viral encephalitis and start acyclovir.
C) Admit for bacterial meningitis and start antibiotics.
D) Discharge to home with close follow-up tomorrow at 8 a.m.

Discussion

The correct answer is B. The probable diagnosis in this setting is herpes simplex encephalitis. Her CSF results are consistent with a viral process and are not consistent with bacterial meningitis (due to the normal glucose and only lymphocytes in the differential). Given the mortality of herpes simplex encephalitis (30%–70%), all patients in whom the diagnosis is suspected should be started on acyclovir 10 mg/kg q8h IV empirically (with appropriate dosage adjustments for renal failure), while further confirmatory testing is pending (CSF PCR for the herpes simplex virus). Treatment should be for a minimum of 10 days and has been advocated (with little evidence to support it) to be as long as 21 days. It is important to recognize that the EEG and CT may be normal in herpes simplex encephalitis, particularly early in the disease. On CT, one may see evidence of temporal lobe hemorrhage and/or hypodensity in the temporal lobes. EEG can show either periodic lateralized epileptiform discharges or focal slowing in the temporal lobes. Temporal lobe changes may be even more prominently visualized on MRI, and this may be of benefit in cases in which the diagnosis remains unclear. Even with prompt, appropriate treatment, only 38% of patients returned to normal or near normal neurologic functioning at 2 years.

Objectives: Did you learn to . . .

- Recognize the clinical presentation of and the laboratory findings in viral encephalitis?
- Initiate appropriate treatment in a patient with a presumptive diagnosis of herpes encephalitis?

CASE 11

A 70-year-old male presents to your office as a new patient. He is with his wife, who assists in providing the history. His appetite is reduced, and he has lost 10 pounds in the past 6 months. His only medication is aspirin, and he has no significant past medical history. On exam, his vital signs are normal, and he is in no acute distress. His gait is slow, and he takes 8 steps to turn. He has retropulsion (takes 2 steps backward when you pull him from behind). There is a resting tremor in both hands but more prominently in the right. You find cogwheel rigidity in both arms as well. His cognitive screening tests are normal.

The most likely diagnosis is:

A) Essential tremor.
B) Parkinson disease.
C) Normal pressure hydrocephalus (NPH).
D) Progressive supranuclear palsy.
E) Stroke.

Discussion

The correct answer is B. This patient most likely has Parkinson disease. Answer A is incorrect because essential tremor is typically worsened by activity and is not associated with the other neurologic findings seen in this patient. Answer C is incorrect. The classic triad of NPH includes urinary incontinence, gait ataxia, and dementia. Answer D might be a consideration, but there is no specific finding of progressive supranuclear palsy here (eg, aggressive course, more severe axial rigidity, and downward gaze paresis). Stroke is quite unlikely to present in this insidious fashion with generalized findings. However, there is a controversial entity called "vascular parkinsonism" in which lacunar infarcts of the basal ganglia are thought to cause parkinsonism.

Which of the following is NOT a common feature of idiopathic Parkinson disease?

A) Rigidity.
B) Extraocular movement paresis.
C) Bradykinesia.
D) Loss of postural reflexes or gait disturbance.

Discussion

The correct answer is B. There are four cardinal features of Parkinson disease: tremor, bradykinesia, rigidity, and postural instability. Two or more of these features should be present to make the diagnosis. The tremor of Parkinsonism is a resting tremor (as opposed to the postural, intention or action tremor) and is most common in the hands. Rigidity (answer A) is described as increased resistance to passive movement and may be reinforced by having the patient open and close the fist on the opposite hand. Cogwheel rigidity is a ratchet-like sensation noted when testing a limb with concurrent tremor. Bradykinesia (answer C) may be observed by monitoring the speed and amplitude of movements. Gait disturbance (answer D) with reduced stride length and stooped posture is a common finding but generally occurs later in the course of the disease. Postural reflexes and ability to rise from a chair are also impaired. Postural reflexes may be tested by retropulsion.

* *

You are fairly certain that your patient has Parkinson disease.

What else might you find with idiopathic Parkinson disease?

A) Micrographia.
B) Extraocular movement paresis.
C) Apraxia.
D) Autonomic dysfunctions.
E) Alien limb phenomenon.

Discussion

The correct answer is A. Micrographia, writing in small letters, is associated with Parkinson disease. The others are not. This is important because there are a number of neurologic syndromes that can mimic Parkinson disease. Decreased facial expression (hypomimia) with decreased rate of eye blink and diminished vocal volume (hypophonia) are also common with Parkinson. Other conditions that occur in patients with Parkinson disease include depression, cognitive impairment, and REM sleep behavioral disorder.

 HELPFUL TIP: There are "Parkinson Plus" syndromes, so called because they present with parkinsonian features with another characteristic. Look for these syndromes in those that you believe may have Parkinson disease:

Progressive supranuclear palsy, which is associated with supranuclear gaze palsy and axial rigidity.
Shy-Drager syndrome, which is notable for autonomic dysfunction, including marked orthostatic hypotension.
Cortico-basal ganglionic degeneration, which is associated with apraxia, cortical sensory dysfunction, and the "alien limb phenomenon." Alien limb phenomenon occurs when the patient's arm moves by itself (eg, will reach up to touch the patient's face). The patients do not believe that the limb belongs to them. Spontaneous limb movements also occur when the patient is startled or the limb is touched (anyone see Dr. Strangelove?).

The diagnosis of Parkinson disease is most appropriately made:

A) With a brain MRI.
B) By CSF analysis.
C) Clinically.
D) By a neurologist.

Discussion

The correct answer is C. The diagnosis is based on a history and physical examination that are consistent with Parkinson disease. Additionally, a response to dopaminergic agents is consistent with the diagnosis of Parkinson disease. Answer A is incorrect because there are no findings on neuroimaging that are specific for the diagnosis of Parkinson. Answer B is incorrect because CSF analysis cannot provide the diagnosis. Anwer D is clearly incorrect—do you really need a neurologist for this? The "gold standard" for diagnosis is neuropathologic exam, but you would rather not wait for the autopsy to diagnose Parkinson.

 HELPFUL TIP: Up to 10% of patients with Parkinson disease will have some degree of intention tremor in addition to their rest tremor.

* *

Your patient takes only aspirin, which you know is not a cause of Parkinsonism.

Which of the following medications is frequently associated with a Parkinson-like syndrome in the elderly?

A) ACE inhibitors.
B) HMG-CoA reductase inhibitors.
C) Calcium channel blockers.
D) Metoclopramide.
E) All of the above.

Discussion

The correct answer is D. Metoclopramide is a frequent cause of the misdiagnosis of Parkinson disease in the elderly. Additional medications, such as SSRIs, antipsychotics, and others, can mimic Parkinson disease. **Drug-induced parkinsonism may last for up to 6 months after discontinuation of the offending agent.**

* *

You think it best to initiate treatment in this patient.

Possible treatments of Parkinson disease include all of the following EXCEPT:

A) Levodopa.
B) Pallidotomy.
C) Pramipexole.
D) Donepezil.
E) Selegiline.

Discussion

The correct answer is D. Donepezil is used to treat Alzheimer disease. The initial symptoms of Parkinson disease typically respond well to levodopa and the dopamine agonists. Selegiline is a monamine oxidase B inhibitor and yields modest symptomatic benefits. Dopamine receptor agonists, such as pramipexole (Mirapex), ropinirole (Requip), and bromocriptine, are important medications that may be used in the initial treatment of Parkinson disease.

 HELPFUL TIP: If a patient does not respond to levodopa/carbidopa, question your diagnosis. Parkinson patients should "always" respond to levodopa/carbidopa. Often the response is dramatic and occurs within hours, but sometimes patients will need to take levodopa/carbidopa for longer before a response is seen.

 HELPFUL TIP: Surgical options for advanced Parkinson disease include pallidotomy and deep brain stimulation (DBS). In general, stimulation of the thalamus is used to treat tremor but has little impact on the other symptoms of Parkinson disease (bradykinesia, etc.). Subthalamic nucleus stimulation is more beneficial for ameliorating the other features of Parkinson disease, but may have a less profound impact on tremor.

Which of the following is NOT a common side effect of levodopa?

A) Nausea.
B) Paresthesias.
C) Dyskinesia/dystonia.
D) Hallucinations.

Discussion

The correct answer is B. Paresthesias are not associated with the use of carbidopa/levodopa. The use of carbidopa with levodopa allows the dose of levodopa to be optimized. Carbidopa helps to prevent levodopa-induced nausea (answer A). Dystonia and dyskinesia (answer C) are common with therapy >2 years or at peak dose responses and may necessitate lowering the doses. Psychiatric problems (answer D), including hallucinations and psychosis, can be seen with dopaminergic agonists and levodopa. Other common side effects of levodopa include hypotension, confusion, and other psychiatric disturbances.

 HELPFUL TIP: Levodopa is a dopamine precursor, and carbidopa is a peripheral dopa decarboxylase inhibitor that does not cross the blood-brain barrier. The symptoms of tremor, rigidity, and bradykinesia are initially relieved by levodopa. However, with time, larger doses are required to maintain control of symptoms.

 HELPFUL TIP: One of the dopamine agonists (pramipexole, ropinirole, bromocriptine) can be used to help minimize the dose of levodopa needed, thus minimize the side effects of levodopa.

* *

You decide to start levodopa/carbidopa (Sinemet) and bromocriptine. At the follow-up visit, the patient is doing relatively well on this combination. However, he notices that in the mornings and evenings he tends to be stiff and has difficulty ambulating.

The most appropriate next step is to:

A) Initiate a "drug holiday" to restore the patient's sensitivity to the drug.
B) Add another dopaminergic agent such as ropinirole (Requip).

C) Add a COMT inhibitor such as entacapone (Comtan).

D) Add an anticholinergic agent such as benztropine (Cogentin).

Discussion

The correct answer is C. The patient is experiencing the "wearing-off" phenomenon. There are several ways to address this. One option is to add a drug such as entacapone (Al Capone's brother?). Tolcapone (Tasmar) and entacapone (Comtan) are catechol-O-methyl-transferase (COMT) inhibitors and slow the metabolism of levodopa. COMT inhibitors have no effect on their own and should only be used with levodopa. Another option is to switch the patient from immediate-release carbidopa/levodopa to a sustained-release product (eg, Sinemet CR). The effectiveness of this strategy is not conclusively proven, and there is no benefit from using controlled-release carbidopa/levodopa as the initial agent in Parkinson. Another common approach to the wearing-off phenomenon is altering the dosing of carbidopa/levodopa—either increasing the dose or shortening the interval between doses.

 HELPFUL TIP: Tolcapone (Tasmar) is associated with fatal hepatic necrosis and requires monitoring of LFTs. Thus, entacapone (Comtan) is the preferred drug.

 HELPFUL TIP: Patients with nausea in response to carbidopa/levodopa may need additional carbidopa to control their nausea. This is available from DuPont free of charge. It also helps to take carbidopa/levodopa with food.

* *

When you counsel your patient regarding medication use, you urge him not to stop taking his medication all at once.

Which of the following is NOT a potential adverse effect of abrupt discontinuation of dopaminergic agonists and/or levodopa?

A) Neuroleptic malignant syndrome (NMS).

B) Severe rigidity.

C) Confusional state.

D) Severe dyskinesias.

Discussion

The correct answer is D. Levodopa and dopamine agonists should be tapered. Abrupt discontinuation of these medications may precipitate neuroleptic malignant syndrome (NMS). In addition, abrupt withdrawal is also associated with an acute confusional state separate from the mental status changes seen in NMS. Severe worsening of the patient's parkinsonism is expected, which can result in prominent rigidity. Dyskinesias are frequently seen with dopaminergic agonist/levodopa **therapy**, but are not exacerbated or triggered by **withdrawal** of these agents.

 HELPFUL TIP: Diagnostic criteria for definite NMS include hyperthermia, muscle rigidity, and 5 of the following: mental status changes, tremor, tachycardia, incontinence, labile blood pressure, metabolic acidosis, tachypnea/hypoxia, elevation of creatine kinase, diaphoresis/sialorrhea, and leukocytosis. Treatment includes supportive care as well as the use of bromocriptine and propranolol, although there is limited data to support the use of either agent. **Dantrolene is ineffective.**

* *

A year later your patient returns and seems to be doing well. You ask him about symptoms of Parkinson disease, if he is having any adverse effects of medications, and if he is experiencing any of the Parkinson-associated diseases.

Which of the following is NOT associated with Parkinson disease?

A) Depression.

B) Dementia.

C) REM sleep disorder.

D) Narcolepsy.

E) Decreased visual contrast sensitivity.

Discussion

The correct answer is D. Narcolepsy has not been associated with Parkinson disease. However, excess daytime sleepiness has been associated. This is likely due to a combination of factors, such as sleep disturbance, depression, dopaminergic drugs, and Parkinson disease itself. Depression is commonly seen in Parkinson disease and is reported to occur in up to 41% of patients. Dementia, typically with Lewy bodies, present on pathological analysis, is seen and can affect the decision to proceed with surgical treatment of Parkinson disease, as patients with advanced dementia get less benefit from surgery. Also, REM sleep behavior disorders are seen in Parkinson disease and can be a source of stress for families and caretakers. REM sleep behavior disorder is characterized by acting-out of dreams that can consist of vocalizations as well as active and even violent movements. Typically REM sleep behavior disorder responds to clonazepam. Finally, decreased visual contrast sensitivity can occur with Parkinson disease as well.

 HELPFUL TIP: The dopamine agonists (pramipexole, ropinirole, etc) have been associated with compulsive behavior (sexual compulsion, compulsive gambling, etc). This may explain why some elderly patients like to go to Las Vegas and Atlantic City.

 HELPFUL TIP: Pergolide is no longer on the market because of cardiac valvular fibrosis.

Objectives: Did you learn to . . .

- Identify common features of Parkinson disease?
- Diagnose Parkinson disease?
- Manage a patient with Parkinson disease?
- Understand pharmacotherapy available for Parkinson disease and some of the potential adverse effects of drug therapy?

CASE 12

A 45-year-old left-handed woman who is a busy executive with a Fortune 500 company presents with excessive daytime sleepiness. She is otherwise healthy and takes no medications. How do you approach this problem?

A) Reassure her that it is normal for people to be drowsy under stressful work conditions.
B) Begin zolpidem at night for sleep.
C) Schedule the patient for polysomnography.
D) Discuss the patient's sleep hygiene.
E) Administer modafinil (Provigil) prior to important board meetings.

Discussion

The correct answer is D. It is essential that all patients with complaints of either insomnia or excessive daytime sleepiness have a thorough sleep history taken. Polysomnography may be necessary, but this test—like all diagnostic tests—should be driven by a hypothesis. A history is necessary to develop a hypothesis and determine a test's utility. Starting hypnotic agents (answer B) or stimulant (answer E) without thoroughly investigating the underlying problem may cover up significant, treatable problems and is considered bad form.

Which of the following is NOT an important aspect of a sleep history?

A) Sleeping and waking times.
B) Use of stimulants and alcohol.
C) Sleep interruptions (children, pagers, etc).
D) Work schedule.
E) Listening to "soft rock" ("easy listening" or "adult contemporary").

Discussion

The correct answer is E. Maybe this one was too easy, but we hate "easy listening" music. The Geneva Convention prohibits its use on prisoners of war we've been told. All ranting aside, this tidbit of her history has no bearing on her sleep. Important parts of the sleep history include the sleeping environment (alone, with spouse or other individual, in the daylight hours, etc), nap history, family history of sleep problems, and symptoms of specific sleep disorders (snoring, hypnagogic hallucinations, etc). A medication history is important as well as a history of watching TV in bed, eating in bed, etc, which indicate poor sleep hygiene.

 HELPFUL TIP: One of the favorite parasomnias of the editors is "exploding head syndrome" (this is real, not a joke). Patients have the feeling of popping or explosions occurring in their head as they fall asleep. Another great diagnosis is "moss brain," an archaic term for a type of CNS disease.

Which of the following is NOT part of a typical sleep study?

A) Monitoring of EEG.
B) Monitoring respirations and oxygen desaturations.
C) Evaluating the sleep latency in response to sleep aids, such as zolpidem and trazodone, to maximize effective pharmacologic therapy.
D) Monitoring EMG.
E) Video monitoring of sleep.

Discussion

The correct answer is C. Sleep studies are generally done in the naïve state without the use of medications. All of the rest are true. Answers D and E require special note. Answer D, monitoring EMG, informs the physician about muscle activity during sleep. Answer E, video monitoring and taping, allows the physician to look for problems, such as awakening, evidence of restless leg syndrome, sleep apnea, etc.

In considering a diagnosis of narcolepsy, which of the following is NOT part of the diagnosis?

A) Cataplexy.
B) Sleep paralysis.
C) Hypnagogic hallucinations.
D) Sleep myoclonus.
E) Excessive daytime sleepiness.

Discussion

The correct answer is D. Sleep myoclonus (hypnagogic jerks) are commonly seen in normal people as they begin to fall asleep (witness colleagues at grand rounds with sudden tossing of the head) and is not a part of narcolepsy. Narcolepsy is a disorder characterized by four cardinal traits, although not all need be present to make the diagnosis: cataplexy, excessive daytime sleepiness, sleep paralysis, and hypnagogic hallucinations.

Answer A, cataplexy, is a sudden loss of voluntary muscle control during which the patient may appear to be asleep; however, cataplexy does not have to be accompanied by sleep attacks, and the patient may be aware throughout the attack. Answer B, sleep paralysis, can occur either at the onset of sleep or upon awakening and can be quite frightening to the patient. Answer C, hypnagogic hallucinations, are vivid and typically fearful dreams that occur at the onset of sleep but can also occur upon awakening (hypnopompic hallucinations). Answer E, excessive daytime sleepiness, is a hallmark of narcolepsy and can include sleep attacks as well as persistent drowsiness and "microsleep" (brief intrusions of sleep during a waking state). The complete tetrad of symptoms is seen in only 10% of patients with narcolepsy.

Which of the following is NOT a treatment for narcolepsy?

A) Amitriptyline.
B) Clonazepam.
C) Fluoxetine.
D) Modafinil (Provigil).
E) Sodium oxybate.

Discussion

The correct answer is B. Clonazepam is not a treatment for narcolepsy. Treatment of narcolepsy can be divided into two primary goals. The first goal is to address daytime sleepiness, which is primarily done with stimulants such as modafinil or methylphenidate. The second goal is to reduce the symptoms of cataplexy. This can be accomplished with agents such as tricyclic antidepressants, and to a lesser extent, selective serotonin reuptake inhibitors. Sodium oxybate (aka gamma hydroxy butyrate) can be used for treatment of cataplexy as well as sleep hallucinations and sleep paralysis. Some evidence suggests it may also help with excessive daytime sleepiness. Given its street popularity and abuse potential (including date rape), prescriptions are centrally controlled nationally for this medication at the time of this publication.

* *

After a thorough history, you find nothing to suggest narcolepsy besides daytime sleepiness. Of course, you are considering other diagnoses simultaneously.

Which of the following would NOT suggest a possible diagnosis of obstructive sleep apnea?

A) Difficulty falling asleep.
B) Frequent nighttime arousals.
C) Obesity.
D) Paroxysmal nocturnal dyspnea.
E) Snoring.

Discussion

The correct answer is A. Difficulty falling asleep is not one of the components of obstructive sleep apnea. Snoring, obesity, excessive daytime sleepiness, and paroxysmal nocturnal dyspnea are all associated with obstructive sleep apnea. Some patients will note frequent arousals from sleep with or without accompanied shortness of breath.

 HELPFUL TIP: It is important to note that not all patients with sleep apnea are overweight, and this diagnosis must be considered in all patients with excessive daytime sleepiness or other suggestive symptoms. Small oropharyngeal airway (especially in **thin** women) and gastroesophageal reflux are associated with sleep apnea.

What treatment options would NOT be appropriate to consider in your patient if she has obstructive sleep apnea?

A) Bilevel positive airway pressure (BiPAP).
B) Continuous positive airway pressure (CPAP).
C) Positional therapy.
D) Uvulopalatopharyngoplasty (UPPP).
E) Zolpidem.

The correct answer is E. Sleep aids, including benzodiazepines, do not have a role in the treatment of obstructive sleep apnea and may worsen symptoms. CPAP and BiPAP are both potential treatments. Polysomnography (sleep testing) with titration of CPAP or BiPAP should determine which modality to use and the pressure settings. These should not be arbitrarily set to the "normal settings" for a patient. Positional therapy, avoiding sleeping on one's back, may be effective in some patients. Some techniques for achieving this goal include sewing an object on the back of the pajama shirt that will irritate the patient when he or she rolls onto it. Weight loss, although not mentioned above, can provide improvement in symptoms as well. Surgical therapies including uvulopalatopharyngoplasty can also be considered based upon the patient's symptoms and preferences.

* *

Your patient's sleep study shows that she has restless legs syndrome.

Which would be a FIRST-LINE agent for treatment of restless legs syndrome?

A) Clonazepam.
B) Codeine.
C) Methadone.
D) Pramipexole
E) Tramadol.

Discussion

The correct answer is D. Restless legs syndrome is characterized by an urge to move the lower extremities, due most often to an uncomfortable sensation. This sensation usually occurs during rest and is typically relieved by moving the legs. Dopaminergic agents, either levodopa (eg, Sinemet) or agonists, such as ropinirole (Requip) and pramipexole (Mirapex), are the first-line treatments for restless legs syndrome. Benzodiazepines such as clonazepam and narcotic medications such as methadone and codeine as well as the non-narcotics tramadol and gabapentin have all been reported to be successful alternative therapies for restless leg syndrome.

What other workup would you suggest for this patient once the diagnosis of restless legs syndrome is made?

A) No further workup is indicated, initiate treatment as above.
B) Serum calcium.
C) Serum iron studies, including ferritin.
D) Serum vitamin B_{12}.
E) Serum vitamin B_6.

Discussion

The correct answer is C. Recent studies have shown a link between low iron stores and restless legs syndrome. All patients with restless legs syndrome should have an iron profile performed, and low iron or ferritin levels merit iron supplementation. Other associations are diabetes, pregnancy, end-stage renal disease, Parkinson disease, venous insufficiency, folate deficiency, and caffeine intake (dump that fourth cup of coffee).

 HELPFUL TIP: The editors are skeptical about the sudden "outbreak" of restless legs syndrome now that there are patented drugs with an indication for treating restless legs syndrome. Amazing how drug advertising can influence physicians and the public.

Objectives: Did you learn to . . .

- Take an appropriate sleep history?
- Generate a differential diagnosis for daytime sleepiness?
- Gain familiarity with the diagnostic testing used in a sleep laboratory?
- Identify the presentations of and treatments for common sleep disorders, including narcolepsy, obstructive sleep apnea, and restless legs syndrome?

CASE 13

A 60-year-old right-handed male presents with the complaint of head pain.

Which of the following historical descriptions is of the LEAST value in identifying a specific diagnostic classification for head/face pain?

A) Right-sided, electric, stabbing pain involving primarily the cheek, occurring for seconds to minutes repeatedly throughout the day.

B) Right-sided, electric, stabbing pain involving primarily the throat, tongue, and right ear.

C) Right-sided severe headache involving the orbit and associated with lacrimation and rhinorrhea typically occurring in groups.

D) "Sinus pressure" with a history of sinus headaches responsive to antibiotics in the past.

E) Pattern of severe right-sided "stabbing and boring" headaches that began at approximately 30 years and are alleviated with scheduled indomethacin.

Discussion

The correct answer is D. Sinus headaches are typically a diagnosis of exclusion. Acute sinusitis can cause severe head and face discomfort, but **sinusitis remains a relatively uncommon etiology for recurrent head and face pain. Most countries outside the United States and Canada do not recognize "sinus headaches" as a diagnostic or treatable entity.** The specific headache syndromes described in answers A, B, C, and E are described in more detail in the following discussions.

* *

If this patient gives you the history of right-sided severe headache involving the orbit associated with lacrimation and rhinorrhea typically occurring in groups, which of the following

would you use for initial acute treatment of this headache syndrome?

A) Naproxen.

B) Oxygen.

C) Tylenol.

D) Verapamil.

Discussion

The correct answer is B. The type of headache syndrome described is most consistent with cluster headaches. These are most commonly seen in men and are characterized by exquisite pain, typically centered at the orbit. Conjunctival injection, rhinorrhea, and lacrimation frequently accompany the headache. Pain is often disabling. As the name suggests, the patient tends to have headaches in groups (or clusters). These headaches are more common at night, and REM sleep is thought to be a triggering factor. For acute treatment, conventional headache medications such as DHE and the triptans can be effective. Treatment with high-flow oxygen has also shown significant efficacy as an abortive treatment: typical protocol would be 8 L oxygen on nonrebreather for 15 minutes, with reports of 70% of patients achieving headache relief. Verapamil can be effective for prophylaxis but is not effective as an abortive. Other, more typical migraine prophylactic agents (propranolol, topiramate, indomethacin, valproic acid) have been tried, but no systematic studies have been done to evaluate their efficacy in cluster headaches.

* *

If your patient describes a history of severe right-sided "stabbing and boring" headaches that began at approximately 30 years and are alleviated with scheduled indomethacin.

This would be most consistent with which of the following headache syndromes?

A) Tension headache.

B) Paroxysmal hemicrania.

C) Migraine without aura.

D) Chronic daily headache.

E) Analgesic rebound headache.

Discussion

The correct answer is B. Paroxysmal hemicrania is classically described as a unilateral headache with a stabbing/boring character. Although age of onset can vary greatly, it classically occurs in women in their thirties (although it can be seen in men as well). Patients will have between 2 and 40 episodes during a given day, although they do not cluster together as is typical in cluster headaches. Although autonomic symptoms (rhinorrhea, lacrimation, conjunctival injection, and ptosis) can be seen in a majority of patients, these headaches can be differentiated from clusters by the pattern of recurrence (sporadic throughout the day versus in clusters); significant overlap between the two headache syndromes does exist and differentiation can be difficult. Paroxysmal hemicrania typically is exquisitely sensitive to indomethacin, and response to indomethacin is highly correlated with this diagnosis.

Migraine headaches (answer C) typically do not occur multiple times in 1 day and are usually described as a throbbing pain. Chronic daily headaches (answer D) as well as analgesic rebound headaches (answer E) generally are continuous in nature with limited, if any, periods of time without some degree of headache. Chronic daily headache in the setting of prolonged analgesic use is highly suggestive of analgesic rebound headache. The duration of analgesic therapy necessary to trigger and propagate these headaches remains uncertain. However, it can be as little as 3 times per week.

* *

With further history, your patient describes right-sided, electric, stabbing pain involving primarily the cheek and occurring for seconds to minutes repeatedly throughout the day.

What would be a first-line choice for therapy of this entity?

A) Carbamazepine.
B) Amitriptyline.
C) Ibuprofen.
D) Morphine.
E) Microvascular decompression (Janetta procedure).

Discussion

The correct answer is A. This description is typical of trigeminal neuralgia. Carbamazepine has been shown to be effective in treating trigeminal neuralgia and was used for treatment of this disorder prior to being used for seizures. Tricyclic antidepressants, opioids, and NSAIDs are not first-line agents for treatment. Typically, NSAIDs are of limited, if any, benefit in this setting. Other agents that have been used for treatment

with at least anecdotal reports of benefit include gabapentin, oxcarbazepine, clonazepam, baclofen, phenytoin, and topiramate. Microvascular decompression (the Janetta procedure) can be effective in alleviating pain from trigeminal neuralgia (tic douloureux), which is described in the question. However, medical therapy remains the first-line treatment.

> **HELPFUL TIP:** A unilateral electric, stabbing pain occurring in the tongue, oropharynx, and occasionally extending to the ipsilateral ear has been described; this is known as **glossopharyngeal neuralgia**. Treatment of glossopharyngeal neuralgia is similar to the pharmacologic treatment of trigeminal neuralgia described above. If the patient complains of stabbing eye or temporal headaches lasting seconds, consider the diagnosis of "jolts and jabs" headaches (aka "ice pick" headaches). They occur 40–50 times a day or more and are likely a migraine variant.

Objectives: Did you learn to . . .

• Describe the features of various headache syndromes?
• Initiate treatment for cluster headaches, paroxysmal hemicrania, and trigeminal neuralgia?

CASE 14

A 55-year-old male with a history of diabetes and prostate carcinoma presents to your office with complaints of back pain, groin numbness, and an inability to initiate voiding.

The most likely explanation for these symptoms is:

A) Cauda equina syndrome.
B) Urinary outlet obstruction secondary to prostate carcinoma.
C) Hydroureter and hydronephrosis secondary to urolithiasis.
D) Neurogenic bladder from long-standing diabetes.
E) All of the above are equally likely.

Discussion

The correct answer is A. This is a presentation of cauda equina syndrome. Cauda equina syndrome is caused by compression of the cauda equina at the level of L4 or L5 by a protruding disk, tumor, etc. Symptoms include progressive fecal or urinary incontinence (secondary to inability to initiate voiding), impotence, distal motor weakness, and sensory loss in a saddle distribution. Answer B is incorrect. This patient's symptoms are not likely to be due to urinary outlet obstruction. Urinary outlet obstruction should not be associated with inability to initiate voluntary voiding (although voiding may not work so well) and should not be associated with sensory changes in a saddle distribution. The same is true of answers C and D; neurogenic bladder from diabetes could be a possibility. However, this should not include back pain or perineal numbness.

On examination of this patient you would expect to find:

A) Increased rectal tone.
B) Decreased rectal tone.
C) Normal rectal tone.
D) No rectum.

Discussion
The correct answer is B. Patients with cauda equina syndrome should have decreased rectal tone. If you chose answer D, well, I don't know what to say.

The INITIAL treatment of this patient should include all of the following EXCEPT:

A) Pain management with narcotics.
B) Dexamethasone administered IV.
C) Placement of a Foley catheter.
D) Urgent neurosurgical consultation.
E) Methylprednisolone 30 mg/kg over 1 hour then 5.4 mg/kg/hour for 24 hours.

Discussion
The correct answer is E. This dose of methylprednisolone is indicated for spinal cord injury (eg, from trauma) and not for epidural compression by tumor. **High-dose steroids** have demonstrated no additional benefit in cord compression from tumor when compared to lower-dose steroids. All of the remaining options are correct. Pain management is critical in any patient. Dexamethasone may reduce tumor (and surrounding) edema leading to a reduction in cord compression. A Foley catheter is indicated to treat the patient's urinary retention and, since this is a neurosurgical emergency, urgent neurosurgical

consultation should be obtained (although there is contradictory data about whether early surgical intervention makes any difference). Local radiation may also be used acutely depending on your surgeon, oncologist, etc.

 HELPFUL TIP: The diagnosis of cauda equina syndrome is often delayed for months because many patients initially have incomplete syndromes, including only pain and mild neurologic symptoms. This is unfortunate since outcome depends on the degree of neurologic dysfunction at the time of diagnosis.

Objectives: Did you learn to . . .
• Recognize the clinical presentation of cauda equina syndrome?
• Identify causes of cauda equina syndrome?
• Initiate treatment of a patient with cauda equina syndrome?

 QUICK QUIZ: SEIZURE DISORDERS

Absence seizures are characterized by all of the following EXCEPT:

A) Loss of consciousness.
B) Feeling of déjà vu.
C) Rhythmic lip smacking or eye blinking.
D) Staring spells.
E) Occurrence up to hundreds of times per day.

Discussion
The correct answer is B. Feelings of déjà vu and other psychic phenomenon such as hallucinations are associated with temporal lobe (aka simple partial) seizures.

CASE 15

A 2-year-old female presents to the ED after having a seizure. The parents note that the patient was fine this morning, spiked a temperature to 39.9°C, and then had a 5-minute tonic-clonic seizure which resolved spontaneously. This is her second such episode in 18 months. On arrival, the patient is febrile, lethargic, and looks postictal.

Your next step is to:

A) Reassure the parents that this is a simple febrile seizure.

B) Obtain blood cultures and start ceftriaxone.

C) Perform an LP if the CBC shows leukocytosis and elevated bands.

D) Administer acetaminophen and wait for 2 hours to see if the patient returns to baseline before deciding on further treatment.

E) None of the above.

Discussion

The correct answer is B. This patient **must** be assumed to have meningitis until proven otherwise. Treatment should be started immediately. Answer A is incorrect. This is not a simple febrile seizure by history. The child is postictal and looks ill. While it may end up being a febrile seizure, you cannot make that conclusion at this point. If the child did not look lethargic and was up and running around, no further evaluation or treatment would be needed at this time. Answer C is incorrect for two reasons. First, the CBC may be relatively normal even with meningitis. Second, you do not want to delay antibiotics until the CBC and LP are done. Answer D is incorrect for the same reasons. The standard of care in meningitis is antibiotics within 30 minutes of hitting the door. Waiting to see the patient's response to acetaminophen for 2 hours will clearly put you out of this time window.

* *

You do the right thing and treat the patient with ceftriaxone. The patient does look better in an hour or so and has returned to baseline. She is alert, attentive, and playing with toys. The parents are concerned about whether or not this patient has a seizure disorder. They would like a further evaluation.

Which of the following is indicated now, assuming you decide to evaluate the patient for a seizure disorder?

A) EEG done on the same day.

B) Admission to the hospital and EEG the next day.

C) Serum electrolytes and glucose.

D) Trial of anti-epileptic drug.

E) None of the above.

Discussion

The correct answer is C. The workup of a seizure includes serum electrolytes, calcium, magnesium phosphate, glucose, etc. **This need not be done for someone with a known seizure disorder who has his or her typical seizure and returns to baseline.** In these cases only a drug level of their antiepileptic drug need be done unless there is some change in the seizure type, mental status, etc. Answers A and B are incorrect. The EEG will be positive because of the recent seizure and may not reflect the underlying condition. Thus, waiting a couple of weeks after the seizure will give a better picture of what the brain's innate electrical activity looks like. Answer D is incorrect because we have not yet proven this child has a seizure disorder. Prescribing antiepileptic drugs would be premature.

 HELPFUL TIP: A "stat" EEG can be helpful if you are not sure if a patient is having (or had) an active seizure versus a pseudoseizure. A stat EEG may also be helpful in a patient with mental status changes who you believe may be having nonconvulsive status.

* *

The parents are wondering what to do about treating this patient to prevent further febrile seizures.

Your recommendation to prevent further seizures is:

A) Acetaminophen at the onset of fever.

B) Ibuprofen at the onset of fever.

C) Phenytoin until the child reaches 5 years.

D) Buccal midazolam at the onset of any fever.

E) None of the above.

Discussion

The correct answer is E. None of these will prevent febrile seizures. Phenobarbital **can** prevent febrile seizures but is associated with behavior and learning problems and is generally not recommended. Answers A and B seem like a good idea but do nothing to reduce the occurrence of febrile seizures. Neither answer C nor D is effective. One study suggests that rectal diazepam at the onset of a fever will reduce the occurrence of febrile seizures. However, it is associated with some morbidity (eg, sleepiness, etc) and should be reserved for those with frequent febrile seizures.

* *

The parents have another child at home who has had **one** febrile seizure. He is now 12 months old. The parents want to know his likelihood of having a seizure disorder.

You can let them know that he has APPROXIMATELY:

A) 1%–5% chance of developing a seizure disorder.
B) 10%–15% chance of developing a seizure disorder.
C) 40%–50% chance of developing a seizure disorder.
D) 80%–90% chance of developing a seizure disorder.

Discussion
The correct answer is A. Patients who have a single febrile seizure have approximately a 2%–5% chance of developing a seizure disorder. This is essentially the same risk as the rest of the population.

 HELPFUL TIP: About 50% of patients who have their first febrile seizure <15 months will have a recurrent febrile seizure. This drops to 30% if the first seizure is >15 months. Family history is also involved; 45% of those who have a first-degree relative with febrile seizures will have a second seizure.

BIBLIOGRAPHY

Adams HP Jr, del Zoppo G, Alberts MJ, et al. Guidelines for the early management of adults with ischemic stroke: a guideline from the American Heart Association/American Stroke Association Stroke Council, Clinical Cardiology Council, Cardiovascular Radiology and Intervention Council, and the Atherosclerotic Peripheral Vascular Disease and Quality of Care Outcomes in Research Interdisciplinary Working Groups. *Circulation.* 2007;115(20):e478.

Adams HP, Hachinski V, Norris JW, ed. *Ischemic Cerebrovascular Disease.* New York: Oxford University Press, 2001.

Adams RD, Victor M, Ropper AH, ed. *Principles of Neurology.* New York: McGraw-Hill, 1997.

Bradley WG, Daroff RB, Fenichel GM, Marsden CD, ed. *Neurology in Clinical Practice. Principles of Diagnosis and Management.* Woburn, MA: Butterworth Heinemann, 2000.

Chronicle E, Mulleners W. Anticonvulsant drugs for migraine prophylaxis. *Cochrane Database Syst Rev.* 2004;3:CD003226.

Confavreux C, Suissa S, Saddier P, Bourdes V, Vukusic S. Vaccinations and the risk of relapse in multiple sclerosis. *N Engl J Med.* 2001;344:319.

Disease modifying therapies in multiple sclerosis. Report of the Therapeutics and Technology Assessment Subcommittee of the American Academy of Neurology and the MS Council for Clinical Practice Guidelines. *Neurology.* 2002;58:169.

Jankovic J, Stacy M. Medical management of levodopa-associated motor complications in patients with Parkinson disease. *CNS Drugs.* 2007;21(8):677.

Johnston SC, Nguyen-Huynh MN, Schwarz ME, et al. National Stroke Association guidelines for the management of transient ischemic attacks. *Ann Neurol.* 2006;60(3):301.

Miller AE, Morgante LA, Buchwald LY, et al. A multicenter, randomized, double-blind, placebo-controlled trial of influenza immunization in multiple sclerosis. *Neurology.* 1997;48:312.

Pahwa R. Understanding Parkinson's disease: an update on current diagnostic and treatment strategies. *J Am Med Dir Assoc.* 2006;7(Suppl 2):4.

Practice parameter: evidence-based guidelines for migraine headache (an evidence-based review). Report of the Quality Standards Subcommittee of the American Academy of Neurology, 2000.

Practice parameter: the usefulness of evoked potentials in identifying clinically silent lesions in patient with suspected multiple sclerosis (an evidence-based review). Report of the Quality Standards Subcommittee of the American Academy of Neurology. *Neurology.* 2000; 54:1720.

Silberstein SD, Saper JR, Frederick FG. Migraine: diagnosis and treatment. In: Silberstein SD, ed. *Wolff's Headache and Other Head Pain.* New York: Oxford University Press; 2001:121.

Warden CR, Zibulewsky J, Mace S, et al. Evaluation and management of febrile seizures in the out of hospital and emergency department settings. *Ann Emerg Med.* 2003;41(2):215.

Wyllie E, ed. *The Treatment of Epilepsy, Principles and Practice.* Philadelphia: Lippincott Williams & Wilkins, 2001.

19
Ophthalmology

Emily Greenlee

GLOSSARY OF TERMS

Accommodation: Change in the shape of the lens to compensate for changes in focal length. The term is also used more generally to mean the adjustment of the eye in general to compensate for vision of objects at different distances.

Amblyopia: Unilateral or bilateral loss of vision not attributed to structural abnormality of the eye or visual pathway. This may be a result of strabismus or visual deprivation.

Esotropia: Inward deviation of the eyes when compared to normal.

Exotropia: Outward deviation of the eyes when compared to normal.

Strabismus: A general term that refers to a misalignment of the eyes. Esotropia, exotropia, and hypertropia (one eye deviated upwards) are all examples of strabismus. The term strabismus says nothing about etiology, which can be congenital, neurologic, or muscular.

CASE 1

A mother presents with her healthy 2-month-old male infant. She reports that for the past week his eyes have been noticeably crossed. He appears to fixate with either the right or left eye. She feels that aside from being cross-eyed, he seems to see well. On examination, his eyes are very crossed. When either eye is covered, he fixes and follows with the contralateral eye and appears to have normal motility.

The likely diagnosis in this patient is the following:

A) Pseudoesotropia.
B) Congenital esotropia.
C) Accommodative esotropia.
D) Sixth nerve palsy.

Discussion

The correct answer is B. Esotropia is more common than exotropia. Congenital esotropia is generally found in children <6 months old. Answer C, accommodative esotropia, occurs when there is significant uncorrected farsightedness. It is the most common cause of esotropia in childhood and develops between 6 months and 7 years. It is rare for accommodative esotropia to develop <4 months or >8 years. Pseudoesotropia (answer A) is common in infants due to their flat nasal bridges and medial epicanthal folds, giving an appearance of esotropia. The thing to do here is to shine a penlight in their eyes. When you look at where the light hits the eye, it will be in the same location bilaterally for pseudoesotropia but in different parts of the eye with true esotropia (Figure 19–1; see also color section). You can also use the corneal light reflex to determine if the malalignment is esotropia or exotropia. As a penlight is aimed at the patient, the corneal light reflex should be slightly nasal in each eye for the orthotropic patient (normal alignment). If there is an esotropia, the corneal light reflex will appear to be temporal in one eye. If there is an exotropia, the reflex will appear to be nasal in one eye.

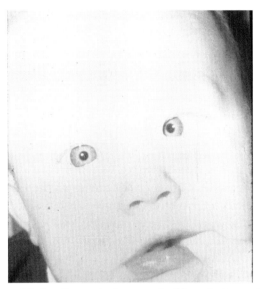

Figure 19–1 Congenital esotropia. Note the large devi-ation with abnormal corneal light reflexes. The corneal light reflex of the left eye appears more temporal than that of the right eye. Therefore, the eye is deviated inwards.

 HELPFUL TIP: It is important to differentiate an esotropia or exotropia from sixth nerve palsy. A sixth nerve palsy affects the lateral rec-tus muscle and the patient will have limited abduction on the affected side.

Which of the following statements is FALSE?

A) Congenital esotropia is nearly always present at birth.
B) Alternating fixation (eg, the ability to fix on an object with either eye) is characteristic of congen-ital esotropia.
C) Patients with congenital esotropia have a normal degree of hyperopia (farsightedness).
D) Patients with a high degree of uncorrected hyper-opia (farsightedness) can develop an accommoda-tive esotropia.

Discussion

The correct answer (and the false statement) is A. Con-genital esotropia presents by the age of 6 months but is rarely present at birth. If true esotropia is observed at birth, it may be due to another neurologic disorder and further evaluation is indicated. Any form of strabismus may result in vision loss, and for this reason, it is important to treat strabismus early in life.

The rest of the answer choices are true statements. Answer B: Patients have two eyes with equal vision, neither is preferred, so they will use both eyes to focus on objects (although not at the same time, of course!). Answer C: Patients with congenital esotropia do have a normal degree of hyperopia for their age (1–2 diopters of hyperopia; +1.00 to +2.00. Answer D: Adaptation for near vision consists of accommodation (change in lens shape), miosis (constriction of the pupil), and conver-gence. This can eventually lead to an accommodative esotropia which can easily be corrected with glasses. After glasses, the patient no longer uses the near response of accommodation and convergence because the glasses are now providing the correction so the eyes straighten. See Figure 19–2; see also color section.

Which of the following is NOT an appropriate treatment for strabismus?

A) Surgical correction if correction of refractive errors does not resolve the strabismus.
B) Full hyperopic spectacle correction.
C) Patching the bad eye.
D) Atropine drops or patching without surgery.
E) Atropine drops or patching plus surgery.

Discussion

The correct answer is C. The goal of the treatment of strabismus is to prevent amblyopia. Amblyopia is com-monly caused by strabismus (ocular misalignment), sig-nificant uncorrected refractive error, or disorders

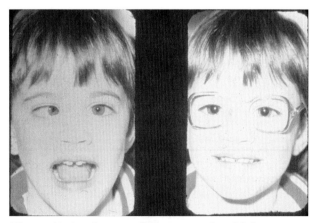

Figure 19–2 Accommodative esotropia with improve-ment when vision is corrected.

which distort images from the eye to the brain (ie, congenital cataracts). The body "turns off" the vision in the bad eye allowing the good eye to work and produce interpretable signals. In addition to surgical treatment (realignment, removal of cataract, etc) one needs to blur the vision in the **good eye** to strengthen the bad eye. This can be done by patching the good eye (not the bad eye as in answer C) or by blurring the vision in the good eye using atropine drops if compliance with a patch is an issue (although eye patches remind kids of pirates and pirates are cool).

In which of the following situations would neuroimaging be necessary?

A) A 6-month-old with long-standing large angle esotropia and equal visual acuity bilaterally.

B) A 5-year-old with +3.00 D OU with recent onset esotropia.

C) A 12-year-old with normal refraction and acute esotropia with diplopia.

D) A newborn with a unilateral congenital cataract and an esotropia.

Discussion

The correct answer is C. **Any unexplained new onset strabismus mandates an evaluation.** The 12-year-old with acute esotropia and diplopia and no evidence of hyperopia requires neuroimaging to rule out any underlying neurologic disorder. The age of the patient is older than that seen with congenital, acquired, or accommodative esotropia. The refraction is normal so this does not fit with accommodative esotropia. Diplopia also suggests acute onset. Further workup is therefore necessary. Answer A is incorrect because this is a classic history for congenital esotropia. Answer B is incorrect because it is consistent with accommodative esotropia. Answer D is incorrect because there is reason for the esotropia—a congenital cataract. None of these would, therefore, require neuroimaging.

 HELPFUL TIP: Acquired strabismus **always** requires a rapid and complete evaluation. It can be caused by tumor, intracranial hemorrhage, botulism, lead poisoning, etc. Any child with strabismus requires a full ophthalmologic examination.

Objectives: Did you learn to . . .

- Describe the nomenclature of strabismus?
- Determine the underlying causes of esotropia?
- Recognize some unusual causes of strabismus which require further workup?
- Describe the risk and treatment of amblyopia?

CASE 2

A 50-year-old Asian female presents to the ED with severe nausea, vomiting, right eye pain, and blurry vision. She reports the symptoms began only a few hours earlier. She has no significant past medical history. On gross examination, her visual acuity is OD 20/200, her right eye is injected, and her right pupil is larger than her left. There does **not** appear to be a relative afferent pupillary defect (RAPD).

 HELPFUL TIP: Interpreting RAPD. The "swinging flashlight test" is used to test for an RAPD. The pupillary response should be equal in both eyes. An RAPD is detected when there is a relative difference in the pupillary response between the two eyes. This occurs when there is optic nerve damage or significant retinal disease (eg, large retinal detachment, retinal artery occlusion, optic neuritis). One will **not** get an RAPD in refractive errors, vitreous bleeds, etc.

With regard to the case above, which of the following would NOT be considered in the differential diagnosis?

A) Trauma secondary to blunt injury from a softball.

B) Central retinal artery occlusion.

C) Contact lens-associated bacterial keratitis.

D) Acute angle closure glaucoma.

E) Anterior uveitis.

Discussion

The correct answer is B. Of these answer choices, only central retinal artery occlusion would have no pain and would result in an RAPD from a diffuse retinal ischemia. All of the others will present with pain and **without** an RAPD. Answer A, blunt injuries, may result in decreased vision secondary to corneal abrasions or edema, intraocular inflammation, hyphema, or retinal injuries. Injury can also cause injection and a traumatic mydriasis (dilation of the pupil). Direct and consensual pupillary reflexes would be normal (no RAPD) unless there was an associated traumatic optic neuropathy or significant retinal damage. Answer D, acute angle closure glaucoma, would cause diffuse injection with a mid-dilated pupil and no RAPD. Answer E, anterior uveitis, would also cause injection, a ciliary flush but no RAPD. There is often asymmetry of the pupils in chronic anterior uveitis secondary to central posterior synechiae (adhesions between the iris and lens).

Which of the following is REQUIRED in order to diagnose acute angle closure glaucoma?

A) Slit lamp.
B) Tonometer.
C) Fluorescein and appropriate UV light.
D) Snellen eye chart.
E) A and B.

Discussion

The correct answer is B. The most important examination technique used to diagnose acute glaucoma is intraocular pressure measurement. This could be a Tonopen, applanation tonometry at the slit lamp, a Schiotz tonometer, etc. Answer A is incorrect. A slit lamp is useful for diagnosing structural problems, iritis, etc. Answer C, fluorescein, is used to diagnose corneal injuries (deepithelized cornea will take up fluorescein). Answer D, a Snellen eye chart, is used to determine visual acuity but is not necessary for diagnosing glaucoma. It is always a good idea to check vision in every patient with eye complaints, however. See Figure 19–3; see also color section.

Which of the following is NOT an associated risk factor of acute angle closure glaucoma?

A) Hyperopia (farsightedness).
B) Asian descent.
C) Male gender.
D) Pharmacologic dilation.
E) Increasing age.

Discussion

The correct answer is C. Associated risk factors for acute angle closure glaucoma are hyperopia, Asian

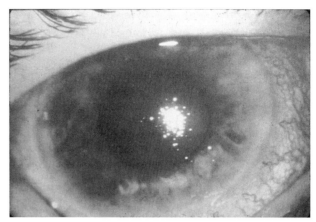

Figure 19–3   Acute angle closure glaucoma. Note the injection, hazy corneal reflex, and mid-dilated pupil.

descent, female sex, and older age. Patients with hyperopia have smaller eyes and more crowded anterior chambers. Females also tend to have smaller eyes. As individuals age, cataracts may lead to an increase in lens size further crowding the anterior chamber predisposing to acute angle closure glaucoma.

 HELPFUL TIP: Pharmacologic dilation may result in an attack of acute angle closure glaucoma.

Which of the following is NOT a presentation of acute angle closure glaucoma?

A) Headache.
B) Abdominal pain.
C) Vomiting.
D) Limitation of extraocular motion.
E) Halos around light.

Discussion

The correct answer is D. Patients with acute angle closure glaucoma can present with all of the above findings except for the limitation of extraocular motion. Severe eye pain and blurred vision may also be noted.

* *

You call the ophthalmologist to see this patient with acute angle closure glaucoma. She is going to be delayed because of traffic.

Which of the following drugs is NOT appropriate to use as a temporizing measure?

A) Topical carbonic anhydrase inhibitors.
B) Topical β-blockers.
C) Topical glycerin.
D) Topical atropine drops.
E) Oral acetazolamide.

Discussion

The correct answer is D. Atropine is **contraindicated** in acute glaucoma since it will dilate the eye, exacerbating the problem. Topical β-blockers and topical or oral carbonic anhydrase inhibitors (eg, acetazolamide) reduce aqueous production and thereby reduce intraocular pressure. In addition to the medications noted above, a topical α_2-adrenergic agonist (eg, brimonidine, apraclonidine) should be given to lower intraocular pressure. Topical glycerin is used to clear the corneal edema. Hopefully, this will serve to temporize while the ophthalmologist is on the way. See Table 19–1.

 HELPFUL TIP: Did you notice that pilocarpine, the classic agent for treating acute glaucoma is absent from the list? Turns out, it doesn't work all that well.

Table 19–1 DRUGS USED FOR ACUTE GLAUCOMA AND HOW THEY WORK

Drug	Mechanism of Action
Topical β-blockers (eg, timolol)	Reduces aqueous humor production
Topical α_2-adrenergic agonists (eg, brimonidine)	Decreases aqueous humor production
Topical carbonic anhydrase inhibitors (eg, dorzolamide, brinzolamide)	Decreases aqueous humor production
Oral carbonic anhydrase inhibito (eg, acetazolamide)	Diuretic **and, more importantly,** decreases the production of aqueous humor
Mannitol (rarely used now for acute glaucoma, mostly OR cases only)	Osmotic diuretic draws aqueous humor from the eye

* *

The ophthalmologist makes it to the hospital and wants to take this patient for surgery.

What is the definitive treatment of choice for acute angle closure glaucoma?

A) Laser peripheral iridotomy (LPI).
B) Trabeculectomy.
C) Tapping of the anterior chamber to lower intraocular pressure.
D) Aqueous suppressants.
E) Surgical iridectomy.

Discussion

The correct answer is A. The treatment goal is to allow the free flow of aqueous so that it does not accumulate behind the iris to push it forward to obstruct the trabecular meshwork. A laser peripheral iridotomy creates a small hole in the peripheral iris that allows aqueous to enter the anterior chamber. As long as this hole remains patent, the patient is no longer at risk for an attack of angle closure, and it is unusual for the hole to close unless there is a history of intraocular inflammation. Answer C, tapping the anterior chamber, can be used before laser therapy in order to clear the cornea so that visualization is better for the procedure. However, it is adjunctive and not a treatment of choice. Also, topical glycerin works well and can accomplish the same goal without being invasive. Answer D, aqueous suppressants are discussed in the previous question. Answer E, a surgical iridectomy, is performed for patients who are unable to sit still for the laser procedure (eg, children, mentally incapacitated).

Which statement is FALSE regarding closed and open-angle glaucoma?

A) The main difference is that the drainage angle (trabecular meshwork) is closed in angle closure glaucoma and open in open-angle glaucoma.
B) Scopolamine and other agents with anticholinergic properties are contraindicated in open-angle glaucoma but not in closed-angle glaucoma.
C) Acute angle closure glaucoma usually occurs in hyperopic individuals while myopia is associated with open-angle glaucoma.
D) The majority of people diagnosed with glaucoma have primary open-angle glaucoma.

Discussion

The correct answer (and false statement) is B. Scopolamine and agents with anticholinergic properties, which would cause dilation of the pupil, are **contraindicated** in those with closed-angle glaucoma (and those with **narrow** angles who may not yet have obstructed). Once peripheral iridotomy is performed, anticholinergics are no longer an issue because the patient is no longer at risk. However, they can be used in those with open angle glaucoma. All of the rest of the statements are correct.

Which of the following does NOT increase a patient's risk for primary open-angle glaucoma?

A) Family history.
B) White race.
C) Elevated intraocular pressure (>21 mm Hg).
D) Age >40 years.
E) Thin corneas.

Discussion

The correct answer is B. Blacks are much more likely to develop open-angle glaucoma than whites. Blacks are also more likely to suffer vision loss from glaucoma. Family history, high intraocular pressures, and thin corneas are all risk factors for the development of open-angle glaucoma. High intraocular pressures lead to optic nerve damage. Thin corneas lead to a falsely low intraocular pressure reading so patients may go untreated for a longer period of time. Minor risk factors include diabetes and myopia (nearsightedness). All patients should be screened for glaucoma as part of their routine eye exam.

Which of the following is typical of early glaucoma?

A) Central vision loss.
B) Peripheral vision loss.
C) Asymptomatic.
D) Decreased contrast.
E) Blurring of vision.

Discussion

The correct answer is C. Most people with early open-angle glaucoma are asymptomatic. This is why screening is so important. A significant number of axons of the optic nerve may be damaged before this manifests itself as visual field loss. Examination of the optic nerve for abnormalities is the best way to diagnose early glaucoma. Later symptoms involve loss of peripheral or central vision.

Which of the following is necessary to diagnose a patient with open-angle glaucoma?

A) Optic nerve head cupping with corresponding visual field loss.
B) Thin corneas.
C) Elevated intraocular pressure.
D) Narrow but open drainage angle.

Discussion

The correct answer is A. Cupping of the optic nerve head is thinning of the neural rim secondary to damage from high intraocular pressure. There should be a corresponding visual field defect consistent with the appearance of optic nerve cupping to diagnose a patient with glaucoma. If there is a thinning of the superior optic nerve, there should be an inferior visual field defect and vice versa. If there is a visual field defect which does not seem to correlate with the extent of optic nerve cupping, further evaluation may be necessary to evaluate for other etiologies of the visual field defect, such as optic nerve compression. In open-angle glaucoma, the mechanism of injury to the optic nerve is thought to be direct mechanical compression.

Answer C is incorrect. **Elevated intraocular pressure does not diagnose open-angle glaucoma.** Elevated intraocular pressure by itself is considered a risk factor for glaucoma. When not accompanied by cupping or visual field loss, it is considered ocular hypertension. Patients with ocular hypertension still need to be monitored for the development of open-angle glaucoma. Answer B, thin corneas, is discussed above. Answer D is incorrect. The drainage angle must be widely open—thus the name "open-angle glaucoma."

 HELPFUL TIP: A variant of open-angle glaucoma is normal-tension glaucoma which shows evidence of cupping and visual field loss at normal intraocular pressures (<21 mm Hg). Patients with lower intraocular pressures who have glaucoma are thought to have a vascular etiology (eg, ischemia) to their optic nerve damage since they also tend to have associated migraines or Raynaud phenomenon.

Which of the following statements regarding glaucoma is true?

A) If treated early enough, normalizing the intraocular pressure can reverse the process of glaucoma and restore sight.

B) The funduscopic exam in patients with glaucoma will generally show small retinal hemorrhages in addition to optic nerve cupping.

C) Papilledema is seen with glaucoma as a result of increased pressure on the optic nerve.

D) All of the above.

E) None of the above.

Discussion

The correct answer is E. Answer B is incorrect. Once there is visual loss, it cannot be restored. Answer C is incorrect. Papilledema is seen as a result of increased **intracranial** not intraocular pressure.

See Figure 19–4 (see also color section) for an image of normal-appearing optic nerves. Compare this figure with Figure 19–5 (see also color section), which shows optic nerve findings in patients with glaucoma. The cup (central depression) of the optic nerve, which represents the axons diving down into the optic nerve, is larger compared with normal. Cupping represents damage to the optic nerve and fewer axons are present.

Objectives: Did you learn to . . .

- Recognize the signs and symptoms of acute angle closure glaucoma?
- Identify risk factors associated with acute angle closure glaucoma?

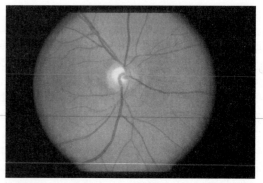

Figure 19–5   Glaucomatous optic nerve. Observe the cupping of the optic nerve head.

- Describe the pathology and basis for treatment for glaucoma?
- Differentiate between angle closure and open-angle glaucoma?
- Describe optic nerve findings in glaucoma?

 QUICK QUIZ: GLAUCOMA AGENTS

Topical α_2-adrenergic agonists, such as brimonidine (Alphagan), lower intraocular pressure by decreasing the production of aqueous humor with a minor effect on aqueous outflow.

Which of the following is NOT considered a potential side effect of these medications?

A) Hypertension.

B) Lethargy.

C) Dry mouth.

D) Apnea in children.

E) Diarrhea.

Discussion

The correct answer is E. α_2-Adrenergic agonists do not cause diarrhea. All of the remaining choices are considered side effects of α_2-adrenergic agonists.

 QUICK QUIZ: GLAUCOMA AGENTS

Topical β-blockers lower intraocular pressure by decreasing aqueous production.

Which of the following is NOT considered a systemic side effect of these medications?

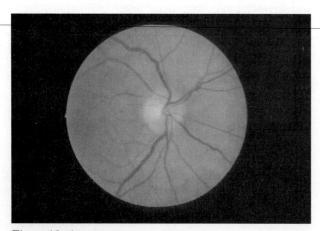

Figure 19–4   Normal optic nerve.

A) Bronchospasm.
B) Bradycardia.
C) Worsening of congestive heart failure.
D) Increased low-density lipoprotein (LDL).

Discussion

The correct answer is D. β-Blockers do not increase LDL. They increase triglycerides and decrease high density lipoproteins (HDL). The message here is that **topical β-blockers can have systemic effects, including congestive heart failure**. Be aware of these, especially in the elderly.

 QUICK QUIZ: VISION LOSS

A 70-year-old white female presents with sudden loss of the upper half of her vision in the left eye. **She reports no pain.** During the past 2 months, she reports a 5-pound weight loss and has been fatigued. Her past medical history is significant for hypertension and type 2 diabetes.

Which of the following is the LEAST likely diagnosis given this history?

A) Retinal detachment.
B) Branch retinal artery/vein occlusion.
C) Optic neuritis.
D) Anterior ischemic optic neuropathy.

Discussion

The correct answer is C. Retinal detachment, branch retinal artery/vein occlusion, and anterior ischemic optic neuropathy all cause **painless** sectorial loss of vision in this age group. **Optic neuritis** usually occurs in a younger age group and is associated with pain and a central scotoma (blind spot).

 HELPFUL TIP: Many patients complain of pain when they move their eyes. Diagnoses to consider include optic neuritis, intraorbital infection/inflammation, and orbital myositis (eg, acute Graves disease, orbital pseudotumor, sarcoidosis, polyarteritis nodosum, systemic lupus erythematosus, dermatomyositis, rheumatoid arthritis, Wegener granulomatosis, etc).

 QUICK QUIZ: ANTERIOR ISCHEMIC OPTIC NEUROPATHY

Which of the following is FALSE about nonarteritic (not related to temporal arteritis) anterior ischemic optic neuropathy (NA-AION)?

A) It is associated with diabetes.
B) It is associated with hypertension.
C) It occurs in patients who are generally younger than patients who have giant-cell arteritis.
D) Inducing nocturnal hypotension is standard therapy in patients with anterior ischemic neuropathy.

Discussion

The correct answer is D. It is important to **avoid nocturnal hypotension.** Thus, avoid antihypertensive medications at nighttime if possible. Occasionally, midodrine needs to be prescribed to support the blood pressure at night. The rest of the statements are true. Think of NA-AION as equivalent to peripheral vascular disease: it is associated with hypertension, smoking, diabetes, etc. Although the age of patients with NA-AION overlaps with that of patients with temporal (giant cell) arteritis, the patients with NA-AION tend to be younger.

CASE 4

A 65-year-old white male presents with complaints of "seeing wavy lines when looking at the doorway or blinds" in his right eye. He feels that this occurred suddenly and has no pain or other ocular symptoms. His past medical history is significant for hypertension. He has a 40-pack-per year smoking history. On examination, his visual acuity is 20/400 in the right eye. He has no RAPD and slit lamp exam reveals that his anterior segment examination is normal. Examination of his right fundus reveals a subretinal hemorrhage involving his fovea.

Which of the following is the most likely cause of this patient's vision loss?

A) Age-related macular degeneration.
B) Acute angle closure glaucoma.
C) Cataract.
D) Diabetic retinopathy.

Discussion

The correct answer is A. This is a typical presentation for age-related macular degeneration (see the Discussion below for more information). Answer B is incorrect because acute angle closure glaucoma presents with pain. Answer C is incorrect because cataracts cause slowly progressive vision loss. Answer D is incorrect. This would be an unusual presentation for diabetic retinopathy, and the patient has no known history of diabetes.

Which of the following statements is FALSE?

A) Age-related macular degeneration is the leading cause of severe central vision loss in individuals >50 years in the U.S.
B) Smoking has been shown to be a risk factor in the development of wet age-related macular degeneration.
C) Age-related macular degeneration is more common in the black population in comparison with other populations.
D) The Age-Related Eye Disease Study has shown a beneficial effect of vitamin E, vitamin C, beta-carotene, copper, and zinc in delaying the progression to wet age-related macular degeneration.
E) The main complaint of wet age-related macular degeneration is metamorphopsia, which is distortion or waviness centrally in the visual field.

Discussion

The correct answer is C. Age-related macular degeneration is more commonly seen in the white population. Answers A and B are correct. Smoking is a risk factor in the progression to wet age-related macular degeneration; age-related macular degeneration is the leading cause of **central** vision loss in individuals >50 years. Answer D is correct. The listed micronutrients are beneficial in preventing dry age related macular degeneration. The same micronutrients delay the progression from dry to wet age-related macular degeneration. Answer E is correct. Patients with age-related macular degeneration complain of distortion and/or waviness in the central visual field.

characterized by drusen (yellow lesions in the outer retinal layers of the macula) or atrophy within the macula. Dry age-related macular degeneration may lead to wet (neovascular) age-related macular degeneration, which is associated with a choroidal neovascular membrane (CNVM). The CNVM is an abnormal growth of blood vessel in the outer layers of the retina which grows in the macula or fovea and affects vision.

What is the purpose of Amsler grid testing?

A) To detect any metamorphopsia (distortion and/or waviness in the central) visual field which may be secondary to macular degeneration.
B) To improve visual functioning through strengthening exercises.
C) To determine the size of any choroidal neovascular membrane.
D) To evaluate if a choroidal neovascular membrane would be amenable to laser treatment.

Discussion

The correct answer is A. Amsler grid testing is done at home by the patient. Its purpose is to determine if there may be a choroidal neovascular membrane causing metamorphopsia.

The Amsler grid is a lined grid with a central fixation spot. The patient is instructed to test each eye separately with proper corrective lenses. The grid is placed approximately 14 inches away from the patient. As the patient fixates on the central dot with one eye only, he/she is asked to note any wavy lines, distortion, or missing areas. The grid detects metamorphopsia and often locates the affected area in relation to the fovea (central fixation spot). To determine if a choroidal neovascular membrane exists, a fluorescein angiogram should be performed. The Amsler grid can also be used in patients taking medications which may be toxic to the eye, such as hydroxychloroquine. It can provide early evidence of retinal toxicity.

 HELPFUL TIP: Dry age-related macular degeneration is the nonneovascular form of age-related macular degeneration. It is

 HELPFUL TIP: There are several treatments available for neovascular age-related macular degeneration. These include laser of the

choroidal neovascular membrane, intravenous injection of photosensitizing drug (verteporfin) followed by nonthermal red light, intravitreal injection of antivascular endothelial growth factor medications, and surgical removal of choroidal neovascular membrane. A combination of beta-carotene, vitamin C, vitamin E, copper, and zinc has been shown to be beneficial in preventing the progression of certain types of dry age-related macular degeneration. All treatments are aimed toward preserving existing vision, not improving vision. In addition, patients should be encouraged to cease smoking.

Objectives: Did you learn to . . .

- Recognize the signs and symptoms of age-related macular degeneration?
- Differentiate between dry and wet age-related macular degeneration?
- Use an Amsler grid for patient self-monitoring?
- Recognize treatment modalities for wet age-related macular degeneration?

CASE 5

A 55-year-old white male with a history newly diagnosed type 2 diabetes mellitus presents for routine evaluation. He has no complaints, including no ocular complaints. On nondilated direct ophthalmoscopic examination, both fundi appear to be normal.

When should this patient be referred for formal ophthalmologic examination?

A) Immediately upon diagnosis.
B) Within 3 months.
C) Within 6 months.
D) Within 1 year.
E) When he develops visual symptoms.

Discussion

The correct answer is A. Patients with type 2 diabetes should be referred for a dilated exam immediately upon diagnosis because they may have been undiagnosed for a long time period and may already have a degree of retinopathy. **For patients with type 1 diabetes**, the recommendation is to refer within 5 years of diagnosis.

What are the common findings seen on direct ophthalmoscopic examination in nonproliferative diabetic retinopathy?

A) Exudates.
B) Cotton wool spots.
C) Dot-blot hemorrhages.
D) Microaneurysms.
E) All of the above.

Discussion

The correct answer is E. Direct ophthalmoscopic examination may reveal all of these findings in nonproliferative diabetic retinopathy. These are caused by the increased fragility of capillaries and arterioles of the retina with diabetes. It cannot, however, evaluate for diabetic macular edema, which can be seen only with a binocular view at the slit lamp with a high-power lens. However, if there are extensive exudates on direct ophthalmoscopy, it is likely that there is macular edema.

What is the main cause of vision loss in NONPROLIFERATIVE diabetic retinopathy?

A) Dot-blot hemorrhages.
B) Macular edema.
C) Cataract.
D) Neovascularization.

Discussion

The correct answer is B. Nonproliferative diabetic retinopathy by definition has no neovascularization (new, fragile blood vessel growth secondary to microvascular disease). The main source of decreased vision is macular edema. Treatment of focal macular edema consists of focal laser to leaking microaneurysms. If the patient has diffuse macular edema a more extensive ("grid laser") pattern is used.

What is the main cause of vision loss in PROLIFERATIVE diabetic retinopathy?

A) Cataract.
B) Macular edema.
C) Vitreous hemorrhage.
D) Neovascular glaucoma.

Discussion

The correct answer is D. Vision loss in proliferative retinopathy occurs when friable neovascular vessels break open and bleed (vitreous hemorrhage). Vision loss can also occur if the neovascular vessels grow over

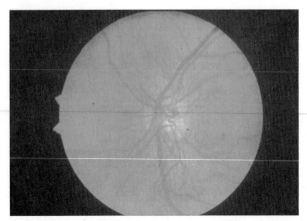

Figure 19–6   Proliferative diabetic retinopathy. Neovascularization of the optic nerve.

the drainage angle of the eye, causing glaucoma. This is far less common than vitreous hemorrhage. See Figure 19–6 (see also color section) for an image of neovascularization. The treatment of proliferative diabetic retinopathy consists of panretinal photocoagulation, which involves lasering the peripheral retina, thereby decreasing the ischemic drive for neovascularization. Treatment of vitreous hemorrhage is observation with head-of-bed elevation until the hemorrhage settles out and clears enough for laser treatment. Vitreous hemorrhages may be caused by other things, such as retinal detachments, so ultrasound is usually performed acutely since one will not be able to see the retina after a significant hemorrhage.

 HELPFUL TIP: Aspirin is safe in patients with neovascularization. The risk of bleeding does not increase significantly. The cardiovascular benefit outweighs the risk to the eye.

Which of the following statements is TRUE?

A) In the U.S. diabetic retinopathy is the leading cause of blindness in individuals >60 years.

B) Intensive glycemic control has been shown to worsen mild or moderate nonproliferative diabetic retinopathy in patients with type 1 diabetes during the first year of treatment.

C) Intensive insulin therapy in patients with type 1 diabetes cannot delay the onset and progression of retinopathy, nephropathy, and neuropathy.

D) Intensive glycemic control in patients with type 2 diabetes cannot reduce the risk of developing retinopathy, nephropathy, and neuropathy.

Discussion

The correct answer is B. Intensive glycemic control in individuals with type 1 diabetes and mild to moderate nonproliferative retinopathy has been shown to **worsen** retinopathy in the first year. Long-term, intensive glycemic control in patients with type 1 and type 2 diabetics reduces the risk of retinopathy. Answer A is incorrect. Diabetic retinopathy is the leading cause of blindness in individuals aged 20–64 years.

Objectives: Did you learn to . . .

● Identify when to refer patients for formal ophthalmologic examination in type 1 and type 2 diabetes?

● Recognize the signs of diabetic retinopathy on direct ophthalmoscopic examination?

● Understand the causes of vision loss in those with nonproliferative and proliferative diabetic retinopathy?

● Describe the basis for treatment of both nonproliferative and proliferative diabetic retinopathy?

CASE 6

A 20-year-old male presents to the ED with complaint of a "bloody eye." He was in a fight earlier in the evening and was hit in the eye ("but you should see the other guy!"and with your luck, you probably will). You examine him and discover the findings in Figure 19–7 (see also color section). His visual acuity in the affected eye is to hand motions. He also has moderate edema of the lids but is able to open his eyes. On slit lamp exam, the pupil appears normal. His motility is full and there is no diplopia.

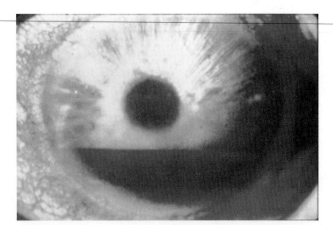

Figure 19–7

What is the MOST important first step in evaluation of this patient?

A) Detection of an RAPD.
B) Patching until the heme clears.
C) Evaluation for possible open globe.
D) Immediate CT scanning to evaluate for an orbital fracture.
E) Surgical anterior chamber washout of the heme.

Discussion

The correct answer is C. This is a hyphema, with blood filling about one-third of the anterior chamber (see Figure 19–7; see also color section). More important is the history of trauma. The first, and most important, step in ocular trauma is to look for evidence of an open or ruptured globe. **There should be no pressure placed on the eye until an open globe in ruled out.** Signs of ruptured globe are 360 degrees of conjunctival chemosis (conjunctival swelling), a shallow anterior chamber, an irregular pupil, or low intraocular pressure. **Intraocular pressure measurements should not be taken until an open globe is ruled out. However, a normal globe pressure does not rule out a ruptured globe.** The leak may be small or may be plugged with choroid. If there is any doubt about whether there is an open globe, ophthalmology should be consulted.

> **HELPFUL TIP:** When evaluating for a ruptured globe, remember that the most common areas of rupture are the limbus (the margin of the cornea where it meets the sclera) and sclera behind the insertion of rectus muscles. This is where the sclera is thinnest.

> **HELPFUL TIP:** A Seidel test can be used to look for an open globe. A moistened fluorescein strip is gently placed at the site of injury. Slit-lamp exam is done with cobalt blue light. If a rupture is present, the fluorescein dye will be diluted by the aqueous, which will appear as a dark stream through the green fluorescein.

Which is NOT a complication of hyphema (bleeding into the anterior chamber)?

A) Corneal blood staining.
B) Glaucoma.
C) Rebleeding.
D) Iris heterochromia.

Discussion

The correct answer is D. Complications of hyphema include rebleeding, which is most common in the first 3–5 days after injury. The hyphema may also stain the cornea, which takes months to clear. Glaucoma may also occur because of clogging of the trabecular meshwork by RBCs, leading to a rise in intraocular pressure. Answer D, iris heterochromia, describes difference in iris coloring (eg, one blue eye and one brown) and can be caused by a retained foreign body (eg, iron) but is more often due to an underlying condition.

Which of the following is the most appropriate treatment for this patient?

A) Treat at home with topical steroids.
B) Hospital admission and IV steroids.
C) Hospital admission and IV antibiotics.
D) Hospital admission and topical antibiotics.
E) Treat at home with topical antibiotics.

Discussion

The correct answer is A. This patient has a hyphema, which is blood in the anterior chamber, usually due to direct trauma. Although the party line in the past was that all of these patients require admission, sending a patient home with instructions to avoid further trauma and vigorous activities is sufficient in **reliable** patients with limited disease. However, **an ophthalmologist should be involved in this decision**. In addition to topical steroids, other potential treatments include cycloplegic agents and perhaps antifibrinolytic agents, such as aminocaproic acid.

Objectives: Did you learn to . . .

- Recognize the complications of ocular trauma?
- Identify the complications of hyphema, especially in the pediatric population?
- Initiate management of a patient with hyphema?

CASE 7

A 27-year-old white male reports irritation and redness of his right eye after hammering on an old iron fence.

He was not wearing safety glasses, and the injury occurred 3 days ago. On exam, his visual acuity is 20/200. His right eye is injected, and his pupil is irregularly peaked to one side upon gross inspection. Slit lamp examination reveals a laceration of his cornea extending to the limbus with a wick of iris occluding the laceration site.

Which of the following is an important aspect of his history in regard to management?

A) Mechanism of injury.
B) Lack of protective eyewear.
C) Length of time since injury sustained.
D) Type of materials involved in the injury.
E) All of the above.

Discussion

The correct answer is E. All of these aspects are important when considering management. Answer A, high-velocity of hammering metal on metal, is concerning for a possible intraocular foreign body. Answer B is important as a preventive measure to avoid future injury. However, even with protective eyewear, metal may be able to injure the eye. Any person involved in mechanics or carpentry should be advised to wear protective eyewear consisting of occlusive goggles. Answer C is important because the delay in seeking treatment may complicate matters, especially if the type of material (answer D) in the eye is organic and can act as a nidus of infection.

* *

You place a Fox shield on this patient and contact the ophthalmologist, who requests a tetanus booster and antibiotics.

What would be the next step in the evaluation and treatment of this patient?

A) Imaging for an intraocular foreign body by orbital CT scanning.
B) Evaluation for an intraocular foreign body by orbital ultrasound.
C) Try to remove the foreign body from the posterior chamber with a magnet.
D) Complete ocular examination, including intraocular pressure and dilated funduscopic examination.

Discussion

The correct answer is A. Given his history, the patient needs to be evaluated for a possible intraocular foreign body. The best imaging modality is with orbital CT scanning. Orbital ultrasound (answer B) would also be appropriate, but for surgical planning, CT scanning is preferred. Answer C is incorrect because it is likely to cause more damage. This type of foreign body removal is best left to an ophthalmologist in the OR. Answer D is incorrect because it would be best to defer intraocular pressure measurements until the extent of the laceration is evaluated since no pressure should ever be placed on a potential open globe.

* *

The patient has a Fox shield placed to protect the eye and undergoes an orbital CT. There appears to be a piece of metal within his vitreous cavity.

Which of the following are inert intraocular foreign bodies?

A) Iron.
B) Copper.
C) Glass.
D) Aluminum.
E) C and D.

Discussion

The correct answer is C. Iron, copper, and aluminum are all reactive species and must be removed from the eye. Glass is inert and may be left in place, depending on the situation and the risk of surgery.

What are signs of a retained IRON intraocular foreign body?

A) Iris heterochromia.
B) Mydriasis.
C) Glaucoma.
D) Retinal degeneration.
E) All of the above.

Discussion

The correct answer is E. All of the above are signs of siderosis caused by a retained iron intraocular foreign body. Given the toxicity to the eye, the foreign body must be removed surgically.

 HELPFUL TIP: Corneal foreign bodies may be removed using a needle after the administration of topical anesthetic. Metallic foreign bodies in the cornea may leave a rust ring around the area of the foreign body which can be removed using an ocular burr. The rust ring may be left in place if it is out of the visual axis because it does not cause any long-lasting problems.

Objectives: Did you learn to . . .

● Recognize the signs of a corneoscleral laceration?
● Manage a corneoscleral laceration in the emergency setting?
● Appreciate the effects of intraocular foreign bodies?
● Manage an intraocular foreign body in the emergency setting?

CASE 8

A 55-year-old farmer presents to the ED complaining of ocular pain and irritation. He reports accidentally splashing ammonia in both eyes. He attempted to rinse his eyes with water prior to coming to the ED. His visual acuity is OD 20/100 and OS 20/80. Both eyes are injected with corneal edema.

What is the immediate first step in the treatment of chemical injuries to the eye?

A) Complete ocular examination, including dilated funduscopic examination.
B) Immediate irrigation with saline until the pH is 7.0.
C) Application of topical glycerin to clear the corneal edema.
D) Topical anesthetic with debridement of surface epithelium.

Discussion

The correct answer is B. Immediate irrigation with normal saline (or water if saline is unavailable) is the initial step even **before** a complete exam. A lid speculum should be placed and topical anesthesia applied. Irrigation may be administered by a handheld bottle or through IV tubing with an irrigation lens. The pH should be checked with a pH strip and irrigation discontinued when the pH reaches 7.0. Any particulate matter should be removed prior to irrigation if it is a reactive substance (eg, ammonium hydroxide crystals) since fluid may dissolve these causing more injury. The upper lid should be everted to check for any particulate matter. A moistened cotton swab may be used to sweep

the superior/inferior fornices to remove any residual debris.

Which of the following is a complication of chemical injuries to the eye?

A) Corneal ulceration.
B) Inflammation.
C) Deepithelialization of the cornea.
D) All of the above.
E) None of the above.

Discussion

The correct answer is D. All of the answer choices are complications of chemical injuries to the eye.

 HELPFUL TIP: Alkali burns tend to be more severe than acid burns. Alkali burns cause ocular surface damage by saponifying fatty acids in cell membranes. Alkaline agents readily penetrate the cornea causing degradation. Acids cause protein denaturation, which creates a barrier to penetration. Therefore, acids cause less tissue destruction. The eye may become insensate from nerve destruction, so absence of burning sensation is not adequate to determine whether further irrigation is needed. **Check the pH as noted above.**

* *

You have copiously irrigated the patient's eyes to a pH of 7. He feels a little better. The ophthalmologist will see him in 3 days and recommends outpatient treatment in the meantime.

Which of the following is NOT a recommended home-going treatment for chemical injuries to the eye?

A) Topical anesthetics.
B) Topical corticosteroids.
C) Tetracycline.
D) Vitamin C.
E) Atropine.

Discussion

The correct answer is A. Topical anesthetics should never be given for treatment of **any** ocular condition.

They are used for evaluation in the acute setting only. Anesthetic abuse results in inhibited epithelial cell division and migration. This may impede healing. Topical corticosteroids are useful in inhibiting polymorphonuclear leukocyte (PMN) degradation of corneal stromal collagen. Steroids are useful in the first 2 weeks of injury but should be prescribed in consultation with an ophthalmologist. Tetracycline chelates calcium which inhibits PMNs, thereby reducing collagenolysis. Vitamin C promotes collagen synthesis. The recommended dosage is 2 g vitamin C per day. Atropine or other topical cycloplegics are indicated for anterior chamber reactions. Intraocular pressure is best controlled by oral carbonic anhydrase inhibitors, avoiding topical glaucoma medication toxicity to the cornea.

Objectives: Did you learn to . . .

- Describe the difference between acid and alkali injuries to the eye?
- Treat a chemical eye exposure in the emergency setting?
- Recognize the complications of chemical eye injuries?

CASE 9

A 25-year-old college student presents with complaints of redness, sensitivity to light, and tearing of her right eye for the past day. She lives in the dorm but reports no exposure to others with a red eye. For the past few days, she has had a sore throat and slight cough. You suspect conjunctivitis ("pink eye").

Regarding conjunctivitis, which of the following statements is FALSE?

A) Gonococcal conjunctivitis presents with severe hyperacute purulent discharge.
B) Adenoviral conjunctivitis generally begins in one eye and spreads to the contralateral eye.
C) An enlarged preauricular node is a sign of allergic conjunctivitis.
D) Toxic conjunctivitis has been associated with the use of topical antibiotics, antivirals, and preservatives.

Discussion

The correct answer is C. There is no enlargement of preauricular nodes with allergic conjunctivitis.

An enlarged preauricular node is a prominent feature of adenoviral conjunctivitis. A prominent symptom of allergic conjunctivitis is itching and often tends to be bilateral. All the other statements are true.

* *

Your patient has no purulent drainage. On examination, her visual acuity is 20/40. Her right eye is diffusely injected and tearing; the left eye appears normal to inspection. She has a slightly tender right preauricular lymph node about 1 cm in size.

What do you recommend as the initial treatment of this patient's conjunctivitis?

A) Symptomatic treatment with artificial tears 4–8 times per day, cool compresses, and strict hygiene to prevent spread to the contralateral eye or to others.
B) Treatment with topical vasoconstrictors/antihistamines QID for 1–2 weeks.
C) Topical antibiotic treatment for 1 week.
D) Administration of topical steroids, artificial tears, and cool compresses.
E) None of the above.

Discussion

The correct answer is A. This patient appears to have viral conjunctivitis which is treated symptomatically. There is no need to treat with topical vasoconstrictors/antihistamines unless there is a significant itching component. It is not bacterial, so no antibiotics are needed. Additionally, prophylactic antibiotics are not necessary since there is rarely a secondary bacterial infection. Occasionally, corneal subepithelial infiltrates will develop which reduce vision. In these patients, topical steroids may be used for 1 week then tapered to prevent significant scarring. However, this is rare. See Figure 19–8 (see also color section) for an image of viral conjunctivitis.

 HELPFUL TIP: Antibiotics have magical powers in viral conjunctivitis. How else can you explain the fact that a single dose of topical antibiotics is enough to get a child back into school or daycare?

If your patient is a part-time nursing assistant at a care facility, how long should she stay away from patient care?

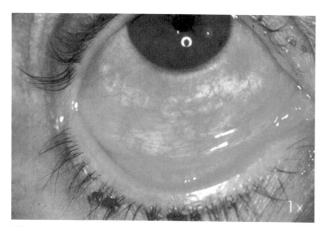

Figure 19–8   Viral conjunctivitis. Viral hemorrhagic conjunctivitis is often epidemic.

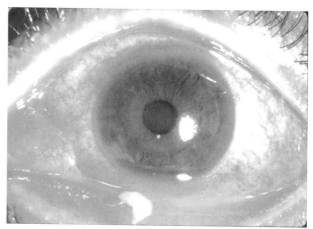

Figure 19–9   Bacterial conjunctivitis. Note the mucopurulent discharge.

A) Two days.
B) Two weeks.
C) Until her eyes are clear.
D) Until she has taken antibiotics for 24 hours.

Discussion

The correct answer is C. Viral conjunctivitis is highly contagious and is thought to be infectious as long as the eye is red and producing discharge. Promote good hand hygiene and avoid contact with others until the eye clears. In many instances, removal from school and/or work is not feasible, but patient education regarding the highly contagious nature of viral and bacterial conjunctivitis remains important.

Which of the following is (are) appropriate in the treatment of acute gonococcal conjunctivitis?

A) Conjunctival Gram stain and culture.
B) Ceftriaxone IM/IV.
C) Saline irrigation.
D) None of the above.
E) All of the above.

Discussion

The correct answer is E. The hallmark of acute gonococcal conjunctivitis is severe purulent discharge which occurs within 12–24 hours of infection. Preauricular adenopathy may also be seen. Management consists of Gram stain of purulent material to document gonococcus, culture, ceftriaxone IM/IV (or spectinomycin if cephalosporin-allergic), eye irrigation, and treatment for possible concurrent chlamydia infection. There is

increasing resistance of gonorrhea to fluoroquinolones, which are no longer recommended as initial therapy. See Figure 19–9 (see also color section) for an image of bacterial conjunctivitis and Figure 19–10 (see also color section) for an image of ophthalmia neonatorum.

Which of the following is NOT indicated in the treatment of allergic conjunctivitis?

A) Cool compresses.
B) Artificial tears.
C) Chronic topical vasoconstrictors/antihistamines.
D) Short-term topical steroids.
E) Diphenhydramine.

Discussion

The correct answer is C. Given the possibility of rebound hyperemia with prolonged use, chronic

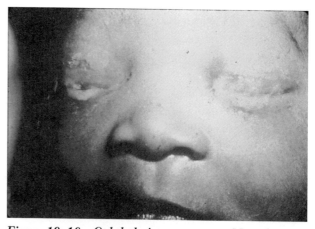

Figure 19–10   Ophthalmia neonatorum. Note the severe mucopurulent discharge.

vasoconstrictors/antihistamines are never indicated. Topical steroids should be reserved for severe cases and tapered over 1 to 2 weeks. Topical NSAIDs, such as ketorolac, and antihistamines, such as levocabastine and olopatadine, may be used to alleviate intense itching but are very expensive.

Objectives: Did you learn to . . .

- Differentiate among viral, bacterial, and allergic conjunctivitis?
- Choose appropriate treatments modalities for the various causes of conjunctivitis?

CASE 10

A 35-year-old white male presents with complaints of pain, tearing, and redness of his left eye. He states that he was hammering metal siding without the use of safety glasses. He has a sheepish look to his injected eye—he knows better but was in a hurry. He feels like a flake of metal may have gotten into his eye. On examination, his left eye is injected and has a small metal fragment lodged in his cornea. His pupil is round and his anterior chamber is formed.

What is the best way to remove the corneal foreign body?

A) Removal with fine-toothed forceps.
B) Removal with a TB needle.
C) Removal with burring.
D) Saline irrigation.

Discussion

The correct answer is B. For distinct foreign bodies lodged within the cornea, a TB or 25-gauge needle should be used. The eye should be anesthetized with topical proparacaine. The tip of the needle is then used to gently lift the foreign body from its bed. If there is a remaining rust ring, a burr may be used to remove it, but this is usually not necessary. Topical bacitracin or erythromycin should be used to prevent infection.

 HELPFUL TIP: **Always** evert the upper eyelid to look for additional foreign bodies. These can be removed using a cotton-tipped swab. Irrigation may also be useful.

Which of the following is FALSE regarding the use of topical fluorescein, which is used to highlight epithelial defects of the cornea?

A) Fluorescein is a nontoxic, water-soluble dye.
B) Fluorescein fluoresces under a cobalt blue filter.
C) Fluorescein exhibits positive staining of epithelial defects.
D) Fluorescein does not penetrate the cornea.

Discussion

The correct answer is D. Fluorescein **does** diffuse through the corneal stroma and causes a green flare in the anterior chamber. Rapid staining of the anterior chamber after the removal of a corneal foreign body suggests a large, deep corneal injury.

* *

After successfully removing the piece of metal, you plan to discharge the patient. Which of the following is NOT considered a treatment for corneal abrasions?

A) Observation alone.
B) Topical antibiotics.
C) Cycloplegics.
D) Topical steroids.
E) Patching.

Discussion

The answer is D. In uncomplicated corneal abrasions in non-contact-lens wearers, observation alone may be indicated. Antibiotics should be used for all contact lens-related abrasions. The patients should also be advised to withhold contact lens use until the abrasion is healed. Cycloplegic agents and topical NSAIDs may be used if there is significant discomfort or traumatic iritis. Patching may also be used PRN for patient comfort but is unnecessary and may increase pain and increase healing time. Topical steroids may inhibit epithelial healing and promote infection and should be avoided.

 HELPFUL TIP: Multiple vertical corneal abrasions suggest a foreign body under the upper lid. Blinking and closing the eye will leave a vertical abrasion on the cornea. Evert the eyelid and sweep the fornices with a moistened cotton swab to remove any residual foreign body.

Objectives: Did you learn to . . .

- Remove a corneal foreign body?
- Use topical fluorescein in corneal abrasions?
- Manage uncomplicated corneal abrasions?

CASE 11

A 65-year-old white male with a history of hypertension, adult-onset diabetes, rheumatoid arthritis, and rosacea presents with chronic complaints of redness, tearing, and irritation OU. He sometimes also has "a film over his vision" which comes and goes. His ocular examination appears normal. He does, however, have an oily tear film with rapid breakup of his tears over his ocular surface. There is evidence of plugging of his meibomian glands (sebaceous glands along his lid margins), but the eyelids are otherwise normal in appearance.

Which of the following is the most likely diagnosis?

A) Meibomian gland dysfunction.
B) Staphylococcal blepharitis.
C) Hordeolum.
D) Chalazion.
E) Seborrheic blepharitis.

Discussion

The correct answer is A. Meibomian glands are the sebaceous glands of the upper and lower eyelids, which are located along the posterior lid margin behind the lashes. These are punctate openings along the lid margin, which become inspissated with thick secretions. This eventually leads to an unstable tear film, creating symptoms of burning, redness, foreign body sensation, and filmy vision. It is considered a form of blepharitis (inflammation of the eyelids). Answers B and E are incorrect. Staphylococcal and seborrheic blepharitis have similar symptoms but involve the anterior eyelid margin at the base of the lashes **(not the meibomian glands as in this patient)**. Both typically have predominant signs of crusting or mattering. Seborrheic blepharitis often has crusting of an oily or greasy consistency. Answers C and D are inflammatory processes, commonly but incorrectly grouped together as "styes." A hordeolum (stye) affects the anterior lid margin glands which become acutely plugged. A chalazion affects the posterior lid margin glands which become plugged and chronically inflamed. Stye is synonymous with hordeolum.

What part of his past medical history is associated with meibomian gland dysfunction?

A) Hypertension.
B) Diabetes.
C) Rheumatoid arthritis.
D) Rosacea.

Discussion

The correct answer is D. Meibomian gland dysfunction is associated with rosacea. Typical findings of rosacea include facial papules, pustules, telangiectasia, erythema, and rhinophyma.

What are other associated findings with both blepharitis and meibomian gland dysfunction?

A) Conjunctival injection.
B) Corneal punctate epithelial staining.
C) Peripheral corneal marginal infiltrates.
D) Eyelid telangiectasia.
E) All of the above.

Discussion

The correct answer is E. All of the above may be seen with both blepharitis and meibomian gland dysfunction.

What treatment do you prescribe for this patient?

A) Observation and reassurance.
B) Daily warm compresses, lid scrubs with dilute baby shampoo, and oral doxycycline or metronidazole.
C) Erythromycin ophthalmic ointment PRN.
D) Daily warm compresses, topical steroids, and frequent use of artificial tears.

Discussion

The correct answer is B. The treatment of meibomian gland dysfunction consists of lid hygiene and doxycycline 50–100 mg QD–BID for 3–6 weeks. The dosage may then be tapered according to symptoms. Gastrointestinal upset and photosensitivity are common side effects of doxycycline. Also, doxycycline is contraindicated in pregnant women and children <10 years. Treatment of staphylococcal blepharitis consists of lid scrubs with dilute baby shampoo and topical bacitracin, erythromycin, or sulfacetamide. Seborrheic blepharitis is often treated with aggressive lid hygiene.

Topical steroids are used only for short duration if there is significant inflammation present and should generally be prescribed by an ophthalmologist.

Which of the following is a common complication of meibomian gland dysfunction?

A) Bacterial keratitis.
B) Preseptal cellulitis.
C) Chalazion.
D) Scleritis.
E) Chronic conjunctivitis.

Discussion

The correct answer is C. Meibomian gland dysfunction can cause a chronic granuloma to form behind the plugged meibomian gland, which is called a chalazion. The inflammation is sterile—unlike a hordeolum (stye), which is a painful purulent abscess. Treatment of a chalazion involves frequent warm compresses and massage. Topical antibiotics are of little value since it is sterile. If these measures fail, an intralesional injection of steroids or incision and drainage is warranted. Hordeola (styes) often resolve spontaneously but warm compresses and massage are often helpful. If there is any evidence of cellulitis, systemic antibiotics are indicated. Drainage using a needle may also be helpful. Topical antibiotics are often not effective.

Objectives: Did you learn to . . .

- Recognize the signs and symptoms of blepharitis and meibomian gland dysfunction?
- Describe the etiologies of blepharitis and meibomian gland dysfunction?
- Differentiate among meibomian gland dysfunction and staphylococcal and seborrheic blepharitis?
- Determine appropriate treatment for blepharitis and meibomian gland dysfunction and the complications of hordeola and chalazion?

CASE 12

A 7-year-old white female presents with painful swelling and redness of her upper and lower lids of her right eye. She reports having a bug bite near her right eye a week ago, which has been very itchy. On examination, her right eyelids are extremely edematous with a well-demarcated area of erythema. Her ocular exam is normal. She has no RAPD, proptosis, or motility deficit.

This presentation is most consistent with:

A) Orbital cellulitis.
B) Preseptal cellulitis.
C) Contact dermatitis.
D) Anaphylactoid reaction to the insect bite.
E) None of the above.

Discussion

The correct answer is B. The presentation of this patient is consistent with preseptal cellulitis which is defined as inflammation/infection anterior to the orbital septum. The septum is a fibrous sheet which extends from the periosteum of the superior and inferior orbital rims and extends into the upper and lower eyelids. This is less dangerous than orbital cellulitis, which occurs posterior to the orbital septum and has the risk of spread of infection into adjacent structures. Orbital cellulitis can be complicated by subperiosteal abscess, cavernous sinus thrombosis, meningitis, or intracranial abscesses. Answer A is incorrect. Infection occurring **posterior** to the orbital septum is called orbital cellulitis. This is characterized by fever, proptosis, restriction of motility, chemosis, and pain on eye movements. Answer C is incorrect. Contact dermatitis should include blistering, scaling, lichenification, etc. Answer D is incorrect because an anaphylactoid reaction is systemic.

Which of the following statements is TRUE?

A) The most common cause of preseptal cellulitis in children is sinusitis.
B) The most common cause of preseptal cellulitis in teens and adults is sinusitis.
C) Orbital cellulitis is most commonly caused by bacteremia from a secondary source (as opposed to direct spread from an adjacent structure).
D) The most common secondary source for orbital cellulitis is otitis media.

Discussion

The correct answer is A. The most common cause of preseptal cellulitis in children is sinusitis. In contrast, teens and adults usually have preseptal cellulitis from a superficial source, such as skin trauma with inoculation.

HELPFUL TIP: Both orbital cellulitis and preseptal cellulitis are commonly secondary to sinusitis. Preseptal and orbital cellulitis may also occur from direct inoculation or bacteremia from a distant source.

The most common pathogen causing preseptal cellulitis from a skin trauma with inoculation is:

A) *Staphylococcus epidermidis.*
B) *Haemophilus influenzae.*
C) *Staphylococcus aureus.*
D) *Streptococcus pneumoniae.*

Discussion

The correct answer is C. *Staphylococcus aureus* is the most common pathogen of preseptal cellulitis from skin trauma. Some may have chosen answer B. Prior to the introduction of the HIB vaccine, children <5 years often had preseptal cellulitis secondary to *Haemophilus influenzae.* However, this is no longer the most common pathogen. Most cases of preseptal and orbital cellulitis in children are caused by Gram-positive cocci. Orbital cellulitis in children is usually caused by a single organism. In contrast, adults with orbital cellulitis frequently have polymicrobial infections including Gram-positive cocci, *H. influenzae*, and anaerobes. Mucormycosis should be suspected in diabetics and immunocompromised individuals.

Which of the following is TRUE?

A) Preseptal cellulitis usually requires no imaging.
B) Preseptal cellulitis and orbital cellulitis **MAY** both require CT imaging of the orbit and sinuses.
C) Orbital cellulitis requires imaging only to determine extent of orbital inflammation/infection and to evaluate for underlying sinusitis.
D) All cases of preseptal and orbital cellulitis should be treated with IV antibiotics.

Discussion

The correct answer is B. In contrast to preseptal cellulitis, orbital cellulitis causes proptosis, motility restriction, chemosis (swelling of conjunctiva), or pain on eye movements. In preseptal cellulitis, the eye itself is typically uninvolved. Answer A is incorrect. Both preseptal cellulitis and orbital cellulitis require CT imaging of the orbit and sinuses. In preseptal cellulitis, imaging is warranted if no direct inoculation site is identified to rule out underlying sinusitis. In orbital cellulitis, additional scanning is warranted if no improvement occurs within 24-48 hours because a subperiosteal abscess may form, requiring surgical drainage. Answer D is incorrect. Mild preseptal cellulitis in the older compliant patient may be treated with oral antibiotics as an outpatient. In severe cases of preseptal cellulitis, the patient should be admitted and treated with IV antibiotics. Answer C is incorrect. **All patients with orbital cellulitis** should be treated inpatient with broad-spectrum IV antibiotics until a suspected pathogen can be confirmed and selected antibiotics can be used.

Objectives: Did you learn to . . .

- Differentiate between orbital and preseptal cellulitis?
- Recognize conditions that predispose patients to these processes?
- Manage orbital and preseptal cellulitis?

CASE 13

A 67-year-old white man with a history of coronary artery disease, hypertension, and peripheral vascular disease presents with the sudden onset of painless loss of vision OD several hours ago. He states he was watching TV when "things went black" in his right eye. He notes that this happened a few times before but his vision always returned to normal after a couple of minutes. On examination, he has light perception vision, the presence of an RAPD, and a normal anterior segment of the eye. Upon funduscopic exam, the fundus appears diffusely white with a reddish hue within the macula (Figure 19–11; see also color section).

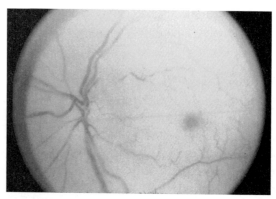

Figure 19–11

The patient's history and examination are most consistent with which of the following?

A) Central retinal vein occlusion (CRVO).
B) Anterior ischemic optic neuropathy (AION).
C) Central retinal artery occlusion (CRAO).
D) Choroidal ischemia.

Discussion

The correct answer is C. A central retinal artery occlusion is characterized by acute painless loss of vision. The ischemia and edema of the retina cause diffuse whitening. There is a cherry-red spot in the macula which is the normal choroidal circulation amidst the ischemic retina (see Figure 19–11; see also color section). The extensive ischemia causes an RAPD and significant visual loss. His previous history of recurrent episodes of loss of vision which returned to normal is consistent with amaurosis fugax.

In a patient with this history, irreversible retinal damage occurs after what time frame?

A) 10 minutes.
B) 30 minutes.
C) 60 minutes.
D) 90 minutes.

Discussion

The correct answer is D. Amaurosis fugax, or transient monocular blindness, is typically caused by carotid disease. It is often described as a curtain or shade coming over the vision. It lasts from a few seconds to 15 minutes. If occlusion is complete for >90 minutes, irreversible retinal damage and visual loss ensue. Patients should seek medical care immediately. Patients with a history of amaurosis fugax should be evaluated for carotid and cardiac disease, which frequently means carotid Dopplers and echocardiography.

Treatment for central retinal artery occlusion includes all of the following EXCEPT:

A) Thrombolytics.
B) Digital compression/decompression of the globe.
C) Oxygen.
D) Increasing blood carbon dioxide levels (eg, rebreathing).
E) Acetazolamide.

Discussion

The correct answer is A. Therapy for central retinal artery occlusion is aimed at dislodging the embolism, maintaining retinal viability, and reducing intraocular pressure (to increase the pressure gradient between the artery and the eye). This can be accomplished by digitally compressing then decompressing the eye with a finger (to dislodge the embolism), oxygen (which will increase oxygen delivery), increasing serum carbon dioxide levels (thus dilating intracranial arteries), and acetazolamide (to reduce intraocular pressure).

Comparing central retinal *artery* occlusion with central retinal *vein* occlusion, which of the following is TRUE?

A) Central retinal artery occlusion is more likely to be associated with giant cell arteritis.
B) The main feature of both is retinal whitening with a cherry-red spot.
C) Central retinal vein occlusion usually results from atherosclerotic thrombosis while central retinal artery occlusion results from hyperviscosity syndromes and hypercoagulable states.
D) An RAPD is characteristic of central retinal artery occlusion but is not seen with central retinal vein occlusion.

Discussion

The correct answer is A. Giant cell arteritis is seen in 1%–2% of central retinal artery occlusion. However, a more limited anterior ischemic retinopathy is generally seen with giant cell arteritis. If a patient presents with symptoms of central retinal artery occlusion, but no embolus is visualized, he/she should be asked about symptoms of giant cell arteritis. Answer B is incorrect because only central retinal artery occlusion is associated with retinal whitening and a cherry-red spot. The appearance of a central retinal **vein** occlusion is one of tortuous dilated veins, optic nerve edema, and intraretinal hemorrhages/edema. Answer C is incorrect because central retinal **artery** occlusion is usually caused by atherosclerotic thrombosis or emboli while central retinal **vein** occlusion is associated more with hyperviscosity syndromes (eg, polycythemia) and hypercoagulable states (eg, protein C deficiency) in younger patients. In older patients with central retinal vein occlusions, main risk factors include vasculopathic states such as hypertension and diabetes. Answer D is incorrect because an RAPD can be seen with either syndrome. There is always an RAPD with a central retinal artery occlusion due to the diffuse level of ischemia. An RAPD may or may not be seen with a central retinal vein occlusion depending on the level of ischemia.

 HELPFUL TIP: Other causes of central retinal artery occlusion include vasculitis, such as in giant cell arteritis, or blood dyscrasias. Other causes of central retinal vein occlusions include increased intraorbital or intraocular pressure, glaucoma, blood dyscrasias, lupus anticoagulant, antiphospholipid antibody, and protein C deficiency. See Figure 19–12 (see also color section) for an image of the retina in central retinal vein occlusion.

Further evaluation and treatment of a central retinal artery occlusion include all of the following EXCEPT:

A) Anterior chamber tap and fluid removal.
B) Topical timolol.
C) Immediate ESR/CRP.
D) Carotid Doppler/cardiac echography/ECG.
E) Orbital MRI/MRA.

Discussion
The correct answer is E. There is no need for orbital imaging in the management of a central retinal artery occlusion. All of the other answer choices are important management steps (see Discussions above). In addition, blood pressure, fasting blood sugar or glycosylated hemoglobin, CBC, and PT/PTT should be

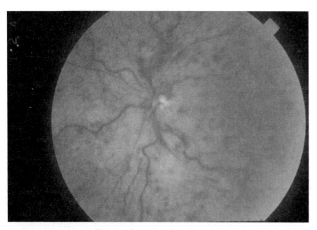

Figure 19–12   Central retinal vein occlusion. Note the dilated tortuous veins, optic disc edema, and retinal hemorrhage/edema.

done. If there is a suspicion of giant cell arteritis, an ESR/CRP should be checked. Other tests might include a rheumatoid factor, syphilis serology, serum protein electrophoresis, and antiphospholipid antibodies. A similar workup is warranted in central retinal vein occlusion, except there is no need to search for an embolic source with a carotid Doppler and cardiac echography.

Objectives: Did you learn to . . .

● Recognize the symptoms of vascular disorders of the eye?
● Differentiate between central retinal artery and vein occlusions?
● Describe some causes of ocular vascular occlusions?
● Determine the appropriate systemic workup for artery and vein occlusions?

CASE 14

A 40-year-old white female presents to your ED with complaint of seeing "little floating black spots" in her vision in the left eye. She also notes little sparks of light in the temporal periphery of the left eye. She noted this while shopping today and denies any history of trauma. On examination, there is no RAPD (she has normal direct and consensual pupillary reflexes). Visual fields to confrontation demonstrate peripheral vision loss in the left eye. Dilated examination reveals pigmented cells within the vitreous, and peripheral retinal examination reveals billowing grey folds. The macula appears normal, and her vision is 20/20.

Which of the following is the most appropriate step in the management of this patient?

A) Place a patch over the left eye.
B) Refer to an ophthalmologist immediately.
C) Lower blood pressure acutely with IV labetalol.
D) Apply timolol solution to the affected eye.
E) Offer reassurance and see her lawyer in court.

Discussion
The correct answer is B. This patient is presenting with urgent ophthalmologic disease. She has classic symptoms of retinal detachment—flashing lights, visual field disruption, and floaters. Also, the majority of her vision is still intact. In her current state, she has a high likelihood

of retaining good vision. Prognosis for retinal detachment depends on the closeness of the detachment to the macula, its location, progression, and history of preexisting retinal conditions. None of the other treatments listed does anything for retinal detachment. Answer A is rarely indicated in the ED. Answer C is treatment for hypertensive retinopathy. Answer D is for glaucoma. Answer E is just plain wrong in this case.

Risk factors for retinal detachment include all of the following EXCEPT:

A) Glaucoma.
B) Aphakia.
C) Myopia.
D) Trauma.
E) Prior ocular surgery.

Discussion

The correct answer is A. Glaucoma is not a risk factor for retinal detachment. Both myopia (nearsightedness) and aphakia (surgical removal of lens) are risk factors. Trauma and previous surgery also predispose to retinal detachments. Most individuals with retinal detachment are >50 years. As people age, the vitreous detaches from the posterior wall of the eye which can tug on the retina causing a tear.

Objectives: Did you learn to . . .

- Suspect retinal detachment in patients presenting with "floaters" and "flashes"?
- Identify patients who are at risk for retinal detachment?

CASE 13

A 55-year-old white male with type 2 diabetes mellitus presents with complaint of a gradual decrease in vision in both eyes. He notes glare with oncoming headlights while night driving. Despite this, he feels that he is able to read better without his bifocals.

Which of the following is the most likely cause of this patient's complaints?

A) Retinal detachment.
B) Cataracts.
C) Glaucoma.
D) Diabetic retinopathy.

Discussion

The correct answer is B. Progressive visual loss and glare while driving at night are common complaints caused by cataracts. The eye exam can confirm the diagnosis, as most significant cataracts are easily visualized. The red reflex is diminished bilaterally, and a haze of gray is observed over the lens. Symptoms of retinal detachment are more acute. Glaucoma and diabetic retinopathy are less likely, but could also be present. Eye pressure and a dilated eye exam should be completed.

All of the following conditions and medications are risk factors for cataract formation EXCEPT:

A) Corticosteroids.
B) Trauma.
C) Radiation.
D) Calcium channel blockers.
E) Diabetes mellitus.

Discussion

The correct answer is D. All of the other answer choices are associated with cataract formation. Other risk factors include age, tobacco, alcohol, and sunlight (so wear your shades).

Of all of the patients with cataracts below, which one has an indication for cataract surgery?

A) A patient with no visual complaints with a visual acuity of 20/50.
B) A patient with complaints of glare and inability to drive at night with a visual acuity of 20/40.
C) An older patient with a history of a unilateral **congenital** cataract and best-corrected visual acuity of 20/100.
D) A patient with right monocular diplopia that resolves with new spectacle correction.

Discussion

The correct answer is B. There is no strict visual acuity which determines the appropriate timing of cataract surgery although most consider 20/40 or worse a cutoff. If there are significant lifestyle limitations secondary to visual disability from a cataract, then cataract surgery is indicated. Answer C is incorrect. An older person with a history of congenital cataracts and poor best-corrected visual acuity most likely suffered from amblyopia; therefore, cataract surgery is unlikely to benefit such a patient. Answer D is incorrect. Monocular diplopia (double vision from one eye only) is an indication for cataract surgery, but if new spectacle correction improves the diplopia, then cataract surgery is not necessary.

Complications of cataract surgery include which of the following?

A) Endophthalmitis.
B) Retinal detachment.
C) Glaucoma.
D) Hemorrhage.
E) All of the above.

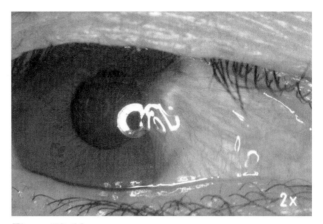

Figure 19–13

Discussion

The correct answer is E. Current-day cataract surgery is typically done by phacoemulsification with an intraocular lens implant. Phacoemulsification is an ultrasound method of fragmenting and aspirating the cataract. Although associated with fewer complications than older large-incision cataract surgery techniques, the potential complications mentioned above still exist. Additional complications include wound leaks, uveitis, macular edema, retained lens material, and vitreous loss.

Objectives: Did you learn to . . .

- Identify patients at risk for cataract development?
- Recognize the symptoms and visual disability in those with progressive cataracts?

 QUICK QUIZ: SOMETHING ON THE EYE

A patient presents to your clinic without vision symptoms but complains of a growth in his eye (Figure 19–13; see also color section). The growth is painless and has been present for several years but is now becoming very obvious. Strangers tend to stare.

This growth is most likely due to:

A) Systemic inflammatory illness.
B) Exposure to UV light and dust.
C) Foreign body granuloma.
D) Trauma to the sclera and cornea with scarring.
E) Any of the above can lead to this finding.

Discussion

The correct answer is B. This is a pterygium, an overgrowth of conjunctival tissue, which is a result of recurrent exposure to UV light and high winds with dust. It is of no clinical significance unless it encroaches on the visual field or causes cosmetic distress. It is characterized by crossing onto the cornea as opposed to a pinguecula, which has a similar appearance but does not infringe upon the cornea.

 QUICK QUIZ: PAINFUL EYE

A 40-year-old patient presents with a painful, red area on the eye (Figure 19–14; see also color section). He notes the gradual onset of severe pain of a boring nature with pain in the periocular area as well. He has a history of rheumatoid arthritis.

What is the diagnosis?

A) Episcleritis.
B) Pterygium.

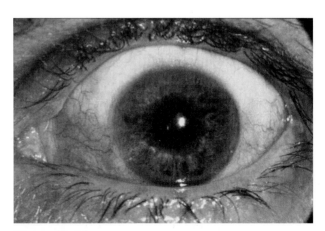

Figure 19–14

C) Scleritis.
D) Pingueculitis.
E) Epidemic hemorrhagic conjunctivitis.

Discussion

The correct answer is C. This is scleritis. Notice the erythema and inflammation which differentiates it from a pterygium. The erythema and inflammation is not originating from fibrovascular tissue as in the pterygium. It is deep beneath the conjunctiva in the sclera. Scleritis may also be nodular in nature or diffuse. Scleritis can be easily mistaken for episcleritis which may appear similar. Episcleritis is inflammation of the overlying episcleral tissues which are more superficial than the sclera. However, patients with episcleritis do not have the severity of pain noted with scleritis, and the inflammation and erythema are generally not as intense. Pingueculitis appears as yellowish, slightly raised nodules in which are found in the same area as are pterygiums. Scleritis is an ophthalmologic emergency and should be referred.

QUICK QUIZ: OPHTHALMOLOGY

A 70-year-old white female presents for her routine medical evaluation. She reports no problems, but on review of systems she states that she has had a gradual decrease in vision in the right eye over the past several months. She had successful cataract surgery of both eyes 3 years ago. After the surgery, she had 20/20 vision OU. Now on examination, her vision is OD 20/50 and OS 20/20. She has no RAPD. The slit lamp exam of her anterior segment of both eyes reveals intraocular lens implants behind her irides. There seems to be a hazy membrane behind her lens implant.

The most likely diagnosis is which of the following?

A) Posterior capsular opacity.
B) Endophthalmitis.
C) Retinal detachment.
D) Posterior uveitis.
E) Intraocular lens dislocation.

Discussion

The correct answer is A. Months to years after successful cataract surgery, patients may experience a gradual decline in their vision due to an opacification of the posterior capsule behind their intraocular lens implant. During cataract surgery, most of the normal capsule of the lens remains and holds the intraocular lens implant. In successful cataract surgery, only the anterior portion of the capsule is removed and a bowl of capsule remains. The posterior portion of this capsule may become hazy over time caused by the proliferation of residual lens epithelial cells. The patient does not have any symptoms of infection or inflammation and reports no flashes or floaters which would eliminate most of the other choices. An intraocular lens dislocation is rare and is usually seen in the setting of trauma. Treatment is laser capsulotomy.

CASE 14

A 56-year-old white male with a history of hypertension and diabetes presents with complaints of double vision and pain for the past 2 days. On exam, his vision is OD 20/50 and OS 20/25. He has a larger pupil with an RAPD OD. The lid of his right eye is slightly lower than the left. His right eye is deviated slightly temporally and inferiorly, and he has difficulty adducting and elevating the eye.

The most likely diagnosis is which of the following?

A) Graves disease.
B) Horner syndrome.
C) Third nerve palsy.
D) Myasthenia gravis.

Discussion

The correct answer is C. The case presented is a typical scenario of a third nerve palsy. Patients with a third nerve palsy present with diplopia (from ocular muscle paralysis), ptosis, and a dilated pupil. Recall that the ocular muscles are innervated by CN 3 except for the lateral rectus (CN6) and the superior oblique (CN4), so the eye will be "down and out" in a third nerve palsy. **Often the pupil is spared in diabetics. Pupil involvement should prompt an investigation for an intracranial aneurysm.** Answer A, Graves disease, may present with motility deficits and compression of the optic nerve resulting in an RAPD. However, Graves is less likely in this patient because it should present with lid retraction and proptosis, not ptosis. Graves also may cause restriction of the medial and inferior rectus muscles which causes difficulty abducting and elevating the eye. Answer B, Horner syndrome, may present with ptosis but the affected side would have miosis (and not mydriasis as in this patient), and it does not present with motility deficits. Answer D, myasthenia gravis, may present with ptosis and motility deficit but these finding are usually elicited with fatigue and are variable.

The workup of this patient should involve:

A) Cerebral angiography.
B) CT/CTA.
C) MRI/MRA.
D) Orbital ultrasonography.

Discussion

The correct answer is C. Although cerebral angiography has long been the gold standard in detecting cerebral aneurysms, the first-line and less invasive diagnostic test is MRI/MRA.

CASE 15

A 55-year-old white female comes in complaining of eye irritation/redness bilaterally, but left greater than right. On examination, her vision is OD 20/30, OS 20/50. She has no RAPD. Motility of her eyes shows a very mild upward gaze deficit of both eyes. Her eyes look bulgy and red (OS>OD). The sclera of her eyes is quite exposed since her eyes protrude so much. There is punctate staining of her corneas with fluorescein. The remainder of her anterior segment exam looks unremarkable.

The patient's presentation is most consistent with the diagnosis of:

A) Viral conjunctivitis.
B) HSV keratitis.
C) Scleritis.
D) Graves disease.

Discussion

The correct answer is D. The most common cause of unilateral and bilateral proptosis (protrusion of eyes) is Graves disease. Patients may be hyperthyroid (most common), euthyroid, or hypothyroid. They often present with proptosis, lid retraction, and diplopia. These findings are due to lymphocytic infiltration of extraocular muscles causing restriction in motion in the opposite direction. The most common muscle affected is the inferior rectus, followed by the medial rectus, causing restriction when their antagonist muscles are active (eg, elevation and abduction deficits). Occasionally, the muscles can become so enlarged that they cause a compressive optic neuropathy causing an RAPD. The proptosis and lid retraction can cause corneal exposure which this patient has and is the likely cause of her decreased vision as seen by her corneal staining.

The best way to definitively diagnose Graves ophthalmopathy in this patient is:

A) Orbital MRI.
B) TSH, free T4.
C) Orbital CT.
D) Visual field testing.

Discussion

The correct answer is C. The best way to diagnose Graves ophthalmopathy is by orbital CT scanning with axial and coronal cuts. Orbital ultrasound is another way to determine if there is infiltration of the extraocular muscles or optic nerve compression. Because some patients can be euthyroid, TSH and free thyroxine (T4) are not diagnostic; however, these tests will be necessary in the workup of this patient. Visual field testing is performed in Graves patients when there is a suspicion of compressive optic neuropathy.

Objectives: Did you learn to . . .

- Recognize the presentation of third-nerve palsy?
- Recognize the presentation of Graves ophthalmopathy?

BIBLIOGRAPHY

Alward WLM. Glaucoma: *The Requisites in Ophthalmology.* St Louis: Mosby, 2000.

Amaurosis Fugax Study Group. Current management of amaurosis fugax. *Stroke.* 1990;21:201.

Bressler SB. Age-related macular degeneration. Focal Points: Clinical Modules for Ophthalmologists. *American Academy of Ophthalmology.* 1995;13(2).

Diabetes Control and Complications Trial Research Group. The effect of intensive treatment of diabetes on the development and progression of long-term complications in insulin-dependent diabetes mellitus. *N Engl J Med.* 1993;329:977.

Diabetes Control and Complications Trial Research Group. Progression of retinopathy and intensive versus conventional treatment in the Diabetes Control and Complications Trial. *Ophthalmology.* 1995;102:647.

Executive Committee for the Asymptomatic Carotid Atherosclerosis Study. Endarterectomy for asymptomatic carotid stenosis. *JAMA.* 1995;275:1421.

Hayreh SS, Kolder HE, Weingeist TA. Central retinal artery occlusion and retinal tolerance time. *Ophthalmology.* 1980;87:75.

Hayreh SS, Podhajsky P, Zimmerman MB. Role of nocturnal arterial hypotension in optic nerve head ischemic disorders. *Ophthalmologica.* 1999;213:76.

Lee AG, Brazis PW. *Clinical Pathways in Neuro-ophthalmology: An Evidence-based Approach.* New York: Thieme, 2003.

North American Symptomatic Carotid Endarterectomy Trial Collaborators. Beneficial effect of carotid endarterectomy in symptomatic patients with high-grade carotid stenosis. *N Engl J Med.* 1991;325:445.

Pediatric Eye Disease Investigator Group. The clinical spectrum of early-onset esotropia: experience of the Congenital Esotropia Observational Study. *Am J Ophthalmol.* 2002;133;102.

Preferred Practice Patterns Committee, Retina Panel. Diabetic Retinopathy. American Academy of Ophthalmology; 1998.

Putterman AM, Stevens T, Urist MJ. Nonsurgical management of blowout fractures of the orbital floor. *Am J Ophthalmol.* 1974;77:232.

Rubin PAD, Bilyk JR, Shore JW. Management of orbital trauma: fractures, hemorrhage, and traumatic optic neuropathy. Focal Points: Clinical Modules for Ophthalmologists. *American Academy of Ophthalmology.* 1994;12(7).

Shields MB. *Textbook of Glaucoma.* 5th ed. Baltimore: Lippincott Williams & Wilkins, 2005.

United Kingdom Prospective Diabetes Study Group. Intensive blood-glucose control with sulphonylureas or insulin compared with conventional treatment and risk of complications in patients with type 2 diabetes (UKPDS 33). *Lancet.* 1998;352:837.

United Kingdom Prospective Diabetes Study Group. Tight blood pressure control and risk of macrovascular and microvascular complications in type 2 diabetes: (UKPDS 38). *Br Med J.* 1998;317:703.

Acknowledgment. Photographs were provided by the University of Iowa Department of Ophthalmology. Special thanks to Dr. James Folk and Dr. Young Kwon for their photograph contributions.

20

Otolaryngology

Jason K. Wilbur and Mark A. Graber

CASE 1

A 2-year-old is brought to your office by her mother who is concerned that she has been pulling at her left ear since late last night and has a fever of 101.3°F. She has been drinking normally, but she was not interested in breakfast this morning. She has had recurrent bouts of these symptoms, the last of which was 9 months ago. Each time the symptoms resolved with one "shot." There is no report of vomiting or diarrhea. She is alert and interactive. She has some evidence of mucoid discharge from her nares bilaterally.

Each of the following findings is diagnostic of acute otitis media EXCEPT:

A) Profuse, purulent ear discharge without other evidence of otitis externa.

B) Air-fluid level behind the tympanic membrane (TM) with marked redness of the TM and poor movement with pneumatic otoscopy.

C) Bulging, thickened yellow and red TM that does not move well with pneumatic otoscopy.

D) Bubbles in fluid behind the TM with impaired mobility of the TM on pneumatic otoscopy.

E) Yellow, opaque TM, poor movement with pneumatic otoscopy, and substantial ear pain.

Discussion

The correct answer is D. Suspected ear infections drive many parents to bring their children to a family physician. Distinguishing between acute otitis media (AOM) and otitis media with effusion (OME) is a daily task for most of us, but not a trivial one. It is important that we do this well, so that antibiotics are not overprescribed, leading to increased emergence of resistant organisms and side effects from unnecessary treatments. A TM may be inflamed (ie, erythematous) due to something other than AOM. Likewise, there may be fluid in the middle ear that is not infected, otherwise known as otitis media with effusion (OME). In order to diagnose AOM, you need evidence of fluid in the middle ear **and** inflammation. Middle ear effusion is diagnosed by: (1) bubbles and/or air-fluid level behind the TM; (2) **two** or more of the following: decreased or absent movement with pneumatic otoscopy, opacification of the TM, discoloration of the TM (yellow, white, blue). These findings get you to OME but not AOM. To diagnose AOM, you will need to have OME with evidence of acute inflammation, such as marked pain, thickened and/or bulging TM, and reddened TM. For these reasons, answers B, C, and E are examples of AOM. Answer A, purulent otorrhea without evidence of otitis externa, would be the one exception where you can diagnose AOM without even seeing the TM. Answer D was the exception because there is evidence of OME without inflammation.

HELPFUL TIP: Do not believe a red ear drum. By itself, redness of the TM has a 15% positive predictive value for diagnosing AOM. That's terrible! **Use pneumatic otoscopy** which is the standard of care for diagnosing AOM. **Tympanometry** is an alternative to pneumatic otoscopy. Of course, you still need to look in the ear.

* *

Your patient's left TM is opaque, red, and immobile upon pneumatic otoscopy.

All of the following factors increase her risk for developing otitis media EXCEPT:

A) She attends day care.
B) Her mother smokes inside the house.
C) The patient is a female.
D) Patient still uses a pacifier.

Discussion

The correct answer is C. The following are known risk factors for the development of AOM: day-care attendance, smoking inside the home, **male gender**, pacifier use, children in developing countries, age between 6 and 18 months, and lack of breast-feeding.

Which of the following findings is reliably found in patients with acute otitis media?

A) Fever.
B) Ear pulling.
C) Irritability.
D) Rhinitis.
E) None of the above.

Discussion

The correct answer is E. None of the above is reliably found in patients with AOM. Other unreliable factors include vomiting, diarrhea, and cough. The presence or absence of any of these findings is **not** helpful in making the diagnosis of otitis media. Although ear pain is a symptom of inflammation, it is a relatively weak predictor of AOM and must be accompanied by other findings as listed above. On the other hand, **pneumatic otoscopy or otoscopy plus tympanometry is the way to make the diagnosis,** but always be certain that you have a good seal or you run the risk of a false-positive finding.

 HELPFUL TIP: Patients with AOM who are ≥2 years may be observed rather than treated with antibiotics. They should meet the following criteria: fever <39°C, mild otalgia, immunocompetent, and follow-up assured within 48–72 hours. Analgesics should be given regardless.

* *

This patient has not had any problems with otitis media for at least 9 months, has not been on antibiotics during that time, is not in day care, and has no allergies. You elect to treat her with an antibiotic.

Which of the following is the most appropriate treatment for this patient?

A) Amoxicillin 40 mg/kg/day divided TID.
B) Amoxicillin 80-90 mg/kg/day divided BID.
C) Ceftriaxone 50 mg/kg IM once.
D) Azithromycin 10 mg/kg for 1 day then 5 mg/kg for days 2–5.
E) Amoxicillin/clavulanate 40–80 mg/kg/day divided BID.

Discussion

The correct answer is B. Amoxicillin is the first-line treatment of AOM. The dose is 80–90 mg/kg/day in all patients whether antibiotic-naïve or not. More broad-spectrum (and expensive) drugs, such as ceftriaxone, amoxicillin/clavulanate, azithromycin, etc, should be reserved for patients who fail initial therapy with a first-line drug or have a penicillin allergy.

 HELPFUL TIP: You can treat children >6 years with a 5-day course of amoxicillin. Amoxicillin/clavulanate should be reserved for treatment failures.

 HELPFUL TIP: No antibiotic has proven superior to amoxicillin in the treatment of otitis media. Other antibiotics will work but are more expensive and/or have greater side effects.

Which of the following statements best characterizes the role of antibiotics in the treatment of acute otitis media?

A) Antibiotics have been shown to reduce suppurative complications of otitis media, such as mastoiditis, in developed countries.
B) The majority of patients with otitis media benefit from the use of antibiotics.

C) The use of antibiotics in otitis media reduces hearing loss and benefits language development.

D) With or without antibiotics, approximately 75% of children have resolution of symptoms after 7 days.

E) All of the above are true.

Discussion

The correct answer is D. The benefit of antibiotics for most children with AOM is marginal (NNT is ~12); thus, the option exists to observe and not give antibiotics in children ≥2 years who have mild symptoms, are not immunocompromised, and have good follow-up. The rest of the statements are incorrect. Antibiotics do **not** reduce suppurative complications in **developed** countries, but they do seem to prevent suppurative complications in developing countries where sanitation and health care access are not optimal. Answer B is incorrect. The number needed to treat (NNT) with antibiotics is up to 12 in order to benefit one individual, and this benefit is limited to a 6% absolute reduction of pain at days 2–7 (21% versus 15%). Answer C is incorrect. In developed countries, suppurative complications are rare and treating with antibiotics does not impact these outcomes in any way.

> **HELPFUL TIP:** Acute otitis media is usually caused by *Streptococcus pneumoniae, Haemophilus influenzae, Moraxella catarrhalis,* and various viruses. Most cases are viral, and the majority—bacterial or viral—resolve spontaneously.

* *

You prescribe amoxicillin for 10 days and suggest acetaminophen for comfort. A few days later, the patient's mother calls to say that she is no better. You ask her to come in to clinic for evaluation.

When treating acute otitis media, which of these individuals should be considered a treatment failure and switched to another antibiotic?

A) A patient with a fever that continues at 24 hours after starting an oral antibiotic.

B) A child who is still tugging at his ear 5 days into a course of antibiotics.

C) A symptomatic child who still has a bulging, red, immobile tympanic membrane 3 days after starting antibiotics.

D) A child who continues to have rhinorrhea 1 week after starting antibiotics.

E) All of the above.

Discussion

The correct answer is C. You should consider switching to a different antibiotic in patients who remain symptomatic at 3 days **and who continue to have positive findings on pneumatic otoscopy**. Symptoms are not enough: they are unreliable. Remember, because most of these are viral infections, antibiotics are not doing much good. Answer A is incorrect because 24 hours is not sufficient to determine if a particular antibiotic will be effective. Answer B is incorrect because patients pull at their ears for a number of reasons, not just otitis media. Answer D is incorrect. If you chose this one, back to microbiology 101! Rhinorrhea does not respond to antibiotics and is most likely not bacterial in origin.

> **HELPFUL TIP:** There is no consensus regarding the antibiotic choice for amoxicillin failures. Amoxicillin/clavulanate and ceftriaxone are acceptable alternatives as are TMP/SMX, azithromycin, and clarithromycin. The number needed to harm is approximately 8 with amoxicillin/clavulanate; the diarrhea is often more distressing than the otitis.

* *

She returns with persistent pain and fever after taking amoxicillin for 3 days. On exam, you find evidence of persistent AOM. You switch the patient to your favorite second-line antibiotic. You see her back in 2 weeks for ear check and find complete resolution. The mother asks what she could do to avoid these troublesome infections in the future.

All of the following have been shown to reduce the incidence of recurrent otitis media EXCEPT:

A) Antibiotic prophylaxis.

B) Conjugate pneumococcal vaccine **and/or** influenza vaccine.

C) Tympanostomy tubes.

D) Tonsillectomy.

Discussion

The correct answer is D. Primary tonsillectomy has not been shown to reduce the recurrence of otitis media. However, **adenoidectomy with or without tonsillectomy will reduce the rate of recurrent otitis media in patients who already have tympanostomy tubes.** Answer A, the use of antibiotic prophylaxis, will reduce recurrent otitis media. **Antibiotic prophylaxis should be considered in the patient who has had ≥3 episodes of otitis media in 6 months or ≥4 episodes in 12 months.** Reasonable choices for antibiotics include amoxicillin and trimethoprim/sulfamethoxazole. Give one-half of the usual daily dose. This is generally given at bedtime. Often, antibiotics can be stopped during the summer because an upper respiratory infection is the precipitant of most cases of otitis media (remember that the great majority are solely viral). Pneumococcal vaccine (eg, Prevnar) will reduce the risk of recurrence in children with severe and recurrent acute otitis media. The same is true of influenza vaccine. Also recommended to reduce the frequency of AOM: avoid pacifier use, avoid bottle-propping at night, avoid smoke exposure, and breast-feeding for at least the first 6 months of life.

 HELPFUL TIP: Although it is traditionally done, there is no reason to follow up acute otitis media in patients >15 months of age who are asymptomatic. Clearly, if they are still symptomatic, follow-up is warranted.

 HELPFUL TIP: Addition of Cortisporin suspension is appropriate if there is AOM with a ruptured TM (manifested by purulent ear drainage). Other antibiotic drops can be used but are more expensive. No, Cortisporin will not cause hearing loss.

* *

The patient returns 4 weeks later with the mother who says, "She is still pulling at her left ear." There are no other complaints. On exam, you find the left tympanic membrane is without redness or opacity but contains a fluid level. The right ear exam is unremarkable.

What is your next diagnostic step?

A) Pneumatic otoscopy.

B) Hearing test.

C) Tympanostomy.

D) No further diagnosis needed; treat with antibiotic.

Discussion

The correct answer is A. Even though we all think we can do it well, the diagnosis of otitis media is fraught with problems. Pneumatic otoscopy should be done in all patients but especially in those for whom long-term therapy is being considered. Remember that fluid can persist for a month or more after an otitis media.

* *

On your exam, the TM does not move with insufflation. The patient's mother asks you if the child should have tubes placed.

Which of the following is NOT an indication for tympanostomy tubes?

A) Chronic bilateral effusions for >3 months with unilateral hearing loss.

B) Failure of antibiotic therapy to prevent recurrent otitis media.

C) Language delay secondary to otitis media.

D) >20 dB hearing loss bilaterally.

Discussion

The correct answer is A. Patients should meet the criteria listed above before being considered for tympanostomy tubes. Note that this requires that patients also meet the criteria for prophylactic antibiotic therapy (≥3 episodes of AOM in 6 months or ≥4 episodes in 12 months). A modification of answer A is also a criterion: chronic bilateral effusions for >3 months with **bilateral** hearing loss. **Although included as a criterion, there is no evidence that tympanostomy tubes improve language development in the short or long term.**

If fluid persists in the middle ear after acute otitis media, it is termed otitis media with effusion (OME).

Which of the following interventions has proven benefit in patients with OME?

A) Oral decongestants.

B) Oral antihistamines.

C) Prolonged treatment (≥1 month) with oral antibiotics.

D) Oral corticosteroids.

E) None of the above.

Discussion

The correct answer is E. There are not useful medical interventions for persistent OME. Autoinflation ("eustachian tube exercises" or forced exhalation with closed nose and mouth) is often recommended but has not shown a benefit. Patients may benefit from surgical intervention (see discussion about tympanostomy tubes above).

Objectives: Did you learn to . . .

- Diagnose otitis media appropriately?
- Initiate treatment in a patient with otitis media?
- Recognize failed antibiotic therapy and choose a new antibiotic?
- Describe prevention strategies for recurrent otitis media?
- Recognize indications for tympanostomy tube placement?

 QUICK QUIZ: EAR PAIN

Which of the following can cause ear pain?

A) Temporomandibular joint (TMJ) syndrome.

B) Cervical spine degenerative arthritis.

C) Cranial nerve lesions (5, 7, 9, or 10).

D) Bell palsy.

E) All of the above can cause ear pain.

Discussion

The correct answer is E. All of the above can cause ear pain. A more complete list is given in Table 20–1. The main point here is that not all that hurts in the ear is otitis media.

CASE 2

A 23-year-old female college student presents to your clinic complaining of ear pain. She is on the swimming team and notes that this pain occurs during swimming

Table 20–1   CAUSES OF EAR PAIN

- Auricular disease
- Canal disease
  - Otitis externa
  - Foreign body
  - Trauma
  - Eczema
  - Ramsay-Hunt syndrome
- Middle ear disease
  - Otitis media
  - Mastoiditis
  - Ménière disease
- Referred pain
  - Dental disease (eg, abscess)
  - TMJ syndrome
  - Carotidynia
  - Pharyngeal disease (eg, pharyngitis)
  - Cranial nerve lesions (CN V, VII, IX, X)
  - Upper cervical nerve disease, any cause (eg, disk disease)
  - Bell's palsy and other neurologic diseases (eg, trigeminal neuralgia)

season. The pain is increased by motion of the pinnae. The external auditory canal is erythematous, edematous, and exquisitely tender when you try to use the otoscope to examine her TM. There is whitish debris in the external auditory canal.

The most likely organism involved in this patient's disease is:

A) *Streptococcus.*

B) *Haemophilus.*

C) *Moraxella.*

D) *Pseudomonas.*

E) *Parainfluenza.*

Discussion

The correct answer is D. This patient likely has otitis externa. The most common pathogenic organism isolated in cases of otitis externa is *Pseudomonas* followed closely by *Staphylococcus aureus*. However, up to one-third of cases of otitis externa are polymicrobial.

Which of the following is (are) considered first-line treatment for otitis externa?

A) Oral ciprofloxacin.

B) Acetic acid drops.

C) Polymyxin and neomycin combination products.

D) A and C.
E) B and C.

Discussion

The correct answer is E. Otitis externa can be treated with a wide array of topical agents. One option is to acidify the external ear canal. Neither *Pseudomonas* nor *Staphylococcus* species can thrive at an acidic pH. Thus, acetic acid drops (VoSol) can be used. They are cheap and effective. Another approach is to use a topical antibiotic. Polymyxin/neomycin combinations (eg, Cortisporin) are safe and effective. A number of other antibiotic preparations are available. Alcohol-based solutions are another alternative. Answer A is incorrect because oral treatment is not indicated for simple otitis externa.

 HELPFUL TIP: There are a number of much more expensive treatments for otitis externa on the market, including ciprofloxacin otic drops, ofloxacin otic drops, etc. These have no advantage and are very expensive. **There is no treatment advantage to using antibiotics at all. Topical drying agents, alcohols, and acetic acid have as good an outcome as do antibiotics.**

* *

This patient is concerned about recurrences of her otitis externa.

What advice can you give her?

A) Avoid exposure by putting a petroleum jelly (eg, Vaseline) impregnated cotton plug in her ear before swimming.
B) Use a blow dryer on her ear after swimming.
C) Instill a 50/50 mixture of alcohol and vinegar in her ears after swimming.
D) Avoid swimming when she has active disease.
E) All of the above.

Discussion

The correct answer is E. All of the above can be used to minimize disease recurrence.

 HELPFUL TIP: Necrotizing (malignant) otitis externa is a separate entity that occurs primarily in diabetics but also in those with HIV. It is an invasive pseudomonal (95%) cellulitis that causes erythema and tenderness around the ear. It is a true emergency that requires IV antibiotics and surgical consultation.

* *

You treat the patient with neomycin/polymyxin drops, and the symptoms persist and possibly worsen a little after 5 days. The patient has no fever and no signs of cellulitis around the ear.

Of the following possibilities, which is the LEAST likely to explain her persistent symptoms?

A) Resistant organisms.
B) Noncompliance with medical recommendations.
C) Misdiagnosis of otomycosis.
D) Development of contact dermatitis.

Discussion

The correct answer is A. Treatment failures due to antibiotic resistance are uncommon, and antibiotics are not necessary in the treatment of most cases of otitis externa. Several things could explain her persistent symptoms. First, the patient should be questioned regarding compliance (answer B). Is she still swimming despite advice to the contrary? Is she using the drops at least TID and letting them soak into her ear? Another possibility is the development of an allergic reaction, (up to 35% of patients treated chronically with topical neomycin). Patients may also "fail" treatment for otitis externa because of misdiagnosis (answer C). Otomycosis, or fungal infection of the auditory canal, causes redness, discharge, itching, and sometimes pain.

* *

On exam, you note fine, white, cotton-like fibers filling the ear canal along with the other debris. The exam is otherwise unchanged.

What is your next step?

A) Admit for IV antibiotic and antifungal therapy.
B) Clean the ear canal under direct otoscopy and add oral amoxicillin/clavulanate to her medication regimen.

C) Clean the ear canal under direct otoscopy and add topical clotrimazole 1% to her medication regimen.
D) Order CT or MRI of the head and neck to rule out abscess.
E) Refer to an otolaryngologist.

Discussion

The correct answer is C. On exam, you have identified signs of otomycosis. It could be that the otomycosis was present initially or developed in the interval with antibiotic administration. Otomycosis is usually due to *Aspergillosis*; *Candida* represents only 10%–20% of cases. Thorough cleaning of the ear canal is an important part of therapy. A topical antifungal that is active against *Aspergillosis* is recommended (eg, clotrimazole, miconazole, nystatin).

 HELPFUL TIP: Ear wicks are excellent tools for delivery of medication deep into the ear canal but **should be changed daily**.

 HELPFUL TIP: Cortisporin suspension is pH neutral and does not burn. The solution causes more pain with instillation.

Objectives: Did you learn to . . .

- Identify bacterial pathogens implicated in otitis externa?
- Diagnose and treat a patient with otitis externa?
- Recommend prevention strategies for otitis externa?
- Determine why treatment for otitis externa may fail?

CASE 3

A 59-year-old male presents with a 3-week history of hoarseness. He denies sore throat or heartburn. He has had no fevers, night sweats, or weight loss. When he initially presented a week ago, your partner treated him empirically for postnasal drainage. He smokes 2 packs of cigarettes per day and frequently drinks alcohol. On exam, his vital signs are normal. His voice sounds husky. You find no other abnormalities.

The best next step in the management of this patient is:

A) Empiric antibiotic treatment.
B) Empiric proton pump inhibitor treatment.
C) Direct laryngoscopy.
D) Esophagogastroduodenoscopy (EGD).
E) Neck MRI.

Discussion

The correct answer is C. The first concern is to rule out malignancy, so the larynx should be visualized. Direct laryngoscopy is a straightforward office procedure and takes only a few minutes. If the equipment and expertise are not available in your office, referral to an otolaryngologist is appropriate. Although there are no firm guidelines, some authors recommend direct laryngoscopy after 2 weeks of hoarseness in patients who are at risk (>60 years and those who have a history of tobacco and alcohol use). Since laryngoscopy is such an available, low-cost, low-risk procedure, it is hard to justify postponing it for any patient at risk for malignancy.

Answers A and B are incorrect, because further empiric medication trials will only delay laryngoscopy. Antibiotics are not indicated for the lone symptom of hoarseness. In other instances, empiric proton pump inhibitor therapy may be more practical since gastroesophageal reflux is a common cause of vocal cord dysfunction. Answer D is incorrect. In this patient, direct laryngoscopy is preferred to EGD. Answer E is incorrect. Neck MRI is not indicated in the initial evaluation of hoarseness, but it might be used for follow-up after laryngoscopy or to investigate a neck mass.

All of the following are potential causes of hoarseness EXCEPT:

A) Vocal cord mass.
B) Infectious laryngitis.
C) Hypothyroidism.
D) Lung malignancy.
E) A vow of silence.

Discussion

The correct answer is E. Far from being a cause of hoarseness, voice rest is often recommended for patients with hoarseness due to overuse (eg, singers). All of the other options are known to cause hoarseness. Of particular note is answer C: hypothyroidism can

Table 20–2   CAUSES OF HOARSENESS, BASED ON VOICE CHARACTERISTIC, A PARTIAL LISTING

Breathy: Vocal cord paralysis, abductor spasmodic dysphonia, functional dysphonia

Hoarse: Vocal cord lesion, muscle tension dysphonia, reflux laryngitis

Low-pitched: Reinke's edema (edema of the upper tissue layer of the vocal cords seen almost exclusively in smokers), vocal abuse, reflux laryngitis, vocal cord paralysis, muscle tension dysphonia

Strained: Adductor spasmodic dysphonia, muscle tension dysphonia, reflux laryngitis

Tremor: Parkinson disease, essential tremor of the head and neck, spasmodic dysphonia, muscle tension dysphonia

Vocal fatigue: Muscle tension dysphonia, vocal cord paralysis, reflux laryngitis, vocal abuse

From Rosen CA, et al: *AFP* June, 1998.

result in an accumulation of connective tissue elements, basically myxedema, in the vocal cords. Intrathoracic processes such as lung cancer can present with hoarseness (see Helpful Tip below). Table 20–2 lists causes of hoarseness grouped by the change in voice.

 HELPFUL TIP: The laryngopharynx is innervated by the recurrent laryngeal nerve, a branch of the vagus nerve (cranial nerve X). In addition to being fun and interesting medical trivia, knowing the innervation is important because chest malignancy, aneurysms, complications of thoracic surgery, etc, can potentially present with hoarseness.

* *

On direct laryngoscopy, you note a mass lesion on the right vocal cord. You refer the patient to an otolaryngologist. The patient asks if you think that the mass is cancer. Because you are compassionate and also not entirely certain, you try to be more optimistic.

You remind him of risk factors for laryngeal cancer, which include all of the following EXCEPT:

A) Tobacco smoking.
B) Alcohol use.
C) Epstein-Barr virus.
D) Family history of head and neck cancers.
E) Male gender.

Discussion

The correct answer is C. Epstein-Barr virus (EBV) infection is associated with the development of nasopharyngeal cancer, not laryngeal cancer. Additionally, EBV infection has been associated with Burkitt lymphoma (children in Africa), Hodgkin disease, and non-Hodgkin lymphoma. The other answer choices are risk factors for laryngeal cancer. Tobacco and alcohol use are independent risk factors for the development of most types of head and neck cancers (oral, laryngeal, etc), and the two substances may act synergistically in the promotion of these cancers. A family history of head and neck cancer has a weaker association, but the association is still present. Males are 2–4 times more likely to have head and neck cancers in comparison with females.

If this patient is found to have cancer, what pathologic variant is most likely?

A) Adenocarcinoma.
B) Squamous cell carcinoma.
C) Schneiderian papilloma.
D) Neuroblastoma.

Discussion

The correct answer is B. Upon pathologic examination, the great majority of head and neck cancers are found to be squamous cell carcinomas. Adenocarcinoma (answer A) may arise from the gastrointestinal tract and could be seen on laryngoscopy but would rarely occur on the vocal cords. Schneiderian papillomas (answer C) are polyps that arise from the nasal and sinus mucosae, are associated with HPV, and may transform into carcinomas. Neuroblastomas (answer D), which arise from the sympathetic nervous system, rarely occur in the head and neck region.

* *

During your examination of the oropharynx, you also encountered a small, white, indurated plaque on the underside of the tongue. When you scraped the plaque with a tongue blade, nothing happened.

This lesion is most appropriately described as:

A) Squamous cell carcinoma.
B) *Candida albicans.*
C) Leukoplakia.
D) Geographic tongue.
E) Aphthous ulcer.

Discussion

The correct answer is C. Leukoplakia is a premalignant lesion of the oropharynx (~5% will progress to cancer over 10 years). It occurs in response to trauma and/or exposure to irritants and carcinogens, having an especially strong association with smokeless tobacco use. In fact, the lesion **could** be squamous cell carcinoma (answer A), and it should be biopsied. However, it would be premature to diagnose the patient with squamous cell carcinoma, and the lesion is more accurately described as leukoplakia. Answer B, *Candida albicans* lesions, may look like leukoplakia (white plaques on oropharyngeal mucosa), but you should be able to scrape some of the plaques off with a tongue blade (although thrush can be remarkably adherent). Answer D, geographic tongue, is so named because of the meandering white-bordered patches that occur on the dorsum of the tongue. It is most often asymptomatic, and the lesions vary in shape (or completely resolve) over time. Answer E, an aphthous ulcer, is just that—an ulcer, not a plaque. You should not confuse leukoplakia with an aphthous ulcer.

 HELPFUL TIP: Vitamin A and beta-carotene may have a beneficial effect on leukoplakia, with an increased rate of resolution of the lesions. However, beta-carotene likely increases lung cancer in smokers.

You receive a letter from the otolaryngologist that states the patient does indeed have squamous cell carcinoma of the larynx. The patient will be seen in consultation with an oncologist and presented at tumor board. His treatment may consist of surgery, chemotherapy, and/or radiation.

Objectives: Did you learn to . . .

- Generate a differential diagnosis for hoarseness of voice?
- Evaluate a patient with a voice complaint?

- Identify oral lesions, particularly leukoplakia?
- Recognize important issues in the prevention and treatment of head and neck cancers?

CASE 4

A 61-year-old male presents to your office with complaint that over the last few months he cannot seem to understand what people are saying when they are standing to his **left** side. He also has episodes of "dizziness," especially when he changes position from sitting to lying and vice versa. He denies nausea and vomiting. He worked for 30 years in a factory and has had bilateral tinnitus for the last 10 years. He has had no previous hearing problems or evaluation. His past medical history is significant for CAD and hypertension. His takes atenolol, chlorthalidone, and aspirin. There is no family history of ear disease. On exam, both ears are normal in appearance, with normal canals, minimal cerumen, normal TMs with landmarks clearly visible. Weber test is best heard by the patient on his **right** side. Rinne test on both sides was negative (air conduction >bone conduction).

These findings are consistent with which type of hearing loss on the left?

A) Conductive.
B) Sensorineural.
C) Mixed.
D) Unable to tell.

Discussion

The correct answer is B. Hearing can be assessed in the office using the Weber and Rinne tests. The Weber test is performed by putting the tuning fork on the forehead and seeing if the sound lateralizes to one side or the other. In conductive hearing loss (answer A), the sound will be **louder** (ie, the test will lateralize) to the "bad" side (eg, the side with wax occluding the canal). However, in sensorineural hearing loss, the sound will lateralize to the "good" side (eg, the side not affected by a hearing problem). The Rinne test is performed by comparing bone conduction (on the mastoid) to air conduction. Patients will notice poor air conduction versus bone conduction if there is a conductive hearing loss. Normal Rinne tests in both ears suggest that neither ear has conductive loss. This patient has decreased hearing on the **left** and the Weber test lateralizes to the **right**; and these findings point to a problem with sensorineural hearing loss in the **left** ear.

Which of the following is LEAST likely to be responsible for this patient's hearing loss?

A) Ménière disease.
B) Acoustic neuroma.
C) Presbycusis.
D) Otosclerosis.
E) Noise exposure.

Discussion

The correct answer is D. Otosclerosis is a bony overgrowth that involves the stapes and leads to **conductive** loss. Your patient has a sensorineural hearing loss. The other answers are causes of sensorineural hearing loss. Ménière disease (answer A) presents with the classic triad of hearing loss, tinnitus, and vertigo. These manifestations may be temporally separated with hearing loss, tinnitus, and vertigo occurring at different times. Patients with Ménière disease will note fullness in their ear, which resolves with the onset of vertigo. Typically, the vertigo will last for several hours. Sensorineural hearing loss can also be caused by an acoustic neuroma (answer B), a benign tumor that arises from cranial nerve VIII (acoustic nerve), and symptoms include unilateral hearing loss, vertigo, tinnitus, and disequilibrium. Presbycusis (answer C) is one of the most common causes of sensorineural hearing loss and is often thought of as the "normal" hearing loss that is associated with aging. Presbycusis manifests as an inability to hear high frequencies. This leads to problems with speech discrimination, especially in noisy environments (eg, parties, etc). It is typically symmetrical and may be associated with tinnitus. However, it may be unilateral, especially in those who have one ear turned towards noisy equipment in their job. Table 20–3 lists causes of conductive and sensorineural hearing loss.

What is the next step in the evaluation of this patient?

A) Audiogram.
B) Brain stem evoked responses.
C) MRI.
D) Tympanogram.

Discussion

The correct answer is A. An audiogram can further define the air versus bone conductance relationship, check speech discrimination, and define the frequency of hearing loss. Brainstem-evoked responses evaluate the

Table 20–3 CAUSES OF CONDUCTIVE AND SENSORINEURAL HEARING LOSS

Conductive Hearing Loss	Sensorineural Hearing Loss
Trauma: ossicle disruption, TM perforation	Presbycusis
Cerumen in the canal	Ménière disease
Barotrauma	Stroke
Otitis media	Tumor (eg, acoustic neuroma)
Middle ear effusion	Infection (eg, syphilis, CMV, etc)

neural pathways of hearing and, with MRI, could be useful if tumor were higher on the differential. A tympanogram, that evaluates movement of the TM, might be useful if conductive hearing loss were suspected.

 HELPFUL TIP: Brainstem-evoked potentials measure how long it takes an auditory signal to reach the brainstem. If an acoustic neuroma is present, the brainstem-evoked potential will be prolonged. However, the false-negative rate is up to 30%, and brainstem-evoked potentials have been largely replaced by MRI in the diagnosis of acoustic neuroma.

* *

The audiogram confirms sensorineural hearing loss in the left ear. You order an MRI of the posterior fossa to rule out acoustic neuroma. The results are negative. The patient continues to have episodes of vertigo, and the hearing loss on his left side persists. When probed further, he does have an increase in tinnitus during his vertiginous episodes.

You should consider all of the following treatments for this condition EXCEPT:

A) Restrict salt, caffeine, and tobacco.
B) Diuretics (eg, hydrochlorothiazide).
C) Intracochlear injection of gentamicin.
D) Labyrinthectomy or endolymphatic sac shunt.
E) H$_2$-blockers (eg, cimetidine).

Discussion

The correct answer is E. The clinical picture now looks most like Ménière disease—a disease for which there is no cure. Luckily not all patients with Ménière disease will experience worsening of their condition over time, and up to 90% are able to maintain normal daily activities with optimal medical management. Few patients progress to debilitating disease. The mainstays of therapy include diet/lifestyle modification and diuretics. Outside the United States, betahistine, an H_1-blocker, is commonly used, but H_2-blockers have no role in therapy. A more aggressive approach is indicated in patients with more severe disease, and this might include surgery, intracochlear gentamicin (to kill the nerve and reduce vertigo), labyrinthectomy, or endolymphatic sac shunt.

 HELPFUL TIP: Treating Ménière disease can be problematic. Studies of this condition are frequently of poor quality with a significant placebo effect. This, along with spontaneous remissions and exacerbations, limits the usefulness of data about treatment.

 HELPFUL TIP: Consider the role of medications when a patient complains about tinnitus. It can be caused by a number of medications including NSAIDs, calcium channel blockers, diuretics, etc.

Objectives: Did you learn to . . .

- Evaluate a patient with hearing loss?
- Describe differences between conductive and sensorineural hearing loss?
- Generate a differential diagnosis for hearing loss?
- Diagnose and treat a patient with Ménière disease?

 QUICK QUIZ: PERIPHARYNGEAL INFECTION

A 7-year-old female is brought to your office by her concerned parents. Over the last 24 hours, the patient has developed pain in her mouth, drooling, and fever. She refuses to eat. On examination, she is febrile and slightly tachycardic. She has trismus but you are able to see that the sublingual space is swollen and tender. There are no ulcerations. There is well-demarcated erythema, brawny edema, tenderness, and warmth in the submandibular area. Her respirations are normal, and her lung sounds are clear.

What is the next step in the evaluation and management of this patient?

A) Reassurance, oral rehydration, and analgesics.
B) Oral antibiotics.
C) MRI of the head and neck.
D) Intravenous antibiotics.
E) Intubation and mechanical ventilation.

Discussion

The correct answer is D. This patient is presenting with classic signs and symptoms of Ludwig angina (related neither to angina nor to Ludwig von Beethoven). The term Ludwig angina is reserved for infection of the submandibular and sublingual areas. The status of the patient's airway must be addressed first. This patient is stable and her airway appears patent; therefore, answer E is incorrect. Answers A and B are incorrect because patients with Ludwig angina may experience rapid progression of symptoms and should be treated with intravenous antibiotics and observed in the hospital. Answer C is incorrect because the diagnosis of Ludwig angina is clinical. Also, MRI may delay antibiotic treatment and is unlikely to be of any value, unless you suspect the presence of an abscess.

CASE 5

A 30-year-old male comes to your office complaining of a swollen neck. He noticed it 10 days ago when he was stung by a bee on the right side of his anterior neck. The area has continued to enlarge. It is no longer tender. It was erythematous after the sting, but the redness has resolved. He notes no other symptoms. He has just returned from a camping trip in Minnesota. His only medications are atenolol and chlorthalidone for hypertension. On exam you find a 2-cm firm, somewhat tender, enlarged lymph node in the right anterior cervical chain. The node is mobile, nonfluctuant, with no surrounding erythema. There are also shotty anterior and posterior cervical nodes in addition to the larger node. You find no other lymphadenopathy.

What elements of the presentation make malignancy LESS likely?

A) The node is freely mobile.
B) The node is only 2 cm.
C) The node is associated with trauma (bee sting).
D) The node is tender.
E) All of these help to rule out malignancy.

Discussion

The correct answer is A. Nonmalignant nodes are generally <1 cm in size, freely mobile, and rubbery in constancy. Malignant nodes tend to be larger, rock-hard, and fixed. They become immobile secondary to tumor invasion into the surrounding tissues and/or inflammation. Remember that pain in a node is not always indicative of an inflammatory or benign process. Hemorrhage into, or necrosis of, a malignant node can cause capsular distention leading to pain. Answer C is of particular note. This patient's bee sting was quite a while ago and is unlikely to be a useful part of the history unless there is ongoing inflammation. Patients will often attribute a physical malady to something in their lives whether or not it makes sense from a biological and medical perspective. Of course, lymphadenopathy is not the only source of neck masses. Table 20–4 outlines differential diagnosis of neck mass in adults.

What is the next step in the management of this patient?

A) Empiric antibiotics.
B) Observation for 4 weeks.
C) Open biopsy of the node.
D) Fine-needle aspiration of the node.
E) Incision and drainage.

Discussion

The correct answer is B. Patients with lymphadenopathy can be observed for 3–4 weeks unless there is a suggestion of malignancy (eg, fever, night sweats, weight loss, etc). **A 3–4 week delay makes no difference in patient outcome if the node does turn out to be malignant.** If adenopathy does not resolve, further evaluation including biopsy can be done. Open biopsy and fine-needle aspiration each have advantages and disadvantages, but either could be used to obtain tissue.

Table 20–4 DIFFERENTIAL DIAGNOSIS OF NECK MASS IN ADULTS

Congenital anomalies
- Lateral neck: Brachial cysts and fistulae, cystic hygromas, dermoids
- Central neck: Thyroglossal duct cyst, thyroid masses, thymic rests, dermoids

Infection/Inflammation
- Mononucleosis
- Tuberculosis
- Toxoplasmosis
- Cat-scratch disease (*Bartonella henselae*)
- *Staphylococcus*
- *Streptococcus*
- Other viral, bacterial, and fungal infections
- Sialadenitis
- Abscess
- Inflammatory or reactive lymphadenopathy

Neoplasm
- Benign masses: lipoma, hemangioma, neuroma, fibroma
- Malignant masses: mucosal head and neck cancers, lymphoma, thyroid cancer, salivary gland cancer, sarcoma, distant metastases

Trauma
- Hematoma (acute or fibrosed)
- Pseudoaneurysm
- AV fistula

Idiopathic and others
- Metabolic: gout, CPPD (pseudogout)
- Inflammatory pseudotumor
- Castleman disease (a benign lymphoproliferative disorder)
- Kimura disease (a chronic subcutaneous inflammatory condition, cause unknown)

Answer A, empiric therapy with antibiotics, is possibly correct if you suspect a lymphadenitis or a bacterial infection causing secondary lymphadenopathy. However, in this patient there is no tenderness or other signs of infection, arguing against lymphadenitis.

Which of the following tests is NOT helpful in arriving at a diagnosis in a patient with GENERALIZED lymphadenopathy?

A) CBC.
B) Chest radiograph.
C) Glucose, BUN, creatinine.
D) HIV.
E) Heterophile antibody.

Discussion

The correct answer is C. Glucose, BUN, and creatinine are not likely to help you with the diagnosis of generalized lymphadenopathy. Lymphadenopathy in primary care is malignant approximately 1% of the time. The workup should proceed in 3 stages: first, CBC, CXR; second, PPD, HIV, RPR, ANA, heterophile; third: Biopsy. Use your clinical judgment to determine the extent of testing necessary in any individual case.

 HELPFUL TIP: Just like in real estate: location, location, location. Supraclavicular nodes are malignant up to 50% of the time in individuals >40 years.

 HELPFUL TIP: Benign lymphadenopathy is common in young children. In children <5 years presenting for a health maintenance exam, up to 44% have palpable lymph nodes. Occipital and posterior auricular nodes are common in infants but not in children >2 years.

Objectives: Did you learn to . . .

• Describe features of malignant and nonmalignant lymph nodes?
• Evaluate a patient with lymphadenopathy?

CASE 6

A 42-year-old female presents to your office with the chief complaint of 2 days of headache, sore throat, and nasal congestion productive of green mucus. She denies any fever, contact with ill persons, and gastrointestinal symptoms, but she does have a history of seasonal allergies. Her examination is significant for a temperature of 36.8°C, pulse 82, respiratory rate 16, and a blood pressure 124/76 mm Hg. Her posterior oropharynx shows mild erythema and post-nasal drainage, but no exudates. There is nasal mucosal erythema and swelling with clear rhinorrhea. Her neck is supple with no adenopathy. Respirations are clear.

The most likely agent causing her symptoms and the most common cause of acute rhinosinusitis is:

A) Rhinovirus.
B) *Streptococcus pneumoniae.*
C) *Haemophilus influenza.*
D) *Moraxella catarrhalis.*
E) Norwalk virus.

Discussion

The correct answer is A. Viruses are the most common cause of upper respiratory infections (or colds or rhinosinusitis). Up to 50% of colds are caused by the 100 different serotypes of rhinoviruses. Other viruses that commonly cause colds include Coronaviruses, RSV, parainfluenza, and influenza. Norwalk virus typically causes an intestinal illness. The bacteria listed (answers B–D) are associated with infections of the upper respiratory tract, particularly otitis and sinusitis, but are much less common than viruses.

 HELPFUL TIP: Resident bacteria in the nasopharynx include *Streptococcus pneumoniae*, *Haemophilus influenzae*, and *Moraxella catarrhalis*. Although most causes of sinusitis are viral, these bacteria make up the great majority of organisms causing bacterial sinusitis. Sinusitis may also result from extension of dental root infection into the sinus cavity, and these infections are caused by microaerophilic and anaerobic bacteria.

Initial treatment for acute rhinosinusitis include(s):

A) Oral decongestants.
B) NSAIDs.
C) Nasal steroids.
D) Oral antibiotics.
E) A and B.

Discussion

The correct answer is E. Most cases of rhinosinusitis are viral and need only symptomatic treatment. Analgesics and systemic and nasal decongestants are reasonable options. Another option is ipratropium nasal spray that will also help to decrease mucus production. Note that only the first-generation antihistamines with anticholinergic activity (eg, diphenhydramine) will provide any benefit in these patients. Nasal steroids are ineffective acutely.

Which of the following does NOT increase the likelihood that a patient has a bacteria sinusitis?

A) Purulent nasal drainage.
B) Persistence of symptoms for >7 days.
C) Thickened nasal mucosa or effusion on CT scan.
D) Maxillary tooth pain.
E) Unilateral maxillary sinus pain.

Discussion
The correct answer is C. Radiography is particularly poor at diagnosing bacterial sinusitis. Thickened nasal mucosa is only 40%–50% specific for sinusitis. The other problem with imaging is that all patients with an upper respiratory infection will have fluid in the sinuses. Clinical criteria are more helpful in predicting the presence of bacterial sinusitis; thus, answers A, B, D, and E are true statements. Additionally, a biphasic course, sometimes referred to as double sickening, is a good predictor of bacterial sinusitis: if the patient initially improves and then gets worse, consider a secondary infection. Answer A deserves special note because green nasal drainage does not indicate that bacteria are present. Secretions will turn green with a viral illness, as with anything else that concentrates protein in the mucus (eg, anticholinergics).

 HELPFUL TIP: A viral URI can last up to a month. Because 25% of patients with a URI are still symptomatic at 14 days, duration of symptoms alone is not diagnostic of bacterial sinusitis.

 HELPFUL TIP: The (Russian) Empire Strikes Back. There is now a particularly virulent rhinovirus primarily found in Russia that can be fatal. See, maybe all of those Russian leaders did die of bad colds.

* *

The patient is initially convinced that only antibiotics will make her better. Through skillful negotiation, you manage to avoid prescribing antibiotics for what you strongly suspect is a viral infection. Two weeks later, the patient returns. Initially, she improved, but then she developed subjective fever, face pressure, maxillary tooth pain, and copious green nasal drainage. You now suspect that a bacterial sinusitis has developed. The look on her face says, "I told you so." She has no drug allergies.

Which of the following treatments do you offer as first-line therapy?

A) Azithromycin.
B) Trimethoprim/sulfamethoxazole.
C) Prednisone.
D) Ceftriaxone.
E) None of the above.

Discussion
The correct answer is B. Most guidelines addressing the treatment of acute bacterial sinusitis recommend narrow-spectrum antibiotics, like trimethoprim/sulfamethoxazole. Other alternatives include amoxicillin and doxycycline. A 10-day course is usually sufficient, but longer courses may be necessary. Alternatives for patients who do not respond include more broad-spectrum antibiotics (eg, fluoroquinolones, amoxicillin/clavulanate, etc). However, azithromycin and other macrolides may not provide adequate coverage and should be considered third-line agents if used at all. Answer C is incorrect. There is no reason to prescribe steroids here. Answer D, ceftriaxone, might be considered in cases of treatment failure, but oral antibiotics are generally preferred. You should continue to recommend that the patient use decongestants and other symptom-oriented therapies.

 HELPFUL TIP: When you treat sinusitis you are treating an abscess. Drainage is key, including oxymetolazone for limited periods, systemic decongestants, and saline irrigation. **Topical steroids are ineffective acutely for acute sinusitis and are very expensive.**

 HELPFUL TIP: All noses that run are not infectious. Remember allergic rhinitis, vasomotor rhinitis (now termed idiopathic rhinitis), etc. Vasomotor rhinitis is an exaggerated response to stimuli such as cold, recumbency, and air pollution. It can be differentiated from allergic rhinitis by the absence of other allergic symptoms (itching, eye involvement, perhaps asthma, etc) and the absence of eosinophils on Hansel stain of mucus. Other considerations include rhinitis medicamentosum as a result of using topical vasoconstrictors (eg, oxymetazoline and cocaine).

Objectives: Did you learn to . . .

- Describe the most common pathogens involved in rhinosinusitis?
- Recognize clinical signs and symptoms that are more consistent with bacterial sinusitis than viral rhinosinusitis?
- Prescribe treatment for viral and bacterial sinusitis?

CASE 7

A 65-year-old male presents with dizziness that started a few days ago. He reports that he is otherwise healthy and takes no medications.

Which of the following is the best question to ask him in order to elicit a better characterization of his dizziness complaint?

A) "Is the room spinning round and round?"
B) "Do you feel that you are going to faint?"
C) "Can you describe the dizziness using any other words?"
D) "Do you feel as though you are drunk?"

Discussion

The correct answer is C. When you explore a complaint of dizziness, allow the patient to characterize the nature of the dizziness further without putting words into his mouth. This is a good time for that old technique learned in medical school but rarely used in practice: the open-ended question. Avoid using medical jargon (eg, "vertigo") and leading questions. Let the patient find the words to describe the dizziness and then draw your conclusion based on his description. There are essentially 4 types of dizziness: vertigo,

presyncope, imbalance (dysequilibrium), and undifferentiated dizziness. Patients will usually come up with their own terminology that will allow you to categorize their dizziness into one of these 4 types.

* *

The patient describes a sensation of the room spinning, usually lasting less than a minute. Further, this sensation comes on in different positions and has led to a fall which resulted in minor injuries. The patient denies any upper respiratory symptoms, fevers, hearing loss, or tinnitus. He sometimes feels nauseated with the dizziness but has not vomited. He first noticed the dizziness while in bed and rolling over, but it now occurs more frequently and in various positions. Sudden turning of the head definitely exacerbates his symptoms. You are comfortable identifying this as vertigo.

Which of the following is LEAST likely to present with vertigo?

A) Labyrinthitis.
B) Ménière disease.
C) Otitis media.
D) Perilymphatic fistula.

Discussion

The correct answer is C. There are many causes of vertigo, but otitis media should not generally be thought of as one of them (or at least should be a diagnosis of exclusion). Labyrinthitis is probably caused by viral infection and results in severe vertigo that lasts for days. Ménière disease results in episodic vertigo that lasts for minutes to hours. Perilymphatic fistula occurs when perilymph leaks through a tear in the oval window (secondary to a fall or barotrauma including sneezing). Although it often results in vertigo, it is a relatively uncommon cause of vertigo. Perilymphatic fistula may be secondary to trauma and typically resolves on its own.

Which of the following is the best next step in the diagnosis of this patient?

A) Dix-Hallpike maneuvers.
B) Obtain blood for CBC, electrolytes, BUN, and creatinine.
C) MRI brain and brainstem.
D) CT brain.
E) Audiometry.

Discussion

The correct answer is A. A complete evaluation of the patient with vertigo includes examination of the neurologic and cardiovascular systems as well as the ears, eyes, nose, and throat. While performing a physical exam, the Dix-Hallpike maneuver can be a useful tool. In order to perform the maneuver, move the patient rapidly from a seated to a supine position, turning the head to the left or right, and observe for nystagmus. The patient is helped into a seated position, and the maneuver is repeated, turning the head to the other side. If nystagmus occurs within 30 seconds of performing the maneuver, it is considered a positive test. Answer B is incorrect. Laboratory tests are rarely helpful. Answers C and D are incorrect because neuroimaging should be performed only if the history and/or exam indicate the need for it. In this patient, the exam is not even complete yet! Answer E is incorrect because audiometry (although helpful in the diagnosis of Ménière disease) is premature.

* *

Dix-Hallpike maneuver is positive with rotation of the head to the left. The symptoms last for less than 1 minute. The rest of the physical exam is unremarkable.

The most likely diagnosis in this patient is:

A) Labyrinthitis.
B) Benign paroxysmal positional vertigo (BPPV).
C) Vertebrobasilar stroke.
D) Motion sickness.
E) None of the above.

Discussion

The correct answer is B. The history of episodic, positional vertigo and the positive Dix-Hallpike maneuver make BPPV the most likely diagnosis. **The Dix-Hallpike maneuver is not specific for BPPV. The Dix-Hallpike maneuver is designed to discriminate central from peripheral vertigo.** In this patient, the history is probably the most important aspect in making the diagnosis. See Table 20–5 to interpret the Dix-Hallpike maneuver. BPPV is more common in older patients but can occur at any age. Women are more commonly affected than men. BPPV is caused by calcium stone deposition in the posterior semicircular canal.

The other diagnoses listed are less likely. Answer C needs special note. Stroke should be considered in any patient presenting with sudden onset, persistent vertigo and risk factors (eg, hypertension, atrial fibrillation, etc).

Table 20–5   DIX-HALLPIKE MANEUVER

Suggestive of Peripheral Vertigo
- Delayed onset of nystagmus and symptoms
- Nystagmus always in same direction
- Vertigo reflex fatigable after multiple maneuvers
- Nystagmus suppressible by patient

Suggestive of Central Vertigo
- Nystagmus in multiple directions
- No latency to onset of nystagmus
- Reflex not fatigable

However, not every elderly patient with vertigo needs an MRI. If the history is consistent with BPPV, then neuroimaging is not necessary.

You feel comfortable recommending the following treatment EXCEPT:

A) Prednisone.
B) Lorazepam.
C) Meclizine (Antivert).
D) Rehabilitation exercises.
E) Dimenhydrinate (Dramamine).

Discussion

The correct answer is A. Steroids are not likely to improve symptoms in BPPV. Benzodiazepines, anticholinergics, and antihistamines are all employed in treating the symptoms of BPPV. Cawthorne rehabilitation exercises, physical therapy, and physician-directed head positioning (aka Epley maneuvers to move stones out of the posterior semicircular canal) may be successful. Most patients will improve with time, although many will have relapses.

Objectives: Did you learn to . . .

- Describe types of dizziness?
- Generate a differential diagnosis for vertigo?
- Diagnose and treat a patient with benign paroxysmal positional vertigo?

CASE 8

A 15-year-old male wrestler presents to the ED with a nosebleed and a swollen ear. He clearly did not win this round. Prior to coming to the ED, he held pressure to his nose for 30 minutes. He has had nosebleeds before, but none that were this bad. When asked how much blood he lost, his father shrugs and says it was "all over the mat." On examination, you see blood oozing slowly from the anterior nasal septum.

Which of the following is/are sources of anterior epistaxis?

A) Ethmoid artery.
B) Sphenopalatine artery.
C) Kiesselbach arterial plexus.
D) All of the above.
E) None of the above.

Discussion

The correct answer is C. Kiesselbach plexus is a venous collection system in the anterior nose that contains blood from the ethmoid and sphenopalatine arteries. It is the most common site of bleeding. The ethmoid and sphenopalatine arteries supply the posterior area of the nose, and bleeding from these sites is more difficult to control.

What is the best next step in managing this patient's nosebleed?

A) Continue to hold pressure against the septum.
B) Pack the anterior naris with gauze.
C) Spray the mucosal surface with phenylephrine.
D) Apply silver nitrate to the bleeding site.
E) Any of the above can be used.

Discussion

The correct answer is E. Any of the answer choices could be used alone or in combination to try to stop the bleeding. If these methods are not successful, consider electrocautery, laboratory evaluation for signs of bleeding disorders (eg, CBC, PT/PTT), and otolaryngology consultation. Laboratory studies will rarely be helpful.

 HELPFUL TIP: If you pack a patient's nose, leave the packing in place for ≥24 hours. Also, prescribe antibiotics to prevent sinusitis.

* *

With cautery and direct pressure, you were able to stop the bleeding. You now turn your attention to his left ear.

You find a purplish, tender, fluctuant swelling at the left pinna.

The best treatment for this condition is:

A) Analgesics, protection, and observation.
B) Compressive dressing, using a headband.
C) Oral antibiotics.
D) Incision and drainage, leaving the wound open to drain and heal by secondary intention.
E) Needle drainage followed by compressive dressing sutured into the pinna.

Discussion

The correct answer is E. With traumatic auricular hematoma/seroma, fluid collects between the perichondrium and underlying cartilage, predisposing the cartilage to loss of vascular supply and necrosis. In order to avoid "cauliflower ear" deformity, the hematoma or seroma must be evacuated via incision or needle drainage. However, you cannot stop there: a compressive dressing must then be sutured into the pinna, or the fluid is likely to re-accumulate. Answer B is incorrect because compressive dressing alone is insufficient. Answer D is incorrect only because it does not include compressive dressing. Answers A and C are incorrect because taking these actions will delay definitive treatment (and antibiotics are not needed anyway). If the patient were to present late (≥10 days after the injury), he will not benefit from incision and drainage or needle drainage and instead should be referred for otoplasty.

Objectives: Did you learn to . . .
- Evaluate and treat a patient with epistaxis?
- Treat a patient with auricular trauma?

 QUICK QUIZ: MOUTH SORES

A 20-year-old female presents with 3 painful ulcerations on her inner lip and tongue. She has no other symptoms. Although she has never had such sores before, everyone else in her family has had similar mouth sores. She smokes only when drinking wine coolers, which occurs about once per week. She is afebrile, and her exam is otherwise unremarkable.

The most likely diagnosis is:

A) Aphthous ulcers.
B) Behçet disease.

C) Crohn disease.
D) Gluten enteropathy.
E) Squamous cell carcinoma.

Discussion

The correct answer is A. This otherwise healthy young woman with a family history of "similar sores" most likely has aphthous ulcers or "canker sores." The etiology of aphthous ulcers is not well understood, and they are alternatively explained as viral, autoimmune, genetic, traumatic, or due to chemical irritants or other processes. Answer B, Behçet disease, is uncommon in the United States. It is thought to be an autoimmune disease, and it presents with recurrent oral and genital ulcerations and skin and eye lesions among other findings. Answers C and D can both present with isolated oral ulcers but are less common than idiopathic aphthous ulcers. Answer E is incorrect because it is highly unlikely that this young, healthy person has developed cancer.

CASE 9

A 34-year-old male dentist presents to your office with a 1-week history of right facial weakness. He states that he "just woke up this way one morning." He would have come in sooner, but he was busy with his practice and he has felt fine. He has not noticed any other neurologic symptoms. He denies pain, fever, or upper respiratory symptoms. He reports being healthy and taking no medications. On examination, his vital signs are normal. You note that his right eyebrow sags, as does the right corner of his mouth. He cannot close the right eye completely or raise his right eyebrow, and the right nasolabial fold is less prominent than the left. The remainder of the neurologic examination is normal.

The neurologic finding in this patient that most suggests a cranial nerve process (as opposed to a central brain lesion) is:

A) Normal strength in the upper extremities.
B) Inability to smile on the right.
C) Inability to wrinkle the forehead.
D) Normal blood pressure.
E) Normal speech rate and rhythm.

Discussion

The correct answer is C. Partial sparing of the forehead muscles suggests a brain lesion because innervation of the forehead contains crossed fibers from both sides of the brain; a bilateral brain lesion is possible but unlikely. Thus, a dense paralysis is more likely to be peripheral (CN7) since all innervation is knocked out when this is involved. This patient's entire right face, including the forehead, is paralyzed, which suggests a lower motor neuron (CN7) process. Although answers A and E are found in a normal neurologic exam and are reassuring, they are not as helpful in isolating the location of the lesion to a lower motor neuron source. Answer B, lower facial muscle weakness or paralysis, can occur with upper or lower motor neuron disease. Answer D, normal blood pressure, is not helpful.

* *

You tell the patient that you suspect he has Bell palsy. He asks what causes this problem.

Which of the following is the most likely cause of this patient's Bell palsy?

A) Herpes virus.
B) Tick-borne illness.
C) Diabetes.
D) Adenovirus.

Discussion

The correct answer is A. It seems that many cases of Bell palsy are due to reactivation of herpes simplex virus. Other viral etiologies have been implicated as well, including Epstein-Barr virus, CMV, and coxsackievirus. Although answer B, tick-borne illnesses (eg Lyme disease), may cause Bell palsy, these represent a minority of cases. Answer C, diabetes, may put a patient at increased risk of contracting Bell palsy, but it does not cause the disease. Answer D is incorrect because herpes virus is most commonly associated with Bell palsy. Remember mycoplasma as a cause of Bell palsy.

 HELPFUL TIP: Bell palsy is more likely to occur in pregnancy, especially the last trimester and the first week postpartum.

Which of the following treatments is MOST LIKELY to benefit this patient?

A) Acyclovir.
B) Prednisone.
C) Artificial tears and eye patching at night.
D) A and B.
E) None of the above.

Discussion

The correct answer is C. In a patient with Bell palsy and weakness to eye closure, good eye care and protection from trauma must be employed to prevent corneal damage (remember that this patient cannot close his right eye). **The evidence for antiviral therapy is negative; acyclovir likely doesn't work.** There may be some slight benefit to corticosteroid. Steroids are most likely to provide a benefit if started within a few days after the onset of symptoms. Our patient is 1 week out from the onset of symptoms.

* *

You recommend eye care but not medications. Knowing that patients with Bell palsy generally require a lot of reassurance, you discuss the diagnosis in detail, including prognosis.

The patient can expect which of the following?

A) Complete resolution (~100% likelihood) with nearly zero risk of recurrence.
B) Likely resolution (>50% likelihood) with nearly zero risk of recurrence.
C) Likely resolution (>50% likelihood) with ~10% risk of recurrence.
D) High probability (~95% likelihood) of persistent paralysis.

Discussion

The correct answer is C. Most patients will recover, but it may take months. Patients with complete paralysis are more likely to have persistent symptoms, whereas those with partial paralysis usually recover more quickly and completely.

 HELPFUL TIP: Ramsay-Hunt syndrome is the name given to zoster oticus complicated by hemifacial paralysis. If identified early, antivirals may help the patient with Ramsay-Hunt syndrome.

Objectives: Did you learn to . . .

• Differentiate Bell palsy from a central lesion?
• Describe causes of Bell palsy?
• Manage a patient with hemifacial paresis?

 QUICK QUIZ: OH, MY ACHING JAW

A 30-year-old female presents with several months of pain and stiffness in her jaw. When asked to localize the pain, she points to the temporomandibular joints (TMJs) bilaterally. She notes that the pain is worse with stressful situations, driving, and chewing. Her husband complains that she grinds her teeth at night. She is otherwise healthy. On physical examination, you find palpable popping in the TMJs bilaterally, and the remainder of her exam is unremarkable.

You make all of the following recommendations EXCEPT:

A) Start chewing gum daily.
B) Use ibuprofen as needed.
C) Use a bite block at night.
D) Learn relaxation techniques.

Discussion

The correct answer is A. Increased use of the TMJ by chewing gum, is the opposite of what the patient should be doing. Jaw rest is important. This patient's history is consistent with TMJ syndrome. In addition to those described in the case, symptoms of TMJ may include ear pain, headache, limited jaw mobility, and crepitus and tenderness on palpation of the joint. TMJ syndrome may occur unilaterally or bilaterally. No therapy appears to have greater efficacy than another, and many different interventions have been tried, although poorly studied. All of the listed interventions are reasonable. Also, you might recommend a softer diet, hot packs, and TMJ massage.

 HELPFUL TIP: The headache of TMJ may be felt in the sinus region, retro-orbitally, or as an earache. Check for TMJ when patients present with these symptoms.

CASE 10

A 22-year-old female presents to your office with complaint of severe facial pain for the past 3 days. She has poor dentition and you find that on exam there is mandibular swelling and tenderness.

All of the following are causes of mandibular area swelling EXCEPT:

A) Submandibular duct stone.
B) Dental abscess.
C) Retropharyngeal abscess.
D) Ludwig angina.
E) Brachial cleft cyst.

Discussion

The correct answer is C. Retropharyngeal abscesses are generally not visible but present with fever, throat pain, and symptoms due to swelling of the retropharyngeal space (dysphagia, drooling, odynophagia, airway obstruction). All of the other answer choices can cause swelling around the mandible.

Which of the following is NOT true of sialolithiasis (salivary duct stones)?

A) Intermittent swelling of the salivary gland.
B) More than 80% involve the parotid gland.
C) The majority resolve with conservative, non-operative treatment.
D) Antistaphylococcal antibiotics should be used in their treatment.
E) Sialogogues (eg, lemon drops) should be used as part of the treatment.

Discussion

The correct answer is B. **More than 80% of cases of sialolithiasis involve the submandibular gland.** Answer A is true. Swelling tends to occur when patients eat and tends to resolve between meals as saliva slowly makes its way through the duct. Answer C is true. Most salivary duct stones pass spontaneously. Answer D is true. Think of this as an abscess. Antistaphylococcal antibiotics should be used until the stone passes. Answer E is true. Sialogogues such as lemon drops promote saliva formation. The effectiveness is questionable but it is worth a try, and it gives the patient something to do.

Which of the following is considered good practice with regards to salivary duct stones?

A) Patients should be followed up within 2 weeks if the stone does not pass in the office.
B) Stones can be removed using sialolithotomy (using a probe and/or scalpel to nick the outlet).

C) Patients should be referred for lithotripsy if stones do not pass within 4 days.
D) Surgical excision of the duct should be done if the stone does not pass.
E) None of the above is true.

Discussion

The correct answer is B. A probe can be used to "dilate" the duct. Occasionally, the outlet needs to be nicked using a scalpel blade to allow the stone to egress. Answer A is incorrect. Patients should be followed up in 24 hours if the stone does not pass. Answer C is incorrect. Lithotripsy has been used with some good results but is definitely third line. Answer D is incorrect. Excising the duct seems a bit dramatic.

* *

You check the patient's mouth and decide that there is likely a dental abscess, not a salivary duct stone. She needs to have her tooth extracted but the dentist will not be able to see the patient until the morning. She requires antibiotics but is penicillin-allergic.

The antibiotic of choice for this patient is:

A) Erythromycin.
B) Clindamycin.
C) Azithromycin.
D) Levofloxacin.
E) Trimethoprim/sulfamethoxazole.

Discussion

The correct answer is B. Clindamycin is the drug of choice as an alternative to penicillin. The drug used for a dental abscess should cover anaerobes. There is resistance to erythromycin and azithromycin. Neither levofloxacin nor trimethoprim/sulfamethoxazole covers anaerobes.

* *

During your exam, you also noticed a firm nodule in the submental area in the midline. It moves up and down when she swallows. She says that it has been there for years—as long as she can remember.

The most likely cause of this midline nodule is:

A) Submandibular gland infection.
B) Thyroglossal duct cyst.
C) Infected frenulum.
D) Brachial cleft cyst.

Discussion

The correct answer is B. This is likely a thyroglossal duct cyst. The other answer choices are incorrect. Submandibular glands (answer A) and brachial cleft cysts (answer D) are lateral to the midline. The frenulum (answer C) is under the tongue.

* *

You start the patient on clindamycin, but she returns in the morning with severe submandibular swelling and trismus. The tongue is elevated in the mouth and there is brawny edema. She is having difficulty swallowing her secretions and some stridor. You make the diagnosis of Ludwig angina.

The most appropriate treatment in this patient now is:

A) Continue PO clindamycin and add salt water gargles.
B) Continue PO clindamycin and add PO metronidazole.
C) Incise and drain the swollen area under the tongue.
D) Refer immediately for surgical evaluation for possible tracheostomy.
E) Admit for IV fluids and levofloxacin.

Discussion

The correct answer is D. This patient's situation has become fairly desperate overnight while on an appropriate antibiotic. Securing an airway should be your first concern. Unfortunately, patients with Ludwig angina do not respond to local incision and drainage as the swelling is usually diffuse, spreads quickly, and does not result in discreet pus pocket formation until late in the course. She should be admitted for IV fluids, appropriate IV antibiotics (not levofloxacin), and possible tracheostomy. Patients with advancing Ludwig angina do not tolerate endotracheal intubation; thus, an alternative airway is provided with tracheostomy.

CASE 11

A 21-year-old male presents with complaint of a sore throat. His symptoms started 3 days ago. He has had subjective fevers, sweats, fatigue, and mild nausea. He has no cough or rhinorrhea. His temperature is 38.3°C. His vital signs are normal otherwise. He has symmetrically enlarged tonsils with exudates present and tender anterior cervical lymphadenopathy.

What is the most appropriate step in the evaluation and management of this patient?

A) Reassure and recommend salt water gargles.
B) Obtain a routine aerobic culture of the oropharynx.
C) Prescribe penicillin 500 mg BID for 10 days.
D) Prescribe levofloxacin 500 mg daily for 7 days.

Discussion

The correct answer is C. This patient has 4 of 4 signs/symptoms ("Centor criteria") suggestive of streptococcal (group A strep or *Streptococcus pyogenes*) pharyngitis: fever, tender cervical adenopathy, exudative pharyngitis, and lack of other URI symptoms. In this patient, the most appropriate step would be empiric antimicrobial treatment. Answer B, performing a culture, will take a few days and does not add much given the strength of the clinical argument for strep throat. Furthermore, the oropharynx is colonized by many kinds of flora that do not cause disease, and we only really care about group A streptococcus, so a routine aerobic culture is of no value. A rapid assay or a specific "rule-out" culture for group A strep could be done rather than treating based on clinical grounds. Although salt water gargles seem to help reduce the pain of pharyngitis, answer A is incorrect because you would want to do more than that for this patient who likely has strep throat. Answer D is incorrect because levofloxacin and other fluoroquinolones are not indicated for treatment of strep throat.

Following are 3 treatment strategies for the patient you think might have strep throat:

Strategy 1: No testing (or minimal testing). In this strategy, one treats based on clinical symptoms. You look for 4 criteria: fever, exudate, absence of other URI symptoms, tender anterior cervical adenopathy. Treat patients who meet 3 or 4 criteria, and do not treat others. Another approach is to treat patients who meet 4 criteria, do a rapid strep test on those who meet 3 (possibly 2) criteria. Avoid treatment and testing of those with 1 or zero criteria. This has been recommended by the CDC for nonimmunosuppressed patients in the absence of an outbreak of rheumatic fever in the community.

Strategy 2: Testing. Test all patients and treat those with a positive strep screen. Do not culture others.

Strategy 3: For Children. The majority of group A strep pharyngitis occurs in children aged 5–15 years. In this age group, 15%–30% of acute pharyngitis is caused by group A strep. In children, a rapid strep test is considered the standard (although many argue that it is not necessary in the older child). Cultures are optional depending on the reliability of your rapid antigen test. Many would culture **all** rapid strep test negative children and this is an acceptable strategy.

So, now you are quite confused. So is everyone else.

Which of the following is true about antibiotic therapy of streptococcal pharyngitis?

A) Azithromycin is the drug of choice because of resistant streptococci.
B) There is no significant resistance seen in group A β-hemolytic streptococci, and penicillin is still the drug of choice.
C) Cephalexin is the preferred drug because it covers *Haemophilus influenza* which is a frequent coinfector with streptococci.
D) Amoxicillin is preferred for strep throat because it does not cause a rash if the patient happens to have mononucleosis.

Discussion

The correct answer is B. There is no significant resistance among group A β-hemolytic streptococci to penicillin. Thus, penicillin remains the drug of choice despite drug detailing. There is no reason to use **anything else,** except in the case of allergy when **erythromycin** can be used.

 HELPFUL TIP: Penicillin VK can be used BID in streptococcal pharyngitis which increases compliance.

Antibiotics should be started within the following time period to reduce the risk of rheumatic fever from streptococcal pharyngitis:

A) 2 days after presentation.
B) 2–4 days after presentation.
C) 4–6 days after presentation.
D) 6–8 days after presentation.
E) 8–10 days after presentation.

Discussion

The correct answer is E. Antibiotics should be started within **9 days after presentation** to prevent rheumatic

fever, which is the goal when we treat streptococcal pharyngitis. Thus, there really is no reason to hurry treatment.

A patient with streptococcal pharyngitis should be considered infectious and kept out of school for what period after beginning antibiotics?

A) 12 hours.
B) 24 hours.
C) 36 hours.
D) 48 hours.

Discussion

The correct answer is B. Patients should be considered infectious for 24 hours after the initiation of therapy for streptococcal pharyngitis. The risk of transmission is reduced markedly after this point. Unfortunately, the patient is infectious for 3–5 days before he or she becomes symptomatic, so removing the patient for 24 hours after treatment is closing the barn door after the horse is gone.

* *

Which of the following is the most likely cause for his current symptoms?

A) Gonococcal pharyngitis.
B) Infection with a resistant *Streptococcal* organism.
C) Mononucleosis.
D) Recurrent *Streptococcal* pharyngitis.

Discussion

The correct answer is D. Since his symptoms resolved, you either got the diagnosis and treatment right or he had some other self-limited infection. Therefore, it would be unlikely that he had gonococcal pharyngitis or resistant *Streptococcal* organisms. Nonetheless, sexual history is important—even when confronted with pharyngitis; if a patient with exudative pharyngitis is not improving, consider gonococcal disease. Remember that gonococcal disease will be missed for 2 reasons in this scenario: the history is never obtained regarding oral sex, and gonococcus requires Thayer-Martin agar to grow so it will not show up on routine culture. Answer B, resistant *Streptococcus* organisms causing pharyngitis.

HELPFUL TIP: Most causes of throat pain are acute infections (strep throat, other bacterial infections, viral pharyngitis, mononucleosis), but consider other causes as well: carotidynia, viral thyroiditis, mouth-breathing, peritonsillar abscess.

CASE 12

The next patient presents with a sore throat and tender anterior **and** posterior cervical adenopathy. He is febrile and relatively stoic. He has been sick for 2 weeks with significant fatigue and is not getting better. In addition to the adenopathy, you notice left-sided abdominal pain with minimal guarding but no rebound tenderness. You believe that you feel a spleen edge. However, the patient's heterophile antibody (monospot) is negative. You decide to get anti-Epstein-Barr virus (anti-EBV) antibodies.

The results of the anti-EBV antibody test are as follows (VCA is against the capsid): IGM-VCA positive, IgG-VCA negative, Anti-EBV nuclear antigen antibody negative.

How do you interpret these results?

A) The patient has acute EBV infection.
B) The patient has had EBV at least 6 weeks ago.
C) The presence of anti-EBV nuclear antigen antibody indicates the infection occurred within the last 4 weeks.
D) The patient has never been infected with EBV.

Discussion

The correct answer is A. The patient has an EBV infection that started in the last few weeks. Here is why. IGM-VCA is produced acutely and is elevated in the acute infection for 2–4 weeks. Since this patient's IGM-VCA is positive, he has had an acute EBV infection within the past month. IgG-VCA appears around 3–4 weeks and persists for life. Antibodies against the EBV nuclear antigen show up at 6–12 weeks after infection. If this antibody is present in the blood, it suggests that there has not been an acute infection; the infection had to have been at least 6 weeks ago.

Of the following, which does NOT cause a mononucleosis-like syndrome?

A) Acute HIV conversion.
B) CMV.

C) Toxoplasmosis.
D) West Nile virus (WNV).
E) Leptospirosis.

Discussion

The correct answer is D. West Nile virus is characterized by fever, headache, myalgias, back pain, and anorexia lasting 3–6 days. Much less common manifestations are pharyngitis, nausea, vomiting, diarrhea, encephalitis, etc. One thing to note is that WNV may include lymphadenopathy. All the other answer choices can cause a mononucleosis-like syndrome. Other causes of mononucleosis-like syndromes include adenovirus, parvovirus B19 (erythema infectiosum), herpes virus 6 (Roseola infantum), and ehrlichiosis (Asian form only).

 HELPFUL TIP: Depending on the population studied, 1–2% of patients with a mononucleosis-like syndrome who are **heterophile negative** are HIV-positive.

* *

Returning to your patient, you diagnose EBV mononucleosis.

If confirmation of splenomegaly was desired prior to making a determination regarding the patient's ability to play contact sports, what would be your next step to confirm splenomegaly?

A) CT scan chest/abdomen/pelvis.
B) MRI abdomen.
C) Plain radiograph of the abdomen.
D) Ultrasound of the abdomen.
E) Plain film and left lateral decubitus films of the abdomen.

Discussion

The correct answer is D. Ultrasound can provide accurate measurements of spleen size without the need for intravenous contrast material or the added cost of CT or MRI. Unfortunately, normative data regarding spleen size has not been conclusively established for the adolescent population.

If splenomegaly were confirmed in this patient, what would be the generally accepted recommendation with regard to athletic participation?

A) No participation until negative acute titers for EBV.

B) No participation for 6 weeks after the diagnosis is made assuming complete resolution of symptoms.

C) No participation until 3 weeks after the diagnosis is made assuming complete resolution of symptoms and then only noncontact training for another week.

D) Full practice and competition allowed immediately unless abdominal pain occurs.

E) No return to contact sports ever.

Discussion

The correct answer is C. It is generally thought that return to practice or **noncontact training** is safe 3 weeks after the diagnosis of mononucleosis, provided that all other symptoms have resolved. If there are no clinical concerns for splenic enlargement at 4 weeks, the patient may be cleared to return to full competition. This recommendation is based upon the observation that most cases of splenic rupture in athletes have occurred when those athletes returned to competition in <4 weeks from the time of diagnosis.

* *

The patient returns 2 days later and is noting increased pharyngeal swelling and difficulty swallowing. You look into his throat and note "kissing tonsils." There is no stridor but he feels as though there is something in his throat.

What is the best treatment for this patient at this time?

A) Prednisone.

B) Amoxicillin.

C) Clindamycin.

D) Azithromycin.

E) Tonsillectomy.

Discussion

The correct answer is A. Steroids are useful for symptomatic mononucleosis; **however, they should be reserved for patients with significant symptoms.** Antibiotics are not indicated for mononucleosis. Tonsillectomy is also not indicated. The patient likely has paratracheal node swelling as well. In this patient,

admission may be indicated if there is enough potential for airway obstruction.

 HELPFUL TIP: Amoxicillin is not a good choice for treating patients with streptococcal pharyngitis because if you are wrong and the patient has mononucleosis, the patient could develop a rash (it occurs but is less common with penicillin). A rash with mononucleosis does not mean that the patient is allergic to amoxicillin.

What is the approximate sensitivity of the heterophile antibody test (monospot) for mononucleosis within the first 2 weeks of symptoms?

A) 10%

B) 30%

C) 50%

D) 70%

E) >90%

Discussion

The correct answer is D. The sensitivity of the monospot ranges from 60%–80% 2 weeks into the illness. The point here is not the number but that there are heterophile negative mononucleosis syndromes **and** not everyone with EBV mononucleosis will have a positive monospot when tested. However, they should have atypical lymphocytes on WBC differential.

 HELPFUL TIP: The monospot is not as sensitive in children. It will be positive in <40% of children <5 years when they are infected with EBV. However, anti-EBV antibodies will be positive.

Objectives: Did you learn to . . .

- Describe different strategies to approaching the patient with symptoms of *Streptococcal* pharyngitis?
- Treat a patient with *Streptococcal* pharyngitis and recurrent pharyngitis?

BIBLIOGRAPHY

Albino JE, et al. Management of temporomandibular disorders. *J Am Dent Assoc.* 1996;127(11):1595.

American Academy of Pediatrics Subcommittee on Management of Acute Otitis Media. Diagnosis and management of acute otitis media. *Pediatrics.* 2004;113(5):1451-65.

Bisno AL. Diagnosis of strep throat in adults: are clinical criteria really good enough? *Clin Infect Dis.* 2002;35(2):126.

Dykewicz MS. Rhinitis and sinusitis. *J Allergy Clin Immunol.* 2003;111(2 Suppl):S520.

Harrison CJ. The laws of otitis media. *Prim Care.* 2003; 30(1):109.

Lodi G. Interventions for treating oral leukoplakia. *Cochrane Database Syst Rev.* 2001(4):CD001829.

Neff MJ. AAP, AAFP, AAO-HNS release guideline on diagnosis and management of otitis media with effusion. *Am Fam Physician.* 2004;69(12):2276.

Paradise JL, Campbell TF, Dollaghan CA. Developmental outcomes after early or delayed insertion of tympanostomy tubes. *N Engl J Med.* 2005;353:576.

Parnes LS, Agrawal SK, Atlas J. Diagnosis and management of benign paroxysmal postitional vertigo (BPPV). *CMAJ.* 2003;169(7):681.

Rosen CA, Anderson D, Murry T. Evaluating hoarseness: keeping your patient's voice healthy. *Am Fam Physician.* 1998;57(11):2775.

Rosenfeld RM, Brown L, Cannon CR, et al. Clinical practice guideline: acute otitis externa. *Otolaryngol Head Neck Surg.* 2006;134(4 Suppl):S4.

Salinas RA. Corticosteroids for Bell's palsy (idiopathic facial paralysis). *Cochrane Database Syst Rev.* 2002(1): CD001942.

Schwetschenau E, Kelley DJ. The adult neck mass. *Am Fam Physician.* 2002;66(5):831.

Shah R. Otalgia. *Otolaryngol Clin North Am.* 2003;36(6): 1137.

Sullivan FM, Swan IR, Donnan PT. et al. Early treatment with prenisolone or acyclovir in Bell's palsy. *N Engl J Med.* 2007;357:1598-607.

Tusa RJ. Dizziness. *Med Clin North Am.* 2003;87(3):609.

21

Care of the Older Patient

Katrina Cannon and Jason K. Wilbur

CASE 1

An 83-year-old female patient whom you have followed for many years has just been admitted to a nursing home following a short hospitalization. Because of a steady decline in function and lack of family and social support, you and the patient realized that she could no longer safely live alone in her home, and her needs were too great for assisted living. Her medical problems include congestive heart failure, chronic atrial fibrillation, osteoarthritis, and depression. Her current medications are warfarin, furosemide, acetaminophen, calcium carbonate, lisinopril, metoprolol, and fluoxetine. Both the patient and the nursing staff report poor sleep and depressed mood for the last 2 weeks, and the nurses are asking for a sleep aid.

What it the best next step in the management of her insomnia?

A) Add diphenhydramine 50 mg PO HS.
B) Add diazepam 5 mg PO HS.
C) Add amitriptyline 25 mg PO HS.
D) Recommend increased activity during the day, avoidance of naps, warm milk before bed, and waking at the same time each morning.

Discussion

The correct answer is D. There are no great medicines for promoting sleep in elderly nursing home residents. Given the lack of efficacy data of most hypnotics coupled with the known adverse effects, a trial of good sleep hygiene should be undertaken first. Good sleep hygiene generally consists of the following:

eliminate daytime naps, encourage daily activities and a set waking time, increase aerobic exercise (but not within a few hours of bedtime), and maintain a quiet, comfortable sleeping environment. Nighttime rituals, such as meditation and warm milk, may help insomnia and are unlikely to cause any harm. If these initial efforts fail, a low dose of a traditional hypnotic (eg, zolpidem, zaleplon) or trazodone is an appropriate initial choice. Trazodone has fewer anticholinergic effects and effects on blood pressure than other options (nortriptyline, etc) but should still be used with caution and monitoring for adverse effects.

Diphenhydramine (answer A) has powerful antihistaminic and anticholinergic properties that may result in increased confusion. Diazepam (answer B) has an exceptionally long half-life in elderly patients and may cause daytime somnolence. Amitriptyline (answer C) is listed by the Centers for Medicare and Medicaid Services (CMS) as a medication to be avoided in nursing home patients because of high potential for severe adverse drug reactions (falls, constipation, etc).

 HELPFUL TIP: There are many potential causes of sleep disturbance in the nursing home. The following are sources of sleep problems that you may want to investigate or treat empirically: pain, anxiety, depression, delirium, dementia, primary sleep disorders (eg, sleep apnea, restless leg syndrome), environmental issues (eg, alarms, lights).

* *

The nurses implement your recommendation to try sleep hygiene, and over the next month your patient's sleep improves, as does her mood. Unfortunately, she experiences two falls with minor injuries while ambulating in her room. Upon examination, you find normal vital signs, no orthostatic hypotension, and no focal neurologic deficits.

Which of the following is the most appropriate next step?

A) Discontinue warfarin.
B) Employ bed and chair alarms.
C) Obtain a computerized tomography (CT) scan of the head.
D) Reduce or discontinue fluoxetine.
E) Restrict activities and prescribe a wheelchair.

Discussion
The correct answer is D. Falls are usually multifactorial in origin, so simple interventions do not generally solve the problem. SSRIs have been shown (in imperfect studies) to increase the risk of falls in the elderly, so reducing or discontinuing fluoxetine is prudent. She should be monitored for symptoms of depression while her antidepressant therapy is tapered.

Answer A, discontinue warfarin, may be appropriate if she continues to fall but this action is not likely to reduce her frequency of falling. Answer B, use of bed and chair alarms, is helpful when patients have cognitive impairment and cannot remember to ask for help when getting up; however, these devices can act as tethers to further restrict a patient's movement. Likewise, further restriction of activities and mandatory wheelchair use may lead to deconditioning, loss of muscle strength, and an increased risk of falls. Answer C, CT scan of the head, may be warranted if the patient sustained a head injury or had an abnormal neurologic exam.

* *

Over the next year, you observe a steady decline in your patient's function, with a series of falls despite interventions. Ultimately, your patient has a devastating thromboembolic stroke, which results in right hemiparesis and dysphagia. After a short hospital stay, she returns to the nursing home and undergoes therapy. She continues to have difficulty with her swallowing but is able to tolerate thickened liquids without aspirating. She has a 5% weight loss over the next 2 months, and her nurse reports poor oral intake. Her medications are now warfarin, furosemide, acetaminophen, calcium carbonate, and lisinopril.

In this malnourished, elderly nursing home patient, which of the following interventions or diagnostic studies will most likely lead to improvement in her condition?

A) Admit to the hospital and initiate parenteral feeding.
B) Refer for esophagogastroduodenoscopy (EGD).
C) Screen for depression.
D) Add megestrol acetate.
E) Obtain a complete blood count (CBC).

Discussion
The correct answer is C. Depression is one of the most common causes of weight loss in the nursing home patient, and this patient has a history of depression with no treatment in place now. Stroke survivors are also at high risk for depression. Consider using a screening tool, such as the Geriatric Depression scale. A positive screen requires further investigation. Now that she is bedridden falls are not as much of an issue so an SSRI may be appropriate.

Answer A is incorrect. We are not sure of the patient's wishes regarding intravenous nutrition, and more conservative measures should be instituted before considering parenteral nutrition. Answer B is incorrect. Although an EGD may be important at some point if indicated, proceeding to EGD immediately is premature. Answer D, megestrol acetate, has been reported to improve food intake in patients with cancer cachexia, but its value in the nursing home is questionable. Answer E is incorrect. Evidence of chronic infection or anemia could be found on a CBC, but no signs or symptoms of infection (besides weight loss) are present.

 HELPFUL TIP: The initial evaluation of a nursing home patient with weight loss should focus on medication review, gastrointestinal symptoms, dental and mouth problems, swallowing dysfunction, ability to feed oneself, and psychiatric disorders (eg, depression, dementia, or psychosis). Hyperthyroidism, hyperparathyroidism, malignancy, and chronic infection should be considered as causes of weight loss (albeit less likely). Factors associated with aging, such as decreased olfaction, taste, and salivation (and nursing home food) may decrease the enjoyment of eating.

* *

You diagnose depression and initiate treatment. Also, you encourage the nursing staff to observe your patient while eating and assist her if necessary. You add a daily multiple vitamin. Her mood improves slightly and her weight stabilizes. However, over the next 6 months, your patient becomes more withdrawn and spends most of her time in bed. Because of her stroke, she is not very mobile, and she requires assistance with transfers and movement in bed. Ultimately, she develops a skin ulcer on her sacrum. Nursing staff reports a sacral pressure ulcer measuring 3 × 2 cm. There appears to be some interruption of the epidermis, like an abrasion.

According to conventional staging criteria, what stage is this decubitus ulcer?

A) Stage I.
B) Stage II.
C) Stage III.
D) Stage IV.

Discussion

The correct answer is B. Pressure ulcers (in older parlance, decubitus ulcers, pressure sores, bed sores) are caused by unrelieved pressure resulting in damage to underlying tissue. Anatomic areas of concern in bedbound patients include sacrum, coccyx, heels, and occiput. Chair-bound patients are more likely to develop ulcers over the ischial tuberosities. Risk factors for pressure ulcers include advancing age, immobility, moisture (eg, urinary or fecal incontinence), malnutrition, and decreased sensory perception. Ulcers are staged by clinical appearance (Table 21–1).

* *

Because of miscommunication within the nursing home staff, the ulcer goes untended over the weekend. An alarmed nurse calls you to report full-thickness skin loss. You arrange to visit your patient in the evening.

In the meantime, you prescribe what treatment?

A) Foam pad with occluding dressing (eg, Allevyn).
B) Wet-to-dry dressing.
C) Topical antibiotics.
D) Transparent, occlusive dressing (eg, Tegaderm).
E) Chemical enzyme debridement (eg, Accuzyme).

Discussion

The correct answer is A. In treating pressure ulcers, there are several principles to follow: relieve pressure; protect the wound and surrounding skin from further trauma; maintain a clean wound bed; provide a moist wound environment; eliminate dead space; control exudates; ensure adequate nutrition; and diagnose and treat infection. Your patient's ulcer has worsened and is now Stage III. Without further information, a foam dressing is a safe choice for initial treatment of a Stage III ulcer. Foam pads are useful for deeper wounds with moderate exudate and may also protect the wound from further pressure. In most cases, the wound should be kept moist, so wet-to-dry dressings are not appropriate. If moist gauze packing is used, it should be kept moist with intermittent reapplication of saline or changed before drying. From the nurse's report, there is no evidence of necrosis, excessive drainage, or infection, so debridement and antibiotics may not be helpful

Table 21–1 PRESSURE ULCER STAGES

Stage I	Stage II	Stage III	Stage IV
Nonblanchable erythema	Partial thickness skin loss	Full-thickness skin loss	Full-thickness skin loss
Intact skin	Epidermis and/or dermis	Damage or necrosis of subcutaneous tissues, extending to underlying fascia	Extensive destruction, tissue necrosis, or damage to muscle, bone, or supporting structures
Changes in skin temperature, consistency, or sensation	Presents as abrasion, blister, or shallow crater	Presents as deep crater	

at this time. A transparent, occlusive dressing is used for Stage II ulcers, but is insufficient for Stage III or IV. In addition to dressing the wound, you should employ the following measures: repositioning every 1–2 hours, pressure-relieving mattress and cushions, and optimizing nutrition. Consultation with a wound care specialist or a surgeon may be necessary if these measures fail.

 HELPFUL TIP: There is evidence of benefit from electrical stimulation of pressure ulcers, but there is minimal supporting evidence for the use of other adjunctive therapies (ultrasound, hyperbaric oxygen, ultraviolet light, vasodilators, etc).

 HELPFUL TIP: To prevent pressure ulcers, schedule regular and frequent repositioning for bed and chair-bound individuals. Turn at least every 2–4 hours on a pressure-reducing mattress or every 2 hours on a nonpressure-reducing mattress. Also, maintain the head of the bed ≤30 degrees to reduce pressure on the sacral area.

Which of the following statements is NOT true about the evaluation and treatment of pressure ulcers?

A) A pressure ulcer covered by eschar cannot be staged until the eschar is removed.
B) If a pressure ulcer shows no signs of healing over 2 weeks, one should reevaluate wound management strategies and reexamine factors affecting the wound.
C) One should consider osteomyelitis or deep soft-tissue infection in a wound that is not healing.
D) Wound cultures should be obtained routinely to target antibiotics toward the organisms found.
E) In an otherwise clean wound that is not healing as expected, consider empiric therapy with topical antibiotics.

Discussion

The correct answer is D. The routine culturing of pressure ulcers is not recommended. Antibiotics are generally not useful since the organisms found are polymicrobial colonizers and not responsible for infection. This does not hold true for patients with a true infection, and empiric therapy with topical antibiotics is indicated if a wound shows no improvement with good wound care.

Objectives: Did you learn to . . .

- Manage insomnia in elderly nursing home residents?
- Develop an approach to the problem of falls in nursing home residents?
- Identify nursing home residents at risk for malnutrition?
- Develop a treatment plan for malnutrition in the institutionalized elderly?
- Diagnose, evaluate, and manage pressure ulcers in the nursing home setting?

 QUICK QUIZ: VACCINES

A 65-year-old male presents for a routine visit and you recommend pneumococcal vaccination (23-valent polysaccharide vaccine, Pneumovax). Your patient asks what the vaccine is supposed to do.

According to the best available evidence, you are able to say:

A) "This vaccine will reduce your risk of pneumococcal bacteremia."
B) "This vaccine will reduce your risk of pneumococcal pneumonia."
C) "This vaccine will reduce your risk of all types of pneumonia."
D) "This vaccine will reduce your risk of death from influenza."

Discussion

The correct answer is A. The 23-valent polysaccharide pneumococcal vaccine has only been shown effective in reducing the risk of pneumococcal bacteremia. The vaccine does not appear to reduce the risk of pneumonia in general or even pneumococcal pneumonia in particular. Influenza vaccination decreases the risk of death due to influenza, but pneumococcal vaccination does not.

QUICK QUIZ: HORMONES AND AGING

After she saw an advertisement for testosterone treatment to "reverse the aging process," one of your vivacious older female patients asks about testosterone for her husband.

Regarding sex hormone changes associated with aging, which of the following statements is true?

A) Leydig cells in the testes increase with aging.
B) Total testosterone levels increase with aging.
C) Sex-hormone binding globulin levels increase with aging.
D) Follicle-stimulating hormone levels are unchanged with aging.
E) Luteinizing hormone levels decrease with aging.

Discussion

The correct answer is C. Sex hormones in males >40 years demonstrate a decline of total testosterone at a rate of 1%–2% per year. Simultaneously, sex-hormone binding globulin increases, resulting in a sharper decline in bioavailable testosterone. In response to low testosterone, follicle-stimulating and luteinizing hormone levels increase. Leydig cells (responsible for producing testosterone) **decrease** in number. Older males with subphysiologic testosterone levels are at increased risk of sexual dysfunction, osteoporosis, diminished lean body mass, and depression. Although controversial, some experts recommend testosterone supplementation in symptomatic males with low serum testosterone. Testosterone supplementation likely does not improve strength, lean body mass, depressed mood, bone mineral density, and sexual function in aging males with documented low testosterone levels. Side effects of testosterone supplementation in older males include liver dysfunction, hypercholesterolemia, erythrocytosis, prostate tissue growth, acne, gynecomastia, and edema.

CASE 2

A 79-year-old female patient, well known to you from 5 years of treating her hypertension, presents to your office with concerns about her vision and hearing. Over the last year, she has noticed worsening vision in her left eye. She denies eye pain, tearing, and redness. She wears bifocals and last had an eye exam 3 years ago. At that time, she recalls her eye doctor said her vision was "stable." Also, her gynecologist recently retired and she would now like you to assume that care. Which of the following is true regarding common visual problems in older adults?

A) Initial symptoms of macular degeneration include decreased visual acuity and central visual field distortion.
B) Cataracts are less common in the older population than is macular degeneration.
C) Symptoms of open-angle glaucoma are dramatic and manifest early in the disease.
D) Initial symptoms of central retinal artery occlusion include severe pain and sudden loss of vision.
E) If a cataract is detectable on physical exam, it should be removed.

Discussion

The correct answer is A. By 65 years, approximately 1 individual in 3 has some form of eye disease that results in vision loss. The most common cause of blindness in older Americans is age-related macular degeneration (AMD). The disease typically presents with loss of vision in the central field with preservation of peripheral vision. Answer B is incorrect. Cataracts are more common than is macular degeneration. However, the availability of cataract surgery in the United States has reduced cataract-related vision loss in older Americans. Worldwide, cataracts are the leading cause of visual impairment. Cataract surgery is indicated when vision loss due to the cataract is interfering with function not simply because the physician finds it, so Answer E is incorrect. Open-angle glaucoma, the most common form of glaucoma, progresses slowly over time. Significant visual field loss may occur, but is only recognized late in the disease. Central retinal artery occlusion presents with sudden onset of painless monocular blindness (amaurosis fugax). Severe eye pain and loss of vision would be more consistent with acute closed-angle glaucoma.

Which of the following is TRUE of age related macular degeneration (AMD)?

A) Among African Americans, AMD is the most common cause of blindness.
B) Risk factors for AMD are similar to those for cardiovascular disease.
C) Risk factors for AMD are similar to those for cataracts.

D) Only nonexudative ("dry") AMD is amenable to treatment with laser photocoagulation.

E) AMD only affects peripheral vision.

Discussion

The correct answer is B. Risk factors for AMD include age, hypertension, smoking, and previous history of cardiovascular disease. Also, blue eye color and family history appear to predispose individuals to AMD. Answer A is incorrect. Among African Americans, glaucoma—not AMD—is the most common cause of blindness. Answers C and D are incorrect. AMD is divided into nonexudative ("dry") and exudative ("wet") AMD. The exudative type is less common but causes most of the severe vision loss due to AMD. Also, certain patients with exudative AMD benefit from laser photo coagulation, whereas those with nonexudative AMD do not. Answer E is incorrect because AMD causes central visual field deficits.

 HELPFUL TIP: A combination of carotenoids and other antioxidant vitamins may reduce the risk of vision loss in AMD. A multivitamin-multimineral supplement with a combination of vitamin C, vitamin E, beta-carotene, and zinc is recommended for AMD.

* *

Your patient performs poorly on a Snellen eye chart visual acuity test, and you decide to refer her to a local ophthalmologist. She then complains that she is less socially active in the last year. Her son thinks she is depressed because she talks on the phone with him less than she did a year ago. Your patient thinks these problems are related to a loss of hearing.

Regarding presbycusis (age-related hearing loss), which of the following is true?

A) Presbycusis usually results in unilateral hearing loss.

B) Presbycusis usually results in low-frequency hearing loss.

C) Presbycusis usually results in loss of speech discrimination.

D) Presbycusis usually results in major depression.

E) Sensorineural presbycusis does not respond to hearing aid use.

Discussion

The correct answer is C. Presbycusis is present in 33% of patients >65 years. Presbycusis typically presents with symmetric high-frequency hearing loss and loss of speech discrimination; patients complain of difficulty understanding rapid speech, foreign accents, and conversation in noisy areas. Types of presbycusis include conductive, sensorineural, mixed, and central hearing loss. Although some patients may experience depression with hearing loss, the majority do not. Hearing aids are underutilized in presbycusis but are potentially beneficial for most types of hearing loss, including sensorineural hearing loss. Other devices, such as a portable amplifier with microphone and ear piece (eg, PocketTalker), can be used to improve hearing function, especially for one-on-one conversations.

 HELPFUL TIP: Hearing loss, and sensory impairments in general, can be confused with cognitive impairment or an affective disorder. Hearing aids are useful for most patients with presbycusis, but if speech discrimination is <50%, results with hearing aids may be poor.

* *

Your patient asks if medications can cause hearing loss.

Which of the following drugs is NOT associated with sensorineural hearing loss?

A) Ibuprofen.

B) Aminoglycosides.

C) Furosemide.

D) Magnesium salicylate.

E) Acetaminophen.

Discussion

The correct answer is E. All of the drugs except for acetaminophen can cause hearing loss. Cisplatin, aminoglycoside antibiotics, and loop diuretics can all cause hearing loss, as can salicylates (eg, aspirin) and some of the other NSAIDs (eg, ibuprofen, diflunisal) and chloroquine. This list is obviously not exhaustive.

* *

Your patient (79 years) asks, "Do I have to keep getting mammograms and Pap smears?" She relates a history of normal annual mammograms and Pap smears for the past 20 years. She had a hysterectomy for uterine fibromas and has been monogamous with her husband for 55 years. Her sister died of breast cancer.

Consistent with current guidelines, you recommend:

A) Continue Pap smears and pelvic exams yearly.
B) Discontinue mammography but perform clinical breast exams every 2 years.
C) Discontinue pelvic exams but continue Pap smears.
D) Discontinue Pap smears but continue mammography and clinical breast exams at 1–2-year intervals.
E) Discontinue all screening tests/exams.

Discussion

The correct answer is D. Screening decisions in the elderly should be individualized, and the patient's overall health status must be considered. This patient has very little risk of cervical, endometrial, or vaginal cancer (status posthysterectomy for a benign condition, low-risk sexual behavior, and a history of normal exams); therefore, it is reasonable to discontinue Pap smears. Annual pelvic examination is more controversial, with the ACS recommending it as a screening measure for ovarian cancer and the USPSTF recommending against it. Early detection of breast cancer may result in decreased morbidity and mortality. Screening for breast cancer continues to be recommended for women with a 5–10-year life expectancy but the optimal interval in older women is unknown. Healthy older women with risk factors, such as this patient, may receive even greater benefit from screening for breast cancer.

* *

Your patient is an overweight white female with no history of bone fracture. She has never had a bone mineral density test and asks if she should have one. You are unaware of any risk factors in her other than white race and postmenopause status.

What do you tell her?

A) "You are not at risk for osteoporosis and should not be screened."
B) "All women >65 years should be screened for osteoporosis regardless of risk."
C) "Take 1,000 mg of calcium per day to prevent osteoporosis."

D) "Because of your risk factors, you should start a bisphosphonate, vitamin D, and calcium supplementation."
E) "Alcohol use will help decrease your risk of osteoporosis."

Discussion

The correct answer is B. The USPSTF currently recommends bone densitometry screening for all women ≥65 years. The National Osteoporosis Foundation recommends bone densitometry for postmenopausal females with one or more of the following risk factors: family history of osteoporosis, personal history of low trauma fracture, current smoking, or low body weight (<127 lbs.). The preferred method for measuring bone density is dual-energy radiographic absorptiometry (DEXA).

Answers A, C, D, and E are incorrect. Additional risk factors for osteoporosis include female gender, white or Asian race, alcohol abuse, sedentary lifestyle, and poor intake or absorption of calcium and vitamin D. All postmenopausal women should consume 1,200–1,500 mg of elemental calcium per day in divided doses. The optimal amount of vitamin D is 400–800 IU per day. Weight-bearing exercises also strengthen bone. Bisphosphonates are indicated for treatment of osteoporosis and should not be used without a diagnosis. Smoking is associated with osteoporosis. Diabetes, once thought to protect against osteoporosis, may increase the risk of falls and fractures in older adults.

* *

Next, your patient asks whether any of her medications put her at risk for osteoporosis.

Which of the following is LEAST likely to increase the risk of osteoporosis?

A) Glucocorticoids.
B) Anticonvulsants.
C) Sulfonylureas.
D) Loop diuretics.
E) Proton pump inhibitors.

Discussion

The correct answer is C. Sulfonylureas do not have a direct effect on bone mineralization. Glucocorticoids and anticonvulsants are known to increase bone turnover, resulting in increased risk of osteoporosis. Loop diuretics cause renal calcium wasting. Recent evidence has found an association between proton pump inhibitor use and osteoporosis. Additionally, heparin, methotrexate, cyclosporin, and gonadotropin-releasing hormone agonists may increase the risk of osteoporosis. Excessive amounts of levothyroxine can cause increased bone turnover. Thiazide diuretics are protective.

* *

Your patient asks what causes osteoporosis.

Although most osteoporosis in women is primary (idiopathic), which of the following cause(s) secondary osteoporosis?

A) Hypoparathyroidism.
B) Multiple myeloma.
C) Estrogen use.
D) Hyperlipidemia.
E) All of the above.

Discussion

The correct answer is B. Approximately 70% of women have no identifiable cause for osteoporosis and therefore are diagnosed with primary (idiopathic) osteoporosis. Common causes of secondary osteoporosis include chronic corticosteroid use, alcoholism, gastrointestinal disorders, hyperthyroidism, **hyper**parathyroidism (so, answer A is incorrect), multiple myeloma, and primary renal diseases. Estrogen (answer C) will increase bone mineral density. Hyperlipidemia (answer D) is not known to be associated with osteoporosis.

* *

You encourage appropriate vitamin D and calcium intake as well as weight-bearing exercises. You plan to obtain a DEXA scan.

Using DEXA scan results, osteoporosis is defined as:

A) A T-score of 2.5 standard deviations or more below the mean ($\leq$–2.5).
B) A T-score from 1.0 up to 2.5 standard deviations below the mean (–1.0 up to –2.5).
C) A Z-score of 2.5 standard deviations or more below the mean ($\leq$–2.5).
D) A Z-score from 1.0 up to 2.5 standard deviations below the mean (–1.0 up to –2.5).
E) None of the above.

Discussion

The correct answer is A. The T-score compares the patient's bone mineral density to that of young, healthy women. **Osteoporosis** is defined as a T-score of 2.5 standard deviations or more below the mean ($\leq$–2.5). **Osteopenia** is defined as a T-score from 1.0 up to 2.5 standard deviations below the mean (–1.0 to –2.5). Answer C is incorrect. The Z-score compares bone mineral density to that of age-matched controls. Therefore, it does not reflect the bone loss from baseline in a young healthy female, and it is not used for diagnosis. Answer D is incorrect for the same reason.

If you find that your patient has osteoporosis, you may consider using all of the following drugs to treat her osteoporosis EXCEPT:

A) Bisphosphonates (eg, alendronate, risedronate).
B) Estrogens.
C) Progesterone (eg, Provera, Depo-Provera).
D) Vitamin D and calcium.
E) Calcitonin.

Discussion

The correct answer is C. Progesterones are not indicated for the treatment (or prevention) of osteoporosis. In fact, in young, healthy, premenopausal women, they are associated with a decrease in bone mineral density. This is because they suppress estrogen production (as with Depo-Provera). All of the other options are acceptable choices for the treatment of osteoporosis. Calcium (1,200–1,500 mg per day in divided doses) and vitamin D (400–800 IU per day) should be prescribed for everyone with osteoporosis. Bisphosphonates are the treatment of choice, but estrogens/hormone therapy or calcitonin nasal spray are acceptable alternatives with FDA approval for the treatment of osteoporosis.

* *

Before she leaves the office, you present your patient with literature on living wills and durable power of attorney for health care (DPOA-HC).

Which of the following statements is TRUE regarding advance health-care planning?

A) The Joint Commission requires that patients be asked about their advance directives on admission to the hospital.
B) A DPOA-HC can override a patient's decision regarding treatment.
C) Once the patient has signed a living will, no further changes can be made regarding treatment decisions.
D) A DPOA-HC must be a family member or blood relative.

Discussion

The correct answer is A. The Joint Commission requires that patients be asked about their advance directives on admission to the hospital. Advance directives can take many forms but are usually manifest in one of two ways: through a living will or a DPOA-HC. The purpose of a living will is to instruct health-care decision-making in future events when the patient may not be able to communicate his or her wishes. These documents often contain brief clinical scenarios with patient preferences for life-sustaining measures. In contrast, a DPOA-HC is not as limited and can address situations not foreseen in a living will. If the patient becomes unable to participate in health-care decision-making, the DPOA-HC is instructed to exercise substituted judgment, using the patient's previously stated health-care preferences, to help direct future care. The DPOA-HC is appointed by the patient and can be a family member or another adult. The DPOA-HC cannot override a patient's decision in health-care matters because such an action would violate patient autonomy.

 HELPFUL TIP: Although advance directives should be addressed with all patients, it is of particular importance to discuss them in the setting of chronic illness, life-threatening illness, advancing age, and with any deterioration in health status. A patient can change advance care plans whenever he or she wishes, as these decisions may change over time depending on goals of care.

Objectives: Did you learn to . . .

- Identify and implement appropriate preventive health services for older females?
- Diagnose and manage common vision problems in older adults?
- Identify and manage common hearing problems in older adults?
- Discuss issues related to breast and gynecologic cancer screening?
- Define appropriate criteria for osteoporosis screening and identify risk factors?
- Recognize the important and complementary roles of DPOA and advance directives?

 QUICK QUIZ: GERIATRIC PREVENTIVE CARE

Which of the following statements is FALSE regarding preventive health in older adults?

A) Although the optimal interval for vision screening is undetermined, many professional organizations recommend vision and glaucoma screening every 1–2 years in adults >65 years.

B) In women at high risk for breast cancer, tamoxifen reduces the risk of cancer by almost 50%.

C) The American Cancer Society and American College of Obstetrics and Gynecology (ACOG) recommend screening ultrasound for ovarian cancer in all women >60 years.

D) Although Pap smears are not generally recommended for elderly women, the distribution of cervical cancer cases is bimodal, with peaks at 35–39 years and 60–64 years.

Discussion

The correct answer is C. ACOG, the USPSTF, and the American College of Physicians specifically recommend **against** ultrasound screening for ovarian cancer in asymptomatic women. All the other statements are true.

 HELPFUL TIP: ACOG now recommends ultrasound screening for ovarian cancer in all women with ≥2 weeks of unexplained urinary frequency or urgency; pelvic or abdominal pain; early satiety or difficulty eating; and bloating. It is unclear if these guidelines will be beneficial or harmful (unnecessary surgery, etc).

CASE 3

An 82-year-old male patient presents to your office for confusion. His wife reports that he was in his usual state of health until 3 days ago. At that time, he developed abdominal pain and felt feverish. He then began to have a dry, hacking cough. On examination his temperature is 100.3°F and blood pressure is 118/56. He is pale and lethargic but in no acute distress. He is oriented to person only. Other than mild upper abdominal tenderness, there are no additional findings on exam.

This patient appears to have a new onset of confusion. You suspect delirium.

Which of the following is true with regards to delirium and dementia?

A) In delirium it is rare to find an underlying medical cause.
B) A primary feature of delirium is inattention.
C) Dementia is characterized by a fluctuating course.
D) The diagnosis of delirium in the elderly requires that the patient has underlying dementia.

Table 21–2   DSM-IV DIAGNOSTIC CRITERIA FOR DELIRIUM

Disturbance of consciousness with reduced ability to focus attention
Disorientation, memory deficit, or other change in cognition that is not better accounted for by a preexisting dementia
Acute onset with fluctuating course (often changing throughout the day)
Evidence that the disturbance is caused by an underlying medical condition or drug use

Discussion

The correct answer is B. The Diagnostic and Statistical Manual of Mental Disorders (DSM-IV) provides the diagnostic criteria for delirium, which are listed in Table 21–2. Not all signs and symptoms of delirium are present in every delirious patient. Delirium can be confused with dementia, depression, or psychosis. Delirious patients may present as agitated, psychotic, somnolent, or withdrawn. Dementia is typically more chronic in nature with an insidious onset. Dementia progresses over time and usually cannot be reversed. Often delirium is treatable or reversible if the underlying medical condition is identified. Patients with dementia usually have intact attention, whereas delirious patients have markedly impaired attention. Patients with dementia have "poverty of thought," which implies decreased content of their thoughts. Delirious patients may have a rich content to their thoughts, but the thoughts are disordered.

 HELPFUL TIP: Delirium may be either hypoactive or hyperactive, or both, all in the same patient. Many patients with delirium are not identified due to their hypoactive state (these aren't the ones screaming obscenities and yanking IV lines). Elderly patients are more susceptible to delirium, and delirium is sometimes the only identifiable symptom in an elder with an acute illness.

* *

With further history from the patient's wife, you find that he has coronary artery disease, diabetes mellitus type 2, hypertension, and benign prostatic hyperplasia.

Which of the following is the most useful question to elicit risk factors for delirium?

A) "Does the patient have any drug allergies?"
B) "Does the patient use tobacco?"
C) "Does the patient use alcohol?"
D) "Does the patient have edema?"
E) "Does the patient use acetaminophen?"

Discussion

The correct answer is C. Studies have consistently identified the following risk factors for delirium: advancing age, preexisting dementia, underlying structural brain disease other than dementia, uncorrected impairment in vision or hearing, multiple chronic illnesses, polypharmacy, the use of physical restraints, history of alcohol abuse, male gender, and functional impairment.

Although hypoxia (due to myocardial infarction, pulmonary embolus, or any other source) may lead to delirium, tobacco use alone does not predispose a patient to develop delirium. In isolation, knowledge about edema, acetaminophen use, or drug allergies is less helpful. Questioning about alcohol use will help to identify patients who have a tendency to overuse alcohol, putting themselves at risk for delirium.

 HELPFUL TIP: Delirium is characterized by impaired consciousness, whereas dementia is characterized by impaired cognition. However, preexisting dementia greatly increases the risk of delirium, and simply moving a patient with dementia to a new environment can precipitate delirium.

The appropriate evaluation of the patient with delirium includes which of the following?

A) Evaluation of metabolic causes such as electrolytes, glucose, etc.
B) Evaluation for infection such as urinary tract infection, pneumonia, etc.
C) Evaluation of a patient's medications.
D) Evaluation of oxygen saturation.
E) All of the above.

Discussion

The correct answer is E. Causes of delirium are protean, often acting together in a multifactorial manner, and are best considered by a systematic approach. Metabolic causes include electrolyte disturbances, hypoglycemia, and hypoxia. A number of infections may lead to delirium. Neurologic causes include head trauma, meningitis, and vasculitis. Many medications cause delirium, including anticholinergics, antidepressants, sedative-hypnotics, and steroids. Dehydration and prerenal azotemia may lead to delirium. Alcohol intoxication or withdrawal may precipitate delirium. See Table 21–3.

* *

You obtain a number of tests. The chest radiograph shows a left lower lobe consolidation. The abdominal film shows a nonspecific bowel gas pattern. The white blood cell count is 12,700/mm³, blood urea nitrogen 36 mg/dL, creatinine 1.5 mg/dL, and glucose 150 mg/dL. The remainder of the blood counts and chemistries are normal. With the exception of trace ketones, the urinalysis is within normal limits. Cultures will not be available for at least 24 hours. The ECG shows normal

Table 21–3   CAUSES OF DELIRIUM, "WHHH-HIMP" ACRONYM

Wernicke encephalopathy
Hypoperfusion
Hypoglycemia
Hypertensive encephalopathy
Hypoxia
Infection or intracranial bleed
Meningitis or encephalitis
Poisons or medications

sinus rhythm. With the available information, you decide to admit this patient for treatment of delirium due to pneumonia and dehydration.

You are called in the middle of the night for agitated behavior and noncompliance with nursing care. The patient has pulled out his IV and struck a nurse.

You appropriately prescribe which of the following interventions?

A) Administer haloperidol 0.5 mg PO.
B) Administer haloperidol 1 mg IV.
C) Apply physical restraints.
D) Administer morphine 5 mg IV.

Discussion

The correct answer is A. Agitated delirium should be treated quickly, and haloperidol is the treatment of choice. Most of the time, delirium does **not** require pharmacologic treatment. However, this patient is at risk of harming himself and others because of his agitated delirium, so some action must be taken. Agitated delirium causes physiologic and psychologic stress on the patient, results in interference with medical care, and portends a poorer prognosis. The incidence of delirium in hospitalized patients of all ages is 30%, and the incidence in postoperative patients may approach 50%. In older patients, drug clearance decreases, so low doses of antipsychotic medication should be administered initially. (Start low and go slow.) Increasing doses of oral haloperidol can be given every 30 minutes if the patient continues to have agitation.

Answer B is incorrect because IV haloperidol is associated with QT prolongation; PO or IM haloperidol is preferred. Answer C is incorrect; physical restraints may lead to patient injury and may worsen delirium. Restraints should only be applied when absolutely necessary and for as short a duration as possible. Answer D is incorrect because we have no reason to believe the patient is in pain. However, pain can certainly result in agitation, so keep it in mind.

* *

You reflect that primary prevention of delirium is probably more effective than secondary prevention. For this patient, delirium must now be treated, but you try to avoid this complication in your hospitalized older patients.

You know that research has shown a reduction in delirium in hospitalized older patients when which of the following strategies is employed?

A) Increased sedative medication use for sleep-deprived patients.
B) Early mobilization for immobilized patients.
C) Cholinesterase inhibitor (eg, donepezil) therapy for cognitively impaired patients.
D) Physical restraints for combative patients.
E) Music therapy for depressed patients.

Discussion

The correct answer is B, early mobilization for immobilized patients. Identification of risk factors and targeting interventions to reduce or eliminate risk factors can prevent delirium. Because one patient may have a number of risk factors for delirium and because delirium is usually a multifactorial syndrome, a multicomponent intervention strategy is warranted. An often-cited study by Inouye et al demonstrated the effectiveness of this strategy.

In the study, sleep-deprived patients received a warm drink, relaxing music, and back massage at bedtime. Unit-wide noise reduction was implemented as well. Early ambulation and active range-of-motion exercises were employed for bed-bound patients. All patients were encouraged to ambulate. Cognitively impaired patients received orienting stimuli and cognitively stimulating activities. Patients with hearing and visual impairments received portable amplifying devices and visual aids, respectively. Investigators used a protocol for early recognition and treatment of dehydration. There was no specific therapy for depression or combativeness.

Which of the following statements about delirium is true?

A) Bed rails and restraints are effective in preventing injury in the delirious patient.
B) Atypical antipsychotics (eg, olanzapine, risperidone) can be used to treat delirium.
C) Diphenhydramine is a good choice for a sleep aid in patients who are prone to developing delirium.
D) A feeding tube (eg, Dobhoff tube) should be used in the patient who is not eating in order to prevent delirium.
E) None of the above is true.

Discussion

The correct answer is B. Atypical antipsychotics can be used in the treatment of delirium. Answer A is incorrect

because bed rails and restraints increase the risk of injury in the delirious patient. Answer C is incorrect. Diphenhydramine is a particularly poor choice because of its anticholinergic side effects, which can exacerbate or cause delirium. A short-acting sedative agent (eg, zolpidem) or trazodone would be better. Answer D is incorrect, as anyone who has done inpatient work knows. The feeding tube and the Foley are often the first to get yanked!

 HELPFUL TIP: Ethical dilemmas abound in the treatment of delirium. Atypical antipsychotic use in demented patients is associated with increased mortality. Older antipsychotics pose a greater risk for extrapyramidal symptoms when compared with atypicals and may have the same mortality risk. Agitated, delirious patients cannot provide informed consent, so "implied consent" is usually substituted in order to use drug therapy for delirious patients at risk for self-injury and to stabilize critically ill delirious patients.

Objectives: Did you learn to . . .

- Define delirium?
- Describe the signs and symptoms of delirium?
- Distinguish delirium from dementia?
- Identify causes and risk factors for delirium?
- Treat and prevent delirium?

CASE 4

In the early morning hours, a 78-year-old female presents to the ED with complaint of right buttock and hip pain. Several hours before her arrival, she fell in the bathroom of her daughter's home. She recalls standing on a floor mat, leaning her head back to drink a glass of water, and then hitting the ground. She denies loss of consciousness. Her daughter was at the scene quickly and found the patient awake, alert, and moving all extremities. Her vital signs are normal. Other than right hip tenderness, her examination is unremarkable.

Which of the following is most likely to assist you in determining the cause of her fall?

A) CT scan of the head.
B) ECG.

C) Additional history.

D) Serum chemistry profile.

E) CBC.

Discussion

The correct answer is C. If there is an answer choice for "more history," it is usually the right answer. History is one of the most important factors to determine the etiology of a fall. Ten percent of falls in older individuals can result in serious injury, such as a hip fracture or subdural hematoma—both of which can be deadly. Falls in elderly individuals are typically multifactorial in nature. Randomized clinical trials demonstrate a reduction in the occurrence of falls in community-dwelling elders when health-care personnel engage in a multifactorial risk assessment with targeted management. Such an approach requires a thorough history.

All of the following are risk factors for falls in elderly EXCEPT:

A) Use of four or more medications.

B) Orthostatic hypotension.

C) Doing tai chi, which improves balance.

D) Environmental hazards (eg, poor lighting or uneven walking surfaces).

Discussion

The correct answer is C. Doing tai chi has been shown to reduce the risk for falls in the elderly. All of the other answer choices increase the risk for falls. Additional risk factors for falls include history of a fall in the last year; impaired balance and gait; poor vision (acuity <20/60); decreased muscle strength; and syncope or arrhythmia. Still more risk factors include poor lighting, lack of grab bars and handrails, cluttered floor, restraint use, and improper bed height.

During your examination, which of the following physical maneuvers is most likely to assist you in evaluating the risk of future falls?

A) Get-Up-and-Go test.

B) Test for pulsus paradoxus.

C) Osler maneuver.

D) Lumbar spine flexibility test.

E) Test for nystagmus.

Discussion

The correct answer is A. The timed Get Up and Go test is a commonly used method of assessing disability and fall risk in geriatric assessment. From a seated position, the patient is instructed to stand up, walk 3 meters (~10 feet), turn around, and return to her chair. An adult with no disability should be able to complete this test in <10 seconds. Increasingly longer time to perform the test is associated with increasing fall risk. While performing the test, assess the patient's sitting balance, transition from sitting to standing, gait, and steadiness and quickness with turning. While potentially useful in the evaluation, the other tests listed are not directly associated with fall risk.

* *

After a thorough history, you perform a complete workup, including ECG, radiology studies, and appropriate laboratory tests. You find that the fall was caused by environmental factors (poor lighting and a loose throw rug) rather than an organic cause intrinsic to the patient. The patient asks how exercise might help her avoid future falls.

Which of the following is the best answer?

A) Physical therapist supervision is essential to have an effective fall prevention program.

B) In elderly patients, the effect of exercise on falling is unknown.

C) Strength training has a greater effect than balance training on reducing fall risk.

D) Unsupervised balance and strength training is effective in reducing fall risk.

E) Group exercise is more effective than exercising alone to prevent falls.

Discussion

The correct answer is D. There is no particular type of exercise that seems to prevent falls to a greater degree than any other type of exercise. Strength, balance, and gait training all appear to be important. Exercise programs have been shown to benefit elders at risk for falls. Although initial instruction by a therapist may be helpful, a physical therapist need not supervise all exercises. Patients are able to perform exercises targeted toward fall prevention at home, and they do not need to be part of an exercise group. A meta-analysis of the Frailty and Injuries: Cooperative Studies of Intervention Techniques (FICSIT) trials found that combined balance and strength training reduces the risk of falls in community-dwelling elders.

* *

You recommend strength and balance exercises to the patient, but she is worried and says, "My heart's too old for exercise."

You assure her that light exercises are safe and then review normal age-related cardiovascular changes, which include:
A) Reduced ventricular compliance.
B) Reduced maximal heart rate.
C) Reduced response to sympathetic nervous stimulation.
D) Increased atrial filling.
E) All of the above.

Discussion
The correct answer is E. Even in the healthy elderly without signs of vascular disease, there are important changes in the cardiovascular system. Maximum cardiac output is reduced, mostly through reduced maximal heart rate; thus the equation:

$$Maximal\ heart\ rate = 220 - age$$

Additionally, there is reduced response to sympathetic stimulation, with less chronotropic and inotropic response to stress. Reduced ventricular compliance results in increased atrial filling volume and pressure, increased left atrial size, and increased dependence on atrial contraction for ventricular filling. However, endurance training may improve cardiac output, and active older adults have a higher cardiac output compared to sedentary persons of the same age.

* *

Because of her right hip pain, you consider giving the patient an ambulatory device for temporary use. She has good upper extremity strength, can bear some weight on the right, but needs improved stability.

Which of the following devices would be most appropriate in this setting?
A) Wheeled walker.
B) Forearm crutches.
C) Walk cane (hemi-walker).
D) Imperial walker.
E) Multiple-legged cane (quad cane).

Discussion
The correct answer is E. Ambulatory devices are employed with the following goals: improve mobility, decrease the risk of falling, and relieve discomfort associated with acute or chronic musculoskeletal and neurologic conditions. An inappropriately selected device can increase energy expenditure and the risk for falls. Canes widen a patient's base, resulting in increased stability. They are typically used for balance, not weight-bearing. **Multiple-legged canes**—called "quad canes" because of the presence of four tips—provide a more stable base and some weight-bearing, when compared with standard, single-tipped canes. **Walk canes** are useful for patients who require full weight-bearing on one arm, as in a stroke survivor with loss of lower extremity function. **Crutches,** either forearm or axillary, are used for patients who cannot bear any weight on one leg.

Walkers can support a patient's weight, provide lateral stability, and expand a patient's support base. **Standard walkers,** those with four rubber tips, provide the greatest support and are helpful in cases of ataxia. **Front-wheeled walkers** are useful for patients with a fast gait, such as a festinating gait in Parkinsonism. Also, a front-wheeled walker is easier to manipulate than a standard walker. **Four-wheeled walkers** should be used when the patient requires some increased stability but does not need as much weight-bearing as a standard walker would provide. Patients with mild to moderate Parkinson disease may benefit from four-wheeled walkers. In this case, the patient requires only improved stability and slight assistance with bearing weight. Of the available choices, the multiple-legged cane is the best option.

* *

Unfortunately, you do not have access to a multiple-legged cane for your patient. But you do have a supply of adjustable single-tip aluminum canes available.

If you were to provide her with a cane, what method would you use to fit the cane?

A) Allow the patient to fit the cane length to her comfort level.

B) Select a device with a length equal to the distance from the floor to the greater trochanter of the femur.

C) Fit the cane length so that the handle comes to rest at the patient's waist.

D) Select a device with a length equal to the distance from the floor to the fingertips with the arm relaxed.

Discussion

The correct answer is B. You should fit a cane for a patient by selecting a device that reaches from the floor to the greater trochanter of the femur. Another option is to fit the cane so that it reaches the flexor crease of the wrist when the arm is extended to the side. A properly fitted ambulatory device should be comfortable, allowing the patient to stand erect without excessive forward flexion of the spine. Excessive forward flexion occurs when the device is too short and can result in increased risk of falling. Also, to obtain maximum efficiency from the upper extremities, the device should not be too long. The usual recommendation is to have a device fitted so that the elbow is flexed at 15%–30% when the cane is in use. This is done by measuring as noted above.

Objectives: Did you learn to . . .

- Recognize the morbidity associated with falls in older people?
- Evaluate causes and risks of falls in this population?
- Implement appropriate interventions for falling patients?
- Assess gait abnormalities that may lead to falls?
- Select ambulatory devices for appropriate patients?

 QUICK QUIZ: ASSISTIVE DEVICES

If a patient is having difficulty walking due to left-sided leg weakness after a recent stroke, in which hand should a cane be used?

A) Left hand.

B) Right hand.

C) Either hand.

D) No cane should be prescribed; a wheelchair is preferred.

Discussion

The correct answer is B. When a cane is used to support lower leg function limited by weakness or pain, the cane should be used in the hand *contralateral* to the affected side (left side weak, right hand gets the cane). This enables the patient to maintain normal arm swing while advancing the cane and the affected leg at the same time to reduce the weight-bearing forces on the affected limb during the step.

CASE 5

Accompanied by her two daughters, a 69-year-old female presents to your office as a new patient without complaints. Further history from her daughters reveals that the patient was widowed 4 years ago, now lives alone, and has experienced memory loss over the last 2 years. One daughter has taken over the patient's checkbook and is responsible for paying the bills. She has noticed that her mother often wears the same clothes and bathes infrequently—new habits for her. The past medical history includes hypothyroidism and hypertension. Family history is significant for depression and memory problems in the patient's mother prior to her death from "old age." The patient takes chlorthalidone, levothyroxine, and acetaminophen as needed.

Physical examination reveals a thin, elderly female in no distress. She is alert but does not correctly identify the year. She describes her mood as "happy" most of the time. The remainder of the exam is unremarkable. You suspect dementia.

Which of the following is true regarding the diagnosis of dementia?

A) The diagnosis is rarely missed in the primary care setting.

B) To diagnose dementia, impairment in executive function must be present.

C) To diagnose dementia, impairment in memory must be present.

D) Alzheimer disease is a diagnosis of exclusion.

E) Neuroimaging is essential in the diagnosis of dementia.

Discussion

The correct answer is C. One of the necessary components in order to make a diagnosis of dementia is memory impairment.

Answer A is incorrect. In contrast to delirium and depression, the onset of dementia is insidious. Symptoms often go unrecognized for months to years prior to diagnosis. Although the patient may complain of confusion or memory loss, family members are more likely to provide the chief complaint and history. During the initial phases of a dementing illness, patients and family members may attribute cognitive changes to normal aging. In early cognitive impairment, memory symptoms may wax and wane. However, symptoms of dementia can be differentiated from occasional normal lapses based on their increasing severity. For example, it is normal to forget an acquaintance's name, but clearly abnormal to forget a spouse's name.

Answer B is incorrect. Many patients with dementia have impaired executive functioning (eg, judgment, reasoning, planning, etc), but the presence of impaired executive functioning is not a requirement.

Answer D is incorrect, as Alzheimer disease (AD) is diagnosed by a specific set of clinical criteria. DSM-IV provides diagnostic criteria for dementia and AD, making AD a diagnosis of inclusion rather than exclusion.

Answer E is incorrect. Dementia is a clinical diagnosis and does not require neuroimaging for confirmation. Experts and professional medical associations differ in their recommendations regarding the use of neuroimaging in dementia. In general, neuroimaging is recommended if dementia occurs in the following scenarios: onset <65 years, sudden onset, presence of focal neurologic signs, and suspicion of normal pressure hydrocephalus.

* *

You use several office assessment tools to further characterize the memory loss. She scores 23/30 on the Folstein Mini-Mental State Exam, missing orientation and recall items. Clock drawing is grossly abnormal. Her Geriatric Depression Scale is 3/15 (positive screen is ≥5/15). She performs all basic activities of daily living independently, but has voluntarily given up driving and control of her finances.

Regarding assessment tools used in the evaluation of memory loss, which of the following statements is most accurate?

A) The Mini-Mental State Exam (MMSE) evaluates executive function and visual-spatial skills.
B) Formal neuropsychological testing offers no benefit over the MMSE for detecting dementia.
C) The use of a screening tool for depression is not helpful in the evaluation of memory loss.
D) Clock drawing evaluates executive function and visual-spatial skills.

Discussion

The correct answer is D. Clock drawing can be used to evaluate executive function as well as visual-spatial skills. **Clock drawing is a simple test that takes 1 minute or less to perform.** The patient is asked to draw a clock face and set the hands to 2:50 or 11:10. This test requires planning and visual-spatial ability on the part of the patient—two areas that are incompletely evaluated by the MMSE. A normal clock does not rule out dementia, but an abnormal clock is suggestive of cognitive impairment. There are several scoring systems, and the sensitivity and specificity for dementia are as high as 87% and 82%, respectively.

Answers A and B are incorrect. The MMSE is a 30-point scale, with the cutoff for dementia between 24 and 26. The MMSE can be performed in a few minutes and tests memory, orientation, language, construction, and concentration. The MMSE does not test prosody (expressive and receptive inflection of vocalization) or executive function and, as a result, has poor sensitivity for early cognitive impairment in some individuals. Performance on the MMSE is strongly correlated with education; therefore, there may be false-positives in undereducated patients and false-negatives in highly educated individuals. Compared to the MMSE, formal neuropsychological testing assesses a broader array of cognitive functions, and it identifies behavioral abnormalities and assesses mood disorders. It can also help to differentiate between types of dementia. In general, neuropsychological testing is the most sensitive and specific cognitive assessment tool, but it is time-consuming and requires a high level of expertise to administer and interpret. Answer C is incorrect because depression may cause memory problems, especially in the elderly, and a screening test (such as the Geriatric Depression scale) should be administered in the workup of memory concerns. Depression often coexists with dementia, and treatment of depression may improve memory problems.

* *

So far, you have collected the following information on this patient: MMSE score 23/30, impairment in driving and managing finances, disorientation to time, but intact abilities to cook, clean, and care for herself.

Using conventional staging for Alzheimer disease, how would you categorize this patient's dementia?

A) Mild.
B) Moderate.
C) Severe.
D) Terminal.
E) Insufficient information to determine the stage.

Discussion

The correct answer is A. **Mild AD** symptoms include impaired memory, mild personality changes, and mild disorientation. **Moderate AD** symptoms include aphasia, apraxia, insomnia, and increasing confusion. **Severe AD** symptoms include severe memory loss, motor impairment, and loss of some activities of daily living (eg, urinary incontinence, feeding difficulties, etc). Symptoms of **terminal AD** include immobility, dysphagia, and increasing susceptibility to infections. See Table 21–4 for medication management for dementia.

Which of the following findings would most likely cause you to search for a diagnosis other than Alzheimer disease in a patient presenting with memory impairment?

A) Paranoid behavior.
B) Apraxia.
C) Bradykinesia and rigidity.
D) Aphasia and personality changes.

Discussion

The correct answer is C. Bradykinesia and rigidity are features of parkinsonism, which, in the setting of memory loss, should prompt consideration of Lewy body dementia or Parkinson disease. Paranoid behavior, delusions, and hallucinations can all occur with more severe AD. Aphasia, apraxia, and personality changes typically occur later in AD but can be initial complaints in atypical presentations of AD.

In order to diagnose dementia, impairment in memory must be present. Additionally, a patient must display at least one of the following cognitive disturbances: aphasia (language disturbance), apraxia (impaired motor abilities despite intact motor function), agnosia (impaired ability to identify objects despite intact sensation), and disturbance in executive function (eg, planning, judgment, insight). Finally, the diagnostic criteria for dementia require that these cognitive disturbances result in functional impairments that represent a significant change from a previous level of functioning.

* *

Although you suspect AD in this patient, you consider other types of dementia as well.

Table 21–4 MEDICATION MANAGEMENT FOR DEMENTIA

Behavioral Subtype	Acute Management	Long-term Management
Psychosis	Conventional high-potency antipsychotic (CHAP)*	Risperidone, CHAP
Anxiety	Benzodiazepines	Buspirone
Insomnia	Trazodone	Trazodone
Sundowning	Trazodone; consider CHAP, risperidone, olanzapine	Trazodone; consider CHAP, risperidone, olanzapine
Aggression, severe	CHAP, risperidone	Divalproex, risperidone, CHAP
Aggression, mild	Trazodone	Divalproex, SSRIs, trazodone, buspirone

* CHAP includes haloperidol, perphenazine, and fluphenazine. For elderly demented patients, typical doses should be about one-quarter of the usual dose (eg, risperidone 0.25, olanzapine 2.5 mg, or quetiapine 25 mg, haloperidol 0.25–0.5 mg).

Regarding various causes of dementia, which of the following is most accurate?

A) Normal pressure hydrocephalus is recognized by the triad of dementia, headache, and visual field disturbances.
B) Clinical features of Pick disease include memory loss and disinhibition.
C) Alzheimer disease is confirmed by generalized cortical atrophy on CT or MRI of the brain.
D) Diagnostic criteria for Lewy body dementia include cognitive impairment and psychomotor agitation.

Discussion

The correct answer is B. Pick disease, a frontotemporal dementia, is characterized by memory loss and disinhibition. **Frontotemporal dementias** constitute a heterogeneous group of neurodegenerative disorders that have the common pathologic finding of cortical degeneration in frontal areas of the brain. Pick disease is included among these. Typical features of these dementias include an insidious onset and a slowly progressive course. Patients have impairments in judgment and insight. They are disinhibited and socially inappropriate. Patients may present with anxiety, depression, delusions, or emotional indifference. Neuropsychological testing and neuroimaging aid in the diagnosis.

Normal pressure hydrocephalus (NPH) classically presents with dementia, gait ataxia, and urinary incontinence. However, there is no headache; thus answer A is incorrect. When detected early, it responds to ventriculoperitoneal shunting and is thus a reversible cause of dementia. Although neuroimaging will show enlarged ventricles in many patients with NPH, the same findings are also present in some vascular dementias.

Alzheimer dementia is a clinical diagnosis; thus answer C is incorrect. Neuroimaging may be consistent with the diagnosis but has poor sensitivity. Additionally, generalized cortical atrophy can be associated with AD and other conditions. Alzheimer is the most common form of dementia, encompassing about 60% of patients with dementia. Vascular and Lewy body dementias account for about 15%–30%. In many cases, dementia has more than a single cause. Alzheimer and vascular dementias frequently coexist—an entity commonly referred to as "mixed dementia."

Lewy body dementia is characterized pathologically by the presence of Lewy bodies in the brain stem and cortex. Clinical features consist of cognitive impairment, detailed visual hallucinations, fluctuation in alertness, and motor symptoms of parkinsonism (not psychomotor agitation; thus answer D is incorrect).

Which of the following is NOT consistent with the diagnosis of vascular dementia?

A) Diabetes.
B) Tobacco use.
C) Diffuse slowing or normal electroencephalogram (EEG).
D) Normal brain MRI.

Discussion

The correct answer is D. A normal MRI essentially rules out vascular dementia. Features suggestive of vascular dementia include a stepwise deterioration in cognitive function, onset of cognitive impairment with stroke, infarcts and white matter changes on neuroimaging, and focal neurologic findings on examination. There are no well-defined criteria for clinical diagnosis of vascular dementia, and available rating scales have poor predictive value when compared to autopsy as the diagnostic standard. A history of vascular risk factors, such as diabetes, hypertension, and smoking, helps to support the diagnosis.

* *

In order to evaluate for reversible causes for this patient's dementia, you consider ordering laboratory tests.

Which of the following lab tests are NOT indicated in the initial evaluation for reversible causes of dementia?

A) Cyanocobalamin (vitamin B_{12}).
B) Liver enzymes.
C) Complete blood count.
D) Cerebrospinal fluid analysis.
E) Thyroid function tests.

Discussion

The correct answer is D. When evaluating a newly diagnosed case of dementia, one must consider infectious, metabolic, toxic, and inflammatory etiologies. Therefore, the minimal required laboratory tests should include complete blood count, serum glucose and electrolytes, vitamin B_{12}, and renal, liver, and thyroid function tests. Further laboratory tests should be obtained as clinical suspicion indicates. In the appropriate patient,

Table 22–5 LABORATORY EVALUATION OF DEMENTIA

Required Minimum Testing
- Complete blood count
- Serum glucose and electrolytes
- Vitamin B$_{12}$
- Renal function tests
- Liver function tests
- Thyroid function tests

Testing Based on Clinical Suspicion
- Urinalysis
- Urine toxicology screen
- HIV antibody assay
- Cerebrospinal fluid analysis

Other Testing in the Appropriate Setting
- RPR or VDRL
- Neuroimaging (recommended for all patients by some societies)

one might obtain urinalysis, urine toxicology screen, HIV antibody assay, and cerebrospinal fluid analysis. Because of the extremely low incidence of neurosyphilis, routine testing for syphilis is no longer required but should be considered in the appropriate setting. Neuroimaging is not a required part of every workup but may be helpful in some patients (Table 21–5).

* *

You obtain laboratory studies. Blood chemistries, blood counts, thyroid hormone levels, vitamin B$_{12}$ level, and liver enzymes are in the normal range. A noncontrast CT scan of the brain shows nonspecific "age-related" changes. The patient and her family return to discuss the test results. You begin to educate them about AD and dementia in general. The two daughters are concerned that other family members may be at risk for developing AD.

Which of the following is the strongest risk factor for developing AD?

A) Age.
B) Apolipoprotein E 4 (APOE 4) allele.
C) Family history.
D) Head trauma.
E) Low educational level.

Discussion

The correct answer is A. As with many diseases, age is the greatest risk factor for developing AD. In individuals

aged 65 to 69 years, the incidence of AD is 1%. In individuals ≥85 years, the incidence rises to 8%. All of the other answer choices are associated with an increased risk of AD but to a lesser degree than age.

Family history is a risk factor strongly associated with developing AD. By 90 years, almost 50% of individuals who have first-degree relatives with AD will develop the disease. There are genetic risk factors as well. Mutations on chromosomes 1, 14, and 21 are known risk factors for AD. Trisomy 21 is a risk factor for developing AD at an earlier age (often by 50 years). APOE 4 allele increases risk and decreases age-of-onset of AD in a dose-related fashion, with the greatest risk present in persons homozygous for APOE 4. Other risk factors include a history of head trauma, lower educational achievement, female sex, and depression. Hypertension and hyperlipidemia are associated with dementia, and controlling these diseases might reduce the risk of developing dementia in the future, but the evidence is not strong. Possible protective factors include nonsteroidal antiinflammatory drugs.

* *

The patient and family ask about medications to treat AD.

Which of the following statements is TRUE?

A) All studies show that vitamin E supplementation improves cognition and prevents further neuron loss in AD.
B) Ginkgo biloba and cholinesterase inhibitors have a synergistic effect, improving cognition in AD.
C) Cholinesterase inhibitors do not prevent neuron loss in AD.
D) Estrogen replacement therapy is the initial treatment of choice for AD in postmenopausal women.
E) Cholinesterase inhibitors maintain cognition at baseline levels for 2 years after initiation of therapy; after that time, patients decline slowly.

Discussion

The correct answer is C. Cholinesterase inhibitors do not prevent neuron loss. Results with vitamin E have been inconsistent. A recent meta-analysis found a slightly **higher** risk of death in those on high-dose vitamin E (≥400 IU/day), primarily in those with coronary artery disease (Ann Intern Med 142(1):1). Given the low cost and potential benefits of vitamin E, it may still be reasonable to use in combination with a cholinesterase inhibitor in AD at a dose of <400 IU/day if the patient or family are so inclined. There is no strong evidence to support the use of ginkgo biloba in AD. Estrogen replacement therapy is not indicated for the treatment of AD and estrogen may **increase** dementia risk.

As of December 2007, five prescription medications are approved for treatment of AD. Cholinesterase inhibitors (eg, donepezil, rivastigmine, galantamine, tacrine) represent the largest class of available pharmacotherapy used to treat mild to moderate AD. Studies suggest that decline may stabilize for 3–6 months after which there is steady loss of cognition. By 9–12 months, there is no difference in decline between those on therapy and those on placebo. The fifth approved medication is an N-methyl D-aspartate (NMDA) antagonist, memantine (Namenda), used to treat moderate to severe AD. NMDA antagonists work differently from cholinesterase inhibitors, and so the two types of drugs can be prescribed in combination.

* *

You decide to start the patient on a cholinesterase inhibitor.

In your discussion about the medication, you tell the patient and her family:

A) "These drugs are indicated for treating all types of dementia."
B) "These drugs offer no benefit in moderate to severe dementia."
C) "These drugs are proven to reverse memory loss."
D) "These drugs are proven to reduce mortality."
E) None of the above.

Discussion

The correct answer is E. There is no shortage of controversy when it comes to medications for dementia. One thing is certain: there is evidence that cognitive loss and progressive behavioral problems can be slowed with memantine and cholinesterase inhibitors in any stage of dementia. However, whether these changes are clinically significant is arguable. Answer A is incorrect. Mostly, these drugs are used in AD. Their use in Lewy body and vascular dementia is off-label but may be worth a try; there is some data to support cholinesterase inhibitors for these patients. However, there is no evidence to support their use in frontotemporal dementias (eg, Pick disease). Patients with frontotemporal dementias should be treated symptomatically (with antipsychotics, a controlled, low-stimulus environment, etc). Answer B is incorrect. Most studies of cognitive effects of cholinesterase inhibitors have occurred in mild to moderate dementia (MMSE = 10–24). Although there may not be any effect of these drugs on cognition in severe, end-stage dementia, there may be some benefit in patient behavior and function. Answer C is incorrect. In comparison with placebo, cholinesterase inhibitors are found to delay further cognitive and functional decline but do not reverse the process. In cholinesterase inhibitor studies of mild to moderate dementia, there is typically a 3-point difference on the MMSE between treatment and placebo groups at 6 months. This finding is due to a loss of thinking abilities in the placebo group and a delay in that loss in the treatment group. There is no reversal of the disease process. However, long-term use of these medications appears to delay time to nursing home placement. Answer D is incorrect because cholinesterase inhibitors do not affect mortality in patients with dementia.

 HELPFUL TIP: Not every confused elderly person should be put on a cholinesterase inhibitor. Consider the diagnosis, severity of disease, and the goals for the patient.

All of the following are well-recognized side effects of cholinesterase inhibitors EXCEPT:

A) Tachycardia.
B) Nausea, vomiting, and diarrhea.
C) Anorexia.
D) Exacerbation of asthma and COPD.

Discussion

The correct answer is A. All of the above except for tachycardia are well-recognized side effects of the cholinesterase inhibitors. They have a "vagotonic" action, which can cause bradycardia and syncope and worsen cardiac conduction abnormalities. To minimize adverse events, the dose of cholinesterase inhibitor should be increased only after the patient has been on a stable dose for 4–6 weeks. In general, the cholinesterase inhibitors have similar side effect profiles. However, tacrine carries an increased risk of liver toxicity and should be avoided.

> **HELPFUL TIP:** The side effects of cholinesterase inhibitors include nausea, diarrhea, and anorexia, all common in nursing home patients. If your patient is losing weight and not eating, consider discontinuing the cholinesterase inhibitor and see if they improve.

* *

You start the patient on your cholinesterase inhibitor of choice. One year later, the patient returns with her daughter, with whom she now lives. The daughter reports disturbing symptoms that occur nightly. The patient wakes up in the middle of the night and wanders the house, becoming confused and agitated. The daughter states, "I just can't take much more of this."

After inquiring about pain and any changes in health status, your initial recommendation is to:

A) Employ soft restraints only during the night.
B) Consider environmental changes including more daytime structured activities at an adult day-care center.
C) Initiate an antipsychotic before bedtime.
D) Initiate a sedative-hypnotic before bedtime.

Discussion

The correct answer is B. Treating behavioral issues in patients with AD can be very challenging. Further history must explore the possibility of pain-related agitation, decline in comorbid conditions or new health conditions such as occult infection, and any medication changes that may play a role. If a treatable cause is not identified, then environmental change is the best initial recommendation. Adding structured daytime activities may facilitate a better sleep-wake cycle. Adult day-care programs exist that specialize in day care for elderly people including demented patients. Adult day care can provide structured activities during the day, along with respite for the daughter who is obviously asking for extra support. Although medications are sometimes needed, answers C and D are incorrect for initial treatment in this case. Once environmental changes have failed or there are other immediate health risks involved, then medications may be necessary. Antipsychotics currently offer the only drug treatment for behavioral symptoms in dementia; however, there are no great choices. Haloperidol, risperidone, and olanzapine

are used most often. Sedatives, such as benzodiazepines, often result in paradoxical agitation in elderly demented patients. Answer A is incorrect. Restraints should be avoided in most cases, even soft restraints. Although they are sometimes required to prevent harm to the patient or caretakers, restraints are known to result in worsened agitation and an increased risk of fall and injury.

> **HELPFUL TIP:** When patients with Lewy body dementia receive antipsychotic medication for hallucinations, parkinsonian features become much more pronounced. If possible, avoid antipsychotics in these patients.

* *

Over time, as the patient's dementia progresses, you reevaluate end-of-life issues and advance directives. With the support of her family, the patient decides not to have cardiopulmonary resuscitation.

In end-stage AD, which of the following is correct?

A) Malnutrition is the most common cause of death in severely demented patients.
B) Hospitalization for pneumonia in severely demented patients reduces incidence of morbidity and mortality.
C) In advanced AD, gastrostomy tube-feeding prevents aspiration.
D) To increase comfort, dehydrated AD patients should receive intravenous hydration.
E) In advanced AD, treatment of infections with oral and intravenous antibiotics is equally efficacious.

Discussion

The correct answer is E. Hospitalization for demented patients with pneumonia is a wash. The number of patients saved by the use of intravenous antibiotics is offset by an increase in death and functional deterioration as a result of the hospitalization. Thus, on balance, oral and intravenous antibiotics are equally efficacious in the treatment of infections in these patients; therefore, severely demented homebound patients or nursing home residents should be treated in their usual environment rather than hospitalized, if the family agrees.

Answer A is incorrect. The majority of patients with dementia die of infection, not malnutrition. Answer B is incorrect as noted above. Answer C is incorrect. Even in moderate to severe AD, feeding tubes can be useful in the acute setting. But the tube should be removed and natural feeding resumed as soon as the acute event passes. **Permanent gastrostomy tube-feeding is not recommended in patients with severe or terminal dementia. Tube-feeding does not prolong life, prevent aspiration, or promote weight gain in advanced dementia.** Although many patients with advanced dementia are malnourished and dehydrated, these conditions do not appear to cause discomfort.

 HELPFUL TIP: Remember the caregivers! Ask about their health and mood. 25% of caregivers to the elderly are depressed, and older people caring for their disabled spouses have a 63% higher chance of dying than noncaregivers of the same age.

Objectives: Did you learn to . . .

- Identify symptoms, signs, and diagnostic criteria for dementia?
- Describe different types of dementia and how they are diagnosed?
- Evaluate the patient with dementia, considering the potential causes of dementia?
- Describe potential benefits and limitations of current pharmacologic therapy for Alzheimer disease (AD)?
- Describe the natural course of AD?
- Manage a patient with end-stage AD?

CASE 6

A 71-year-old male whom you have known since you started your practice has recently suffered a stroke, resulting in language deficits and right hemiparesis. His medical history is significant for hypertension, hyperlipidemia, ulcer requiring partial gastrectomy (remote), and coronary artery disease. He quit tobacco and alcohol 5 years ago. He is retired and widowed. After a 3-day hospitalization, he appears stable enough for discharge. His medications include aspirin, atenolol, lisinopril, atorvastatin, and acetaminophen. Prior to entering a nursing home to receive skilled nursing care and therapies, the patient wants to know who will pay for the services. He has Medicare parts A and B.

You are able to assure him:

A) Medicare will cover all expenses indefinitely regardless of personal financial resources.
B) Medicaid will cover all of the expenses for the first 100 days of skilled care regardless of personal financial resources.
C) Medicare will cover part of the expenses for the first 100 days of skilled care regardless of personal financial resources.
D) Medicare requires a hospital stay of ≥7 days prior to entering a nursing home for skilled care.
E) Medicaid and Medicare do not cover nursing home expenses under any circumstances.

Discussion

The correct answer is C. Medicare Part A, which provides some health care for patients ≥65 years if they qualify for Social Security benefits, will pay all costs for skilled care for the first 20 days and part of the costs thereafter up to a total of 100 days. This Medicare benefit includes rehabilitation (eg, physical therapy, occupational therapy, speech therapy, etc) and skilled nursing care (eg, nursing home, skilled care facility, rehabilitation hospital) after a hospital stay of at least 3 days. This benefit is contingent upon the patient having an appropriate diagnosis and rehabilitation potential, and continuing to show improvement during the time the benefit is in place. Medicare does not provide extended nursing home coverage. Medicaid will provide extended nursing home care if a person's assets and income are below a certain threshold, which varies from state to state. Note: Although Medicare Part B will pay for physician visits to nursing home patients, Medicare does not pay for nursing or other care directly related to permanently living in a nursing home.

* *

Although he received fairly intensive physical, occupational, and speech therapies, your patient does not regain much function. He has only minimal movement in the right arm and complains of pain in the right shoulder. A radiograph of the right shoulder shows degenerative changes. Despite maximal doses of acetaminophen administered regularly, your patient continues to complain of shoulder pain. You involve physical therapists in his care to reduce the risk of chronic dislocation of the shoulder.

In order to control his pain, which of the following is the most appropriate to add as a scheduled, and presumably chronic, medication?

A) Oxycodone.
B) Gabapentin.
C) Propoxyphene.
D) Aspirin.
E) Naproxen.

Discussion

The correct answer is A. A narcotic pain medication may be the best choice in this situation (chronic pain in a nursing home resident who does not respond to or cannot tolerate acetaminophen; plus he has an ulcer history). Propoxyphene (answer C) has harmful active metabolites that may accumulate in older patients and is ineffective as a pain medication (no better than placebo in multiple studies); therefore, oxycodone is preferred to propoxyphene. Gabapentin (answer B) is indicated for postherpetic neuralgia and is more useful for neuropathic pain (although not very useful there either). Aspirin (answer D) and NSAIDs like naproxen (answer E) must be used with caution in the elderly because of increased risk of silent gastrointestinal bleeding, fatal gastrointestinal bleeding, and renal insufficiency. NSAIDs are typically not first-line agents for arthritis pain in this age group and probably offer no greater pain relief than acetaminophen. Nonpharmacologic modalities should be employed as well, including massage, exercises, and physical therapy.

* *

A nurse calls to report that your patient has developed lethargy, decreased appetite, and a temperature of 37.8°C. Your first thought is, "That's not a fever."

Then you realize that:

A) An elevated temperature in older individuals is most often due to changes in basal body temperature regulation.
B) Oral antibiotics will not be sufficient to treat this infection.
C) Antibiotics will not be necessary to treat this condition.
D) Absence of significant fever in the elderly does not rule out serious bacterial infections.

Discussion

The correct answer is D. Older individuals, especially frail elders and nursing home patients, often have lower basal body temperatures in comparison with younger persons and who may not mount as great a febrile reaction to infection. A temperature >38.1°C in a frail elder is most likely associated with a serious bacterial or viral infection. Absence of significant fever does not rule out serious bacterial infections. Answer C is incorrect. With the available information, it is difficult to say with any certainty if the patient has an infection treatable with antibiotics. If he did, oral antibiotics are often appropriate in the nursing home setting, even when treating pneumonia.

* *

With a decline in his function and a mildly elevated temperature, you plan to evaluate this patient for infection. According to the nursing staff, there are no other residents with apparent infections. Your patient has not developed any focal symptoms (eg, cough, dysuria, diarrhea, site-specific pain).

Which of the following tests will be LEAST helpful?

A) Complete blood count.
B) Urinalysis and microscopic exam of the urine.
C) Stool culture.
D) Chest radiograph.
E) Blood oxygen saturation (pulse oximetry).

Discussion

The correct answer is C. This is not a black-or-white area, but there are some principles and expert opinions to follow. First, know that that the most common infections in nursing home residents originate in the urinary tract, respiratory tract, skin, soft tissue, and gastrointestinal tract. Patient and family wishes regarding care must be known prior to initiating an evaluation, therapy, or hospital transfer. Although the elderly patient may have a serious infection with only slight or even no leukocytosis, a normal white blood cell count on CBC will reduce suspicion for serious bacterial infection. Even without specific urinary symptoms, urinalysis is recommended because of the high incidence of urinary tract infection in this population (but remember that asymptomatic bacteriuria is also common in this setting). Blood oxygen saturation below the normal range may indicate serious respiratory illness; in the setting of hypoxia, a chest radiograph is recommended. If the infection is isolated to one resident and no gastrointestinal symptoms exist, stool culture is unlikely to help.

Regarding infectious diseases in nursing home settings, which of the following is correct?

A) If the influenza vaccine is administered within 24 hours of an outbreak, patients require no further prophylaxis.

B) All residents who are carriers of methicillin-resistant *Staphylococcus aureus* (MRSA) must be treated with appropriate antibiotics.

C) Most cases of bacteremia are caused by infected skin ulcers.

D) New residents should receive a 2-step tuberculin skin test, unless positive in the first test.

E) All residents who are carriers of *Clostridium difficile* must be treated with appropriate antibiotics.

Discussion

The correct answer is D. The incidence of tuberculosis is relatively high in the older population, as is mortality from the disease. Institutionalized elders should be screened for tuberculosis with the 2-step tuberculin skin test. A 2-step test involves repeating the tuberculin skin test 1–3 weeks after an initial negative test (<10 mm induration). Anergy testing is no longer recommended. The test is positive if the induration is ≥10 mm.

Answer A is incorrect. In a nursing home, an influenza outbreak can have devastating results, with a mortality rate up to 30%. In the event of an outbreak, even residents who received the vaccine should receive antiviral prophylaxis (see Chapter 8, Infectious Diseases). Only 50% of nursing home residents will develop an adequate antibody response to the influenza vaccine, and that response takes up to 2 weeks after administration to develop.

Answers B and E are incorrect. Residents who are carriers of MRSA or *C. difficile* will not benefit from eradication if they are not infected. In addition, they may return to a carrier state quickly after antibiotic treatment; therefore, antibiotic treatment of these carrier states is not recommended. Answer C is incorrect because urinary tract infections are the most common cause of bacteremia in nursing home residents.

 HELPFUL TIP: In elderly nursing home residents, a positive response to tuberculin skin testing is most often due to reactivation of old disease. Risk factors associated with reactivation of tuberculosis include: chronic steroid use, diabetes, malignancy, malnutrition, renal failure, and chronic institutionalization.

HELPFUL TIP: Indications for pneumococcal vaccination include patients with chronic illness at high risk for invasive pneumococcal disease (eg, diabetes, chronic pulmonary disease, cardiovascular disease, etc), institutionalization, ≥65 years, immunocompromised state. Patients with an immunosuppressive disorder (eg, HIV, asplenia, renal failure, organ transplant, etc) should have a one-time revaccination at least 5 years after initial as should those who had their first immunization prior to age 65.

* *

Over the next year, the patient has increasing difficulty with cognition. He begins to experience urinary incontinence several times per day, necessitating the use of a pad. A midstream clean-catch urinalysis shows bacteria and white blood cells (2–4 WBC/hpf) but is negative for glucose and nitrites. His postvoid residual bladder volume is 80 cc.

Which of the following is true regarding the potential cause of and therapeutic intervention for urinary incontinence in this patient?

A) The most likely cause is obstruction from the benign prostatic hyperplasia, and an α-blocker will improve the incontinence.

B) The most likely cause is immobility, and scheduled voiding is indicated.

C) Based on the currently available evidence, the most likely cause is detrusor hyperactivity, and an indwelling catheter is indicated.

D) The most likely cause is stress incontinence, and pelvic floor muscle strengthening (Kegel exercises) is indicated.

E) The most likely cause is bacteriuria, and antibiotics will improve the incontinence.

Discussion

The correct answer is B. Urinary incontinence is very frequent in nursing home residents, with a rate of up to 50%. As with many other geriatric syndromes, incontinence is often multifactorial or the result of decreased function. A frequent cause of urinary incontinence in nursing home residents is immobility because of severe physical impairment or dementia or both. In this setting, the initial treatment of choice is prompted voiding every 2 hours when the patient is awake. Also, fluid and caffeine intake should be monitored and adjusted to reduce urine output without causing dehydration.

Answer A is incorrect. Although there is no information about the patient's prostate size, he has a relatively normal postvoid residual volume, making overflow incontinence from outlet obstruction less likely. Answer C is incorrect—or at least the diagnosis of detrusor hyperactivity cannot be made on the basis of current information. The patient has not been fully evaluated with urodynamic tests, so it is difficult to determine whether his incontinence is stress-type or urge-type. If he has urge-type incontinence due to detrusor hyperactivity, an indwelling bladder catheter is not appropriate. Detrusor hyperactivity can often be treated successfully with pharmacotherapy.

Answer D is incorrect. Stress incontinence is less common in men than women, and urine loss is typically associated with increased abdominal pressure (eg, coughing, sneezing, lifting). Answer E is incorrect. The presence of bacteria in the urine is a common finding in nursing home patients. In general, bacteriuria without symptoms—other than incontinence—should not be treated. Studies have demonstrated little or no improvement in incontinence after treating bacteriuria.

 HELPFUL TIP: When urinary incontinence results from obstruction or detrusor hyporeflexia, intermittent bladder catheterization should be employed and chronic indwelling catheters avoided. Appropriate indications for chronic indwelling bladder catheters in the nursing home include: comfort care of the terminally ill, presence of skin wounds contaminated by incontinent urine, and urine retention not practically managed with intermittent catheterization.

* *

Although his urinary incontinence improves, your patient develops difficulty with loose stools and occasional fecal incontinence. The stools are quite watery with no blood or melena. Aside from occasional abdominal cramping, he feels well. He has no new neurologic symptoms.

Which of the following is the most likely cause of fecal incontinence in this situation?

A) Infectious diarrhea.
B) Ulcerative colitis.
C) Decreased anal sphincter tone.
D) Fecal impaction.

Discussion

The correct answer is D. In nursing home residents with limited physical mobility, overflow incontinence due to fecal impaction is most likely. Remember that oxycodone you started earlier? Even with a stool softener and/or a laxative, constipation may result. A fecal impaction can be treated with an enema, stool softeners, laxatives, and dietary changes, but sometimes requires manual disimpaction. Decreased sphincter tone may occur as a result of neurologic insult, but this patient was previously continent of stool. Although infection might be causing incontinence, there are no other symptoms of infection. The onset of inflammatory bowel disease is usually seen in younger populations, often with blood in the stools, making ulcerative colitis less likely.

* *

As a result of your patient's report of physical abuse of another patient by the nursing staff, an investigation is under way in the nursing home.

Reflecting on elder abuse and neglect, you realize which of the following is true?

A) Up to 75% of nursing aides in nursing homes have seen or heard of a resident being abused or neglected.
B) A "dependent elder" is defined as anyone living in a nursing home.
C) Approximately 70% of elder abuse and neglect occurs in nursing homes.
D) There is a universally accepted definition of elder abuse and neglect, which is codified in law in every state.
E) Elder abuse is widely defined as "purposeful physical harm of anyone >65 years."

Discussion

The correct answer is A. In some studies, high rates of mistreatment have been found in nursing homes, with up to 75% of nursing aides witnessing or hearing about acts of abuse. However, it is not known whether nursing home residents are at greater risk than community-dwelling dependent elders. Answer B is incorrect. The definition of dependent elder is not consistent, and may apply to elders who are cognitively impaired, physically debilitated, or financially dependent. Nursing home residents are generally considered dependent; however, living in a nursing home itself is not sufficient to establish that a person is a dependent elder. Answers C and D are incorrect. The study of elder abuse and neglect (also referred to as elder mistreatment) suffers from lack of a universally accepted definition, variations in laws between states, and inherent difficulties in obtaining accurate reports of abuse. Therefore, attempts to determine the incidence of elder abuse and neglect have resulted in wide variations. Answer E is incorrect. Elder abuse may include physical harm, sexual abuse, psychological abuse, neglect, or financial exploitation. Although all states now have laws addressing elder mistreatment, those laws vary between states, and health-care providers are encouraged to know the law in their area.

 HELPFUL TIP: Risk factors for elder mistreatment include older age, cognitive impairment, substance abuse, low socioeconomic standing, minority status, and caregiver stress (probably the most important).

* *

As your patient's cognitive impairment progresses, he becomes more withdrawn and uncooperative with nursing care, such as bathing. A nurse calls to ask, "Shouldn't he be on risperidone or something to improve his behavior?"

According to the Omnibus Budget Reconciliation Act of 1987 (OBRA), antipsychotic medication is indicated for demented patients with:

A) Repetitive, bothersome behavior (eg, name-calling).
B) Continuous crying out and screaming.
C) Uncooperative behavior (eg, refusing to eat).
D) All of the above.

Discussion

The correct answer is B. One goal of OBRA was to decrease the inappropriate use of antipsychotic medications in nursing home residents. In demented patients, antipsychotic medications may be appropriately administered in the following settings: agitated, belligerent acts that present a danger to the patient or other residents; psychotic symptoms (delusions, hallucinations, paranoia); and continuous crying out and screaming (lasting ≥24 hours). Attempts to redirect the patient should always be employed first. You should also attempt to uncover occult causes of agitation, such as infection or pain. Once behavior control is attained, assess whether the antipsychotic can be reduced in dose or discontinued. According to OBRA, **inappropriate** indications for antipsychotic medication include restlessness, uncooperative behavior, poor self-care, and repetitive, bothersome actions.

Objectives: Did you learn to . . .

- Describe some common Medicare/Medicaid reimbursement issues for nursing home care?
- Manage chronic pain in the nursing home?
- Describe an appropriate evaluation for the nursing home resident with fever?
- Recognize infectious disease issues commonly presenting in the nursing home?
- Develop an appropriate strategy for the evaluation and management of urinary and fecal incontinence in nursing home residents?
- Recognize the impact of elder abuse and neglect?
- Implement appropriate measures for agitated behavior in the nursing home?

 QUICK QUIZ: GERIATRIC PHARMACOTHERAPY

Which of the following is true about drug therapy in the elderly?

A) GI absorption is substantially decreased in the elderly.
B) Sedative-hypnotic drugs should be given an 8-week trial without interruption for anxiety in the elderly.
C) Mirtazapine (Remeron) causes anorexia and weight loss in the elderly.
D) As a general rule, the volume of distribution of fat-soluble drugs is increased in the elderly when compared to the volume of distribution in water-soluble drugs.

Discussion

The correct answer is D. The volume of distribution of fat-soluble drugs is relatively increased in the elderly due to a loss of muscle mass and proportionately more fat mass. Therefore, fat-soluble drugs, like diazepam, have a greater relative volume of distribution while water-soluble drugs, like alcohols, will have a relatively smaller volume of distribution. Answer A is incorrect because drug absorption does not change substantially with aging. Sedative-hypnotic drugs should be used only for short-term therapy of 2–4 weeks because of the risk of falls and other adverse effects; this is true for both community-dwelling elders and those in nursing homes. Answer C is incorrect because mirtazapine (Remeron) can increase appetite and lead to weight gain in the elderly. For this reason it can be useful in patients who are depressed and not eating well.

 HELPFUL TIP: Although hepatic function with regard to drug metabolism does not change substantially with age, drugs tend to have decreased elimination in the elderly as a result of decreased renal function. For these reasons, the half-life of many sedative-hypnotic drugs is substantially increased in the elderly.

CASE 7

Your next patient is an 83-year-old male familiar to your clinic, who presents for routine care. He has hypertension, hyperlipidemia, and osteoarthritis. He has been widowed for 10 years and continues to live independently in an apartment in the same town as his daughter. He stopped smoking 30 years ago, but continues to drink alcohol. He denies any problems related to his drinking, but you inquire anyway and ask specifically how much he drinks. His routine includes 3 shots of whiskey per day. He says he likes drinking 1 shot before his daily walk and the other 2 shots after he returns. He finds the routine very motivating and keeps him in shape.

In regard to his drinking behavior, you are aware that:

A) Older adults accumulate significantly lower blood alcohol levels than younger adults due to decreased absorption.

B) Drinking 3 shots per day should not be any concern as long as his liver function tests are normal.

C) Alcohol consumption can reduce the availability of nutrients such as zinc, vitamins A, B_1, B_2, B_6, B_{12}, and folate.

D) The lifetime prevalence of alcoholism for men ≥65 years is <5%, but should still be screened for routinely.

E) The standard screening CAGE questionnaire for problem drinking behavior has not been validated in older adults.

Discussion

The correct answer is C. Alcohol consumption can reduce the availability of nutrients such as vitamins A, B_1, B_2, B_6, B_{12}, zinc, and folate. Patients often present with malnutrition, poor self-care, and alcohol-related illnesses such as anemia, peptic ulcer disease, diabetes, hypertension, liver disease, neuropathy, and mental status changes. Checking for deficiencies may be warranted in this situation depending on your patient's other dietary intake.

Answer A is incorrect. Older adults accumulate significantly higher blood alcohol levels than younger adults. A young adult's blood alcohol level will be approximately 0.03% after "1 drink" (1.5 ounces of distilled liquor, 5 ounces of wine, or 12 ounces of beer), although in a 75-year-old, the level may rise as high as 0.08% which is the legal limit for intoxication in many states. Answer B is incorrect. Drinking behavior should be questioned regardless of liver function tests. Further evaluation of potentially harmful drinking behavior (≥2 drinks/day for women, or ≥3 drinks/day for men) is recommended. The National Institute on Alcohol Abuse and Alcoholism has identified drinking more than 1 alcoholic beverage daily as potential problem drinking in older adults. Answer D is incorrect. The lifetime prevalence of alcoholism for men ≥65 years is >5%, approximately 14% for men and 1.5% for women >65 years. Denial of the problem is more frequent in older patients and impairments in functioning related to alcohol use may not be recognized until serious complications arise. Answer E is incorrect. Diagnosis of alcohol abuse and dependence in older adults is challenging. Brief screening tools such as the CAGE questionnaire (Table 21–6) have been validated in the older population and could be used in this situation. A positive response to any CAGE question suggests problem drinking. In this case, your patient denies any drinking problems and his CAGE screen is negative.

Table 21–6 CAGE SCREENING TOOL FOR PROBLEM DRINKING

C Have you ever felt you should Cut down?
A Does others' criticism of your drinking Annoy you?
G Have you ever felt Guilty about your drinking?
E Have you ever had an "Eye opener" to steady your nerves or get rid of a hangover?

Positive response to any question suggests problem drinking; questionnaire has been validated in older population.

* *

You advise him to cut back to <3 drinks per day and plan to follow up. As you review the patient's basic activities of daily living (ADLs) and instrumental activities of daily living (IADLs), he is independent in all ADLs and most IADLs. He walks daily, eats 3 small meals/day, and maintains a steady weight of approximately 180 lbs (BMI = 25 kg/m²). He manages his own finances, prepares his own meals, but usually has his daughter do the grocery shopping for his convenience. When you ask about transportation, he reports that he drives mostly to get around town to the golf club, social events, and the post office when needed. He denies any vision or hearing problems.

In order to keep him healthy, safe and functional, you appropriately recommend:

A) Indoor walking only.
B) Weight loss.
C) Periodic screening for hearing impairment.
D) Restricted driving.

Discussion
The correct answer is C. The USPSTF recommends screening older adults for hearing impairment by periodically questioning them about their hearing, counseling them about the availability of hearing aid devices, and making referrals for abnormalities when appropriate. Based on the 1996 recommendations, there is insufficient evidence to recommend for or against routinely screening older adults using audiometric testing, but this may be appropriate when hearing problems are identified. The Institute of Medicine recommends one-time audiometric testing for individuals aged 40–59, 60–74, and ≥75 years. In this patient, asking about hearing difficulty and testing with a whispered-voice out of the field of vision is a reasonable approach for hearing screening.

Answer A is incorrect. Daily exercise including walking indoors or outdoors in safe environments (weather permitting) should be encouraged in all age groups. Answer B is incorrect. His current weight is adequate, and he is at risk for malnutrition if he has problem drinking, so he does not need to lose weight. Answer D is incorrect. Safety is a concern due to the increasing number of older drivers, their high crash rate/mile driven, and their increased likelihood of serious injury and death. However, most seniors prefer automobile transportation to keep active in the community and should continue to drive. In this patient, without specific concerns, there is no need to recommend restricted driving.

 HELPFUL TIP: If you are concerned about driving safety, ask direct questions about any recent driving problems, such as minor accidents, traffic violations, getting lost, or difficulty with parking. The legal requirements about a physician's reporting of unsafe older drivers vary from state to state. The AMA has published an excellent guide, *Physician's Guide to Assessing and Counseling Older Drivers* that covers the law in each state (see bibliography for availability).

* *

One month later, your patient's daughter calls to inform you that he fell and broke his left hip while vacationing with the family in California. He had total hip arthroplasty (THA) and is still in the hospital recovering. Now they are trying to make arrangements to bring him home. The discharge planner has identified a local nursing home that can provide rehabilitation, but some of the family would like for him to return to his apartment.

In regards to recovery after hip surgery, you inform the daughter that:

A) Rehabilitation after hospital discharge results in better outcomes for patients with hip fracture.
B) Rehabilitation can only be provided inpatient at a hospital or nursing home, not at home.

C) Surgical repair in elderly patients should be delayed if possible (>72 hours after injury) to reduce 1-year mortality and other complications.

D) Early mobilization after hip surgery is recommended in younger patients, but in older patients weight bearing is usually delayed at least 5 days after surgery to allow proper healing.

Discussion

The correct answer is A. Studies show that rehabilitation immediately after hospital discharge appears to result in superior outcomes for patients with hip fracture or stroke. Answer B is incorrect. Rehabilitation can be provided in either inpatient (eg, hospital or skilled nursing facility) or outpatient settings (eg, clinic, day hospital, or home). For inpatient care, patients must be able to participate in rehabilitation which includes a minimum of 3 hours of therapy 5 days/week. Care usually involves an interdisciplinary team including nurses and skilled therapists. Home-based services can provide part-time or intermittent therapy as prescribed by a physician. Answer C is incorrect. Early surgical repair (<24 hours after fracture) is ideal and has been shown to reduce 1-year mortality and complications such as pressure ulcers and delirium. Delay for medically unstable patients may be necessary. Answer D is incorrect. Early mobilization is the standard of care for both hip and knee arthroplasty in younger and older adults. Weight bearing often begins on the second postoperative day.

* *

Your patient and his daughter agree that rehabilitation locally sounds like the best plan.

The goals of rehabilitation include:

A) Restore function.

B) Help patients compensate for and adapt to functional losses.

C) Prevent secondary complications.

D) Maximize potential for participation in social, leisure, or work roles.

E) All of the above.

Discussion

The correct answer is E. These are all goals of rehabilitation.

* *

The patient returns to the local nursing home for inpatient rehabilitation. Despite wonderful progress with physical therapy, he is unable to ambulate without using a cane. He is frustrated that he cannot walk on his own, and is concerned that all this walking and exercise is going to damage the recently surgically repaired hip joint.

You can tell him that:

A) He does not need to restrict his activity because the hip prosthesis is well-designed for bending, walking, and climbing stairs.

B) His frustration is likely a major depressive disorder and will require medication treatment.

C) He should continue the exercises because the advantages outweigh the low risks of surgical failure.

D) He should not expect full recovery even with exercise because nearly every patient requires an assistive device to walk after THA.

Discussion

The correct answer is C. Whether correction is with screws, partial repair, or complete joint replacement, early weight bearing is usually tolerable with low rates of surgical failure and helps to counteract the poor outcomes clearly associated with prolonged inactivity. As noted in a discussion above, early mobilization and continued exercise are the keys to prevention of further decline and loss of function.

Answer A is incorrect. After THA, patients should avoid certain motions such as bending over to tie shoes and crossing legs when seated. Often times a raised toilet seat is also recommended to reduce the load placed on the hip prosthesis in extreme flexion. Walking and general range of motion exercises should be encouraged as tolerated. Answer B is incorrect. Depression is not uncommon after a disabling injury such as hip fracture. However, this patient's frustration may or may not reflect clinical depression and should be further evaluated before starting medication. Answer D is incorrect. Although hip fractures carry approximately 5% in-hospital mortality and estimated 25% in the year following fracture, about 75% of survivors recover to prior level of function. Up to 50% of these patients require an assistive device, but certainly not everyone.

* *

After 2 more weeks, your patient is now functioning well enough to return home. He can transfer independently and ambulates with a cane for support. Prior to discharge, the rehabilitation team would like to assess his home environment.

The occupational therapy practitioner on the team:

A) Provides a comprehensive assessment wherever the patient is employed based on his/her occupation, which does not typically include the home environment.

B) May provide training for specific adaptive equipment for patients to enhance performance in everyday activities and promote independence.

C) Is a skilled professional who has completed an occupational therapy training program after completion of high school.

D) Is licensed to write prescriptions in most states, primarily for pain control.

Discussion

The correct answer is B. Occupational therapists (OTs) provide training for specific adaptive equipment to enhance performance in everyday activities and promote independence. They also provide guidance to family members and caregivers if needed. Answer A is incorrect. OTs provide home or job-site assessment, regardless or employment status or occupation. Answer C is incorrect. OTs are skilled professionals whose education includes the study of human growth and development with an emphasis on the social, emotional, and physiological effects of illness and injury. One must have a bachelor, master's, or doctoral degree to enter the field of occupational therapy. There are also occupational therapy assistants who generally earn an associate degree and practice under the supervision of a trained OT. Answer D is incorrect because OTs do not have license to prescribe medications.

Objectives: Did you learn to . . .

- Identify and screen for problem drinking in the older patient?
- Promote early rehabilitation after hip fracture repair?
- Describe some aspects of rehabilitative services?

CASE 8

A 68-year-old male arrives at your clinic to establish care. He admits that he does not visit the doctor regularly, but he feels his health has been pretty good since he changed his "bad habits." He did not bring any records, but he knows he has heart disease and high blood pressure. His bad habits included smoking about 1 pack per day for 40 years, but he proudly states he quit

"cold turkey" after a heart attack at 63 years. As far as health-care maintenance, he did have a colonoscopy 5 years ago at his wife's request, and he remembers his last PSA was normal, but he does not recall any type of screening for abdominal aortic aneurysm (AAA).

The US Preventive Services Task Force recommends one-time AAA screening:

A) For all men aged 65–74 years.

B) For all men aged 65–74 years who have smoked >100 cigarettes in their lifetime.

C) For all men aged 65–74 years who have ever smoked >1 pack of cigarettes in their lifetime.

D) For all men ≥65 years if life expectancy >10 years.

E) All male and female current smokers >65 years.

Discussion

The correct answer is B. The USPSTF and a consortium of leading professional organizations currently recommend one-time AAA screening with abdominal ultrasonography for all men aged 65–74 years who have ever smoked (defined as >100 lifetime cigarettes). Answers A and C are incorrect. The USPTF currently does NOT recommend screening men who have never smoked (<100 cigarettes in a lifetime). The American College of Cardiology/American Heart Association guidelines advise screening men >60 years who have a strong family history (parents or siblings) of AAA, but family history is not explicitly considered in the USPSTF guidelines. Answer D is incorrect. Screening is recommended for men aged 65–74 years regardless of life expectancy. The evidence in men >75 years and in women of any age does not support AAA screening, and neither of the above guidelines recommends routine screening in those groups.

* *

At the next visit, your patient returns with copies of his medical records which you have also received and reviewed. He is up to date on his immunizations, colonoscopy, and PSA, but there is no record of AAA screening. He agrees to have the screening ultrasound since the test sounds easy but questions why screening for AAA is necessary.

You inform him that:

A) AAA occurs in approximately 1 in 20 older men who have ever smoked.

B) Rupture of an AAA has a mortality rate of 50%.

C) AAA ruptures cause approximately 1,000 deaths per year in the U.S.

D) Treatment for AAA includes open surgical repair, endovascular repair or surveillance if AAA is <6 cm.

Discussion

The correct answer is A. AAA is a common condition, occurring in approximately 1 in 20 older men who have ever smoked. Answer B is incorrect. Rupture of an AAA is associated with an even higher mortality rate of 80%, hence the importance of screening. Answer C is incorrect. Epidemiologic studies indicate that AAA ruptures cause approximately 10,000–15,000 deaths per year in the U.S. Answer D is incorrect. Treatment for AAA is based upon the aneurysm size, rate of expansion, and symptoms. Asymptomatic patients with aneurysms ≥5.5 cm in diameter should undergo repair, not surveillance. Surveillance for medium-sized aneurysms 4.0–5.4 cm is by ultrasound or CT every 6–12 months and every 2–3 years for aneurysms 3.0–4.0 cm. Earlier repair in men with AAA ≥5.0 cm or women with AAA ≥4.5 cm may be indicated if rate of increase is ≥0.5 cm in 6 months. AAA repair options include open surgical repair or endovascular repair, but the benefits of endovascular repair are still under investigation. Currently, the ACC/AHA guidelines recommend surgical repair for most patients.

* *

The ultrasound shows minimal atherosclerotic disease of the abdominal aorta. Two years later, the patient returns for follow-up at the prompting of his daughter, who has been noticing that he complains about his knees hurting all the time. He has never been interested in surgery, but he would like to try something different. When asked about his pain on a scale of 0 to 10 (0 = no pain and 10 = worst pain possible), he reports pain approximately 2/10 most days, and up to 6/10 after moderate activity. He uses acetaminophen sometimes but does not want to get addicted to pain medicine.

In addition to increasing his dose of acetaminophen, you suggest a topical analgesic such as:

A) The lidocaine patch 5% because it can be applied conveniently anywhere on the body to provide additional knee pain control.

B) The lidocaine patch 5% because it acts locally where applied without achieving clinically significant serum drug levels.

C) Capsaicin because it can be applied topically once per day for effective pain control.

D) Capsaicin because it takes only 1–2 days to achieve a clinical effect.

Discussion

The correct answer is B. Older adults are less likely to be treated adequately for pain in comparison with younger adults. Of nonopioid analgesics, acetaminophen remains the best choice for first-line therapy of mild-moderate pain due to its tolerability. Topical agents such as the lidocaine patch 5% or capsaicin can also provide localized pain control. Topical agents can be very useful pain therapy because they penetrate the skin to act on peripheral nerves and soft tissue directly underlying the application site. These topical agents lack systemic absorption and have limited potential for any clinically significant systemic effect or drug-drug interactions which often is an issue in elderly patients on multiple medications. Answer A is incorrect. The lidocaine patch 5% must be applied directly over the painful area for best results. Answers C and D are incorrect. Capsaicin is dosed on a regular schedule every 6 hours to achieve maximal effect, which generally takes 2–4 weeks.

* *

After making some recommendations, you see the patient 1 month later for a follow-up visit. He reports improved pain control. Today he picked up a coupon at the local drug store for an arthritis pill that contains chondroitin. He wants to know if this might help his knee pain.

You discuss the current evidence and inform him that:

A) Large-scale trials indicate significant symptomatic benefit in osteoarthritis with the use of chondroitin supplements.

B) For patients with severe osteoarthritis only, a clinically relevant benefit is likely and the use of chondroitin should be encouraged.

C) Chondroitin is a large macromolecule that is poorly digested and is potentially unsafe in older patients with any stomach problems.

D) The combination of chondroitin and glucosamine is the most popular supplement sold over-the-counter for joint pain in the U.S.

Discussion

The correct answer is D. The combination of chondroitin and glucosamine is the most popular supplement sold over-the-counter for joint pain in the United States. However, scientific evidence is lacking to support the use of chondroitin to prevent or reduce joint pain associated with osteoarthritis. Answer A is incorrect. In a recent systematic review of 20 trials that compared the effects of chondroitin with placebo or no treatment in patients with hip or knee osteoarthritis, chondroitin had minimal or no effect on joint pain. Answer B is incorrect. For patients with advanced osteoarthritis, a clinically relevant benefit is unlikely. Answer C is incorrect. Chondroitin is a large macromolecule, and only 12%–13% of ingested chondroitin is absorbed into the blood stream. However, multiple studies have found no evidence to suggest that chondroitin is unsafe (except to the sharks that provide the cartilage to make the supplement).

* *

Now that your patient has seen you for a few years, he feels more comfortable in discussing other health concerns such as constipation. He usually has a bowel movement (BM) every 2–3 days, but sometimes he gets hard stools that require excessive straining. His wife tells him to eat more fiber, but he wants to know what else he can do to help "keep regular."

Which of the following statements is true about constipation?

A) The prevalence of self-reported constipation decreases with aging.
B) Patients should be encouraged to defecate before meals when the colonic activity is the greatest.
C) Fiber is a safe, inexpensive approach to improve stool consistency and accelerate colon transit time.
D) Increased caloric intake correlates well with constipation in the elderly.

Discussion

The correct answer is C. Fiber is a safe, inexpensive approach to improve stool consistency and accelerate colon transit time. Increasing fiber is a good first-line approach and should be encouraged. The daily recommended fiber intake is 20–35 grams. Answer A is incorrect because the prevalence of self-reported constipation increases with aging—up to 45% of frail elderly individuals report constipation as a health issue. It is not uncommon for patients and physicians to have

Table 21–7 ROME CRITERIA FOR FUNCTIONAL CONSTIPATION

Two or more of the following should be present for at least 12 weeks of the preceding 12 months:
- Straining for greater than 25% of defecations
- Lumpy or hard stools for greater than 25% of defecations
- Sensation of incomplete evacuation for greater than 25% of defecations
- Fewer than 3 defecations per week
- Manual evacuation or assistance to facil

different clinical definitions of constipation, so further history is helpful to clarify what the patient means by "constipation." The Rome criteria offers a consensus definition of constipation used in clinical trials and may be helpful to further characterize constipation (Table 21–7). Answer B is incorrect. Patients should be encouraged to defecate first thing in the morning or 30 minutes **after** meals when colonic activity is the greatest, and to take advantage of the gastrocolic reflex. Answer D is incorrect. Decreased (not increased) caloric intake correlates well with constipation in the elderly. Constipation in the presence of weight loss, rectal bleeding, and/or iron deficiency anemia should prompt further examination of the colon to exclude cancer.

* *

You rule out secondary causes of constipation and decide that your patient likely has primary transit constipation. You first provide nonpharmacologic recommendations to promote regular bowel habits.

Which of the following options would be the best pharmacologic approach to use on a regular basis in order to help this patient with his constipation?

A) Fiber: psyllium (Metamucil), oat bran, or methylcellulose (Citrucel).
B) Stool softener: docusate calcium (Surfak) or docusate sodium (Colace).
C) Stimulant laxative: senna (Senakot), castor oil, or bisacodyl (Dulcolax).
D) Enema: tap water, sodium bisphosphonate, or soap enema.
E) Prokinetic agent: Tegaserod (Zelnorm) 5HT4 agonist.

Discussion

The correct answer is A. Primary causes of constipation fall into 3 categories: (1) normal transit constipation, (2) slow transit constipation, and (3) anorectal dysfunction. There is no evidence-based guideline for the preferred order of using different types of laxatives. Supplemental fiber helps improve stool form and frequency and is a good first step. Psyllium also has the benefit of reducing lipids and improving glucose control in diabetics.

Answer B is incorrect. While stool softeners are commonly prescribed and may be helpful, studies indicate that stool softeners alone are not superior to psyllium. Answer C is incorrect. Stimulant laxatives, when used in recommended doses, are unlikely to harm the colon if used for short duration. However, stimulant laxatives may cause electrolyte imbalance or abdominal pain. Answer D is incorrect. Enemas should only be used in acute situations and with caution due to the risk of colonic perforation. Large-volume enemas can result in hyponatremia, while enemas containing phosphate can lead to hyperphosphatemia, especially in patients with renal insufficiency. Answer E is incorrect. Prokinetic agents stimulate propulsion along the gastrointestinal tract. The 5HT4 agonist tegaserod (Zelnorm) improves symptoms of constipation in adults but is not approved for individuals >65 years and is currently available only under restricted use.

HELPFUL TIP: There are many secondary causes of constipation, most commonly medications and coexistent medical conditions such as diabetes, hypothyroidism, scleroderma, and amyloidosis.

Objectives: Did you learn to . . .

- Screen for abdominal aortic aneurysm?
- Provide the safe and effective treatment for osteoarthritis pain?
- Identify and treat constipation in the older patient?

BIBLIOGRAPHY

Allman RM, Goode PS, Patrick MM, et al. Pressure ulcer risk factors among hospitalized patients with activity limitation. *JAMA*. 1995;273(11):856-70.

American Geriatrics Society, British Geriatrics Society, and American Academy of Orthopaedic Surgeons Panel on Falls Prevention. Guidelines for the prevention of falls in older persons. *J Am Geriatr Soc*. 2001;49(5):664.

American Medical Association/National Highway Traffic Administration/US Department of Transportation; June 2003. Physician's Guide to Assessing and Counseling Older Drivers. Available at: http://www.ama-assn.org/ama/pub/category/10791.html, last updated Feb 26, 2007. Accessed May 24, 2007.

American Occupational Therapy Association. Available at: http://www.aota.org/featured/area6/index.asp. Accessed November 22, 2007.

American Psychiatric Association. *Diagnostic and Statistical Manual of Mental Disorders (DSM-IV)*. 4th ed. Washington, DC: American Psychiatric Association, 1994.

Barnes A. Legal issues in geriatric medicine and gerontology. In: Hazzard WR, Blass JP, Ettinger WH Jr, et al., eds. *Principles of Geriatric Medicine and Gerontology*. 4th ed. New York: McGraw-Hill, 1999:545.

Bentley DW, Bradley S, High K, et al. Practice guidelines for evaluation of fever and infection in long-term care facilities. *Clin Infect Dis*. 2000;31:640.

Bergstrom N, Allman RM, Alvarez OM, et al. Treatment of pressure ulcers. Clinical Practice Guidelines No. 15. Rockville, MD: US Department of Health and Human Services, Public Health Service, Agency for Health Care Policy and Research. Dec. 1994. AHCPR Pub. No. 95-0653.

Fine PG, Herr KA. Efficacy, safety, and tolerability of pharmacotherapy for management of persistent pain in older persons. *Annals of Long-Term Care*. 2006;14(3):25.

Geldmacher DS. Alzheimer's disease: current pharmacotherapy in the context of patient and family needs. *J Am Geriatr Soc*. 2003;51(5):S289.

Gruenewald DA, Matsumoto AM. Testosterone supplementation therapy for older men: potential benefits and risks. *J Am Geriatr Soc*. 2003;51:101.

Inouye SK, Bogardus ST, Charpentier PA, et al. A multicomponent intervention to prevent delirium in hospitalized older patients. *N Engl J Med*. 1999;340:669.

Loue, S. Elder abuse and neglect in medicine and law: the need for reform. *J Legal Med*. 2001;22:159.

Mehr DR, Tatum PE. Primary prevention of diseases in old age. *Clin Geriatr Med*. 2002;18(3):407.

Podsiadlo D, Richardson S. The timed "Up & Go": a test of basic functional mobility for frail elderly persons. *J Am Geriatr Soc*. 1991;39(2):142.

Reichenbach S, et al. Meta-analysis: chondroitin for osteoarthritis of the knee or hip. *Ann Intern Med*. 2007;146:8;580.

Ross GW, Bowen JD. The diagnosis and differential diagnosis of dementia. *Med Clin North Am*. 2002;86(3):455.

Schwartz RS, Buchner DM. Exercise in the elderly: physiologic and functional effects. In: Hazzard WR, Blass JP, Ettinger WH Jr, et al, eds. *Principles of Geriatric Medicine and Gerontology*. 4th ed. New York: McGraw-Hill, 1999;143.

Tariot PN. Medical management of advanced dementia. *J Am Geriatr Soc.* 2003;51(5):S305.

Tinetti ME. Preventing falls in elderly persons. *N Engl J Med.* 2003;348(1):42.

U.S. Preventive Services Task Force. Screening for abdominal aortic aneurysm: recommendation statement. *Ann Intern Med.* 2005;142:198.

Van Hook FW, Demonbreun D, Weiss BD. Ambulatory devices for chronic gait disorders in the elderly. *Am Fam Physician.* 2003;67(8):1717.

Watson YI, Arfken CL, Birge SJ. Clock completion: an objective screening test for dementia. *J Am Geriatr Soc.* 1993;41(11):1235.

Wuillen DA. Common causes of vision loss in elderly patients. *Am Fam Physician.* 1999;60(1):99.

Zoorob R, et al. Cancer screening guidelines. *Am Fam Physician.* 2001;63(6):1101.

Care of the Surgical Patient

22

Mark A. Graber

CASE 1

You are covering the ED on a Saturday night. You see an intoxicated male who was in a bar fight, which he lost. He then decided to beat up the only thing he could to prove his manliness. He punched a window putting his hand and arm through the glass. His parents did not believe in immunizations, so he has never had a primary tetanus series.

Exam reveals a puncture wound over the second metacarpophalangeal (MCP) joint on the right hand caused during the fight. There are also puncture wounds further up the arm caused when he hit the window. He cannot adduct his thumb or oppose it with his ring finger. The rest of his neurovascular exam is intact. The puncture wounds that are on the proximal forearm appear contaminated with foreign material.

Which of the following is the most appropriate management option for the laceration over his second MCP joint?

A) Antibiotics for 5 days, leave the wound open to drain.
B) Closure with nylon suture and antibiotics for 5 days.
C) Closure with silk suture and antibiotics for 5 days.
D) Orthopedic consult to explore the joint capsule.

Discussion

The correct answer is D. This is the classic "clenched fist" injury that occurs when a clenched fist hits a mouth and/or tooth. While it looks benign, these injuries have a high likelihood of becoming infected, especially if the joint capsule is penetrated. Copious irrigation and exploration of the joint capsule are indicated.

 HELPFUL TIP: Use a syringe with a 30-gauge needle and methylene blue to enter the joint capsule. If there is resistance when you try to inject methylene blue, the joint capsule has not been violated. If the methylene blue flows freely from the syringe and into the wound, it is likely that the joint capsule has been penetrated and operative irrigation and repair are indicated.

* *

Along with the orthopedist, you explore the wound, use methylene blue, and decide there is no joint capsule penetration. It is time to irrigate this wound.

Your solution of choice is:

A) Povidone-iodine (eg, Betadine) mixed 50/50 with saline.
B) Normal saline.
C) Tap water.
D) Hydrogen peroxide.
E) B and C.

Discussion

The correct answer is E. Either normal saline **or** tap water can be used to cleanse the wound. The infection rate is the same regardless of which is used. As a matter of style, however, we usually use saline in the United States. Answers A and D are incorrect. Both povidone-iodine and hydrogen peroxide (as well as alcohol) are toxic to tissues and should not be put in the wound. Povidone-iodine can be used to cleanse intact skin, however.

* *

You now turn your attention toward his other wounds. A radiograph shows no evidence of foreign body (glass). However, you are still suspicious that there may be glass in the wound.

Which of the following is the procedure of choice at this point to identify a foreign body?

A) CT scan.
B) Fluoroscopy.
C) Ultrasound.
D) Divining rod.

Discussion

The correct answer is C. Ultrasound is effective at detecting foreign bodies in wounds, entails no radiation, and has a higher success rate than fluoroscopy. CT is not indicated at this point. Divining rod, well, that is up to you.

* *

No foreign body is found on exploration or ultrasound. You are deciding what to do with this wound since the patient cannot oppose his thumb and ring finger.

Inability to oppose the thumb is associated with:

A) Median nerve injury.
B) Radial nerve injury.
C) Ulnar nerve injury.
D) All of the above.

Discussion

The correct answer is A. To test for median nerve injury, test flexion of the interphalangeal thumb joint and opposition of the thumb and fifth finger. The radial nerve innervates the extensors of the hand and is tested by testing extension of the wrist and fingers. Patients with a radial nerve injury have a wrist drop. The ulnar nerve innervates (most of) the intrinsic muscles of the hand. Test for ulnar nerve injury involves abducting and adducting the fingers (spread the fingers apart and then hold them together).

* *

Even though the patient grew up in a family that did not believe in immunizations, the patient now prefers not to die of lockjaw and wants a tetanus immunization.

The BEST regimen for this patient is:

A) Tetanus immune globulin followed by a tetanus toxoid at the same time.
B) Tetanus immune globulin followed by a tetanus toxoid in 2 weeks.
C) Tetanus toxoid now followed by a second booster in 2 weeks.
D) Tetanus toxoid now followed by a second booster in 2 months.

Discussion

The correct answer is A. In a patient who has not had a primary series and who likely has a contaminated wound, tetanus immune globulin should be given with simultaneous administration of tetanus toxoid (at a different site from the immune globulin). If the patient has had a primary series, tetanus booster is indicated if it has been 10 years since the last booster **or** the patient has a suspect wound and it has been >5 years since the last immunization.

 HELPFUL TIP: Tdap (tetanus, diphtheria, and pertussis) should be given once during the teen years even if the patient has already received a Td booster. Other indications for Tdap include health-care workers, aged 19–64 years, who have direct patient contact (these patients should get one dose of Tdap), and those who have close contact with an infant <12 months.

Objectives: Did you learn to . . .

- Perform a neurologic exam of the hand for radial, median, and ulnar nerve injury?
- Manage tetanus boosters/Tdap boosters/tetanus immune globulin in patients with a potentially contaminated injury?
- Evaluate and manage a "clenched fist" injury and joint space violation?

QUICK QUIZ: PAIN CONTROL

Which of the following is the correct starting dose of morphine for moderate to severe pain such as an acute abdomen or long bone fracture?

A) 0.1 mg/kg IV.
B) 1 mg/kg IV.
C) 2 mg IV, reassess, and repeat every 30 minutes.
D) 2 mg IV repeated to a total of 5 mg IV within 30 minutes.

Discussion

The correct answer is A. Morphine should be given at a dose of 0.1 mg/kg or approximately 10 mg IV in an adult. Lower doses are likely to be ineffective, and the traditional 2 mg IV dose is almost homeopathic.

QUICK QUIZ: PAIN CONTROL

Which of the following drugs will give the most rapid pain control when given IV?

A) Fentanyl (Sublimaze).
B) Hydromorphone (Dilaudid).
C) Meperidine (Demerol).
D) Morphine.

Discussion

The correct answer is A. Fentanyl has a peak effect at 3–5 minutes. This is followed by meperidine at 5–7 minutes, morphine at 20 minutes, and hydromorphone at 15–30 minutes. Thus, to get rapid control of pain, fentanyl is the preferred agent. Meperidine is the least preferred agent because of drug interactions (MAO inhibitors, SSRIs) and toxic metabolites (normeperidine can cause agitation and seizures).

CASE 2

You get a call from one of your diabetic patients that he is having difficulty urinating and has quite a bit of pain in the perineal area. He has not felt well for several days and was running a low-grade fever. He went to his chiropractor 2 days ago when he only had pain and swelling. He now notes that his temperature is higher (he doesn't have a thermometer but is feeling warm). You suggest that he present to your office.

* *

Exam reveals an obese male who waddles into the office because of pain in his scrotal area. Vitals: BP 150/100, pulse 112, respirations 20, temperature 39.0°C. Other significant findings include a swollen scrotum which is bright red and tender to touch. You do not have extended laboratory access in your office, but a urine dipstick is negative for blood and leukocyte esterase. His blood sugar, which is usually fairly well controlled, is 320 mg/dL.

Your next step for this patient is which of the following?

A) Start the patient on nafcillin for MSRA and streptococcal coverage and follow up with the patient in the morning.
B) Refer the patient to a surgeon on an emergent basis.
C) Begin amoxicillin/clavulanate and follow up with the patient in the morning.
D) Start an IV, give a single dose of ceftriaxone, followed by oral amoxicillin/clavulanate for 10–14 days.

Discussion

The correct answer is B. This likely represents Fournier gangrene. The systemic symptoms of fever, tachycardia, and elevated blood sugar make this the most likely diagnosis. The treatment is emergent and surgical. For this reason, antibiotics are inappropriate as a sole therapy. Answer A is incorrect because nafcillin does not cover MRSA.

Fournier gangrene is best described as:

A) Necrotizing fasciitis.
B) Necrotizing cellulitis.
C) Caused by aerobic bacteria.
D) Secondary to streptococci.

Discussion

The correct answer is A. Fournier gangrene is a form of necrotizing fasciitis. This is termed type 1 necrotizing fasciitis and is caused by mixed aerobic and anaerobic bacteria. Answer B is incorrect. Necrotizing cellulitis is isolated to the superficial skin; Fournier gangrene involves tissue including the fascia. Answer C is incorrect because, as noted above, Fournier gangrene is caused by mixed aerobic and anaerobic bacteria. Answer D is incorrect. **There is necrotizing fasciitis secondary to** streptococci (see Discussion below); however, it is a different infection from the organisms that cause Fournier.

Which of the following is NOT a risk factor for Fournier gangrene?

A) Diabetes.
B) Immunosuppression.
C) Varicella infection.
D) End-stage renal disease.

Discussion

The correct answer is C. Varicella infection **is** a risk factor for **type II necrotizing fasciitis**, which is a different entity. Type II necrotizing fasciitis is caused by group A streptococcus. Generally, patients with type II necrotizing fasciitis are not diabetic or otherwise immunocompromised. Other risk factors for type II necrotizing fasciitis include IV drug use, penetrating trauma, and blunt trauma.

* *

The surgeon evaluates the patient and asks your opinion on the antibiotic regimen.

What do you recommend for this patient with necrotizing fasciitis?

A) Penicillin and clindamycin.
B) Clindamycin and metronidazole.
C) Cefotaxime and metronidazole.
D) Ticarcillin clavulanate (Timentin) **or** ampicillin clavulanate (Unasyn) plus metronidazole.
E) C or D.

Discussion

The correct answer is E. As noted above, Fournier gangrene is a mix of aerobic and anaerobic bacteria. Answers A and B will cover anaerobes and some Gram-positive organisms. However, aerobic and Gram-negative coverage is lacking. More broad-spectrum antimicrobial coverage is needed in this patient.

 HELPFUL TIP: IVIG has been used in necrotizing fasciitis caused by *Clostridium* species as well as in those with streptococcal fasciitis. While there is a suggestion of benefit, the data are incomplete and more study is warranted. Hyperbaric oxygen has also been used but suffers from the same lack of data.

* *

The patient has a wide excision of necrotic tissue. After surgery he becomes hypotensive and tachycardic (BP 90/50, pulse 128), and his serum lactate is 8 mg/dL.

What is the most appropriate next step in his management?

A) Start IV dopamine to stabilize his blood pressure.
B) Start IV norepinephrine to stabilize his blood pressure.
C) Start IV saline to stabilize his blood pressure.
D) Start IV albumin to stabilize his blood pressure.

Discussion

The correct answer is C. This patient is likely hypovolemic secondary to third spacing and/or sepsis and needs volume. The lactate of 8 mg/dL suggests that he has hypoperfusion with poor tissue oxygenation (although it could also be secondary to necrotic tissue). Administration of dopamine (or other vasopressors) will not increase peripheral circulation and may decrease tissue oxygenation by increasing vascular tone and decreasing perfusion. Albumin has not demonstrated any advantage over crystalloids in almost any circumstance—post paracentesis of >5 liters is the exception. Mortality of necrotizing fasciitis approaches 30% even with the best care.

 HELPFUL TIP: The thinking about sepsis has changed dramatically in the past several years. Pressors are out. Fluid is in. It is clear that fluid reverses tissue hypoperfusion and tissue hypoxia much more than pressors. The septic patient should get an infusion of normal saline until the serum lactate begins to drop. In general, a serum lactate of >4 mg/dL indicates the need for a central line and ICU care.

* *

The patient is given 4 liters of normal saline and his lactate drops to 3 mg/dL. Four hours later, however, his lactate is up to 6 mg/dL although his blood pressure remains stable at 105/70 with a pulse of 95.

What is your next step?

A) More normal saline; the patient is still in shock.
B) No more fluid except normal saline for maintenance plus insensible loss to maintain a neutral fluid balance.

C) IV or PO glucose to allow aerobic metabolism.
D) Switch to D5-1/2 NS to both give fluid and calories.

Discussion

The correct answer is A. This patient is still in shock. Shock is not defined by an absolute pulse or blood pressure but rather by tissue hypoperfusion. The increasing lactate in this patient reflects tissue hypoperfusion and thus the need for more fluid. You do not want to put the patient into CHF. Again, make sure there is not additional necrotic tissue that needs surgical removal as this could cause an elevated lactate.

 HELPFUL TIP: The other type of necrotizing fasciitis is type 2. The predominant organism here is group A streptococcus, and it responds well to clindamycin. It occurs in otherwise normal hosts and may occur as a result of varicella or other skin disruption. Type 1 necrotizing fasciitis generally occurs in patients with an underlying illness (eg, diabetes, vascular disease, etc) and is known by its putrid odor. Type 2 necrotizing fasciitis occurs in any population.

Objectives: Did you learn to . . .

- Diagnose and treat Fournier gangrene?
- Differentiate between types of necrotizing fascitis?
- Prescribe appropriate fluids and pressors in septic shock?

 QUICK QUIZ: CA-MRSA

Which of the following regimens is appropriate for the treatment of community-acquired MRSA (methicillin-resistant *Staphylococcus aureus*)?

A) Amoxicillin/clavulanate (Augmentin) plus rifampin.
B) Cephalexin (Keflex).
C) Doxycycline **or** TMP/SMX (eg, Bactrim, Septra).
D) Erythromycin **plus** rifampin.

Discussion

The correct answer is C. The treatment for MRSA is abscess drainage (if an abscess is present) and antibiotics. Doxycycline 100 mg BID **or** TMP/SMX-DS **two**

tablets BID are considered appropriate treatments for community-acquired MRSA. Some would add rifampin to these regimens. However, rifampin alone is not advisable because of rapid development of resistance. Note that this is a different organism than is hospital-acquired MRSA, which generally requires vancomycin due to greater resistance to a wider array of antimicrobials.

 HELPFUL TIP: **Vancomycin is not a preferred drug for treating staphylococcus.** Inpatient mortality rates are higher in patients with staphylococcal infections treated with vancomycin than with other antibiotics. So, if you have a sensitive organism (methicillin-sensitive *Staphylococcus aureus*), change antibiotics to something other than vancomycin, such as nafcillin or ampicillin/clavulanate—or whatever the susceptibilities indicate.

 QUICK QUIZ: ANTIBIOTIC COVERAGE

Which of the following organisms is (are) not *generally* covered by TMP/SMX?

A) *Staphylococcus aureus*.
B) Streptococci strains.
C) *Escherichia coli*.
D) Enterococcus.
E) B and D.

Discussion

The correct answer is E. Neither streptococci strains nor enterococci strains are sensitive to TMP/SMX. This has implications for the treatment of MRSA. Cellulitis (one of the manifestations of MRSA) can be from either staphylococci or streptococci strains. So, unless you are confident that you have MRSA (abscess formation, etc), TMP/SMX is not a great choice for cellulitis. Doxycycline, on the other hand, does cover streptococci strains. We know that some *E. coli* are resistant. However, most are still sensitive.

CASE 3

You are working in a rural ED when you get a call that a 62-year-old farmer has been trapped between a tractor and a silo while loading silage. It seems to have pinned his legs and pelvis, but from the waist up he is fine. Nonetheless, the ambulance crew places the patient in a collar and on a backboard and transports him to the ED.

The patient is in significant pain from his lower extremities and pelvis. His blood pressure is initially 105/65 with a pulse of 115. Primary survey is unremarkable although he is still boarded and collared.

Which of the following most clearly reflects the approach to this patient's pain?

A) Use IV meperidine (Demerol) for pain control.
B) Use IV morphine for pain control.
C) Use IV fentanyl (Sublimaze) for pain control.
D) Pain medications are contraindicated now given the patient's overall condition.

Discussion

The correct answer is C. Fentanyl generally has a negligible affect on blood pressure (although one should never say "never"). Both morphine and meperidine tend to lower a patient's blood pressure, so they are relatively contraindicated in this patient with a marginal blood pressure or hypotension. Those who chose answer D have been hanging around old-time surgeons too long. It is unconscionable to withhold pain medication.

* *

Further exam shows that the patient's pelvis is unstable. As you recall, a fractured pelvis can lead to significant blood loss.

In the short term what is the best way to approach this?

A) Pressors (eg, dopamine) plus fluids.
B) Pelvic binder.
C) Fluids (normal saline).
D) Activated factor VIIa (NovoSeven).
E) Embolization by interventional radiology (45-minute delay).

Discussion

The correct answer is B. A pelvic binder will significantly reduce bleeding in an unstable pelvis fracture. Answer A is incorrect because in trauma dopamine is not indicated when the problem is hypovolemia (see above). Answer C is incorrect. We really want to stop the bleeding. While normal saline is a good choice for resuscitation fluids, we want to tamponade the bleeding

and not just chase our tails with fluids. Of course, the patient would receive fluids, but the most important step is the binder. Answer D is incorrect. Activated factor VIIa **may** prove to have a role in trauma, but it is not going to be the primary modality to stop bleeding. Additionally, it has a number of adverse effects including increased thromboembolic phenomenon (PE, DVT, etc). Finally, interventional radiology (answer E) will likely be needed at some point. They are quite good at stopping bleeding vessels. However, the delay time during which you are watching the patient bleed is unacceptable.

* *

You appropriately place a pelvic binder, which tamponades the bleeding. The patient's blood pressure stabilizes. You now turn to other issues. This patient will clearly need a Foley catheter.

Relative contraindications to placement of a Foley catheter include which of the following?

A) Blood at the meatus.
B) Gross hematuria.
C) High riding prostate.
D) Gross blood from the rectum.
E) A and C.

Discussion

The correct answer is E. Both blood at the meatus and a "high riding prostate" (ever wonder what it is riding on?) signify the possible disruption of the urethra. Thus, since one does not want to place the catheter in the wrong place, like the peritoneal space, catheterization is relatively contraindicated. Answer B, gross hematuria, can be from the kidney and is not a contraindication to catheterization.

* *

You find blood at the urethral meatus. The patient complains that he needs to void.

Your options at this point include which of the following?

A) Urethrogram to document an intact urethra.
B) Performance of suprapubic cystotomy using ultrasound guidance.
C) Use a coudé catheter to catheterize the urethra.
D) Placement of a bladder catheter via the urethra but using a wire guide (such as with a central line).
E) A and B.

Discussion

The correct answer is E. One could perform a urethrogram using a water-soluble dye (eg, Gastrografin) to document the urethra is intact and if so place a standard Foley. One could also do a suprapubic cystotomy using ultrasound guidance. Answers C and D are incorrect. A coude catheter is used to bypass a stricture (prostate or otherwise) and would be no safer than a regular catheter in this patient. Likewise, a wire could end up anywhere and should not be used in this patient.

 HELPFUL TIP: If you feel uncomfortable doing a formal cystotomy, a central line with balloon placed into the bladder can be used as a temporizing solution.

* *

You now turn your attention to his leg. He is complaining of severe leg pain that seems out of proportion to the degree of injury. The calf is tender with increased pain on passive stretch.

Which of the following is true?

A) Since the patient has excellent pulses, a compartment syndrome is not likely.
B) Compartment syndrome is defined as compartment pressures of >15 mm Hg.
C) Compartment syndrome is only associated with significant crush injuries or fractures.
D) Pain out of proportion to the injury is a red flag for compartment syndrome.

Discussion

The correct answer is D. Pain out of proportion to the injury is a red flag for compartment syndrome. Answer A is incorrect because pulses can be maintained until there is significant increase in compartment pressures and significant injury to muscle and nerves. Answer B is incorrect because it is difficult to define a specific cut-off for compartment syndrome. Some patients tolerate higher pressures and others cannot tolerate 30 mm Hg (normal compartment pressure is zero). However, when the pressure gets above 20–30 mg Hg, strong consideration should be given to the presence of compartment syndrome. Answer C is incorrect.

Compartment syndrome can be due to a number of factors including electrical injury, excessive muscle use, tetany, reperfusion after ischemia, etc.

 HELPFUL TIP: Traditionally, we are taught the "5 Ps" of compartment syndrome: pulselessness, paresthesia, pallor, pain, and paralysis. But this is misleading. Pain may be the only symptom. By the time the others are present, there may be significant disruption of vascular supply and extensive injury.

* *

You decide that it is likely that this patient has a compartment syndrome.

Which of the following labs will be the most helpful in treating this patient?

A) CBC.
B) Urinalysis and microscopic exam.
C) Glucose.
D) Sodium.
E) PT/PTT.

Discussion

The correct answer is B. One of the major complications of compartment syndrome is rhabdomyolysis, which manifests as a urine dipstick positive for blood but with a negative microscopic exam for red blood cells. The positive dipstick is picking up myoglobin in the urine. This can be confirmed by a serum CPK. CBC, glucose, sodium, and coagulation studies may be appropriate depending on the clinical situation but are not useful in establishing the presence of myoglobinuria.

 HELPFUL TIP: Myoglobin can be measured in the urine. However, many laboratories have stopped doing this test favoring the positive dipstick/negative microscopic exam approach. Additionally, **there can be false-negative dipstick findings.** Thus, check a CPK as well if rhabdomyolysis is a consideration.

* *

The patient has a positive dipstick for blood with no red blood cells on microscopic exam (presumptive myoglobinuria). A follow-up serum CPK is 32,000 IU/L. You make the diagnosis of rhabdomyolysis and decide to check additional laboratories.

Which of the following are typically found in rhabdomyolysis?

A) Elevated calcium, decreased phosphate.
B) Decreased potassium, elevated phosphate.
C) Elevated phosphate, decreased calcium.
D) Any of the above combinations may be seen.

Discussion

The correct answer is C. In addition to an elevated CPK, other laboratory findings in rhabdomyolysis include hyperphosphatemia, hyperkalemia, hypocalcemia, hyperuricemia, and hypoalbuminemia. **Hypocalcemia** is the most common laboratory abnormality, present in approximately 70% of patients.

The most common adverse consequence and greatest danger of rhabdomyolysis is:

A) Disseminated intravascular coagulation.
B) Acute renal failure.
C) Seizure from hypocalcemia.
D) Acute gout from hyperuricemia.
E) Cardiac arrhythmia from hyperkalemia.

Discussion

The correct answer is B. Myoglobin precipitates in the renal tubules causing acute renal failure. Answer A, DIC, can occur but is rare. Answer C, seizures from hypocalcemia, have not been reported in this condition nor has answer D, gout. The potassium elevation from rhabdomyolysis generally does not reach a level sufficient to cause arrhythmias.

The primary treatment for rhabdomyolysis is:

A) Mannitol infusion.
B) Saline infusion.
C) Furosemide.
D) Dialysis.

Discussion

The correct answer is B. The most important treatment for rhabdomyolysis is saline infusion with alkalinization of the urine. Answer A, mannitol, can be used to increase urine flow, but this treatment is secondary to good hydration and urine alkalinization. Answer C, furosemide, is not used in rhabdomyolysis. Loop diuretics will acidify the urine and are contraindicated. Answer D, dialysis, is what we are trying to avoid using saline.

 HELPFUL TIP: In patients with rhabdomyolysis, try to maintain urine output of 200–300 cc/hour for an adult. Alkalinize the urine using sodium bicarbonate. Remember that in order to alkalinize the urine, you have to maintain an adequate serum potassium level otherwise the body will reabsorb potassium in exchange for hydrogen ions causing urine acidification.

* *

The patient is able to maintain urine output after you institute saline.

What treatment you suggest for the underlying compartment syndrome?

A) Fasciotomy.
B) Immobilization and traction.
C) Hot packs and elevation of the affected limb.
D) Ice and elevation of the affected limb.

Discussion

The correct answer is A. The treatment of compartment syndrome is fasciotomy. A rapid surgical or orthopedic consultation is critical in the treatment of compartment syndrome.

* *

The patient does well and everyone is happy.

Objectives: Did you learn to . . .

- Recognize manifestations of compartment syndrome and understand that compartment syndrome can be present with pain alone?
- Identify patients at risk for compartment syndrome and rhabdomyolysis?
- Manage compartment syndrome?
- Diagnose and treat rhabdomyolysis?

CASE 4

A 60-year-old female presents to your office for severe abdominal pain. She reports that she developed vague left lower quadrant abdominal pain yesterday. This morning she awoke from her sleep with severe, diffuse abdominal pain, anorexia, and vomiting. On examination she is lying very still. Temperature is 38.4°C, pulse 106, respirations 16, blood pressure 100/62. She has dry mucous membranes. Her abdomen has diminished bowel sounds and is rigid with involuntary guarding and rebound tenderness greatest in the left lower quadrant. On pelvic examination, she is exquisitely tender on the left with a palpable mass. There are no masses on rectal examination, and her stool is negative for occult blood.

Laboratory tests include a negative urine pregnancy (she's 60 but can you be too careful?), WBC 25,500/mm^3, HCT 32%, platelets 450,000/mm^3, Na 142 meq/L, K 3.2 meq/L, BUN 24 mg/dL, and Cr 1.0 mg/dL. Abdominal x-ray demonstrates free air under the diaphragm.

Based on the information available, the most likely diagnosis in this patient is:

A) Diverticulitis.
B) Pelvic inflammatory disease.
C) Appendicitis.
D) Ovarian torsion.
E) Abdominal aortic aneurysm.

Discussion

The correct answer is A. The most likely cause of this patient's symptoms is diverticulitis. Answer B is incorrect because pelvic inflammatory disease (PID) is unlikely in a 60-year-old female. Also, the clinical presentation and pelvic exam findings are more consistent with diverticulitis than PID. Answer C is incorrect because appendicitis is unlikely since the pain is present on the **left** side, not the right side as one would expect with appendicitis. Answer D is incorrect because ovarian torsion is unlikely in a postmenopausal female unless there is a malignancy. Additionally, the pain of ovarian torsion should be colicky rather than constant and there should be no peritoneal signs (at least until the ovary is necrosed). Answer E is incorrect. Abdominal aortic aneurysm is unlikely because of the exam findings here: there is no pulsatile mass, the patient is normotensive, there is fever, and you can palpate a left lower quadrant mass. However, in older patients presenting

with abdominal pain, you must always keep the diagnosis of abdominal aortic aneurysm in mind.

 HELPFUL TIP: A palpable aorta need not be present on abdominal exam for there to be an aortic aneurysm with dissection. Maintain a high degree of suspicion.

Which of the following is true regarding this patient's disease process?

A) The majority of patients with this disease will develop symptoms at some time.
B) The condition is associated with a high malignant potential.
C) The condition has peak incidence of occurrence in the sixth, seventh, and eighth decades of life.
D) The condition primarily affects the ascending colon.

Discussion

The correct answer is C. Diverticu**losis** is an acquired disease that peaks in the sixth, seventh, and eighth decades with estimated 50% of octogenarians having the condition. Answer A is incorrect. Most individuals are asymptomatic from the disease process with only 10%–20% developing symptomatic diverticu**litis**. Acute diverticulitis has a variety of presentations. Peridiverticular inflammation occurs when a fecalith becomes entrapped in a diverticular wall resulting in a localized contained microperforation. Pain is typically acute and located in the left lower quadrant. Examination may reveal only a mildly tender abdomen without any masses. Peridiverticular abscess and phlegmon result in worsening left lower quadrant abdominal pain, and often a mass is palpable.

All of the following physical exam findings indicate peritonitis EXCEPT:

A) Murphy sign.
B) Rovsing sign.
C) Involuntary guarding.
D) Rebound tenderness.

Discussion

The correct answer is A. Peritonitis is inflammation of the peritoneum. It can be aseptic, bacterial, or viral.

Most commonly, peritonitis results from bacterial contamination of the peritoneum after injury to an abdominal viscus. In this patient's case, generalized peritonitis occurs because either an inflamed section of the colon ruptured or a phlegmon ruptured. Pain due to peritonitis is usually severe and associated with anorexia and emesis. The patient will often have fever, tachycardia, leukocytosis, signs of dehydration, and electrolyte abnormalities.

Answer A, Murphy sign, is tenderness to palpation of the right subcostal region during deep inspiration and is associated with biliary colic and cholecystitis but does not indicate peritonitis. Answer B, Rovsing sign, is pain at the disease site when palpating another site, classically a finding in appendicitis; the area of peritoneal inflammation has increased pain when palpating elsewhere on the abdomen. Answers C and D, involuntary guarding and rebound tenderness, are classic findings in peritonitis.

> **HELPFUL TIP:** Epiploic appendagitis (yes, it is spelled correctly) can mimic both appendicitis and diverticulitis. It generally presents similarly to appendicitis but on the left. It occurs mostly in individuals in their thirties. It occurs when there is torsion or infarction of an epiploic appendage on the peritoneal aspect ("outside") of the colon. Diagnosis is by CT scan and it generally resolves on its own.

* *

You have identified free air on x-ray, indicating a ruptured viscus.

The best film for identifying free air in the abdomen is:

A) A flat plate abdomen.
B) An upright abdomen.
C) A left lateral decubitus film of the abdomen.
D) An upright chest radiograph.

Discussion

The correct answer is D. An upright chest radiograph is the best x-ray film for identifying free air in the abdomen. CT is more sensitive but is not available in all situations and is expensive.

While you are waiting for the surgeon to arrive, which of the following is the LEAST important part of appropriate preoperative management?

A) Maintaining the patient in an NPO state.
B) Administration of antibiotics to cover Gram-negative bacteria.
C) Administration of antibiotics to cover Gram-positive bacteria.
D) Administration of antibiotics to cover obligate anaerobic bacteria.

Discussion

The correct answer is C. The treatment of Gram-positive organisms is the least important part of treatment for this patient. Initial treatment of perforated diverticuli should include fluid replacement and electrolyte correction. A urinary catheter can be placed in order to monitor fluid balance if appropriate. Empiric antibiotic therapy should be provided based on the most likely pathogens. Perforations of the appendix, diverticuli, and other parts of the colon account for >80% of the causes of acute bacterial peritonitis. Distal small bowel and colonic perforations should include coverage for Gram-negative bacteria, such as *E. coli*, and obligate anaerobe pathogens, such as *B. fragilis*. Examples of possible regimens include single-agent treatment with second-generation cephalasporin versus an aminoglycoside with metronidazole or ampicillin/sulbactam. A number of antibiotic combinations are appropriate.

* *

The patient undergoes surgery with a partial bowel resection and primary reanastomosis. Two months following your patient's surgery, she presents with complaint of abdominal pain. The pain is crampy and intermittent. Further history reveals a 24-hour history of vomiting, abdominal bloating, and low-grade fever. She reports her last bowel movement was 2 days ago and denies any flatus over the last 24 hours. On examination, her temperature is 37.1°C, pulse 105, respirations 12, and blood pressure 158/60. Her abdomen is slightly distended, diffusely tender to palpation without rebound or guarding, and has hyperactive bowel sounds. On flat-plate and upright views of the abdomen, there are dilated loops of small bowel and multiple air fluid levels.

Which of the following is true regarding this patient's current disease process?

A) She most likely has a closed-loop small bowel obstruction.
B) She most likely has an extramural source of obstruction.
C) Dilated loops of bowel are defined as bowel loops >5 cm in diameter on plain film.
D) Both partial and complete bowel obstructions reveal no colonic gas on plain film.

Discussion

The correct answer is B. This patient most likely has an external source of obstruction. Bowel obstructions are divided into two classes: mechanical and functional (aka pseudoobstruction, ileus, or neurogenic obstruction). Mechanical obstructions are further classified into both their location and etiology. Possible etiologies include intraluminal bodies (eg, gallstone ileus or foreign body), intramural lesions (eg, tumor or intussusception), and extramural lesions (eg, adhesions).

Obstructions can be further divided into open- and closed-loop. Open-loop obstructions have an outlet for gas and secretion relief (eg, vomiting), whereas closed-loop obstructions block both inflow and outflow to an area. Closed-loop obstructions, like bowel torsion or volvulus, cause acute, severe abdominal pain.

Bowel obstruction presents with crampy, intermittent abdominal pain, vomiting, distention, and obstipation. History often includes previous abdominal surgery. Depending on the degree of obstruction and its duration, there may be hyperactive bowel sounds, high-pitched bowel sounds, or decreased/absent bowel sounds. An upright abdominal plain film or lateral recumbent abdominal film confirm diagnosis with findings of dilated loops of small bowel (bowel >3 cm in diameter) on the flat plate and air-fluid levels on the upright or decubitus film. **CT scan is more sensitive for obstruction than are plain films and will often reveal the source of the obstruction.** However, CT should be reserved for patients in whom the diagnosis is unclear. Patients with a complete small bowel obstruction will lack air in the colon on plain film. However, remember that air can be introduced into the rectum during a rectal exam.

Which of the following is (are) a cause of ileus?

A) Burns.
B) Spinal cord injury.
C) Hypokalemia.
D) Pneumonia.
E) All of the above can cause an ileus.

Discussion

The correct answer is E. All of the above can cause an ileus. Additional causes include: peritonitis, pancreatitis, uremia, narcotics, etc.

HELPFUL TIP: Adynamic ileus with colonic distension (aka acute colonic pseudoobstruction, Ogilvie syndrome) may respond to neostigmine 2 mg IV. Remember that cholinergics such as neostigmine may cause increased salivation, lacrimation, respiratory secretions, and muscle weakness leading to possible death. Proper dosing is important for avoiding these adverse effects.

* *

You diagnose small bowel obstruction, which you believe is most likely related to adhesion formation after hemicolectomy.

Which of the following is a FALSE statement regarding the management of bowel obstruction?

A) Initial treatment orders should include NPO, nasogastric decompression, intravenous fluid resuscitation, and electrolyte replacement as needed.
B) This patient should undergo emergent surgical intervention.
C) If she has fever or leukocytosis, she should undergo surgical intervention.
D) If she requires surgery, broad-spectrum antibiotics to cover anaerobes and Gram-negative aerobes should be administered perioperatively.

Discussion

The correct answer is B. Peritoneal adhesions account for more than half of all small bowel obstructions. Up to 80% of episodes of small bowel obstruction caused by adhesions resolve without surgical intervention. Initial treatment includes restricting oral intake, intravenous fluid resuscitation with normal saline, and electrolyte correction.

The other answer choices are true statements. Almost all patients require nasogastric decompression to relieve pain and prevent passage of swallowed air. The goal is to prevent small bowel strangulation. Patients can be safely observed if there is no evidence of strangulation. Indications of strangulation include rapidly progressing abdominal pain or distention, development of peritoneal findings, fever, diminished urine output, leukocytosis, hyperamylasemia, metabolic acidosis, and persistent obstruction. **Complete** bowel obstruction should always be treated surgically. Also, patients with *de novo* obstruction (eg, no history of laparotomy) usually require surgical intervention. If surgery is necessary, broad-spectrum antibiotics that cover anaerobes and Gram-negative aerobes should be administered perioperatively to reduce wound infection and abdominal sepsis rates.

Which of these patients with a small bowel obstruction can be safely observed?

A) A patient with a fever and a partial small bowel obstruction.
B) A patient with localized abdominal pain and a partial small bowel obstruction.
C) An afebrile patient with a closed-loop obstruction.
D) All of the above.
E) None of the above.

Discussion
The correct answer is E, none of the above. See Discussion of the question above.

 HELPFUL TIP: Remember that patient-controlled analgesia is the most effective modality for treating pain in the postoperative patient. Side effects of narcotics may include urinary retention in addition to constipation or respiratory depression.

Objectives: Did you learn to . . .

● Assess abdominal pain and recognize an acute abdomen?
● Provide appropriate peri-operative management for gastrointestinal surgery?
● Identify and treat small bowel obstruction after abdominal surgery?

CASE 5

A 52-year-old female presents to your office as a new patient and requests a "100,000 mile tune-up." She has not seen a physician in over 10 years and has one

complaint today. She has a bulge in her right groin that occurs when she lifts heavy objects and when she coughs. She denies any episodes of severe, persistent pain, redness in the area, fever, or abdominal pain. On physical examination, she is an obese female with normal vital signs. When you ask her to perform a Valsalva maneuver, you can palpate a bulge in the right groin.

Which of the following is true regarding this bulge?

A) Because she is a female, it most likely represents a femoral hernia.
B) Surgery is required in all such cases as soon as possible.
C) The larger the bulge, the more likely it is to become incarcerated.
D) Hernias are the most common cause of bowel obstruction in someone without prior abdominal surgeries.

Discussion
The correct answer is D. Among patients who have not had abdominal surgery, hernias are the most common cause of bowel obstruction. When patients with a history of abdominal surgery are included, hernias are the second most common cause of bowel obstruction overall. Answer A is incorrect. Hernias in the groin can be direct inguinal, indirect inguinal, or femoral. In both men and women, the most common type is an indirect inguinal hernia, though femoral hernias are more common in women than men. Direct inguinal hernias are rare among women. Answer B is incorrect because the surgical repair of hernias is elective. Surgery is absolutely indicated in cases of incarceration, but the incarceration rate is 5% initially and drops to 1% per year after 4–6 months. A risk-benefit analysis is recommended, especially in older patients with comorbid conditions. Answer C is incorrect. Larger hernias are **less** likely to incarcerate. Incarceration is defined as a loop of bowel slipping into a hernia and becoming entrapped. Strangulation occurs when the incarceration is so severe that it results in compromised blood supply to the incarcerated bowel.

 HELPFUL TIP: Recent data confirm that hernia repair is elective as long as there is no incarceration. Reportedly, 31% of patients have continued pain after repair and 6% report pain severe enough to interfere with activities.

To reduce her chances of having recurrent herniation after surgery, you advise her to:

A) Be on bed rest before the operation.
B) Lose weight before the operation.
C) Burst and taper steroids before the operation.
D) Pursue an aggressive weight loss program after the operation.

Discussion

The correct answer is B. Obesity is associated with recurrent herniation after hernia repair, so obese patients should be instructed to lose weight before surgery. Other factors associated with hernia recurrence are smoking, steroid use, and infection. Answers A, C, and D are incorrect because they may **increase** the risk of hernia recurrence after repair.

* *

Your patient mentions that her 6-month-old grandson has a bulge at his navel.

Regarding hernias in infants and children, which one of the following statements is most accurate?

A) Umbilical hernias in infants require repair if not closed by 1 year of age.
B) A scrotal sac that is translucent with a bright light is likely a hydrocele.
C) Omphaloceles occur to the right of the umbilicus.
D) White infants have the highest rate of umbilical hernias.

Discussion

The correct answer is B. A scrotal sac that is translucent is generally a hydrocele. A hydrocele is a fluid collection in the tunica vaginalis of the scrotum or processus vaginalis in the inguinal canal. Hydroceles can either be present at birth or develop later. Clinically, a hydrocele transilluminates with a bright light. It is important to remember that this finding can also be observed with an incarcerated inguinal hernia. Answer A is incorrect. Most umbilical hernias in infants close spontaneously within the first 2–3 years. Because of this, operative repair is not recommended <3–4 years. Answer C is incorrect. An omphalocele is a defect in the anterior abdominal wall through which intraabdominal contents are extruded. It is seen at the base of the umbilicus (not to the right), and the organs are covered with a membrane. A neonate with a herniation of intraabdominal contents to the right of the umbilicus may have gastroschisis. Omphalocele and gastroschisis require surgical repair. Answer D is incorrect. Umbilical hernias occur in 4%–9% of white infants and 25%–50% of black infants. They rarely pose any threat to the infant.

Objectives: Did you learn to . . .

*   Describe the clinical presentation and appropriate management of hernias?
*   Make recommendations to reduce hernia recurrence in patients undergoing hernia repair?
*   Describe hernia presentations in infants and children?

CASE 6

A 24-year-old male presents to your clinic with a 5-day history of rectal bleeding. For several years, he has had hard stools but has developed rectal bleeding in the last few days. In addition he has severe, intermittent, crampy abdominal pain which he thinks is due to constipation. He reports a mild fever.

On examination, temperature is 37.9°C, pulse 95, respirations 12, and blood pressure 108/78. His abdomen is nontender. He has no guarding or rebound tenderness. Anoscopy reveals gross blood and two internal hemorrhoids.

Regarding hemorrhoids in general, which of the following is true?

A) Patients with hemorrhoids most commonly complain of perianal burning, itching, swelling, and pain.
B) A grade III hemorrhoid can be reduced manually.
C) If a patient <50 years with rectal bleeding is found to have hemorrhoids on examination, further studies are not indicated.
D) Because they are above the dentate line, strangulated internal hemorrhoids are not painful.

Discussion

The correct answer is B. Grade III hemorrhoids can be reduced manually. Hemorrhoids are normal vascular structures in the anal canal; however, the venules can become engorged and symptoms such as pain, bleeding, and itching may result. Two types of hemorrhoids exist: external hemorrhoids derive from the inferior hemorrhoidal plexus below the dentate line, and internal hemorrhoids derive from the anal cushions above the dentate line. Internal hemorrhoids occur on the left lateral, right anterior, and right posterior anal walls and are classified into Grades I–IV. Grade I hemorrhoids slide below the dentate with straining but not through the anus. Grade II protrude the anus but spontaneously reduce, whereas Grade III hemorrhoids must be manually reduced. Grade IV internal hemorrhoids cannot be reduced. Answer A is incorrect because most patients with symptomatic hemorrhoids present with painless rectal bleeding. Answer C is incorrect. You should consider further evaluation (eg, flexible sigmoidoscopy, colonoscopy, etc) in patients <50 years who present with rectal bleeding, even if hemorrhoids are present and are the likely source of bleeding. In patients >50 years with rectal bleeding, a full colonoscopy is routinely recommended to rule out any cancerous process. Answer D is incorrect. Although most internal hemorrhoids do not cause pain, strangulated internal hemorrhoids are very painful and can become necrotic and gangrenous, requiring emergent surgery.

Which of the following would you NOT consider as a treatment for this patient's hemorrhoids?

A) Psyllium.
B) Dicyclomine.
C) Warm sitz baths.
D) Short course of topical hydrocortisone.
E) Increased water intake.

Discussion
The correct answer is B. Dicyclomine (Bentyl, Antispas) is not indicated. Dicyclomine is an anticholinergic and will contribute to constipation—exactly what you want to avoid in hemorrhoids. Answer A and E are the primary modes of treatment. Psyllium, as well as a diet high in fiber and water, will reduce straining and thus reduce intraabdominal pressure. Answer C, warm baths or showers, have been shown to reduce anal canal pressures (40°C). Answer D, a short course of topical hydrocortisone (eg, Anusol HC), may be of benefit. Long-term topical steroids are contraindicated. Finally, good hygiene and analgesia should be prescribed as needed.

 HELPFUL TIP: Most symptomatic hemorrhoids respond to conservative measures and surgery should not be performed unless conservative measures fail or other indications exist (eg, strangulation).

Which of the following is TRUE about treating hemorrhoids surgically?

A) Irritable bowel syndrome is a relative contraindication to hemorrhoid surgery.
B) It is best to ligate all hemorrhoids in a single office visit.
C) Band ligation results in sloughing of hemorrhoid in 1–2 weeks.
D) Following excision, thrombosed external hemorrhoids should be closed to prevent bleeding.

Discussion
The correct answer is C. Rubber-band ligation generally results in the sloughing of the hemorrhoid in 1–2 weeks. Answer A is incorrect. Inflammatory bowel disease—not irritable bowel syndrome—is a relative contraindication to the surgical treatment of hemorrhoids. Other contraindications to office-based hemorrhoidectomy procedures include bleeding diathesis, pregnancy and the period immediately postpartum, anorectal fissures, active anorectal infections, AIDS or other immunodeficient states, portal hypertension, rectal wall prolapse, and anorectal tumors. Complications of hemorrhoidectomy include pain, significant bleeding with sloughing, thrombosis of external hemorrhoids, and very rarely sepsis with pelvic cellulitis. Answer B is incorrect. Although evidence is scarce, standard of care dictates that only one hemorrhoid be ligated in a single office visit (because of concerns about excessive tissue necrosis). Answer D is incorrect. Patients who present with external hemorrhoids that are painful, tender, swollen, with bluish discoloration have thrombosis. If the patient presents within 48 hours of thrombosis, the thrombus should be expressed. It is specifically important **not** to close the hemorrhoid once the clot is expressed. A small ellipse of the hemorrhoid should be removed to facilitate continued drainage and prevent re-accumulation of clot.

* *

You prescribe conservative treatment for your patient's hemorrhoids, and since he does not return for his next scheduled appointment, you assume he is doing well. You see him again 6 months later. He reports that he had indeed healed. Although he still takes psyllium, he began having painful bowel movements with blood-streaked stool 2 days ago. Upon examination of the anus, you find a fissure.

All of the following findings would lead you to consider Crohn disease EXCEPT:

A) Posterior midline fissure.
B) Painless fissure.
C) Multiple fissures.
D) Nonhealing fissure.

Discussion

The correct answer is A. The posterior (dorsal) midline is where solitary fissures, unrelated to inflammatory bowel disease, are typically located. Fissures in any other location should raise suspicion for Crohn disease. Answers B, C, and D are also suggestive of Crohn disease.

In a patient with an uncomplicated, initial anal fissure, what do you recommend for first-line therapy?

A) Lord dilation.
B) Botulinum toxin injections.
C) Topical nitroglycerin.
D) Oral psyllium.
E) Oral nifedipine.

Discussion

The correct answer is D. All of the options may be employed for treating anal fissures. However, in patients with an uncomplicated, initial anal fissure, it seems prudent to initiate conservative therapy (eg, psyllium, dietary fiber, water, warm soaks, etc) prior to proceeding to more invasive measures. Most fissures will respond to conservative measures. Generally, healing takes 2–4 weeks. In addition to the treatments listed, topical diltiazem and topical nifedipine are also used as are various surgical approaches. Answer A, Lord dilation requires special note as a relatively arcane procedure for stretching the anal sphincter muscle (under anesthesia, we hope!).

* *

You note that this patient's fissure is deep, ulcerating, and located at the left lateral aspect of the anus. Given this examination, you are concerned about Crohn disease. You briefly consider what you know about inflammatory bowel disease (IBD).

Which of the following is true of IBD?

A) Ulcerative colitis is primarily a diagnosis of young males.
B) Crohn disease can be isolated to colonic disease.
C) Ulcerative colitis is generally associated with deep colonic ulcerations and transmural inflammation while those of Crohn disease are more superficial.
D) Crohn disease is more common in blacks and ulcerative colitis is more common in whites.

Discussion

The correct answer is B. Crohn disease can be isolated to the colon. Answer A is incorrect because ulcerative colitis is evenly distributed between men and women with a similar incidence in each. Answer C is incorrect. Crohn is associated with deeper ulcerations and transmural inflammation leading to fistulae and strictures, etc. Answer D is incorrect. In general, inflammatory bowel disease is more common in whites than nonwhites. See Chapter 7, Gastroenterology for more on Crohn disease.

Objectives: Did you learn to . . .

- Characterize hemorrhoids based on location?
- Grade internal hemorrhoids based on severity?
- Manage hemorrhoids with conservative and surgical treatment?
- Treat an uncomplicated anal fissure?
- Recognize anal fissures as potential signs of Crohn disease?

CASE 7

A 58-year-old female presents to your clinic for a lump found on routine breast self-exam. Her older sister died from breast cancer, and she is very concerned about the possibility of breast cancer in herself. She never misses her monthly breast exam and notes she has never felt this lump before. She first noticed the lump 2 weeks ago, and it has not changed in size or consistency since that time. She has had mammograms yearly since 40 years of age that have always been normal. She denies any weight loss or fatigue and reports being postmenopausal for the last 5 years. She previously took combination hormone replacement therapy, which she discontinued last year.

On examination, her breasts appear symmetrical with no skin abnormalities. The nipples are symmetric in size, shape, and color without retraction or discharge. You palpate a small, pea-sized thickening in upper outer quadrant of the right breast. This is the lump that she noticed 2 weeks ago. It is fixed to the deep aspect of the chest wall, so you have a hard time delineating whether the borders are smooth.

Regarding breast lumps, which one of the following statements is FALSE?

A) Abnormal screening mammography is the most common presentation of breast carcinoma.
B) Cysts are most common in premenopausal women.
C) A history of fibroadenoma is associated with an increased risk of breast cancer.
D) A radiographic oil cyst is pathognomonic for fat necrosis.

Discussion

The correct answer is A. The most common presentation of breast carcinoma is a breast lump felt by the patient. Breast masses can be cysts, fibroadenomas, thickened areas with fibrocystic change, fat necrosis, and carcinoma. Only one-third of breast masses palpated by a patient and one-fifth palpated by a physician are found on further surgical evaluation. Answer B is true. Cysts primarily present when women are premenopausal and are uncommon in the postmenopausal state, unless the woman is taking hormone replacement. Cysts are well demarcated, mobile, and firm. The diagnosis is confirmed with aspiration of non-bloody fluid followed by complete resolution of the mass. Fibroadenomas occur between 20 and 50 years and are described as firm, rubbery, and mobile. They can be confirmed by characteristic findings on ultrasound and fine needle aspiration if necessary. Answer C is true. While historically believed to be entirely benign, fibroadenomas are associated with a small but significant increased risk for breast cancer. Answer D is true. A radiographic oil cyst (a circumscribed mass of mixed soft-tissue density and fat with a rim that is often calcified) is due to fat necrosis, which occurs in areas

of the breast that have been subject to trauma, surgery, infection, or radiation therapy. About 50% of the time fat necrosis has no precipitant. It is most common in the superficial aspects of pendulous breasts of obese women. When an oil cyst is seen radiographically, no further workup is needed.

* *

Your patient is concerned about her family history of breast cancer. She asks about genetic testing.

You are able to tell her that the BRCA 1 gene is associated with which of the following?

A) Breast cancer.
B) Uterine cancer.
C) Ovarian cancer.
D) A and B.
E) A and C.

Discussion

The correct answer is E. The BRCA (**BR**east **CA**ncer) 1 and 2 genes are related to familial breast cancer and BRCA 1 is also associated with an increased risk of ovarian cancer. They are not associated with uterine cancer. The usefulness of testing for these genes in primary care is questionable, and they **cannot** be relied upon for general screening or diagnostic purposes.

* *

You are suspicious that this patient's mass may be cancer, and you order **mammography and ultrasound**. However, these studies show no mass. When your patient returns to discuss her test results, you examine her again. The mass is still palpable.

The next best step in management of this patient is:

A) Breast exam and mammogram every 6 months.
B) Breast exam and mammogram every 3 months.
C) Referral to a surgeon to consider excisional biopsy.
D) Ultrasound-guided biopsy.
E) Return to normal screening.

Discussion

The correct answer is C. A palpable mass that is suspicious for cancer **cannot** be ignored even in the presence of negative radiologic studies. No other option is acceptable, nor would any other option be defensible if this patient were to develop overt breast cancer. Answer D would be a viable option if a mass were identified on ultrasound, but none was.

* *

When making diagnostic decisions regarding breast masses, age matters.

Which of the following is NOT TRUE about how a diagnostic evaluation should proceed?

A) In women <40 years, lesions that appear benign on ultrasound may be followed simply by a repeat examination in 3 months.

B) In women >40 years, lesions that appear benign on ultrasound and cytological analysis need no follow-up.

C) In women >40 years where a lesion is palpated but not seen on mammogram or ultrasound, excision should follow if clinical suspicion dictates.

D) In women >40 years who have a palpable lesion and desire definitive removal, no further testing is necessary prior to excisional biopsy.

Discussion

The correct answer is B. Women >40 years should be followed up in 3 months even with negative cytology. Clinical diagnosis of carcinoma has accuracy of 60%–85%. Extent of workup, however, is driven by clinical suspicion. Radiologic studies should be ordered as indicated. A needle biopsy either by fine-needle aspirate (FNA) or core needle biopsy is the next step in evaluation of solid tumor masses. Needle diagnosis offers the advantages of being simple, quick, inexpensive, relatively noninvasive, highly available, and an accurate way of diagnosing atypical cells.

Because of the risk for carcinoma, algorithms for workup of solid tumors differ for women <40 years and those ≥40 years. Women <40 years who desire observation should be evaluated by ultrasound and/or FNA. If either is suspicious, surgical excision should be performed. If there is a negative FNA, the patient can be followed up in 3 months.

In women ≥40 years, palpable masses should further be evaluated by ultrasound and mammography. If the lesion cannot be identified radiologically, it should be removed by excision if clinical suspicion dictates. If the lesion appears benign by radiography, it can be followed by FNA. Those with atypia on FNA should be referred for excision. If the lesion appears benign both radiologically and cytologically, it still warrants further follow-up in 3 months by clinical exam. Answer D is correct. All women with a palpable breast mass who desire an excisional biopsy can proceed directly to definitive removal, regardless of age.

* *

You perform an FNA which the cytopathologist reads as "probable malignancy." You recall from previous visits that the patient's older sister had breast cancer. Additionally, your patient went through menopause at 53 years, and used HRT for 5 years. You obtain further history, including a history of menarche at 14 years and that the patient has never been pregnant.

Which of these factors does NOT contribute to an increased risk of breast cancer in THIS patient?

A) Her nulliparity.
B) Her age at menarche.
C) Her family history.
D) Her age at menopause.
E) Her history of hormone replacement.

Discussion

The correct answer is B. The risk of breast cancer is roughly associated with the lifetime exposure to estrogen. This patient's age at menarche is in the mid to late age range and is thus **not** a risk factor for breast cancer. Younger age at menarche (eg, 10 years) is associated with an increased risk of breast cancer. Nulliparity and greater age at first pregnancy are associated with an increased risk, as is greater age at menopause. A history of a first-degree relative with breast cancer is a strong risk factor. Finally, as demonstrated in the Women's Health Initiative, estrogen/progesterone replacement therapy (HRT) is associated with an increased risk of breast cancer.

* *

While you wait for definitive pathology results, you consider the different types of breast cancer that this patient might have.

Regarding various types of breast cancer, all of the following are true EXCEPT:

A) Cystosarcoma phyllodes tumors are not always malignant.

B) Infiltrating lobular carcinoma is the most common histological type of invasive breast carcinoma.

C) Paget disease of the breast clinically appears eczematous.

D) Sarcomas, lymphomas, melanomas, and angiosarcomas are all possible causes of cancer in the breast.

Discussion

The correct answer is B. Infiltrating **ductal (not lobular)** carcinoma is the most common histological type of invasive breast cancer. Invasive breast carcinoma includes a wide variety of histological diseases. Infiltrating **ductal** carcinoma accounts for 65%–80% of breast cancers, whereas infiltrating **lobular** carcinoma is the second most frequent, accounting for 10% of breast cancers. Answer A is true. Cystosarcoma phyllodes tumors, which have a clinical presentation similar to fibroadenomas but are more rapidly growing, may be either malignant or benign. Yet the malignant nature of cystosarcoma phyllodes is sometimes difficult to determine on cytology, and the lesions may require a wide excision. Answer C is true. Paget disease of the breast, is a rare form of breast cancer with eczematous changes of the nipple, including itching, erythema, and nipple discharge. Answer D is true. Many other malignancies may occur in the breast, including sarcomas, lymphomas, melanomas, and angiosarcomas.

* *

The pathology results are final and show infiltrating ductal carcinoma. Your patient will see a breast surgeon next week. As you await the results of surgery, you consider her prognosis.

All of the following are favorable prognostic indicators in breast cancer EXCEPT:

A) Hormone receptor negative.
B) Absence of axillary nodal involvement.
C) Low-grade tumor.
D) Pure tubular, mucinous, or medullary histological types.
E) Tumor size <1 cm.

Discussion

The correct answer is A. Patients whose tumors are hormone receptor **negative** have a worse outcome than do patients whose tumors are hormone receptor positive. Answer B, absence of axillary nodal involvement, is a better prognostic factor than the presence of nodal involvement. Axillary lymph node status is the single most important predictor of overall survival in breast cancer. Answer C, low-grade tumor, is also a good prognostic factor. Answer D, patients with a single cell type have a better prognosis as well. Answer E is true. A very useful predictor of tumor behavior is tumor size, and tumor size <1 cm is a positive prognostic sign.

Objectives: Did you learn to . . .

- Generate a differential diagnoses for breast masses?
- Evaluate a patient with a breast mass?
- Identify risk factors for breast cancer?
- Describe several types of breast cancers?
- Describe factors that are used to establish prognosis in breast cancer?

 QUICK QUIZ: BREAST CANCER RISK

A 50-year-old female presents for a routine physical. She wants to know her risk of developing breast cancer. You want to give her a more accurate picture, and you decide to use the Gail Model.

When taking her history, you must ask about which of the following?

A) Number of first-degree relatives with breast cancer, current age, age at menopause, number of breast biopsies, and age at first live birth.
B) Number of first-degree relatives with breast cancer, current age, age at menopause, and number of children.
C) Number of first-degree relatives with breast cancer, current age, age at first menstrual period, and number of children.
D) Number of first-degree relatives with breast cancer, current age, age at first menstrual period, number of breast biopsies, and age at first live birth.

Discussion

The correct answer is D. The Gail Model is a computer program that estimates a woman's chance of developing breast cancer. Factors that affect the score include the number of first-degree relatives with breast cancer, current age, age of first menstrual period, number of breast biopsies, and age at first live birth. For example, if this 50-year-old patient had menarche at age 11, first live birth of a child at age 30, one first-degree relative with breast cancer, and no breast biopsies, her 5-year risk of breast cancer is 2.1% and her lifetime risk is 18.3%. This tool may be useful in patients who are candidates for tamoxifen for breast cancer prophylaxis. The National Cancer Institute maintains a website for the Gail Model calculation, located at http://bcra.nci.nih.gov/brc/q1.htm.

CASE 8

An orthopedic colleague asks you to consult on a 64-year-old male prior to an elective total hip replacement. The surgery is scheduled for 3 months from now. The patient is a smoker with diabetes mellitus type 2 and has recently had a cardiac catheterization that showed significant, but nonbypassable, coronary disease. He is asymptomatic and is able to walk stairs without difficulty. The surgeon would like some preoperative recommendations.

You would recommend all of the following EXCEPT:

A) The patient should stop smoking 4 weeks before surgery.
B) The patient should have preoperative and postoperative β-blockers if the pulmonary status allows it.
C) The patient should have a chest radiograph done.
D) The patient should have his hemoglobin/hematocrit drawn.
E) The patient should have his creatinine measured.

Discussion

The correct answer is A. Paradoxically, unless patients stop smoking ≥8 weeks before surgery, the risk of adverse pulmonary outcomes is increased. The cause of this phenomenon remains unclear but may occur because the cilia are able to mobilize material in the lungs. Answer B is true. The use of pre-, intra- and postoperative β-blockers is well supported for patients with coronary artery disease. One of the most serious intraoperative events is a myocardial infarction. β-blockers have been shown in multiple studies to reduce this risk and to improve outcomes if the patient has an elevated risk for a myocardial infarction. Although answers C, D, and E are true, a lot of other routine preoperative assessment is not supported in the literature but is recognized as the standard of care. See Tables 22–1 and 22–2 for the appropriate workup of the preoperative patient.

Which of the following is (are) effective for the prevention of postoperative deep venous thrombosis (DVT)?

A) Early mobilization.
B) Enoxaparin 30 mg subcutaneously every 12 hours.
C) Enoxaparin 40 mg subcutaneously every 24 hours.
D) Heparin 5,000 units subcutaneously every 12 hours.
E) All of the above.

Discussion

The correct answer is E. All of the modalities listed above can prevent the development of DVT. Aspirin and low-dose warfarin (target INR 1.5) are also effective but less so than heparin or enoxaparin. Intermittent leg compression and graded compression stockings are effective as well, but without the risks associated with the use of heparin and other anticoagulant/antiplatelet agents.

Table 22–1 PREOPERATIVE STUDIES AND THEIR INDICATIONS

Tests	Indications
Bun/Creatinine	>60 years or history renal, cardiac, or vascular disease
CBC/H&H	Possible hematologic or infectious process, significant blood loss predicted
Coagulation studies	Stigmata of liver disease, history of coagulopathy, possible DIC, anticoagulation, alcohol abuse
ECG/CXR	As indicated by history and physical (eg, exacerbation of pulmonary disease with cough, etc)
Electrolytes	Diuretic use, history of renal or cardiac disease, possible dehydration by history or physical
Glucose	Diabetics, obese patients, undergoing vascular procedures, other reason for increased glucose (eg, steroids)
Liver enzymes	History of liver disease or stigmata of liver disease
Urine β-hCG	If indicated by history
Urinalysis	Pregnancy, diabetes, urologic surgery, symptomatic patients

Table 22–2 MAYO CLINIC PREOPERATIVE GUIDELINES

Age	Studies Indicated
<40 years	No routine preoperative evaluation required
40–59 years	ECG, creatinine, and glucose
≥60 years	ECG, chest radiograph, CBC, creatinine, glucose

 HELPFUL TIP: Many experts recommend heparin dosed at 5,000 U SQ q 8 hours instead of q12 hours. This dosing is more effective but is associated with more bleeding. Balance these two considerations when you decide whether to use q 8 hour or q 12 hour heparin.

* *

The patient undergoes his hip replacement and his postoperative ECG is normal. Four hours after surgery, he develops mild respiratory distress, a fever, and cough. On chest x-ray, there is a right lower lobe infiltrate. There is no evidence of fluid overload.

Which of the following is the most likely cause of this patient's fever and infiltrate?

A) Pneumococcus.
B) Gram-negative organisms.
C) Atelectasis.
D) Aspiration pneumonitis.
E) Aspiration pneumonia.

Discussion

The correct answer is D. In the hours after surgery, an aspiration **pneumonitis** would be the most likely cause of this patient's current findings. Aspiration pneumonitis occurs when there is aspiration of gastric contents with a pH of <2.5. In order for aspiration pneumonitis to develop, the volume of aspirate needs to be at least 1–4 mL/kg of stomach contents. Aspiration pneumonitis develops over a matter of hours. In contrast, pneumococcal (answer A) and Gram-negative (answer B) pneumonias generally develop several days after surgery (unless a subclinical pneumonia was present at the time of surgery). Aspiration **pneumonia** (answer E) is caused by anaerobes and mixed flora and

develops slowly over days to a week. Answer C, atelectasis requires special note. **Atelectasis does not cause fever.** Both atelectasis and fever occur frequently in the post-operative period, but their occurrence together is most likely due to chance. The old adage about atelectasis and fever has been shown to be untrue. Thus, in the postsurgical patient with fever, look for another cause besides atelectasis.

Of the following, which generally IS NOT a cause of post-operative fever in the first 48 hours?

A) Malignant hyperthermia.
B) Surgical "trauma" (eg, cutting through muscle).
C) Wound infection.
D) Hyperthyroidism.
E) Drug fever.

Discussion

The correct answer is C. Wound infections generally are not found in the first 48 hours after surgery. All of the rest can be found either immediately after surgery (malignant hyperthermia, hyperthyroidism, drug fever) or soon thereafter (fever from surgical trauma secondary to the release of cytokines). Table 22–3 summarizes the causes of postoperative fever.

* *

The patient's chest radiograph is consistent with aspiration pneumonitis (infiltrate in the right lower lobe).

Which of the following statements is NOT TRUE with regards to aspiration pneumonitis?

A) It can progress to ARDS.
B) Patients with aspiration pneumonitis present with fever, dyspnea, bronchospasm, and hypoxia.
C) It should be treated with antibiotics that cover for anaerobes.
D) It tends to resolve in approximately 7 days.

Discussion

The correct answer is C. Aspiration **pneumonitis** is a chemical process that is unrelated to infection. Thus, aspiration pneumonitis does not need to be treated with antibiotics at all (although it usually is as a practical matter—since it is difficult to differentiate from pneumonia). The rest of the answer choices are true statements.

Table 22–3 CAUSES OF POSTOPERATIVE FEVER

Immediate (within hours of surgery)
- Drugs or blood products: generally hypotension, rash, etc
- Trauma from surgery or before surgery: evident from history
- Malignant hyperthermia: within 30 minutes of anesthesia induction but may be hours out

Acute (first week after surgery)
- Nosocomial infections or extension of a preoperative infection
- *C. difficile* infection
- Intubation
- Aspiration
- UTI: especially if chronic indwelling or urologic manipulation
- Surgical site infection generally >1 week, if cause fever but may occur in 1st week, but group A *Streptococcus* and *Clostridium* may occur within hours of surgery
- Also: pancreatitis, alcohol withdrawal, PE, MI, thrombophlebitis, gout

Subacute (1–4 weeks after surgery)
- IV and central catheter site infections
- Antibiotic-associated diarrhea, including *C. difficile* infection
- Drug fever: β-lactams, sulfa, heparin, etc.
- DVT, PE, fat emboli from long bones, liposuction, acute chest syndrome (SSA)

HELPFUL TIP: The term **aspiration pneumonia** is defined differently in different parts of the literature. When you read about aspiration pneumonia, be sure you know which definition the authors are using, because the description of the disease and the treatments vary. Some authors use the term to include all pneumonias caused by aspiration. Many of the cases included in this definition are caused by many of the same organisms that cause community-acquired pneumonia, including *Pneumococcus, Haemophilus influenzae,* etc. Patients tend to have a fever and infiltrate, etc, which develop within 2 days of the aspiration. For these patients, the appropriate antibiotics include agents to cover hospital-acquired organisms, especially Gram-negative organisms, including *Pseudomonas*.

Other authors describe aspiration pneumonia as anaerobic infections that result from aspiration. Patients have a more indolent course, with onset of symptoms over days to weeks. Generally, these patients have purulent sputum, with lower lobe involvement most common. The upper lobes may be involved if the patient aspirates while recumbent. Patients may have a polymicrobial infection including *Peptostreptococcus, Fusobacterium, Bacteroides,* and *Prevotella.* Patients are treated with antibiotics such as clindamycin, ampicillin/sulbactam, or amoxicillin/clavulanate (metronidazole as a single agent is avoided because of high failure rate).

* *

You treat the patient with fluids and tracheal suction. However, he remains febrile and tachycardic at about 128 bpm. There is no evidence of dehydration at this point and he seems euvolemic.

Which of the following would be the most appropriate first step in the treatment of tachycardia in this postsurgical patient?

A) Oral or rectal aspirin.
B) Oral or rectal acetaminophen.
C) IV β-blockers.
D) IV fluids.

Discussion
The correct answer is B. The **initial** treatment for this patient is acetaminophen. Reducing the fever and metabolic stress will result in a reduction of the heart rate. Answer A is incorrect because this patient is post-surgical. Giving aspirin, an antiplatelet agent, may result in increased postoperative bleeding. Answer C, IV β-blockers, can be used and would be appropriate if the patient was having ischemic symptoms and needed an immediate reduction in pulse. Answer D, IV fluid, is incorrect in this patient who is already well hydrated (as stipulated in the question). Note that IV fluids **are** appropriate in postoperative tachycardia if the patient is dehydrated.

* *

The patient's pulmonary status has improved. The surgeon notices that the patient has hyperkalemia and thrombocytopenia. The patient is on a number of drugs postoperatively. She is wondering which of these drugs is causing the problem.

You let her know that the most likely cause is:

A) β-blockers.
B) Albuterol.
C) Aspirin.
D) Morphine.
E) Heparin.

Discussion

The correct answer is E. Heparin can cause both hyperkalemia and thrombocytopenia (HITTS: heparin induced thrombocytopenia thrombosis syndrome). Hyperkalemia is caused by heparin's ability to block the aldosterone system and usually requires prolonged heparin use (although in diabetics and those with renal failure it may occur more rapidly because of poor reserve). Thrombocytopenia is caused by the development of antiplatelet antibodies and occurs 5–10 days after the start of heparin therapy and is associated with thromboembolic phenomenon. Platelets can get as low as 30,000/microliter. Stop the heparin and anticoagulate with a nonheparin agent (eg, bivalirudin). A nonimmune-mediated thrombocytopenia also occurs in up to 20% of individuals who receive heparin. This occurs within the first 4 days of heparin administration with a nadir of 100,000 platelets per microliter and there are no clinical consequences.

Answer A is incorrect because β-blockers cause neither hyperkalemia nor thrombocytopenia. Answer B, albuterol, can cause **hypokalemia** (as can other catecholamines) by driving potassium intracellularly. However, albuterol does not cause **hyperkalemia** or thrombocytopenia. Answers C and D are incorrect because neither aspirin nor morphine is associated with hyperkalemia or thrombocytopenia.

 HELPFUL TIP: Heparin can also cause a postoperative fever.

* *

After you stop the patient's heparin, the thrombocytopenia and hyperkalemia begin to resolve. You start the patient on intermittent leg compression.

Which of the following is TRUE about the use of heparin in patients with a history of heparin-induced thrombocytopenia?

A) The use of low-molecular-weight heparin is contraindicated in patients with a history of heparin-induced thrombocytopenia.
B) Heparin can be reintroduced once the patient is treated with steroids.
C) The use of lepirudin and argatroban are contraindicated in the treatment of heparin-induced thrombocytopenia.
D) Heparin can be used during cardiopulmonary bypass despite a previous history of a thrombocytopenic reaction to heparin.
E) None of the above.

Discussion

The correct answer is D. Heparin can be used during cardiopulmonary bypass despite a previous history of heparin-induced thrombocytopenia. The theory is that the development of enough antibodies to reproduce thrombocytopenia takes several days and patients will generally be on cardiopulmonary bypass for only a matter of hours. Thus, heparin can be used during cardiopulmonary bypass even if there is a history of prior heparin-induced thrombocytopenia.

Answer A is incorrect. Low-molecular-weight heparins, especially danaparoid, have been used successfully in patients with a history of heparin-induced thrombocytopenia. There is only about a 5% cross-reactivity between unfractionated heparin and danaparoid in vivo. Answer C is incorrect. The treatment of patients who need anticoagulation after heparin-induced thrombocytopenia includes lepirudin and argatroban. These two agents are direct thrombin inhibitors which do not cross-react with heparin.

 HELPFUL TIP: Drugs that raise the gastric pH (H₂-blockers, proton pump inhibitors) increase the risk of postoperative pneumonia. Normally, the acid pH of the stomach prevents colonization with pathogenic bacteria. This defense is compromised when the stomach pH rises. Thus, infection with aspiration is more likely.

Objectives: Did you learn to . . .

- Perform a preoperative medical evaluation?
- Generate a differential diagnosis for postoperative fever?
- Diagnose and treat aspiration pneumonitis?
- Recognize some complications of heparin use?
- Employ appropriate DVT prophylaxis measures?
- Manage a patient with heparin-induced thrombocytopenia?

QUICK QUIZ: ANESTHESIA FOR SURGERY

Regarding anesthesia evaluation both preoperatively and intraoperatively, which one of the following is NOT TRUE?

A) Therapeutic beta blockade should be administered preoperatively in vascular surgery patients who have underlying cardiac disease in order to reduce perioperative and long-term risks of cardiac events.
B) Minimum potassium before proceeding with elective CABG surgery should be 3.5 meq/L.
C) ASA Class IV designation includes patients who have well-controlled major systemic disease.
D) Risks of anesthesia include allergic drug reactions, failure to intubate and provide adequate oxygenation and ventilation, nerve damage, and malignant hyperthermia.

Discussion

The correct answer is C. ASA (American Society of Anesthesiologists) Class IV includes patients who have a systemic disease that is life threatening and **not** well-controlled. All the other options are true. Answer B is a true statement. A recent study of more than 2,000 perioperative elective CABG patients showed perioperative arrhythmias and need for cardiac resuscitations increased in patients with serum potassium levels <3.5 meq/L. Answer D is a true statement. Anesthesia risks include allergic drug reactions, failure to intubate and provide adequate oxygenation and ventilation, nerve damage, and malignant hyperthermia, among others. Mortality rate from anesthesia is surmised to be about 1–2 per 10,000 patients. The ASA classification system is outlined in Table 22–4.

CASE 9

A 60-year-old male patient of yours is planning to undergo coronary artery bypass graft (CABG). After you perform a physical exam and laboratory tests, you discuss his case with the surgeon. She asks if you will help to manage him postoperatively, and you agree. She then asks if you are aware of his risk of arrhythmia during the postoperative period.

You appropriately and correctly reply:

A) "His risk for atrial fibrillation is less than it would be if he were undergoing valve replacement simultaneously with CABG."
B) "Of the potential arrhythmias, he is most likely to encounter bradycardia requiring pacing."
C) "Nonsustained ventricular tachycardia is highly unlikely in this setting."
D) "Keep his potassium low, around 3.0 meq/L, and he will be less likely to experience tachyarrhythmias."
E) "Heart rhythm, schmart rhythm. He's too old for arrhythmias."

Table 22–4 ASA PHYSICAL STATUS CLASSIFICATION

Class	Description	Risk of Operative Mortality
I	Healthy individual	<0.1%
II	Patient with mild systemic disease	0.5%
III	Patient with severe systemic disease that is controlled	4.4%
IV	Patient with severe systemic disease that is uncontrolled and a threat to life	23.5%
V	Patient who is unlikely to survive for 24 hours, with or without surgery	50.8%

Discussion

The correct answer is A. With CABG, the risk of postoperative atrial flutter or fibrillation is around 30%. That risk almost doubles when valve replacement is accomplished simultaneously with CABG. Answer B is incorrect because bradyarrhythmias occur less frequently than tachyarrhythmias. Answer C is incorrect. Nonsustained ventricular tachycardia is extremely common in the immediate postoperative period. Answer D is incorrect. Plasma potassium levels < 3.5 meq/L are associated with an increased risk of tachyarrhythmias. Answer E is incorrect, not to mention insensitive! Older patients are more likely to experience arrhythmias in this setting.

All of the following factors are associated with a lower incidence of mortality in patients undergoing CABG EXCEPT:

A) Aspirin in the postoperative period within 48 hours of surgery.
B) Perioperative β-blocker administration.
C) Female gender.
D) Higher volume of CABG procedures performed at a given hospital.

Discussion

The correct answer is C. Female gender may actually be associated with a higher incidence of mortality, presumably related to smaller diameter of coronary arteries. The other statements are true. Early postoperative aspirin use is associated with lower mortality, as is perioperative β-blockade. Institutions that perform a larger number of procedures generally have a lower mortality rate, which is especially true for higher risk patients (eg, more severe disease, older, greater number of comorbidities).

* *

Your patient does well postoperatively. He is 2 weeks out from his surgery and presents to your office complaining that he has "the flu." He reports a temperature of 99°–100°F and some chest pain when he takes a deep breath. You obtain a chest x-ray that shows postoperative changes with small bilateral pleural effusions that were not present at discharge.

Regarding this patient, all of the following are true EXCEPT:

A) These signs and symptoms are suggestive of postpericardiotomy syndrome.
B) If this condition is left untreated, it has a high incidence of mortality.

C) One out of four treated patients will go on to have future recurrences of the condition.
D) Treatment should include either nonsteroidal antiinflammatory agents or steroids.

Discussion

The correct answer is B. This patient has signs and symptoms of postpericardiotomy syndrome (Dressler syndrome). Postpericardiotomy syndrome can occur with any cardiac surgery. The typical presentation is as follows: a few weeks or months following surgery, the patient develops a flu-like illness with low-grade fever and chest pain (usually described as a peristernal aching, pressure, or pleuritic pain). Both pericardial and pleural effusions can develop (although the pericardium is usually left open). Episodes last between 3 weeks and 3 months. Treatment includes nonsteroidal antiinflammatory agents and sometimes steroids for 4–8 weeks. Without treatment, the illness will eventually self-resolve. One-quarter will go on to have recurrences in the next 3 years.

Objectives: Did you learn to . . .

- Identify factors that may reduce mortality rates in patients undergoing CABG?
- Recognize and manage complications of CABG?

CASE 10

A 15-year-old male presents to your office with a 3-day history of diarrhea and right lower quadrant abdominal pain. He has tenderness in the right lower quadrant with guarding and rebound. He remains afebrile and has been hungry, scarfing down 5 waffles for breakfast. The patient has no other significant history. You decide that this patient might have appendicitis, so you draw some labs. The white blood cell count is normal (7,500/mm³), as is the urinalysis.

Which of the following is true about appendicitis?

A) A normal white cell count effectively rules out the diagnosis of appendicitis.
B) The majority of patients with appendicitis present with fever.
C) The absence of anorexia effectively rules out appendicitis.

D) A fecalith is found on radiograph in the majority of patients with appendicitis.

E) None of the above.

Discussion

The correct answer is E. None of the above is true. Discussing these in order: 10% of patients with appendicitis have a normal white cell count; a minority of patients with appendicitis present with fever (15% in one study); only 75% of patients with appendicitis complain of anorexia; and a radiographic fecalith is found in only a small minority of patients.

Which of the following is specific for appendicitis?

A) Obturator sign.

B) Psoas sign.

C) Rovsing sign.

D) Tenderness at McBurney point.

E) None of the above is specific for appendicitis.

Discussion

The correct answer is E. None of the above is specific for appendicitis. An obturator sign is present if there is pain on internal and external rotation of the hip. The obturator sign can be seen with any pelvic abscess that is in contact with the hip area, but is more commonly seen with a retrocecal abscess. The psoas sign is pain on use of the psoas muscle (eg, lifting the leg at the hip), and it can be seen with any inflammatory process that is in contact with the psoas muscle, including a psoas abscess. Rovsing sign is when pain increases in an area of peritonitis when the abdomen is palpated elsewhere. For example, in a patient with appendicitis, right lower quadrant pain will be increased with palpation of the **left** lower quadrant. This is indicative of peritonitis in the area that has increased pain, but it is not specific for appendicitis. Tenderness at McBurney point can be seen in a number of processes including appendicitis, ileitis, any process in the cecum, urinary tract infection, etc.

Which of the following is true about the treatment of pain in the acute abdomen?

A) Early treatment with morphine will obscure the proper diagnosis.

B) Treatment with pain medication invalidates informed consent.

C) Early treatment of pain with morphine is safe except in children.

D) Ketorolac is preferred for patients who may undergo a surgical procedure.

E) None of the above is true.

The correct answer is E. None of the above is true. Early treatment of pain in the acute abdomen actually **improves** diagnostic accuracy in both children and adults. Ketorolac is not a good choice because of its antiplatelet effects, which increase the risk of bleeding intraoperatively.

* *

Although you have thought a lot about his potential problem, you have not done anything more for the 15-year-old with abdominal pain!

The test most likely to help you arrive at a diagnosis in this patient is:

A) Erythrocyte sedimentation rate (ESR).

B) C-reactive protein (CRP).

C) Abdominal ultrasound.

D) Abdominal CT scan.

E) Colonoscopy.

Discussion

The correct answer is D. The test most likely to be helpful in arriving at a diagnosis in this patient is a CT scan of the abdomen looking at the appendix. Answers A and B are incorrect. Both the CRP and the ESR are nonspecific markers of inflammation and are not helpful in the diagnosis of appendicitis. Answer C, an ultrasound, can be used. However, it is not as sensitive as a CT scan. Ultrasound can be useful in the female patient in whom other diagnoses need to be ruled out, such as ovarian pathology. But, when looking specifically at the appendix, CT is preferable. Answer E, colonoscopy, is not particularly useful in the diagnosis of appendicitis but could be used for other purposes such as looking for inflammatory bowel disease once appendicitis is ruled out by CT.

 HELPFUL TIP: Not all patients need a CT scan. Those with obvious appendicitis should go directly to the OR. CT should only be used in patients in whom the clinical diagnosis is equivocal. **There is some long-term risk from radiation exposure, so CT should not be done without a good indication.**

If this patient's CT scan is positive for appendicitis, the likelihood that he will have a normal appendix removed at appendectomy is:

A) 5%
B) 10%
C) 15%
D) 20%

Discussion

The correct answer is C. Unfortunately, the false-positive rate (of taking normal patients to the OR) has not really changed with CT scan. The negative laparotomy rate is still about the same as it was in the pre-CT era. The negative laparotomy rate has gone down in men and the young but has increased in the elderly and in women. Also, CT may contribute to a delay in therapy and an increased rate of rupture prior to surgery.

In general, which of the following is true about appendicitis?

A) Pain is in the right upper quadrant in the majority of pregnant women with appendicitis.
B) Atypical presentations are more common in the elderly patient than in other groups.
C) Patients with a retrocecal appendix generally present with well-localized tenderness and signs of peritoneal irritation.
D) All of the above.

Discussion

The correct answer is B. Symptoms tend to be atypical in the elderly. In fact, elderly patients may have appendicitis with a normal white count, poorly localized pain, and absence of fever. Answer A is incorrect. Despite classic teaching, patients who are pregnant tend to have "typical" symptoms with right lower quadrant pain. This is especially true in the first half of pregnancy. Certainly the appendix can be displaced cephalad but the majority will still have right lower quadrant pain. Answer C is incorrect. Patients with retrocecal appendicitis will commonly complain of a dull ache. However, signs of peritoneal irritation may be minimal or absent.

 HELPFUL TIP: Some patients have recurrent appendicitis. These patients will present with multiple episodes of "typical" appendicitis, which resolve during observation. When the appendix is finally removed, it is frequently scarred down.

Objectives: Did you learn to . . .

- Describe the findings in acute appendicitis?
- Diagnose appendicitis and determine how ancillary tests are best used in the patient presenting with signs and symptoms of appendicitis?
- Manage a patient with appendicitis?

CASE 11

A 72-year-old male presents to your office for a 3-month history of episodic abdominal pain. It is primarily located in the epigastric region and radiates to the back. It occurs both during the night and day and lasts about 1 hour. His past medical history is significant for a 5-year history of diabetes. He takes glyburide, atorvastatin, and aspirin. He has no previous surgical history. You are concerned about an aortic aneurysm and obtain an abdominal ultrasound. The ultrasound reveals a normal aorta but the technician notes several stones in the gallbladder. You are concerned that this patient may have symptomatic cholelithiasis.

Which of the following is true of his risk for gallstones?

A) This patient has an increased risk of cholesterol stones because he is diabetic.
B) This patient's risk of gallstones would have peaked in his fourth decade of life.
C) This patient's risk of gallstones is increased because of his atorvastatin use.
D) This patient's risk for cholesterol stones is lower because of his advanced age.

Discussion

The correct answer is A. Diabetic patients have an increased risk of gallstones when compared to the general population. Other associations include female gender, family history, obesity, and certain medical illnesses including hyperlipidemia, cystic fibrosis, short bowel syndrome, parenteral nutrition, hemolytic anemia (eg, sickle cell) and history of terminal ileum resection. Answer B is incorrect because the risk of gallstones increases linearly with age. Answer C is incorrect. Atorvastatin and other statins are not associated with an increased risk of gallstone formation, but clofibrate and other fibrates are. Answer D is incorrect. Cholecystectomy rates for symptomatic gallstones increases after the fourth decade of life, and increasing age is associated with an increased risk.

Which of the following statements is FALSE regarding the evaluation of the gallbladder?

A) Ultrasound will find pericolic fluid in only 50% of patients with cholecystitis.
B) A HIDA scan can be positive (eg, no tracer in the duodenum) in the absence of cholecystitis.
C) ERCP has an attendant risk of pancreatitis.
D) The absence of disease on ultrasound effectively rules out gallbladder disease.

Discussion

The correct answer is D. Although ultrasound is highly sensitive for stones (≥95%), it will miss some. Answer A is a correct statement as are B and C. A HIDA (hepatic iminodiacetic acid) scan can be abnormal (eg, no tracer in the duodenum) in cholecystitis but also in any other condition in which the common duct is blocked including a common duct stone or tumor. Additionally, if there is liver disease (which may prevent the uptake of HIDA into the gallbladder), a full gallbladder, gallbladder dysfunction, or spasm of the sphincter of Oddi, one can have a false-positive scan (eg, no tracer in the duodenum).

> **HELPFUL TIP:** CT is not a very sensitive study for gallstones. Ultrasound is the study of choice for diagnosing gallstones (sensitivity is 25% for CT versus 95% for ultrasound).

Regarding different types of gallstones, all of the following are true EXCEPT:

A) Cholesterol stones are associated with obesity and hyperlipidemia.
B) Black pigment stones are associated with cirrhosis.
C) Brown pigment stones are associated with liver fluke infection.
D) Blue pigment stones are associated with being an avid fan of the St. Louis Blues hockey team.

Discussion

The correct answer is D. Although beer-swilling hockey fans might be prone to developing gallstones, there are no studies that show this. Besides, blue pigment stones do not exist. All the other answer choices are true. Stone types include cholesterol, black pigment,

and brown pigment stones. Cholesterol stones are associated with advancing age (due to decreased synthesis of bile salts from cholesterol), hyperlipidemia, diabetes, obesity, and living in the Western hemisphere. Black pigment stones contain calcium bilirubinate, calcium carbonate, and calcium phosphonate. They are associated with hemolytic diseases, Crohn disease, ileal resection, cirrhosis, and total parental nutrition (TPN). Brown stones are observed more often in East Asia and are associated with liver fluke infection.

> **HELPFUL TIP:** Recent literature has shown that cholecystokinin infusion can decrease stones associated with TPN by preventing the biliary stasis that leads to calcium bilirubinate formation. This is generally not a problem in patients on short-term TPN.

* *

You refer the patient to your favorite surgical consultant for evaluation for cholecystectomy. However, before his surgery appointment, you see him again in the ED. He presents with fever, nausea, vomiting, and anorexia for the last 48 hours. His exam is significant for temperature 38.9°C, mild tachycardia and tachypnea, and a normal blood pressure. He is tender in the right upper quadrant and has an associated Murphy sign. He has no jaundice or palpable right upper quadrant mass.

Laboratory values include WBC 14,800/mm³, ALT 58 IU/L, AST 64 IU/L, alkaline phosphatase 45 IU/L, total bilirubin 1.5 mg/dL (mildly elevated liver enzymes and bilirubin), amylase 95 IU/L, and lipase 52 IU/L (normal amylase and lipase).

Your working diagnosis is now:

A) Acalculous cholecystitis.
B) Acute calculous cholecystitis.
C) Pancreatitis.
D) Ascending cholangitis.

Discussion

The correct answer is B. The clinical presentation, exam, and laboratory data point toward acute cholecystitis. Answer A is incorrect because **acalculous** cholecystitis occurs more often in critically ill hospitalized patients, and you already know that this patient has stones, so his cholecystitis is by definition **calculous** in nature. There must be no gallstones detected on ultrasound to diagnose acalculous cholecystitis. Answer C is incorrect. His pancreatic enzymes are normal (although one can certainly have pancreatitis with a normal amylase and lipase). Answer D is incorrect. Patients with ascending cholangitis usually have markedly elevated transaminases and an obstructive laboratory pattern (eg, elevated bilirubin, alkaline phosphatase, and pancreatic enzymes).

Regarding the differential diagnosis of complicated cholelithiasis, which of the following is true?

A) Empyema of the gallbladder is primarily a disease of the elderly and carries a high mortality rate due to associated Gram-positive sepsis.
B) Emphysematous cholecystitis occurs primarily in elderly diabetics as a late complication of miliary tuberculosis.
C) The most common consequence of gallbladder perforation is generalized peritonitis.
D) The triad of Charcot (jaundice, fever, and right upper quadrant pain) is associated with cholangitis.

Discussion

The correct answer is D. The classic triad of Charcot (jaundice, fever, and right upper quadrant pain) is associated with cholangitis, but it is **not** seen in the majority of cases, probably due to earlier detection of cholangitis. Nonetheless, it can be helpful if present. Answer A is incorrect because patients generally develop a Gram-**negative** sepsis. Answer B is incorrect because emphysematous cholecystitis is not a complication of miliary TB, but it can occur with anaerobic cholecystitis. Miliary TB rarely affects the gall bladder. Answer C is incorrect. The most common consequence of gallbladder perforation is a localized, walled-off abscess. Additionally, a cholecystenteric fistula may form between the gallbladder and the duodenum or jejunum. Stones can then pass into the bowel. Stones >2 cm in diameter are likely to lodge in the terminal ileum, a process termed gallstone ileus.

Generally, patients with cholecystitis typically have a prior history of biliary colic. Pain with acute cholecystitis is similar except is often more severe, longer lasting (>24 hours), and associated with anorexia, nausea, vomiting, fever, elevated white count (12,000–15,000), right upper quadrant guarding, and a positive Murphy sign

(arresting inspiration when palpating the gallbladder). **Murphy sign is only 65% sensitive (less in the elderly). Additionally, 38% with confirmed cholecystitis have neither leukocytosis nor fever.** About 15% of the time there is associated jaundice and 20% of the time there is a palpable mass in the right upper quadrant. Biliary pancreatitis can occur when there is blockage of the ampulla of Vater, and cholangitis occurs when there is ductal stone obstruction and biliary infection. Emphysematous cholecystitis occurs primarily in elderly male diabetics; gas-producing bacteria, most commonly *Clostridium perfringens*, results in gas in the gallbladder and causes a severe sepsis.

* *

Given the physical findings, leukocytosis, and mild elevation of transaminases, you conclude that this patient has cholecystitis.

Which of the following should NOT be considered in the management of this disease?

A) Initial treatment includes hospitalization with intravenous fluid resuscitation.
B) Possible antibiotic regimens include a third-generation cephalosporin, second-generation cephalosporin with metronidazole, or an aminoglycoside with metronidazole.
C) Most episodes of cholecystitis are caused by a single organism with enterococcus predominating.
D) If early cholecystectomy is not chosen as initial treatment, it should be performed late (at least 6 weeks after diagnosis).

Discussion

The correct answer is C. The initial treatment of cholecystitis includes hospitalization and intravenous fluid resuscitation. Most cholecystitis episodes are sterile, but because of the inability to determine which are secondarily infected, patients are routinely treated with antibiotics. Acceptable antibiotic regimens include a third-generation cephalosporin, second-generation cephalosporin with metronidazole, or an aminoglycoside with metronidazole. While enterococcus is frequently encountered, it is rarely a solitary pathogen and does not required specific targeted antimicrobial therapy. Definitive therapy for cholecystitis is cholecystectomy. Controversy surrounds whether cholecystectomy should be performed acutely or be delayed. Generally, shorter hospitalizations and better outcomes are found with early cholecystectomy.

Objectives: Did you learn to . . .

- Identify risk factors for gallstones?
- Recognize complications of gall bladder disease?
- Manage a patient with symptomatic gallstones and cholecystitis?

CASE 12

A 64-year-old male presents to the ED complaining of chest pain. He reports that he has had intermittent pain in the left subcostal area for the last 2 days. He denies any nausea, vomiting, diaphoresis, or radiation of symptoms. He does admit to a 6-month history of increasing shortness of breath both at rest and with exertion. In addition he reports an intermittent productive cough that has been worse over the last two weeks. He has lost about 15 pounds over the last 6 months. Past history is significant for a 100-pack-per-year history of tobacco. Otherwise, he has not been to a physician in over 10 years.

On your physical exam, he is afebrile, pulse is 105, respiratory rate 28, blood pressure 124/76, and oxygen saturation of 86% on room air. Cardiac exam shows a regular rhythm without murmur, gallops, or rub. Lung exam reveals dullness to percussion at the bilateral bases with decreased breath sounds throughout. Cardiac monitoring is significant only for sinus tachycardia. Chest x-ray shows large bilateral pleural effusions that layer-out on decubitus views. You initiate 4 liters of oxygen by nasal cannula and decide to perform a thoracentesis for both therapeutic and diagnostic measures. See Chapter 3, Pulmonary for discussion of differentiating exudate from transudate, technique of pleuracentesis, etc.

* *

You perform a pleuracentesis. The fluid you obtain is grossly bloody. Further analysis shows >300,000 RBC/mm³. Given that the patient has no history of trauma you are primarily concerned with pulmonary embolism or malignancy as a source for the bloody effusion. A spiral CT of the chest is obtained that demonstrates a mass in the left lower lobe without evidence of pulmonary embolism. You discuss these findings with the patient, telling him that they are consistent with lung cancer. You admit him for further evaluation and treatment of his dyspnea.

Which of the following statements is FALSE regarding this patient's lung cancer?

A) Most patients with lung cancer will have a symptomatic pleural effusion at some point in the course of their illness.
B) This patient most likely has adenocarcinoma.
C) If workup for distant metastasis is negative, this patient remains a surgical candidate.
D) Evaluation for distant metastases includes brain imaging and a bone scan.

Discussion

The correct answer is C. Once tumor has spread to the pleura, it is considered stage IIIB, and there is no benefit of surgical intervention. Since most lung cancers are found late, most are not amenable to surgery. Answer A is a true statement. More than 50% of patients with lung carcinoma will have a pleural effusion at some point in their disease. Answer B is a true statement. Adenocarcinoma is the most common type of lung cancer comprising 30%–40% of all lung cancers. Answer D is a true statement. Evaluation for distant metastases should include a head CT (the most common location for metastases) and a bone scan (vertebral spread is especially common).

 HELPFUL TIP: When a pleural effusion is grossly bloody and there is no history of trauma or pulmonary infarction, the likelihood of lung cancer is >90% with a prognosis of only 3–11 months.

Which of the following is true about lung cancer?

A) It is the leading cause of cancer death in women.
B) It is surpassed only by prostate cancer as a cause of cancer death in men.
C) It is surpassed only by cervical cancer as a cause of cancer deaths in women.
D) Deaths from breast, prostate, and colorectal cancer combined exceed the number of deaths from lung cancer.

Discussion

The correct answer is A. Lung cancer has exceeded breast cancer as the number one cause of cancer deaths in women. Of particular note is answer D. Deaths from lung cancer **exceed** the number of deaths from breast, prostate, and colorectal cancer **combined**.

* *

On the second day of his hospital stay, your patient's pleural fluid cytology returns consistent with adenocarcinoma.

Given this finding, which of the following statements is TRUE regarding tumor classification, prognosis, and recommended treatment?

A) The most common site for metastasis is bone.
B) The preferred treatment is chemotherapy and local radiation.
C) Thoracentesis has a high success rate in preventing the recurrence of pleural effusion.
D) This patient is likely to develop a second primary lung cancer in the next year.

Discussion

The correct answer is B. The preferred treatment is chemotherapy and radiation. Resection is (generally) not indicated in a patient with a malignant pleural effusion. Recall, however, that radiation can be poorly tolerated in patients with a malignant pleural effusion. The resulting radiation pneumonitis can negate any benefit.

Answer A is incorrect because the most common site of metastases is the brain. Answer C is incorrect. Although thoracentesis may help acutely with symptoms, the effusion tends to re-accumulate. Answer D is incorrect because it is not likely that there will be another **primary** tumor in the next year. This risk is only 2%–3%. Besides, this patient has a dismal prognosis, with a life expectancy <1 year.

* *

The cardiothoracic surgeon performs repeat thoracentesis with chest tube placement. Your patient tolerates the procedure well. Since the surgeon is at your hospital only every other day, he asks you to manage the chest tubes the following day.

What statement represents proper chest tube management?

A) A tube that shows no water fluctuations when placed on "water seal" should have wall suction increased to attempt to reopen.
B) Initial postoperative setting of a chest tube is most often –100 cm H_2O.

C) Unless there is major injury to the lung, continuous bubbling of the water seal chamber most likely represents an apparatus leakage.
D) If a purse-string was placed during initial placement of the chest tube, tightly tying the purse string when pulling the chest tube is enough to prevent pneumothorax.

Discussion

The correct answer is C. Continued bubbling in the water seal chamber suggests that there is a leak in the system. Theoretically, once the pleura are drained of air, there should be no further bubbling. Air leakage is seen as air bubbles that increase with increased intrathoracic pressure (eg, cough, Valsalva maneuver, and positive pressure ventilation). Continuous air leakage may be due to a large tear in the lung parenchyma, bronchopleural fistula, or an apparatus leak. Answer A is incorrect. A tube that is nonfunctional should be removed. Increasing the suction will not re-open it. Answer B is incorrect. Initial suction should be –20 cm H_2O. Answer D is incorrect because an occlusive dressing, such as petrolatum gauze, should be placed over the former chest tube site once the tube is removed. A chest tube can be removed when the following criteria are met: fluid drainage is <150 cc/day, the lung is fully expanded on chest x-ray, and no air leak is present in the water seal chamber. Typically, chest tubes are first placed to "water seal" for 6–24 hours to see if the patient will tolerate having the tube removed.

Objectives: Did you learn to . . .

- Evaluate a patient with a lung mass?
- Describe types of lung cancer and determine an appropriate treatment for a patient with lung cancer?
- Manage a patient with a chest tube in place?

CASE 13

A 28-year-old white male who was the restrained front-seat passenger of a vehicle traveling in excess of 60 mph is brought to the ED via ambulance. The driver of the vehicle was found dead at the scene. Ambulance personnel report it took 5–10 minutes to extricate the patient. On arrival, he is mumbling incoherently. He is initially able to give his name, but he is slurring his words. He denies any medical problems, medications, or allergies.

Vitals signs include temperature of 35.5°C, pulse 148, respirations 35, blood pressure of 65/30, and oxygen saturation of 81% on 100% oxygen by face mask. On exam, he is in severe respiratory distress. Lung sounds are absent on the right and diminished on the left. Heart sounds are muffled. You determine that this patient needs immediate treatment for a pneumothorax.

Which of the following is most appropriate at this time?

A) Perform needle decompression on the left.
B) Perform needle decompression on the right.
C) Place a chest tube on the left.
D) Place a chest tube on the right.
E) Perform a chest radiograph and act on the basis of the results.

Discussion

The correct answer is B. The combination of hypotension, hypoxia, and absent breath sounds suggests a tension pneumothorax. Immediate decompression of the affected hemithorax should be performed by placing a large-bore (14- or 16-gauge) needle through the chest wall to relieve intrathoracic pressure. Traditionally this was accomplished by placing a needle in the second intercostal space at the midclavicular line. However, due to high risk of mediastinal vascular injuries, current practices recommend placing the needle in the traditional location for chest tube—that is, the fifth or sixth intercostal spaces at the midaxillary line. Of necessary note is answer E. Tension pneumothorax **should never** be diagnosed on a chest radiograph. It is a true emergency that requires treatment on the basis of clinical exam.

* *

His vital signs and oxygen saturation improve with needle decompression. You place a chest tube and give boluses of normal saline through 2 peripheral IVs. Then, the patient is placed in external fixation device for his femur fracture. Operating room fixation is deferred secondary to unstable medical status. He is admitted to the intensive care unit on a respirator with C-collar following negative FAST examination (Focused Assessment with Sonography for Trauma, a sonographic evaluation to rule out fluid in perihepatic, perisplenic, pelvic, and pericardial spaces).

* *

Repeat chest x-ray in the ICU shows the endotracheal tube and chest tube in appropriate positions. Several rib fractures are noted. There are "fluffy infiltrates" in the left chest that were not present on initial trauma chest series.

Which of the following is true of this condition?

A) It occurs in <25% of patients with significant blunt trauma to the chest.
B) Treatment includes aggressive intravenous steroid and fluid administration.
C) The condition starts to resolve in 48–72 hours.
D) Treatment includes appropriate antibiotics.

Discussion

The correct answer is C. This condition, pulmonary contusion, begins to resolve in 48–72 hours. However, 2–3 weeks may be required for complete resolution. Answer A is incorrect. Pulmonary contusion occurs in up to 70% of trauma patients with **significant** blunt chest trauma. It is usually, but not always, associated with fractured ribs. There may also be a flail segment noted. A chest x-ray demonstrates an infiltrative pattern over the affected area usually about 1 hour post-trauma, but as long as 6–7 hours later. The condition results in a ventilation-perfusion mismatch and is associated with hypoxemia and an increased A-a gradient. If a patient is able to maintain oxygenation and ventilation, intubation may not be required. Answers B and D are incorrect. Treatment currently involves only intubation as necessary, observation, and tincture of time.

* *

You elect to proceed with pulmonary artery catheter placement due to the severity of this patient's condition. Overnight he begins to decompensate. The nurse pages you with his vital signs and Swan-Ganz readings: temperature 37.0°C, pulse 100, respirations 20 (ventilator set at 14), blood pressure 82/30, PCWP 24 mm Hg (normal 5–15), cardiac index 2.0 L/min/m^2 (normal 2.5–3.5), SVR 2000 dyne-sec/cm^2 (normal 1000–1500), and oxygen delivery of 700 ml/min (normal 900–1200).

What is the cause of shock now?

A) Hypovolemic shock.
B) Neurogenic shock.
C) Cardiogenic shock.
D) Septic shock.

Discussion

The correct answer is C. This patient appears to be in cardiogenic shock (elevated pulmonary capillary wedge

Table 22–5 CATEGORIZATION OF SHOCK BY PHYSIOLOGIC PARAMETERS

Type of Shock	Systemic Vascular Resistance	Pulmonary Capillary Wedge Pressure	Oxygen Consumption (based on venous gas)	Cardiac Output
Hypovolemic	Increased	Decreased	Decreased	Decreased
Cardiogenic	Increased	Increased	Decreased	Decreased
Distributive (sepsis, neurogenic)	Decreased	Decreased or normal	Increased	Increased
Obstructive (PE, vena caval obstruction, tension pneumonthorax)	Increased	Low left, high right	Decreased	Decreased

pressure, decreased cardiac index). Cardiogenic shock may be caused by myocardial failure, valve failure, dysrhythmias, and tamponade. Treatment is directed at the underlying disorder. See Table 22–5 for measurements in each type of shock.

 HELPFUL TIP: Note of caution: There is no good evidence to support the use of Swan-Ganz catheters in seriously ill patients. In fact, all of the evidence suggests **worse** outcomes with Swan-Ganz monitoring than without (from sepsis, thrombosis, etc). Be very circumspect before electing to use Swan-Ganz catheters.

* *

Part of the injuries sustained by this patient includes burns to the abdomen and back.

Which of the following statements is FALSE regarding burn wound management in general?

A) The Parkland formula for fluid resuscitation calls for 2–4 mL/kg/% body surface area burned with half of the volume in the first 8 hours and the other half over the next 16 hours.

B) Escharotomy should be performed on all partial-thickness burns.

C) Patients with chemical burns should be treated first with at least 30 minutes tap water irrigation.

D) Prevention of wound infection via topical antimicrobial agents, such as silver sulfadiazine cream, or via silver-coated dressings is the standard of care.

Discussion
The correct answer is B. Escharotomy is not necessary unless there is a full-thickness wound which is circumferential and compromising vascular supply. The thinking about this is changing and some suggest escharotomy of all **full-thickness** burns. Answer A is a true statement about the Parkland formula. Answer C is a true statement with the addendum that **any particulate matter should be brushed off prior to irrigation. Water may activate some substances such as sodium hydroxide.** Answer D is a true statement.

 HELPFUL TIP: Fluids are required for adults with >15% total body surface area (TBSA) burns (second- or third-degree) and >10% for children ≤10 years. For adults the "Rule of 9's" is used to determine TBSA affected. Body surface area is estimated as follows: the head, each arm, front of each leg, and back of each leg count for 9% BSA each; the front and back of the trunk each count for 18%; the remaining 1% BSA is accounted for by the genitalia. TBSA affected in children and adolescents should be based on age-specific charts. Both affected and unaffected BSA should be calculated to assure accurate estimation.

HELPFUL TIP: The Parkland formula was designed to assure adequate hydration in burn patients as reflected by urine output (in the patient with functioning kidneys, of course). Adjust fluids appropriately to maintain adequate hydration without inducing congestive heart failure.

Which of the following is TRUE regarding fluid administration in burn and dehydrated patients?

A) A peripheral line will deliver fluid more rapidly than a central line of an equivalent gauge.

B) Albumin is the fluid of choice in the treatment of burns and should be considered for all patients with significant fluid deficits.

C) D5 1/2 normal saline is the preferred fluid for fluid resuscitation in patients other than burn patients.

D) All of the above are true.

E) None of the above is true.

Discussion

The correct answer is A. A peripheral line will deliver fluid more rapidly than a central line of an equivalent gauge, according to Poiseuille law (flow is directly proportional to tube radius and inversely proportional to tube length). The **shorter** the catheter, the more quickly fluid is delivered (think of a short traffic jam as opposed to a longer one on the same-sized road). Answer B is incorrect. Albumin is not helpful and may increase adverse outcomes in trauma. Answer C is incorrect. Normal saline—or lactated Ringer if you are a surgeon—are the fluids of choice in treating dehydration. Remember that lactated Ringer is slightly hypotonic and thus may worsen cerebral edema. There is no evidence favoring lactated Ringer over normal saline.

Objectives: Did you learn to . . .

• Approach a trauma patient with an understanding of advanced trauma life support principles?

• Identify and manage a patient with a tension pneumothorax?

• Describe various types of shock and how they are differentiated?

• Treat a patient in shock?

• Manage a patient with significant burns?

 QUICK QUIZ: SURGERY

Carbonized particles in the nasal cavity and/or posterior pharynx should suggest:

A) The need for excision of the perichondrium in the nose to prevent underlying cartilage injury from avascular necrosis.

B) Inhalational injury to the lungs.

C) Ingestion of a large amount of particulate matter.

D) The need to check carboxyhemoglobin levels.

E) B and D.

Discussion

The correct answer is E. Carbonaceous material in the nares or oropharynx should suggest the possibility of an inhalation injury. Given that this is related in the inhalation of combusted material, a carboxyhemoglobin level should be considered.

CASE 14

A 48-year-old female arrives at the ED via ambulance after witnesses saw her vomiting large volumes of blood in a local convenience store before collapsing to the floor. She is barely communicating and cannot provide any history. Ambulance personnel have placed 2 large-bore IVs and started normal saline boluses. Just as you start your initial evaluation, she has a large volume hematemesis. You are concerned about her depressed mental status and the severity of her illness and decide to intubate her. After intubation, the chest wall rises symmetrically and the lungs sound clear. Her heart sounds are distant, and she is tachycardic (pulse 120). Her blood pressure is 80/40 mm Hg. Her oxygen saturation is 78%.

The standard of care in detecting esophageal intubation is:

A) Auscultation.

B) Radiograph.

C) End tidal CO_2.

D) Oxygen saturation.

E) None of the above.

Discussion

The correct answer is C. The standard of care is the end tidal CO_2. All of the others are notoriously unreliable.

However, they should all be done. If you think you hear breath sounds but the oxygen saturation is not rising and end tidal CO_2 is low, you are probably in the esophagus.

The end tidal CO_2 can be falsely negative (detecting no CO_2) in which of the following situations?

A) Ingestion of carbonated soft drinks.
B) Intubation in the posterior pharynx above the cords.
C) Nasotracheal intubation.
D) During cardiac arrest.

Discussion

The correct answer is D. The end tidal CO_2 requires that there be gas exchange in the lungs. If there is no gas exchange, the CO_2 will be low. This may be the case during cardiac arrest. Answer A can cause a **false-positive**. Carbon dioxide in the stomach will give a positive end tidal CO_2 with an esophageal intubation. The same is true of answer B. If the patient is breathing spontaneously, the CO_2 will be elevated even when the ET tube is above the cords. Answer C, nasotracheal intubation, should have no effect on end tidal CO_2.

* *

You order laboratory studies that include a CBC, basic metabolic profile, liver chemistries, amylase, lipase, and coagulation studies. In addition, you type and cross for 6 units of packed red blood cells. The nurses have already contacted the gastroenterologist on call, and she is on her way. You decide to perform nasogastric lavage.

Which of the following statements is FALSE regarding nasogastric lavage?

A) Nasogastric lavage may be negative even in the presence of an upper GI bleed.
B) Nasogastric lavage should not be attempted in obtunded patients until they are intubated.
C) Iced fluid should not be used to lavage patients with an upper GI bleed.
D) The placement of an NG tube is contraindicated in patients who may have variceal bleeding.

Discussion

The correct answer is D. Varices **are not** a contraindication to the use of an NG tube. Studies suggest that an NG tube does not increase bleeding. Both A and B are true statements. Lavage **should not** be done in patients who are obtunded or otherwise unable to protect their own airway unless they are intubated. **If the patient has**

obvious bleeding in the vomitus, NG lavage is not necessary unless it is to clear stomach contents in order to perform endoscopy or to prevent vomiting. It adds nothing to the management of the patient with an upper GI bleed except confirming the diagnosis. Remember that false-negative NG aspirates occur with intermittent bleeding and bleeding beyond the ligament of Treitz. Note that insertion of an NG tube is not contraindicated in the obtunded patient in order to clear the stomach. However, lavage, where you are introducing large amounts of fluid that can be aspirated, is contraindicated. C is a true statement. Iced lavage fluid should not be used in patients with a GI bleed. The cooler temperature that results from the ice inhibits hemostasis and can increase bleeding.

 HELPFUL TIP: Other contraindications to gastric lavage include known ingestion of hydrocarbons and caustic agents, such as alkalis and acids.

* *

While your nurse is performing the lavage, you perform a secondary physical examination on the patient. The most obvious finding is a markedly jaundiced state. Other pertinent findings include a 6-cm scalp laceration, which continues to actively bleed, moderate ascites, and lower extremity edema. After lavaging nearly 5 liters of isotonic fluid, the patient's aspirate continues to be bloody. Her vitals are remaining steady now but have shown no sign of improvement. Initial emergent labs have returned: Na 142 meq/L, K 3.2 meq/L, Cl 106 meq/L, CO_2 18 meq/L, BUN 40 mg/dL, Cr 0.8 mg/dL, glucose 110 mg/dL, WBC 7,000/mm^3, Hb 9.8 g/dL, HCT 29%, Plt 62,000/mm^3, INR 3.0, PTT 48, albumin 2.4 g/dL, AST 76 IU/L, ALT 39 IU/L, Bili 3.5 mg/dL, amylase 210 IU/L, lipase 24 IU/dL. The gastroenterologist is still 5–10 minutes away.

In considering what to do next, which of the following would be most appropriate?

A) Address presence of platelet dysfunction by transfusing with a ten-pack of platelets.
B) In order to accurately assess degree of volume depletion, place a central venous pressure catheter or Swan-Ganz catheter and bladder catheter.

C) Regardless of the gastroenterologist, central line placement should be priority at this time because fluid resuscitation is the primary concern.
D) Emergent gastric tamponade should be attempted with a Foley catheter.
E) None of the above is a great idea right about now.

 HELPFUL TIP: An elevated BUN can be indirect evidence of a GI bleed in patients with liver disease. The digestion of blood leads to the elevated BUN.

Discussion

The correct answer is E. None of the above is a particularly good idea right about now. Looking at them one by one: Answer A is incorrect because a platelet count of 62,000 is adequate for hemostasis (although you would not be faulted for giving platelets). A platelet count of <50,000 is considered an indication for platelet transfusion in an actively bleeding patient. Answers B and C are incorrect because coagulopathy (INR 3.0) is a **relative** contraindication to central line placement. It can be done but is not needed at this point. Recall from above that peripheral catheters will deliver more fluid more rapidly when compared to central catheters. Thus, two large-bore, peripheral IVs are the access of choice. Answer D is incorrect because gastric tamponade with a Foley is like trying to stop a leak in the Hoover dam with putty: it won't work. You may want to give vitamin K and fresh frozen plasma to reverse her coagulopathy, however.

Other effective methods for controlling upper GI variceal bleeding that improve outcomes include all of the following EXCEPT:

A) Variceal ligation.
B) Sclerotherapy.
C) TIPS procedure.
D) Vasopressin.

Discussion

The correct answer is D. Vasopressin, while achieving initial control of bleeding in up to 60% of patients, has essentially **no** effect on rebleeding and **no effect on mortality**. This may be because of splanchnic and other ischemia caused by vasopressin. More bad news, octreotide also does not have any effect on mortality unless combined with variceal ligation. Variceal ligation and sclerotherapy both reduce mortality. Additionally, a TIPS procedure (transjugular intrahepatic portosystemic shunt) has been shown to effectively stop bleeding by reducing portal pressures. It also reduces **acute** mortality. Unfortunately, a recent review showed no evidence of long-term advantage.

* *

You consider a central line.

Which of the following techniques is associated with the highest rate of infection?

A) External jugular.
B) Internal jugular.
C) Femoral vein.
D) Subclavian vein.

Discussion

The correct answer is C. Infection is more likely with cannulation of the femoral vein. This makes intuitive sense given its location. Subclavian veins have a higher risk of complication such as arterial injury, hemothorax, pneumothorax, and lung injury. Thoracic duct injury is most common with left internal jugular cannulation. **Ultrasound guidance of central lines is rapidly becoming the standard of care.**

The gastroenterologist arrives and you explain the situation. Vitals at this time include a temperature of 36.8°C, pulse 105, respirations 14 (ventilator dependent), blood pressure 85/40, and oxygen saturation of 92%. The gastroenterologist plans to attempt endoscopy with sclerotherapy, but would like to have the general surgeons available for back-up in case emergent operative intervention becomes necessary. As you prepare to contact the surgeon you recall risk stratification for cirrhotic patients is via the Child-Pugh classification system.

Which of the following statements is FALSE regarding the Child-Pugh scoring system?

A) The Child-Pugh scoring system can be used to predict the risk of variceal bleeding.
B) The 5 criteria used in the Child-Pugh classification are ascites, encephalopathy, albumin, bilirubin, and INR.
C) The Child-Pugh scoring system can be used to determine the outcome of hepatic encephalopathy.
D) A patient with a serum bilirubin of 3.5 mg/dL may have the same Child-Pugh score as a patient with a serum bilirubin of 25 mg/dL.

Discussion

The correct answer is C. The Child-Pugh scoring system does not predict the course of hepatic encephalopathy. The other statements are true. The Child-Pugh classification includes evaluation of ascites, history of encephalopathy, albumin, bilirubin, and INR. Answer A is true because the Child-Pugh score can be used to predict the risk of variceal bleeding as well as the surgical risk and the overall mortality in patients with liver disease. Answer D is true because there is a ceiling to the Child-Pugh scoring system for each parameter, and the same score is given for all bilirubin levels above 3 mg/dL.

The Child-Pugh classification as a global battery of tests can help to more accurately assess degree of cirrhosis, need for transplant (minimum score of 7), mortality rate from variceal bleed, and surgical candidacy for both cirrhotic and malignant liver disease (Table 22–6).

Class A is defined as having 5–6 points, class B is 7–9 points, and class C is 10–15 points. The 1- and 2-year survival in patients with class C disease is 45% alive at 1 year and 35% alive at 2 years.

Class A patients have an operative mortality of 1% while class B and C have operative mortalities of 3%–10% and 30%–50%, respectively. In patients with hepatomas, no class B or C patients survived 3–5 years following resection, although approximately 40% of class A patients survive for 5 years.

 HELPFUL TIP: In severely ill patients, a history of encephalopathy may not be obtainable. This is OK. Severely ill patients can still be a Child-Pugh Class C (the worst class) even with a "1" for hepatic encephalopathy.

 HELPFUL TIP: An easier system is the MELD (Model for End-stage Liver Disease) score. A number of calculators are available; here is one: www.unos.org/resources/MeldPeldCalculator.asp?index=98.

Objectives: Did you learn to . . .

- Manage a patient with a massive upper gastrointestinal bleed?
- Determine if an endotracheal tube has been placed correctly?
- Recognize the uses and limitations of gastric lavage?
- Recognize the uses and limitations of central line placement and Swan-Ganz catheter placement?
- Evaluate a patient with liver disease, using the Child-Pugh score and the MELD score?

 QUICK QUIZ: INTUBATION

Which of the following is NOT a contraindication to a nasotracheal intubation?

A) Patient is not breathing.
B) Patient is anticoagulated or has had TPA.
C) Midface trauma.
D) History of a septoplasty.
E) All of the above are contraindications.

Discussion

The correct answer is D. All of the rest are contraindications to nasotracheal intubation. Specifically, it is not possible to do a nasotracheal intubation in a non-breathing patient. Patients who are anticoagulated may

Table 22–6   CHILD-PUGH CLASSIFICATION SYSTEM

Points Assigned	1	2	3
Encephalopathy	None	Low-grade	High-grade
Ascites	None	Slight	Moderate-Large
Bilirubin	1–2 mg/dL	2–3 mg/dL	>3 mg/dL
Albumin	>3.5 g/dL	2.8–3.5 g/dL	<2.8 g/dL
INR	<1.7	1.8–2.3	>2.3

bleed profusely after a nasotracheal intubation, and midface trauma suggests the possibility that the tube could end up in the brain. **Although the standard of care, two studies have failed to show a difference between CNS complications with orotracheal versus nasotracheal intubation. Nonetheless, avoid nasotracheal intubation in midface trauma, except as a last resort, or you will get dinged if there is a complication.**

CASE 15

You are seeing a 33-year-old resident at a large university hospital setting where medical care is provided free to him. He is about to complete his Family Medicine residency and wants to "get his money's worth" of free procedures before he leaves. He has scheduled a full afternoon of procedures with you, including toenail removal, excision of a mole on his neck, and a cartilage ear piercing for his new job as a cruise ship doctor.

He has had trouble with recurrent pain and inflammation on his left great toe at the medial side. On exam you identify onychocryptosis (ingrown nail). He has tried soaks, growing past the skin, and regular paring—all without success.

Regarding nail removal in this patient, which one of the following statements is FALSE?

A) The great toe is the most commonly affected toe for onychocryptosis.

B) If the patient chooses partial nail removal, about 25% of the nail should be removed on the affected side.

C) Phenol should be placed for no longer than 10 seconds to the germinal tissue to prevent necrosis.

D) When removing the nail, an upward twist of the hand to the medial side should be performed.

Discussion

The correct answer is C. Phenol can be left in place for 3 minutes. Ingrown toenails almost exclusively affect the great toe on either the medial or lateral side. Partial or full nail removal should be implemented when conservative measures have failed. Besides ingrown nails (onychocryptosis), onychomycosis (fungal infection of the nail), recurrent paronychia (nail fold inflammation), and onychogryposis (deformed, curved nail) are all indications for partial or full nail removal. If recurrent ingrown nails have occurred, germinal tissue

can be ablated with phenol on a cotton swab held in place for 3 minutes, and afterwards the phenol should be neutralized with alcohol.

* *

Next, he complains about a small regular mole on his neck that he repeatedly cuts while shaving. He would like to have it removed in whatever way you deem best. The lesion is raised above the skin. Although it is mildly irregular in appearance from the repeated trauma of shaving, there is no evidence of atypia.

Which of the following is NOT a correct statement regarding removal of this lesion?

A) Curettage or shave biopsy would be ideal for this sort of lesion.

B) If sutures are required, 6-O nylon would be ideal in this location.

C) If a punch biopsy is performed, skin should be held taut perpendicular to the angle of the mandible (the natural skin lines of the neck).

D) In this location, both shave and punch techniques require closure by suture approximation.

Discussion

The correct answer is D. Various types of skin lesion removal exist: punch biopsy, shave biopsy, curettage biopsy, and elliptical excisional biopsy. Punch biopsy involves taking a full-thickness sample in skin areas except for the eyelids, lips, or penis. Skin should be held taut perpendicular to the natural skin tension lines and punch instrument is rotated through the skin. The site is closed with either a single interrupted or vertical mattress suture. Shave biopsy is indicated for removal of elevated skin lesions where complete thickness removal is unnecessary. Shave should be made from both lateral edges into center to avoid cutting too deep. No suturing is necessary. Curettage biopsy entails a method of removing lesions that also does not require full thickness sampling. A Fox dermal curettage is used to scrape away unwanted tissue followed by electrical or chemical cautery for hemostasis. Finally, elliptical excision is used when full dermal thickness excision is necessary. Contraindications to skin biopsy include infection at the site or coagulopathy.

* *

Your patient is a little embarrassed to be seen at the mall getting his ear pierced, and asks if you could pierce it for him. He is considering a standard lobe pierce versus an auricular cartilage piercing.

Which one of the following statements is TRUE in regards to counseling and technique?

A) Eczema at the site is a contraindication to piercing.

B) Auricular cartilage piercing should only be performed by a trained physician.

C) Ears should be pierced from the posterior to anterior site.

D) Ear piercing involves boring a 20-gauge needle to the marked site.

E) Ear piercing is contraindicated in nerds.

Discussion

The correct answer is A. Eczema in the area is a contraindication to piercing. Other contraindications include infection, previous keloid formation, immunodeficiency, and coagulopathy. Auricular cartilage piercing is prone to infection and generally least advisable—although it certainly is popular. All of the other answer choices are not true. Answer E requires special note, as nerds can be made hipsters simply by piercing their ears.

 HELPFUL TIP: Auricular cartilage piercing is prone to infection with destruction of the cartilage. Pseudomonas is a common pathogen and oral fluoroquinolones are indicated as treatment.

Objectives: Did you learn to . . .

- Describe techniques and indications for toenail removal?
- Describe various skin biopsy techniques?
- Identify contraindications to ear piercing?

BIBLIOGRAPHY

American College of Surgeons. *Advanced Trauma Life Support for Doctors: Student Course Manual.* 7th ed. Chicago: American College of Surgeons, 2004.

Cameron JL. *Current Surgical Therapy.* 9th ed. St Louis: Mosby, 2007.

Deziel DJ, et al. *Rush University Review of Surgery.* 3rd ed. Philadelphia: W.B. Saunders, 2000.

Graber MA, et al. *The Family Practice Handbook.* 5th ed. Philadelphia: W.B. Saunders, 2006.

Mulholland MW, et al. *Greenfield's Surgery: Scientific Principles and Practice.* 4th ed. Philadelphia: Lippincott Williams & Wilkins, 2006.

Lawrence PF. *Essentials of General Surgery.* 3rd ed. Philadelphia: Lippincott Williams & Wilkins, 2000.

Marino PL, et al. *The ICU Book.* 3rd ed. Philadelphia: Lippincott Williams & Wilkins, 2006.

Pfenninger JL, Fowler GC. *Procedures for Primary Care Physicians.* 2nd ed. St Louis: Mosby, 2003.

Sabiston DR Jr. *Textbook of Surgery: The Biological Basis of Modern Surgical Practice.* 15th ed. Philadelphia: WB Saunders, 1997.

Scott-Conner, CEH, Dawson DL. *Operative Anatomy.* 2nd ed. Philadelphia: Lippincott Williams & Wilkins, 2003.

Alison C. Abreu

CASE 1

You are seeing a 48-year-old female who presents with a 3-month history of low mood, low energy, poor concentration, and irritability. She has lost interest in most things she had enjoyed and has also noticed a 20-pound weight gain. She has been having frequent headaches, has been short tempered, and has noticed that it is hard to wake up in the morning. She reports no thoughts of suicide but has wondered if death would be a relief. She says she has felt restless for a while and feels that she is a bad person. Her mother suffered from depression. She does not consume alcohol or any other substances. She is divorced and has no children.

You think that this patient may meet criteria for a depressive disorder.

Which of the following is NOT a criterion for the diagnosis of major depressive disorder?

A) Low mood.
B) Presence of suicidal ideation.
C) Decreased appetite.
D) Anhedonia.
E) Irritability.

Discussion

The correct answer is E. The presence of irritability, although often seen with depressive disorders, is not used to make the diagnosis. All of the other answer choices listed are part of the criteria in the *Diagnostic and Statistical Manual of Mental Disorders*, 4th ed. (DSM-IV). Special emphasis must be placed on the presence of depressed mood and decreased interest, one of which must be present in order to diagnose major depressive disorder (MDD). The criteria for the diagnosis of a major depressive episode are 2 weeks or more of depressed mood **or** loss of interest **or** anhedonia **AND** 4 of the following: (1) significant change in weight or appetite, (2) insomnia or hypersomnia, (3) psychomotor agitation or retardation, (4) fatigue or loss of energy, (5) feeling worthless or (6) excessive guilt, poor concentration, (7) recurrent thoughts of death, suicidal ideation, attempt or plan.

 HELPFUL TIP: Two acronyms to help clinicians remember the DSM-IV criteria; are SIGECAPS and SPACEDIGS. The only difference between the two is that the latter includes **D**epression while it is assumed in the former.

Sleep	**S**leep
Interest	**P**sychomotor changes
Guilt	**A**ppetite
Energy	**C**oncentration
Concentration	**E**nergy
Appetite	**D**epression
Psychomotor changes	**I**rritability
Suicidality	**G**uilt
	Suicide

Which one of this patient's symptoms is considered a symptom of ATYPICAL depression?

A) Hypersomnia.
B) Low mood.
C) Anhedonia.
D) Psychomotor retardation.
E) Irritability.

Discussion

The correct answer is A. The typical vegetative symptoms of depression include poor sleep, reduced appetite and decreased libido. Patients with **atypical depression** have hyperphagia, hypersomnolence, and mood reactivity (a depressed mood that can brighten rapidly when positive changes occuar) among other symptoms.

* *

You begin to explain the nature of depression to this patient.

Which of the following epidemiological statements is NOT true?

A) The average American has about a 16 % chance of developing depression over his or her lifetime.
B) Approximately 7% of Americans suffer depression each year.
C) Women are five times as likely to get depression as men.
D) The incidence of depression is increasing in younger cohorts.
E) Divorced people are more likely to be depressed.

Discussion

The correct answer is C. Women are **twice (not 5 times)** as likely to have depression as are men. The rate becomes equal in the elderly with elderly men being at a higher risk of suicide than elderly women. Depression is a chronic illness that often begins early in life and is recurrent with significant morbidity and mortality. The lifetime prevalence of MDD is 16% with 6.6% of adults suffering from MDD in any given year. Being divorced is a risk factor for depression.

* *

Your patient reveals that she has also noticed being more anxious and fears going to work. You tell her that anxiety is common with depression.

In what percentage of patients with depression does anxiety coexist (not necessarily meeting DSM-IV criteria for an anxiety disorder)?

A) 1%
B) 30%
C) 70%
D) 95%

Discussion

The correct answer is C. A sizeable majority of patients with depression—up to 70%—also develop significant anxiety, manifesting in the form of psychomotor agitation, motor tension, excessive worry, etc. In fact, 60% of patients with a lifetime diagnosis of MDD have had a **diagnosable anxiety disorder**; while up to 66% of patients with a diagnosis of MDD within the past year also had a diagnosis of anxiety disorder. Only in about 14% of patients did the diagnosis of MDD precede the diagnosis of anxiety disorder.

* *

This patient's situation is not unusual for your practice.

What is the prevalence of major depressive disorder in primary care patients?

A) 1–2%
B) 5–10%
C) 25–30%
D) 45–50%
E) 100%

Discussion

The correct answer is B. Up to 5%–10% of primary care patients meet criteria for MDD and about twice that many (10%–20%) have "minor" depression.

Which of these epidemiological statements about depression in primary care is true?

A) Most depressed patients (~80%) seek their care from primary care physicians.
B) Only about 50% of patients with depression are recognized by their primary care physician.
C) Only about 50% of patients diagnosed with MDD receive adequate treatment.
D) The United States Preventive Task Force (USPTF) recommends screening all primary care patients for depression.
E) All of the above.

Discussion

The correct answer is E. Most depressed patients seek care from their primary care physician. However, only 50% of these are recognized and diagnosed appropriately.

Reasons for this are myriad and include decreased severity of presentation in primary care settings when compared to presentations to an emergency department or psychiatrist. Other reasons include somatic presentations (multiple medical complaints without a physiologic basis); lack of time for the busy clinician; patient reluctance to admit to depressive symptoms; and lack of systematic screening. Given the prevalence of depression in primary care (up to 10%) and the substantial morbidity and mortality resulting from it, the USPTF recommends screening for all primary care patients. Of the roughly 50% of patients with MDD who are correctly diagnosed, only 40% are adequately treated, meaning that 4 out of 5 patients with depression are not adequately treated!

> **HELPFUL TIP:** There are several brief self-rating depression scales that can be used for screening (eg, Beck Depression Inventory, Primary Care Evaluation of Mental Disorders, Patient Health Questionnaire, Zung Depression Scale, etc). A two-question patient screen may be as effective for screening as these more extensive scales. Simply ask:
>   Over the past 2 weeks, have you often felt down, blue, or in the dumps?
>   Over the past 2 weeks, have you lost interest in most activities or things that used to bring you pleasure?
> A positive answer to either of those two questions should prompt a more thorough evaluation of depression. A negative answer to both effectively rules out depression in most patients.

* *

You realize that it is also important to focus on the social history in patients with depression.

Which of the following is associated with a DECREASED risk of depression?

A) Unemployment.
B) Poverty.
C) Being unmarried.
D) Family history.
E) Black race.

Discussion

The correct answer is E. Factors associated with an increased risk of depression include **female gender**

(2X risk), unemployment, poverty, being unmarried (single or divorced), having a family history of depression, a recent childbirth or pregnancy, medical comorbidities, lack of social support, and substance use. Protective factors include marriage, black race, and being retired.

* *

You believe that your patient is suffering from an episode of major depression, and you decide to initiate treatment with an antidepressant.

Following the first episode of depression, what is her risk of relapse?

A) <1%
B) 25%
C) 50%
D) 75%
E) >99%

Discussion

The correct answer is C. The incidence of relapse following the first episode of depression is roughly 50%; this can be reduced by two-thirds by continuing antidepressant medications chronically. Following the second episode, the risk of relapse is roughly 75%, increasing to 90% after the third episode. In order to reduce the risk of relapse, most authorities recommend antidepressant therapy for 6–12 months after remission of symptoms in patients with their first episode of depression. Some patients probably benefit from indefinite medical therapy, including those with a severe first episode (eg, significant suicide attempt); patients with a psychotic depression; patients with three or more episodes (as their risk approaches 100%); elderly patients with their first episode of depression; and possibly those with a strong family history of depression.

* *

You choose a serotonin reuptake inhibitor (SSRI) and tell your patient to contact you if she suffers from adverse effects.

Which of the following is NOT a typical adverse effect of SSRIs?

A) Nausea.
B) Headaches.
C) Restlessness.
D) Insomnia.
E) Urinary retention.

Discussion

The correct answer is E. Urinary retention is not seen with SSRIs. The other four answer choices are typical adverse effects of SSRIs. The anticholinergic effect of urinary retention is typical of the tricyclic antidepressants (TCAs). For SSRIs, most of the adverse effects are transient and time limited, and most patients can tolerate them. Sexual dysfunction and gastrointestinal problems are also common. Akathisia can also occur as can (rarely) dystonic reactions.

* *

Your patient returns to see you 2 weeks after starting her SSRI and reports that she has not noticed any benefit from the medication.

Which of the following statements is most accurate?

A) The antidepressant is not going to work, so she should switch medicines to one of the same class.
B) The antidepressant is not going to work, so she should switch medicines to another antidepressant from a different class.
C) It is too early to judge the efficacy of the antidepressant now.
D) Antidepressants begin working within 3–4 days.
E) Going up on the dose is not an option at this time.

Discussion

The correct answer is C. Antidepressants begin to exert their **biological** effects immediately with increases in neurotransmitters but the effects on mood are not apparent for about 2–4 weeks. As such, it is premature to abandon this medication. Increasing the dose **or** giving it at least 2 weeks more at the current therapeutic dose are the best options.

* *

You increase the medication dose, and the patient returns to see you in another 2 weeks. This time, she is feeling better and more energetic. People at work are beginning to notice her improved attitude, and her sleep has become more refreshing now. She wants to know how long she should stay on the medication.

The correct answer is:

A) At least 1 month.
B) At least 2 months.
C) At least 4–6 months.
D) At least 2 years.
E) Forever.

Discussion

The correct answer is C. Different organizations recommend different durations of treatment but the shortest recommended course is 4–6 months, with most authorities treating for 6–12 months after recovery.

Objectives: Did you learn to . . .

- Diagnose major depressive disorder?
- Appreciate the epidemiology and course of depression?
- Recognize features of atypical depression?
- Initiate treatment for depression?
- Identify adverse effects of SSRIs?

CASE 2

You are assessing a 45-year-old professional male who has a history of MDD in his early twenties but has fully recovered since then. He recently suffered an uncomplicated anterior wall myocardial infarction (MI). His wife mentions that she thinks he is depressed. He is tired all the time, has poor sleep, a poor appetite, and he has been irritable. He has also been tearful and blames himself for his MI (too many burgers . . . with cheese and bacon). He is willing to consider the diagnosis of depression because he remembers having suffered from it before. He also knows a history of MDD puts him at risk of medical illnesses.

Which of the following illnesses is more prevalent in patients with MDD?

A) Coronary heart disease.
B) Cerebrovascular disease.
C) Diabetes mellitus.
D) Osteoporosis.
E) All of the above are more prevalent in depressed patients.

Discussion

The correct answer is E. **It is unclear if patients with depression are more likely to have these illnesses as a result of the depression or the reverse; patients with these illnesses are more likely to be depressed.** Depressed patients have an average of 3.4 more chronic conditions than nondepressed patients. Patients with depression are more likely to have MIs, strokes, diabetes, and osteoporosis. At least two studies have now linked a lifetime history of MDD to an increased risk (1.2–3 times) of early menopause.

* *

You know that some of this patient's symptoms could be secondary to his medical illness.

Which one of the following symptoms, if present, is the MOST SPECIFIC for depression?

A) Sleep problems.
B) Appetite difficulties.
C) Psychomotor agitation.
D) Low energy.
E) Excessive preoccupation with death.

Discussion

The correct answer is E. In the acronym SPACE DIGS, the last four letters stand for symptoms that are specific for depression and more independent of somatic illnesses. These symptoms are **D**epressed mood, loss of **I**nterests, inappropriate **G**uilt, and thoughts of **S**uicide (DIGS). The presence of any of these symptoms should lead you to suspect depression.

 HELPFUL TIP: Although depression can often be precipitated by a stressor, it can also arise with no precipitating factor, and the response to treatment is independent of whether it is "reactive" (identifiable stressor present) or "endogenous" (no identifiable stressor).

Which of the following statements is NOT true about depression post-MI?

A) Major depression is an independent risk factor for post-MI mortality.
B) Minor depression is an independent risk factor for post-MI mortality.
C) Minor depression is more prevalent than major depression post-MI.
D) Treating depression improves cardiac outcomes in post-MI patients.
E) Approximately half of the people who sustain an MI have symptoms of depression afterwards.

Discussion

The correct answer is D. In the post-MI period, major depression prevalence is almost 20%, and minor depression is about 27%. Concurrent major depression elevates mortality risk after MI by a factor of 3.5, which is the same degree of risk as CHF. Patients with a mood disturbance (eg, minor depression) also have a higher incidence of mortality. Although treatment of depression has been shown to improve some medical outcomes (eg, HbA1c levels in diabetics), this is not the case in cardiovascular disease. Treatment of depression does not change mortality or morbidity after an MI.

 HELPFUL TIP: There is some recent data suggesting that SSRIs may reduce recurrent events in the depressed post-MI patient. It may have to do with their antidepressant effect or, perhaps, their antiplatelet effect. The data is not the most robust, however.

 HELPFUL TIP: Patients suffering strokes also have an elevated risk of depression with approximately 33% of poststroke patients meeting criteria for MDD; there is a similar correlation of depressive symptoms to stroke mortality.

* *

You decide to recommend treatment to this patient.

Which of the following therapies would NOT be a good choice for treating his depression?

A) Bupropion (Wellbutrin).
B) Interpersonal psychotherapy (IPT).
C) Nortriptyline.
D) Paroxetine (Paxil).
E) Sertraline (Zoloft).

Discussion

The correct answer is C. Tricyclic antidepressants should be avoided in patients with cardiovascular disease because of their arrhythmogenic potential (eg, torsade de pointes). The safety of SSRIs has been demonstrated in a number of studies in cardiac patients. Also, bupropion has been proven safe in this population. Psychotherapy, particularly IPT and Cognitive Behavior Therapy (CBT), has also proven effective in this population.

HELPFUL TIP: Consider a baseline ECG in all patients for whom you consider tricyclics to evaluate the QT interval. If the QT is prolonged at baseline, it predisposes patients to tricyclic-induced arrhythmias.

Objectives: Did you learn to . . .

- Diagnose depression occurring with an acute medical illness?
- Recognize the impact of depression on other medical conditions?
- Treat a post-MI patient with depression?

 QUICK QUIZ: PSYCHIATRIC DIAGNOSIS

A 44-year-old patient of yours has come to see you multiple times for low mood. She does not have trouble with energy, sleep, concentration, or appetite. She tells you, "I've been depressed for as long as I can remember." You have tried treating her with 2 different SSRIs, but she had trouble with side effects and did not notice much improvement in her mood.

Which of the following is the best diagnosis for this patient?

A) Adjustment disorder.
B) Bipolar affective disorder.
C) Dysthymia.
D) Major depressive disorder.
E) Premenstrual dysphoric disorder.

Discussion

The correct answer is C. Dysthymia is best understood as long-term, low-level depressive symptoms that do not meet criteria for major depressive disorder. Dysthymic symptoms include depressed mood most days for at least 2 years and 2 or more of the following 6 symptoms: appetite change, sleep disturbance, low energy or fatigue, low self-esteem, concentration difficulties, and hopelessness. In order to diagnose dysthymia, the person cannot be free of the symptoms for >2 months during the first 2 years. Treatment is the same as for depression with primary care efficacy studies showing response to SSRIs and psychotherapy. Many people with dysthymia may also experience 1 or more episodes of MDD in their lifetime (often called "double depression").

CASE 3

A 34-year-old female presents to your clinic for treatment of depression. She reports a lifelong history of low-level depressive symptoms that have worsened over the past 6 months since she lost her job. She also suffers from inadequately controlled diabetes mellitus (Hb A1C 8.0 %) and has been diagnosed with a personality disorder in the past. She drinks 3–4 beers everyday and has been arrested for driving while intoxicated twice. On questioning, you realize she has a moderately severe level of depression. She is not suicidal so you decide to initiate treatment as an outpatient with close follow-up.

Which of these factors does NOT contribute to a poor outcome when treating depression?

A) Chronic depressive symptoms.
B) Female gender.
C) Personality disorder.
D) Comorbid medical conditions.
E) Alcoholism.

Discussion

The correct answer is B. Even though females are twice as likely to get depressed as males, gender does not seem to influence treatment response. The presence of any of the other factors listed reduces the chance of a successful response to treatment.

* *

In choosing an antidepressant for this patient, you would like to use one with a high success rate. However, you know that the success rates for most antidepressants are fairly similar.

What are the chances of this patient's failing to respond to the first antidepressant chosen?

A) <1%
B) 10–20%
C) 30–40%
D) 60–70%
E) 90–95%

Discussion

The correct answer is C. Studies have consistently shown an antidepressant response rate of somewhere between 60%–70% with 30%–40% failing to respond, regardless of what antidepressant is tried. When unpublished studies are included, the failure rate for SSRIs approaches 50%.

> **HELPFUL TIP:** 50% of patients who do not respond to an initial SSRI will respond to another drug in the same class. So, changing to another SSRI is reasonable in a patient who has failed one SSRI. Is this observed effect due to differences between drugs, pharmacodynamics, or just longer treatment? No one knows.

* *

You start a different drug, venlafaxine (Effexor). Ten days later, your patient calls you just to say that the new medicine seems no better and her sleep is even worse. She started taking the medication in the morning because she thought it might be interfering with her sleep. She tends to lie in bed for 2 hours before falling asleep.

In addition to recommending good sleep hygiene and increased exercise, you prescribe:

A) Trazodone.
B) Zolpidem.
C) Lorazepam.
D) Phenobarbital.

Discussion

The correct answer is A. Trazodone is often added to help with insomnia and boost serotonergic activity. For depression, it is preferred to benzodiazepines unless anxiety is a significant issue. Phenobarbital should be avoided. Zolpidem might be a consideration, but trazodone is preferred in patients with depression.

> **HELPFUL TIP:** Indications for psychiatric referral include:
> - Failure of medical treatment
> - Imminent suicidality
> - Severe depression for which hospitalization is thought to be necessary
> - Diagnosti clarification or treatment recommendation
> - Comorbidities which make treatment response less likely
> - Patient requests referral

* *

After switching to venlafaxine and titrating up to the maximum dose, your patient's symptoms are now coming under control. When you see her next, she describes a 20-minute episode of chest tightness, dyspnea, diaphoresis, and extreme anxiety. You believe that she suffered a panic attack. You wonder if you should alter your diagnosis.

In which of the following disorders do panic attacks NOT occur?

A) Panic disorder.
B) Major depressive disorder.
C) Generalized anxiety disorder.
D) Social phobia.
E) None of the above.

Discussion

The correct answer is E. Panic attacks are a cluster of symptoms signifying anxiety and are not a disorder by themselves. As such, they can be part of any affective syndrome and are frequently seen in a variety of syndromes including those mentioned above. The presence of a single panic attack in a person with a depressive disorder should not necessarily lead to a new diagnosis.

Objectives: Did you learn to . . .

- Identify risk factors for a poor outcome when treating depression?
- Assess the likelihood of a successful outcome in a patient with depression?
- Generate alternative methods for treating resistant depression?

CASE 4

A 41-year-old female comes to your office with complaint of difficulty trusting people, irritability, low mood, and recurrent nightmares. Her symptoms started when she was a teenager following the death of her parents in a house fire. She was rescued by firefighters but has never been able to forgive herself for surviving when her parents died. She has not been able to form close relationships, and she is seeking help because of renewed nightmares. They were common in the first 2 years following the incident but had faded away until recently. Continuing news reports of terrorist activities and bombings have brought all of this back to the forefront again. She sometimes wakes up in a fright after dreaming that her own house is on fire. She is afraid to go near any bright lights or fireworks displays. When she is forced to be in the presence of fires, she frequently notices palpitations, dyspnea, and a sense of doom.

What is the patient's primary diagnosis?

A) Major depressive disorder.
B) Generalized anxiety disorder.
C) Panic disorder.
D) Posttraumatic stress disorder.
E) Dysthymia.

Discussion

The correct answer is D. The patient's symptoms are characteristic of posttraumatic stress disorder (PTSD), which arises after one has been exposed to a situation in which one's life or "physical integrity" is in danger.

Which of the following is NOT necessary for a diagnosis of PTSD?

A) The patient needs to experience, witness, or be confronted by a potentially lifethreatening event, or an event threatening the physical integrity of the patient or others.
B) The patient must respond with intense fear, horror, or helplessness.
C) Symptoms have to be present for more than 1 month.
D) The patient must be involved in combat.
E) The patient must meet a specified number of symptoms.

Discussion

The correct answer is D. Although PTSD is common among military veterans, there is no specified criterion that the patient must have been in combat. To meet criteria for PTSD, the patient must have been exposed to an event that is threatening to the integrity or life of the patient or another. Such events are as varied as combat, rape, assault, cancer, or an intensive care unit stay. The patient then has recurrent intense fear, helplessness, or horror that lasts for more than 1 month. Symptoms occurring within 4 weeks of the event and lasting for at least 2 days but <1 month can qualify for the diagnosis of acute stress disorder.

Which of the following is NOT a part of PTSD?

A) Nightmares.
B) Flashbacks.
C) Hypervigilance.
D) Fear of death.
E) Difficulty maintaining relationships.

Discussion

The correct answer is D. Fear of death is not a criterion. Symptoms of PTSD are divided into 3 clusters. To meet the symptom criteria for PTSD, the patient needs 1 symptom from the first cluster, 3 from the second, and 2 from the third.

The **first cluster** involves reexperiencing a previous traumatic experience (eg, flashbacks, nightmares, psychological distress in response to triggers that evoke the experience).

The **second cluster** involves avoidance of stimuli associated with the trauma (efforts to avoid thoughts, feelings, or conversations associated with the trauma; efforts to avoid activities, places, or people that arouse recollections of the trauma; inability to recall an important aspect of the trauma); a numbing of general responsiveness (markedly diminished interest or participation in significant activities; feeling of detachment or estrangement from others; restricted range of affect; a sense of a foreshortened future).

The **third cluster** involves persistent symptoms of increased arousal, such as difficulty falling or staying asleep, irritability or outbursts of anger, difficulty concentrating, hypervigilance, or an exaggerated startle response.

Which of the following is TRUE of treatment for PTSD?

A) There is no effective treatment.
B) There are no FDA-approved medications
C) Most patients spontaneously remit.
D) Though treatment is often effective, most patients do not achieve cure.
E) Atypical antipsychotics have no role in treatment.

Discussion

The correct answer is D. Symptom improvement, but not cure, is the norm. Paroxetine and sertraline are FDA approved for the treatment of PTSD, although data supports the efficacy of other agents including the other SSRIs, MAOIs, TCAs, and nefazodone. Case reports suggest that prazosin, the α-blocker, can be useful for nightmares, and atypical antipsychotics have been found useful as adjunctive treatment. Psychotherapy can be helpful and benzodiazepine use should be limited because of the high risk of dependency in this population and the lack of efficacy as monotherapy.

Objectives: Did you learn to . . .

- Recognize risk factors for PTSD?
- Diagnose PTSD?
- Treat PTSD?

CASE 5

A 29-year-old female presents to you for a second opinion, and brings a large stack of medical records with her. She says that this is more like a "fourth or fifth opinion." Although you find many negative diagnostic studies in her record, she is sure that her many symptoms must have some physical cause. Over the last few years she has had chronic headaches, multiple joint pains, and intermittent abdominal and chest pains. She has diarrhea and bloating on occasions, but upper endoscopy, colonoscopy, CT scans, and other studies have not revealed an etiology. She reports severe anxiety that has worsened with the onset of "seizures" in the last year (and you note that brain MRI, EEG, and neurologic exam at the time did not support a seizure disorder). Additionally, she complains of some vague weakness and numbness and thinks that she might have had a stroke. Finally, she complains of pain with sexual intercourse. Nothing she does improves any of these symptoms. Further review of her records shows a variety of diagnoses from different physicians: "chronic pain syndrome," "chronic fatigue," "fibromyalgia," "irritable bowel syndrome," "premenstrual syndrome," and others.

Which of the following is the most likely primary diagnosis?

A) Hypochondriasis.
B) Somatization disorder.
C) Generalized anxiety disorder.
D) Factitious disorder.
E) Conversion disorder.

Discussion

The correct answer is B. Typically, patients with unexplained symptoms see many doctors, have numerous tests, and often undergo a variety of procedures. At the outset, it is important to consider a primary psychiatric disorder, but a thorough and appropriate evaluation into possible organic causes should be completed before a psychiatric diagnosis is reached. Many times patients with unexplained symptoms will ultimately be diagnosed with a somatoform disorder (of which answers A, B, and E are all types).

This patient presents with somatization disorder, which by definition must have 4 pain symptoms: 2 gastrointestinal symptoms, 1 sexual symptom, 1 pseudoneurological symptom. Also, in order to diagnose somatization disorder, the complaints must have started <30 years, have no identifiable organic basis, and not be intentionally feigned.

Answer A is incorrect. Hypochondriasis is characterized by a preoccupation that one has some sort of serious disease based on misinterpretation of bodily cues. Answer C is incorrect because anxiety is present but totally overshadowed by the somatic complaints. Answer D, factitious disorder, is diagnosed in patients who intentionally produce symptoms (eg, overdosing on insulin, injecting feces into the bloodstream) to assume the "sick role." Answer E is incorrect. With conversion disorder, patients present with sudden onset of anatomically implausible neurologic symptoms (eg, whole body numbness, bilateral deafness, etc).

* *

You believe that this patient has somatization disorder.

You begin by saying:

A) "Relax. This is all in your head."
B) "Your pain isn't real. But your psychiatric illness is. It's called somatization disorder."
C) "You have a number of symptoms that are very real but cannot be explained by our investigations. The evidence suggests that you do not have any life-threatening illnesses. You have a well-defined disorder, and other patients have similar problems."
D) "You have a lot of very serious symptoms. But my physical exam is inconsistent with your complaints. Basically, I don't believe a word you're saying. The sooner that you admit to falsifying these symptoms, the sooner I can start helping you."

Discussion

The correct answer is C. In patients with somatization disorder, it is best to use an honest but gentle approach.

Most patients feel better if they have a name for an illness, but using the term "somatization disorder" may actually be detrimental. It is important to affirm the patient's symptoms (these are real problems) and to try to find some common language to use to describe what he or she is feeling. Patients may not be receptive to your interpretation initially, but repeating the discussion at subsequent visits and focusing on normal diagnostic tests may help them accept the diagnosis.

* *

Next, you discuss a plan of action with this patient.

You recommend:

A) A multidisciplinary approach, utilizing many different specialty services.
B) Starting an SSRI.
C) Starting electroconvulsive therapy (ECT).
D) Monthly visits with you and limited diagnostic testing and specialty consultation.
E) Referral for exploratory laparotomy.

Discussion

The correct answer is D. It is best to have patients with somatization disorder establish regular clinic visits, typically with one provider. Unscheduled visits to the ED should be discouraged unless first discussed with the primary provider. Patients should be allowed to discuss all of their complaints, and a physical exam should be performed at every office visit. These measures will let the patients know that their concerns are being taken seriously. Lab tests, radiographs, and consultations should be limited, with the clinician using his or her best judgment as to when such diagnostic tests are indicated. Answers B and C are incorrect because SSRIs and ECT are not accepted therapy for somatization disorder.

 HELPFUL TIP: In patients who are willing to be referred to psychiatry, individual psychotherapy, cognitive behavioral therapy, and group therapy may be beneficial.

Objectives: Did you learn to . . .

- Recognize and describe various somatoform disorders?
- Generate an appropriate plan for a patient with somatization disorder?

CASE 6

A 21-year-old college student presents to your office for evaluation. She complains of feeling stressed out. She is taking classes full-time and is also in one of the military reserve units at the college. One weekend each month, she must attend drill which involves handling weapons. Although she did not have problems handling the weapons initially, she now gets very emotional and upset when she thinks about having to use them at the next drill weekend. She is nervous and is afraid that she might accidentally fire a weapon. She knows that her fears are silly and she has been telling herself to "just get over it." Last weekend, at drill, she suddenly felt that she was going to have a heart attack. She developed tightness in her chest, her heart was racing, and she felt unable to breathe. Although the symptoms eventually abated, the episode made her even more alarmed, and now she is worried that it will happen again and she will have a heart attack. She comes to see if you can help.

Which of the following is UNNECESSARY for the initial workup?

A) Take more medical, psychiatric, and family history.
B) Order an echocardiogram.
C) Perform a physical exam.
D) Order thyroid function tests.

Discussion

The correct answer is B. Given the information you have so far, an echocardiogram is not indicated and is rarely used as part of a primary workup. When it comes to test questions, never say no to more history (unless you are supposed to be managing a patient's airway). A complete history and physical exam are essential in the evaluation of this new patient. Thyroid abnormalities can be a cause of some of these symptoms, including palpitations and chest tightness.

* *

She has no prior psychiatric history, but her mother is taking medication for depression. While taking her social history, you ask questions regarding substance abuse.

Use of which of the following substances might explain her symptoms?

A) Nicotine.
B) Alcohol.

C) Caffeine.

D) Herbal weight loss medication.

E) Any of the above.

Discussion

The correct answer is E. Many substances can cause symptoms like this patient has. These include stimulants, such as caffeine and nicotine, and some herbal weight loss products containing ephedra (*Ma Huang*). Withdrawal from hypnotics like alcohol can also lead to similar symptoms.

* *

She does not smoke, drinks alcohol occasionally, and drinks coffee on weekday mornings before class. Her physical exam is normal. Her mental status exam is remarkable for a neutral mood, a restricted and anxious affect, but no suicidal thoughts and no psychotic symptoms. The laboratory tests you order are normal. You are leaning towards a psychiatric diagnosis at this point, specifically an anxiety disorder.

Which of the following is NOT an anxiety disorder?

A) Panic disorder.

B) Obsessive-compulsive disorder.

C) Posttraumatic stress disorder.

D) Generalized anxiety disorder.

E) Delirium.

Discussion

The correct answer is E. Delirium, while it may present with features similar to an anxiety disorder, is a cognitive disorder. Anxiety disorders are the most common form of mental illness in the United States, affecting about 19.1 million people or 13% of the adult population. They include answers choices A through D as well as social anxiety disorder (social phobia), specific phobias, acute stress disorder, anxiety disorder not otherwise specified, and anxiety disorders that are judged to be secondary to a medical condition or a substance.

* *

Of the listed anxiety disorders, you think she has developed panic disorder and that she has been having panic attacks.

Which of the following would NOT be a typical symptom of a panic attack?

A) Palpitations.

B) Diaphoresis.

C) Syncope.

D) Dyspnea.

E) Dizziness.

Discussion

The correct answer is C. The symptoms of a panic attack are those associated with an activation of the "fight-or-flee response," or the overactivation of the sympathetic nervous system. Typical symptoms include palpitations, sweating, trembling, dyspnea, a sense of smothering, fear of dying, chest pain, nausea, dizziness, numbness and tingling, and derealization or depersonalization. It would be rare for a patient to actually lose consciousness from a panic attack (though they may feel they might), and actual syncope should force one to look for an alternate diagnosis.

 HELPFUL TIP: Hyperventilation can cause cerebral vasoconstriction and secondary cerebral hypoxia resulting in syncope. However, this is pretty unusual.

* *

To make your diagnosis of panic disorder, the patient needs to meet specific DSM-IV criteria.

Which of these is NOT a criterion for panic disorder?

A) Recurrent and unexpected panic attacks.

B) At least 1 month of worry about having more attacks.

C) Worry about the implication of the attack or its consequences (dying, "going crazy," etc).

D) Change in behavior related to the attacks.

E) Predictable panic attacks that occur in response to cues.

Discussion

The correct answer is E. The criteria for panic disorder do not include predictable panic attacks in response to cues. After patients have had repeated panic attacks, they often develop phobic avoidance of places, objects, or events associated with their symptoms (agoraphobia). This is a symptom that indicates very severe panic disorder. Patients often scout out routes of escape before going to places that might provoke an attack.

HELPFUL TIP: The vast majority of patients with panic disorder present with somatic complaints rather than cognitive or mood symptoms. Patients are often misdiagnosed initially. Consider panic attacks in patients presenting with the appropriate somatic symptoms.

* *

Your patient is worried that these attacks will keep occurring.

How would you best describe the prognosis for panic disorder?

A) It is easily curable in most patients.
B) There is no effective treatment for it.
C) Most patients do not improve over time.
D) It is a recurrent or chronic illness.
E) None of the above.

Discussion

The correct answer is D. Panic disorder is a recurrent or chronic disease in most patients. Answers A and C are incorrect. Although panic disorder is not easily curable, almost all patients will improve over time, but very few attain complete remission even with medical treatment. Relapse is common.

* *

The patient is, of course, very concerned about future panic attacks. She asks what to do when another occurs.

You advise her to do all of the following EXCEPT:

A) Move to a quiet area.
B) Slow down her breathing.
C) Reassure herself that she is not dying.
D) Breathe into a brown paper bag.
E) Avoid stimulants like caffeine or nicotine.

Discussion

The correct answer is D. Although commonly observed in popular lore, breathing into a paper bag is not recommended. Breathing into a brown paper bag can have the opposite effect of that intended—the patient may continue hyperventilating with CO_2 building up, which may contribute to more panic symptoms. All of the other answer choices are reasonable recommendations

for a patient suffering from panic attacks. Educating the patient on hyperventilation and helping her consciously slow her breathing may help abort the panic attack. Quiet rooms and reassurance can also help.

* *

You begin to discuss treatment options with this patient.

Which of the following is NOT an effective treatment for panic disorder?

A) Benzodiazepines such as clonazepam (Klonopin).
B) Bupropion (Wellbutrin).
C) Psychotherapy such as cognitive-behavior therapy.
D) SSRIs such as fluoxetine (Prozac).
E) Tricyclic antidepressants such as imipramine.

Discussion

The correct answer is B. Bupropion is not effective for anxiety disorders. Evidence abounds to support the efficacy of TCAs, benzodiazepines, SSRIs, and monoamine oxidase inhibitors (MAOIs). Psychotherapy has been found to be as effective as medications for the treatment of mild to moderate panic disorder and can be used in combination with medications for more severe cases. A benzodiazepine with an SSRI or TCA may be particularly effective. Studies have shown that no class of medications is superior, and medication choice is based on safety, adverse-effect profile, tolerability, co-morbid illnesses, history of substance use, cost, etc. SSRIs are frequently considered first line.

* *

As you decide on the medication and dosage, you remember a journal article on common mistakes made by physicians treating panic disorder in the community.

Which of these is NOT one of the common mistakes made in the treatment of panic disorder?

A) Starting the SSRI too high.
B) Not increasing the medication dose high enough.
C) Underutilization of benzodiazepines.
D) Too rapid a titration.
E) Often using medications not proven to work with panic disorder.

Discussion

The correct answer is "C." Far from being underutilized, **benzodiazepines are often overprescribed.**

While effective for panic disorder, problems with tolerance, dependence, and abuse limit benzodiazepines as long-term agents for panic disorder. Patients with panic disorder are extremely sensitive to medication side effects and are likely to suffer from jitteriness and restlessness if started at too high a dose of an SSRI. In order to reduce the chances of precipitating jitteriness and restlessness, a lower dose of SSRI (about half the starting dose used to treat depression) is usually recommended. The same problems can occur with rapidly increasing doses of SSRIs, so "start low and go slow," increasing the dose every 2–4 weeks to reach the maximum allowable dose.

> **HELPFUL TIP:** If using benzodiazepines for panic attacks or panic disorder, use longer half-life agents such as clonazepam or diazepam. Shorter half-life drugs can be prescribed for aborting panic attacks if needed. Taper benzodiazepines as soon as possible. Avoid them in patients with severe personality disorders and substance abuse.

* *

Your patient says, "I know another female in the reserve who has something similar, but I've never noticed the guys to have a problem. Is this just something that happens to women?" You tell her a bit about gender differences in anxiety disorders.

Which of these statements is NOT true about the gender ratio of the following anxiety disorders?

A) Generalized anxiety disorder affects more women than men in a 2:1 ratio.
B) Obsessive-compulsive disorder affects men and women equally.
C) Posttraumatic stress disorder affects men more than women in a 2:1 ratio.
D) Social anxiety disorder affects men and women equally.

Discussion
The correct answer is C. Many affective illnesses (mood and anxiety disorders) including depression and some anxiety disorders are biologically sexist; women are more likely to be affected than men. All of the options listed are correct except "C", which inverts the true ratio.

Objectives: Did you learn to . . .

- Evaluate patients with anxiety symptoms?
- Recognize panic attacks and diagnose panic disorder?
- Initiate treatment for panic disorder?
- Describe some epidemiologic issues with anxiety disorders?

CASE 7

You have a 34-year-old male patient who has started sustained-release bupropion (Wellbutrin SR) 150 mg BID for depression. He reports partial but not total resolution of his symptoms. He also thinks that the medication is causing some side effects.

Which of the following is the most likely adverse effect attributable to this medication?

A) Insomnia.
B) Sexual dysfunction.
C) Weight gain.
D) QT prolongation.
E) Increased smoking.

Discussion
The correct answer is A. Bupropion is associated with vivid dreams and insomnia. Taking the second dose no later than 4 p.m. can help reduce the likelihood of this side effect. Unlike most other antidepressants, bupropion is not associated with sexual dysfunction or weight gain. In fact, it has been associated with weight loss in the short term, and patients who quit smoking are less likely to gain weight if they are taking it. Bupropion can cause dry mouth and nausea, which are usually self-limited. It does not cause QT prolongation, unlike TCAs. Bupropion appears to curb the cravings for nicotine. It lowers the seizure threshold and should be avoided in patients with epilepsy.

* *

This patient is relatively healthy and takes no other medications, giving you a wide number of options for treatment. In other words, you did not have to think too hard before starting bupropion.

In which of the following disease states would bupropion be contraindicated?

A) Hypertension.
B) Severe depression.

C) Bulimia nervosa.

D) Bipolar depression.

E) Borderline personality disorder.

Discussion

The correct answer is C. Bupropion is contraindicated in patients with anorexia nervosa or bulimia nervosa (an increased risk of seizures is found in both diseases) or a current or past seizure disorder. Additionally, bupropion must be avoided in patients taking MAOIs. It is as effective as the other antidepressants, and it can be used in bipolar disorder and severe depression.

* *

You decide to switch his medication from bupropion to citalopram (Celexa).

Which is the best way to accomplish this switch?

A) Stop the bupropion immediately and then wait 2 weeks before starting citalopram.

B) Taper the bupropion over 2 weeks to avoid a discontinuation syndrome, and then start the citalopram.

C) Start citalopram immediately, and then taper the bupropion over several days.

D) Start citalopram now, then taper off the bupropion 2 weeks later if he is doing well.

Discussion

The correct answer is C. Unlike SSRIs which can cause a withdrawal syndrome, bupropion can be discontinued with a minimal taper. A brief taper may avoid a sudden rebound of depressive symptoms while the new agent is started. Answer A is incorrect. Bupropion can be taken with an SSRI. However, answer D is incorrect because it is preferable to stop the bupropion rather than continue it indefinitely while taking another medication. A single effective agent is generally preferred.

Objectives: Did you learn to . . .

- Use bupropion appropriately?
- Identify adverse effects of bupropion?
- Recommend strategies to transition from bupropion to another antidepressant?

 QUICK QUIZ: PSYCHIATRIC DIAGNOSIS

A 22-year-old college student who moved to your town from Lagos, Nigeria, last month is referred to you by his academic advisor for concerns that he may be depressed. Although he speaks English well, he does not know anyone in town. His family is still in Lagos, and he does not anticipate returning to see them anytime soon because of his busy course schedule and the cost of travel. He has not made many friends yet. He enjoys watching soccer in his spare time, but he is not sleeping well, and he feels quite homesick.

Which of the following is the most appropriate diagnosis at this time?

A) Major depressive disorder.

B) Adjustment disorder.

C) Bipolar affective disorder.

D) Dysthymia.

E) None of the above.

Discussion

The correct answer is B. Adjustment disorder is the development of emotional or behavioral symptoms in response to identifiable stressor(s) occurring within 3 months of the onset of the stressor(s). The symptoms or behaviors must be clinically significant, such that either the patient's distress is in excess of what would be expected from exposure to the stressor, or there should be impairment in social or occupational/academic functioning. The patient's symptoms cannot be due to bereavement (a separate diagnosis). Once the stressor (or its consequences) is terminated, the symptoms should resolve within 6 months. Treatment depends upon the level of distress and can range from supportive care to active intervention with medications, therapy, or hospitalization.

CASE 8

An 85-year-old woman is brought to the ED by her daughters because she has been acting strangely lately. Her house is a mess, even though for most of her life she has been quite fastidious. She has been calling her daughters at odd hours of the night, upset, and insisting that her youngest daughter is stealing her money. During the day, she goes outside of her house in her nightgown and housecoat, again quite unlike her usual customs. Four months ago, her husband of 58 years was diagnosed with a brain tumor. His condition has deteriorated quite rapidly, and he is now in a nursing home, and does not recognize his wife or daughters. Because of these events, the daughters have attributed your patient's odd behavior to the stress she is under. But as her symptoms have continued to worsen, they are now quite concerned and decide they must bring her in for evaluation.

In the ED, the patient is dressed in her housecoat and slippers and appears disheveled. She is lying on a cart, but she keeps trying to get up and leave. She is angry at her two daughters who are with her, and she is uncooperative with the physical exam. When you ask her about what has been happening, she appears distrusting, and her answers do not make sense.

Which of the following diagnoses is LEAST likely now?

A) Delirium.
B) Dementia.
C) Bereavement.
D) Psychotic depression.
E) Alcohol abuse.

Discussion

The correct answer is C. Although your patient's husband is gravely ill and she is grieving, her symptoms are more severe than what is expected for bereavement. Bereavement is a normal process, but it does not include severe impairment in social or occupational functioning, nor does it include paranoid delusions or other psychotic symptoms. All of the other diagnoses listed could result in the severity of symptoms described in this case.

Which of the following tests is indicated in the evaluation of this patient's behavior changes?

A) Chest x-ray.
B) Urinalysis.
C) Complete blood count.
D) B$_{12}$ levels.
E) All of the above.

Discussion

The correct answer is E. A thorough medical workup is warranted in the patient with "mental status changes" (eg, delirium, new onset psychotic symptoms, etc). Several medical problems—infection, hypoxia, myocardial infarction, to name a few—can cause the symptoms the patient is experiencing and must be ruled out.

In this patient who you believe has psychotic depression, all of the following are appropriate management options at this time EXCEPT:

A) Discharge with referral for outpatient psychotherapy.
B) Admission to a psychiatric unit.
C) Electroconvulsive therapy.
D) Psychiatric consultation.

Discussion

The correct answer is A. Psychotherapy is not an appropriate single therapy for psychotic depression—especially in this patient, whose symptoms are so severe. Answer B is appropriate, as the patient may benefit from hospitalization. Answer C is appropriate. Electroconvulsive therapy (ECT) is effective in treating psychotic depression and is often indicated if safety is of immediate concern or an early response is needed. Answer D is appropriate. In general patients with psychotic depression should be referred to a psychiatrist, due to the severity of the illness.

* *

You determine that your patient's symptoms are severe enough for hospitalization. Her daughters agree, but the patient is adamantly opposed and insists on returning to her home.

How would you proceed?

A) Call hospital security and make plans to hospitalize her. After all, she appears quite ill and cannot care for herself. When she is well, she will understand that it was the right plan.
B) Discharge her home, asking her daughters to take turns staying with her until she is better.
C) Follow state-dictated protocol to attempt to obtain a legal order for hospitalization against her will.
D) Follow national protocol (New World Order Directive 55.12.A) to attempt to obtain a legal order for hospitalization against her will.
E) Make a medical determination that she is not competent, allowing you to hospitalize her despite her objection.

Discussion

The correct answer is C. Each state has its own laws that govern how an involuntary hospitalization process is conducted. If the patient poses an imminent threat to self or others, the law generally allows involuntary hospitalization for a brief period of time until a court hearing is held. Involuntary hospitalization is also allowed if the patient is unable to care for herself and she is suffering from a mental illness that renders her incapable of making health care decisions. Answer D is incorrect. There are no national laws governing involuntary hospitalization. Answer B is incorrect. Because of the severity of this patient's symptoms, it would be inappropriate to simply discharge her to the care of her daughters.

* *

You have admitted the patient under a 72-hour hold, and you are discussing treatment options with the psychiatrist, who thinks that ECT might be appropriate. You are concerned about cognitive problems in this patient.

All of the following are associated with an increased risk of memory loss with ECT EXCEPT:

A) Concomitant lithium use.
B) Bilateral electrode placement.
C) High stimulus doses.
D) History of seizure disorder.

Discussion

The correct answer is D. Seizure disorder is not associated with an increased risk of memory loss with ECT. ECT is known to cause transient problems with memory loss. This usually manifests with the patient having trouble remembering events that occur around the time of the ECT. Most of the memory complaints completely resolve within a few months of completing ECT. However, some situations may increase the risk of memory loss, including concomitant lithium use, bilateral electrode placement (unilateral is safer), and a higher stimulus dose.

* *

In further discussions with the patient and her family, you try to explain ECT and dispel some myths.

All of the following are potential complications or adverse effects of ECT EXCEPT:

A) Delirium.
B) Nonsustained ventricular tachycardia.
C) Headache.
D) Dementia.
E) Fatigue.

Discussion

The correct answer is D. Although transient memory loss and even delirium can occur after ECT, it does not cause dementia. A number of cardiac rhythm disturbances can occur and are more likely in patients with cardiac disease. However, these are self-limited and generally minor (eg, premature ventricular contractions, atrial premature complexes, nonsustained ventricular tachycardia). Headache and fatigue are common after ECT.

Objectives: Did you learn to . . .

- Recognize abnormal behavior and generate an appropriate differential diagnosis?
- Evaluate a patient with new cognitive and behavioral problems?
- Determine when involuntary hospitalization is appropriate and how it might be undertaken?
- Discuss potential adverse effects of ECT?

⧗ QUICK QUIZ: PSYCHIATRIC DIAGNOSIS

A 47-year-old female presents to your clinic in tears, requesting your help. She cannot stop crying, her sleep is poor, and she feels terribly lonely. She tells you that last week, her mother had a stroke. She survived, but is now in a nursing home and suffering from Broca aphasia. Your patient describes her mother as her "best friend." She has not had trouble with depression or other mental illness in the past.

Which of the following is the most likely diagnosis?

A) Bereavement.
B) Adjustment disorder.
C) Major depressive disorder.
D) Bipolar affective disorder.
E) Dysthymia.

Discussion

The correct answer is A. Bereavement is a natural reaction to the loss of a loved one. Some of the symptoms may mimic those of a depression and making the diagnosis can be complicated. The duration and expression of bereavement also differs among different cultural groups and sub-groups, further complicating the diagnostic process. Generally, a diagnosis of MDD is not given unless the symptoms of depression are present 2 months after the loss.

CASE 9

You get a call from a patient complaining of "not feeling well and getting worse" over the past 3 days. She has had electrical sensations in her upper extremities and head and also complains of dizziness and malaise. She has not traveled anywhere recently and has not been near any sick people. She takes no medications since she stopped her antidepressant a few days ago. She thought that she did not need the medicine anymore since she felt better after taking it for 9 months.

Which of the following is the most likely diagnosis?

A) Influenza.
B) Bupropion discontinuation syndrome.
C) SSRI discontinuation syndrome.
D) Serotonin syndrome.
E) Hypertensive crisis.

Discussion

The correct answer is C. A discontinuation syndrome (also known as withdrawal syndrome) has been associated with SSRIs when they are suddenly stopped or doses are missed or reduced. This is especially common with paroxetine. The symptoms described above are typical of the discontinuation syndrome, particularly the paresthesias which patients often describe as an "electric shock." Bupropion is not associated with a withdrawal syndrome. None of the other options have such characteristic symptoms.

Which of the following symptoms would be unusual in the patient with SSRI discontinuation syndrome?

A) Dizziness.
B) Nausea.
C) Lethargy.
D) Somnolence.

Discussion

The correct answer is D. The other options are the most commonly reported symptoms in patients experiencing the discontinuation syndrome. Insomnia—not somnolence—is a common problem. Symptoms can be divided into two main clusters: somatic and psychological. Patients usually have clusters of symptoms rather than isolated symptoms. See Table 23–1.

Table 23–1 SYMPTOMS OF SSRI DISCONTINUATION SYNDROME

Somatic Symptoms
- Disequilibrium (eg, dizziness, vertigo, ataxia, tremor)
- Gastrointestinal symptoms (eg, nausea, vomiting, anorexia)
- Flu-like symptoms (eg, fatigue, lethargy, myalgias, chills, headache)
- Sensory disturbances (eg, paresthesias, sensations of electric shock)
- Sleep disturbances (eg, insomnia, vivid dreams)

Psychological Problems
- Anxiety/agitation
- Crying spells
- Irritability
- Overactivity
- Depersonalization
- Decreased concentration/slowed thinking
- Confusion and memory problems

Which of the following statements is FALSE regarding discontinuance of SSRIs?

A) Symptoms usually begin within a few days of stopping the SSRI.
B) The symptoms rarely last longer 2 weeks and are self-limited.
C) Restarting the medication takes about 2 weeks to relieve symptoms.
D) The longer the patient has been on the medication, the more likely the risk of a discontinuation syndrome.

Discussion

The correct answer is C (which is false). Symptoms can be noticeable in some patients with just one missed dose (especially with paroxetine [Paxil]) but typically develop within 2 days of medication discontinuation. The syndrome is uncomfortable but usually self-limited, lasting <2 weeks. Restarting the medication will lead to cessation of symptoms within 24 hours in virtually all cases. The risk of discontinuation increases with length of therapy, particularly when the patient has been on an SSRI >7 weeks.

Which SSRI is LEAST likely to cause a discontinuation syndrome?

A) Fluoxetine.
B) Sertraline.

C) Paroxetine.

D) Citalopram.

E) Fluvoxamine.

Discussion

The correct answer is A. The risk of withdrawal increases with **shorter** half-lives. The half-life of fluoxetine is about 4–6 days while its active metabolite, norfluoxetine has a half-life up to 16 days, making it highly unlikely that fluoxetine would cause a discontinuation syndrome in most patients, as it effectively acts as its own taper. Fluvoxamine (with a half-life of 15 hours) and paroxetine (21 hours) have the shortest half-lives and are most likely to cause the discontinuation syndrome. To minimize the risk of withdrawal syndrome, taper off SSRIs when stopping them.

 HELPFUL TIP: Discontinuation syndrome is likely a hyposerotonergic state; therefore, all serotonergic agents can cause a serotonin withdrawal. These agents include SSRIs, MAOIs, TCAs, venlafaxine (Effexor), and mirtazipine (Remeron), but not bupropion.

* *

Your patient restarts her SSRI and feels better. She has questions about antidepressants in general, wondering if she is taking the right one. As you start to discuss benefits and risks of different medications, you remind yourself about some important issues. For example, all SSRIs are not the same.

Which SSRI has the most anticholinergic activity?

A) Fluoxetine.

B) Paroxetine.

C) Sertraline.

D) Citalopram.

E) Escitalopram.

Discussion

The correct answer is B. With the exception of paroxetine, SSRIs do not possess appreciable anticholinergic activity.

Which of the following SSRIs is LEAST likely to have drug-drug interactions?

A) Fluoxetine.

B) Paroxetine.

C) Citalopram.

D) Sertraline.

E) Fluvoxamine.

Discussion

The correct answer is C. Citalopram and its stereoisomer, escitalopram, have relatively clean profiles with no major interactions with any of the cytochrome P450 enzymes. Sertraline is also an attractive option if drug-drug interactions are a concern. The other three have significant drug-drug interactions that have clinical importance.

Mirtazapine (Remeron) is commonly associated with the following side effects EXCEPT:

A) Sedation.

B) Weight gain.

C) Dizziness.

D) Lycanthropy.

E) Increased triglycerides.

Discussion

The correct answer is D. Lycanthropy is the ability to transform into a werewolf. Although close in behavior to antisocial personality disorder, lycanthropy is not caused by mirtazapine but rather by the bite of another lycanthrope. Mirtazapine is a potent antihistamine and an α_1-adrenergic agonist, potentially leading to orthostatic hypotension. Sedation is present in over 50% of patients taking the drug, while weight gain is reported in 12%. It can also lead to increased triglycerides. Paradoxically, the side effect of sedation lessens with increasing doses. It is a great antidepressant for patients who have lost their appetite or weight and in low doses for those with insomnia. Typical doses range from 15–60 mg per day.

Which of the following antidepressants has a black box warning about hepatic failure?

A) Nefazodone (Serzone).

B) Bupropion.

C) Paroxetine (Paxil).

D) Nortriptyline.

E) Phenelzine (Nardil).

Discussion

The correct answer is A. Nefazodone is a 5-HT_{2A} receptor antagonist and is an effective antidepressant with sedative properties. It has significant inhibitory effects on CYP3A4 and has several significant drug interactions as a result. In the recent past, several cases of hepatic failure have been reported with this drug, leading to a black box warning on the package insert and limiting its clinical use. None of the other antidepressants listed have had such problems.

Venlafaxine has been noted to cause all of the following side effects EXCEPT:

A) Increased blood pressure.
B) Dizziness.
C) Dry mouth.
D) Weight gain.
E) Sexual disturbance.

Discussion

The correct answer is D. Venlafaxine blocks both norepinephrine and serotonin reuptake and has minimal activity on the cholinergic, histaminergic, and alpha-receptors. There is a dose-related increase in blood pressure, with a mean elevation of 10–15 mm Hg in diastolic pressure at doses of ≥300 mg in up to 10% of patients. There is a slight increase in pulse, as well. Answer D is incorrect. Weight loss is a common complaint. Venlafaxine generally has the same side effect profile as the SSRIs, potentially causing sexual dysfunction, dizziness, and dry mouth. Patients can have a significant withdrawal from venlefaxine and should be tapered off of it slowly.

 HELPFUL TIP: Venlafaxine (Effexor) and duloxetine (Cymbalta) are toxic in overdose and now cause as many deaths as TCAs (at least in England). They cause QT and QRS prolongation in overdose. Treatment is the same as the treatment of TCA overdose (bicarbonate, etc) although data is limited.

You decide to switch the patient to fluoxetine and she does well.

Objectives: Did you learn to . . .

• Identify SSRI discontinuation syndrome?
• Recognize important antidepressant interactions?
• Describe adverse effects of various antidepressants?

 QUICK QUIZ: MAOIs

You are seeing a new patient with a history of recurrent major depression. Many years ago a different physician put him on phenelzine (Nardil), which you recognize as having potentially serious food and drug interactions. You are considering switching him to an SSRI.

How long after an MAOI is discontinued can an SSRI be started?

A) 1 day.
B) 3 days.
C) 7 days.
D) 14 days.
E) SSRIs and MAOIs can be given together.

Discussion

The correct answer is D. Because of significant drug-drug interactions (see next discussion), SSRIs should not be started until 2 weeks after discontinuation of an MAOI.

 QUICK QUIZ: MAOIs

What is the drug-drug interaction of concern with SSRIs and MAOIs?

A) Serotonin syndrome.
B) Tyramine crisis.
C) Anticholinergic crisis.
D) Hypertensive crisis.
E) Stevens-Johnson syndrome.

Discussion

The correct answer is A. Serotonin syndrome is caused by an excess of serotonin and can be caused by drug-drug interactions involving serotonergic agents including SSRIs, buspirone, meperidine, dextromethorphan, triptans etc. It is characterized by hyperreflexia, diarrhea, flushing, and autonomic instability. It can be fatal. As a result, the concurrent use of an SSRI and MAOI is absolutely **contraindicated**. Hypertensive crisis occurs when foods containing tyramine (eg, aged cheese and cured meats) interact with MAOIs to release catecholamines, causing hypertension, headaches, nausea, and diaphoresis. In severe cases, it can lead to strokes or death. Anticholinergic crisis is discussed in the Emergency Medicine chapter. Stevens-Johnson syndrome is an autoimmune dermatological disorder that leads to desquamation of mucosal surfaces and is not associated with antidepressant use (although it can be seen with other drugs).

CASE 10

A 43-year-old male who you started on citalopram 4 weeks ago returns for a follow-up visit. He feels better but complains of delayed ejaculation. You consider changing him to an antidepressant that is less likely to cause sexual dysfunction.

Which of the following would you AVOID?

A) Nefazodone.
B) Bupropion.
C) Mirtazapine.
D) Trazodone.
E) Nortriptyline.

Discussion

The correct answer is "E." Sexual dysfunction is a common side effect of most psychotropics. There are few controlled data to guide us as to how to approach this issue, but sildenafil (Viagra) is effective in antidepressant-induced sexual dysfunction. Unlike all of the other options, nortriptyline—and other TCAs—frequently cause sexual dysfunction.

* *

Your patient wonders if there is a more "natural" alternative to citalopram.

Which herbal product has some data supporting its use in mild to moderate depression?

A) Kava-kava.
B) Valerian.
C) Butterbur.
D) St. John's wort.
E) Saw palmetto.

Discussion

The correct answer is D. St John's wort, (*Hypericum perforatum*), has been widely used in Europe for decades as an antidepressant and has data supporting its efficacy in mild-to-moderate depression. However, two well-done trials in the United States failed to find

efficacy for this product, making its use still a subject of debate.

 HELPFUL TIP: St John's wort is a known inducer of the P450 enzyme, reducing the efficacy of oral contraceptives. It has also been associated with decreased efficacy of antiretrovirals, cyclosporine, digoxin, theophylline, and warfarin.

* *

This patient is also having sleep difficulties and asks what herbal therapy he might be able to use.

Which of the following is an herbal alternative to benzodiazepines for anxiety and insomnia?

A) Valerian.
B) St. John's wort.
C) Saw palmetto.
D) Ginseng.
E) Gingko.

Discussion

The correct answer is A. Valerian (*Valeriana officinalis*) has been touted to have anxiolytic properties, similar to benzodiazepines, and its mechanism of action is thought to be similar (eg, inhibition of GABA). It appears to be safe and has the same drug interactions and contraindications as benzodiazepines. The other options are not known to affect sleep to a significant degree.

 HELPFUL TIP: Kava-kava is advertised as an anxiolytic but should generally be avoided. Kava-kava (*Piper methysticum*) has been reported to cause liver damage, in some cases leading to liver transplant or eventual death.

Objectives: Did you learn to . . .

● Develop approaches to the problem of sexual dysfunction with antidepressants?
● Recognize herbal therapies that might be employed in treating symptoms of depression?

QUICK QUIZ: PSYCHIATRIC DIAGNOSIS

A 31-year-old patient comes in to your office with complaint of several years of low mood and irritability. He is a writer, but he has been having trouble for the past few years with getting his work done. Every once in a while, he will have a few weeks where he is quite productive, staying awake for days at a time on a caffeine-fueled writing marathon. He feels that these "high" episodes have enabled him to keep his job as a professor at the local liberal arts college. In between these episodes, several students have complained to his department head that he is late to lectures, slow at returning papers and tests, and hard to contact when they have questions. He finds himself angry with the students for being so demanding.

Which of the following is the most appropriate diagnosis?

A) Major depressive disorder.
B) Adjustment disorder.
C) Generalized anxiety disorder.
D) Bipolar affective disorder.
E) Dysthymia.

Discussion

The correct answer is D. There are two types of bipolar disorder, type I and type II. Both are characterized by episodes of mood elevation. The main difference between types I and II is symptom intensity and duration of the manic episodes.

Patients with **bipolar I disorder** must have had at least 1 episode of mania: a distinct period of abnormally and persistently elevated, expansive, or irritable mood, lasting at least 1 week (or any duration if hospitalization is necessary). In addition, there must be at least 3 of the following symptoms concurrently: (1) inflated self-esteem or grandiosity, (2) decreased need for sleep, (3) more talkative than usual, (4) flight of ideas or racing thoughts, (5) distractibility, (6) increased goal-directed activity or psychomotor agitation, and (7) excessive involvement in pleasurable activities that have a high risk for negative consequences/impulsivity. The episode must cause impairment in occupational or social functioning and cannot be substance induced.

Patients with **bipolar II disorder** have had at least one episode of hypomania: a distinct period of persistently elevated, expansive, or irritable mood, lasting for at least 4 days, which is clearly distinct from the usual, non-depressed mood. During the hypomanic episode, at least 3 of the manic symptoms listed above must be present, although the episode is not severe enough to cause marked impairment in occupational or social functioning, require hospitalization, or include psychotic symptoms. Although patients with bipolar disorders often have depressive episodes as well as manic or hypomanic episodes, depression is not required for the diagnosis of bipolar disorder.

CASE 11

You are seeing a 28-year-old patient whose first child you delivered a month ago. She comes to your clinic with her son for his one-month well child check. She has a question about breast-feeding, but otherwise tells you that things are going well. You observe, however, that she seems tired and is less animated than usual. She is gentle with her infant, but her face doesn't seem to light up with the glow that you often see with new mothers.

Which of the following best explains your observations?

A) Sleep deprivation.
B) Marital discord at home.
C) Post-partum depression.
D) Thyroid dysfunction.
E) Any of the above.

Discussion

The correct answer is E. Your patient's symptoms could result from any of these problems and more, including, difficulty with role adjustment, anemia, etc.

* *

You want to gather more information to see if there is a pathological process underlying her behavior.

You would do all of the following EXCEPT:

A) Ask her to fill out an Edinburgh Postnatal Depression Scale (EPDS).
B) Order thyroid function tests.
C) Order a sleep study.
D) Ask more questions about how things are at home and how she is coping.
E) Ask about a previous history of depression.

Discussion

The correct answer is C. There are many other more likely problems here than a sleep disorder, and a sleep study is unlikely to be helpful. The EPDS is a validated self-rated scale that is useful for detecting post-partum depression. It has symptoms that have been adjusted for this particular population. Hypothyroidism can always mimic depression and might need to be ruled out. A thorough history is always essential.

The incidence of postpartum depression is approximately:

A) 1%
B) 10%
C) 30%
D) 50%

Discussion

The correct answer is B. Approximately 7 in 10 women suffer from "baby blues," postpartum symptoms which can manifest as mood swings, anxiety, fatigue, and sadness occurring within a few days of delivery and lasting only a week or so. However, postpartum depression affects up to 10% of women, and symptoms can appear anywhere from weeks to months after birth. The diagnosis is often missed because many mothers are ashamed to admit feeling unhappy at a time when they think (and society tells them) that they should be happy. Physicians may focus on the infant's physical health and miss assessing the mother-baby interaction.

* *

In obtaining more history, you realize that this patient was having some troubles with depression even during her pregnancy.

When is the most common time for pregnancy-related depression to occur?

A) At conception.
B) First trimester.
C) Second trimester.
D) Third trimester.
E) Postpartum.

Discussion

The correct answer is D. A large epidemiological study from the United Kingdom followed pregnant women prospectively throughout the course of their pregnancies and found that the **incidence of depression was higher in the third trimester than it was in the postpartum period**. This suggests the need for the physician to begin to inquire about symptoms earlier.

 HELPFUL TIP: Pregnancy does not treat depression. For some reason, it had been assumed that a woman's depression would abate during pregnancy. Studies in the last several years have disproved this myth.

* *

If you had been aware of her depression earlier and wanted to prescribe an antidepressant during her pregnancy, you would have been cautious, prescribing a Pregnancy Safety Category B drug.

Which of the following antidepressants is Category B in pregnancy?

A) Fluoxetine.
B) Bupropion.
C) Nortriptyline.
D) Mirtazapine.
E) None of the above.

Discussion

The correct answer is E. None of the above, and no antidepressant, is category B for pregnancy. All of the above are category C.

Risks associated with SSRI use during pregnancy include all of the following EXCEPT:

A) Irritability of the neonate.
B) Preterm delivery.
C) Low birth weight.
D) Persistent pulmonary hypertension.
E) Tetralogy of Fallot.

Discussion

The correct answer is E. A number of adverse effects have been associated with SSRI use in pregnancy, including neonatal irritability, low birth weight, and preterm labor. A recent meta-analysis of studies examining neonatal outcomes when women took antidepressants during pregnancy showed that infants exposed to SSRIs during the second half of pregnancy (ie, >20 weeks' gestation) had an increased risk (2% absolute risk) of developing persistent pulmonary hypertension, a potentially life-threatening condition, after birth. SSRIs have not been linked to development of tetralogy of Fallot.

If you had decided to prescribe an antidepressant medication for her during pregnancy, which one of the following would have been LEAST desirable?

A) Fluoxetine.
B) Paroxetine.
C) Sertraline.
D) Nortriptyline.
E) Citalopram.

Discussion

The correct answer is B. Although no antidepressant medication has been shown to be risk-free when used during pregnancy, paroxetine is the only antidepressant medication listed that is Category D in pregnancy, due to the increased incidence of cardiac anomalies (mainly atrial and ventricular septal defects) in infants who were exposed in utero.

Objectives: Did you learn to . . .

- Recognize the high incidence of depression and depressive symptoms in the postpartum period?
- Diagnose postpartum depression?
- Treat depression in the pregnant and postpartum patient?

CASE 12

A couple you have known for some time brings in their 7-year-old son, Jimbo, to your clinic because his behavior has changed over the past month. His school performance has worsened, and he has started to get into fights at school. He is not eating as well and is having frequent nightmares. He now has frequent headaches and stomachaches and clings to his mother when it is time to go to school. The parents cannot understand what is going on and report no antecedent trauma.

Which of the following is the most likely diagnosis?

A) Major depressive disorder.
B) Posttraumatic stress disorder.
C) Adjustment disorder.
D) Bereavement.
E) Normal childhood difficulties anticipated with being named Jimbo.

Discussion

The correct answer is A. Up to 3% of children and 8% of adolescents suffer from depression. DSM-IV criteria are the same as in the adult, except **irritability can be substituted for the depressed mood requirement** in children. PTSD is unlikely as there is no antecedent trauma. Adjustment disorder is not likely since there have been no major changes in the child's regimen, and bereavement is not likely since there have been no losses in the child's life. The patient's symptoms are clearly not part of normal childhood, even if his name is Jimbo.

 HELPFUL TIP: Bullying at school and other social problems need to be investigated in this child and any other presenting with symptoms of depression.

Which of the following statements is NOT true about depression in children?

A) Abuse or neglect increases the risk of depression.
B) Having a depressed parent increases the risk of being a depressed child.
C) The clinical course is roughly the same as in adults.
D) "Masked" symptoms, such as abdominal pain, are more common in children than the typical symptoms of depression, such as sleep disturbance.
E) Male and female children are equally affected by depression.

Discussion

The correct answer is D. Although clinicians should be aware of age-appropriate manifestations (Table 23–2), symptoms of depression are similar in children and adults. Typical symptoms of depression are more common in children than are "masked" symptoms such as stomachaches and fear of leaving home. The risk of depression is higher in children of depressed parents, particularly those whose mothers are depressed, and the rates increase dramatically as children become adolescents. Abuse and neglect increase the risk. The clinical course in young people is roughly the same as in adults. Male to female ratio is 1:1 in children, and girls develop an increasing incidence as they grow older; and by puberty, the ratio approaches the 2:1 female:male ratio seen in adults.

Table 23–2 COMMON MANIFESTATIONS OF DEPRESSION IN CHILDREN

Increased irritability, anger, or hostility
- Being bored
- Reckless behavior
- Outbursts of shouting, complaining, unexplained irritability, or crying
- Poor school performance
- Fear of death
- Alcohol or substance abuse
- Frequent nonspecific physical complaints such as headaches, muscle aches, stomachaches, or fatigue

Depression in Children and Adolescents, National Institutes of Health Publication No. 00-4744 (http://www.nimh.nih.gov/publicat/depchildresfact.cfm).

* *

You tell the family about Jimbo's prognosis.

Which of the following statements regarding prognosis is FALSE?

A) Childhood MDD confers a 2–4-fold increase in risk for adult MDD.
B) 25% of adolescents with MDD develop substance abuse disorders.
C) Almost 50% of children with MDD will attempt suicide sometime in their life.
D) Roughly 20% of adolescents have suffered at least one episode of MDD by 18 years while 65% report transient symptoms of depression.
E) After the initial episode, only 10% will suffer a relapse.

Discussion
The correct answer is E. Between 50% and 66% (**not 10%**) will have a recurrence within 5 years after resolution of their first episode. The other statements are all true. Treating MDD in children might reduce some of the negative outcomes and improve the prognosis, so every effort should be made to aggressively identify and treat these patients. In children and adolescents, the mean depression episode length is 7–9 months with remission typically occurring over 1.5–2 years.

 HELPFUL TIP: The risk of suicide is very high among depressed youths. It is the third leading cause of death in the 15–24-year age

group, and children with MDD have a 4–5-fold higher lifetime incidence of suicide attempts than nondepressed children. Estimated 20% of adolescents have suicide ideation each year, and 5%–8% attempt suicide each year.

* *

You recommend treatment for Jimbo.

Which of the following therapies has NOT shown efficacy in childhood depression in randomized controlled trials?

A) Fluoxetine.
B) Sertraline.
C) Cognitive behavioral therapy.
D) Venlafaxine.
E) Interpersonal therapy.

Discussion
The correct answer is D. The manufacturers of venlafaxine sent out a "Dear Doctor" letter recommending that venlafaxine not be used in children <18 years because it lacks efficacy data, and it has an increased incidence of emotional lability. The bottom line is that fluoxetine is probably the SSRI of choice in children, followed by sertraline. **However, the NNT is 10 to benefit 1 child.** Avoid paroxetine since it may be associated with a higher suicide risk. TCAs should be avoided because of lack of efficacy and potential suicide risk. Cognitive behavioral therapy and interpersonal therapy have been shown to be effective in children and adolescents.

 HELPFUL TIP: Adverse effects of medication in children are similar to those in adults and include insomnia, fatigue, headaches, and nervousness. Slowing of growth has been reported, and studies addressing this issue are underway. The long-term impact on personality and the developing brain are unknown.

Objectives: Did you learn to . . .
- Increase your awareness of childhood depression?
- Diagnose depression in children?

- Describe the natural history of depression in children?
- Generate an appropriate treatment plan for children with depression?

CASE 13

Tommy is a 9-year-old male who has been having difficulty with his behavior since he started first grade. He is often fidgety and squirming in his chair and has difficulty remaining in his seat. He talks out of turn, is often "on the go," and is not liked by the other children because he intrudes into games and has a hard time waiting his turn. He is the product of an uncomplicated pregnancy and has no significant past medical history.

What is the most likely diagnosis?

A) Attention-deficit hyperactivity disorder (ADHD).
B) Adjustment disorder.
C) Oppositional defiant disorder (ODD).
D) Conduct disorder (CD).
E) Nonverbal learning disorder.

Discussion

The correct answer is A. The symptoms of ADHD according to DSM-IV are given below. Answer B, adjustment disorder, is incorrect because there is no history of a significant life event. Answers C and D are incorrect. ODD and CD are characterized by aggressive behavior and a disregard for rules and adults. This is not given as part of Tommy's history. Answer E is incorrect. Nonverbal learning disorder presents with school performance problems and may be associated with ADHD but would not be directly responsible for this patient's hyperactivity.

For the diagnosis of ADHD patients must meet one of the following criteria:

1) At least six symptoms of inattention for at least 6 months that is maladaptive and inconsistent with level of development
   - Careless mistakes, poor attention to details
   - Cannot sustain attention
   - Does not seem to listen
   - Poor follow through on tasks
   - Difficulties with organization
   - Avoids or dislikes tasks that require sustained attention

- Often loses things required for a task (notebooks, pens, etc)
- Easily distracted from a task

2) Six or more of the following hyperactive-impulsive symptoms for 6 months, which is maladaptive and inconsistent with level of development.

Hyperactivity symptoms

- Fidgets or squirms in seat
- Leaves seat in classroom at inappropriate times
- Hyperactivity in inappropriate settings
- Cannot play or relax quietly
- Always in motion
- Talks too much

Impulsivity symptoms

- Blurts out answer before questions completed
- Trouble waiting for turn in games, school, etc.
- Interrupts others (verbally, in games, etc)

Additionally, the following are required:

- Must be present before age of 7 years!
- Impairment in two settings (home, work, school, worship, etc)
- Clinically significant impairment in social, academic or occupational spheres
- Symptoms are not due to another problem (developmental delay, personality disorder, mood disorder, etc)

Which of the following is FALSE about ADHD?

A) It affects 3%–7% of children.
B) There are genetic and environmental influences on the risk of developing ADHD.
C) Males are more likely to have ADHD than females.
D) The incidence of ADHD has increased over the years.
E) Comorbid disorders are not common.

Discussion

The correct answer is E. Comorbid disorders are very common in ADHD with conduct disorder, oppositional defiant disorder, depression, anxiety, learning disabilities, and mental retardation being the most frequent. ADHD affects 3%–7% of children and its incidence has almost doubled over the past decade. Heritability is similar to that for schizophrenia and bipolar disorder. Imaging studies generally show volumetric changes and decreased frontal region activation. Alcohol and tobacco exposure in utero have both been linked to at least a two-fold increase in risk. Males are 3–6 times more likely to be diagnosed with ADHD than females.

Which of the following statements is NOT TRUE of the prognosis and treatment of Tommy's ADHD?

A) The natural history of ADHD is that 33% of children will outgrow the symptoms, 33% will have the same frequency and intensity of symptoms, and 33% will have residual symptoms which are subclinical.
B) Tommy has a 70%–80% chance of responding to stimulants.
C) If Tommy is treated with stimulants, his risk of drug abuse is halved.
D) Tommy is at increased risk of getting into accidents.
E) Behavior therapy is effective for reducing ADHD symptoms.

Discussion

The correct answer is E. Unfortunately, intensive behavior therapy has been shown to be ineffective. The breakdown of the prognosis for children with ADHD symptoms is that roughly 33% will experience complete symptom resolution, 33% will get some improvement, and 33% will remain ill with the disorder. Stimulants, which are first-line therapy, will work in 70%–80% of the patients. If a patient does not respond to the first stimulant, he still has a 70%–80% chance of responding to a second stimulant. Children treated with stimulants are half as likely to abuse substances as those who were not treated. Children with ADHD are at risk for impulsive behavior and risk-taking which leads to substance abuse, accidents, etc.

* *

You decide to start Tommy on methylphenidate.

Which of the following is NOT true about treatment with methylphenidate?

A) It improves handwriting.
B) Optimal dosing is 0.6–1 mg/kg/day.
C) It can cause reduced growth.
D) Short-term memory is not affected.
E) Tommy might get along better with his classmates.

Discussion

The correct answer is D. Stimulants do improve short-term memory in patients with ADHD. The other

Table 23–3   STIMULANT EFFECTS

Effects of Stimulants on Motor Response
- Reduce activity to normal
- Decrease excessive talking, noise and disruption in the classroom
- Improve handwriting
- Improve fine-motor control

Effects of Stimulants on Social Skills
- Reduce off-task behavior in classroom
- Improve ability to play and work independently
- Decrease intensity of behavior
- Reduce bossiness with peers
- Reduce verbal and physical aggression
- Improve (but not normalize) peer social status
- Reduce noncompliance, defiance, and oppositional behavior with adults
- Parents and teachers become less controlling and more positive

Effects of Stimulants on Cognitive Ability
- Improve ability to sustain attention, especially in boring tasks
- Reduce distractibility
- Improve short-term memory
- Reduce impulsivity
- Increase amount of academic work completed
- Increase accuracy of academic work

Side effects
- Lack of appetite
- Decreased growth, especially initially
- Insomnia
- Headaches and stomachaches
- Irritability
- Tachycardia or blood pressure increase (rare)
- Muscle tics or switches (rare)
- Psychosis or delirium (rare)

answer choices are true. Do you think this is why doctors have notoriously bad handwriting? Stimulants have a widespread effect on multiple domains, as listed in Table 23–3.

* *

Tommy's father is happy with his son's response to methylphenidate and wonders if he too would benefit from a similar medication. He recalls being in trouble ever since grade school for talking "out of turn" and always being put in detention. He was always restless and fidgety but this has improved as he aged. He has a hard time at work sitting through meetings, as he tends to daydream, and he has numerous fights with his wife because she accuses him of not listening to her. He has been unable to get promoted because he cannot pass the exams he has to take, but he thinks that he is smart enough. He says that he just cannot concentrate.

Which of the statements below would NOT be consistent with an adult presenting with ADHD?

A) Adults present with the same core symptoms as children but in a different fashion.
B) Adults are less likely to have overt hyperactivity symptoms compared to children.
C) Adults often present when their children are diagnosed.
D) Adults are less likely to smoke than same-age persons without ADHD.
E) Adults often seek professions that allow them to use their symptoms to their advantage.

Discussion

The correct answer is D. Adults present differently from children, but have the same core symptoms of hyperactivity, inattention, and impulsivity. Many adults are diagnosed with ADHD only when their children have been diagnosed or when increasing difficulty at work or at home leads them to seek help. Often, comorbidities drive them to seek help, and the primary diagnosis of ADHD is made only incidentally. Adults typically present seeking help for their inattention and concentration difficulties, as overt hyperactivity lessens with age. Some adults compensate by taking part in careers that reward their intellectual curiosity, endless energy, and desire for change. Table 23–4 compares adult with child presentations of ADHD.

 HELPFUL TIP: Adults may have residual symptoms that do not meet full criteria for ADHD at the time of evaluation. **A clear history of symptoms starting in childhood (<7 years according to DSM-IV) must be present to diagnose an adult with ADHD. There is no such thing as adult-onset ADHD.** Confirmation of the history can be obtained from collateral sources, including old school reports and family members.

* *

You decide to treat Tommy's father with medication. He would prefer not to have a stimulant, and he asks if there are other options for treatment.

Which of the following medications would you recommend?

A) Fluoxetine.
B) Bupropion.
C) Mirtazapine.
D) Phenelzine.
E) Risperidone.

Discussion

The correct answer is B. In addition to stimulants, which are also first-line agents in adults, there are a variety of medications that can be used to treat ADHD, although most studies are undertaken in children and most of these medications are not FDA approved for treating ADHD. Second-line agents include the antidepressants bupropion, desipramine, imipramine, and

Table 23–4   PRESENTATIONS OF ADHD SYMPTOMS IN CHILDREN AND ADULTS

Children	Adults
Hyperactive child: squirms, cannot stay in his seat, constantly on the go	Hyperactive adult: has subjective inner restlessness, trouble relaxing
Impulsive child: blurts out answers, interrupts others, talks incessantly	Impulsive adult: speeding tickets, car crashes, impatient, smokes more, higher divorce rate, higher substance use rate, and overeating
Inattentive child: does not follow through, is forgetful, does not listen Fewer enter college and graduate, compared to children their age without ADHD	Inattentive adult: often late for appointments, forgets anniversaries, has difficulty with work meetings; problems with focusing, planning, organizing and completing tasks at home and at work; advances more slowly at work than peers; misplaces keys, glasses, an other items; may forget to pay bills, pick up the kids on time, etc.

nortriptyline. The α-blockers guanfacine and clonidine are also used, mostly as an adjunct in children with concomitant conduct disorder or sleep problems. Stimulant side effects are similar in adults and the restriction necessitated by their controlled status may lead to patients preferring other options. Remember that a history of substance abuse or psychotic disorder is almost always a contraindication to stimulant use.

> **HELPFUL TIP:** Atomoxetine (Strattera) is the first nonstimulant drug approved for ADHD (it is a selective norepinephrine reuptake inhibitor) and the only drug approved for adult ADHD. It is not a controlled prescription, having no apparent abuse potential. However, no direct comparative studies exist between stimulants and atomoxetine, so its place in therapy is not yet well-defined. Maximum efficacy of atomoxetine is achieved in a few weeks (rather than immediately, as with stimulants). Atomoxetine has a similar side effect profile to the stimulants.

Objectives: Did you learn to . . .

● Recognize childhood and adult presentation of ADHD?
● Prescribe efficacious treatments for ADHD?
● Recognize side effects and advantages of various medications for ADHD?

CASE 14

A man calls your office because he is concerned that his wife of 2 years is acting strangely. She has not slept for most of the past week, staying up at night cleaning the house and calling random people in the phone book. She even went out and spent $3,000 on a dress that left nothing to the imagination and went out dancing all night. He becomes more upset when he reveals that his wife was seen kissing another man on the dance floor. You ask him to bring his wife in as soon as possible.

That afternoon you find a provocatively dressed 30-year-old female sitting in your office and laughing giddily as her husband gives most of the intelligible history. She keeps reaching over to touch you on the leg as you interview her. You find her hard to understand because she talks so fast. You manage to catch something about "winning Miss America."

What is the most likely diagnosis?

A) Mania.
B) Psychosis.
C) Agitated depression.
D) Anxiety disorder.
E) ADHD.

Discussion

The correct answer is A. Mania is the correct diagnosis. None of the other conditions can fully explain the abnormal elevation in mood and the subsequent behavior changes. The symptoms of distractibility, expansive mood, grandiosity, increased goal-directed activity, increased pleasurable activity with potentially painful consequences (eg, sexual activity with multiple partners, gambling, shopping sprees), decreased need for sleep, and pressured speech are consistent with a diagnosis of mania. Symptoms have to be present for at least 1 week or must be severe enough to require hospitalization. There must be a marked impairment in social or occupational functioning or psychotic features. These symptoms should not be due to substance use.

> **HELPFUL TIP:** Manic episodes lasting >4 days but <7 days are classified as "hypomanic episodes."

Which of the following statements is TRUE regarding bipolar illness?

A) Bipolar 1 is characterized by mania and recurrent MDD.
B) Bipolar 2 is characterized by mania and dysthymia.
C) Bipolar 1 is characterized by hypomania and recurrent MDD.
D) None of the above is true.

Discussion

The correct answer is A. Bipolar 1 is characterized by mania and MDD, which is usually recurrent. Answer B is incorrect. Bipolar 2 is characterized by recurrent MDD and hypomania, **not** mania and dysthymia. In other words, the major distinction between bipolar 1 and 2 is the greater severity of manic episodes with bipolar 1.

Regarding the epidemiology of bipolar illness, which of the following statements is FALSE?

A) The prevalence of bipolar 1 is ~1.5%.
B) Many patients are misdiagnosed initially with depression.
C) Untreated suicide rate is almost 20%.
D) Women are twice as likely to be affected as men.
E) Suicide risk is highest in the depressed or mixed state.

Discussion

The correct answer is D. Unlike depression, bipolar illness affects males and females equally. Bipolar 1 affects approximately 1.5% of the population, while bipolar 2 affects almost double that number. Untreated, nearly 20% will commit suicide—a rate about 20 times that of the general population. Risk is highest in depressed states or the mixed states (both mania and depression present at the same time). Bipolar disorder typically has its onset in early adulthood, although it can begin in childhood or adolescence. Depression is present 20%–30% of the time, even with ongoing maintenance treatment. Over half of bipolar patients are initially misdiagnosed with depression, and the average patient is only accurately diagnosed after 5 years of symptoms.

 HELPFUL TIP: Up to 50% of people with bipolar disorder have concomitant alcohol abuse or dependence.

* *

You want to start a medication for this patient.

Which of the following would NOT be an appropriate treatment choice for her mania?

A) Lithium.
B) Olanzapine.
C) Divalproex.
D) Carbamazepine.
E) Buspirone.

Discussion

The correct answer is E. Lithium was the first medication approved for treatment of bipolar mania and depression. It reduces the incidence of recurrence of mania, hypomania, and depression by approximately 66%. Lithium has a significant anti-suicide effect with an estimated 8–9-fold reduction in risk. It is dosed at nighttime or twice daily. Lithium has a narrow therapeutic window, and there are a number of drug-drug interactions.

Both divalproex and olanzapine have FDA approval for treatment of acute mania and appear to be somewhat effective in the prevention of recurrent episodes. However, only lithium and lamotrigine (Lamictal) are FDA approved for bipolar treatment and maintenance. Tegretol is a second-line agent that is also effective, but side effects limit its use. Buspirone is modestly effective in treating generalized anxiety disorder and may be used as an augmenting agent with some antidepressant medications to treat depression, but it is not effective in the treatment of bipolar disorder.

* *

You decide to start lithium.

Which of the following is a well-recognized side effect of lithium?

A) Diabetes.
B) Hypothyroidism.
C) Immunosuppression.
D) Abnormal hair growth.

Discussion

The correct answer is B. Patients who take lithium should have their thyroid function monitored. Also, lithium can affect electrolyte levels, so check serum electrolytes periodically. As lithium has a narrow therapeutic window, serum lithium levels should be measured as well, with a goal of 0.6–1.0 meq/L.

Which of the following drugs or drug classes does NOT alter lithium levels?

A) NSAIDs.
B) Diuretics.
C) ACE inhibitors.
D) ARBs.
E) Narcotics.

Discussion

The correct answer is E. Lithium is cleared by the kidneys. Anything that can cause a change in renal function can affect lithium levels. NSAIDs, diuretics, ACE inhibitors, and ARBs can all affect renal function.

Objectives: Did you learn to . . .

- Recognize and diagnose bipolar disorder?
- Initiate treatment for bipolar disorder?
- Describe some potential adverse effects of treatment for bipolar disorder?

CASE 15

A 20-year-old white female gymnast presents to you because she has missed her period for 6 months. She feels cold all the time and has noticed that when she crosses her legs, she gets pins-and-needles sensations down her leg. She had a stress fracture of her right tibia 5 years ago but denies any other medical history. She denies being sexually active and the review of systems is positive for frequent heartburn, constipation, and fatigue. Which of the following diagnoses would NOT be in your differential?

A) Pregnancy.
B) Hyperthyroidism.
C) Malignancy.
D) Anorexia nervosa (AN).
E) All of the above should be included in the differential.

Discussion

The correct answer is E. All the answers should be part of a reasonably broad differential diagnosis in this young woman. In patients presenting with weight loss and a possible eating disorder, you should eliminate medical causes of weight loss, using history, physical exam, and appropriate labs. Despite her denial of sexual activity, a pregnancy test is a necessary part of the evaluation, since pregnancy is the most common cause of amenorrhea in this population. Hyperthyroidism and malignancy can present with vague complaints similar to this patient's. Likewise, anorexia nervosa can give rise to this patient's constellation of symptoms.

* *

As you take more history, you realize that this patient is a very finicky eater. She is a strict vegan and restricts her calories to <1000 per day in order to stay in shape. She is 5 feet 3 inches tall and weighs only 100 pounds, but she thinks she is overweight.

Which of these additional findings would you expect on physical exam?

A) Bradycardia.
B) Hypertension.
C) Adnexal mass.
D) Clonus.
E) Proptosis.

Discussion

The correct answer is A. Common physical findings in weight loss, and specifically AN, include emaciation, sunken cheeks, hypotension, bradycardia, lanugo, mottled teeth, and dry or yellow skin. Peripheral edema may develop during weight gain or when laxative or diuretic abuse is stopped. Murmurs can occasionally be auscultated.

Patients with anorexia nervosa may present with:

A) Paresthesias.
B) Cold intolerance.
C) Constipation.
D) Fatigue.
E) All of the above.

Discussion

The correct answer is E. All of the above are symptoms of anorexia nervosa (AN). These are common symptoms seen in starvation. Answer A is not intuitive but is true. Loss of fat allows for greater exposure of superficial nerves, so the act of crossing the legs or sitting down on a hard chair can cause paresthesias.

 HELPFUL TIP: Patients with AN rarely have insight into the illness and often deny that weight loss is a problem. These patients are often perfectionists and overachievers who are sensitive to criticism and come from families with conflict. Weight loss is a method of control and is seen as a significant achievement.

 HELPFUL TIP: The word "anorexia" in anorexia nervosa is a misnomer, as loss of appetite is exceedingly rare in this illness. Patients are hungry but voluntarily restrict their caloric intake. The initial weight loss may be precipitated by appetite loss caused by depression, medical illness, dieting, or stressful life event.

Which would be an expected laboratory finding in this patient?

A) Leukocytosis.
B) Hyperkalemia.
C) Increased amylase.
D) Decreased cholesterol.
E) Erythrocytosis.

Discussion

The correct answer is C. Amylase may be increased as a result of purging behavior (and thus salivary stimulation). Answers A and E are incorrect. Leukopenia, not leukocytosis, with a mild, normochromic, normocytic anemia is a common hematologic finding, although the CBC may be normal. Answer B is incorrect. There is usually whole-body depletion of potassium, zinc, magnesium, and phosphate. Answer D is incorrect, as cholesterol is often elevated (as are BUN and liver enzymes). This cholesterol elevation is neither intuitive nor well-understood but is observed to occur in patients with AN. See Table 23–5 for medical complications of AN.

* *

In order to increase your patient's motivation to comply with medical recommendations, you describe some of the adverse effects of excessively low weight.

Table 23–5 SELECTED MEDICAL COMPLICATIONS OF ANOREXIA NERVOSA

Neurologic	Seizures Peripheral neuropathy Cortical atrophy Cognitive impairment
Cardiovascular	Bradycardia Orthostatic hypotension Heart failure ECG changes: low-voltage, nonspecific ST segment changes, QT prolongation
Endocrine	Amenorrhea Euthyroid sick syndrome Osteopenia/osteoporosis Growth retardation
Fluids and electrolytes	Dehydration Metabolic alkalosis Hypokalemia Hypomagnesemia Hypocalcemia
Gastrointestinal	Elevated liver enzymes Constipation Esophagitis Mallory-Weiss tears Parotid gland hypertrophy
Dermatologic	Lanugo Brittle nails and hair Acrocyanosis Dry, scaly skin
Hematologic	Bone marrow suppression

All of the following abnormal findings will resolve when an adequate body weight is regained EXCEPT:

A) Bradycardia.
B) Muscle wasting.
C) Osteoporosis.
D) Infertility.
E) Euthyroid sick syndrome.

Discussion

The correct answer is C. Patients with AN are usually young and therefore experience some of their lowest weights at the same time they are expected to reach peak bone mass. Bone mass later in life is the result of peak bone mass and subsequent bone loss. If a patient becomes osteopenic or osteoporotic when she is young, she will remain so as she ages. Return to good nutrition will not add bone mass that has been lost. All of the other physical changes listed should return to normal with return to a normal weight.

Which of the following is the most appropriate next step in the management of this patient?

A) Tell her to stop gymnastics, withdraw from classes, and go to live with her mother.
B) Start an antidepressant.
C) Admit her to the hospital.
D) Consult psychiatry and nutrition specialists.

Discussion

The correct answer is D. This patient is most likely to benefit from a coordinated plan involving a multidisciplinary team, including primary care, psychiatry, and nutrition. Answer A is incorrect, as it is a dramatic reaction that does not address the patient's primary problem, and the patient is unlikely to comply with it. Answer B is incorrect. An antidepressant may be helpful in patients with a clearly defined depressive or anxiety disorder. However, the use of antidepressant therapy for AN has not been successful, and certain antidepressants are associated with weight loss. Answer C, hospitalization, is not likely to be beneficial at this point. The utility of hospitalization has been difficult to determine in AN. Commonly accepted reasons for hospital admission include the following: severe low weight (70%–75% of ideal body weight); severe bradycardia (<40 bpm) or cardiac arrhythmia; marked symptomatic hypotension or syncope; acute psychiatric emergency (threatened suicide); significant dehydration or electrolyte disturbances; acute food refusal; and failed intensive outpatient therapy.

* *

As you plan to involve psychiatric and nutritional services, you continue your discussion of eating disorders with this patient.

Which of the following statements is NOT TRUE about the epidemiology of eating disorders?

A) At least 90% of eating disorder patients are female.
B) Rates are higher in industrialized, Western nations.
C) A family history of depression increases the risk of females developing eating disorders.
D) Male wrestlers have a higher risk of eating disorders than the average male.
E) Mortality rates in anorexia nervosa are insignificant.

Discussion

The correct answer is E. AN is characterized by a high incidence of mortality, one of the highest in psychiatry. It must be taken very seriously. Up to 10% of hospitalized patients die from direct effects of starvation, refeeding syndrome, suicide, or electrolyte imbalance leading to cardiac arrhythmias. At least 90% of eating disorder patients are female with prevalence rates higher in certain groups, such as models, actresses, athletes, and dancers. Western, industrialized societies endorse thinness and dieting as an ideal for women, resulting in higher rates of eating disorders. At normal body weights, **over 40% of 9- and 10-year-old American girls believe they are overweight** and consider dieting as an option! Eating disorders are distinctly uncommon in poorer countries where starvation is widespread and there is no cultural endorsement of thinness. Answer C is true. A family history of depression or obesity increases risk of an eating disorder by 2- to 5-fold, with a family history of depression alone increasing the risk about 5-fold. Answer D is true. In males, wrestlers have a higher prevalence of eating disorders because of weight requirements in their sport. In men, body shape and not necessarily absolute body weight is the typical focus of concern.

 HELPFUL TIP: There are two subtypes of AN: restrictive and binge/purge. Therefore, a patient who binges and purges (through forced emesis, laxatives, etc) does not necessarily have bulimia.

 HELPFUL TIP: Comorbidities are prevalent in eating disorder patients and include MDD (50%–75%), anxiety disorders, obsessive-compulsive disorder, and substance abuse. Personality disorders are also prevalent with the anxious, sensitive, rigid, and perfectionistic types predominating (Cluster C).

* *

In your discussions of eating disorders, your patient asks about bulimia and how you distinguish between AN and bulimia.

Which of the following statements is NOT true when comparing patients with AN and bulimia nervosa (BN)?

A) BN is more prevalent than AN.
B) BN patients are more likely to be normal weight than AN patients.
C) The prognosis for AN is better than that for BN.
D) BN patients are more likely to have esophageal tears.
E) Medications are effective in BN but not in AN.

Discussion

The correct answer is C. BN has a better prognosis than AN, with only 20% of women still meeting diagnostic criteria 5–10 years after initial presentation. BN is more common than AN, with the prevalence increasing just like it has with AN. Answer B is true. Patients with BN are usually close to normal weight. However, they show several stigmata: loss of dental enamel and chipped teeth with cavities; enlarged parotid salivary glands with elevated serum amylase from repeated vomiting episodes; menstrual irregularities; bradycardia and hypotension; and decreased metabolic rate. Rare complications include esophageal tears or gastric rupture due to gastric dilatation (not as likely in AN). Answer E is true. Treatment for BN involves the same principles as AN. However, serotonergic agents are useful, including SSRIs, TCAs, MAOIs, and trazodone. These agents reduce binge eating and bulimic symptoms whether patients are depressed or not.

 HELPFUL TIP: The mean age of onset of eating disorders is 17 years, with very rare onset in women >40 years (although recurrence can occur in this age group).

Objectives: Did you learn to . . .

- Evaluate a young person with a suspected eating disorder?
- Diagnose anorexia nervosa?
- Recognize medical complications of eating disorders?
- Distinguish between anorexia nervosa and bulimia nervosa?
- Initiate appropriate treatment and referral for a patient with an eating disorder?

QUICK QUIZ: EATING DISORDERS

In order to be diagnosed with bulimia nervosa according to DSM-IV, a patient must meet all of the following criteria EXCEPT:

A) Recurrent purging via self-induced vomiting.
B) Recurrent binge eating.
C) Symptoms are present at least twice per week for at least 3 months.
D) Self-evaluation is unduly influenced by body shape and weight.

Discussion

The correct answer is A. For the diagnosis of bulimia nervosa, self-induced vomiting need not be present. Rather, some sort of compensatory behavior must be present during bulimic episodes. This behavior might include vomiting, but is not limited to vomiting, and may also include laxative or diuretic use, fasting, or excessive exercise. Also, there are purging and non-purging subtypes of BN. Answers B, C, and D are required for the diagnosis of BN. BN affects about 1%–3% females (usually white) and 0.1%–0.3% males. Comorbidities of depression, anxiety, substance abuse, and personality disorders are also common. Dramatic, unstable personality traits (Cluster B) predominate in this illness unlike the sensitive, rigid (Cluster C) personality traits in AN.

QUICK QUIZ: EATING DISORDERS (OR, HOLD THE PIE FOR NOW, PLEASE)

A previously healthy 17-year-old female is hospitalized for anorexia nervosa. She has her weight rapidly restored with intravenous fluids and a 3,000 Kcal/day diet. She rapidly gains 10 pounds in her first 2 days and seems to be doing well. However, when you round the next morning, she is nonresponsive. Physical exam reveals evidence of JVD, pulmonary rales, and lower extremity edema.

What is the most likely cause of this patient's apparent congestive heart failure (CHF)?

A) Previously undiagnosed heart disease.
B) Refeeding syndrome.
C) Suicide attempt by SSRI overdose.
D) Myocardial infarction.

Discussion

The correct answer is B. The scenario described fits with the clinical picture caused by refeeding syndrome. Refeeding syndrome occurs when rapid expansion of the circulating volume overwhelms the cardiovascular system's ability to adapt, leading to CHF. It also involves changes in electrolytes and glucose. It typically occurs in malnourished patients. Prevention involves careful monitoring of electrolytes including magnesium, phosphorus, potassium and calcium, while advancing caloric intake in a small, linear fashion and keeping track of volume status. Answers A and D are incorrect as the patient is unlikely to have significant heart disease given her age and gender. Answer C is unlikely because suicide attempts by SSRIs do not generally lead to cardiac abnormalities like those described above.

 HELPFUL TIP: See Table 23–6 for warning signs that an agitated patient may become violent. For most of us, these warning signs may seem intuitive. And they are. The trick is paying attention to them and addressing them. See Table 23–7 for ways to calm the agitated patient (although in the editors' experience nothing beats IM haloperidol and IM lorazepam).

QUICK QUIZ: PHYSICIAN HEAL THYSELF?

Which of the following is true about physicians' risk of suicide compared to the general population?

A) Female physicians have a risk of successful suicide equal to male physicians.
B) Physicians are more likely to be depressed than the general population.
C) Female physicians are more likely to attempt suicide than the general female population.
D) Medical students and residents are less likely to be depressed than the general population.

Table 23–6 WARNING SIGNS THAT AN AGITATED PATIENT MAY BECOME VIOLENT

Hyperactivity: pacing or other increase in psychomotor activity

Loud, angry, or profane speech

Increased muscle tension, manifested by clenched jaw, fist, rigid posture, gripping chair, sitting on chair edge, etc

Intoxication

Suspicious, angry, or irritable affect

Breathlessness, tachycardia, diaphoresis, pupillary dilation, visibly palpitating temporal arteries

Uncooperativeness with requests

Door-slamming, chair-toppling, or other form of property destruction

Grabbing objects that could be potential weapons

Verbal or physical threats

The clinician's response to the patient: if you feel anxious, take it seriously and be alert to possible danger

Table 23–7 TECHNIQUES TO CALM THE AGITATED PATIENT

Remove the patient to a quiet and nonstimulating environment.

Keep a distance from the patient and avoid physical contact.

Identify exits and alarms.

Maintain non-threatening demeanor and stance.

Keep your hands at your side where they are easily visible.

While maintaining steady eye contact, speak in a steady but authoritative voice, using the patient's name with each sentence.

Avoid sudden jerky movements and remain calm.

Have familiar faces nearby if possible.

Show the patient concern but tell him that violence is not acceptable and you are willing to work with him if he calms down.

There is strength in numbers. Have other personnel nearby to help if necessary.

Call for help from police or security if needed. A backup system, which has been tested, should be in place.

Consider antipsychotics, such as haloperidol (available in oral and parenteral forms), risperidol (available in liquid), etc. A benzodiazepine may be used as an adjunct, but should **not** be used alone.

Mechanical restraints may be employed if absolutely necessary.

Figure out **why** the patient is agitated (eg, take history, perform mental status exam, order appropriate tests, etc).

Discussion

The correct answer is A. In the general population, women have 2–4 times more suicide attempts than men, while men are 4 times more likely than women to be successful. However, among physicians, the rate of successful suicide in men and women is equivalent. This occurs despite the fact that female physicians have fewer attempts than the general female population. Physicians have roughly the same rate of depression as the general population, while medical students and residents have a higher rate than the general population (15%–30% versus 16% in the general population). Other factors for suicide risk (in addition to being a physician) are noted in Table 23–8.

 QUICK QUIZ: SUICIDE RISK

You have a colleague who is depressed and has transient thoughts of suicide. Which of the following would suggest that he should be hospitalized today?

A) He thinks about suicide only infrequently.

B) He has not formulated a plan to commit suicide.

C) He has updated his will within the past few days.

D) He is willing to follow up in clinic tomorrow.

E) He has given away his guns.

Discussion

The correct answer is C. If a person admits to suicidal ideation, ask the following questions to assess his level of risk and to determine whether or not he should be hospitalized.

How often does he think about suicide?

Does he have a concrete plan? And if so, is it plausible?

Is he giving away treasured belongings, updating his will, making final plans, etc?

Is he in danger of acting on his thoughts?

Why has he not attempted suicide yet? What keeps him from doing it?

Does he have access to harmful means (eg, guns, drugs, etc)?

Table 23–8   FACTORS AFFECTING SUICIDE RISK

Risk factors
- Living alone (particularly first year alone)
- Loss of spouse or separation
- Alcohol use
- Having access to a gun or lethal means
- Loss of activity, job, property, or capabilities
- Mild/minimal cognitive impairment
- Paranoia
- Hopelessness
- Anxiety
- Older white male
- Personal or family history of suicide attempt or completion
- Urban dweller

Protective factors
- Effective treatment for mental and physical disorders
- Social and family support
- Coping skills
- Resilience
- Religious faith
- Lack of access to lethal means

 QUICK QUIZ: PSYCHOTROPIC DRUGS

Which of these antidepressants can be administered once weekly?

A)   Paroxetine (Paxil).
B)   Buspirone (Wellbutrin).
C)   Fluoxetine (Prozac).
D)   Escitalopram (Lexapro).
E)   Venlafaxine, sustained release (Effexor-SR).

Discussion

The correct answer is C. Fluoxetine has a long enough half-life that it can be administered once a week. You don't need to prescribe the "long-acting" fluoxetine. Any fluoxetine can be dosed once weekly.

CASE 18

You are on call and have been paged to see a 21-year-old female who has just overdosed on a handful of acetaminophen because her boyfriend left her after their most recent fight. She has had similar overdoses

three times in the past (they fight a lot). According to a friend, she has a history of tumultuous relationships. In the ED, she is combative and yelling, "I'm so angry that I'm still alive!" She has a blood alcohol level of 106 mg/dL.

What is the most likely primary diagnosis?

A)   Antisocial personality disorder.
B)   Bipolar affective disorder.
C)   Major depressive disorder.
D)   Borderline personality disorder.
E)   Somatization disorder.

Discussion

The correct answer is D. This patient's history is consistent with a diagnosis of borderline personality disorder (BPD). Persons with BPD often have stormy relationships, characterized by extremes of emotional intensity (eg, "love-hate" relationships). You might also consider depression as a diagnosis here, but the history does not support major depressive disorder. However, concomitant depression is common in patients with BPD. A, B, and E are not supported by the clinical presentation. BPD is mostly a diagnosis of females (over 90%). Characteristics are listed in Table 23–9.

 HELPFUL TIP: A personality disorder (PD) is an enduring pattern of relating to the world in ways which are inflexible, ineffective, and markedly different from cultural norms. PDs cause distress or functional impairment and start by adolescence in most people. The prevalence rate of personality disorders varies widely across studies, with borderline personality disorder being the most prevalent of all.

* *

Your patient's boyfriend storms into the ED and demands to see her. He has "love" and "hate" tattooed on his knuckles. The nurse recognizes him immediately as a frequent visitor. Apparently, he has been in the ED on multiple occasions for injuries sustained from fights. Your patient pulls you aside to tell you that she is afraid of him, saying, "I just worry when he gets mad. He went to jail for beating and raping his last girlfriend." The nurse also informs you that he is suspected of stealing narcotics from a pharmacy in town. You call security.

Table 23–9 CHARACTERISTICS OF BORDER-LINE PERSONALITY DISORDER

Fears of abandonment

Unstable and intense relationships

Unstable sense of self

Impulsivity

Suicidal behavior, threats or gestures or self-mutilation (cutting is often a feature of borderline personality disorder)

Significant mood reactivity

Chronic feelings of emptiness

Intense anger outbursts

Transient stress-related paranoid ideation or dissociation

Table 23–10 CHARACTERISTICS OF ANTI-SOCIAL PERSONALITY DISORDER

Recurrent criminality

Deceitfulness shown by repeated lying, use of aliases, or conning others

Impulsivity

Irritability and aggression

Reckless disregard for safety

Consistent irresponsibility, failing to fulfill financial obligations or work

Lack of remorse

Childhood conduct disorder and person now at least 18 years

Which of the following personality disorders is most likely in this man?

A) Paranoid personality disorder.
B) Histrionic personality disorder.
C) Schizotypal personality disorder.
D) Antisocial personality disorder.

Discussion

The correct answer is D. Antisocial personality disorder (ASPD) is primarily seen in males, and of the options given, it is the only personality disorder that really fits. ASPD is quite prevalent in prison populations. Answers A and C are incorrect because these are Cluster A disorders, which are characterized by strange rather than violent behavior. Answer B is incorrect. Histrionic personality disorder shows attention-seeking and seductive behavior. Although patients with ASPD can be charming, they also use violence and threats to achieve their purposes. Characteristics of ASPD are listed in the Table 23–10.

Besides borderline personality disorder, which other personality disorder increases the risk of *completed suicide* the most?

A) Paranoid personality disorder.
B) Histrionic personality disorder.
C) Schizotypal personality disorder.
D) Avoidant personality disorder.
E) Antisocial personality disorder.

Discussion

The correct answer is E. In addition to BPD, ASPD is the other personality disorder most likely to be seen in completed suicides.

Considering the current psychiatric diagnosis classification system, under what axis will you classify this patient and her boyfriend in terms of their personality disorders?

A) Axis I.
B) Axis II.
C) Axis III.
D) Axis IV.
E) Axis V.

Discussion

The correct answer is B. The current psychiatric classification system is listed in Table 23–11.

 HELPFUL TIP: Impulsivity is a risk for completed suicide. Even though patients may not want to die, an impulsively taken overdose or other suicide attempt may inadvertently lead to death. This is why patients with borderline personality disorder and anti-social personality disorder have a high risk of completed suicide.

Table 23–11 CURRENT PSYCHIATRIC CLASSIFICATION SYSTEM

Axis I. Major psychiatric disorders (eg, depression, schizophrenia, etc)

Axis II. Personality disorders and mental retardation
- Cluster A: "the **weird** cluster"—patients are aloof, act strange, and prefer to be alone. Paranoid, schizoid, and schizotypal personality disorders are included here.
- Cluster B: "the **wild** cluster"—patients have significant problems with mood lability, impulsivity, or are preoccupied with being admired for their sexuality or intelligence. Borderline, antisocial, histrionic, and narcissistic personality disorders are included here.
- Cluster C: "the **whiny** cluster"–patients are clingy, sensitive, and rigid. Avoidant, dependent, and obsessive-compulsive personality disorders are included here.

Axis III. General medical conditions potentially relevant to understanding the psychiatric disorders.

Axis IV. Psychosocial and environmental factors that may contribute to the patients' distress (eg, homelessness, recent divorce, etc).

Axis V. Global Assessment of Function, a 0–100-point scale for assessing the individual's overall level of functioning in the physician's judgment.

Table 23–12 ACRONYMS FOR SUICIDE RISK ASSESSMENT

NO HOPE	SAD PERSONS
No framework for meaning	**S**ex–male
Overt change in clinical condition	**A**ge–older
Hostile interpersonal environment	**D**epression
Out of hospital recently	**P**revious attempt
Predisposing personality factors	**E**thanol abuse
Excuses for dying to help others	**R**ational thought loss
	Social support lacking
	Organized plan
	No spouse
	Sickness

You have a frank discussion with your patient about suicide.

Which of the following is NOT a true statement about suicide in the general population?

A) Medical diagnoses can increase the risk of suicide.
B) Over 90% of people who commit suicide have a mental or substance abuse disorder.
C) Older Americans are at higher risk of suicide.
D) The rate of successful suicides has increased over the years.
E) Suicide is one of the top 10 causes of death in the U.S.

Discussion

The correct answer is D. The rate of completed suicide has stayed stable over time. Answer A is a true statement. Medical diagnoses can be risk factors for suicide, especially chronic pain, chronic illness, terminal illness, or recent surgery. Older Americans commit suicide at a rate four times that of the general population

with a peak incidence at 75 years for men and 60 years for women. Answer E is a true statement. Suicide is the seventh leading cause of death in the United States and the third leading cause of death in those aged 15 to 24 years. There are two acronyms that are useful for assessing suicide risk: NO HOPE and SAD PERSONS. See Table 23–12.

 HELPFUL TIP: 75% of older Americans who commit suicide have seen their primary care physician within the preceding four weeks and 39% within the same week. Up to half of successful suicides have made a prior attempt.

Objectives: Did you learn to . . .

- Identify borderline and antisocial personality disorders?
- Classify personality disorders?
- Assess suicide risk?

CASE 19

A 21-year-old man presents to your clinic because his girlfriend dragged him in. He just started his first year in college but quit 2 days ago because he feels that "they are all out to get me." He has not been sleeping because he thinks he might be murdered in his sleep.

He tells you that the FBI has bugged your office and, therefore, does not want to answer your questions.

Which of the following would you NOT expect to find on mental status exam?

A) Delusions.
B) Hallucinations.
C) Lack of insight.
D) Decreased psychomotor activity.
E) Poverty of speech.

Discussion

The correct answer is D. The patient described is acutely psychotic. You would expect him to have increased psychomotor activity. All of the other options would also be anticipated findings in this patient. Common symptoms of psychosis include delusions, hallucinations, psychomotor agitation, flight of ideas, nonsensical speech and behavior, lack of insight into one's behavior, and lack of judgment.

All of the following are potential causes of this patient's psychosis EXCEPT:

A) Substance abuse.
B) Alcohol withdrawal.
C) Bipolar disorder.
D) Bereavement.

Discussion

The correct answer is D. Bereavement may result in mild delusions and sometimes hallucinations regarding the bereaved subject, but it should not cause overt psychosis. Moreover, there is nothing in the history here to support a diagnosis of bereavement. Causes of psychosis are listed in Table 23–13.

 HELPFUL TIP: Psychosis is a symptom and not a diagnosis and should prompt a search for an etiology. Some of the causes are potentially life threatening.

* *

The patient relaxes and becomes cooperative, and you are able to obtain a history and perform a physical exam. He denies drug use or medical illnesses. Your patient thinks he is going "crazy" and admits that he has been having these symptoms "for a while" but did

Table 23–13 CAUSES OF PSYCHOSIS

Potentially life-threatening causes
- Meningitis or encephalitis
- Hypoxemia
- Hypertensive encephalopathy
- Wernicke encephalopathy
- Intracranial bleed
- Drug withdrawal, intoxication, or reaction to prescribed drugs

Other medical causes
- Metabolic disorders (eg, hyperglycemia, hyponatremia, etc)
- Neurologic disorders
- Nutritional deficiencies (eg, pellagra, beriberi, pernicious anemia, etc)
- Industrial exposure to toxins

Psychiatric causes
- Schizophrenia or schizophreniform disorders
- Brief psychotic disorder
- Mood disorders including bipolar disorder and psychotic depression
- Schizoaffective disorder
- Dementia
- Delirium
- Delusional disorder

not want to tell anybody, for fear of being institutionalized. Your physical exam and labs are unremarkable.

Which of the following diagnoses is the most likely cause of this patient's psychosis?

A) Schizophrenia.
B) Psychotic depression.
C) Delirium.
D) Drug intoxication.
E) Dementia.

Discussion

The correct answer is A. Schizophrenia is a heterogeneous group of disorders characterized by the following: positive symptoms (delusions, hallucinations, disorganized behavior, disorganized speech); negative symptoms (poverty of speech, anhedonia, affective flattening, avolition, asociality); mood symptoms (dysphoria, suicidal thoughts, hopelessness); and cognitive symptoms (attention and memory deficits and difficulty with abstract thinking). It is the most common of the psychotic disorders. A negative laboratory evaluation and physical exam makes drug intoxication unlikely, while this patient's ability to converse with you and give a history makes delirium and dementia unlikely. Psychotic depression is unusual in young people, but rather more commonly seen in older patients with severe depression.

Which of the following statements is NOT true about schizophrenia?

A) Nearly 50% attempt suicide with a 10% success rate.

B) Lifetime prevalence is 1% worldwide, consistent across cultures.

C) Schizophrenia is a disease of late adolescence or early adulthood.

D) Men are more likely to be affected than women.

E) Risk of relapse is at least 50% after successful treatment in patients who do not remain on antipsychotic maintenance therapy.

Discussion

The correct answer is D. Schizophrenia has a worldwide prevalence of approximately 1%, which is true for all cultures, countries and both genders. It generally begins in late adolescence or early adulthood, and onset >50 years is rare and should prompt the search for other etiologies to explain the psychosis. Men have a slightly earlier age of onset (early 20s) than women (late 20s), but men and women are affected equally by the illness. The course is variable with some patients having exacerbations and remissions (although full remissions are rare), while others remain chronically ill. Approximately 50% of patients who develop schizophrenia have a family history of schizophrenia. Suicide attempts are common, usually the result of depression or a response to command hallucinations, paranoid delusions, or agitation. Nearly 50% will attempt suicide, while about 10% will be successful. After successful treatment of the first episode, approximately 50% will relapse if not on maintenance medication.

Which of the following medication options is the proper treatment choice?

A) Olanzapine (Zyprexa).

B) Risperidone (Risperdal).

C) Haloperidol (Haldol).

D) Aripiprazole (Abilify).

E) Any of the above.

Discussion

The correct answer is E. All of the antipsychotics listed are first-line treatment choices for schizophrenia. Most psychiatrists have replaced older "typical" agents like haloperidol with newer "atypical" agents (eg, risperidone, olanzapine) because of better tolerability and possibly increased benefit for negative symptoms. However, the newer agents are significantly more expensive than the older agents. Also, many atypicals cause significant weight gain, and some have been linked to new-onset diabetes. The CATIE trial, a recent large study that compared several newer antipsychotic medications to perphenazine, an older antipsychotic, measured outcomes associated with antipsychotic use including efficacy and tolerability. This study showed that tolerability had a significant impact on medication compliance, and it also demonstrated that for some patients, an older antipsychotic may still be a good option. Of the newer agents, aripiprazole (Ability) and ziprasidone (Geodon) are less associated with weight gain.

Which of the following is TRUE of the course of schizophrenia?

A) Positive symptoms usually occur first.

B) Negative symptoms are easier to treat than positive symptoms.

C) Negative symptoms often look like depression.

D) Schizophrenia is not typically associated with brain changes.

E) Family therapy is not helpful in this illness.

Discussion

The correct answer is C. Negative symptoms often precede the development of the positive symptoms by many years, are often non-specific, and can be mistaken for depression. A typical history is that of a normal young man who begins to fail classes and avoid his old friends as he gets to the end of high school. This is often mistaken for teenage rebellion, depression, or drug use until the onset of positive psychotic symptoms of hallucinations or delusions several years later. Answer B is incorrect. Negative symptoms are chronic and are resistant to treatment with all currently available antipsychotics. Antipsychotic drugs modulate dopamine and/or serotonin and are much better at treating positive symptoms. Answer D is incorrect, as brain imaging may reveal enlargement of cerebral ventricles and decreased brain volume. However, these findings are neither sensitive nor specific enough to have much value in diagnosis. Answer E is incorrect. A large body of literature supports the fact that family therapy, especially directed at support and psychoeducation, reduces the risk of relapse. Recent evidence indicates that individual cognitive behavioral therapy can also be effective.

Objectives: Did you learn to . . .

- Recognize psychosis and its causative diagnoses?
- Treat psychosis?
- Recognize schizophrenia and understand its epidemiology and prognosis?

CASE 20

A 33-year-old factory worker comes to your clinic complaining of sleep difficulty since he moved to the "graveyard shift." He complains of falling asleep at work and having difficulty sleeping during the day.

Which of the following is the most likely diagnosis?

A) Narcolepsy.
B) Circadian rhythm sleep disorder.
C) Obstructive sleep apnea.
D) Primary insomnia.

Discussion

The correct answer is B. This patient suffers (as do most residents and a significant number of physicians) from a circadian rhythm sleep disorder, which is defined as a sleep disruption leading to excessive sleepiness when the patient wishes to be awake or insomnia when the patient wishes to be asleep. It occurs as a result of a mismatch between the biological circadian rhythm and the person's environment. He does not give a history consistent with narcolepsy or obstructive sleep apnea, and primary insomnia is a diagnosis of exclusion.

* *

He asks your advice on how to treat his sleeplessness.

What would be the best advice to offer at this time?

A) Have him sleep at work.
B) Have him take naps throughout the day.
C) Tell him to quit his job.
D) Recommend bright light at night before going to work.
E) Prescribe stimulants for when he is at work.

Discussion

The correct answer is D. This patient's circadian rhythm disturbance might also be called a "phase-advance" type sleep disorder (early sleep onset with insomnia at the desired sleep period). Such problems respond best to bright light in the evening to keep one awake during the time the individual would usually be asleep. Light boxes are available commercially and should provide white light at 2,500 lux or more. The light should be fairly close to the patient's eyes, and a bit off to the side. The other options are not likely to be helpful if this patient wants to keep his job.

If this patient wished to use a nutritional or herbal supplement, which of the following would you recommend?

A) Melatonin.
B) Kava-kava.
C) Gingko.
D) Ginseng.
E) St. John's wort.

Discussion

The correct answer is A. There is some evidence to suggest that melatonin can help with circadian rhythm disorders. Melatonin should be taken at the time of day the patient wants to sleep. In this case, you should advise him to take it in the morning. The doses used for circadian rhythm disturbances are much less than the dose used for primary insomnia, typically 0.5 mg or less, compared to 3 mg. The other herbal supplements have no evidence for use in sleep disturbances except for kava-kava which is too dangerous to recommend.

Which of the following is NOT a delayed sleep phase type of circadian rhythm sleep disorder?

A) Readaptation to day work from night work.
B) West-to-east jet lag.
C) East-to-west jet lag.
D) All of the above are considered delayed sleep phase circadian rhythm sleep disorders.
E) None of the above is considered a delayed sleep phase circadian rhythm sleep disorder.

Discussion

The correct answer is C. Delayed sleep phase involves a persistent pattern of late sleep onset and late morning awakening. West-to-east jet lag and readapting to day shift after working night shift also cause similar problems. "C" does not cause a delayed sleep phase disturbance. East-to-west jet lag causes the opposite problem, advancing sleep phase so that persons are sleepy early in the evening but then awake early in the morning. A potentially effective treatment for delayed sleep phase would include prescribing a bright light in the morning and melatonin in the afternoon.

Objectives: Did you learn to . . .

- Recognize circadian rhythm disorders?
- Recommend treatment for circadian rhythm disorders?

 QUICK QUIZ: BECAUSE YOU WILL FORGET IT WITHOUT REPETITION.

A 70-year-old male presents with memory loss that has been progressive over the years. He often has fluctuating attention and is rigid with bradykinesia. He frequently experiences visual hallucinations.

Which of the following is the most likely diagnosis?

A) Alzheimer disease.
B) Dementia with Lewy bodies.
C) Parkinson disease.
D) Vascular dementia.
E) Frontotemporal dementia.

Discussion

The correct answer is B. Dementia with Lewy bodies (DLB) shares many features in common with Parkinson disease (PD). These features include parkinsonian motor symptoms, such as bradykinesia, rigidity, and tremor. Both PD and DLB are characterized histologically by the presence of Lewy bodies. However, in DLB, Lewy bodies are diffusely spread in the cortical regions and brainstem, whereas in PD, Lewy bodies are primarily present in the subcortical nuclei. Fluctuating cognition that resembles delirium, visual hallucinations, and an exquisite sensitivity to the adverse effects of neuroleptics all characterize DLB. There is a lack of response of dopaminergic agents with DLB but cholinesterase inhibitors offer a modest benefit.

 QUICK QUIZ: DEMENTIA

A 65-year-old man with a history of hypertension, diabetes, and peripheral vascular disease has been noted to have abrupt deterioration in his cognitive ability following an episode of disorientation and word-finding difficulty 1 month ago.

Which of the following is the most likely diagnosis?

A) Alzheimer disease.
B) Dementia with Lewy bodies.
C) Parkinson disease.
D) Vascular dementia.
E) Frontotemporal dementia.

Discussion

The correct answer is D. Vascular dementia (previously known as multi-infarct dementia) is caused by vascular disease and, next to Alzheimer and Lewy body dementias, is one of the most common causes of dementia. It classically presents with an abrupt onset followed by step-wise deterioration of cognitive function. Medical comorbidities are common, including diabetes, hypertension, and obesity. Evidence of vascular disease is usually present on clinical exam with focal neurological signs, such as are seen after a stroke involving motor areas. Imaging typically shows infarctions of periventricular and deep subcortical white matter, presenting as white matter hyper-intensities on T_2 weighted MRI. Treatment includes modifying vascular risk factors, and some authors recommend cholinesterase inhibitors.

CASE 21

A 37-year-old female patient returns to see you for follow-up of depression. You last saw her a month ago, and at that time she was experiencing her third relapse of recurrent major depression. She had been in remission for 3 years prior, and until 2 years ago she had been taking sertraline 150 mg daily, a regimen that she had found effective during an 18-month course of treatment. At her visit last month, you assessed her symptoms with the Patient Health Questionnaire-9 (PHQ-9), and her score at that time was 21. You reinstituted sertraline at 50 mg daily for 2 weeks and then 100 mg daily, which she is currently taking. She reports compliance with her medication, and she reports having mild nausea if she takes it on an empty stomach. She feels the medication is somewhat sedating, but she says the sedation is not as much of a problem for her in the daytime as long as she takes the sertraline at night. At her visit today, her PHQ-9 score is 17. She denies having thoughts of death or suicide.

Which of the following options is LEAST appropriate to recommend to your patient at this time?

A) Continue sertraline 100 mg daily and return for follow-up in 1 month.

B) Continue sertraline 100 mg daily, add weekly cognitive behavior therapy, and return for follow-up in 1 month.

C) Increase sertraline to 150 mg daily.

D) Stop the sertraline and start citalopram 20 mg daily.

E) Continue sertraline 100 mg daily and add bupropion SR 150 mg BID, return for follow-up in 1 month.

Discussion

The correct answer is D. At the current visit, the patient has been taking sertraline for 1 month and has been at the present dose for 2 weeks. It can take up to 6–8 weeks for an antidepressant medication to reach its full effect, so it is reasonable to maintain the medication at its present dose and reassess in 1 month. Answer choices B, C, and E are more appropriate options for the patient. Combination treatment with cognitive behavior therapy and an antidepressant medication has been shown to be more effective for treating depression than either treatment strategy alone. The STAR*D trial, a multisite randomized controlled trial funded by the National Institutes of Mental Health (NIMH), used algorithms with aggressive titration of antidepressant medication, including sertraline with a target dose of 150 mg daily. As this patient previously responded to sertraline 150 mg daily, it is reasonable to increase the dose of sertraline now to 150 mg daily. The STAR*D trial also found that many patients who did not respond to an initial antidepressant regimen did respond to either a dose increase, addition of an augmentation agent (buspirone, bupropion, or triiodothyronine), or switch to a different antidepressant. Adding an augmentation agent, since she has had a partial response to the current regimen, is a reasonable option. Switching to a new antidepressant at this time is not indicated.

Which of the following statements is NOT true regarding the PHQ-9?

A) The PHQ-9 is a clinician-administered questionnaire to evaluate for symptoms of major depression.

B) It takes 3–5 minutes to complete the PHQ-9.

C) A score of 10 or more on the PHQ-9 is a positive screen.

D) The PHQ-9 can be used to screen for depression as well as to monitor symptom severity over time.

E) The PHQ-9 does not assess for suicide risk.

Discussion

The correct answer is A. The PHQ-9 is a patient-administered, 9-item questionnaire that takes 3–5 minutes to complete. It can be used to screen for major depression as well as to monitor symptom severity over time. A score >10 is considered a positive screen, while a score <5 is considered to be negative or in remission. The maximum score is 30. While the PHQ-9 does ask about the presence of "thoughts of death or dying," it does not assess whether someone is at low or high risk for suicide attempt.

Objectives: Did you learn to . . .

- Develop strategies to treat resistant depression?
- Describe a widely used depression assessment tool, the PHQ-9?

BIBLIOGRAPHY

American Foundation for Suicide Prevention Available at www.afsp.org/physician.

Diagnostic and Statistical Manual of Mental Disorders. 4th ed., Text Revision. Washington, DC: American Psychiatric Association, 2000.

Hendin H, Davis M, Detre T, et al. Confronting depression and suicide in physicians: A consensus statement. *JAMA.* 2003;289:3161.

Hendrick V, Smith LM, Suri R, et al. Birth outcomes after prenatal exposure to antidepressant medication. *Am J Obstetric Gynecology.* 2003;188:812.

Khan A, Khan S, Kolts R, Brown WA. Suicide rates in clinical trials of SSRIs, other antidepressants, and placebo: analysis of FDA reports. *Am J Psychiatry.* 2003;160:790.

Kulin NA, Pastuszak A, Sage SR, et al. Pregnancy outcome following maternal use of the new selective serotonin reuptake inhibitors. *JAMA.* 1998;279:609.

Lieberman JA, Stroup TS, McEvoy JP, et al. Effectiveness of antipsychotic drugs in patients with chronic schizophrenia. *N Engl J Med.* 2005;353:1209.

Nemeroff CB, Schatzberg AF. *Recognition and Treatment of Psychiatric Disorders: a Psychopharmacology Handbook for Primary Care.* Washington, DC: American Psychiatric Press, 1999.

Rush AJ, Trivedi MH, Wisniewski SR, et al. Acute and longer-term outcomes in depressed outpatients requiring one or several treatment steps: a STAR*D report. *Am J Psychiatry.* 2006;163:1905.

Schatzberg AF, Haddad P, Kaplan EM, et al. Serotonin reuptake inhibitor discontinuation syndrome: A hypothetical definition. *J Clinl Psychiatry*. 1997;58:5.

Stahl SM. Essential *Psychopharmacology of Depression and Bipolar Disorder*. Cambridge University Press, Cambridge UK, 2001.

Szymanski ML, Zolotor A. Attention deficit/hyperactivity disorder: management. *Am Fam Physician*. 2001;64:1355.

Uncapher H; Arean PA. Physicians are less willing to treat suicidal ideation in older patients. *J Am Geriatr Soc* 2000;48:188.

Varley CK. Psychopharmalogical Treatment of Major Depressive Disorder in Children and Adolescents. Editorial. *JAMA*. 2003;290:1091.

Wagner KD, Ambrosini P, Rynn M, et al. Efficacy of sertraline in the treatment of children and adolescents with major depressive disorder: two randomized controlled trials. *JAMA*. 2003;290:1033.

Wisner KL, Gelenberg AJ, Leonard H, et al. Pharmacologic treatment of depresision during pregnancy. *JAMA*. 1999;282:1264.

24

Nutrition and Herbal Medicine

Philip Gregory

CASE 1

A 59-year-old male presents for follow-up. He is well-known to you, receiving chronic anticoagulation with warfarin for a mechanical aortic valve. His protime and INR have been in the therapeutic range for years. When asked, he denies taking any other medications. He has had no new medical problems and is feeling well.

Today his INR is 6.2 (therapeutic range 2.5–3.5). You inquire about dietary changes, focusing on foods rich in vitamin K.

Which of the following is true regarding vitamin K?

A) Vitamin K is a water-soluble vitamin.
B) Broccoli and olive oil are good sources of vitamin K.
C) Vitamin K deficiency results in a hypercoaguable state.
D) Warfarin reduces the absorption of vitamin K.
E) Vegetarians are at risk for developing vitamin K deficiency.

Discussion

The correct answer is B. Vitamin K is a fat-soluble vitamin present in leafy green vegetables such as spinach and cabbage and in other foods such as milk, butter, bacon, and vegetable oils. Olive oil and broccoli are particularly rich in vitamin K. Therefore, vegetarians are not at high risk for developing vitamin K deficiency. Vitamin K deficiency causes a hypocoaguable state resulting in a reduction in clotting factors and elevated prothrombin time and INR, leading to poor clotting ability and hemorrhage. Warfarin does act on vitamin K, but by reducing conversion of vitamin K to its active form rather than reducing absorption.

You would be more likely to suspect vitamin K deficiency in this patient if he also suffered from which of the following conditions?

A) Crohn disease.
B) Irritable bowel syndrome.
C) Hepatitis C.
D) Coronary artery disease.

Discussion

The correct answer is A. Vitamin K deficiency can occur with chronic small bowel disease, after small bowel resection, and with use of broad-spectrum antibiotics. Microorganisms in the bowel synthesize vitamin K, and use of broad-spectrum antibiotics reduces the numbers of these organisms. The majority of vitamin K is absorbed in the distal small bowel, and any disease affecting this area—including Crohn and celiac diseases—can reduce the absorption of the vitamin. Irritable bowel syndrome is a functional disease not associated with impaired absorption.

* *

Upon more direct questioning, the patient denies any changes in his diet but admits to starting a vitamin therapy program recently. He has no clue what he is taking and calls his wife to find out what the products contain. You suspect that he is taking excessive doses of vitamins that may affect his INR.

Large doses of which of the following vitamins are most likely to result in an increased INR in patients taking warfarin?

A) Vitamin A.
B) Vitamin C.
C) Vitamin D.
D) Vitamin E.
E) Zinc.

Discussion

The correct answer is D. Large doses of vitamin E (>400 mg/day) can interfere with vitamin K metabolism and platelet function, resulting in increased prothrombin time and therefore increased INR in some patients. In patients who take warfarin, starting a high-dose vitamin E supplement should be done cautiously. Extra monitoring of INR and/or warfarin dose adjustments may be needed. See Table 24–1 for supplements that can affect the INR.

The other answer choices are unlikely to affect the INR. Vitamin A (answer A) consumed in quantities exceeding 10 times the Recommended Daily Allowance (RDA) for several months may cause alopecia, ataxia, glossitis, and hepatotoxicity. Vitamin C (answer B) is usually well-tolerated but large doses can cause nausea, diarrhea, and abdominal pain. Excessive intake of vitamin D (answer C) may cause hypercalcemia, hypercalciuria, nausea, vomiting, myalgia, and bone demineralization. Zinc (answer E) toxicity manifests as anemia and depressed immune function.

Table 24–1 COMMON VITAMINS AND HERBALS THAT INTERACT WITH WARFARIN (PARTIAL LIST)

Warfarin Interaction	Vitamin/Herbal
Increased INR and increased risk of bleeding	Danshen
	Dong quai
	Fish oil
	Garlic
	Ginkgo
	Policosanol
	Vitamin E
Decreased INR and decreased risk of bleeding	Coenzyme Q10
	St. John's wort
	Vitamin K

 HELPFUL TIP: In comparison with water-soluble vitamins (B complex, C), fat-soluble vitamins (A, D, E, and K) are more likely to accumulate, resulting in toxicity.

* *

The patient learns that the vitamin therapy he currently takes has large amounts of vitamin E, but no vitamin K. You counsel him to discontinue this supplement, hold a dose of warfarin, and continue on the same dose. You ask him to come back next week for another prothrombin time/INR. Before leaving, he asks about taking a multivitamin.

From available evidence, you are able to tell him:

A) "Most multivitamins do not contain enough vitamin E to cause a problem."
B) "Multivitamins should be standard preventive medicine and have a well-described role in improving health."
C) "Iron supplements are recommended for middle-aged males."
D) "Folic acid and B vitamins should be taken by everyone to reduce homocysteine."

Discussion

The correct answer is A. Most multiple vitamins contain <400 IU of vitamin E and usually will not cause a problem. A fairly well-balanced North American diet provides the necessary nutrients to avoid vitamin deficiency syndromes. Supplementation with multivitamins is usually not necessary unless there are dietary intake deficiencies related to an unbalanced diet. Taking a multivitamin generally has **not** been linked to improved health status. Average adult males generally have adequate iron stores and should not receive supplemental iron due to the potential for exacerbating undiagnosed iron storage disease. While folate, vitamin B_6, and vitamin B_{12} lower serum homocysteine levels, there is no evidence that this intervention is helpful in reducing disease burden or improving health.

Regarding vitamin and mineral supplementation, all of the following statements are true EXCEPT:

A) Folate supplementation during pregnancy is recommended to decrease the risk of neural tube defects.

B) Calcium and vitamin D supplementation in postmenopausal females is recommended to reduce the risk of osteoporosis and fractures.

C) Vitamin D supplementation in elderly patients may reduce the risk of falls.

D) Vitamin E supplementation in elderly patients may reduce the risk of cardiovascular disease.

Discussion

The correct answer is D. It is a false statement because vitamin E supplementation has not been shown to reduce the risk of cardiovascular disease and may be associated with an increased risk of all-cause mortality at doses >400 IU per day.

The others statements are true. Answer A has plenty of evidence to back it up. Folate supplementation is universally recommended during the prenatal period and should be started even before pregnancy actually occurs. Answer B is widely recommended although the evidence for calcium reducing fracture risk is weak. As for answer C, one meta-analysis has concluded that vitamin D supplementation in older adults is associated with decreased fall risk (Bischoff-Ferrari, et al, JAMA 2004).

> **HELPFUL TIP:** In general, daily multiple vitamins do not contain large enough doses of vitamins to result in toxicity.

Objectives: Did you learn to . . .

- Describe symptoms, signs, and causes of vitamin K deficiency?
- Identify common vitamins and herbals that interact with warfarin?
- Recognize symptoms of fat-soluble vitamin toxicities?
- Identify benefits, risks, and limitations of vitamin supplementation?

QUICK QUIZ: SUPPLEMENTS TO BREAST MILK

A 6-month-old male infant presents for routine health exam and immunizations. His mother is a strict vegan and has been nursing him exclusively. She has not introduced any foods and she wants to keep breast-feeding him primarily for at least the next 6 months. She takes no medicines and no supplements of any kind.

This breast-fed patient should have supplementation of all of the following EXCEPT:

A) Vitamin B_{12}.

B) Vitamin C.

C) Vitamin D.

D) Iron.

Discussion

The correct answer is B. Vitamin C supplementation is not required. Children breast-fed by strict vegan mothers should have vitamin B_{12} supplementation. Vitamin D is now recommended for all breast-fed infants. Iron is recommended for all breast-fed infants ≥6 months who are not eating iron-fortified foods. There are a variety of liquid multiple vitamins to choose from (eg, Poly-Vi-Sol).

CASE 2

A 34-year-old female presents to your office with concerns about weight gain. She has gained over 100 pounds since she graduated from high school. She tearfully reveals that the weight gain has come despite "not eating much." She walks for exercise, but is unable to quantify her walking.

She denies chronic illnesses. Her only surgery was a tubal ligation after her last child. She smokes 10 cigarettes per day and is unwilling to quit due to fears of further weight gain. She drinks alcohol once or twice per week, never consuming more than 3 beers. The review of systems is positive for a dry cough, bilateral knee pain, and fatigue.

On physical examination, you find an afebrile female with an elevated blood pressure (142/94 mm Hg). She is 5 feet, 3 inches tall and weighs 231 pounds. Her body mass index (BMI) is 41 kg/m^2. You find trace pitting edema at the ankles bilaterally. There is increased pigmentation in the folds of the neck and the knuckles. The remainder of the exam is unremarkable. The patient realizes that she is overweight and asks, "How bad am I?"

Regarding definition and classification of obesity, which of the following is true?

A) Obesity is defined as BMI ≥25 kg/m^2.

B) Severe obesity is defined as BMI >30 kg/m^2.

Table 24–2 DEFINITION OF WEIGHT STATUS BY BMI

Weight Status		BMI (kg/m²)
Underweight		<18.5
Normal		18.5–24.9
Overweight		25.0–29.9
Obese	Class I	30.0–34.9
	Class II	35.0–9.9
	Class III	≥40.0

C) Underweight is defined as BMI <20 kg/m².
D) Obesity is defined as BMI ≥30 kg/m².

Discussion

The correct answer is D. Obesity is defined by BMI ≥30 kg/m²; therefore, all the other answer choices are incorrect. See Table 24–2.
BMI calculation:

$$BMI\ (kg/m^2) = weight\ (kg)/[height\ (m)]^2$$

Example: weight = 110 pounds (50 kg), height = 59 inches (1.5 m), therefore

$$BMI = 50/(1.5)^2 = 22.2\ kg/m^2$$

 HELPFUL TIP: In American adults, the combined prevalence of obesity and overweight (BMI ≥25 kg/m²) is 60% for men and 51% for women. Now that's an epidemic!

* *

You ask her about medications, focusing on those related to obesity.

All of the following drugs are associated with weight gain and an increased risk of obesity EXCEPT:

A) Olanzapine.
B) Metformin.
C) Amitriptyline.
D) Valproic acid.
E) Glipizide.

Discussion

The correct answer is B. Metformin may help diabetic patients lose or maintain weight and, therefore, is not associated with worsening obesity. See Table 24–3 for a list of medications associated with weight gain.

Which of the following tests is most likely to uncover a treatable cause of obesity.

A) Refer for a sleep study.
B) Check urinary free cortisol level.
C) Draw blood for thyroid stimulating hormone level.
D) Draw blood for fasting glucose level.
E) Draw blood for fasting lipid profile.

Discussion

The correct answer is C. Because of her obesity, this patient is also at risk for sleep apnea, diabetes, hypertension, and hyperlipidemia. These concerns will need to be addressed. However, her chief complaint is weight gain. Although in most overweight patients a cause for weight gain is not found, the physician is obligated to

Table 24–3 DRUGS ASSOCIATED WITH WEIGHT GAIN (NOT AN EXHAUSTIVE LIST)

Class	Specific Agents
α-blockers	Prazosin, doxazosin, terazosin
Anticonvulsants	Valproate, carbamazepine, gabapentin
Antidepressants	Tricyclics (eg, amitryptiline), monamine oxidase inhibitors
	Selective serotonin reuptake inhibitors (SSRIs) in some patients
Antihistamines	Cyproheptadine, diphenhydramine
Antipsychotics	Olanzapine, thioridazine, haloperidol, risperidone
β-blockers	Propranolol, metoprolol, atenolol
Diabetes drugs	Insulin, sulfonylureas, thiazolidinediones
Steroid hormones	Corticosteroids, oral contraceptives, estrogen, progesterone, testosterone

search for potentially treatable causes of weight gain, including hypothyroidism. The symptoms of hypothyroidism are often nonspecific and include weight gain and fatigue. The physical exam findings of edema and acanthosis nigricans (hyperpigmentation of the neck folds and knuckles) are often seen in obese patients.

 HELPFUL TIP: Complications of obesity include heart disease, type 2 diabetes, hypertension, stroke, hyperlipidemia, gallbladder disease, reduced fertility, increased risk of certain cancers (prostate, colon, breast, endometrial), and emotional distress.

The finding of acanthosis nigricans is most likely related to which of the following diseases in this 34-year-old patient?

A) Skin cancer.
B) Diabetes.
C) Hemochromatosis.
D) Colon cancer.
E) Hypertriglyceridemia.

Discussion
The correct answer is B. Acanthosis nigricans, classically described as velvety hyperpigmentation in skin creases (axilla, back, neck, flexor aspects of arms), is associated with a number of diseases. Acanthosis nigricans occurs in insulin resistance syndromes, commonly in patients with type 2 diabetes. It is also associated with other endocrine abnormalities, including Cushing disease and hypothyroidism. Acanthosis nigricans can be an external sign of internal malignancy, most commonly gastrointestinal cancers. However, this patient is at lower risk of colon cancer than diabetes given her age, weight gain, and lack of other signs and symptoms of cancer. Hemochromatosis, hypertriglyceridemia, and skin cancer are not directly associated with acanthosis nigricans.

* *

You find that the patient's thyroid function is normal. After consultation with a nutritionist and a prescription for exercise, she returns 3 months later. Her weight is 222 pounds. Tearfully, she tells you that she barely eats and needs something more to help her lose weight.

Which of the following is the most appropriate next step?

A) Prescribe L-thyroxine.
B) Refer to surgery for gastric bypass.
C) Prescribe ephedrine and caffeine.
D) Prescribe sibutramine (Meridia, Reductil).
E) Prescribe paroxetine (Paxil).

Discussion
The correct answer is D. Drug therapy is considered appropriate as an add-on to lifestyle management for people with a BMI $\geq$30 kg/m^2, or a BMI $\geq$27 kg/m^2 who already have a comorbid condition such as diabetes, hypertension, hyperlipidemia, etc. Of the choices listed, sibutramine is the most appropriate. Sibutramine is an adrenergic/serotonergic agent indicated for treatment of obesity. This medication shows modest weight loss (3–5 kg over 1 year) compared to placebo. The starting dose of sibutramine is 10 mg per day, with a maximum dose of 15 mg per day. The most common adverse effects include dry mouth, constipation, and insomnia. Sibutramine should be avoided in patients with a history of coronary artery disease, cardiac arrhythmias, and stroke.

Because this patient's thyroid function is normal, L-thyroxine (answer A) is inappropriate. Although some patients with a normal thyroid hormone level are convinced that they are truly hypothyroid, euthyroid patients should not receive thyroid hormone because of risks of osteoporosis, atrial fibrillation, etc. Although bariatric surgery (answer B) may be indicated in the future, it is premature to refer her for surgery now. Ephedrine and caffeine (answer C) act as stimulants, increasing heart rate and blood pressure, and should be avoided in patients with hypertension or prehypertension. The effect of paroxetine (answer E) on weight is unpredictable, and the medication is not indicated for weight loss.

 HELPFUL TIP: Rimonabant is an endocannabinoid receptor antagonist that is used to treat obesity in Europe. It appears to be effective. As of the writing of this book, it has been reviewed by the FDA but not approved in the U.S. because of concerns about increased risk of suicidality and seizures with rimonabant.

Which of the following weight loss drugs results in gastrointestinal side effects in up to 40% of patients who use it?

A) Orlistat (Alli, Xenical).
B) Sibutramine (Meridia, Reductil).
C) Phentermine (Adipex-P, Ionamin).
D) Leptin.

Discussion

The correct answer is A. Orlistat is a lipase inhibitor that functions in the intestines and prevents the absorption of about 30% of dietary fats. Due to its mechanism of action, orlistat is associated with gastrointestinal side effects in 40% of patients taking the drug. The most bothersome potential adverse events include fecal incontinence and abdominal pain. Orlistat should be taken with meals. The prescription dose is 120 mg three times per day. Weight loss is modest: 3–4 kg over 1 year compared to placebo. The other drugs listed are used to treat obesity, but do not have the same gastrointestinal effects as orlistat.

 HELPFUL TIP: The OTC dose of orlistat (Alli) is one-half the dose of the prescription strength. However, it is equally effective (or ineffective) at this lower dose.

* *

You initiate a medication to help her lose weight and refer her to a weight loss program that focuses on overall lifestyle modification. When she returns in 3 months, her weight is 235 pounds, and she is very frustrated.

You appropriately recommend which of the following?

A) Adding a second drug for weight loss.
B) Referral to psychiatry.
C) Referral to bariatric surgery.
D) Referral to plastic surgery.

Discussion

The correct answer is C. This patient now meets accepted indications for bariatric surgery. A consensus conference held by the National Institutes of Health recommended that surgery be considered for patients with a BMI >40 kg/m^2 or in patients with a BMI >35 kg/m^2 who have serious medical problems that should improve with weight loss. After an unsuccessful trial of more conservative therapy, surgery can be considered. Patients selected for surgery must be motivated and well informed. In appropriately selected patients, the risks of complications of obesity should outweigh the risks associated with surgery. Several types of surgery are employed, including gastric bypass and vertical banded gastroplasty.

The other answer choices are not appropriate now. Adding a second drug for weight loss (answer A) has not been shown to improve the rate of success. Referral to psychiatry (answer B) is unlikely to achieve the desired results. Referral to plastic surgery (answer D), presumably for lipectomy, should take place only after bariatric surgery has been completed and long-term weight loss has been achieved.

* *

The patient undergoes a successful operation. You see her in follow-up 6 months later. Her weight is 198 pounds, and you congratulate her. However, she complains of epigastric and right-sided abdominal pain which typically occurs after a meal. She denies diarrhea, constipation, emesis, and fevers.

Which of the following studies will most likely arrive at the diagnosis?

A) Stool culture.
B) Complete blood count (CBC).
C) Right upper quadrant ultrasound.
D) Abdominal radiograph.
E) Abdominal CT scan.

Discussion

The correct answer is C. Gallbladder disease is a common complication of bariatric surgery and of rapid weight loss. The history is consistent with cholelithiasis, and ultrasound is the diagnostic procedure of choice. The etiology of abdominal pain in this patient is not as likely to be infectious, so a stool culture and CBC are not the best diagnostic tests (although you almost certainly would be checking a CBC). In any patient with a history of abdominal surgery presenting with abdominal pain, it is important to consider intestinal obstruction, which could be evaluated initially with a radiograph. However, the history is more typical of gallbladder disease.

HELPFUL TIP: Drug therapy and surgery are no substitute for basic lifestyle modifications, including an appropriately calorie-restricted diet and regular aerobic exercise. These lifestyle approaches should be continued during drug treatment and after surgery.

HELPFUL TIP: Bariatric surgery appears to improve health outcomes when done on the appropriate patients. The incidence of diabetes, etc is reduced after bariatric surgery.

Objectives: Did you learn to . . .

- Define normal weight, overweight, and obesity?
- Appropriately evaluate the obese patient?
- Recognize goals and methods of treating obesity?
- Describe indications for and complications of bariatric surgery?
- Recognize complications that occur as a result of obesity?

QUICK QUIZ: VITAMIN DEFICIENCIES

A 63-year-old male presents to the office after his daughter came home for the holidays and found him confused. At first she thought he was drunk, but after a day without alcohol, the confusion persisted. According to the daughter, the patient drinks about half of a bottle of vodka per day and has done so for years. Although the patient is not able to give much of a coherent history, you are able to determine that he has developed shortness of breath and leg edema. His appetite has been poor for "a long time" and he may have lost some weight although he is not sure.

Physical examination reveals a malnourished, disoriented male who appears older than his stated age and is disheveled. He is mildly tachycardic, but his other vital signs are normal. He has bibasilar crackles on lung exam, 2 + pedal edema, hepatomegaly, and spider telangiectasias.

What is your first action to take with this patient?

A) Administer D50 IV.
B) Administer thiamine IV.

C) Administer vitamin B$_{12}$ IM.
D) Administer niacin orally.
E) Administer folate orally.

Discussion

The correct answer is B. This patient almost certainly has thiamine (vitamin B$_1$) deficiency and appears to be symptomatic. In the United States, thiamine deficiency is most often seen in malnourished alcoholics. Early symptoms of thiamine deficiency are vague—anorexia, fatigue, irritability. Thiamine deficient patients may progress to beriberi (wet or dry), possessing symptoms of heart failure and/or neuropathy (motor and sensory). Other possible manifestations of thiamine deficiency include Wernicke encephalopathy (ataxia, nystagmus, mental status changes, etc) and Wernicke-Korsakoff syndrome (Wernicke syndrome plus additional memory loss and confabulations). Treatment is to administer thiamine IV and then to continue oral supplementation. Thiamine should be given before glucose-containing solutions (eg, D50) if possible. However, this traditional sequence is not necessary if the patient's glucose is so low as to be dangerous. Save the patient first—worry about procedure later.

HELPFUL TIP: Other micronutrient deficiencies that occur in alcoholic patients: niacin deficiency resulting in pellagra (dermatitis, diarrhea, and dementia); folate deficiency resulting in macrocytic anemia; vitamin B$_{12}$ deficiency (generally due to problems with GI absorption rather than as a direct effect of alcoholism) resulting in anemia, neuropathy and dementia.

CASE 3

A 58-year-old female presents to your office with concerns about osteoporosis. A review of her medical history shows a bone density T-score of –1.8 from 2 years ago, suggesting moderate osteopenia. Medical history is also significant for mild untreated hyperlipidemia with total cholesterol of 210 mg/dL, LDL of 140 mg/dL, and HDL of 45 mg/dL. Triglycerides are within the normal range. She had a partial thyroidectomy 15 years ago and currently takes levothyroxine 88 micrograms/day. Otherwise she takes no other medications.

Based on the evidence, which of the following supplements is most appropriate for this patient?

A) Calcium.
B) Calcium plus vitamin D.
C) Vitamin D.
D) Ipriflavone.

Discussion

The correct answer is B. Postmenopausal women should take 1,200–1,500 mg/day of calcium. Vitamin D is also appropriate and many women do not get enough. Postmenopausal women should receive 400–800 IU/day of vitamin D.

Ipriflavone is a semisynthetic isoflavone produced from soy isoflavones. There is evidence that it can prevent bone mineral density loss when used with calcium in postmenopausal women, but it has not been shown to reduce fracture rates. There are also concerns that it might cause lymphocytopenia in some patients.

* *

You counsel her to take 1,500 mg of elemental calcium per day.

In order to improve GI absorption of calcium, you recommend:

A) Taking 1,500 mg at one time with a meal.
B) Taking 1,500 mg at one time an hour before eating.
C) Taking 1,500 mg in 3 divided doses with meals.
D) Taking 1,500 mg in 3 divided doses on an empty stomach.
E) Taking 1,500 mg with her levothyroxine.

Discussion

The correct answer is C. Calcium is best absorbed when taken with food. Theoretically, GI absorption of calcium is limited, and for that reason divided dosing in 500–600 mg aliquots is recommended. Patients should take levothyroxine separately from their calcium. If taken together, calcium reduces levothyroxine absorption. This is also true of iron and levothyroxine.

* *

She then asks you about her cholesterol levels and whether taking soy would be helpful. A friend told her that older women should take soy to prevent heart disease, breast cancer, and osteoporosis.

Which of the following is appropriate to tell this patient?

A) Soy isoflavone supplements are preferred for reducing lipid levels.
B) Dietary soy protein is not associated with a reduced risk of developing heart disease in Western women.
C) Soy protein is as effective as a statin for lowering cholesterol.
D) Soy isoflavones are an acceptable alternative to calcium and vitamin D for preventing osteoporosis.

Discussion

The correct answer is B. Soy protein can modestly reduce lipid levels in some patients but has been shown not to affect important outcomes such as heart attack or death in Western women. Soy isoflavone supplements have not been shown to reduce lipid levels. Soy protein is not nearly as effective as statin drugs (eg, atorvastatin, simvastatin, etc). Soy protein or soy isoflavone supplements are not an appropriate alternative to calcium and vitamin D. See Table 24–4.

* *

Your patient is hoping you can settle a bet. She asks about her younger sister who is going through menopause and started taking black cohosh. Her sister swears the black cohosh helps her hot flashes, but your patient thinks it's "all in her head."

Regarding the use of black cohosh for the treatment of perimenopausal vasomotor symptoms, you tell her:

A) Black cohosh is equivalent to hormone replacement therapy.
B) Black cohosh is equivalent to placebo.
C) Black cohosh is not good for vasomotor symptoms but does promote liver health.
D) Black cohosh is only effective when taken as part of a multibotanical supplement.

Discussion

The correct answer is B. Hormone therapy with estrogen (for women posthysterectomy) or estrogen/progestin is the most effective therapy for vasomotor symptoms of menopause. Black cohosh is not equivalent to hormone replacement. Answer C is of special note because black cohosh has been associated with hepatotoxicity—far from liver health. Answer D is

Table 24–4   OVERVIEW OF THE EFFECTIVENESS OF SOY

Condition	Effectiveness Data	Comment/Recommendation
Breast cancer	Higher intake of soy in the diet is associated with decreased risk of breast cancer. But most research limited to Asian populations. May not apply to Western populations. No clinical trials.	Unknown benefits in Western populations. Data are not strong enough to recommend dietary soy for this use.
Hyperlipidemia/ Cardiovascular disease	Consuming soy protein in place of other protein sources might modestly reduce lipid levels. Does not apply to soy isoflavone supplements. No evidence that eating soy improves outcomes such as death or heart attack. Population research shows no decreased risk of these outcomes in Western women.	Substituting dietary soy for other proteins is acceptable, but only modest benefit expected; not an alternative to mortality- or cardiovascular event-reducing therapies such as statins.
Osteoporosis	Consuming dietary soy protein might improve bone mineral density in postmenopausal women and possibly reduce fracture risk; however, not all evidence is consistent.	There is possible benefit to adding soy protein to the diet, but benefit is likely to be modest at best. Soy is not a substitute for calcium and vitamin D.

incorrect; black cohosh alone or in combination with other botanicals has not been shown to be effective in treating menopausal symptoms.

 HELPFUL TIP: Soy protein integrated into the diet is not harmful and is acceptable for women who want to try it. But it should not be relied upon in place of proven therapies.

Which of the following natural products could be recommended for lowering cholesterol?

A) Fish oil.
B) Psyllium.
C) Garlic.
D) Policosanol.

Discussion

The correct answer is B. Taking a psyllium supplement (eg, Metamucil) 10–12 grams daily can modestly reduce total cholesterol by up to 14% and LDL by up to 10%. Fish oil (answer A) is effective for lowering triglycerides, but not total cholesterol or LDL cholesterol. Garlic (answer C) was long considered effective for modest reduction of cholesterol, but the most recent evidence shows that garlic does not

significantly reduce cholesterol in most people. Similarly, policosanol (answer D) was once considered effective for reducing cholesterol, but evidence is inconsistent. The most reliable evidence shows that it is ineffective.

What percentage of Americans use alternative therapies?

A) 10%
B) 20%
C) 30%
D) 40%
E) 60%

Discussion

The correct answer is D. Eisenberg et al did a prevalence study of the use of complementary and alternative medicine therapies (CAM) that was published in 1993 and updated in 1998. The percentage of telephone respondents who reported using such therapies increased from 33.8% to 42.1%. Overall, 12% of the U.S. population used herbal products. Most were used for chronic conditions such as anxiety, depression, back pain, and headaches. Only 40% of patients informed their physicians of their use of these therapies. Examples of unconventional therapies used include:

Relaxation

Self-help groups

Chiropractic

Biofeedback

Massage

Energy healing

Imagery

Hypnosis

Homeopathy

Spiritual healing

Lifestyle diets

Acupuncture

Herbal medicine

Exercise

Megavitamins

Prayer

Coining

* *

At least 15 million patients take alternative medications in addition to prescription medications, sometimes with adverse outcomes.

Which of these is NOT a reason that patients use alternative therapies?

A) They believe they are safer than medications.

B) Conventional medicine is too technical or impersonal.

C) Prescription medicines are too expensive.

D) Cultural practices.

E) They didn't like the shark in Jaws and therefore use shark cartilage in an attempt to rid the oceans of sharks.

Discussion

The correct answer is E. Many patients use alternative therapies including herbals for various reasons, some of which are listed above. Other reasons cited include perceived physician apathy, difficulty with physician access, fear of medication side effects, and belief that medications lack efficacy and the fact that they are not natural. Many patients do not inform their physicians about their use of these products, mistakenly believing that natural means safe. Unfortunately, there is a large demand for shark cartilage including as chondroitin sulfate. Shark populations have been severely stressed as a result.

What is the current status of the regulation of natural therapies?

A) The FDA does not have a regulatory role with regards to natural therapies.

B) Natural products have to be proven safe and effective in order to be marketed in the United States.

C) Natural therapies are regulated by the Department of Health and Human Services.

D) As long as they contain the ingredients claimed, natural therapies can be marketed in the United States.

E) None of the above.

Discussion

The correct answer is A. The FDA has no regulatory role with regards to natural therapies. They are classified as dietary supplements and not medications. All of the rest are incorrect. Answer B is incorrect because natural therapies need not be proven safe and effective in order to be marketed (witness the use of ephedra). Answer D is incorrect. There is no quality control on natural therapies in the United States. Products may contain varying amounts of the advertised therapy or, in some cases, none at all. There are data suggesting that **most** products for sale do not contain what they advertise and in other cases, contain prescription drugs such as warfarin, steroids, alprazolam, and diethylstilbestrol, etc.

 HELPFUL TIP: The FDA can remove products if it can show that they are hazardous. This is a slow and laborious process as evidenced by how long it took to remove ephedra from the U.S. market.

 HELPFUL TIP: Patients who use herbals should be warned that the products may not contain what they claim and that they take the products at their own risk.

Which of the following is NOT a way for physicians to help their patients who want to use herbal products?

A) Advise patients never to use any products.

B) Inquire nonjudgmentally if patients are using any herbs, vitamins, dietary supplements, or other OTC products.

C) Recommend pregnant and lactating patients avoid them.

D) Inform patients that the FDA does not regulate them.

E) Inform patients about what is known of the product and document your conversation.

Discussion

The correct answer is A. Telling patients not to use any alternative products is judgmental and patient will be unlikely to comply or to even disclose their use of such products to the physician. Patients who should be warned to avoid herbal therapies include pregnant and lactating women (unless there is good safety data), children, immunocompromised patients, and those on medications that have a narrow therapeutic index and problematic drug-drug interactions (eg, warfarin and digoxin).

A partial list of unsafe alternative remedies follows:

- Hepatotoxicity: chaparral, germander, life foot
- Carcinogenic: borage, calamus, coltsfoot, comfrey, life root, sassafras
- Miscellaneous toxicity: Ma-huang, Licorice, poke root

Which herbal product would you recommend for a 45-year-old patient of yours with a history of coronary artery disease (CAD) *and* depression that would address both problems?

A) St. John's wort.
B) Omega-3 fatty acids.
C) Valerian.
D) Ginkgo.
E) Grapefruit juice.

Discussion

The correct answer is B. Fish oil, specifically omega-3 fatty acids, has been epidemiologically linked in numerous studies to a reduction in the incidence of depression, bipolar illness, CAD, and sudden death. Several controlled studies have established the efficacy of omega-3 fatty acids in CAD, and it is now recommended as an option for treating patients with CAD and hypercholesterolemia. An alternate way to get omega-3 fatty acids is to eat fish rich in omega-3-fatty acids such as mackerel, tuna, salmon, sardines, at least twice weekly. None of the other answer choices has been shown to be effective in CAD and depression, though St. John's wort may be helpful in mild depression, grapefruit juice may be

helpful in reducing cholesterol (although **grapefruit juice interacts with multiple medications),** and ginkgo has some antiplatelet effect and is touted for helping with vascular disease.

Which of the following is NOT affected by grapefruit juice?

A) Tacrolimus.
B) Itraconazole/Ketoconazole.
C) Benzodiazepines.
D) Clopidogrel.
E) Aspirin.

Discussion

The correct answer is E, aspirin. All of the other drugs interact with grapefruit juice. Grapefruit juice is a potent CYP 3A4 inhibitor and can interact with numerous medications including some calcium channel blockers, carbamazepine, those listed above, and others. This underscores the importance of knowing the alternative medications your patient might be using.

Which of the following herbs has been promoted as being effective for memory problems and peripheral circulatory problems?

A) Gingko biloba.
B) SAM-e.
C) Ma-huang.
D) Glucosamine.
E) None of the above.

Discussion

The correct answer is A. Ginkgo biloba is one of the most popular herbal products and is possibly effective for mild memory loss, dementia, and peripheral circulatory disorders. Ginkgo can have antiplatelet effects so should be used with caution or not at all in patients taking aspirin. Side effects include GI disturbances, headaches, and dizziness. Answer B, SAM-e is used for arthritis and depression and has been shown to be "likely effective." Answer C, Ma-huang, is ephedra and is used to increase energy and promote weight loss. Answer D, glucosamine, has not been shown to be effective for osteoarthritis. Most of the data are of poor quality.

Which herbal product has aldosterone-like properties and can cause a pseudohyperaldosteronism?

A) Ma-huang.
B) Ginseng.
C) Licorice.
D) Melatonin.
E) None of the above.

Discussion

The correct answer is C. Licorice (*Glycyrrhiza* spp.) has aldosterone-like effects and can lead to fluid retention, hypertension, and hypokalemia. Thus, it should not be combined with other potassium-wasting drugs such as non-potassium-sparing diuretics. It is also contraindicated in patients with severe liver disease and in pregnant patients (may induce premature labor).

Which of the following diseases is NOT supposedly treated by S-Adenosylmethionine (SAM-e)?

A) Depression.
B) Fibromyalgia.
C) Cirrhosis.
D) Osteoarthritis.
E) The urge to watch grade-B 1950s monster movies.

Discussion

The correct answer is E. SAM-e is "likely effective" to treat depression and osteoarthritis. It is "possibly effective" in fibromyalgia and there is insufficient evidence to rate its use in cirrhosis. SAM-e is contraindicated in bipolar patients as it can induce mania. SAM-e can possibly interact with antidepressants, including MAOI inhibitors, leading to serotonin syndrome. GI disturbance is the only notable side effect.

Which of these is useful in the treatment of migraine headaches?

A) St. John's wort.
B) Valerian.
C) Ginger.
D) Feverfew.
E) Saw palmetto.

Discussion

The correct answer is D. Feverfew is "possibly effective" to treat migraine headaches. Answer A, St. John's wort is useful for depression. **However, there are major interactions between St. John's wort and a number of other drugs including cyclosporine, nevirapine, and**

digoxin. Answer B, valerian root, is useful for insomnia. Answer C, Ginger, is used for nausea. Answer E, Saw palmetto, is used for benign prostatic hypertrophy and is "likely effective."

Which of these is NOT potentially useful for women with pregnancy-related nausea and vomiting?

A) Ginger.
B) Acupressure.
C) Vitamin B_6.
D) Doxylamine.
E) Black cohosh.

Discussion

The correct answer is E. Ginger is "possibly effective" to treat nausea and vomiting in pregnancy, postoperative vomiting, and vertigo. Vitamin B_6 (pyridoxine) and doxylamine, an antihistamine, have been shown singly and together to be safe and effective in pregnancy-related nausea and vomiting. In the past, this combination was marketed as Bendectin. However, this drug has been removed from the U.S. market because of inappropriate litigation. Doxylamine is available in the United States as a sleep aid (Unisom) and can be used with vitamin B_6. Acupressure has no known adverse effects and there is some suggestion of efficacy. **Black Cohosh can stimulate uterine contractions and has no known efficacy for nausea and vomiting in pregnancy and so is contraindicated in pregnancy.**

CASE 4

A 51-year-old patient of yours is about to have a scheduled cholecystectomy. He is in otherwise good health and is taking the following herbs and supplements.

Which would you recommend he stop taking before surgery because of association with prolonged bleeding time?

A) Valerian.
B) Ginseng.
C) Vitamin B complex.
D) Echinacea.
E) Ginkgo biloba.

Discussion

The correct answer is E. Ginkgo biloba may have antiplatelet properties and has been associated with a prolonged bleeding time. Thus, it should be stopped prior to planned surgery. Other herbal products that have antiplatelet effects include garlic, feverfew, and fish oil.

CASE 5

One of your patients who often uses complementary and alternative medicine comes into your office with several days of rhinorrhea, sore throat, and ear pain. Your exam reveals a viral upper respiratory infection. He asks you to recommend an alternative remedy.

Which of these are (purported) alternative remedies for the common cold?

A) Echinacea.
B) Zinc.
C) Vitamin C.
D) All of the above.
E) None of the above.

Discussion

The correct answer is D. The three choices above have the reputation of helping alleviate the symptoms of the common cold. The efficacy of all of these is questionable, however.

CASE 6

A 79-year-old male presents to your clinic with complaints of urinary retention, dribbling, and decreased stream. Your exam reveals an enlarged prostate. He asks for an herbal recommendation. What herb has been shown to help with symptoms of benign prostatic hyperplasia (BPH)?

A) Saw palmetto.
B) Butterbur.
C) Valerian.
D) Ginkgo biloba.
E) Ginseng.

Discussion

The correct answer is A. Saw palmetto, *Serenoa repens*, a plant common in Florida, is promoted as having antiandrogenic properties, and there are some data to support its efficacy in BPH. It is "likely effective" although there are some negative studies. Adverse

reactions include rare gastric complaints. Though there is some claim that it helps impotence, there is very little data to support that. Butterbur is promoted for allergic rhinitis. Valerian is a hypnotic and anxiolytic. Ginkgo biloba and ginseng are discussed above.

CASE 7

Since the Women's Health Initiative results came out regarding hormone replacement therapy, several women have contacted your office for alternatives to hormone replacement therapy (HRT) for treatment of menopausal symptoms of hot flashes.

Which of the following could you recommend?

A) Garlic.
B) Black cohosh.
C) Chamomile.
D) Feverfew.
E) None of the above.

Discussion

The correct answer is B. Black Cohosh (*Actea racemosa*), a plant native to North America, is used for premenstrual symptoms, painful menstruation, and hot flashes. **It has some estrogenic effects so should not be used in patients with uterine cancer or breast cancer.** It has been shown to be effective in a few trials but most of the trials have methodologic problems. One common preparation is Remifenin, 40 mg BID. This preparation has the best efficacy data. With the possible exception of an interaction with tamoxifen, no other drug interactions have been found. In clinical studies, GI disturbances have been the most frequently cited significant side-effect. It appears safe for short-term use (up to 6 months) but long-term safety has not been assessed. It should not be used in pregnancy because of its potential ability to stimulate uterine contraction.

 HELPFUL TIP: Although vitamin E and herbal products like phytoestrogens, wild yam, and primrose oil claim efficacy in treating menopausal symptoms, rigorously designed clinical trials performed to date have not confirmed their efficacy.

CASE 8

A 17-year-old male patient of yours comes to your office for a preparticipation physical. He is a little smaller than most of his classmates and has heard that creatine supplementation can help him increase muscle mass and improve his performance. Which of the following is NOT true about creatine?

A) Creatine exists primarily in skeletal muscle.
B) It causes weight gain by increasing muscle mass.
C) It is ineffective in boosting performance in aerobic exercise.
D) It can lead to increased creatinine levels in patients with normal renal function.

Discussion

The correct answer is B. Creatine monohydrate is a naturally occurring protein in the body that exists primarily in skeletal muscle. High levels of creatine are thought to enhance the ability to renew ATP for short bursts of energy. It appears to be effective for enhancing muscle performance during repeated bouts of **brief, high-intensity exercise** but is ineffective for other types of exercise. It does not improve performance in aerobic exercise neither does it benefit older adults seeking to build muscle mass. It also does not appear effective for increasing endurance or for improving performance in highly trained athletes, but its use is widespread amongst athletes, both amateur and professional. It causes weight gain by increasing water retention and not by increasing muscle mass.

* *

Creatine can cause elevated creatinine levels in patients with normal renal function as creatine is metabolized to creatinine. A complication is that creatine has been linked to renal dysfunction in some cases.

Which of these is NOT a disease that creatine is purported to treat?

A) CHF.
B) Neuromuscular disease.
C) Mitochondrial cytopathies.
D) Muscular dystrophies.
E) Diabetes.

Discussion

The correct answer is E. Creatine is also promoted for CHF, neuromuscular diseases, mitochondrial cytopathies,

and various muscular dystrophies. Oral creatine may improve exercise tolerance **in patients with CHF** but has no effect on ejection fraction. Intravenous creatine seems to improve ejection fraction temporarily. When used orally, it seems to **marginally** improve muscle strength and daily-life activity in adults and children with various muscular dystrophies in the **short term.** There is no evidence of its efficacy in the treatment of diabetes. It appears to be safe when used orally and in appropriate doses though high doses raise the concern of adverse hepatic, renal, or cardiac function. Side effects include gastrointestinal pain, nausea, and diarrhea, and muscle cramping.

CASE 9

A 51-year-old female patient of yours with knee osteoarthritis comes to your office because she has seen commercials on television advertising a product containing glucosamine and chondroitin sulfate, which was touted as being effective for osteoarthritis. She has been using naproxen with symptom relief but has had heartburn and is worried about the potential for bleeding. Moreover, she likes the idea of using something natural. She asks for your advice.

Which of the following is true about the use of glucosamine sulfate and/or chondroitin sulfate for osteoarthritis?

A) The combination is more effective than either product alone.
B) Glucosamine is effective in improving symptoms of osteoarthritis.
C) Glucosamine may lower blood sugars.
D) Chondroitin can help patients with coagulation disorders.
E) Chondroitin is "possibly effective" in osteoarthritis.

Discussion

The correct answer is E. Glucosamine sulfate is a glycoprotein that occurs naturally in the body but is available commercially as a synthetic product or from marine exoskeletons. It is not effective in osteoarthritis. Side effects are generally mild and gastrointestinal in nature including nausea, heartburn, diarrhea, and constipation.

Patients at risk for diabetes, hyperlipidemia, and hypertension should use this product cautiously as glucosamine can increase both blood glucose and insulin levels. It can increase blood sugars by impeding glucose-induced insulin secretion and impairing the insulin-induced glucose uptake by skeletal muscle.

Chondroitin sulfate is a glycosaminoglycan made from animal and fish cartilage. It is "possibly effective" in osteoarthritis although there are both positive and negative studies. It is a minor component of the low-molecular-weight heparin, danaparoid, so there is the concern of possible anticoagulant activity. This has not been shown in studies but because of this concern, it should be used with caution (or not at all) for patients on antiplatelet or anticoagulant agents or those with bleeding disorders. It is generally well-tolerated but can cause epigastric pain and nausea in some patients. Dosing is typically 200–400 mg 2–3 times daily. Although chondroitin sulfate and glucosamine sulfate are frequently sold together in combination products, no evidence supports the notion that both are better than either alone.

Objectives: Did you learn to . . .

- Understand the prevalence of alternative therapy use?
- Appreciate the various indications for various herbal products and the evidence base for them?
- Recognize herbs considered safe and those considered unsafe?
- Recognize problematic drug interactions?

BIBLIOGRAPHY

DeMaria EJ. Bariatric surgery for morbid obesity. *N Eng J Med.* 2007;356:2176.

Dickerson LM, Carek PJ. Drug therapy for obesity. *Am Fam Physician.* 2000;61(7):2131.

Fletcher RH, Fairfield KM. Vitamins for chronic disease prevention in adults. *JAMA.* 2002;287:3127.

Gartner, LM, Morton, J, Lawrence, RA, et al. Breastfeeding and the use of human milk. *Pediatrics.* 2005;115:496.

Jellin J, Gregory P, eds. *Natural Medicines Comprehensive Database.* Stockton, CA: Therapeutic Research Faculty, 2007.

Kasper DL, et al. *Harrison's Principles of Internal Medicine.* 15th ed. New York: McGraw-Hill, 2001;461.

Lyznicki JM. Obesity: assessment and management in primary care. *Am Fam Physician.* 2001;63(11):2185.

Newton KM, Reed SD, LaCroix AZ, et al. Treatment of vasomotor symptoms of menopause with black cohosh, multibotanicals, soy, hormone therapy, or placebo: a randomized trial. *Ann Intern Med.* 2006;145:869.

North American Menopause Society. Management of osteoporosis in postmenopausal women: 2006 position statement of The North American Menopause Society. *Menopause* 2006;13:340.

Russell RM. Vitamin and trace mineral deficiency and excess. In Braunwald E, Fauci AS, Kasper DL, et al. *Harrison's Principles of Internal Medicine.* 15th ed. New York: McGraw-Hill, 2001;461.

Scott G. Calcium and vitamin D supplementation: Who needs it? *Prescriber's Letter.* 2007;14:Detail-Document #230304.

25

Substance Abuse

Mark A. Graber

CASE 1

A 70-year-old female is brought into the clinic by her daughter because of concerns about her mother's sleeplessness, isolation, weight loss, falls, and anxiety over the past year. In addition, since the patient has been staying at her daughter's home the past 3 days, she began vomiting, hallucinating, perspiring profusely, and wanted to return to her own home. The patient has no history of medical problems. She is disheveled, confused, diaphoretic, and tremulous. Her blood pressure is 162/110 mm Hg, pulse is 120, and temperature is 38.5°C. She blames her symptoms on being unable to have a cigarette. She also blames her daughter's nagging. When asked about alcohol use, the patient's daughter says she has had a cocktail every evening since she retired from her job last year, and that this helps her to sleep.

Which of the following best describes the patient's current clinical condition?

A) Alcohol withdrawal.
B) Alcohol intoxication.
C) Alcohol tolerance.
D) Alcohol abuse.
E) Alcohol dependence.

Discussion

The correct answer is A. The patient presents tachycardic, hypertensive, and febrile, with diaphoresis, tremors, vomiting, and hallucinations. All of these findings are included in the diagnostic criteria for alcohol withdrawal. Answer B is incorrect. Acute intoxication is characterized by slurred speech, unsteady gait, nystagmus, and impaired memory and judgment. Answers C, D and E are incorrect and are discussed later in this case.

The criteria for alcohol withdrawal include: (1) The patient has stopped or reduced a previously heavy alcohol intake **and two** of the following within hours or days: Autonomic hyperactivity (hypertension, sweating, tachycardia, etc), hand tremor, insomnia, nausea or vomiting, hallucinations, agitation, anxiety, or grand mal seizures. (2) one must have significant impairment in functioning with the withdrawal **and** no other illness causing the symptoms.

Which class of drugs would you choose to treat the symptoms of alcohol withdrawal?

A) Benzodiazepines.
B) Antipsychotics.
C) Antibiotics.
D) Alcohol.
E) Phenytoin.

Discussion

The correct answer is A. The treatment of choice is metabolic support and the tapering use of benzodiazepines to decrease physical distress and to prevent major withdrawal (delirium tremens) from occurring. Thiamine, folate, magnesium, and other vitamin supplements are often given prophylactically. β-Blockers can be used to blunt the tachycardic and hypertensive response but will not prevent the occurrence of seizures or delirium tremens. Answer D is incorrect. Although alcohol will work to prevent withdrawal, it has a fairly short half-life, and you generally do not want to endorse the use of alcohol in a patient with an alcohol use problem.

What would be the best approach to evaluating this patient for alcoholism?

A) Ask her the average amount she drinks.
B) Ask her how often she drinks.
C) Ask her how frequently she gets drunk.
D) Ask what her family and friends say about her drinking.
E) Order a complete laboratory workup.

Discussion

The correct answer is D. The defense mechanism of denial is so strongly evident in alcoholism that the best approach is to explore how alcohol affects her life, rather than direct questions about drinking behavior. Information from family and friends may provide a more accurate account of the problem. Laboratory workups cannot be relied upon to make the diagnosis. The CAGE questionnaire is a brief and useful screening tool, employed effectively in the primary care setting. A positive answer to 2 or more questions is very sensitive and specific for an alcohol use disorder. It consists of asking the patient the following 4 questions.

Have you ever

C: felt that you should **Cut down** on your drinking?

A: been **Annoyed** that people criticized your drinking?

G: felt bad or **Guilty** about your drinking?

E: taken a drink first thing in the morning (**Eye Opener**) to get rid of a hangover or steady your nerves?

 HELPFUL TIP: Compared to the CAGE questionnaire, longer and more time-intensive tests offer better sensitivity and specificity. Two popular alcohol screening questionnaires are the Alcohol Use Disorders Identification Test (AUDIT) and the Michigan Alcohol Screening Test (MAST). However, the CAGE questionnaire is practical and easy to incorporate into practice.

 HELPFUL TIP: Unfortunately, you cannot always trust the family's history either. They may be enabling the alcoholic's addiction.

* *

Upon further questioning, you begin to uncover a long history of heavy drinking.

Which of the following statements about this patient's situation is true?

A) Cerebellar degeneration is uncommon.
B) She is at risk for developing peripheral neuropathy.
C) Alcoholic "fatty liver" is irreversible.
D) She is at decreased or normal risk for heart disease.
E) Immune function should remain relatively intact.

Discussion

The correct answer is B. Peripheral neuropathy can be seen in 10% of heavy drinkers as a result of vitamin deficiencies and the direct impact alcohol has on nerve function. Answer A is incorrect because cerebellar degeneration—suggested by ataxia and nystagmus—occurs as a result of alcohol overuse. Answer C is incorrect because alcoholic "fatty liver" will reverse with abstinence from alcohol. Answer D is incorrect. **Heavy drinking raises blood pressure and levels of triglycerides, increasing risk of myocardial infarction.** Answer E is incorrect. Heavy drinking lowers the white blood cell count and interferes with specific aspects of the immune system; for example, it compromises T-cell function.

* *

This patient reports to you that she has needed to drink increasing amounts of alcohol to help her fall asleep.

The need for increasing amounts of alcohol is an example of:

A) Intoxication.
B) Dependence.
C) Tolerance.
D) Relapse.
E) Abuse.

Discussion

The correct answer is C. Tolerance is defined as the need for increasing amounts of a drug to achieve the same effect, or a diminishing effect from the use of the same amount of a drug. Answer A is incorrect. Intoxication is a characteristic syndrome of maladaptive behavior or psychological changes that occurs with substance use, which is drug-specific, and reverses when the drug use is discontinued. Answer D is incorrect. Relapse involves restarting use of the drug after being abstinent for a while.

The criteria for substance abuse and dependence include:

1) **Dependence:** substance use with impairment or distress with 3 of the following within one year: tolerance, withdrawal, need for increasing amounts of substance, unable to cut down, significant time spent obtaining consuming or recovering from substance use, persistent use despite knowledge of adverse effects.

2) **Substance abuse:** substance use with impairment or distress with 1 of the following within one year: substance use impairs job, school or home, use in hazardous circumstances (eg, alcohol when driving), recurrent legal problems, continued use despite having persistent or recurring interpersonal problems.

Which of the following lab test results are you most likely to find in this patient?

A) Microcytic anemia.
B) Low ferritin.
C) Decreased serum triglycerides.
D) Hyperglycemia.
E) Increased gamma-glutamyltransferase (GGT).

Discussion

The correct answer is E. Elevated GGT is considered to be the most sensitive indicator of alcohol intake and is often present along with elevation of the alanine and aspartate transaminases (ALT and AST). The classic AST:ALT ratio in active alcohol abusers is 2:1. Remember, however, that these laboratory findings are **not specific** for alcohol use and can be caused by medications and other illnesses.

The other answers are incorrect. Patients with alcoholism typically have **macrocytic anemia, elevated serum triglycerides, and hypoglycemia.** Ferritin is often **increased** in active alcohol users.

* *

You have ordered liver function tests, but the results will not be available until the next day.

Which of the following medications would be indicated to prevent delirium tremens in a patient with hepatic impairment?

A) Alprazolam (Xanax).
B) Chlordiazepoxide (Librium).

C) Diazepam (Valium).
D) Lorazepam (Ativan).
E) Clonazepam (Klonopin).

Discussion

The correct answer is D. Benzodiazepines that are metabolized by the cytochrome P450 system will build up in the presence of liver disease, so using those with intermediate half-lives and no active metabolites is essential. Only lorazepam, oxazepam, and temazepam meet these criteria. Answer B is incorrect. Although chlordiazepoxide is often used to prevent symptoms of alcohol withdrawal, it is hepatically metabolized and has an exceptionally long half-life and, therefore, should be avoided in patients with liver problems. Alprazolam is too short-acting to use in this patient.

* *

You are considering whether or not this patient has delirium tremens (DT).

Which of the following statements is true of DT?

A) The majority of patients with alcohol withdrawal develop DT if not treated.
B) Visual hallucinations are uncommon in DT.
C) Symptoms of DT could easily be confused for dementia.
D) Her last drink would need to be about one week ago for her to have DT.
E) Autonomic instability is present in DT.

Discussion

The correct answer is E. Autonomic instability with elevated pulse, blood pressure, and fever are common in DT. Answer A is incorrect. Minor withdrawal symptoms are quite common, but DT develops in only 3%–5% of patients undergoing alcohol withdrawal. Answer B is incorrect. Visual hallucinations are **common** in DT; auditory hallucinations are less likely. Answer C is incorrect. Withdrawal **delirium** typically presents acutely over a matter of hours or days while in **dementia,** the cognitive decline is over a course of months to years. Additionally, autonomic instability is not a feature of early dementia. Answer D is incorrect because the risk for DT usually peaks 72 hours after the last drink.

Which medication would be the best choice for DT in a patient who is vomiting profusely and who has no IV access?

A) Diazepam (Valium).

B) Alprazolam (Xanax).

C) Chlordiazepoxide (Librium).

D) Lorazepam (Ativan).

E) Clonazepam (Klonopin).

Discussion

The correct answer is D. Lorazepam is absorbed well intramuscularly. This makes it a good choice for the vomiting patient. Diazepam is **not** well absorbed IM and thus should not be used in patients without an IV.

 HELPFUL TIP: The IV form of lorazepam can also be administered sublingually to speed absorption.

Delirium tremens carries a fatality rate of:

A) <1%

B) 5%

C) 10%

D) 25%

E) 50%

Discussion

The correct answer is B. Prior to modern treatment, the incidence of mortality reached almost 40% per episode. The other answer choices are incorrect.

Which of the following does NOT predispose to developing DT?

A) Prior episodes of DT.

B) Pneumonia.

C) GI bleed.

D) Female gender.

E) Hepatic failure.

Discussion

The correct answer is D. Female gender does not predispose an individual to DT. All the other answer choices do predispose an individual to DT.

Which of the following is NOT a complication of alcoholism?

A) Dementia.

B) Pancreatitis.

C) Hypermagnesemia.

D) Megaloblastic anemia.

E) Marchiafava-Bignami disease.

Discussion

The correct answer is C. All of the above, with the exception of hypermagnesemia, are associated with alcohol abuse. Several require special note. Alcoholic dementia may be related to direct effects of alcohol on the brain or to nutritional deficiencies. **Hypo**magnesemia is a complication of alcoholism. Hypomagnesemia may decrease the response to thiamine administration. **Marchiafava-Bignami** disease is demyelination and/or necrosis of the corpus callosum and the adjacent white matter. It presents with dementia, dysarthria, spasticity, and inability to ambulate. It can occasionally be seen in nondrinkers as well.

 HELPFUL TIP: Elderly patients with alcohol problems often go unrecognized. Have a high index of suspicion in patients with signs and symptoms such as labile hypertension, insomnia, legal or marital problems, frequent falls and injuries, headaches or blackouts, and vague GI complaints.

Which of the following statements is FALSE about alcohol use disorders?

A) Most patients who develop alcohol disorders do so by their mid-twenties.

B) The lifetime prevalence of alcoholism is between 14%–24%.

C) Alcoholism is frequently comorbid with other psychiatric illnesses.

D) Alcohol abuse is 5 times more frequent in males than in females.

E) About 30% of patients with alcohol abuse meet the DSM-IV criteria for major depressive disorder.

Discussion

The correct answer is A. Most people who develop alcohol use disorders do so by their late-thirties, **not** their mid-twenties. The rest are true statements. Especially noteworthy is Answer C. It is estimated that 50% of all people with alcohol abuse have a comorbid Axis I diagnosis. For example, 50%–60% of people with bipolar illness have problems with alcohol abuse or dependence. Answer E is a true statement. **Although over 80% of patients with alcohol use disorders complain of depressive symptoms, only 30% meet criteria for major depressive disorder.** A useful way to approach patients who complain of depression along with their alcohol abuse is to obtain a longitudinal history to see which came first. If it is impossible to tease out, observe for 1–3 weeks off alcohol. If depression is still present without alcohol use, it is prudent to treat with an antidepressant. Be careful when treating alcohol abusers with antidepressants: active substance use severely reduces the efficacy of these drugs.

 HELPFUL TIP: Substance use rates are highest in individuals between 18 and 25 years. Much of this is experimentation that will end as the individual matures. Some, of course, will go on to chronic abuse.

 HELPFUL TIP: **The best way to deal with alcohol withdrawal is PRN doses of IV diazepam.** The traditional "Librium taper" requires more drug and more time in the hospital. Diazepam is long enough acting that once a patient's symptoms are controlled, they often will not need a second dose of drug. But treat them IV PRN for symptoms. Phenytoin is generally ineffective for the prevention of alcohol-related seizures.

* *

The patient agrees to go to Alcoholics Anonymous (AA).

All of the following describe the 12-step recovery model EXCEPT:

A) Close and prolonged peer support.
B) Use of program of specific activities and fellowship as important components of recovery.
C) A one-time, sliding-scale initial membership fee.
D) A goal of abstinence.
E) Sponsorship of others in the group.

Discussion

The correct answer is C. Twelve-step membership is free of charge. Sponsorship of one another is of utmost importance. More information about AA can be found in the ethics chapter.

* *

Your patient's family asks about AlAnon, the companion program to Alcoholics Anonymous, that helps and supports those who have an alcoholic in their lives.

Attendance at AlAnon meetings provides all of the following EXCEPT:

A) Anonymity.
B) Sponsors.
C) Employee assistance programs for the workplace.
D) Active listening and support.
E) Education.

Discussion

The correct answer is C. AlAnon does not participate in employee assistance programs in the workplace. The rest are true. AlAnon adheres to the principle of anonymity, provides sponsors to participants in need, etc.

Objectives: Did you learn to . . .

- Recognize signs and symptoms of alcohol withdrawal?
- Describe diagnostic criteria for alcohol withdrawal?
- Identify adverse effects of heavy alcohol use?
- Differentiate between substance abuse and dependence?
- Treat alcohol withdrawal?
- Recognize how denial of the illness plays a role in the assessment of substance abuse?
- Identify laboratory abnormalities observed in alcohol abuse and understand the limitations of laboratory studies?

 QUICK QUIZ: ALCOHOL

A 50-year-old divorced white male presents to your clinic in an agitated state, complaining of nausea, vomiting, and double vision. He smells of alcohol, has gross bilateral hand tremors, and is disheveled. He is picking at his shirtsleeves and is oriented to name only. On physical exam, he has lateral nystagmus and an ataxic gait. Vital signs include: Blood pressure 160/92 mm Hg, pulse 100, and respirations 20. Labs are drawn, and his GGT is moderately elevated.

Which of the following is the most likely cause of his symptoms?

A) Wernicke encephalopathy.
B) Normal pressure hydrocephalus.
C) Dementia.
D) Stroke.
E) Alcohol withdrawal.

Discussion

The correct answer is A. Wernicke encephalopathy is the result of thiamine deficiency and can occur in alcoholics and other patients with poor nutrition. See the next question for a description of the clinical findings. Note that several symptoms of Wernicke can mimic withdrawal (agitation, etc). However, as noted in the question, this patient is still intoxicated.

 QUICK QUIZ: WERNICKE

The triad of Wernicke encephalopathy includes all of the following EXCEPT:

A) Ataxia.
B) Nystagmus.
C) Incontinence.
D) Confusion.

Discussion

The correct answer is C. Wernicke encephalopathy may present with the classic triad of ataxia, confusion, and nystagmus. Patients may be incontinent due to alcohol use, but it is not a major feature of Wernicke encephalopathy. The majority of patients, however, do not present with the triad; most present with confusion alone.

 QUICK QUIZ: JUST SAY NO.

What is the most abused illicit substance in the United States?

A) Marijuana.
B) Cocaine.
C) Methamphetamine.
D) Heroin.
E) LSD.

Discussion

The correct answer is A. Marijuana is the most common illicit substance used, outstripping the use of all other illicit substances combined.

CASE 2

A 28-year-old married, pregnant patient and her mother are presenting for a follow-up appointment. At the appointment today, the patient's mother shares that her daughter has been drinking alcohol during her pregnancy. The daughter is very annoyed when confronted with her use of alcohol and will not give specific information about it, but she does admit to drinking. She does not agree to quit during her pregnancy nor to be referred for substance abuse evaluation.

* *

You discuss some of the effects alcohol might have on the developing fetus, including fetal alcohol syndrome (FAS). The diagnosis of FAS requires specific manifestations in 3 areas.

The 3 areas are:

A) At least 2 facial anomalies, retardation of growth <20th percentile, and little motor activity.
B) At least 2 facial anomalies, retardation of growth <10th percentile, and central nervous system problems that may include tremulousness, hyperactivity, attentional deficits, or mental impairment.
C) At least 3 facial anomalies, retardation of growth <20th percentile, and poor sucking reflexes.
D) Small size, hyperactivity, and 1 generalized facial anomaly.

Discussion

The correct answer is B. The diagnosis of fetal alcohol syndrome requires in utero exposure to alcohol and at least 2 facial anomalies, retardation of growth below the 10th percentile, and central nervous system problems that may include tremulousness, hyperactivity, attentional deficits, or mental impairment. The other answer choices are incorrect.

 HELPFUL TIP: The rate of FAS is 59 per 1,000 live births when the children of women who abused alcohol during pregnancy are studied. **FAS is the leading cause of mental retardation in the Western Hemisphere**; children with this disorder have an average IQ of 68–70.

Symptoms and signs of FAS may be detected at what point after birth?

A) Within 12 hours.
B) >Week 1.
C) At 1 month.
D) At 3 months.
E) >1 year.

Discussion

The correct answer is A. Soon after birth, the neonate may display symptoms of withdrawal, including tremulousness, inconsolability, vomiting, poor feeding, etc. The characteristic cluster of facial/physical malformations include short palpebral fissure, a short upturned nose, a hypoplastic upper lip, and a diminished philtrum, are evident within 12 hours of birth. Other principal features are central nervous system dysfunction, growth deficiency at birth, joint and limb abnormalities, and heart defects.

* *

In addition to FAS, you discuss some of the potential problems seen with more limited in utero exposure to alcohol.

What are the criteria for fetal alcohol effects (FAE)?

A) Small size, prematurity, hyperactivity, learning disabilities.
B) Inability to complete tasks, very active, very excitable.
C) Facial malformations, heart defects, hyperactivity.
D) Growth deficiency <10th percentile, learning disabilities.
E) Congenital cardiac anomalies, growth deficiency <10th percentile, facial malformations.

Discussion

The correct answer is A. Knowledge continues to increase regarding the more subtle effects of maternal drinking, such as that seen with "social" alcohol use. FAE can occur with even moderate drinking during pregnancy. The abnormalities commonly observed with FAE include small size, prematurity, hyperactivity, and learning disabilities.

In which stage of pregnancy does the teratogenic action of alcohol cause facial malformations?

A) During the embryonic phase, at the eighth week after conception.
B) During the third week of pregnancy.

C) During the late first trimester.
D) During the second trimester.
E) During the third trimester.

Discussion

The correct answer is B. **Facial malformations occur with the use of alcohol during the third week.** Organs and limbs appear most susceptible to the effects of alcohol during the embryonic phase, which is completed by the eighth week after conception, at a time when most women are first confirming the pregnancy. Alcohol exposure during any stage of development may effect brain development or function.

You are able to convince this patient to reduce and eventually eliminate her use of alcohol; she delivers a healthy-appearing newborn whom she names Harley.

Objectives: Did you learn to . . .

- Identify problem drinking in a pregnant patient?
- Approach a patient with alcohol abuse in pregnancy?
- Describe the findings of fetal alcohol effects and fetal alcohol syndrome?

CASE 3

A 60-year-old female presents to your office and is determined to stop smoking. She has a history of schizophrenia treated with clozapine (Clozaril) and a 43-year history of smoking up to 2 packs of cigarettes per day. She asks you what is available to help her stop. You tell her that nicotine replacement therapy, bupropion (Zyban), and varenicline (Chantix) are currently approved aids for patients who want to stop smoking.

* *

You want to offer her a nicotine replacement therapy (NRT) that is easy to use, has few side effects, and provides steady blood levels of nicotine over the whole day.

Which NRT do you choose?

A) Nicotine patch.
B) Nicotine gum.
C) Nicotine nasal spray.
D) Nicotine inhaler.
E) Nicotine suppositories.

Discussion

The correct answer is A. There are benefits and drawbacks to each of the smoking cessation aids. Like other NRT, the nicotine patch is available without prescription. It is applied to the skin daily and provides a steady release of nicotine through the skin. For a patient with a heavy, long smoking history, begin with the 21-mg patch and taper to the 7-mg patch over a 3-month period. Some of the drawbacks of the patch include slower release of nicotine, the potential for skin irritation, insomnia, and vivid dreams. Some of these side effects can be reduced by having the patient rotate application sites daily (to avoid skin irritation) and removing the patch before bedtime.

Nicotine gum (answer B) is an ion-exchange resin that releases nicotine for absorption through the buccal mucosa with only 30% bioavailability in the rest of the GI tract. Side effects include mouth and throat soreness, jaw fatigue, hiccups, and undesirable taste. There are advantages of nicotine gum: it involves an active coping mechanism (chewing, placing the gum in one's mouth, etc) and is more likely than the patch to delay weight gain. The nasal spray (answer C) delivers 0.5 mg nicotine per dose and is sprayed 1–2 times per hour for a maximum of 5 sprays per hour and 40 sprays per day. Most of the nicotine nasal spray side effects are attributable to its route of use—nasal and throat irritation, rhinorrhea, sneezing, etc. The oral inhaler (answer D) provides an active delivery of nicotine similar to the nasal inhaler, and its side effects are also a consequence of its route of delivery—throat irritation and coughing. There are no nicotine suppositories (answer E). Finally, varenicline, a nicotine receptor agonist is also available to help with smoking cessation.

Which of the following is the most significant side effect of varenicline (Chantix)?

A) Desire to commit violence or commit suicide.
B) Desire to watch endless reruns of Godzilla movies.
C) Leukocytosis.
D) Urinary retention.

Discussion

The correct answer is A. There is an FDA warning about the possibility of suicidal or homicidal ideation with varenicline. This is not good, especially in someone who already has a psychiatric disorder. Other common side effects include flatulence, nausea, headache, and insomnia.

* *

Although this patient does not mind spending $6–$7 per day on cigarettes, she does not want to pay much for something to help her quit.

Which treatment is the most expensive?

A) Nicotine patch.
B) Nicotine gum.
C) Nicotine nasal spray.
D) Nicotine inhaler.
E) Varenicline.

Discussion

The correct answer is E. Varenicline costs approximately $130.00 per month on drugstore.com. The nicotine products are less expensive, in the range of $60–$80 per month.

Which of the following medications might you also prescribe to aid this patient in smoking cessation?

A) Naloxone.
B) Metoprolol.
C) Haloperidol.
D) Bupropion.

Discussion

The correct answer is D. Bupropion is marketed as the antidepressant Wellbutrin and the smoking cessation aid Zyban. It reduces the symptoms of nicotine withdrawal by blocking dopamine in the brain's reward center, and this mechanism is thought to result in reduced nicotine craving. Studies have shown that people who use bupropion doubled their chances of quitting smoking. Its effect appears to be additive to that of NRT. Its effect on smoking cessation is independent of its antidepressant effect, as shown by its equal efficacy in depressed and nondepressed patients. One of the advantages of bupropion is its ability to prevent the weight gain that occurs in most people when they stop smoking. Bupropion should be started at a dose of 150 mg daily for 3 days then increasing to 150 mg twice daily, if the patient is tolerating the drug. The patient should be advised to stop smoking during the second week of treatment.

Common side effects of bupropion include all of the following EXCEPT:

A) Insomnia.
B) Nausea.

C) Suicidal ideation.
D) Tremor.
E) Anxiety.

Discussion

The correct answer is C. Suicidal ideation is not a side effect of bupropion. All the other answer choices are potential side effects.

Which of the following is a contraindication to the use of bupropion?

A) Current use of an MAO inhibitor.
B) Breast-feeding.
C) Seizure disorder.
D) Eating disorder.
E) All of the above.

Discussion

The correct answer is E. All of the above are contraindications to the use of bupropion. Other contraindications include alcoholism (because of seizure risk), pregnancy, and anything that will lower seizure threshold (eg, head trauma, intracranial mass, etc).

* *

This patient is also curious as to whether, at age 60 and with an 86-pack-year history, there is any reason to quit.

How long does it take to reduce the risk of having a heart attack by 50% after one stops smoking?

A) 24 hours.
B) 6 months.
C) 1 year.
D) 10 years.
E) 15 years.

Discussion

The correct answer is C. Twenty minutes after quitting smoking, blood pressure drops and the temperature of hands and feet increases to normal. After 24 hours, the risk of heart attack begins to decrease. After 1 year, the risk of heart attack is 50%. After 5 years, stroke risk is reduced to that of a nonsmoker. After 10 years, the risk of dying from lung cancer is about 50% of a person who continues to smoke. After 15 years, the risk of coronary heart disease approaches that of a nonsmoker.

* *

Your patient expresses concern that she will fail in this attempt to quit smoking. She confides that she has tried to quit on several earlier occasions.

On average, how many attempts are made to quit smoking before a person succeeds?

A) 2
B) 6
C) 10
D) 16

Discussion

The correct answer is B. It takes an average of 6 attempts at quitting before success.

 HELPFUL TIP: Unfortunately, none of these cessation aids has a great track record of success. You can find numbers all over the board. With NRTs, an estimated 15% of patients will be tobacco-free at 1 year. With bupropion, the number is closer to 23%. Varenicline has an estimated 23% 1-year abstinence rate. Counseling may increase the success rate, and all smokers should be urged to quit at every appointment.

* *

This patient has been on clozapine (Clozaril) for control of her psychosis.

The combination of clozapine and bupropion should be used with caution because:

A) Both may lower the seizure threshold.
B) Both may cause hypertension.
C) Bupropion may interfere with the metabolism of clozapine.
D) Severe gastrointestinal symptoms could occur.
E) A psychotic episode could be precipitated.

Discussion

The correct answer is A. Both drugs may lower the seizure threshold. Hypertension should not be a concern. Bupropion does not interfere with the metabolism of clozapine, cause severe gastrointestinal symptoms, or precipitate psychotic episodes.

* *

After your discussion, the patient wants to quit "cold turkey." You gently explain that going from 40 cigarettes per day to zero might be hard on her.

All of the following are symptoms of nicotine withdrawal EXCEPT:

A) Increased appetite.
B) Dysphoria.
C) Tachycardia.
D) Insomnia.
E) Irritability.

Discussion

The correct answer is C. Nicotine withdrawal is associated with **decreased** heart rate. In addition to the above, trouble concentrating and restlessness are common symptoms.

Objectives: Did you learn to . . .

* Employ pharmacotherapy in the treatment of tobacco addiction?
* Enumerate the physiological advantages of smoking cessation at any age?
* Recognize signs and symptoms of nicotine withdrawal?

 QUICK QUIZ: ALL IN THE FAMILY

A known risk factor for substance abuse is being the child of an alcoholic.

Which of the following characteristics is NOT true of the children of alcoholics?

A) They experience earlier onset of problem drinking.
B) They experience earlier pregnancies.
C) They have less stable family involvement.
D) They experience poor academic and social performance in school.
E) They have more antisocial behavior.

Discussion

The correct answer is B. There are no data to suggest early pregnancy as a characteristic. Twin, adoption, and half-sibling studies and studies of familial versus non-familial alcoholism indicate that children of alcoholics have 4 times the risk for developing alcoholism. They also have worse school performance, more antisocial behavior, and less stable family situations.

CASE 4

A 35-year-old intoxicated female presents to your office requesting that she be started on disulfiram (Antabuse). She is otherwise healthy and recently has begun to drink in response to the death of her sister. Before this, she was a teetotaler.

Disulfiram acts by inhibiting:

A) Lactic dehydrogenase.
B) Gastric dehydrogenase.
C) Aldehyde dehydrogenase.
D) Dopamine betahydroxylase.
E) None of the above.

Discussion

The correct answer is C. Disulfiram inhibits aldehyde dehydrogenase, the enzyme that catalyzes the oxidation of acetaldehyde to acetic acid. If alcohol is ingested after inhibition of this enzyme, blood acetaldehyde levels rise, resulting in the characteristic symptoms of the disulfiram-ethanol interaction.

Disulfiram should not be administered until the patient has been abstinent from alcohol for how long?

A) 4 hours.
B) 12 hours.
C) 24 hours.
D) 48 hours.
E) 72 hours.

Discussion

The correct answer is B. A minimum of 12 hours should have elapsed before giving disulfiram to avoid the disulfiram-alcohol reaction. Of course, this depends on how much they were drinking.

 HELPFUL TIP: Disulfiram is absorbed slowly from the GI tract and is eliminated slowly; therefore, a patient should wait at least 1 week after stopping disulfiram before returning to drinking.

If the patient consumes alcohol while taking disulfiram, which of the following is MOST LIKELY to occur?

A) Respiratory depression.
B) Hypertension.
C) Nausea.
D) Cardiovascular collapse.
E) Convulsions.

Discussion

The correct answer is C. The disulfiram-ethanol interaction generally includes flushing of the skin, nausea, palpitations, hypotension, sweating, blurred vision, and dizziness. Rarely, in more severe reactions, respiratory depression, cardiovascular collapse, convulsions, and death may occur. The severity of the reaction is typically dose related and depends on the amount of alcohol ingested.

Common side effects of disulfiram include which of the following?

A) Hypotension.
B) Peripheral neuropathy.
C) Insomnia.
D) Nausea.
E) Depression.

Discussion

The correct answer is B. Drowsiness, hepatotoxicity, rashes, hypertension, peripheral neuropathy, metallic after-taste, and optic neuritis may occur with disulfiram use. These effects are independent of alcohol ingestion.

 HELPFUL TIP: A large number of cases of hepatitis have been reported with usage of disulfiram; therefore baseline liver enzymes should be obtained prior to starting disulfiram and approximately 2 weeks after initiation of treatment. Occasionally, a rash may occur early on. The rash can be treated with antihistamines and the drug can be continued.

* *

After a discussion, the patient thinks that disulfiram is the "one thing that might work." She tries it, but at follow-up, she is not having much success. She continues to drink heavily and (thankfully) has been non-compliant with taking disulfiram regularly. She reports strong craving for alcohol.

As an alternative to disulfiram, you decide to prescribe:

A) Naltrexone (Revia).
B) Naloxone (Narcan).
C) Nortriptyline.
D) Nitroprusside.

Discussion

The correct answer is A. Naltrexone is FDA approved for the treatment of alcoholism. As an opioid antagonist, it blocks the euphoric effects of alcohol. Topiramate (Topamax) can also be used to decrease the craving for alcohol. However, it is not FDA approved for this indication. None of the other drugs listed is used to treat alcohol abuse and dependence.

* *

This patient recalls something about using compost to treat alcoholism. You realize she means acamprosate (Campral).

Which of the following is true about acamprosate?

A) It is contraindicated in those with renal impairment/renal failure
B) At one year, acamprosate is no better than placebo in preventing relapse of alcoholism.
C) The combination of acamprosate and naltrexone is no more effective than either alone.
D) Drug reps will tell you that all of these medications are great and that you should prescribe them.
E) All of the above.

Discussion

The correct answer is E. All of the above are true. Unfortunately, at 1 year none of these drugs is significantly better than placebo.

 HELPFUL TIP: In case we didn't make the point clear above, disulfiram (Antabuse), naltrexone (Revia), and acamprosate (Campral) are not particularly effective drugs in the long term, with success rates no greater than placebo.

Objectives: Did you learn to . . .

- Describe the mechanism of action of disulfiram?
- Recognize side effects of disulfiram?
- Describe the alcohol-disulfiram reaction?
- Prescribe other medical therapies for alcohol use disorders?

CASE 5

A 25-year-old comatose female presents to the ED with pinpoint pupils and respiratory depression.

Which of the following is the most likely cause of coma?

A) Blood alcohol level of 200 mg/dL.
B) Cocaine overdose.
C) Methadone overdose.
D) Benzodiazepine withdrawal.
E) PCP intoxication.

Discussion

The correct answer is C. The classic triad of opioid overdose consists of coma, respiratory depression, and pinpoint pupils (miosis). Certain patients may have atypical presentations, and the triad may not always be present in opioid overdose. Miosis is particularly variable, often not being seen in those with meperidine and propoxyphene; and coingestions, such as sympathomimetics and anticholinergics, can also prevent miosis. Answer A is incorrect. A patient with a blood alcohol level of 200 mg/dL would likely be ataxic, but alcoholic coma typically occurs at blood levels >400 mg/dL and depends upon the level of tolerance. Stimulant overdose presents with dilated pupils. Alcohol and PCP intoxication more likely present with nystagmus and not constricted pupils.

What is the minimum amount of time that you should observe a patient who has overdosed on methadone?

A) 1 hour.
B) 4 hours.
C) 12 hours.
D) 36 hours.
E) 72 hours.

Discussion

The correct answer is D. Methadone has a long half-life (up to 60 hours) and therefore a patient who has overdosed on methadone should be monitored for at least 36–48 hours.

How many doses of naloxone (Narcan) 0.4 mg would be needed in a patient with an overdose of a large quantity of methadone?

A) 1
B) 2
C) 3
D) 4
E) >5

Discussion

The correct answer is E. Naloxone hydrochloride, a pure opioid antagonist, reverses the central nervous system effects of opioid overdose. An initial IV dose of 0.4 mg reverses symptoms within 2 minutes. However, the half-life in adults is 30–90 minutes. Therefore, multiple doses of naloxone may be needed, and patients need to be observed even if they respond symptomatically to a dose of naloxone.

* *

Through eyewitness history, you are able to determine that this patient did indeed overdose on an opioid.

Which of the following statements would most likely be FALSE concerning this patient?

A) Hyperthermia would be present.
B) Cardiac arrhythmias such as bradycardia can be present.
C) Pulmonary edema can be present.
D) Track marks might be present.

Discussion

The correct answer is A. Hypothermia would be more likely with opioid intoxication. Answer B is true. The patient can become bradycardic. Answer C is true. The patient can develop noncardiogenic pulmonary edema as a result of heroin and other opioids. This is likely due to prolonged hypoxemia although the mechanism isn't entirely clear. Answer D is obviously true in a patient who injects drugs.

* *

You discover that the patient has been on a methadone maintenance program, but then she lapsed and overdosed on heroin. Her urine drug screen returns positive for opioids.

What would be the next most appropriate course of action?

A) Detoxify the patient off methadone as an outpatient.
B) Contact the authorities to have the patient arrested.
C) Contact the patient's methadone maintenance clinic for dose increase.
D) Notify the patient of her positive urine drug screen and let her know you are not surprised by the result, as methadone is metabolized to heroin.
E) Have the patient committed to a substance abuse treatment facility.

Discussion

The correct answer is C. That this patient has relapsed into heroin use may mean that her methadone dose is too low for maintenance. This can lead to additional heroin use. The other answer choices are incorrect. Answer D is of particular note. Methadone is metabolized to morphine and not heroin.

 HELPFUL TIP: High-dose methadone can lead to QT prolongation and torsade de pointes.

Methadone is typically prescribed for opioid maintenance therapy:

A) Once daily.
B) Twice daily.
C) Three times daily.
D) Three times weekly.
E) Once monthly.

Discussion

The correct answer is A. Methadone has an elimination half-life of up to 60 hours (range 15–60 hours). Therefore, once-daily dosing is appropriate for the treatment of narcotic addiction. The advantage here is that the medication can be given under direct observation.

 HELPFUL TIP: Methadone should be dosed every 6–8 hours when used for pain control. It may not reach a steady state for 3–5 days.

* *

After she regains consciousness, the patient informs you that she is 20 weeks' pregnant.

Regarding pregnancy and usage of opioids, which of the following would most likely have the best outcome?

A) Continuing the patient on methadone.
B) Withdrawing the patient from all opioids in the first trimester (too late for this one).
C) Withdrawing the patient from all opioids in the second trimester.
D) Withdrawing the patient from all opioids in the third trimester.

Discussion

The correct answer is A. Opioid withdrawal in a pregnant woman can cause fetal distress and low birth weight. To continue the patient on methadone has 2 advantages: it will prevent opioid withdrawal in the patient and the fetus and, hopefully, it will also prevent a patient relapse into heroin use.

Objectives: Did you learn to . . .

• Recognize symptoms and signs of overdose with opioids and other illicit drugs?
• Use methadone for opioid addiction?
• Treat a pregnant patient with opioid addiction?

CASE 6

A 40-year-old female is admitted through the ED, arriving via ambulance from a smaller hospital. The local physician called to report that her friends said that she had "shot up a lot of meth." She is known to use her son's Ritalin prescription on a regular basis. She appears frightened and anxious. She is uncommunicative, rocking back and forth on the exam table, and picking at her skin trying to remove imaginary bugs. She becomes angry easily and lashes out at staff in the ED.

A reasonable differential diagnosis for this patient would include all of the following EXCEPT:

A) Schizophrenia.
B) Drug-induced psychosis.

C) PCP, hallucinogen, or cocaine intoxication.

D) Diabetes.

E) Delirium tremens.

Discussion

The correct answer is D. Though hypoglycemic patients can certainly become confused, diabetes is the least likely cause of these symptoms. Although there is a history of amphetamine use in this patient, the other answer choices should not be eliminated out of hand.

* *

The urine drug screen is positive for amphetamines.

The following are all symptoms of amphetamine use EXCEPT:

A) Tachycardia

B) Hypertension.

C) Perspiration or chills.

D) Weight gain.

E) Psychomotor agitation.

Discussion

The correct answer is D. Weight loss, not weight gain, can be anticipated in the amphetamine user. All of the other symptoms can be seen as a result of amphetamine use. Symptoms can progress to confusion, arrhythmias, seizures, dystonias, or coma.

 HELPFUL TIP: Stimulant use can cause coronary artery occlusion and severe hypertension. Myocardial infarction with stimulant use should be treated like any other MI. Hypertension should be treated with α- and β-blockers.

 HELPFUL TIP: Chronic methamphetamine use is associated with widespread dental caries and gingival disease that can result in the loss of many or all teeth. "Meth mouth," as this is commonly called, is probably caused by prolonged periods of poor dental hygiene, xerostomia, high-calorie food and drink, and tooth grinding.

Which of the following does NOT address the needs of this patient during withdrawal?

A) Provide a secure environment.

B) Provide regular meals and snacks.

C) Make sure the patient is awakened if she spends excess time sleeping.

D) Consider giving a benzodiazepine if the patient remains anxious.

E) Provide education as an intervention towards change.

Discussion

The correct answer is C. Amphetamine withdrawal requires sleep, nutritious food, and a safe place until the unstable state improves. The patient should be allowed to sleep. Stimulant abusers often stay up for a week or more and then crash and sleep for days during withdrawal. Antipsychotic medications and benzodiazepines may be administered if needed.

Objectives: Did you learn to . . .

● Recognize the signs and symptoms of amphetamine intoxication?

● Appropriately treat a patient with amphetamine intoxication and withdrawal?

CASE 7

A 15-year-old male is brought into the ED by his neighbor who found the boy passed out in his backyard with a bag full of glue nearby. He had difficulty rousing the boy. Currently, the patient is lethargic with slurred speech and difficulty walking. When his parents arrive, they are shocked, as their son has been a "good kid." They had no idea he was using any drugs. Of course, he bought lots of tubes of "model glue" but they never saw any completed models.

The signs and symptoms of inhalant use include all of the following EXCEPT:

A) Dizziness.

B) Slurred speech.

C) Unsteady gait.

D) Smell of solvents or glue.

E) Dilated pupils.

Discussion

The correct answer is E. Inhalant intoxication is identified by impaired judgment, impaired social interaction, and aggressive behavior often leading to altercations. Higher doses can lead to lethargy, psychomotor retardation, stupor, or coma. Dilated pupils are seen in anticholinergic toxicity and other drugs (eg, sympathomimetics) but not with inhalants.

All of the following are considered inhalants used by abusers except:

A) Kerosene.
B) Cleaning solvent.
C) Gasoline.
D) Spray paint.
E) Glue.

Discussion

The correct answer is A. Kerosene is not volatile enough to be abusable. The rest can be abused by inhalation.

 HELPFUL TIP: The acute intoxicant effect of volatiles generally lasts approximately 30 minutes. Gasoline is an exception, intoxication from gasoline can last for up to 6 hours.

Withdrawal from inhalants includes all of the following EXCEPT:

A) Onset of symptoms 24–48 hours after use has stopped.
B) Transient hallucinations.
C) Diaphoresis.
D) Confusion.
E) Intense hunger.

Discussion

The correct answer is E. Intense hunger is not a sign of withdrawal. Rather, the patient may be nauseated. All of the other answers are signs of withdrawal.

All of the following can result from chronic solvent or hydrocarbon inhalation EXCEPT:

A) Chronic brain injury.
B) Muscle weakness.
C) CNS microhemorrhages and secondary seizures.
D) Erythrocytosis.
E) Liver and renal damage.

Discussion

The correct answer is D. Solvents and hydrocarbons can cause all of the effects listed above except for erythrocytosis. In fact, one can see bone marrow suppression as a result of chronic inhalant use.

Risk factors for inhalant abuse include all of the following demographic factors EXCEPT:

A) Female.
B) Age 13–15 years.
C) Low socioeconomic state.
D) Native American.
E) Poor school performance.

Discussion

The correct answer is A. Males, not females, are more likely to abuse inhalants. Inhalant users tend to be of lower socioeconomic status, younger (age 13–15 years), and have difficulty in school. There is an increased incidence of inhalant abuse among Native Americans.

 HELPFUL TIP: "Sniffing" is when fumes are inhaled directly from a source container or the substance is placed into a bag and inhaled from the bag. "Huffing" is when the substance is placed on a rag and then inhaled with the rag placed over the nose and mouth.

Objectives: Did you learn to . . .

- Identify some types of inhalants abused?
- Recognize the symptoms of inhalant abuse?
- Describe the demographics of inhalant abuse?

CASE 8

A 40-year-old male who has been smoking marijuana daily for the past 20 years would like to quit his marijuana habit. He wants to apply for a new job, and a drug screen is part of the application process. He makes an appointment with you to discuss what he can expect when he quits and how long will it be until his drug screen is negative.

All of the following are symptoms of marijuana intoxication EXCEPT:

A) Euphoria.
B) Sensation of slowed time.
C) Increased mental alertness.
D) Increased appetite.
E) Dry mouth.

Discussion

The correct answer is C. Marijuana intoxication decreases mental alertness although it can reportedly enhance the senses. When inhaled, intoxication peaks after 10–30 minutes and lasts approximately 3 hours.

How long can marijuana (THC) be detected in the urine?

A) 30 days if used regularly; 2–7 days if used occasionally.
B) 2 weeks.
C) One week for females; 2 weeks for males.
D) 24–48 hours.
E) It cannot be detected in urine samples.

Discussion

The correct answer is A. This patient will have to stop smoking marijuana for a minimum of 30 days before applying for the job if he wants to assure his urine drug screen will be negative. The drug can be present in hair samples for an extended period of time—anywhere from 1–6 months.

Which of the following is associated with marijuana use?

A) Increased violence.
B) Poor academic performance.
C) Increased lung cancer risk.
D) Cognitive difficulties.
E) All of the above.

Discussion

The correct answer is E. Additionally, marijuana has been associated with the development of gum disease. Other risks of marijuana use include testicular atrophy and an avolitional syndrome characterized by severe apathy and melancholy. Marijuana can also cause psy-

chosis and a withdrawal syndrome characterized by irritability, insomnia, and anxiety.

Which of these is NOT one of the claimed benefits of marijuana?

A) Pain reliever.
B) Anxiolytic.
C) Antiemetic.
D) Appetite stimulator.
E) Antidepressant.

Discussion

The correct answer is E. The use of marijuana has been shown to worsen depression. Marijuana has been used successfully for pain, nausea, glaucoma, etc.

 HELPFUL TIP: There may be an association between marijuana use and schizophrenia (see Lancet 2007 Jul 28; 370:319). However, causality has not been proven and other studies take exception with the results of this study.

Objectives: Did you learn to . . .

- Recognize the symptoms of marijuana intoxication?
- Describe the symptoms of marijuana withdrawal?
- Anticipate effects of marijuana use?

QUICK QUIZ: DUDE, WHAT WAS IN THAT POT?

A 20-year-old male is brought by the police into the ED because of severe agitation after smoking what he thought was crack cocaine. He exhibits slurred speech, ataxia, circumoral numbness, and horizontal nystagmus.

Which of the following substances is most likely causing his symptoms?

A) Cannabis (THC).
B) Heroin.
C) Methamphetamine.
D) Phencyclidine (PCP).
E) Nicotine.

Discussion

The correct is D. PCP (aka "angel dust") intoxication is characterized by agitation, impulsiveness, nystagmus, hypertension, tachycardia, numbness, ataxia, and perceptual distortions. Intoxication begins 5 minutes after use and peaks in 30 minutes. PCP-induced psychosis is the most common PCP-induced disorder and may mimic a schizophrenic psychotic episode. PCP may be added to other drugs unbeknownst to the user.

BIBLIOGRAPHY

Anderson CE, Loomis GA. Recognition and prevention of inhalant abuse. *Am Fam Physician.* 2003;68(5):869.

Connors GJ, Donovan DM, DiClemente CC. *Substance Abuse Treatment and the Stages of Change: Selecting and Planning Interventions.* New York: Guilford Press, 2004.

Enoch MA, Goldman D. Problem drinking and alcoholism: diagnosis and treatment. *Am Fam Physician.* 2002;65(3):441.

Johnson BA, et al. Topiramate for treating alcohol dependence: a randomized controlled trial. *JAMA.* 2007; 298(14):1641.

Maisto SA, Connors GJ, Dearing RL. *Alcohol Use Disorders.* Cambridge, MA: Hogrefe and Huber Publishing, 2007.

National Institute on Drug Abuse. Accessed at www.nida.nih.gov on February 8, 2008.

Winslow BT, Voorhees KI, Pehl HA. Methamphetamine abuse. *Am Fam Physician.* 2007;76(8):1175.

26

Ethics

Janeta F. Tansey

CASE 1

A 54-year-old married female, Charlene, has insulin-dependent diabetes and has seen you for her care for the last 7 years. In the last year she has developed diabetic retinopathy and neuropathy. To your great frustration, Charlene continues to resist the recommended lifestyle changes required to control her diabetes.

She is a casual, friendly, woman known as the "candy lady" in her neighborhood where she lives with her husband of 30 years. She loves children and volunteers at the local elementary school, where she is well known for a quick smile, a reassuring hug, and a piece of candy in her large pockets. She is noted during most of her appointments to be munching on M&M's—her favorite candy. She has had dietary consults and many education-oriented doctor appointments but says, "I know I shouldn't eat the way I do, but I just don't have the heart to change who I am, even if it does help my eyes and legs. Who I am is about what I eat and do."

You are wonder about Charlene's capacity for decision-making, given her frank noncompliance with care, even in the setting of serious complications of her diabetes.

All of the following variables are necessary in decision-making capacity EXCEPT:

A) Ability to communicate a choice.
B) Voluntary choice.
C) Understanding of the variables involved in the decision.
D) Family agreement that the patient is competent.
E) Ability to appreciate the personal impact of choices.

Discussion

The correct answer is D. Family concerns need to be addressed but family agreement has nothing to do with determining a patient's competence. All of the other answer choices are important elements to determine decision-making capacity (DMC). One additional necessary element for DMC is the ability to reason about the options in the setting of personal values.

What is the MOST relevant piece of information in Charlene's account that suggests that her capacity is intact?

A) Therapeutic alliance with you despite noncompliance with treatment recommendations.
B) Integration into community relationships, including a stable marriage and responsibilities in the elementary school.
C) Expression of placing perceived self-identity as a higher priority than control of diabetes and its complications.
D) Awareness that her dietary choices are associated with symptoms of eye disease and neuropathy.
E) Flagrant disregard for medical recommendations by eating candy while at her appointment.

Discussion

The correct answer is C. Although several of these variables are relevant in assessing DMC, the capacity for DMC is typically thought of in a step-wise fashion, starting with ability to communicate a choice, then basic understanding of the variables, then ability to appreciate the personal impact of choices, and finally the ability to reason about the options while considering personal values. This last step is the most complicated, but also the most strongly indicative that DMC is intact.

Which of the following statements is TRUE about DMC?

A) Patients who have been found legally incompetent do not have DMC.
B) A patient's DMC may vary according to the circumstances of the situation.
C) A minor's DMC is not clinically relevant since there is a surrogate who bears the responsibility for decision-making.
D) DMC should not be evaluated in cases in which the patient makes an unconventional choice.
E) Patients with psychiatric disease, who are committed to a treatment facility, do not have DMC.

Discussion

The correct answer is B. DMC is not an all-or-none distinction, but can vary widely from case to case or setting to setting. Answer A is incorrect. Patients who have been declared legally incompetent or who have been legally and involuntarily committed may still have a measure of DMC. Moral theory typically urges clinicians to consider the wishes and reasoning of their patients as morally and clinically relevant, regardless of the placement of a legal guardian or the state as a surrogate decision-maker. DMC may ultimately be overridden in certain kinds of legal circumstances, but it should not be done lightly as it suggests a fundamental denial of patient autonomy. As a result, many patients with psychiatric illness (answer E) still have the right to make choices, even with diagnoses such as schizophrenia. Answer D is incorrect. A patient's making unconventional choices can be a marker that DMC capacity is not intact but does not automatically lead one to this conclusion (eg, Jehovah Witness and blood transfusions; to refuse blood is unconventional but DMC may be intact). Answer C is incorrect. Although minors technically cannot make many health-care choices, their wishes should be taken into consideration as they are often able to articulate a preference.

* *

Charlene continues to have a slow decline over time but remains in good spirits despite the complications of her uncontrolled diabetes. One day her husband brings her to the ED. He had found her in the bathroom,

unconscious, and called an ambulance. She has had a stroke and remains unresponsive, on ventilation in the ICU. Her prognosis is poor.

What are appropriate considerations for making a treatment decision about end-of-life care for Charlene?

A) Oral statements to her husband about her end-of-life care.
B) Her husband's wishes for her care as designated health-care proxy.
C) Written advance directives.
D) Oral statements to her physician about her end-of-life care.
E) All of the above.

Discussion

The correct answer is E. Written advance directives are considered the most binding, although all of these issues are relevant in making end-of-life decisions.

Which of the following statements is used to describe medical futility?

A) No worthwhile goals of care can be achieved.
B) The likelihood of success is very small.
C) The patient's quality of life is unacceptable.
D) The prospective benefit is not worth the resources required.
E) All of the above.

Discussion

The correct answer is E. All of the above meanings have been explicitly or implicitly drawn into discussions about medical futility. For this reason, many theorists have objected to use of the term "futility" as a justification for decisions and urge clinicians to be precise about the concerns that arise in a given patient's clinical situation. Another definition of futility is trying to make it through this book and pass the recertification test.

* *

After discussion with her husband, you decide to discontinue ventilation. Charlene dies.

This intervention is appropriately considered:

A) Active, nonvoluntary euthanasia.
B) Physician-assisted suicide.
C) Withholding medical intervention.

D) Withdrawing medical intervention.
E) The principle of double effect.

Discussion

The correct answer is D. Withdrawing medical intervention means discontinuing an intervention that has already been used, although the disease state itself results in death with the intervention's discontinuation. Although the answer might seem intuitive to you, many persons (including physicians) do not recognize the differences among these various interventions.

Active euthanasia (answer A) is when the physician both supplies the means of death and is the final human agent in the events leading to the patient's death (eg, the physician administers the lethal drug). Whether or not active euthanasia is voluntary, involuntary, or non-voluntary depends on the decision-making capacity of the patient. Assisted suicide (answer B) occurs when the physician provides the means of death but the patient carries out the act, such as taking an overdose of phenobarbital. Withholding medical intervention (answer C) means not initiating care for a disease state such that the disease itself results in death. The principle of double effect (answer E) is an ethical theory that suggests that if there is an unintended bad outcome (eg, death) while pursuing an intended purpose (eg, pain relief), there is diminished moral responsibility for the unintended outcome. This principle is sometimes used to justify the use of high-dose opiates or sedatives in patients with intractable pain, even when the unintended effect is respiratory depression and death.

Which case is typically cited as a legal precedent for withdrawing a medical intervention, that results in death from the underlying disease?

A) Cruzan.
B) Tarasoff.
C) M'Naghten.
D) Quinlan.

Discussion

The correct answer is D. Ann Quinlan, a 22-year-old woman in a persistent vegetative state, was unlikely to regain consciousness and was on a ventilator. The father asked for the ventilator to be withdrawn, but the physicians refused. The New Jersey Supreme Court ruled that refusing care, including use of surrogate decision-makers, is a right justified by an individual's right to privacy. The court held that if there is "no reasonable possibility" of recovery, the medical intervention (ventilation in this case) may be withdrawn.

Cruzan is a similar case but has had more complicated effects in the state court systems. In *Cruzan*, the Missouri Supreme Court ruled (and the U.S. Supreme Court affirmed) that the state has an interest in protecting incompetent patients—in this case Nancy Cruzan who was in a persistent vegetative state and receiving tube feedings—from family decisions to discontinue or withhold treatment. The implications have been variable from state to state in the degree to which family or clinicians need to show the court that the patient would not have wanted life-sustaining treatment. This has largely spurred the interest in written advance directives.

The **Tarasoff** case has to do with the duty to warn a third party when a patient poses an imminent and serious threat to an identified third party. **M'Naghten** (sometimes spelled McNaughton) is the case of a patient found not guilty of the actions performed by reason of insanity.

Which of the following statements is TRUE concerning the role of law in life-sustaining interventions?

A) Courts must be involved in decisions regarding incompetent patients.
B) Life-sustaining treatment may be withheld only if patients are terminally ill or permanently unconscious.
C) Physicians may face criminal charges for providing appropriate palliative care and not treating the underlying disease.
D) The most prudent legal advice is to continue treatment in medically futile cases.
E) The law presents few barriers to physicians withholding life-sustaining interventions.

Discussion

The correct answer is E. Sometimes physicians inappropriately provide treatment to patients who have made their end-of-life choices clear and have stated that they do not want prolongation of life. Respecting the patient's prior wishes will **not** result in legal liability for the physician, but the converse is not true; one can be legally liable for treating a patient who does not want treatment (eg, transfusing a Jehovah Witness patient who refused transfusion). Answer A is incorrect. After a patient is declared incompetent, the courts no longer need to be involved, as a legal surrogate is appointed by the court to make decisions for the patient. Answer B is incorrect as treatment may be withheld at any time at the request of a competent patient.

Objectives: Did you learn to . . .

- Evaluate a patient's decision-making capacity?
- Recognize how decision-making capacity may vary based on the patient and the clinical setting?
- Identify some ethical issues in end-of-life care?
- Describe medical futility and understand its importance in making ethical decisions?

CASE 2

Robert, a 27-year-old married nurse from your hospital, is referred to your ED for an urgent evaluation by his supervisor. In the past 2 weeks, it has been noted that he is increasingly distressed while at work, with occasional tearfulness, distractibility, and irritability.

During the initial assessment, Robert reveals that there is a specific reason that he has been so preoccupied. He indicates that 2 weeks ago he was jailed for operating a vehicle while intoxicated and that he feels ashamed. He is afraid that his coworkers have read about it in the newspaper, although no one on his floor has indicated that this is the case. This is his first legal infraction of any kind and he describes it as humiliating.

On further questioning, Robert indicates that he uses alcohol regularly. Although it has not overtly affected his work as far as he can tell, it has caused significant marital strife. He reports that his pattern is to stop by the bar on the way home from work to "relax and let go of the hospital stuff that I worry about." He typically drinks 3 beers and then drives home, where he continues to drink beer throughout the evening. He notes that his wife and children complain that he is emotionally absent and even irritable with them, but he says that his family simply does not understand the stress of the workplace and his need to "forget about it for a few hours." He and his wife have started arguing lately about his alcohol use, especially since the driving charge. He takes special exception to her stating that he is an "alcoholic."

As you take the history, Robert begins to be more guarded in his responses and more restricted in his affect. Suddenly, he blurts out, "I don't think I'm an alcoholic, but I don't want you to put anything in my record about any of this stuff! And I want you to tell my supervisor that there are some personal problems going on at home and that I'll be fine in a few days."

Which of the following statements is TRUE about your obligation with regards to documentation in the chart?

A) You are obligated to document the visit as it occurred so far as the medical facts are concerned, including the concern about alcohol abuse.
B) You can enter incorrect information into the chart in order to protect the patient.
C) You are under no obligation to document anything said and can withhold information from the chart at the patient's request.
D) Hospital administration or legal counsel should be involved if information is going to be purposefully left out of the chart.

Discussion

The correct answer is A. The ethical principles of beneficence, nonmaleficence, and justice drive the decision here. A patient may legitimately ask for non-active medical problems (eg, distant history of sexual abuse) to be withheld from current documentation of an active problem (eg, allergic rhinitis). However, a patient **cannot** legitimately ask to have information withheld from the record if that information is pertinent to an ongoing condition currently being evaluated and treated. In this case, Robert is receiving care simply by virtue of being seen in the ED and disclosing the chief complaint and its associated variables. It is important for you to be forthcoming in explaining why the information may not be withheld from the medical record and also in reassuring him that non-relevant medical information will be omitted from the record if he feels that this is necessary. For example, the specifics of the argument with a wife need not be detailed beyond the comment that there is nonviolent marital conflict over the patient's alcohol use—important because it supports an alcohol abuse disorder. Furthermore, many institutions have specific policies on managing sensitive medical information and there may be a formal mechanism for increasing the security of the patient's medical record.

Why is protection of confidentiality important in medical practice?

A) It shows respect for patient autonomy.
B) It helps prevent stigmatization and discrimination against patients based on private medical issues.

C) It helps solidify trust within the physician-patient relationship.

D) It helps establish a boundary between the physician-patient relationship and the rest of the medical system.

E) All of the above.

Discussion

The correct answer is E. The physician-patient relationship is a long-honored tradition in medicine which is increasingly fragile in a medical system with numerous competing obligations. Nevertheless, it is prudent to remember the aspect of the Hippocratic Oath which states, "What I may see or hear in the course of the treatment . . . , which on no account one must spread abroad, I will keep to myself, holding such things shameful to be spoken about." This is not only important to the tradition of medicine itself, but to the physician-patient relationship. There is no doubt that loss of confidentiality may cause harm to the patient when others are in possession of confidential medical information. Such harms may be as overt as denying medical coverage for certain genetic conditions or as subtle as devaluing a person seen waiting to see the psychiatrist.

Which of the following are legally protected exceptions to the rule of maintaining patient confidentiality?

A) Reporting tuberculosis to public officials without patient consent.

B) Warning a third party at risk of imminent and serious bodily harm from the patient, without patient consent.

C) Reporting a patient's alcohol abuse to a work supervisor without the patient's consent.

D) A and B.

E) All of the above.

Discussion

The correct answer is D. Under current national and state laws, physicians are mandatory reporters of some infectious diseases and of intent to harm another. In most other cases, provision of medical information without the patient's written consent is not legally protected although there may be cases in which it is felt to be morally justifiable. Physicians need to weigh violations of patient confidentiality very carefully, even

when legally sanctioned. Ethicists typically agree that if a physician is going to compromise a patient's confidentiality for an overwhelming moral obligation that, in respect for patient autonomy, the patient needs to be notified. In many situations in which a physician hopes to communicate confidential information to a third party even when the patient is unwilling, a process of education and negotiation with the patient occurs such that respect for autonomy is acknowledged while simultaneously making the patient aware of competing moral obligations.

 HELPFUL TIP: Having a faxed or mailed report containing a patient's confidential medical information misdirected to an unintended recipient is *not* legally protected. Be cautious about transmission of patient information.

Which of the following interferes with protecting patient confidentiality in the medical structure?

A) Involvement of managed care organizations in patient care and medical payments.

B) Electronic records and transmissions.

C) Group practices and/or teaching hospitals with multiple care providers.

D) A and B.

E) All of the above.

Discussion

The correct answer is E. While individual physicians and patients continue to prize the tradition of respect for confidentiality, the multiple players in health care make it nearly impossible to restrict all information to the dyad of physician and patient. Insurance companies will not provide payment without at least information about the diagnosis, and notably, insurance companies are not legally bound by the same legal and ethical codes of conduct regarding patient privacy. Electronic records and transmissions by e-mail, cellular phones, faxes and other means are much more easily accessed by the curious or unintended recipients who have no reason to have confidential information. Open waiting rooms and multiple providers of care mean that larger and larger numbers of the community are aware that a patient is being seen in certain clinics for certain purposes. Although patient records are not often considered a confidentiality issue, once information is in written form, it is more difficult to control who might, either now or in the future, have access to the details of the report. For this reason, some physicians try to err on documenting only that which is considered absolutely necessary to patient care, although the distinction between the "absolutely necessary" and unnecessary can be a difficult line to draw in the sand, especially without the ability to appreciate how multiple variables may play out in the patient's future medical care.

* *

Robert is asking you to be deliberately deceptive with the supervisor. You disagree with this.

Which of the following is FALSE?

A) Trust in the physician-patient relationship depends on allowing the patient to make such a directive about communication with outside persons.
B) A physician who establishes a precedent for deception may be expected to practice deception in a future situation in which the harms greatly outweigh the benefits.
C) A physician who deceives may undermine general trust in the profession.
D) B and C.
E) None of the above.

Discussion

The correct answer is A. Another way of phrasing the question is, "What drives a physician to be honest even when what the patient really wants is not honesty?" Will the patient trust you more if you are deceptive for him? Will this help him (aside from allowing him to keep his job)?

The physician-patient relationship is generally not considered an adequate reason to lie to a third party about the nature of a patient's illness and treatment. There has been concern that a physician who deceives a third party, even in the immediate interest of the patient's confidentiality or other concerns, establishes himself or herself as a physician who may not be trustworthy in other matters. A patient may not consider this at the time a deception is requested. These kinds of ripple-effects from the decisions of an individual physician can affect the profession in general, ultimately producing fears that physicians will take the self-serving path rather than the higher moral ground.

* *

You tell Robert that he has alcohol dependence and then provide education about the diagnosis and treatment options. You recommend outpatient treatment in

Alcoholics Anonymous and a chemical dependency program. Robert agrees, more for the sake of his family stability than because of any true insight into the severity of his problem. You then arrange for follow-up with one of your partners (you've been selected as a contestant on the next *Survivor* and get to escape to a tropical island).

At the next appointment, Robert meets his new physician, Dr. Pincus. At this appointment, Robert indicates that he did attend two AA meetings, but was very uncomfortable with the aspect of the 12-step program that requires acknowledging a "higher power." Robert indicates that he is an atheist and secular humanist, believing that the locus of self-control comes from within the individual human spirit. He has refused to continue in AA due to his rejection of its theistic foundation. He has had no further legal problems and reports that work is still going fine, with diminished irritability once he resolved in his mind that his coworkers were unaware of his previous driving violation. However, he continues to drink 6-9 alcoholic beverages per night and admits that he occasionally needs a shot of whisky in the morning to "make sure I don't lose it with all the work stress." He also works a night shift about once per week and does use approximately the same amount of alcohol before beginning the night shift, although he denies being intoxicated while on the job on these nights ("6 beers just gets me started"). He doesn't think this is a problem because "things are quiet at night and everyone just helps each other keep the patients comfortable." He reports that his family is satisfied with the decrease in consumption and that he considers the matter of alcohol abuse resolved.

Dr. Pincus has had her own problems with alcohol in the past. She has had a rocky course over the past many years but found AA to be very helpful. She has become very active in her Jewish synagogue and community, where she receives support and is accountable to her friends. Her own alcohol history has been marked by difficulty with alcohol bingeing, such that when she starts to drink, she drinks to intoxication. Only with aggressive honesty at a professional-group AA as well as a substance abuse protocol through the state board of medical examiners, does she feel that she's been able to remain completely abstinent for the last 4 years.

Dr. Pincus is considering revealing to Robert some of her own struggles as a health-care professional with a substance abuse disorder. She believes that this will help him reevaluate the role of AA in sobriety and the importance of very tight control of alcohol consumption to prevent relapsing illness.

Self-disclosure is best described as involving the ethical issues of:

A) Deception and nondisclosure.
B) Privacy and boundaries.
C) Informed consent.
D) Impaired colleagues.
E) Autonomy.

Discussion

The correct answer is B. There are explicit and implicit boundaries that exist between a physician's private experiences and the physician-patient relationship. One of these boundaries has to do with preventing physician needs and private matters from encroaching into the visit in a way that is not therapeutic to the patient and does not respect the physician's boundaries. While it would appear that Dr. Pincus has therapeutic reasons—for Robert, not for herself—for crossing the boundary of self-disclosure, both physician motivation for self-disclosure and the immediate and potential effects of the self-disclosure need to be weighed very seriously before private matters are revealed. If there is even a potential of harm, crossing the boundary in this way should be considered a violation of professional norms.

How could Dr. Pincus appropriately respond to Robert's refusal to participate in AA on the basis of his religious impulse?

A) "AA is still shown the best intervention for preventing relapsing alcohol use. I hope you can go and get something out of it without acknowledging your acceptance of the 'higher power' explicitly."
B) "AA has important group support from others who understand how difficult it is to stop using alcohol. It is not meant to be religious, but rather a community of care."
C) "I have found both AA and a theistic worldview to be very helpful in understanding my own powerlessness to control some of my behaviors. Would it be helpful to you to hear more about this?"
D) "I understand how the religious aspect of AA is inconsistent with your own philosophy. Would you be willing to investigate nonreligious group meetings for alcohol abusers?"
E) "AA's 'higher power' can be understood as yourself and is not intended as a theistic conception."

Discussion

The correct answer is D. AA is an example of a prescribed treatment that involves an active religious component. AA's second step involves acknowledgment of a higher power, traditionally invoking a specific monotheistic conception of the divine as a necessity to surrendering the illusion of control. In the interest of respecting a patient's religious rights in a diverse community and of optimizing treatment options, it would be disrespectful and ineffective to have the patient participate in AA while ignoring the second step of the program and the foundational philosophy of AA. While there are fewer studies about the efficacy of nonreligious alcohol treatment groups, it is appropriate to respect Robert's beliefs by investigating nonreligious alternatives. As to answer A, the Cochrane database concludes, "No experimental studies unequivocally demonstrated the effectiveness of AA."

Whether or not self-disclosure of one's own religious beliefs is appropriate is an important question. As mentioned in the discussion in the question above, it is very important for the physician to measure the intent of the disclosure. Also, physicians need to be exquisitely sensitive to the power differential that exists between a physician and patient such that strong individual viewpoints might become threatening or coercive in the physician-patient relationship. In certain religious traditions, sharing one's faith is an important step, demonstrating courage and integrity; nevertheless, physicians should be strongly cautioned to pay heed to the virtue of practical wisdom and the unique circumstances of the medical relationship that makes proselytizing most often inappropriate. A better strategy, if a physician feels that a patient might be seeking additional spiritual or philosophical direction, is to ask open-ended questions and then make an appropriate referral to pastoral care or a spiritual counselor who will be sensitive to the issues the patient has raised as relevant.

Which of the following is true about intervening with an "impaired colleague," like Robert?

A) Impairment should only be reported to a state licensing board if the colleague's patients are placed at known and documentable risk.
B) Because alcohol abuse is a confidential matter, it is inappropriate for a treating physician to report a colleague's impairment to a licensing board.
C) Removing a colleague from direct patient care or increasing supervision during patient care are reasonable first step interventions for a colleague who

is actively engaged in substance **treatment** (eg, a report has already been made).

D) It is preferable to contact a state licensing board directly as opposed to discussing the matter with the patient or institutional administration. This protects both the reporter and the colleague from unnecessary negative repercussions.

E) None of the Above.

Discussion

The correct answer is C. Legal statutes on reporting impaired colleagues vary from state to state, with some state laws making physicians mandatory reporters of impaired physician colleagues, while others simply recommend reporting. Furthermore, state laws are even less prescriptive with regards to non-physician health professionals with impairments. Any impairment should be treated seriously, preferably with support from the institution's administration. It is imperative to protect patients from harm. Although reporting the impaired colleague may result in anger and disappointment from the colleague or even supervisors who are reluctant to tackle such a difficult question, physicians should consider the needs of vulnerable patients and the patients' rights to adequate care.

Confidentiality adds an additional ethical dimension when an impaired colleague reveals his or her impairment to his treating physician. In an effort to respect patient autonomy, physicians will often urge impaired colleagues to report themselves as well as voluntarily engage in treatment protocols. Many states have less restrictive policies for treatment and monitoring for impaired colleagues who self-report. If a physician intends to report her patient's impairment without the consent of the patient, the physician is obligated to be truthful with the colleague about her intentions and rationale for reporting.

A colleague may be impaired in her practice by which of the following?

A) Substance use.
B) Major depression.
C) Dementia.
D) Deficits in fund of knowledge.
E) All of the above.

Discussion

The correct answer is E. Any one of these, whether acute or chronic, does not imply global impairment in medical practice. However, each may have many implications for a colleague's medical practice. Special attention should be given to the colleague's actual and possible consequences in practice, given her specific job requirements and compensatory skills/supports, while assessing the presence and degree of impairment.

Objectives: Did you learn to . . .

- Identify which items are required for inclusion in the medical record?
- Recognize the importance of patient confidentiality and understand when confidentiality might be broken in order to fulfill other ethical obligations?
- Recognize obstacles to protecting patient confidentiality?
- Describe the importance of individual and societal trust in individual physicians and the medical profession as a whole?
- Describe the ethical principles involved in self-disclosure?
- Identify an impaired colleague and determine how to best intervene?

CASE 3

Anne is a 19-year-old single female presenting for her first prenatal visit. She is G1P0, and roughly 10 weeks' gestation by last menstrual period. She is new to your practice. Anne has had no medical care at this facility and no physician appointments since childhood. In collecting the past medical history, Anne reveals that she has had several first-degree female relatives who have been diagnosed with breast and/or ovarian cancer: her mother, two maternal aunts, and a maternal grandmother. A great aunt died young of unknown causes. Anne is unsure of the workup that they had, but there was significant morbidity and mortality as a result of the illnesses. Anne only recently became aware of this family history when her mother and aunts were diagnosed in the last 5 years. When you ask if she has discussed genetic risks for breast cancer, Anne replies, "No."

Anne has been in a stable relationship with her boyfriend, Jordan, since they were juniors in high school. They cohabitate and are engaged to be married, but have not set a wedding date. Anne has completed high school and has been working in telemarketing while applying to art schools. The pregnancy was not planned, but she and Jordan are thrilled, even if "a little nervous," about having a baby.

You are concerned about the BRCA1 and BRCA2 genes. In families with a high incidence of breast and ovarian cancer, mutations in BRCA1 are associated with an 85% lifetime risk of developing breast cancer and a 50% risk of ovarian cancer.

You wonder if this is the best time to bring up genetic concerns with Anne, given Anne's concurrent transition with an unplanned pregnancy.

Which of the following is (are) true about disclosure?

A) Nondisclosure is not justifiable due to fears that a patient will be distressed by the information, unless disclosure might cause death (eg, suicide at hearing a diagnosis of cancer).

B) Regardless of the consequences, nondisclosure could be considered deception and would be morally wrong on the basis of this intrinsic feature.

C) Disclosure is important because it respects patient autonomy and optimizes a patient's ability to make an informed choice.

D) Nondisclosure may be a sign of paternalism rather than beneficence.

E) All of the above.

Discussion

The correct answer is E. There are a variety of moral theories used to comment on whether or not deception or nondisclosure is morally appropriate. Most theorists rely on the principle of respect for patient autonomy, such that a person who has incomplete information is not able to act freely in making a choice for herself. "Consequentialism" is also a commonly used moral theory, suggesting that it is not the intrinsic nature of the act itself but the consequences that follow that determine whether the act is good or evil (as in "the end justifies the means"). In virtue ethics, by comparison, the nature and motivation of the act is very important as a reflection of the physician's character and habits. In virtue ethics, deception is morally blameworthy because it is comparable to lying or deceit. In virtue ethics, motivation is also an important issue to judge the goodness of the action. Answers B and C make reference, in part, to virtue theory.

Which of the following statements is FALSE regarding testing for genetic conditions?

A) Informed consent for genetic testing should be taken more seriously and formally than other kinds of blood testing, such as obtaining a hemogram.

B) Physicians should ask patients what they would do with the different possible outcomes of the genetic test before the test is performed.

C) Physicians should make a recommendation regarding genetic testing guided by evidence-based medicine and the patient's specific narrative and values.

D) Physicians should urge patients to disclose positive results to relatives or spouses if the information is pertinent medically or emotionally to these third parties.

E) Physicians should never disclose genetic information to a third party without the consent of the patient.

Discussion

The correct answer is E. Genetic testing differs from other blood tests because of multiple actual and potential risks, including personal effects on the patient and her family, as well as discrimination by employers or insurers. There is a shortage of formally trained genetic counselors, and patients rely on their physicians not only to help guide their decision-making about whether or not to perform the test, but also what to do with the information obtained. Because such testing has profound medical and/or psychosocial effects on the patient and family, a discussion about disclosure should happen both before and after the test is obtained.

Confidentiality is important for many reasons, not only in establishing and maintaining a good physician-patient relationship and respecting patient autonomy, but also because of the potential discriminations and misuses of genetic information in today's culture. However, when the risk of harm to another related person is high and the patient refuses to disclose important genetic information, there may be adequate cause to break confidentiality in order to prevent serious harm to the third party; therefore, answer E is a false statement.

 HELPFUL TIP: Many diagnostic and screening tests (eg, HIV antibody, PSA, biopsies, etc) should be approached in this way, assuring that the patient has a clear understanding of the implications of the test, including further diagnostic testing, therapies, and prognosis.

* *

You decide to disclose the possibility of genetic risk factors to Anne at the first prenatal visit and also discuss the risk of passing genes to the fetus. Anne seems overwhelmed and asks to bring Jordan to the next visit to discuss this further. When Anne returns with her fiancé, you discuss your concerns about the BRCA1 and 2 genes and why Anne's family history is suspicious. Jordan says, "I think you should be tested right away Anne. This would totally change our future." Anne replies, "What are you saying? Will you leave me if I have the gene? I can't raise this baby by myself."

Which of the following statements is (are) appropriate to consider in promoting the patient's best interests?

A) Patients are vulnerable.
B) Physicians have expertise that patients lack.
C) Patients rely on their physicians.
D) Physicians and patients often agree on what constitutes a patient's best interests, although they may differ in the way they plan to meet those interests.
E) All of the above.

Discussion

The correct answer is E. The nature of a relationship between physician and patient may have as many permutations as there are individuals. However, it is important to appreciate the position of the patient and the need that has pushed her to seek care. Patients are vulnerable in many ways, and the vulnerability is enhanced by limited access to technologic and scientific information. When external variables, such as Jordan's comment and Anne's response, come into play, physicians should pay attention to this narrative and take some responsibility for establishing and maintaining a supportive network even outside of the office. This is particularly important as physicians give patients information about difficult choices. While physicians and patients may often be able to negotiate a mutually acceptable alternative, active dialogue is important. Supports and advocates who are familiar with the patient's values and wishes can be an important adjunct to medical decision-making, as long as there is no material or psychological conflict of interests. Physicians should not adopt a completely hands-off policy in decision-making; rather, physicians should pay attention to supporting the patient with real options and evidence-based variables in a noncoercive, empowering relationship.

* *

Anne decides not to have the test, but to have an elective abortion "in case I passed on the gene to the baby."

For the sake of argument, you are philosophically opposed to elective abortions in this scenario, but you would consider abortion an appropriate intervention if the fetus tests positive for the gene by chorionic villus sampling.

What is the best ethical option for you at this point?

A) Explain that you are personally uncomfortable with abortion, but in deference to Anne's legal rights, you will make a referral to another physician who is willing to provide the elective abortion.
B) Refuse to perform or make a referral for the abortion.
C) Refer to a pro-life counseling agency.
D) Tell Anne, for reasons that you do not feel comfortable disclosing, you will no longer be able to care for her.
E) Perform the elective abortion, despite personal convictions, out of respect for the law and patient autonomy.

Discussion

The correct answer is A. Abortion is a fiercely contentious topic in the United States. Under the 1973 *Roe v. Wade* decision and in subsequent rulings such as *Planned Parenthood v. Casey*, the Supreme Court has affirmed a woman's legal right to abort a fetus. Physicians have responsibilities that should transcend views about a physician's own moral values, such as ensuring that informed consent is practiced and that the patient has medical care available. Informed consent requires a physician to provide the necessary information about the various medical choices available and to assess the patient's emotional needs. Coercion and failure to disclose clinically relevant information is inappropriate; for example, a referral to a pro-life group without informing the patient of the counseling center's position (when known) is a form of manipulation and failure to disclose. Abandoning the patient without a simple explanation is disrespectful, although the physician should be careful not to coerce her in other ways while revealing personal values/beliefs.

Physicians should note that in some states there have been rulings requiring physicians to participate in elective abortions if working in a public aid clinic or in an area with limited physician resources where transfer of care is not an option. Some physicians or institutions (such as Catholic hospitals with clear policies influenced by theological statements) have practiced conscientious objection and been subject to discipline of various forms, including legal sanction. Physicians should be mindful of competing moral values, seeking support and professional guidance in difficult moral and legal cases such that they can act with integrity and purpose in their roles as physicians and moral agents.

* *

Three years later, Anne is seen in a new clinic. She had the abortion. Anne is now an art student and is married to Jordan. Since her last clinic visit, Anne has had a prophylactic mastectomy following a positive test for the BRCA1 gene. She has also had an elective tubal ligation. Anne wants to consider in vitro fertilization and has a friend, Jessica, who is willing to donate ova. They put 18 embryos into cold storage, using Jessica's ova and Jordan's sperm. Anne has 6 embryos implanted, with the result of two fetuses that are carried to term. Anne decides that she does not want any more children and contacts the lab to discard the remaining embryos, eliminating storage costs. The lab agrees and sells the embryos to a private lab, where stem cell research is underway.

Which statement is NOT true about stored tissue samples?

A) The embryos are considered Anne's property only as long as she claims them.

B) Samples used for research purposes are potentially identifiable by third parties as belonging to Jessica and Jordan.

C) Tissue samples may only be used for their initial intended purpose, after which time they must be destroyed.

D) Third parties, such as research labs, upon discovering genetic anomalies in tissue samples, have no legal obligation to find and inform Anne, Jordan, and/or Jessica.

E) Embryos sold to a private lab may be used to establish germ lines via destruction of the embryo.

Discussion

The correct answer is C. At the time of publication, there is ongoing discussion about how to regulate use of tissue samples. While it might seem that this is an ethical question far removed from the purview of the family physician, patients in family practice clinics are very frequently targeted for various research protocols due to their regular follow-up and easy accessibility.

Patients donating tissue samples often give little thought to what happens to those tissues after they are obtained. In many cases, tissues are banked indefinitely after the initial research is conducted, with various identifiers linked to the tissue potentially including the donor's gender, geographic location, educational level, family history, or other private information. Although efforts are made to respect the privacy of the donor, it has been established that there are ways to track down the donor using even the limited identification information associated with the stored sample. Such means are especially facilitated by the wide availability of personal information via the Internet.

Tissue samples may be collected for one purpose, but later used for another. Tissue samples are very important in research and are often the limiting factor for studies, but should informed consent include asking donors for permission for each and every lab test run on the tissue sample? At what point, if any, does the tissue sample become the sole property of the lab? In the example of embryos, discarded embryos are sometimes sold to private labs; parents using IVF technology are often unaware that such embryos may be used to establish a stem cell line from which genetically identical embryos can be created using nuclear transfers. Such stem cell lines are highly lucrative for research purposes, and there has been discussion, for example, of whether parents should be compensated in some manner when a lab sells their discarded embryos or a research facility develops a product using the embryonic stem cells.

 HELPFUL TIP: Family physicians should continue to serve as advocates for their patients. You can do so by investigating the policies and procedures of research groups prior to allowing access to patients and by taking some responsibility for the informed consent process when patients are volunteering to participate in research.

Which of the following are concerns about the consequences of human somatic cell nuclear transfer, commonly called human cloning in the lay literature?

A) Will cloning result in increased miscarriages and deformed fetuses, due to limitations of current technology to perform nuclear transfer?

B) Will cloning result in a culture pre-occupied with "designer babies"?

C) Will cloning result in a culture that devalues persons with disabilities?
D) Will cloning increase reproductive options for same-sex couples, diminishing value of traditional settings for reproduction?
E) All of the above.

Discussion

The correct answer is E. All the above choices have been raised as concerns, although there are many more arguments on both sides of the discussion about the relative risks and benefits.

Objectives: Did you learn to . . .

- Describe the ethical issues regarding disclosure?
- Appreciate the many competing interests involved in genetic testing?
- Identify patient and physician factors that affect the patient-physician relationship?
- Find an ethical and acceptable way to disagree with a patient and continue to ensure that patient's health care?

QUICK QUIZ: ETHICAL DILEMMA

A 20-year-old college female is brought to the ED by two friends who found her passed out, naked, disheveled, and obviously traumatized in her dorm room. The patient has very little memory of events but thinks that she was raped. After an appropriate history and physical exam using a "rape kit," you conclude that there is evidence of nonconsensual vaginal penetration including the presence of semen. The patient tearfully states that she has never had sexual intercourse before and does not want to get pregnant but is Catholic and believes abortion is morally wrong.

What can you tell her?

A) "I think that the Pope is coming around on this topic."

B) "You have to go with your belief system regardless of the consequences."
C) "You could consider an antifertility drug (eg, high-dose OCP) because the conception would be nonconsensual and you are highly unlikely to be pregnant right now."
D) "Catholic doctrine justifies abortion if the fetus is a product of a rape."
E) "Call your priest tomorrow and tell me what you decide."

Discussion

The correct answer is C. Although abortion is not justified under any circumstances in Roman Catholic doctrine, the use of antifertility drugs after rape is supported by Catholic bioethical reasoning: the patient is not an autonomous decision-maker in the process of attempting to conceive and the likelihood of conception at this point is very low.

Answers A, B, and E are neither appropriate nor sensitive. Although this is a case addressing an ethical issue with regard to one specific religion and physicians cannot be held responsible for knowing all the nuances of different religious doctrines, we can and should be sympathetic to the patient's view and attempt to understand her ethical dilemma and assist in resolving it.

BIBLIOGRAPHY

American Medical Association. Code of Medical Ethics, updated 2003, Available at http://www.ama-assn.org/ama/pub/category/2503.html.

Beauchamp TL, Childress JF. *Principles of Biomedical Ethics.* 4th ed. New York: Oxford University Press, 1994.

Campbell A, Gillett G, Jones G. *Medical Ethics.* 3rd ed. South Melbourne, Australia: Oxford University Press, 2001.

Lo, B. *Resolving Ethical Dilemmas: A Guide for Clinicians.* 2nd ed. Philadelphia: Lippincott, Williams & Wilkins, 2000.

Smith HL, Churchill LR. *Professional Ethics and Primary Care Medicine.* Durham, NC: Duke University Press, 1986.

27

End-of-Life Care

Michelle Weckmann and Richard C. Dobyns

CASE 1

A 68-year-old male patient of yours is admitted to the hospital for a COPD exacerbation. This is his third admission for respiratory problems within the last year. His nurse asks if he is an appropriate candidate for hospice care.

Which of the following would allow your patient to receive hospice benefits under Medicare?

A) His cardiac ejection fraction is 15%, and he is dyspneic with minimal exertion (NYHA class III heart failure).
B) He agrees to a do not resuscitate (DNR) status in the event of cardiorespiratory failure.
C) An Apache score of 12.
D) His FEV_1 is <30% of predicted.
E) His dyspnea is worsening despite optimal medical management.

Discussion

The correct answer is E. In the past few years, Medicare has attempted to make hospice more accessible and easier for physicians and patients to use. If your patient has a terminal disease and he has declining function, worsening symptoms, or worsening laboratory tests, he or she probably qualifies for hospice. Answer A, a low cardiac ejection fraction, is a criterion for heart disease **but must be accompanied by dyspnea at rest**. Answer B is incorrect. Despite popular belief, a hospice patient need not agree to a DNR status upon receiving the hospice benefit; however, hospice agencies are permitted to have different admission

criteria and some require a DNR status for admission. Answer C is incorrect. Apache scores are used to estimate severity and survival in hospitalized patients and are not used to determine hospice eligibility. Answer D is incorrect. In the recent past, criteria were more stringent. Now, a specific measure of COPD severity (eg, FEV_1 <30% of predicted) is not necessary.

 HELPFUL TIP: Although prognosis may be the most difficult task a physician faces, an attempt at prognosis in patients with a terminal illness may help them. If you determine a patient has ≤6 months to live, he or she is appropriate for hospice, regardless of diagnosis.

Which statement reflects one aspect of the hospice/palliative care philosophy?

A) The hospice philosophy affirms life and only facilitates death when that death is inevitable.
B) Palliative care treatments do not include aggressive medical treatments such as radiation therapy, IV fluids, or interventional radiologic procedures.
C) The physician who provides hospice care should be available to terminal patients and their families at all times during the dying process.
D) Ameliorating pain through cure of the causative illness is a major goal of palliative care.
E) A death that occurs after the patient's suffering has been alleviated is a success.

Discussion

The correct answer is E. One of the goals of hospice care is symptom control, which should be relieved as quickly as possible. Answer A is incorrect because hospice does not facilitate death but rather works to make life meaningful and comfortable for the terminal patient. Answer B is incorrect because the goal of palliative care is to prevent and relieve suffering (this is the definition of palliative care, which is why answer D is incorrect). Palliative and hospice care seeks to support the best possible quality of life for patients and their families, regardless of the stage of a disease or the need for specific medical interventions. Any intervention, including the modalities listed in answer B, can be considered palliative if the intention is to relieve pain or suffering rather than cure disease. Local radiation, for example, can be an excellent palliative treatment to relieve pain and other symptoms. Answer C is incorrect because hospice is comprised of many individuals including nurses, health aides, chaplains, etc, who are available to assist the patient and family. Care is directed by the primary physician who is expected to be available by phone or have coverage when another member of the hospice team (typically the nurse) has concerns. The primary care physician need not be directly available 24/7.

The Medicare home-hospice benefit includes which of the following?

A) The hospice benefit covers all services related to the admitting illness as long as they are provided by the hospice.
B) The hospice benefit, similar to the Medicare home care benefit, requires that the patient be home-bound.
C) Respite care within an acute hospital setting is provided once every 6 months.
D) Hospice entry requires that the patient cannot live alone (must have an on-site primary caregiver).
E) A per diem rate is paid to the licensed hospice program regardless of the level of services provided.

Discussion

The correct answer is A. The Medicare hospice benefit requires that all care related to the primary admitting illness is covered by the hospice agency. However, Medicare affords individual hospice agencies wide latitude in determining which modalities they wish to use to treat the symptoms of a particular illness. This can lead to perceived differences in the care individual hospice agencies offer. For example, one agency might allow blood transfusions for the relief of dyspnea, while another agency covers only the use of medications such as morphine or lorazepam for dyspnea. In both cases, the hospice agency is conforming to Medicare's requirement by offering a treatment intended to relieve the symptom of dyspnea. Medicare also covers acute hospitalizations related to the primary illness if they are necessary for acute symptom management. Answer B is incorrect because in contrast to Medicare's requirement for the home care benefit, a hospice patient does not need to be homebound. The Medicare hospice benefit does have a provision for up to 5 nights (6 days) of respite care. The requirements are that the respite needs to be provided in a setting where there is a registered nurse available 24 hours, and the patient needs to have been in a home setting (which includes assisted living) where there is a breakdown in the primary caregiver. Respite care can be offered as frequently as needed, which makes answer C incorrect. Answer D is incorrect because Medicare does not require that the patient have a primary caregiver in the home to receive the hospice benefit; however, an individual hospice agency may require a primary caregiver before enrolling a patient. Answer E is incorrect because Medicare pays the hospice organization a stratified per diem rate depending on the level of care the patient requires.

* *

Your patient's family inquires more about hospice care. They ask which other services are covered.

The Medicare hospice benefit includes coverage for all of the following expenses EXCEPT:

A) Medications related to symptom management.
B) Chaplain services.
C) Home health aid services.
D) Room and board for a patient living in a nursing home.
E) Bereavement services.

Discussion

The correct answer is D. All of the other answer choices are services covered under the Medicare hospice benefit. A patient living in a nursing home **is eligible** for hospice care, but the cost of room and board for the nursing home is not paid by the hospice benefit. In some special circumstances, nursing home care will be paid for a short duration (eg, when a hospice patient uses the 5-night respite care benefit).

* *

You believe that your patient has <6 months to live. The local hospice medical director reviews the case and agrees. The patient is dyspneic at rest, requires 24-hour oxygen by nasal cannula, and has an FEV_1 <30% predicted. He wishes to avoid further hospitalization and has elected to have a DNR status. His family wants to know what you can do when he becomes severely dyspneic.

Which of the following is appropriate palliative treatment for severe dyspnea in this patient?

A) Intubation and ventilation.
B) Morphine.
C) Scopolamine.
D) Buspirone.

Discussion

The correct answer is B. Morphine and other opioids are indicated for palliation of dyspnea in respiratory failure. Despite concerns about opioids worsening respiratory function in end-stage COPD, one randomized-controlled trial and one meta-analysis have concluded that oral morphine improves dyspnea in this patient population. Keep in mind that the goal is to alleviate the symptom of dyspnea and **not** to reduce incidence of mortality. Answer A is clearly incorrect, as this patient has chosen hospice care and a far less aggressive stance toward life-prolonging measures. Answer C is incorrect. Scopolamine is used to reduce pharyngeal secretions but is not likely to relieve dyspnea in this patient. Answer D is incorrect. Although anxiety and dyspnea often occur together with anxiety leading to worsening dyspnea and vice versa, buspirone (BuSpar) is a weak anxiolytic and has no direct effect on dyspnea.

How does morphine relieve dyspnea?

A) It acts centrally to reduce the subjective feeling of breathlessness.
B) It acts locally as a bronchodilator.
C) It acts locally to reduce inflammation in the bronchioles.
D) It strengthens diaphragmatic excursions.

Discussion

The correct answer is A. Morphine acts centrally to reduce the subjective feeling of dyspnea. Also, morphine is known to reduce preload and peripheral vas-

cular resistance and thus is occasionally employed in treating dyspnea due to heart failure. Answers B and C are incorrect because morphine does not have any known direct effects on human lung tissue, although animal models suggest a possible local effect and some physicians advocate using nebulized morphine or fentanyl for dyspnea. Answer D is incorrect because morphine reduces the respiratory rate and tidal volume (reduced diaphragmatic excursions).

 HELPFUL TIP: Benzodiazepines may be used in combination with narcotics for added relief of dyspnea and anxiety. The patient should be monitored for excessive sedation and respiratory depression.

Objectives: Did you learn to . . .

- Identify appropriate patients for end-of-life care, particularly for the Medicare hospice benefit?
- Describe the features of the Medicare hospice benefit?
- Recognize and treat patients with end-stage respiratory disease?

 QUICK QUIZ: PAIN RELIEF

A 30-year-old male patient you have known for several years was diagnosed with metastatic melanoma several months ago. He presents now with intermittent, severe headaches associated with nausea. A head CT scan performed last week showed 3 metastatic foci with surrounding edema. He currently takes maximum doses of acetaminophen and large doses of morphine.

Which of the following is the BEST choice to recommend to him now?

A) Neurosurgical consultation.
B) Dexamethasone.
C) Sumatriptan.
D) Ibuprofen.
E) Increased morphine doses.

Discussion

The correct answer is B. Corticosteroids are the preferred therapy for headaches caused by increased intracranial pressure from edema, as is presumably the case here. Corticosteroids reduce edema surrounding tumor and thus relieve symptoms. Whole brain or stereotactic radiation therapy, alone or in combination with corticosteroids, may also be used as palliative therapy for multiple brain metastases. Answer A is incorrect because neurosurgical consultation for craniotomy should be reserved for patients who fail other interventions or who present with rapidly worsening symptoms. Answers C and D are incorrect. Sumatriptan and ibuprofen should not be used to treat increased intracranial pressure. Answer E, increased morphine doses, may be required, but corticosteroids are typically employed first.

CASE 2

A 74-year-old female was diagnosed with adenocarcinoma of the colon 3 years prior to beginning hospice care. She has known metastases to her liver and pelvis. She complains of a cramping pain in her abdomen and a "deep pain" in her groin. She is currently receiving morphine sulfate 10 mg PO every 4 hours (except when asleep) and acetaminophen 650 mg PO TID. She says that her pain is 4 out of 10 on a numeric pain scale. Her past medical history includes hemorrhage secondary to a gastric ulcer four years ago (*H. pylori* negative on biopsy).

Which of the following pain control strategies is a good first step for improving this patient's pain?

A) The likely source of her pain is neuropathic; add gabapentin.
B) Add a strong NSAID such as ketorolac (Toradol) to her current regimen.
C) Add a COX-2 inhibitor (eg, Celebrex) to maintain the narcotic-sparing effect.
D) Decrease the dose of morphine and add octreotide to decrease GI secretion and motility.
E) Maximize the dose of acetaminophen to 1,000 mg every 6 hours.

Discussion

The correct answer is E. The patient is on a suboptimal dose of acetaminophen and this is by far the safest drug for this patient. **Increasing** (not decreasing) this patient's morphine would also be a good choice (main reason that answer D is incorrect). Answer A is incorrect because her pain is better described as visceral or somatic rather than neuropathic. Gabapentin will likely do nothing for this patient and is not the first choice in

neuropathic pain (try a tricyclic antidepressant first). Answer B is incorrect because **ketorolac is the most toxic of the NSAIDs** and is contraindicated in a patient who has had a GI bleed. In addition, ketorolac is the NSAID with the highest rate of associated renal disease. If you were to add an NSAID, ibuprofen would be a reasonable choice—as long as GI protection went along with it. Answer C is incorrect. A COX-2 inhibitor is not the best choice for this patient. COX-2 inhibitors do have gastric toxicity and **the long-term safety advantage of COX-2 inhibitors versus ibuprofen is marginal if it exists at all.** Answer D is incorrect because octreotide will do nothing for this patient (although it can be used to reduce secretory diarrhea).

 HELPFUL TIP: For patients who require chronic narcotic pain medication, avoid the use of combination drugs (eg, Percocet, Lortab, etc). These drugs are more difficult to titrate, and the acetaminophen content limits their ceiling doses.

* *

To determine which medications are appropriate for treating pain, it helps to know the type of pain the patient has.

A patient with metastatic colon cancer may suffer from which type(s) of pain?

A) Neuropathic pain.
B) Visceral pain.
C) Soft tissue/bone pain.
D) Pain from increased intracranial pressure.
E) All of the above.

Discussion

The correct answer is E. It is important to understand that various cancers can cause different types of pain, and that these different pains may be approached with different treatments. Physiologic pain is separated into four categories: soft tissue or bone pain, neuropathic pain, visceral pain, and the pain of increased intracranial pressure.

* *

Soft-tissue/bone pain is also called somatic pain, and the musculoskeletal pain (eg, sports injuries, fractures, etc) everyone experiences is an example of that category of pain. **Neuropathic pain** is described as burning and results from nerve damage, inflammation, and compression. **Visceral pain** includes pain from capsular distention (eg, liver enlargement from metastases, colicky pain from the colon, etc). Depending on where a metastasis or primary tumor is located, it may cause somatic pain (eg, bone tumors), neuropathic pain (eg, Pancoast tumor), visceral pain, or **headache pain from increased intracranial pressure**.

 HELPFUL TIP: Avoid using meperidine (Demerol). It has toxic metabolites that may cause agitation and seizures. Meperidine can also interact with a number of drugs to cause serotonin syndrome.

* *

You add celecoxib (Celebrex), but she develops epigastric pain and discontinues the medication herself (Hah, told you so . . .). You decide to increase her morphine dose.

Which of the following statements is true?

A) IV morphine is 10–20 times more potent than is oral morphine.
B) Naloxone should be given when patients near death demonstrate confusion, decreased responsiveness, a slowed respiratory rate, and cool extremities.
C) Patients exhibiting a local rash or intense pruritis at the site of morphine administration must be given an alternate narcotic.
D) Tolerance to morphine does not occur in patients with terminal illness so any increased analgesic need is due solely to unmet pain.
E) Renal and hepatic insufficiency both contribute to the accumulation of morphine and its metabolites.

Discussion
The correct answer is E. Patients with renal and hepatic insufficiency can accumulate metabolites of morphine, some of which are helpful in pain control and others which may have an anti-analgesic effect. Answer A is incorrect because intravenous morphine is 3–5 times as potent as oral morphine. Answer B is incorrect. Patients who are within several days or hours of death often exhibit pallor, peripheral vasoconstriction, apneic episodes, and obtundation as part of the

physiologic process of dying. Counseling the family and the dying patient is preferable to administering naloxone—an unnecessary pharmacologic intervention that may result in more harm than good. Answer C is incorrect. Local histamine release is a known effect of IV morphine administration. Histamine-mediated skin changes proximal to the IV infusion site of morphine do not represent a contraindication to future morphine use. Diphenhydramine can be used to counter morphine-related histamine effects, such as rash, itching, and hypotension. Answer D is incorrect. Patients do develop tolerance to the effects of morphine.

 HELPFUL TIP: "The hand that writes the narcotic writes the laxative." Start patients on a regimen to prevent constipation when initiating narcotics. Think about the bowel regimen each time you increase the narcotic dose. It will save you and them a lot of grief in the long run.

 HELPFUL TIP: Methylnaltrexone is a narcotic antagonist that has recently been approved for the treatment of narcotic induced constipation in palliative care patients.

Which of the following statements is NOT true regarding the appropriate use of narcotics in end-of-life situations?

A) Delirium can be improved with narcotic dosage reduction and/or the addition of narcotic-sparing analgesics (eg, acetaminophen).
B) If oral morphine cannot be swallowed, a parenteral route must be used.
C) Dosage conversion from one narcotic to another is affected by the type of narcotic used and the route of administration.
D) Transdermal narcotic delivery products are expensive, have a slow onset of action, and have erratic absorption.
E) There is no preestablished ceiling dosage for narcotics, and you may increase the narcotic dose until adverse side effects occur.

Discussion
The correct answer is B. Concentrated oral morphine solutions have sufficient bioavailability across the buccal mucosa that makes swallowing unnecessary for delivery.

Therefore, parenteral routes of administration are unnecessary in most cases. Answer A is true. Delirium is a common and disturbing finding toward the end-of-life, and it can be precipitated or exaggerated by narcotics. On the flip side, untreated pain can also cause delirium and in these patients the delirium improves when narcotic doses are escalated. Acetaminophen is the safest narcotic-sparing analgesic, and its adjuvant action **may** allow for narcotic dosage reduction without a loss of overall analgesia. In the appropriate patient, NSAIDs may also be used. Answer C is true. When a patient who is chronically taking one narcotic switches to another, a dose adjustment calculation must be made. You cannot switch milligram for milligram. Also, some authorities recommend that after the calculation, you slightly reduce the dose of the new narcotic due to tolerance to the previous narcotic. (Refer to narcotic dose conversion charts available in pharmaceutical texts and handbooks.) Answer D is true. Transdermal fentanyl patches, though convenient, have fluctuating bioavailability over the 3 days that each patch is worn, and doses of an alternative narcotic for breakthrough pain should be available. The fentanyl patches are expensive and have a slow onset of action so that fentanyl patches should never be used alone as an initial treatment for acute pain. Answer E is true. Because of the extraordinarily wide dosage range of narcotics, the ceiling dosage cannot be calculated or assumed. Rather, analgesic requirements allow for continual increase unless adverse side effects clearly undermine the use of the drug.

 HELPFUL TIP: There is no consistent relationship between blood levels of morphine and analgesic effects. This is because of tolerance, individual variability in drug effect, etc. Thus, there is no single "right" dose. You should titrate morphine to the desired effect while watching for side effects.

* *

You increase the morphine dose considerably over a 2-week period but your patient continues to have crampy abdominal pain. A colleague suggests you try adding another medication to the currently scheduled morphine.

You choose which of the following drugs?

A) Nalbuphine (Nubain).
B) Methadone.
C) Butorphanol (Stadol).
D) Fentanyl patch (Duragesic).

Discussion

The correct answer is B. Methadone is a potent opioid and may help reduce the tolerance to other narcotics. Answers A and C are incorrect and should not be used in combination with chronic narcotics. Nalbuphine is a partial opioid agonist, and butorphanol is an opioid agonist/antagonist. Answer D is incorrect. Fentanyl is less desirable than methadone because a fentanyl patch still has the same opioid receptor antagonistic effects at high doses as morphine and is much more expensive.

 HELPFUL TIP: Because methadone also interacts at the NMDA receptors, it is the narcotic of choice when treating neuropathic pain, which often responds poorly to other narcotics.

* *

You decide to add methadone.

Which of the following statements is FALSE regarding the use of methadone?

A) Methadone can be legally prescribed for pain and addiction by a physician with a current Schedule II DEA license.
B) Methadone is more easily absorbed by those with bowel problems than is sustained-release morphine.
C) The half-life of methadone is 22 hours.
D) Methadone may be useful for neuropathic pain because it inhibits receptors in the dorsal horn of the spine.
E) Methadone is primarily excreted in the stool and thus drug dosages do not need to be modified in those with mild to moderate renal disease.

Discussion

The correct answer is A. Methadone **can** be prescribed for pain control by physicians with a schedule II DEA license but **cannot** be prescribed for opiate withdrawal or maintenance without a special license. The other answer choices are true statements. Because it has such a long half-life, sustained-release preparations are unnecessary. Sustained-release morphine may pass unabsorbed in patients with a short or dysfunctional gut, whereas methadone would be absorbed. Methadone is primarily excreted into the gastrointestinal tract. Patients with liver disease should have doses adjusted. However, those with renal disease may tolerate "normal" doses since renal excretion is a minor part of methadone's elimination.

 HELPFUL TIP: Methadone is difficult to titrate because of the long half-life. Thus, the patient may need both methadone and morphine to be used for breakthrough pain while you get the dose of methadone correct. Methadone is dosed q8h for pain relief, not q12h or QD as when used for narcotic withdrawal. Remember that methadone can cause torsade de pointes.

Which of the following statements is true regarding the use of the fentanyl patch?

A) The fentanyl patch is not as effective on the skin of cachectic patients because of lack of subcutaneous fat.

B) The fentanyl patch can be titrated upward in dosage every 24 hours in patients with escalating pain.

C) Due to delayed onset of the fentanyl patch alternate analgesia must be provided for 12–23 hours after first application.

D) Fentanyl will continue to be absorbed from subcutaneous tissue into the blood for up to 4 hours after patch removal.

Discussion
The correct answer is C. A previously administered opioid should not be discontinued immediately upon placing the first fentanyl patch. Answer A is incorrect because there is no evidence to support that a certain amount of subcutaneous fat is necessary. Answer B is incorrect because the delayed action of the patch requires that dosage adjustment occur every 48–72 hours. Answer D is incorrect because fentanyl continues to be delivered up to 12 hours after patch removal.

 HELPFUL TIP: The published conversion data from morphine to fentanyl patch is broad and often leads to underdosing (eg, 135–224 mg of morphine = 50 mcg patch in the PDR). We suggest using approximately 2 mg oral morphine/24 hour to 1 microgram fentanyl patch. Thus a patient requiring 140 mg of oral morphine every day should be switched to a 75 microgram fentanyl patch.

* *

As time goes on, the patient has other concerns including constipation, weight loss of 20 pounds over 2 months, sleeplessness, nausea, and anxiety. In addition she expresses how her loss of functional abilities is a hardship for her and her adult daughter who serves as her primary caregiver. Her guilt over losing her health is a continual source of frustration and anger.

What is true regarding her social and emotional pain?

A) It will not affect the patient's analgesic requirements.

B) It will likely complicate treatment compliance.

C) Active treatment of emotional sources of pain should occur after the physical source has been addressed and treated.

D) Prophylactic antidepressants in patients within 6 months of death decrease the probability of developing depression.

Discussion
The correct answer is B. Compliance, always an issue, is especially compromised in those dying patients whose social, spiritual, and emotional problems are not effectively addressed. Similarly, analgesic control of somatic pain is complicated when social, emotional, and spiritual sources of pain exacerbate the patient's response and perception to her somatic pain. Concurrent treatment of all sources of pain is necessary. Antidepressant therapy in dying patients who do not have clinical depression offers no prophylaxis against the development of depression.

* *

You estimate your patient's life expectancy to be ≤2 months. Her frailty has progressed to the point where she is bedbound and utterly dependent for all her activities of daily living. You have made some adjustments, and she is now taking the following medications:

Hydromorphone (Dilaudid) 20 mg PO Q 4 hours

Acetaminophen 1000 mg PO TID

Sorbitol 30 cc PO TID

Metoclopramide 20 mg PO TID

* *

She is comfortable on these doses of drugs but continues to need morphine for breakthrough pain.

Which of the following is the most appropriate medication adjustment to make at this time?

A) Hydromorphone → scheduled **controlled**-release morphine.

B) Hydromorphone → scheduled **immediate**-release morphine.

C) Hydromorphone → scheduled controlled-release morphine and immediate-release morphine PRN.

D) Acetaminophen → immediate-release morphine.

E) Acetaminophen → nortriptyline.

Discussion

The correct answer is C. A patient who has reached a stable dose of short-acting narcotic, such as hydromorphone, should subsequently be switched to a long-acting narcotic agent. An immediate-release medication should be available for acute or breakthrough pain. There is no reason to change the acetaminophen. Nortriptyline is sometimes useful as an adjuvant medication and is particularly helpful when treating neuropathic pain, but it would be additional rather than a substitute for acetaminophen.

* *

The hospice nurse calls you. Your patient is at home and has become restless with slow respirations (6/minute) along with paroxysmal coughing and gagging with a large amount of secretions.

The following are all appropriate orders for this patient EXCEPT:

A) A subcutaneous infusion pump and syringe to provide medications and, if necessary, fluids.

B) Lorazepam 1–2 mg PO or SL Q 1 hour PRN.

C) Scopolamine transdermal patches changed every 3 days.

D) Midazolam 0.4–4 mg subcutaneously (SC) Q 1 hour PRN.

E) Naloxone 2 mg SC Q 2 hours PRN.

Discussion

The correct answer is E. Naloxone is a potent opioid receptor antagonist. Although the sudden change in the patient's status could be partly due to narcotic accumulation, the risks of naloxone antagonism are significant and include severe pain, cardiac arrhythmias, and seizures. Holding or reducing the next dose of opioids is a safer approach. Answer A is correct. A subcutaneous infusion pump may allow effective administration of medications and fluids in patients who cannot tolerate oral administration. The use of hydration at the end-of-life is debatable. Withholding of fluids and nutrition has strong merit, but the evidence is not compelling enough to declare that fluid infusion is futile or possibly harmful in this setting. In addition, dehydration is a common cause of delirium at the end-of-life and her confusion may improve with gentle hydration. It is more important to review the patient's goals and only administer fluids if that is consistent with her goals. Answer C is correct. Scopolamine patches have been shown to decrease oral/pulmonary secretions that lead to the "death rattle" in the final days and hours of life. Such treatment benefits the patient and her grieving family and friends. Answers B and D are correct. They may also be useful. Benzodiazepines have the potential to reduce anxiety, agitation, and insomnia; however, any benzodiazepine can worsen confusion and cause delirium. In addition, benzodiazepines with an extended half-life (eg, diazepam, chlordiazepoxide) should be avoided due to the potential for toxic accumulation.

Objectives: Did you learn to . . .

- Define major physiologic pain categories?
- Describe the pharmacology of pain control?
- Prescribe narcotic pain medications and adjuvant therapies?
- Identify emotional, social, and spiritual symptoms and recognize how they can affect pain management?

QUICK QUIZ: THE SUBCUTANEOUS ROUTE

Regarding the subcutaneous administration of fluids and medications, which of the following statements is TRUE?

A) Not >500 cc of saline per day can be given by hypodermoclysis (subcutaneous administration).

B) Only medication with low lipid solubility can be delivered via subcutaneous administration.

C) Subcutaneous administration is preferred to IV administration in many cases, especially if the patient deems the IV too invasive.

D) In general, subcutaneous administration dosage conversion is closer to oral dosage than to IV dosage.

Discussion

The correct answer is C. There is ample evidence to support the use of the subcutaneous route. Adverse events such as local irritation, pulmonary edema, and local edema are the same or fewer with subcutaneous administration as compared to intravenous administration. In general, most drugs used in end-of-life care can be given subcutaneously. Answer A is incorrect. Evidence demonstrates that up to 1,500 cc of crystalloid solution can be given subcutaneously in a 24-hour period with limited adverse effects. Experience suggests that even greater volumes can be given. Answer B is incorrect. Lipid solubility is not a clinically relevant aspect of bioavailability during subcutaneous administration. Answer D is incorrect. Subcutaneous doses are, generally, very close to the IV dose of a drug. As with IV administration, the onset of action is more rapid than with enteral dosing.

CASE 3

You assume care for the 84-year-old father of one of your patients. The father has severe dementia, suspected to be caused by Alzheimer disease and cerebrovascular disease. You visit him in the nursing home where he has resided for 5 years. His last Folstein Mini-Mental Status Examination was 18 out of 30 2 years ago when the nurses say he was much more functional. He is largely bedbound but can be placed into a sitting position for eating in the "full assistance" dining room. He is fully incontinent and makes repetitive poorly intelligible utterances. He has two stage 2 pressure ulcers and carries the diagnoses of congestive heart failure, coronary artery disease, and a number of other medical conditions, none of which has resulted in any clear decompensation during his 5 years in the facility. He has lost 20 lbs in the last 6 months (BMI now is 21 kg/m^2).

What would be the best recommendation for weight gain in this patient?

A) Megestrol.
B) Nutritional supplements (eg Ensure milkshakes).
C) Dronabinol.
D) Sertraline.
E) Feeding tube.

Discussion

The correct answer is B. The most effective means to maintain weight in elderly patients with dementia is hand feeding, which is expensive and often problematic in nursing homes with limited staff. When hand feeding is not effective, nutritional supplements are the least invasive alternative and are modestly effective in promoting weight gain in elderly patients with dementia. However, remember that weight gain does not affect the rate of cognitive decline and will not improve his dementia or his overall prognosis. Answer D is incorrect because sertraline is not an appetite stimulant. SSRIs like sertraline are associated with weight loss. Answers A and C have been used as appetite stimulants with limited degrees of success. Megestrol (Megace) is minimally effective in improving appetite and increasing weight in patients with cancer cachexia and weight loss related to AIDS, but there is limited evidence that it is effective in geriatric patients. Dronabinol is one of the active ingredient in marijuana. It increases appetite and improves nausea, but again the studies are small and exploratory in nature and focused mainly on patients with AIDS and cancer. Answer E is incorrect. A feeding tube is invasive with a number of side effects, and although it may improve caloric intake it does not necessarily extend life, increase weight, or reduce the incidence of pressure ulcers or aspiration.

* *

The nursing staff asks you if the patient is appropriate for hospice care.

What is your response?

A) "The life trajectory of terminally demented patients is unclear. If his cardiac disease decompensates, then I'll make the referral."
B) "Good idea, but he does not meet Medicare Hospice Benefit criteria because he needs to lose more weight."
C) "You bet. The history of steep functional decline is the best predictor of death, and he is declining by many measures."

D) "You all (the nursing home staff) can provide end-of-life services without hospice."

E) "No dice. Pressure ulcers result from poor nursing care, not dementia, and are never a reason for referral to hospice."

Discussion

The correct answer is C. Predicting death in patients with dementing illness is difficult, which is why it is one of most underutilized diagnoses for referral to hospice care. But the extrapolation of the patient's loss of basic functions over time seems to best predict death. To wait until a more predictable organ system failure occurs (eg, heart failure) is not an appropriate method for making a referral to hospice and results in unnecessary delay in hospice care, so answer A is incorrect. Answer B is incorrect because the policy for reimbursement under the Medicare Hospice Benefit has broadened to include unexplained weight loss in the context of a terminal condition, including dementia. Answer D is incorrect because most nursing homes welcome the additional support afforded by hospice referral. Answer E is incorrect for two reasons. First, the nurses should not be blamed for all pressure ulcers. Patients with terminal dementia are at high risk for pressure ulcers due to malnutrition, incontinence, immobility, and inability to interpret sensory input. Also, the presence of stage 3 or 4 pressure ulcers, which suggest a loss of the patient's self-protective mechanism, correlate with impending death and are included in the current Medicare Hospice Benefit policy. However, this patient has a stage 2 ulcer, so he is not quite there yet. He qualifies on other grounds: decline of function and weight loss in the setting of terminal dementia.

* *

The patient is enrolled in hospice, and 3 months later you are called by the nursing home because of an acute condition change. When you see the patient, he is unresponsive, with labored breathing and mottled feet.

All of the following can be signs of impending death EXCEPT:

A) Cheyne-Stokes breathing.
B) Fever.
C) Cyanosis and mottling.
D) Increased urine output.
E) Talking to someone who is already dead ("Mother, I can see you . . .").

Discussion

The correct answer is D. Most dying patients have a **decrease** in urinary output prior to death. The other answer choices describe changes that are commonly seen in patients who are actively dying. Respiratory changes that occur when a patient is actively dying include Cheyne-Stokes breathing, terminal secretions (death rattle), and periods of apnea. Dying is often accompanied by decreased circulation, resulting in cool extremities and mottling. It is not uncommon for a dying patient to have a fever in the last 24–48 hours of life, typically thought to be secondary to aspiration pneumonia or urosepsis. It is not uncommon for someone who is dying to talk about going on a journey or talk about seeing someone who is dead. This is typically believed to be part of the normal dying process and in the absence of other symptoms should not be confused with delirium.

 HELPFUL TIP: Delirium is very common (up to 85%) in the last few days of life. If the symptoms are distressing to the patient or family, it is best treated with an antipsychotic such as haloperidol.

* *

You need to call the son to tell him of his father's decline.

Which of the following should you say when giving the son an update?

A) "There have been some changes in your father's condition. I think you should go and see him. Call me if you have any questions."

B) "Good news, your dad will soon be out of his misery and released from this mortal coil."

C) "I'm afraid I have some bad news for you regarding your dad. Would you like to talk over the phone or meet at my office later today to discuss it?"

D) "Your dad is dying. If you want to see him alive, you had better go today."

E) Don't call at all. Ask the nurse to inform the son of his father's condition.

Discussion

The correct answer is C. This statement gives a warning shot and allows the person who will receive the bad news some control by allowing him to determine how and where he wants to receive the bad news. Answer A avoids giving the bad news at all. Answer B is flippant, lacks compassion, and uses euphemisms. Answer D is inappropriately blunt. Answer E avoids having the discussion at all and is appropriate only if you will be unable to reach the son in a timely fashion. A common format for giving bad news is the SPIKES six-step protocol (Table 27–1).

Table 27–1 SPIKES SIX-STEP PROTOCOL FOR GIVING BAD NEWS

S Setting. An inappropriate setting can make it difficult to give bad news effectively. Make sure the physical setting is as conducive as possible by trying to ensure privacy, involving significant others, sitting down, connecting with the patient (eye contact, hand holding), ensuring enough time, and minimizing interruptions.

P Patient's perception. Ask about the patient and/or family's knowledge and understanding of the current medical illness.

I Invitation. Ask what information the patient wants to receive. Some patients do not want to hear bad news themselves; in this case, the patient may want you talk to family or friends first.

K Knowledge. Give the medical facts in a straightforward manner using vocabulary and language appropriate to the patient's level. Avoid medical jargon and do not be excessively blunt (ie, avoid saying things such as, "You have very bad cancer and unless you do something you will die."). Give the information in small chunks and frequently assess what the patient has understood. When possible start off with a warning shot (eg, "Unfortunately, I have some bad news for you.").

E Exploring/empathy/emotion. A patient's emotional reaction can vary and is often hard for a physician to experience. An empathetic response can be helpful. This can be fostered by allowing silence after breaking the bad news and watching and listening for the emotion. When you have identified the emotion it can be helpful to name it and determine what caused it. Then make an empathetic statement such as, "I'm sorry. I know this isn't what you wanted to hear."

S Strategy/summary. After the emotions have been addressed, it is helpful to review what has been said and agree on a plan. Consider asking the patient if he wants to discuss treatment options at this time or wait until a future meeting. Receiving bad news can be overwhelming and patients often forget the details of what is said. It is important to have clear, well defined, timely follow-up such as, "Go home and talk with your family. I will see you (and family) back tomorrow, and we can discuss specific treatment options and answer your questions at that time."

 HELPFUL TIP: Do not use phrases such as, "I'm afraid there is nothing more we can do for you." This leaves patients and family feeling abandoned. It is better to be specific, such as, "I am afraid that I don't have any treatments that will cure your cancer but there is still a lot I can offer to help to keep you comfortable in the time you have left." This assures the patient and family that there is still something to be done and that you will not abandon them.

* *

Breaking bad news is difficult in person and even more difficult over the phone.

Which of the following suggestion is NOT recommended when breaking bad news over the phone?

A) Take time to prepare what you are going to say and find a quiet place to make the call.
B) If no one answers the phone, it is acceptable to leave a message detailing the bad news.
C) Identify yourself and avoid answering any direct questions until you are sure of the identity of the person you are talking to.
D) Ask if the person is alone.
E) Speak clearly and slowly, allow time for questions; be empathetic.

Discussion
The correct answer is B. When breaking bad news over the phone, use steps similar to breaking bad news in person (SPIKES protocol).

Obtain the full name, address, and phone number(s) of the person/s you are calling. Write down the key information you need and review what you will say and find a quiet or private area with a phone. Don't delay in making the call. When you call, clearly identify yourself and confirm you are able to speak with the patient or the person closest to the patient (ideally, the health-care proxy or the contact person indicated in the chart). Avoid responding to any direct question until you have verified the identity of the person with whom you are speaking. Ask if the contact person is alone. Do not give death notification to young children. If you do not have a prior relationship with the person to whom you are speaking, ask what they know about the patient's condition. Allow time for questions; be empathetic and ask if you can contact anyone for them. Assess their emotional reaction and follow up as indicated. Never deliver the news of a dire diagnosis or death in the form of voice mail. Instead, leave specific contact information.

> **HELPFUL TIP:** When you need to inform a family that a patient has died use words such as "dead" or "died." Avoid euphemisms such as "expired," "passed away," or "didn't make it" which can be misinterpreted.

Objectives: Did you learn to . . .

- Generate a management plan for a patient with weight loss due to a terminal disease?
- Identify potentially reversible causes of nausea and vomiting?
- Describe the proper steps for breaking bad news?

QUICK QUIZ: NAUSEA

A patient has advanced ovarian carcinoma with ascites and enterocolonic fistulae. She is nauseated but has no symptoms or signs of bowel obstruction. You suspect that the nausea is caused by the patient's underlying disease.

Which of the following drugs is the best initial choice for treatment of this patient's nausea?

A) Octreotide.
B) Metoclopramide.
C) Diphenhydramine.
D) Ondansetron (Zofran).
E) Aprepitant (Emend).

Discussion

The correct answer is B. For idiopathic, intractable nausea and vomiting in terminally ill patients, start with an antiemetic that has antidopaminergic action. Metoclopramide is convenient because it can be given orally, IV, IM, or subcutaneously. Also, metoclopramide has central and peripheral anti-dopaminergic properties and is the best first agent for nausea secondary to presumed GI dysmotility. Haloperidol, prochlorperazine, or

chlorpromazine could be used as well but are more appropriate agents for nausea due to chemotoxicity (haloperidol and prochlorperazine) or inflammation (chlorpromazine). Answer A is incorrect. Octreotide works by slowing the gastrointestinal tract, and its main use is found in patients with nausea and vomiting due to malignancy-related intestinal obstruction. Answer C is incorrect because diphenhydramine alone is a weak antiemetic, used mostly for motion sickness. Although the drugs may help, answers D and E should not be your first choice. Ondansetron, which is now generic and much less expensive than it once was, is a serotonin receptor ($5-HT_3$) antagonist and finds its primary application in treating nausea due to chemotherapy or radiation, but it is effective for other types of nausea. Aprepitant is a neurokinin-1 (NK1) receptor antagonist that is most effective when used with a serotonin receptor antagonist (eg, ondansetron and others) and a corticosteroid to prevent chemotherapy-induced nausea. Aprepitant should not be used alone and is very expensive.

> **HELPFUL TIP:** The combination of metoclopramide and a corticosteroid can be very effective. Lorazepam is also often effective for nausea. Remember that elderly and demented patients may become agitated with metoclopramide administration. Also, extrapyramidal side effects can occur with a frequency that is dose-dependent.

BIBLIOGRAPHY

Baile et al. SPIKES: a six-step protocol for delivering bad news: application to the patient with cancer. *Oncologist.* 2000;5(4):302.

Cervo FA, et al. To PEG or not to PEG: a review of evidence for placing feeding tubes in advanced dementia and the decision-making process. *Geriatrics.* 2006 Jun;61(6):30.

Donner B, et al. Direct conversion from oral morphine to transdermal fentanyl. *Pain.* 1996;64:527.

Faxén-Irving G, et al. The effect of nutritional intervention in elderly subjects residing in group-living for the demented. *Eur J Clin Nutr.* 2002 Mar;56(3):221.

Jacox A, Carr DB, Payne R, et al. Management of Cancer Pain. Clinical Practice Guideline No. 9. AHCPR Publication N. 94-0592. 1994:8.

Medical Guidelines for Determining Prognosis in Selected Non-cancer Diseases. 2nd ed. Arlington, VA: National Hospice Organization, 1996.

Reuben DB, et al. The effects of megestrol acetate suspension for elderly patients with reduced appetite after hospitalization: a phase II randomized clinical trial. *J Am Geriatr Soc.* 2005;53(6):970.

Schonwetter RS. *Hospice/Palliative Care Training for Physicians; A Self-Study Program.* American Academy of Hospice and Palliative Care Medicine, 1998.

Schonwetter R. Hospice and Palliative Medicine: Core Curriculum and Review Syllabus. 1999:7.

Storey P, et al. *Hospice and Palliative Medicine; Core Curriculum and Review Syllabus.* American Academy of Hospice and Palliative Care Medicine, 1998.

Vandekieft G: Breaking bad news. *Am Fam Physician.* 2001;64(12).

www.cancer.gov/cancerinfo/pdq/supportivecare/pain/healthprofessional/.

www.eperc.mcw.edu/ff_index.htm.

28
Evidence-Based Medicine

Elizabeth C. Clark

INTRODUCTION

Disclaimer: The first vignette is not medical and is meant to help you think about principles and equations employed in evidence-based medicine. If you must, consider "cell phone reception" a disease. Read on; you'll see what we mean.

All of the numbers in this chapter are figments of our imaginations and have no basis in reality. The numbers are used for instruction only and should not be assumed accurate for a given disease. Table 28–1 is here for reference. You may want refer to it as you work your way through the chapter.

CASE 1

A new technology has been developed that can tell whether a cell phone will have reception in a given area with a given carrier. It is known as the "reception-o-meter." Needless to say, the cell phone companies are trying hard to suppress this new technology. In comparison with the gold standard of turning on your cell phone and checking whether you have reception or not, the new test has a sensitivity of 90% and a specificity of 95% for all carriers.

Based on this information, what is the likelihood that your cell phone will have reception if the test says you will for a given carrier?

A) 90%
B) 95%
C) 93%

D) 82%
E) There is not enough information to make this calculation.

Discussion

The correct answer is E. If you tried to answer this question and found that you couldn't, good for you! As you discovered, you are missing one important piece of data. In order to answer this question you need to know the positive predictive value (PPV) of the test, and in order to calculate the PPV, you need 3 pieces of data: the sensitivity of the test, the specificity of the test, and the prevalence of the condition, which in this case is the prevalence of having cell phone reception (in other words, the true amount of cell phone reception in a given area).

CASE 2

You are currently in Los Angeles attending a CME course where the reception for carrier X is 99%. You check your "reception-o-meter" and it says you have coverage.

What is the likelihood that your cell phone actually will have reception if you try to make a call?

A) 99.9%
B) 99%
C) 98%
D) 95%
E) None of the above.

Table 28–1 USEFUL EQUATIONS

Sensitivity: True Positives/(true positives + false negatives)

Specificity: True Negatives/(true negatives + false positives)

False-positive Rate: 1 – specificity

False-negative Rate: 1 – sensitivity

Positive Predictive Value: True Positive/(true positive + false positive)

Negative Predictive Value: True Negative/(true negative + false negative)

Discussion

The correct answer is A. In order to answer this question, you can use Bayes theorem or set up 2×2 tables. We're fans of the 2×2 table because we hate having to memorize equations and we can reason through a 2×2 table if we remember a few simple rules about how they work. See Table 28–2.

Here's the 2×2 table method. Begin by drawing a 2×2 table and fill in what you know. To set this up correctly, you have to remember the following equations:

$$\text{Sensitivity} = a/(a + c)$$
$$\text{Specificity} = d/(b + d)$$
$$\text{Positive predictive value (PPV)} = a/(a + b)$$
$$\text{Negative predictive value (NPV)} = d/(c + d)$$

You also have to remember how to include population prevalence in the table.

Now we add the real numbers to the table. Here's what it looks like before (left side) and after (right side) adding the population prevalence (Table 28–3).

Sometimes people get confused about how population prevalence is shown in the table. On the left side, it is easy to see how the sensitivity and specificity fit in the table. Remember that we are using 90% sensitivity

and 95% specificity. If we assume an equal number of people have reception and an equal number do not (100 each are nice, round numbers, selected randomly), we multiply by the sensitivity to get the total in cell "a" and subtract "a" from the total population with reception to get the total for cell "c." We then also multiply by the specificity to get the total in cell "d" and subtract "d" from the total population without reception to get the total for cell "b."

To convert to a 99% prevalence (as we have for carrier X in this question) we start with a larger baseline population, as shown on the right side (10,000 is often plenty, and, yes, this number is also selected randomly and for ease), and we multiply by the prevalence to get the sub-population totals (99% prevalence × 10,000 = 9,900 with reception; 1% × 10,000 = 100 without reception). Once we have the subpopulation totals, then we multiply by the sensitivity and the specificity to get the exact cell numbers as we did in the left side (9900 × 90% sensitivity = 8910 for cell a, 9900–8910 = 990 for cell c (or alternately 9910 × 10% will get the same result for cell c); 100 × 95% specificity = 95 for cell d; 100 – 95 = 5 for cell b).

Once the table is filled in, these numbers can then be used to calculate the PPV, using the equation above. In this case,

$$a/(a + b) = 8910/8915 = 99.9\%$$

For those who prefer the Bayes theorem method, here is how this approach is done. Bayes theorem shows the relationships between sensitivity, specificity, prevalence, positive predictive value, and negative predictive value. The equation for PPV, derived from Bayes theorem, is shown, as is the calculation based on the numbers from the question. Number of True Positives

$$PPV = \frac{\text{Number of True Positives}}{\text{Number of True Positives + Number of False Positives}}$$

$$PPV = \frac{\text{Sensitivity} \times \text{prevalence}}{(\text{Sensitivity} \times \text{prevalence}) + [(1 - \text{specificity}) \times (1 - \text{prevalence})]}$$

$$= \frac{0.9 \times 0.99}{(0.9 \times 0.99) + [0.05 \times 0.01]} = 99.9\%$$

What is the likelihood of not having coverage if the reception-o-meter indicated that you did not have coverage?

Table 28–2 SAMPLE 2 × 2 TABLE

Test	Disease	
	+	–
+	A (true positive)	B (false positive)
–	C (false negative)	D (true negative)
Total	A + C	B + D

Table 28–3   TELEPHONE SERVICE AVAILABILITY BASED ON THE RECEPTION-O-METER

Before Adding Actual Prevalence					After Adding Actual Prevalence				
		Actual Reception					Actual Reception		
		+	–				+	–	
Test	+	90	5		Test	+	8910	5	
Reception	–	10	95		Reception	–	990	95	
Total		100	100		Total		9900	100	
		(50% prevalence)					(99% prevalence)		

A) 95%
B) 90%
C) 50%
D) 9%
E) None of the above.

Discussion

The correct answer is D. The question asks for the negative predictive value (NPV)—the likelihood of not having coverage if the reception-o-meter is negative. This also can be derived from Bayes theorem or calculated using a 2×2 table. For those of you who prefer the Bayes theorem method, the equation for NPV, derived from Bayes theorem, is shown, as is the calculation based on the numbers from the question.

$$NPV = \frac{\text{Number of true negatives}}{\text{Number of true negatives} + \text{number of false negatives}}$$

$$NPV = \frac{\text{Specificity} \times (1 - \text{prevalence})}{[\text{Specificity} \times (1 - \text{prevalence})] + (1 - \text{sensitivity})}$$

$$= \frac{0.95 \times 0.01}{(0.95 \times 0.01) + 0.10} = 8.7\% \text{ (which rounds to 9\%).}$$

For the 2×2 table method, begin by drawing a 2×2 table and fill in what you know. For this question, the table is identical to the table for the previous question. The numbers can be used to calculate the NPV, using the equation

$$d/(d + c), \text{ or } 95/(95 + 990) = 8.7\%$$

Although it takes a little time to set up the table, once you have the table, you can use it to calculate other values as well.

CASE 3

You are in rural Russia where you were invited to help with a community effort to fight multidrug-resistant TB. Here cell phone reception is 10% for Carrier Y. You check your reception-o-meter and it says you have reception.

What is the likelihood that your cell phone will have reception if you try to make a call?

A) 91%
B) 83%
C) 67%
D) 16%
E) None of the above.

Discussion

The correct answer is C. You can use the 2×2 method or the Bayes theorem methods Here's what our 2×2 table looks like (Table 28–4).

To convert to 10% prevalence, start with a large baseline population and multiply by the prevalence to get the subpopulation totals (10% prevalence × 10,000 = 1,000 with reception; 90% × 10,000 = 9000 without reception). Once you have the subpopulation totals, multiply by the sensitivity and the specificity to get the exact cell numbers: 1,000 × 90% sensitivity = 900 for cell a; 1000 – 900 = 100 for cell c (or alternately 1,000 × 10% will get the same result for cell c); 9,000 × 95% specificity = 8,550 for cell d; 9000 – 8550 = 450 for cell b.

Table 28–4   2 × 2 TABLE OF TELEPHONE RECEPTION IN RURAL RUSSIA

Before Adding Actual Prevalence				After Adding Actual Prevalence			
		Actual Reception				Actual Reception	
		+	−			+	−
Test	+	90	5	Test	+	900	450
Reception	−	10	95	Reception	−	100	8550
Total		100	100	Total		1000	9000
		(50% prevalence)				(10% prevalence)	

These numbers can then be used to calculate the PPV, using the equation above. In this case, the equation is

$a/(a + b) = 900/(900 + 450) = 66.7\%$ (rounds to 67%).

Using Bayes theorem, the equation is as follows.

$$PPV = \frac{(\text{Sensitivity} \times \text{prevalence})}{(\text{Sensitivity} \times \text{prevalence}) + [(1 - \text{specificity}) \times (1 - \text{prevalence})]}$$

$$= \frac{0.9 \times 0.1}{(0.9 \times 0.1) + [0.05 \times 0.9]} = 66.7\%$$

What is the likelihood of having coverage if the reception-o-meter said you did not have coverage?

A) 50%
B) 40%
C) 30%
D) 1%
E) None of the above.

Discussion

The correct answer is D. Again, you can use the 2×2 method or Bayes theorem. The 2×2 table for this question is the same as it was for the previous question. However, unlike previously, you are asked for the likelihood of reception if the reception-o-meter said there was no reception. In other words, you have been asked to calculate the false-negative rate (FNR) for this scenario. The equation for the FNR is below.

$$FNR = \frac{\text{False negatives}}{\text{False negatives} + \text{true negatives}} \text{ or } \frac{c}{c + d} = \frac{100}{100 + 8550} = 1\%$$

You were not asked to calculate it, but there is also a false-positive rate (FPR), which is shown below.

$$FPR = \frac{\text{False positives}}{\text{False positives} + \text{true positives}} \text{ or } \frac{b}{a + b} = \frac{450}{450 + 900} = 33\%$$

CASE 4

Research published in a well-respected medical journal looked at screening for lung cancer using a new method. The researchers reported that patients who were screened and had lung cancer detected lived longer after diagnosis than people who were not screened.

Which is true?

A) This shows that screening is effective in prolonging survival.
B) This may be an example of lead-time bias.
C) This may be an example of verification bias.
D) Well-respected medical journals (and board review books) are always right.

Discussion

The correct answer is B. This may be an example of lead-time bias. Screening is intended to diagnose disease earlier than without screening, hopefully allowing for interventions that prevent or slow the progression of the disease. Without screening, the disease may be discovered only after symptoms develop when it may be too late to intervene. Screening, however, can also give the appearance of longer survival, even though in reality no additional life has been gained. Here's an example. Mr. X has the test, is diagnosed with disease, receives treatment, and dies 5 years later. Mr. Y is in

Table 28–5   COMMON TYPES OF BIAS

Bias Type	Effect
Selection bias	Occurs when subjects selected for the study do not represent the population. This is avoided by having large, representative samples.
Confounding bias	Occurs when two or more factors are associated with the outcome and only the one being studied is accounted for (eg, being a Cubs fan is associated with annoying behavior, but being a Cubs fan is also associated with public intoxication which is also associated with annoying behavior; therefore, if we don't account for the drunkenness—confounding variable—we may wrongly say being a Cubs fan *causes* annoying behavior).
Length time bias (**not** lead time)	Occurs because screening tests are more likely to find slow-growing tumors rather than those that are rapidly growing. This can bias results in favor of screening because more slow-growing cancers with a good prognosis will be found with a screening test.
Compliance bias	Occurs because study volunteers and persons who are willing to undergo screening tests are more likely to be compliant. Compliant patients have better outcomes.

the control group, develops symptoms, is diagnosed with disease, receives treatment, and dies 1 year later. Mr. X and Mr. Y both die at age 65 of the same disease. Did Mr. X have more survival time or just more "disease time"? This is called lead-time bias, and it may be avoided by using age-specific mortality rates rather than survival time from diagnosis. Answer C, verification bias, occurs when patients with a negative test are not evaluated with the gold standard test. See Table 28–5 for more types of bias found in studies.

CASE 5

As part of a quality control study, the hemoglobin A1c values of diabetic patients at two clinics are compared.

In a study of 4,000 patients, it is found that the mean hemoglobin A1c value in group 1 is 7.4% and the mean hemoglobin A1c value in group 2 is 7.6%. The authors did the correct statistical test and found a *P* value of 0.04 for this comparison.

Based on this information, you conclude:

A) Group 1 is significantly different from group 2: Reject the null hypothesis.
B) Group 1 is not significantly different from group 2: Don't reject the null hypothesis.
C) Group 1 is not significantly different from group 2: Reject the null hypothesis.
D) Group 1 is significantly different from group 2: Don't reject the null hypothesis.

Discussion

The correct answer is A. To answer this question, you have to know what the usual cutoff for significance is for a *P*-value, and you also have to know what a null hypothesis is. A null hypothesis is the hypothesis that there is not a significant difference between two groups being compared to each other. By setting up null hypotheses in this way we can then search for proof that the null hypothesis is incorrect. Tests of significance are a method of looking for proof that a null hypothesis is incorrect. The *P*-value gives you the probability that the results of the study occurred by chance alone. A *P* value of 0.04 means that if the study results were untrue, we would expect to see these results only 4% of the time (occurring as they did by chance). By convention, a *P* value of ≤0.05 is considered significant. Thus, when you have a *P* value of <0.05, you have evidence that the null hypothesis is false and can therefore reject it.

Objectives: Did you learn to . . .

- Describe sensitivity and specificity?
- Construct a 2×2 table and/or employ Bayes theorem?
- Calculate positive and negative predictive values?
- Calculate false-positive and false-negative rates?
- Recognize forms of bias in research studies?
- Define *P* value and null hypothesis?

CASE 6

Cervical cancer is a disease in which early detection can make a great difference in disease progression. One screening procedure for this disease is the Papanico-laou (Pap) smear. To assess the competency of technicians who read the Pap smear slides, a local lab checked their technician's work against patient records.

A total of 1,000 Pap smears were read. Of these, 100 patients had cervical abnormalities based on biopsy (gold standard). Of this group, 75 had abnormal (positive) Pap smears and 25 had negative Pap smears. There were 900 women without disease. Of these 900 women, 200 had positive Pap smears and 700 had negative Pap smears. **These numbers are for example only; they are not real data, and do not reflect the actual sensitivities and specificities of these tests.**

Using the data above, which of the following is true about this survey of Pap smear technicians?

A) False-negative rate is 20%.
B) False-positive rate is 15%.
C) The sensitivity of the Pap test is 75%.
D) The specificity of the Pap test is 98%.
E) The prevalence of cervical cancer in this sample is 7.5%.

Discussion

The correct answer is C. The sensitivity of the test is 75%. Setting up the data in a 2×2 table (Table 28-6), we are able to answer the question.

Sensitivity: Probability that a patient with the disease will have a positive result (eg, how many patients with the disease are misclassified as not having the disease).

Sensitivity = (TP/[TP + FN])= 75/100 = 0.75 or 75% sensitive.

Specificity: Probability that a patient without the disease will have a negative test (eg, how many patients without the disease are misclassified as having the disease).

Table 28–6   2×2 TABLE FOR PAP SMEARS AND CERVICAL DISEASE

Pap Test Result	Cervical Disease	No Cervical Disease
Positive	True Positive (TP) = 75	False Positive (FP) = 200
Negative	False Negative (FN) = 25	True Negative (TN) = 700
Total	TP + FN = 100	FP + TN = 900

Specificity = (TN/[FP + TN])= 700/900 = 0.777 or ~78% specific

False-Negative Rate: patient has the disease but the test is negative.

False-Negative Rate = (FN/(TP + FN)) = 25/100 = 25% false-negative rate; also calculated as 1– sensitivity

False-Positive Rate: the patient has a positive test but does not have the disease.

False-Positive Rate = (FP/(FP + TN)) = 200/900 = 0.22 or 22% false-positive; also calculated as 1– specificity

Prevalence of the disease: the proportion of individuals who have the disease at any time.

Prevalence = ([TP + FN]/Total Population) = 100/1000 = 10% or prevalence of 100 per 1,000 people

Given the above results of the Pap smear screening tests and if the prevalence of cervical abnormalities among women is 10%, then applying Bayes theorem, we find:

A) The positive predictive value is 27%.
B) The negative predictive value is 96%.
C) The positive predictive value is 0.999.
D) Unable to solve the problem with data provided.
E) A and B.

Discussion

The correct answer is E. The prevalence of a disease is the proportion of individuals who have the disease at a given point in time ([TP+FN]/ (Total Population) = 0.1 or 10%).

The **positive predictive value** of a test is **the probability that a disease exists given a positive test result** = TP/(TP + FP) or 75/275 = 27%. So, a patient with a positive test result has only a 27% chance of having the disease because there are so many false positives.

The **negative predictive value** of a test is the probability of no disease given a negative test result (TN/ [FN + TN]) = 700/725 = 96%. So, a patient with a negative test has a 96% chance of **not** having the disease. This is because there are few false negatives compared to the size of the overall population. If, for example, there were 200 false negatives in the same population the negative predictive value would only be 700/900 = 78%. This is because there are so many false negatives.

* *

Recall that 100 women out of 1,000 had positive biopsies and thus had the disease regardless of what the Pap test said.

How does the pretest probability of cervical abnormalities among women compare with the posttest probability?

A) Posttest probability is about 3 times greater than the pretest probability.
B) Pretest probability is 3 times greater than the posttest probability.
C) Posttest probability is 10 times greater.
D) Pretest probability is 10 times greater.
E) The pretest and posttest probabilities are equal.

Discussion

The correct answer is A. The pretest probability is given above as 100/1,000 or 10%. We know that 10% of the population has the disease.

The posttest probability is the positive predictive value. Remember from above the **positive predictive value** of a test is the probability that a disease exists given a positive test result: TP/(TP + FP) or 75/275 = 27%. Comparing the two results, pretest probability of 10% and posttest probability of 27%, we find that the posttest probability is about 3 times greater than the pretest probability. If answer E were correct and the pretest and posttest probabilities were equal, there would be no point in doing the test.

Objectives: Did you learn to . . .

• Define and calculate sensitivity and then apply it to data interpretation?
• Define and calculate specificity and then apply it to data interpretation?
• Calculate positive and negative predictive values?
• Apply Bayes theorem to determine the utility of a test?

CASE 7

Chest x-rays are often used in diagnostic testing of tuberculosis. Two thousand patients enrolled in a study

and of those, 26 had tuberculosis and 1,974 did not. All the subjects had chest x-rays and the results were provided. Of the 26 subjects with tuberculosis, 21 had positive chest x-rays and 5 had negative chest x-rays. There were 1,974 subjects without tuberculosis, and of these, 10 had positive chest x-rays and 1,964 had negative chest x-rays.

A subject in the study has a positive chest x-ray and becomes your patient.

What is the posttest probability that he has tuberculosis given that his x-ray is positive?

A) 68%
B) 30%
C) 55%
D) 81%
E) Unable to solve the problem with data provided.

Discussion

The correct answer is A. Set up the data in a 2×2 table, and you should be able to answer the question (Table 28–7):

The posttest probability or positive predictive value of a test is the probability that a disease exists given a positive test result (TP/ [TP + FP] or 21/31 = 68%).

The same clinic day, another patient in the study presents to your office with a negative chest x-ray and asks what chance is there that she does not have tuberculosis?

A) 88%
B) 99%
D) 75%
D) 23%
E) Unable to the solve problem with data provided.

Table 28–7   2×2 TABLE OF TUBERCULOUS AND RADIOGRAPH

X-ray	Tuberculosis	No Tuberculosis
Positive	True Positive (TP) = 21	False Positive (FP) = 10
Negative	False Negative (FN) = 5	True Negative (TN) = 1964
Total	TP + FN = 26	FP + TN = 1974

Discussion

The correct answer is B. The negative predictive value of a test is the probability of no disease given a negative test result (TN/ [FN + TN] or 1964/1969 = 98%).

Given that 26 patients of 2,000 have tuberculosis, what is the prevalence of tuberculosis in this sample of patients?

A) 5 per 100,000.
B) 2.6 per 100,000.
C) 26 per 100,000.
D) 1,300 per 100,000.
E) 1.3 per 100,000.

Discussion

The correct answer is D. The prevalence of a disease is the proportion of individuals who have the disease at a specific time ([TP + FN]/[TP + FN + FP + TN] or 26/2,000 = 1.3% = 1,300/100,000).

 HELPFUL TIP: A **type I** error occurs when an association or difference is found when none exists. For example, a *P* value of 0.05 is considered statistically different. This means, however, that 5% of the time, the same conclusion would be produced by chance alone. By contrast, a *P* value of 0.005 means that there is only a 0.5% chance that the conclusion is mistaken and occurred by chance.

 HELPFUL TIP: A **type II error** occurs when there are not enough subjects in a study to show a true association or difference although one exists. For example, in a study of lorazepam versus diazepam for seizures, twice as many patients had their seizures stop with lorazepam. However, the conclusion of the study was that there was no difference between the two drugs. This is because there were not enough subjects for this to reach statistical significance. Inclusion of an additional 100 subjects would have made this reach statistical significance.

Objectives: Did you learn to . . .

- Calculate and apply positive predictive value to clinical scenarios?
- Calculate prevalence of disease in a given population?
- Describe the significance of *P* value and type I error?
- Recognize a type II error?

CASE 8

The number of falls that occurred in 9 Boston nursing homes in November–April 2005 was reported as: 127, 104, 103, 81, 86, 117, 89, 97, and 95.

What is the median number of falls among the nursing home residents?

A) 89
B) 103
C) 97
D) 117
E) 96

Discussion

The correct answer is C. Data are most commonly investigated at their center—where the observations have a tendency to cluster (ie, measures of central tendency). Three common measures of central tendency are mean, median, and mode (see following examples). To calculate the median in a set of data with n observations where n is odd, the median is the middle value ($(n + 1)/2$; in our case, since there are 9 observations, the mean is $(9 + 1)/2 = 5$). If n was even, the median is the average of the 2 middle values, that is, the average of observations ($n/2$) and ($n/2$) + 1. To find the median in our sample, first rank the observations:

81, 86, 89, 95, 97, 103, 104, 117, 127

Take the number of observations and add 1 because there is an odd number of observations and divide by 2 ($[n + 1]/2$ or $[9 + 1]/2 = 5$). The fifth-ranked number of falls, the median, is 97.

What is the mean of falls among the nursing home residents, rounded to the nearest whole number?

A) 89
B) 100
C) 97
D) 101
E) 98

Discussion

The correct answer is B. In a set of data with *n* observations, find the mean by summing the total observations and divide by *n*

$$(81 + 86 + 89 + 95 + 97 + 103 + 104 + 117 + 127)/9$$
$$= 99.89$$

 HELPFUL TIP: The mean is sensitive to extreme observations (eg, if there are data points 1, 1, 1, 1, 1, and 100, the mean is 21 even though the majority of observations are 1). When outliers like this occur or when the data is not symmetrically distributed, the median may be the best measure of central tendency.

What is the mode of falls among the nursing home residents?

A) 89
B) 99.89
C) 117
D) 101
E) Unable to the solve problem with data provided.

Discussion

The correct answer is E. **The mode of a sample is the observation that occurs most frequently.** In the data provided, there is no unique mode because all the observations occur only once. However, if you were checking daily fall rates in one nursing home and they were 1, 2, 3, 3, 2, 3, 2, and 3 the mode would be 3 (since this is the observation that occurs most frequently).

 HELPFUL TIP: If the data distribution is symmetric (eg, normally distributed), then it is a unimodal distribution. Data may have more than one mode (ie, bimodal, trimodal, etc).

Objectives: Did you learn to . . .

• Calculate the mean, mode, and median in a data set with an odd number of data points?
• Apply these measures of data to the analysis of data?

 QUICK QUIZ: EVIDENCE-BASED MEDICINE

Which of the following statements is true?

A) Specificity is the most important test characteristic when trying to find a very dangerous disease.
B) As sensitivity increases, specificity decreases.
C) Specificity need not be considered as long as a test is sensitive enough.
D) As sensitivity increases, specificity increases.

Discussion

The correct answer is B. As sensitivity increases, specificity decreases. This makes intuitive sense. The more cases you detect, the more false positives you will have. Ideally, we would like to have a diagnostic screening test with both high sensitivity and high specificity. In reality, there is an inherent trade-off between sensitivity and specificity—as sensitivity increases, specificity decreases and vice versa. Answer A is incorrect. Generally, when it is very dangerous not to detect disease, it is important to have a highly sensitive test (one that will find "all" cases) with an acceptable specificity. Answer C is incorrect. This is why we do both an ELISA and a Western Blot when trying to detect HIV. The ELISA is very sensitive (picks up the great majority of HIV cases) but is not very specific (categorizes a lot of patients who **do not have the disease** as positive). The Western Blot is more specific and filters the true positives from the false positives found on the screening test (the ELISA).

 QUICK QUIZ: MEDIAN BLOOD PRESSURE

On postoperative day 1, a patient recovering from hip replacement had 6 blood pressures taken. The systolic blood pressures reported were: 175, 136, 210, 161, 175, and 145.

What is his median systolic blood pressure?

A) 161
B) 168
C) 175
D) 117
E) 170

Discussion

The correct answer is B. To calculate the median here, the equation is slightly different from that employed to calculate the median when there are an odd number of data points. To find the median in this sample, first rank the observations: 136, 145,161,175,175, 210.

To calculate the median in a set of data with n observations where n is even, the median is the average of the 2 middle ranks:

$$[(n/2) + ((n/2) + 1)]/2 = (3rd\ measure + 4th\ measure)/2$$
$$= (161 + 175)/2 = 168$$

What is the mean systolic blood pressure of this patient?

A) 161
B) 167
C) 175
D) 171
E) 201

Discussion

The correct answer is B. In a set of data with n observations, find the mean by summing the total observations and divide by n (136 + 145 + 161 + 175 + 175 + 210)/6 = 167.

What is the mode of the systolic blood pressure for this patient?

A) 175
B) 161
C) 171
D) 155
E) Unable to the solve problem with data provided.

Discussion

The correct answer is A. The mode of a sample is the observation that occurs most frequently. In the data provided, 175 occurs twice, which is the most frequent observation.

Objectives: Did you learn to . . .

• Calculate the mean, mode, and median in a data set with an even number of data points?
• Apply these measures of data to the analysis of data?

CASE 9

One common and debilitating complication of diabetes is neuropathy. In a study of diabetic patients, one group had routine therapy and an experimental group had intensive therapy. The first group, routine therapy, had 10% of patients develop neuropathy. The second group, intensive therapy, had 2% of patients develop neuropathy.

Using the data above, how many diabetic patients need to be treated with intensive therapy to prevent one the development of one case of neuropathy?

A) 10
B) 11
C) 8
D) 12.5
E) 25.5

Discussion

The correct answer is D. The question asks, "What is the number needed to treat (NNT)?" In this question, the absolute risk reduction is 8% (10% in control group versus 2% in the treated group). The NNT is the number of patients who need to be treated to prevent one adverse outcome. To calculate this, we need to know a few key terms:

ARR = **A**bsolute **R**isk **R**eduction = control group event rate – experimental group event rate

CER = the **C**ontrol group **E**vent **R**ate

EER = the **E**xperimental group **E**vent **R**ate

NNT = 1/ARR

Using the values given above, ARR = 10% – 2% = 8% and NNT = 1/0.08 = 12.5.

CASE 10

The anticlotting properties of aspirin are well-studied. In a trial studying the long-term outcome of stroke patients, 1% of patients on long-term aspirin therapy developed new onset of strokes and 50% of patients without aspirin therapy developed new strokes.

Using the data above, how many stroke patients need to be treated with aspirin therapy to prevent 1 new stroke?

A) 2
B) 8
C) 10
D) 12
E) 25

Discussion

The correct answer is A. Again, the NNT is the number of patients who need to be treated to prevent 1 adverse outcome. NNT = 1/ARR where ARR = CER – EER. Using the values given above, 50% – 1% = 49% = ARR and NNT = 1/0.49 = 2.

CASE 11

In a pharmaceutical study, Group A is the placebo group and Group B is the group that received the new drug. Data were gathered on Groups A and B and confidence intervals were calculated. Side effect rates were calculated as a percentage of each group.

Which of the following grouping comparison statistics are significantly different?

A) Group A confidence interval 30%–46% and Group B confidence interval 44%–88%.

B) Group A confidence interval 10%–30% and Group B confidence interval 44%–88%.

C) Group A confidence interval 0.1%–0.3% and Group B confidence interval 0.1%–0.3%.

D) Group A confidence interval 88%–90% and Group B confidence interval 88%–90%.

E) None of the above is statistically significant.

Discussion

The correct answer is B. The confidence interval is a range of possible high to low values of data. The true mean is likely to be in the specified range. So, if the relative risk of an adverse outcome is 2 and the confidence interval is –2 to 10 (usually identified by "CI 95% = –2 to 10"), this means that there may be up to 10 times the risk of an adverse outcome **or** 2 times **less** a risk of an adverse outcome. In general, the larger the study group, the narrower the confidence intervals. When you have a large study, you are more likely to get closer to the true value.

Answer B is correct because there is no overlap when comparing the confidence intervals between two groups. When there is an overlap of confidence intervals, as in the other options, the groups are not statistically significantly different. In answer A the true mean value of Group A could lie anywhere between 30%–46% (it could be 45%), and the true mean value of Group B could lie anywhere between 44%–88% (it could also be 45%); therefore, the groups have no statistically significant difference.

 HELPFUL TIP: Confidence intervals are usually given as "CI 95%" which means that there is a 95% probability that the true mean value will be within the confidence interval. When looking at confidence intervals for relative risk, relative benefit, etc, remember that if the CI 95% crosses 1, there is no difference between the groups. Thus, CI 95% 0.8–10 is consistent with a 0.8 times risk or a 10 times risk (or benefit). However, because the CI 95% crosses 1, there is no real difference between the groups.

 HELPFUL TIP: Confidence intervals (CI) are useful when determining the magnitude of a treatment effect. For example, if a relative risk has CI 95% 1.2–1.4, this means there is a very small difference (0.2 to 0.4 times) between the two groups, even though it is statistically significant. **Something that is statistically significant may not be clinically significant.** On the other hand, if the relative risk has a CI 95% 10 – 20, this is a major difference between the groups. This means that one group has a 10 – 20 times greater risk (or benefit depending on what is being studied) than does the other group.

* *

In a clinical trial testing a new provider order entry (POE) technology at a university hospital, relative and absolute risk reduction is discussed. A group of family practice residents at the hospital used the traditional hand-written orders during their intern year and averaged 7 medication errors per year. In the FP residents' second year, POE was instituted (which alerted physicians to medication errors before finalization of orders) and the group's medication errors dropped to an average of 4 per year.

Which of the following statements is true?

A) The relative risk reduction is 43% and the absolute risk reduction is 3 in medication errors.

B) The relative risk reduction is 57% and the absolute risk reduction is 3 in medication errors.

C) The relative risk reduction is 43% and the absolute risk reduction is 4 in medication errors.

D) The relative risk reduction is 57% and the absolute risk reduction is 4 in medication errors.

E) The relative risk reduction cannot be calculated with the information given and the absolute risk reduction is 3 in medication errors.

Discussion

The correct answer is A. POE compared to no POE (the control group) results in a 43% relative decrease in the risk of a medication error—from 7 to 4 errors per year (3/7 = 43%). The difference in the number of medication errors before and after POE is 3 errors (7 − 4 = 3), which is the absolute reduction in the risk of a medication error.

CASE 12

Mr. Handsome Q. Drugrep has come to tell you all about HappyLuckyGolden Drug (HLGD) which is newly indicated for the treatment of the Dreadful Yucks. As a primary care doctor, you are concerned about better treatment for this disease. Current standard treatment involves ChemoRAdical Pharmacotherapy (CRAP). Cure rates with CRAP are only about 10%. Mr. Drugrep has a study that shows HLGD has a 12% cure rate versus placebo. He's very excited and expects HLGD to be the new standard of care.

To his argument, you appropriately respond:

A) "Wow. HLGD is clearly superior to CRAP."
B) "Hmm. HLGD is statistically no different from CRAP."
C) "Wow. HLGD is clearly superior to placebo."
D) "Do you have free samples of HLGD? Where's lunch?"
E) "I need more information before I can make an informed decision."

Discussion

The correct answer is E. You need more information. Before coming to market, a drug manufacturer must demonstrate safety and efficacy of a drug. The new drug may or may not be compared to another currently available treatment. Without a study comparing HLGD to CRAP, you cannot say anything about how these drugs compare, even if HLGD looks better versus placebo. Answer C is incorrect because the placebo results have not been given.

* *

You ask Mr. Drugrep for more information. He proudly tells you the drug study involved 10,000 subjects with the Dreadful Yucks, randomly assigned to placebo (5,000) or HLGD (5,000). All of the subjects completed the trial. At the end of 1 year, 400 subjects on placebo were cured and 600 subjects on HLGD were cured.

He correctly tells you that:

A) The number needed to treat is 10,000.
B) The number needed to harm is 10,000.
C) The relative benefit of HLGD versus placebo is 50% greater cure rate.
D) The absolute benefit of HLGD versus placebo is 50% greater cure rate.

Discussion

The correct answer is C. When you look at drug studies, benefit is often stated as "relative benefit" or relative risk reduction. In this question, 600/5,000 patients benefit from HLGD and 400/5,000 benefit from placebo; thus, 200 more patients are cured with HLGD, 200/400 = 0.5 = 50% relative benefit of the drug. The absolute benefit is only 4% (12% cure with HLGD vs. 8% cure with placebo). For the NNT in this example, think about the previously given equation: NNT = 1/ARR, where ARR = CER − EER. The control group, the placebo, had a risk reduction of 8% (92% still had disease); and the experiment group had a risk reduction of 12% (88% still had disease). So, the ARR =12% − 8% = 4%, and NNT = 1/0.04 = 25. Number needed to harm (NNH) cannot be calculated with the information available because the adverse event rate is not known.

In real life, there are often more dramatic examples of how relative and absolute risks differ. It may be stated there is a 50% reduction in complications of diabetes using Drug A versus placebo. However, when translated into patients, this could be 1/1,000 complications of diabetes in the drug group versus 2/1,000 complications of diabetes in the placebo group. This is a 50% relative decrease in adverse outcomes but in fact may be clinically meaningless. The **absolute** risk reduction is 1/1,000 or 0.1%! This ploy is often used to make drug studies look good. Thus, anytime you are looking at a new drug, ask for the **absolute risk reduction and the number needed to treat (NNT) and the number needed to harm (NNH).**

* *

Mr. Drugrep tells you that the adverse event rate for HLGD is only 1%. Aren't you impressed? But he frowns a little when you want to know the number needed to harm.

To calculate NNH you ask him for:

A) The types of adverse events that occurred in the treatment group.
B) The number of adverse events that occurred in the control group.

C) The percentage of adverse events with standard treatment.

D) The cure rate in the treatment group.

Discussion

The correct answer is B. **Adverse effects** of a drug will often be reported as an absolute number, and here it is 1%. So, the conclusion you are given by the pharmaceutical industry may be: **50% reduction in disease and only a 1% risk of side effects of the drug.** Both of these statements are true. However, they could just as easily be reversed and still be true. That's why we need to know the NNH. It is nice to compare apples to apples. When you ask Mr. Drugrep, he tells you that the adverse event rate in the placebo group was 0.5%. Here's the calculation:

$$NNH = 1/ARI$$

ARI (absolute risk increase) = risk in experiment group – risk in control group

Using the numbers in this question: ARI = 1 – 0.5 = 0.5; NNH = 1/0.5 = 2.

So, for HLGD, the NNT is 25 and the NNH is 2. By the way, the adverse event in question is disfiguring, painful ear hair growth. You will have to treat 25 patients with HLGD to cure 1 case of the Dreadful Yucks; but with every 2 patients you treat, 1 will have an adverse event. Demand NNT and NNH: how many patients who take the drug will benefit and how many will be harmed?

Objectives: Did you learn to . . .

- Employ confidence intervals in the analysis of data?
- Analyze data using risk reduction and relative benefit?
- Understand the importance of absolute risk reduction, number needed to harm, and number needed to treat when clinically applying data from a study?

CASE 13

Mounting paperwork and electronic medical record hassles have played a role in your decision to make a career change. You have found a nice academic job with a research focus—minimal patient care, 10 weeks of vacation, no paperwork. Your work centers on reducing the risk of stroke in patients who have survived one stroke.

This is an example of which category of prevention?

A) Primary prevention.
B) Secondary prevention.
C) Tertiary prevention.
D) Quaternary prevention.

Discussion

The correct answer is C. The idea behind primary prevention, a big interest in primary care, is to prevent a disease from occurring at all by removing its cause (eg, influenza vaccine to prevent illness from influenza). Primary prevention may occur in the health-care setting but is often in the domain of public health. Secondary prevention detects disease at an early stage so that intervention can prevent progression (eg, Pap smears to detect dysplasia prior to cancer declaring itself). Your new job will be to study tertiary prevention: the reduction in complications and mortality due to disease after it is recognized. There is no such thing as quaternary prevention.

CASE 14

You plan to study 2 groups of patients (A and B) to see if variable XYZ makes any difference in death or recurrent stroke. Subjects in Group A had a stroke and then had another stroke or died a year later. Subjects in Group B had a stroke but were alive with no recurrent stroke at the time of the study. You assess the presence of XYZ in each group.

This type of study is called a:

A) Prospective study.
B) Case-control study.
C) Cohort study.
D) Randomized, controlled study.

Discussion

The correct answer is B. A case-control study, like this one, will look at select subjects who are categorized based on outcome and try to find associations with certain variables. Case-control studies do not follow subjects over time, and therefore are not prospective. Cohort studies look at groups over time to find an association between a variable and an outcome. The variable in question is not under the researcher's control. An example of a cohort study might be one looking at the association between two different diets (eg, high-protein versus high-carbohydrate) and the development of type 2 diabetes. The prototypical medical experiment is the randomized, double-blind, controlled trial, in which the researcher has control over exposure to a variable and studies its effect on an outcome. In general, the strength of trial design goes: experimental study > cohort study > case-control study > cross-sectional study. Unfortunately, not all conditions can be studied under a controlled experiment.

* *

You are concerned about numerous confounding variables in your study population. Never fear!

Your trusty statistician recommends the following in order to minimize confounding:

A) Multivariate analysis.
B) Careful calculation of *P*-values.
C) Matched controls and subjects.
D) A and B.
E) A and C.

Discussion

The correct answer is E. Confounders can be a serious threat to any study. Confounders result from extrinsic factors—things that may affect the outcome and are also associated with the variable but are not accounted for in the study. A study may find an association between long-haul truck driving and lung cancer. If tobacco use was not accounted for in this study, the results of the study would be meaningless. Tobacco is a confounder. It is always advisable to look at a study with an eye for which confounder might be missing. Confounding can be limited by a study design that anticipates confounders and matches controls and subjects (answer C). Also, multivariate analysis (answer A) is a statistical method that allows for adjustment of known confounders. Answer B is incorrect because *P* value has nothing to do with confounding but will tell you whether the results should be considered significant or not.

* *

When you review the literature, you find that there are a number of small studies looking at the effect of intervention XYZ on stroke victims. You even find a meta-analysis.

If this is a well done meta-analysis, you should find all of the following EXCEPT:

A) Statistically confirmed heterogeneity between the included studies.
B) A thorough search for all valid studies.
C) An evaluation of whether estimates change with varying assumptions.
D) The exclusion of poor quality studies.
E) The studies included measure the same underlying effect.

Discussion

The correct answer is A. Hopefully a meta-analysis would confirm *homogeneity* between studies. Although there is controversy regarding the appropriate use of meta-analyses, they are often used to study various outcomes by combining smaller studies. A meta-analysis is a systematic review that combines the results of previous studies to evaluate the magnitude or direction of an effect or to evaluate the effect on a subgroup. All valid studies looking at similar outcomes should be included and poor quality studies excluded. A number of statistical maneuvers are done with meta-analyses, including an evaluation of whether estimates will change if study assumptions change.

Objectives: Did you learn to . . .

- Define different types of prevention?
- Define different study types?
- Identify and account for confounding?
- Describe some characteristics of a meta-analysis?

BIBLIOGRAPHY

Fletcher RH, Fletcher SW, Wagner EH. *Clinical Epidemiology: The Essentials.* 2nd ed. Baltimore: Williams & Wilkins, 1988.

Friedland DJ, Go AS, Davoren JB, et al. *Evidence-Based Medicine.* New York: McGraw-Hill, 1998.

Gordis L. *Epidemiology.* Philadelphia: WB Saunders, 1996.

Pagano, Marcello and Gauvreau, Kimberlee. *Principles of Biostatistics.* 2nd ed. Australia: Duxbury Thomson Learning, 2000.

29

Patient-Centered Care

Oladipo Kukoyi, Jason K. Wilbur and Mark A. Graber

INTRODUCTION

This chapter deals with cultural competency and patient safety. Because not all black patients are from America (and thus are not African Americans), the authors have elected to use the term black in this chapter as inclusive of African Americans as well as those individuals who are of African descent but may be from another country.

CASE 1

A young couple who immigrated to your town from Bosnia come to your clinic because they are expecting their first child. The wife is 23 years old, in her first trimester, and without any medical problems. She speaks no English and her husband speaks only a little. However, if he uses his limited English and some hand gestures, you feel that you could conduct an interview with them. Your recent completion of the course, Advanced Life Support for Cultural Competence, enables you to deal with such a situation. You recall how cultural competence is defined.

Cultural competence is defined as:

A) Learning about multiple cultures.
B) Being able to speak multiple languages.
C) Taking diversity classes.
D) Adopting a set of cultural behaviors and attitudes that enable you to deliver effective medical care to people of different cultures.
E) Hiring staff from a variety of different cultures.

Discussion

The correct answer is D. Although the other answer choices are laudable goals, they do not define cultural competency. Cultural competence is a set of behaviors and attitudes that aims to help health-care providers deliver better care to patients from different cultures.

* *

You rack your brain trying to remember why cultural competence is important to you. You remember a few ways that being culturally competent could help you.

Which of these is NOT one of them?

A) It allows efficient use of time and resources.
B) It increases the chance of providing services that are consistent with patient needs.
C) It might improve health outcomes for minority patients.
D) It might improve patient retention.
E) It is less expensive in the long run.

Discussion

The correct answer is E. Cultural competence allows you to use your time and resources efficiently so that you can provide the services your patient wants and needs. This can lead to improved health outcomes for your patients and increased patient satisfaction, allowing you to retain more minority patients. Unfortunately, no studies so far show that it can reduce your practice's costs.

* *

Pondering this, you decide to try and provide culturally competent care to this nice couple in front of you.

Which one of the following is NOT a step in providing culturally competent care?

A) Understanding your own culture.

B) Understanding others' cultures.

C) Accepting every cultural practice as equally valid even when against best medical practices.

D) Understanding how your patients' cultural beliefs affect their attitude towards health care.

E) Adapting your way of working to provide optimal care.

Discussion

The correct answer is C. The goal of cultural competence is provide better health care for patients from different cultures. Some of the specific things this goal calls for include:

- Being respectful of cultural differences
- Learning about other cultures
- Being aware of the health impact of cultural beliefs and practices
- Being sensitive to patients' needs
- Using interpreters when necessary
- Adapting to provide optimal care

An easy way to remember this is Berlin and Fowkes' LEARN model:

Listening to the patient's perspective

Explaining and sharing one's own perspective

Acknowledging differences and similarities between these two perspectives

Recommending a treatment plan

Negotiating a mutually agreed-on treatment plan.

 HELPFUL TIP: Although learning about and respecting patients' different cultural beliefs is vital, good care does not call for accepting practices that are detrimental to your patient's health. There are potential ethical dilemmas that can arise when traditional Western medicine intersects with a culture that has radically different health beliefs. The point here is that there is no simple "trump."

* *

Now that you are ready to proceed with care for your patient, the question of language comes up. Should you use the husband to interpret or not?

To help guide you, you call your hospital compliance officer who tells you that:

A) It is Federal Law that you must provide an interpreter for patients who need it, at your own cost if necessary.

B) It is Federal Law that patients must provide their own interpreters at their own expense.

C) Most insurance companies reimburse for interpreter services.

D) Using family and staff to translate rarely reflects current best practice.

E) There are no privacy concerns when using non-professional interpreters.

Discussion

The correct answer is A. The 2000 census found that more than 46 million adults (~14% of the U.S. population) speak a non-English language at home while >10% of the U.S. population is foreign born. When the health-care professional does not speak the primary language of the patient, loss of important information, misunderstanding of physician instructions, and poor shared decision-making can occur. Title VI of the 1964 Civil Rights Act requires health-care professionals to provide translation services for patients who need them, at the physician's cost if necessary. Failure to do so would qualify as discrimination and could be prosecuted. Unfortunately, most insurance companies do not reimburse for these services. Interpreters can be scarce and costly. As a result, many physicians use any help they can get for translation, including staff members and family members who are bilingual. This leaves room for error. Using a family member as an interpreter makes it hard for the patient to disclose private information they do not want known by the family. Professional interpreters have been trained and certified although ad hoc interpreters often have no formal training and can make translation errors.

Regarding health care, language barriers may result in:

A) Increased risk of intubation for children with asthma.

B) Greater nonadherence to medication regimens.

C) Higher resource use in diagnostic testing.

D) Increased risk of drug complications.

E) All of the above.

Discussion

The correct answer is E. Language barriers have been associated with all of the following: worsened health status; lower likelihood of having a usual source of medical care; lower likelihood of being given a follow-up appointment after ED visit; greater nonadherence to medication regimens; increased risk of drug complications; impaired patient understanding of diagnoses, medication, and follow-up; worsened health status; lower patient satisfaction; longer medical visits; higher resource use in diagnostic testing; increased risk of intubation for children with asthma; greater risk of being assigned more severe psychopathology; and increased risk of leaving the hospital against medical advice.

What is the proper way to use an interpreter?

A) Address all questions to the interpreter.
B) Address questions to the patient while looking at the interpreter.
C) Address questions to the patient while facing the patient.
D) Address questions to the interpreter while facing the patient.

Discussion

The correct answer is C. The physician should speak to and look at the patient. Failure to look at the patient while asking questions may be interpreted as rude and should be avoided. Remember that nonverbal communication is important even when a common language is not shared. The physician should speak clearly and give the interpreter time to translate questions and answers. The physician should periodically pause and ensure that the patient understands the questions that are being asked. One way to do this is by asking brief, close-ended questions.

* *

You remember from medical school that there was disagreement regarding the degree to which a medical interpreter should function as a cultural advocate.

Which of the following would be the most effective preencounter instructions for your interpreter to facilitate communication between you and your patient?

A) "Translate word-for-word all that the patient and I say. You may repeat phrases, but do not rephrase anything."
B) "When clarifying, explaining, or culturally translating concepts, make sure that you are "transparent," that is, let both parties know what you are doing and saying and why."
C) "Be sure to culturally translate whenever you think it is appropriate."
D) "If the patient doesn't seem to understand, go ahead and explain it in other words. Understanding is more important than how things are said."

Discussion

The correct answer is B. Ideally, an interpreter would do an exact translation. However, many concepts do not translate literally or they have different meanings depending on the context. Good interpreters are often aware when the health-care provider and the patient do not have the same understanding of an event, concept, or plan. In this case, the translator should let each party know exactly what has been communicated. This feedback to each party is important so that the interpreter's moral values are not projected onto the patient and unduly influence decisions made by the patient. Transparency is thus critical.

* *

You remember that low literacy is associated with poor outcomes.

Which of the following statements is NOT true?

A) Patients with low literacy have a 50% increased risk of hospitalization.
B) Only 50% of patients take medications as directed.
C) Low literacy is a stronger predictor of a person's health than race.
D) Low literacy is only an issue among minorities and immigrants.

Discussion

The correct answer is D. Poor health literacy skills are a stronger predictor of health status than a person's race, age, income, socioeconomic status, or employment. This relationship holds across different racial and cultural groups. Unfortunately, up to 90 million people in the United States have low-literacy skills and many are ashamed to share this with their physicians. This can lead to noncompliance because patients cannot read prescriptions and other instructions. It is not surprising, then, that low-literacy patients have an increased risk of hospitalization. To help combat this problem, the American Medical Association (AMA) Foundation has launched The Ask Me 3 program (www.askme3.org). The Ask Me 3 program urges doctors to make sure their patients ask and understand the answers to 3 simple questions: What is my main problem? What do I need to do? Why is it important for me to do this? Other suggestions to improve communication include asking the patient to repeat instructions back to the physician; using basic, nonmedical language when talking to patients; and allowing patients to talk uninterruptedly at the beginning of the visit.

* *

You are interested in doing your part to help decrease problems with health literacy. You recently heard that the American Academy of Pediatrics has an office-based intervention to improve reading capability in young children called Reach Out and Read.

Which of the following is/are true about reading and Reach Out and Read?

A) It is a program of primary prevention of reading problems that is evidence based.

B) Physicians model reading out loud during the well-child visit.

C) Free age- and development-appropriate books are given to children between 6 months and 5 years at their well-child visits.

D) All of the above.

Discussion

The correct answer is D. Between 10%–40% of low-income children have no books at home. A quarter of college-educated parents do not read to their young children daily. Reach Out and Read is summarized by the acronym SAFER.

Show the book early in the visit, **S**hare the book with the child, modeling the reading for the parents.

Ask the parents about reading; **A**ssess the child's development and the parent-child relationship.

Give **F**eedback about what you observe the child does; give **F**eedback about parents' attitudes and interactions with the child.

Encourage the parents to read daily to the child; **E**xplain about literacy development.

Refer to the library and literacy programs; **R**ecord in the chart what you did.

Other than giving a book and briefly reading to the child, you need not do all the activities at each visit.

 HELPFUL TIP: The National Center for Cultural Competence at Georgetown University has identified 6 compelling reasons that healthcare providers should incorporate cultural competency into their practice. They are:

- To respond to current and projected demographic changes in the United States
- To eliminate long-standing disparities in the health status of people of diverse racial, ethnic, and cultural backgrounds
- To improve the quality of services and health outcomes
- To meet legislative, regulatory, and accreditation mandates
- To gain a competitive edge in the marketplace
- To decrease the likelihood of liability/malpractice claims

CASE 2

You are seeing a 67-year-old black male for the first time in your clinic. He claims to be healthy but has not seen a physician for over 30 years. He says, "Doctors—I try to avoid them. My wife made me come today." You tell him you are going to take a history and then perform a physical exam on him. After you are done, you tell him you recommend age-appropriate screening exams for colon and prostate cancer. The patient politely declines both. You try to explain the importance of screening to him.

Which of the following statements about screening is FALSE?

A) Prostate cancer is a leading cause of death in black males.

B) Colon cancer is a leading cause of death in black males.

C) There is clear evidence that screening for colon cancer lowers incidence of mortality in black males.

D) There is clear evidence that screening for prostate cancer of black males saves lives.

E) Prostate cancer disproportionately affects black males.

Discussion

The correct answer is D. There is no firm evidence that screening for prostate cancer lowers incidence of mortality from the disease (although there is some information to suggest this might be true). Prostate cancer is the seventh leading cause of death overall in the United States, and the burden of prostate cancer varies among racial and ethnic groups. **Black males have about a 60% higher incidence and a 2-fold higher mortality rate from prostate cancer in comparison with white males.** In comparison with white men, mortality from prostate cancer is 35% lower in non-white Hispanics and 40% lower in Asian Americans and Pacific Islanders.

* *

Your patient now agrees to colon cancer screening but still declines prostate cancer screening. Your exam also revealed an elevated BP of 160/90 with no abnormal cardiac, lung, or other organ system findings.

Assuming you confirm this elevated BP reading at subsequent visits, which of the following antihypertensives would you recommend?

A) Hydrochlorothiazide.
B) Ramipril.
C) Amlodipine.
D) Atenolol.
E) Losartan.

Discussion
The correct answer is A. Although diuretics are a good choice for most patients with hypertension, they are an especially good choice in blacks. Diuretics are particularly effective in blacks, who tend to have extremely salt-sensitive hypertension. Blacks are more likely than other hypertensive patients to have low renin levels, which makes them **less likely to respond to ACE inhibitors.** β-**Blockers also tend to be less effective in black patients.**

* *

Your patient agrees to your medication choice but he wants to know if the research on which you based your choice included black people. You can confidently say yes, knowing that the ALLHAT trial specifically addressed the issue of generalizability by making sure that approximately 33% of the 33,357 subjects were black. However, you know this has not always been true in scientific research. You know that minorities are very underrepresented in research data on which we base our treatment choices.

Which of the following is NOT a reason why there are few minorities in research studies?

A) Past history of abuse leading to mistrust of the health-care system.
B) Lack of representation of minorities in the medical profession.
C) Discrimination.
D) Overrepresentation of minorities in lower socioeconomic status.
E) Minorities are more likely to volunteer for studies but are generally excluded.

Discussion
The correct answer is E. Minorities' contact with the medical system has been fraught with abuse in the past. Possibly the most egregious example of this is the Tuskegee Syphilis Study in the 1930s in which black men with syphilis were recruited for a naturalistic study of the disease. More than 400 black men with syphilis were recruited with 200 men without syphilis as controls. There was no informed consent, and they were told the lie that spinal taps (done for research) were a form of treatment. It was soon apparent that the death rate among those with syphilis was about twice as high as it was among the controls. When penicillin was found to be effective as a cure for syphilis in the 1940s, the participants were neither informed nor offered treatment, so the naturalistic study could continue.

These and other examples of past mistreatment by the medical community constitute a significant source of distrust for minority patients, who are less likely to participate in research. There have also been overt and subtle discriminatory barriers against minority participation in clinical trials. Minorities are more likely to be poor and undereducated, and research subjects are generally more educated and of higher socioeconomic status. Finally, there is a significant underrepresentation of minorities in the medical profession. For example, even though blacks comprise 13% of the population, they are only 4% of the physician population. All these problems lead to difficulties recruiting minority participants for research trials.

What percentage of Americans belongs to a minority group?

A) 15%
B) 20%
C) 25%
D) 34%
E) 41%

Discussion

The correct answer is D. According to the 2006 U.S. Census estimates, 34% of Americans are ethnic minorities, up from 31% in 2000 and 24% in 1990. Yet, only 10% of physicians are from minority groups. This is problematic. The lack of minority physicians leads to a discrepancy in health care access. Data shows minority physicians are more likely to serve minority patients and are more likely to serve in urban, underserved areas (where there tends to be greater concentration of underprivileged patients).

 HELPFUL TIP: Black physicians are 5 times more likely to treat black patients and Hispanic physicians 2.5 times more likely to treat Hispanic patients, in comparison with non-black and non-Hispanic physicians, respectively. Minority physicians are also more likely to serve Medicaid patients and those without insurance.

 HELPFUL TIP: Patients of all races consistently rate their relationships with their physician better when their physician is of the same ethnic background.

Which of the following statements is NOT true?

A) Patients living in a disadvantaged neighborhood have an increased incidence of coronary artery disease.

B) Patients living in inner city, disadvantaged neighborhoods have an increased incidence of asthma.

C) Minority patients who are not economically deprived have the same incidence of disease as those who are economically deprived.

D) Very low income black children have a higher incidence of asthma than white children of the same social economic status.

E) Patients from disadvantaged neighborhoods not only have a higher risk of developing most cancers, but are also less likely to receive aggressive treatment once diagnosed.

Discussion

The correct answer is C. Patients living in disadvantaged neighborhoods have increased incidences of coronary artery disease, most cancers (lung, colon, cervical), diabetes, arthritis, accidents, adverse birth outcomes, **and** asthma. They also get less care and less aggressive care (except for limb amputations in diabetics) for their ailments and are less likely to have care that adheres to treatment guidelines. Minority patients who are economically well off tend to have better health than poorer members of their ethnic group, although their health is still worse than that of comparable white populations.

In care of black patients, all of the following principles are helpful to keep in mind EXCEPT:

A) Family relationships are extremely important.

B) Religion often has a role in the patient's life.

C) It is expected that physicians will call patients by their first name.

D) Food is an important part of black culture.

E) Nonverbal communication is often as important as what is said.

Discussion

The correct answer is C. Blacks often maintain extended family ties and view health care as a family responsibility. Therefore, physicians should consider enlisting the family's help in taking care of an ill family member.

Religion is often an important aspect in black culture and members of the clergy are highly respected in the community. Churches are very helpful for community outreach efforts and evidence exists that using churches to conduct preventive care services, such as immunizations and screening programs for illnesses, leads to better patient compliance with preventive guidelines. Some patients may view illness as a test of one's faith, and it is prudent for the physician to acknowledge and respect the patient's beliefs and perception of illness to the extent that it influences their seeking or receiving healthcare.

Poorer blacks have little choice but to eat what is available at a lower cost. This means our advice to patients to eat a well-balanced diet with fresh fruit, lean meat, and fresh vegetables may be met with a deaf ear. Advice about simple changes in diet including substituting fish or chicken for red meat in dishes, eating more inexpensive vegetables, modifying cooking techniques, and changing to a vegetable-based rather than a meat-based diet may be more likely to meet with success.

Communication is important, with blacks being particularly attentive to nonverbal aspects of communication such as body language and voice inflection. Respect is emphasized in the culture and patients often like to be addressed by their formal titles and not their first names or appellations like "honey" or "sweetie" which are generally condescending. Asking patients permission to call them by their first names is appreciated.

Blacks often prefer information using real-life examples, rather than cold, dry data or written messages. A nice summary of general principles to keep in mind when taking care of blacks is found in an article on Preventive Care for African-Americans by Witt et al. The principles are:

- Gaining trust and understanding the historical distrust of the health-care system
- Understanding and employing the kinship web in decisions regarding screening and treatment
- Involving the church in developing and delivering prevention and care messages
- Asking patients the meaning of words or phrases
- Asking patients about the use of alternative medicines and herbs
- Tailoring messages about prevention to depictions of real-life situations
- Paying attention to body language and other non-verbal communication

 HELPFUL TIP: Unfortunately, fresh produce is often not available in inner cities and low-income areas. This makes dietary change especially difficult.

CASE 3

Two Cuban friends present to your office seeking a family physician to take care of their general health needs. They are both Cuban but although one is white, the other is black.

Which of the following assumptions is correct?

A) Hispanic people are of one race.
B) Hispanic people can all speak English.
C) Hispanic people share a common language.
D) Hispanic people are not American.
E) Hispanic people all like to be called Latino.

Discussion
The correct answer is C. The term Hispanic denotes an ethnic group who share in common some cultural practices with Spanish as their primary language.

However, they comprise a significantly diverse group who may or may not speak English, may be of any race, hail from different countries of origin, have differing histories, socioeconomic status, and cultural identity. Some feel the term Hispanic is derogatory, reflecting their European ancestry, and may prefer the term Latino. Thirteen percent of the overall U.S. population is now Hispanic, and they are the largest ethnic group in the United States having increased by 58% during the 1990s. Despite the diversity represented within the Latino culture, there exist certain values that are shared. As with black cultures, Latinos have strong family ties with families tending to be large and extended. Families serve as the main source of support and often share in decision making. Physicians with a warm beside manner who demonstrate appropriate respect (especially to the elderly) are appreciated. Immigrants from Latin America usually come to the United States for economic or political reasons. Latinos come from a broad spectrum of socioeconomic backgrounds and enter a variety of living conditions in the United States, which has an enormous impact on immigrant and public health.

 HELPFUL TIP: Despite alarmist paranoia from some parts of our political spectrum, second-generation Latino immigrants are as likely to speak English as were prior waves of immigrants from European countries.

Which of the following statements is FALSE regarding health issues affecting the Latino community?

A) Infectious diseases are common.
B) Fear of deportation prevents some from seeking health care.
C) Lack of insurance can be a potent barrier to accessing health care.
D) Moving to the U.S. can paradoxically raise the risk for habits that lead to illness such as obesity and diabetes.
E) Elderly Latinos have a higher mortality than their white counterparts.

Discussion
The correct answer is E. Recent immigrants are often prone to infectious diseases because of inadequate housing, sanitation, and/or immunizations. Reasons why

Latino patients may not get vaccinated include disbelief in the need for the vaccine, being unaware of the vaccine, lack of patient education by a health-care provider, lack of transportation, and financial restrictions.

Immigrating to the United States can result in poorer nutrition, obesity, a sedentary lifestyle, and an increase in smoking and risky sexual behavior in Latinas (Hispanic women). This translates, in part, into a 2-fold increased incidence of diabetes in Latinas. For Latino males, there is an increased risk of drug abuse, alcohol abuse, tobacco use, and driving under the influence. These risks increase the longer the patient lives in the United States.

Latinos often fail to get preventive health care. For example, they have a lower rate of screening for diabetes and hypertension than blacks or whites. Some avoid presenting for health care because they fear being discovered by immigration authorities. Others are hindered by the lack of insurance. Complementary and alternative practices are also common. Even though they are less likely to access health care, older Hispanics seem to have a life expectancy similar to or greater than same-age whites in the United States and they have lower incidence of mortality from cardiovascular diseases, cancer, and chronic illnesses. The risk of diabetes, however, is higher. This phenomenon has been described as "selective immigration," and implies a predilection for healthier individuals to immigrate to this country.

* *

You get into a discussion on race with your new patients, and they point out several things to you that you had not thought of before.

Which of the following is true about race?

A) It is a valid biological construct.
B) It is interchangeable with ethnicity.
C) All members of a certain culture are the same race.
D) It is a purely social construct.
E) It has no importance in American history, especially not Civil War history.

Discussion
The correct answer is D. Race is a much politicized and emotionally charged topic in the history of the United States. Since the late eighteenth and early nineteenth centuries, attempts have been made to validate race as biologically based in order to justify discriminatory practices. However, the Human Genome Project demonstrated conclusively that there is **no** biological basis for race. Humans share over 99.9% of their DNA, and one cannot tell a member of one race from another on the basis of genetics.

Answer B is incorrect. Although race and ethnicity are often used interchangeably, they are not necessarily equivalent. Race is an arbitrary social construct that is given to people based on visual appearance, while ethnicity refers to people with a common country of origin, a shared ancestry, or a common historical past. Culture refers to a specific set of values, beliefs, and customs shared by members of a community. Answer C is incorrect. People from the same culture can be of different races so one can have white and black Hispanics from Cuba, for example. Answer E is incorrect. One need only listen to the news to see that race continues to play an important and often divisive role in American life.

Which of the following health outcome disparities statements is FALSE?

A) White Hispanics have a higher incidence of breast and colorectal cancer.
B) Clinicians may order fewer diagnostic tests if they do not understand a patient's description of symptoms.
C) Clinicians may overcompensate by ordering more tests when they do not understand what their patients are saying.
D) Minority children are more likely to be evaluated and reported for suspected abuse even after controlling for likelihood of abusive injury.
E) Blacks have the highest colorectal cancer mortality rates.

Discussion
The correct answer is A. The **incidence** of colorectal and breast cancer is lower in white Hispanics than in other whites and blacks. However, this does not translate into less significant disease. There are significant disparities in health-care quality and outcomes for minorities compared to nonminorities, even when controlling for possible confounding factors such as income, education, and insurance. **Although Hispanics have a lower incidence of the above-named cancers, they have a similar mortality when compared to non-Hispanics.** The rest of the statements are true. Of note is answer E. Blacks have the highest colorectal cancer mortality rates. Also of note is answer D. When toddlers of different races present with similar

fractures, minority toddlers are significantly more likely to be reported for suspected abuse, even after controlling for age, insurance status, and likelihood of abuse. This is a reflection of bias and stereotyping.

 HELPFUL TIP: Minority patients are significantly less likely to have their pain treated by physicians. There are few, if any, pharmacies in poor, inner-city areas that have narcotics available for patients with a prescription. This adversely affects the pain management of minority patients even further.

* *

In general, mortality rates among racial and ethnic minorities are higher for cancer, heart disease, diabetes, stroke, kidney failure, and HIV/AIDS. Minority groups are also disproportionately affected by asthma, lead poisoning, accidents, homicides, and other environmental health concerns. Some minorities experience higher infant mortality rates and are less likely to receive timely prenatal care. There are many other examples of health-care disparities that exist between majority and minority groups (Table 29–1).

 HELPFUL TIP: Although perhaps not overtly racist, data suggests that unconscious biases can affect our care of patients. A well-known study in the *NEJM* in 1999 found that, all things being equal, physicians were 60% less likely to refer black women for cardiac catheterization than men and white women. Hopefully, awareness of this unconscious bias can mitigate its effect so that better care will be provided to all patients.

PRESCRIPTION ERORS

You are on the board of your hospital's therapeutics and safety committee and you have been asked to address the issue of medication errors. Mrs. X, a 72-year-old patient with diabetes who was hospitalized for an acute myocardial infarction had died from what seems to be a sudden cardiac event. This was unexpected as she was recovering rather well. One of the nurses on the floor had told her supervisor that Dr. Watters, your partner, had written an order for 6 U of insulin but the new nurse, fresh

Table 29–1 HEALTH-CARE DISPARITIES AMONG MINORITY GROUPS

- Infant death rates for blacks are twice that of whites.
- Heart disease mortality rates are 40% higher in blacks in comparison with whites.
- Hispanics are almost twice as likely as whites to die from diabetes and are more likely to be obese and have high blood pressure than are non-Hispanic whites.
- Blacks are 13% less likely to undergo coronary angioplasty and 33% less likely to undergo bypass surgery than are whites.
- Only 7% of black and 2% of Hispanic preschool children hospitalized for asthma are prescribed routine medications to prevent future hospitalizations in comparison with 21% of white children.
- The length of time between an abnormal screening mammogram and follow-up diagnostic testing is more than twice as long for Asian Americans, Hispanics, and blacks in comparison with whites.
- Minorities are less likely to get immunizations, mammograms, and other preventive care, even when paid for by Medicare.
- There are higher rates of non-insurance and lack of physicians in minority communities, that lead to reduced access to primary care.
- Minorities are less likely to get heart catheterizations, CABG, dialysis, lung cancer surgery, and organ transplants.
- Blacks have 55% higher mortality rate and 6-year shorter life expectancy in comparison with whites.
- Several studies show the deleterious effect of discrimination on health outcomes, including increasing the risk of diabetes, hypertension, depression, and preterm birth independent of other risk factors.

out of nursing school, had misread this as 60 U of insulin and had proceeded to give the patient that amount, precipitating the hypoglycemic event that was to lead to the fatal event. The nurse is distressed as she thought she was only following orders. Around your office, Dr Watters' handwriting is a thing of legend: many pharmacists have had to call to double-check his prescriptions.

Which of the following would have been the MOST effective way to prevent the type of error that occurred?

A) The nurse should have called to confirm the dose of insulin before giving it.

B) "U" should have been written out as "units."

C) Computerized orders would have helped in this instance.

D) Having a clinical pharmacist as part of the team could have helped catch the error and prevent it from happening.

E) All of the above.

Discussion

The correct answer is E. It is estimated that between 44,000 and 98,000 deaths annually are attributable to medical errors, most of which are preventable. Though the numbers have been challenged, it is unarguable that medical errors continue to contribute to adverse outcomes in our patients. One of the large contributors to this is medication errors, and one of the leading causes of medication errors is the use of dangerous abbreviations and dose designations. The use of "U" as above has been reported in the literature to be very problematic as it can easily be misread as a zero or a four, leading to up to 10-fold overdoses which can have terrible consequences in patients using insulin.

Which of these is NOT recommended as a way to prevent prescription errors?

A) Computerized order entry systems.

B) A brief notation of the purpose for the prescription.

C) Metric system for all therapies except those like insulin and vitamins that use standard units.

D) Inclusion of age, and when appropriate, weight of the patient.

E) A trailing zero after a decimal.

Discussion

The correct answer is E. Nurses and pharmacists may not see the decimal point and thus give an inappropriately large dose of medication.

Which of these is prohibited by HIPAA?

A) Calling out patients' names in the waiting room.

B) Leaving a message on a patient's answering machine.

C) Releasing health information to a specialist without patient authorization if that information is to be used for purposes of treatment, payment, or health operations.

D) Faxing patient information.

E) None of the above.

Discussion

The correct answer is E. Since April 14, 2003, when the Health Insurance Portability and Accountability Act went into effect, many physicians have been confused as to what they can and cannot do under the HIPAA law. Physicians can still call out patients' names in the waiting room as long as you don't go into particulars of their presenting complaint in front of other people. You may leave a message on a patient's answering machine if the patient has authorized you to do so. You may fax information once you verify the fax number is correct—but you can only fax to persons the patient designates or consents to. You may also have your patients sign in at the front counter but again, you must avoid identifying their presenting problem. Finally, HIPAA gives physicians broad leeway in sharing information with other physicians provided the information is used for treatment, payment, and healthcare operations. You must give a notice of your privacy practices to the patients and ask them to sign a form acknowledging receiving the notice or make a good-faith effort to get them to sign it.

BIBLIOGRAPHY

Cultural Competence Compendium: Section IV. Underserved and underrepresented racial, ethnic, and socioeconomic groups. American Medical Association Available at: http//wwwama-assn.org/ama/pub/category/2661.html.

Diaz Jr. VA. Cultural factors in preventive care: Latinos. Primary Care; *Clinics in Office Practice.* 2002;29(3).

Institute of Medicine. Unequal treatment: confronting racial and ethnic disparities in health care. Available at: http://books.nap.edu/books/030908265X/html/.

National Center for Cultural Competence. Available at: http://www.georgetown.edu/research/gudc/ncc6.html.

Recommendations to Correct Error-Prone Aspects of Prescription Writing, NCCMERP Council Recommendation, adopted Sept. 4, 1996, Available at: http://www.nccmerp.org.

Rodriguez MA. Cultural and linguistic competence: improving quality in family violence health care interventions. *Clinics in Family Practice.* March 2003.

Witt D, Brawer R, Plumb J. Cultural factors in preventive care: African-Americans. Primary care; *Clinics in Office Practice.* 2002.29(3).

Yarnall KSH et al. Primary care: Is there enough time for prevention? *Am J Public Health.* 2003;93:635. Available at: http://www.acgme.org.

30

Final Examination

Mark A. Graber and Jason K. Wilbur

This is your final exam. See how you do.

1. Which of the following is a contraindication to use of sulfasalazine in Crohn disease?

A) Aspirin allergy.
B) Heme positive stools.
C) Fever.
D) Platelet count <100,000.

See p. 265.

2. Which of the following tests is the MOST sensitive for the diagnosis of bacterial overgrowth syndrome (of the GI tract)?

A) Breath urea test.
B) Breath xylose test.
C) Breath hydrogen test.
D) CLO test.

See p. 268.

3. Which of the following is the most appropriate treatment for menorrhagia in a 42-year-old female hypertensive smoker?

A) Low androgenic progesterone oral contraceptive.
B) Progesterone IUD (eg, Mirena, Progestasert).
C) Copper T IUD.
D) Low estrogen oral contraceptive.

See p. 512.

4. Which of the following must be present to make the diagnosis of pelvic inflammatory disease?

A) Adnexal pain.
B) Elevated WBC count.
C) Elevated CRP.
D) Temperature of >38°C.

See p. 525.

5. This ECG shown on page 887 represents an:

A) Inferior wall MI.
B) Anterior wall MI.
C) Inferolateral MI.
D) Normal ECG.

See p. 105.

6. The most appropriate initial treatment for this rhythm in a stable patient, shown on page 888, is:

A) Amiodarone.
B) Adenosine.
C) Diltiazem.
D) Lidocaine.

See p. 97.

7. The criteria for lone atrial fibrillation include all of the following EXCEPT:

A) Absence of hypertension.
B) Absence of diabetes.
C) Absence of *acquired* valvular heart disease.
D) Age <65 years.

See p. 72.

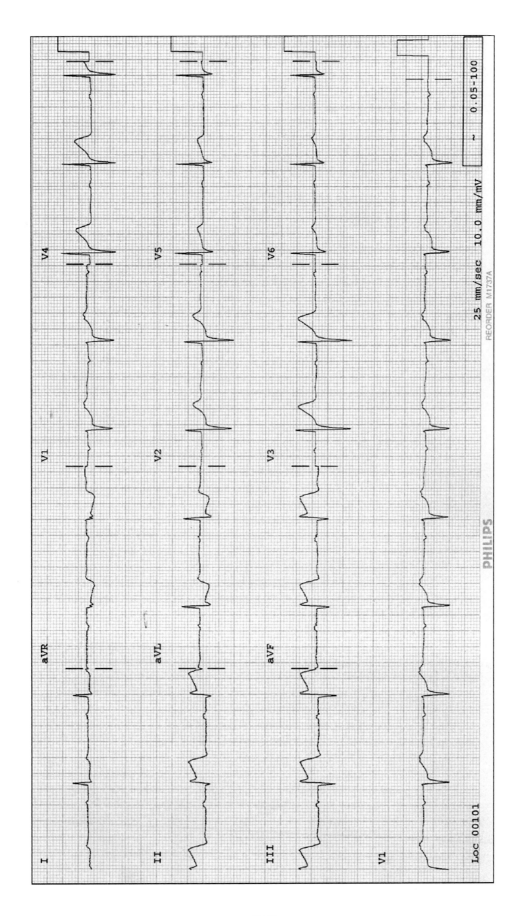

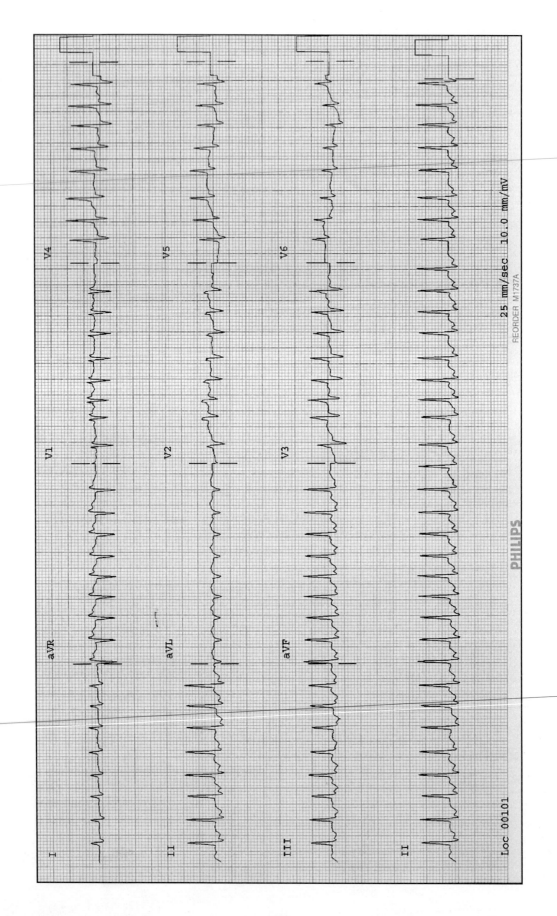

8. Which of the following is the preferred antiplatelet drug for treating chest pain in the ED?

A) Aspirin 81 mg PO.
B) Aspirin 325 mg PO.
C) Clopidogrel 75 mg PO.
D) Clopidogrel 300 mg PO.
E) 2B/IIIA glycoprotein inhibitor.

See p. 49.

9. Which of the following is NOT a contraindication to the use of tPA in MI?

A) Blood pressure of >180/110.
B) Noncompressible vascular puncture (eg, subclavian line).
C) Major surgery within 3 weeks.
D) Menstrual bleeding.

See p. 53.

10. In a patient with coronary artery disease, or >20% risk of cardiac disease in the next 10 years, what is the recommended LDL goal?

A) <130 mg/dL.
B) <110 mg/dL.
C) <100 mg/dL.
D) There is no LDL goal if the HDL is >50 mg/dL.

See p. 59.

11. Your patient has an elevation of his liver function tests after starting an HMG-CoA reductase inhibitor. When would you stop this patient's HMG-CoA reductase inhibitor?

A) Doubling of LFTs.
B) Tripling of LFTs.
C) Quadrupling of LFTs.
D) Only when there is biopsy evidence of bridging fibrosis.

See p. 59.

12. Which of the following is NOT an *absolute* contraindication to cardiac exercise testing?

A) Unstable angina.
B) Recent pulmonary embolism.
C) Active pericarditis.
D) Left bundle branch block.

See p. 62.

13. Which of the following does NOT improve cardiovascular mortality in CHF?

A) Digoxin.
B) Spironolactone.
C) ACE inhibitors.
D) β-Blockers.

See p. 78.

14. In general, what will happen with an innocent flow murmur during a Valsalva maneuver?

A) It gets louder.
B) It gets softer.
C) It is unchanged in volume.
D) The sound becomes more harsh.

See p. 485.

15. In a study of drug A, 50% of patients in the treatment arm benefit versus 25% in the placebo group. What is the number needed to treat (NNT)?

A) 2
B) 4
C) 6
D) 8

See p. 871.

16. The most common cause of erythema multiforme is:

A) Herpes zoster.
B) Streptococcal pharyngitis.
C) Genital herpes.
D) Rhus exposure (poison ivy).

See p. 599.

17. Topical tretinoin (Retin-A) is most effective in what kind of acne?

A) Cystic/nodular.
B) Inflammatory papular.
C) Pustular.
D) Comedonal.

See p. 596.

18. Which of the following is true regarding isotretinoin (Accutane)?

A) Women should be on one form of birth control before using this drug.
B) Pregnancy should be avoided for 3 months after discontinuation of this drug.
C) Monthly pregnancy tests should be done on women who are sexually active with men.
D) Isotretinoin may increase the HDL.

See p. 597.

19. Which of the following statements is true regarding gastric lavage in a patient with a toxic ingestion?

A) Gastric lavage should be done if it has been <4 hours after the ingestion.
B) Gastric lavage should be done until the returned material is clear (maximum of 10 L).
C) Gastric lavage is associated with esophageal injury and aspiration.
D) Gastric lavage is indicated for petroleum distillates within 1 hour of ingestion.

See p. 1.

20. Ipecac:

A) Should not be used, period.
B) Can be used if the ingestion may cause mental status changes.
C) Is effective if used within 30 minutes of an ingestion.
D) Is available OTC in U.S. pharmacies.

See p. 1.

21. Which of the following is NOT seen with an anticholinergic overdose?

A) Dry, flushed, skin.
B) Miosis.
C) Confusion.
D) Low-grade fever.

See p. 6.

22. Which of the following is NOT a cause of an elevated anion gap acidosis?

A) Methanol and other ingestions (eg, salicylate).
B) Diabetic ketoacidosis.
C) Uremia.
D) GI bicarbonate loss.

See p. 9.

23. Reperfusion of extremities in hypothermia can cause all of the following EXCEPT:

A) Acidosis.
B) Hypokalemia.
C) Paradoxical central temperature drop.
D) Arrhythmia.

See p. 25.

24. Which of the following statements is true?

A) A negative pregnancy test effectively rules out ectopic pregnancy.
B) Absence of an adnexal mass effectively rules out ectopic pregnancy.
C) Any women of reproductive age with a uterus in the ED with abdominal pain is pregnant until proven otherwise.
D) The HCG should double every 5 days early in a normal pregnancy (eg, when one is worried about an ectopic pregnancy).

See pp. 31–32.

25. Which of the following is NOT included in the drug cocktail for the unconscious patient?

A) Glucose.
B) Thiamine.
C) Naloxone (Narcan).
D) Flumazenil (Romazicon).

See p. 3.

26. Which of the following is indicated in the child with croup (laryngotracheobronchitis)?

A) Amoxicillin.
B) Azithromycin.
C) Dexamethasone.
D) Oral theophylline.

See p. 45.

27. What is the appropriate course of action after treating a child with croup with inhaled epinephrine?

A) Admission for observation.
B) Admission if room air oxygen saturation is ≤95%.
C) Observation for 12 hours followed by discharge if stable.
D) Observation for 2 hours followed by discharge if stable.

See p. 46.

28. Which of the following is the ONE BEST drug indicated for dyspnea in the terminally ill patient who wishes to be DNR?

A) Buccal scopolamine.
B) Lorazepam or other benzodiazepine.
C) Morphine or other opiate.
D) Nebulized lidocaine.

See p. 851.

29. Which of the following is the ONE BEST drug to reduce headache and confusion secondary to CNS tumor?

A) Acetaminophen.
B) Dexamethasone.
C) Morphine.
D) Sumatriptan.

See pp. 851–852.

30. What blood level of morphine is the most appropriate when treating pain from a terminal cause?

A) 1 micrograms/dL.
B) 5 micrograms/dL.
C) 10 micrograms/dL.
D) Blood levels are irrelevant to ascertain the appropriate dose of morphine in the terminally ill.

See p. 854.

31. How frequently should methadone be dosed when used for pain control in the terminally ill?

A) Q 12 hours.
B) Q 8 hours.
C) Q 4 hours.
D) Methadone should not be used for pain management in the terminally ill.

See p. 855.

32. Which of the following statements is true about a gastric feeding tube in the demented elderly?

A) It increases the patient's quality of life.
B) It should be used as a comfort measure only.
C) It reduces mortality.
D) It does nothing to improve quality of life but can cause complications.

See p. 857.

33. Which of the following statements is true about the treatment of gastroesophageal reflux disease (GERD)?

A) Treatment of *H. pylori* is effective in curing GERD.
B) Treatment should always start with a proton pump inhibitor.
C) Surgical options (eg, fundoplication) are often suboptimal with patients still requiring medication.
D) Esomeprazole is vastly superior to omeprazole.

See p. 251.

34. Which of the following statements is true regarding Barrett esophagus?

A) All patients with GERD should have an endoscopy to stage their disease vis-à-vis Barrett esophagus.
B) Barrett esophagus is a change from the normal columnar epithelium to squamous epithelium.
C) Barrett esophagus is present in >50% of patients with GERD.
D) Barrett esophagus can regress with adequate treatment of GERD.

See p. 252.

35. Which of the following is NOT a component of CREST syndrome?

A) Calcinosis.
B) Renal failure.
C) Esophageal dysmotility.
D) Sclerodactyly.

See p. 254.

36. Which of the following histories in a patient with GERD is most concerning for serious underlying disease?

A) Food bolus impaction on two separate occasions.
B) Dysphagia to liquids followed in several months with dysphagia to solids.
C) Reflux of undigested food at night.
D) Halitosis.

See p. 250.

37. Which of the following is an appropriate test of cure for *H. pylori*?

A) Stool antigen test done 1 month after finishing treatment.
B) Serum antibody test done 3 months after finishing treatment.
C) CLO test done 1 week after finishing treatment.
D) Breath urea test done 1 week after finishing treatment.

See pp. 258–259.

38. NSAIDs can cause ulceration in:

A) Stomach.
B) Duodenum.
C) Colon.
D) All of the above.

See p. 259.

39. Which of the following is the MOST specific test for gluten enteropathy (nontropical sprue)?

A) Antiendomysial IgA antibody.
B) Tissue transglutaminase antibody.
C) Antigliadin antibody.
D) Breath hydrogen test.

See p. 269.

40. *C. difficile* colitis has been linked to all of the following EXCEPT:

A) Hospitalization.
B) Use of fluoroquinolones.
C) Use of PPIs.
D) Use of H_2-blockers.

See p. 297.

41. Which of the following is the one best screening test for hepatitis C?

A) Quantitative HVC PCR.
B) Hepatitis C antibody.
C) RIBA.
D) Qualitative HVC PCR.

See p. 272.

42. Which of the following is a relative contraindication to treatment for hepatitis C with interferon?

A) Fever.
B) Severe depression.
C) Severe osteoarthritis.
D) Severe eczema.

See p. 273.

43. Routine prenatal screening in the first trimester includes all of the following EXCEPT:

A) Blood type and antibody screen.
B) Hepatitis B surface antigen.
C) HIV antibody.
D) MSAFP (maternal serum alpha-fetoprotein).
E) Rubella antibody.

See p. 492.

44. A 25-year-old G5P4 female at 26 weeks' gestation presents to labor and delivery with abdominal pain. The pain is sharp or tearing and located in her lower abdomen. She has not had any contractions. She began to have vaginal spotting before she came in. Her pregnancy has been complicated by tobacco use and hypertension. What is the most likely diagnosis?

A) Cervical cancer.
B) Normal labor.
C) Placenta previa.
D) Placental abruption.
E) Uterine rupture.

See p. 493.

45. An 18-year-old G0 female presents for a physical exam and her first Pap smear. She has recently started sexual activity and has one lifetime partner. The results of the Pap smear show low-grade squamous intraepithelial lesion (LSIL). In accordance with guidelines, you recommend:

A) Immediate colposcopy.
B) Immediate referral for excisional procedure.
C) Return in 12 months for Pap smear.
D) Return in 3 months for Pap smear.
E) Return in 6 months for colposcopy and Pap smear.

See p. 544.

46. A 48-year-old female presents with menopausal symptoms. She has had a total hysterectomy but her ovaries are intact. She would like to know the benefits and risks of taking estrogen-only hormone replacement therapy. You tell her that estrogen-only HRT is associated with:

A) Decreased risk of breast cancer.

B) Decreased risk of ovarian cancer.

C) Increased risk of colon cancer.

D) Increased risk of osteoporosis.

E) Increased risk of stroke.

See p. 529.

47. **A 22-year-old G2P2 female is ready to leave the hospital on postpartum day 2 after NSVD, but she develops lower abdominal pain and fever. She denies urinary symptoms. She reports constipation and moderate lochia. Her temperature is 38.8°C. She had prolonged rupture of membranes and prolonged labor, and the placenta was removed manually. The most appropriate course of action now is:**

A) Discharge with acetaminophen for fever and follow up in 2 days.

B) Discharge with amoxicillin and follow up in 2 days.

C) Keep the patient in the hospital and obtain cultures for gonorrhea and chlamydia.

D) Keep the patient in the hospital and start IV gentamicin and clindamycin.

E) Manual exploration of the uterus for retained placenta.

See pp. 496–497.

48. **The USPSTF recommends screening for osteoporosis in:**

A) All adults ≥65 years.

B) All men ≥75 years.

C) All women ≥65 years.

D) All women at onset of menopause.

E) Women ≥50 years who smoke.

See p. 696.

49. **A 79-year-old male presents with his wife with complaint that he has been more forgetful over the past month. The patient agrees and complains of forgetting where he put things, where the car is parked, and names of acquaintances. Also, he is more irritable and angers easily. He has trouble sleeping, and he has lost 5 pounds. He is healthy and takes no medications. He has poor eye contact, a blunted affect, and poor concentration. His vitals and physical exam are** otherwise normal. **He can recall 3 items and draw a clock with no difficulty. The most likely cause of his symptoms is:**

A) Delirium due to metastatic carcinoma.

B) Delirium due to underlying systemic infection.

C) Dementia due to Alzheimer disease.

D) Dementia due to stroke.

E) Depression.

See p. 691.

50. **Which of the following statements is true?**

A) An elevated troponin is always indicative of cardiac ischemia/infarct.

B) Troponin rises before CPK and stays elevated for a longer period of time.

C) Pulmonary embolism and renal failure are two causes of an elevated troponin.

D) CPK is overall the most sensitive (but not specific) cardiac marker for cardiac ischemia.

See p. 49.

51. **Which of the following is NOT a class 1 indication for tPA in a patient with an acute myocardial infarction?**

A) >1 mm ST elevation in 2 or more contiguous leads.

B) Pain <10 hours.

C) Age <75 years.

D) New complete bundle branch block and typical history suggestive of MI.

See p. 54.

52. **An 80-year-old female nursing home resident with dementia recently started refusing medication and slapping at the staff when they try to bathe her. The nurse at the care center calls to request something for her agitation. As the safest and most effective intervention, you recommend:**

A) A behavior log to track when the agitation occurs and what might be causing it.

B) Haloperidol 1 mg IV prior to bathing and medication administration.

C) Haloperidol 1 mg PO BID.

D) Restraints with bathing.

E) Risperdal 0.5 mg PO QHS.

See p. 710.

53. Delirium in the hospitalized elderly patient can be prevented by implementing all of the following interventions upon admission EXCEPT:

A) Ensuring patient has access to usual aids (hearing aids, glasses, etc).
B) Early mobilization.
C) Lorazepam 1 mg QHS.
D) Noise reduction at night.
E) Orientation stimuli.

See p. 701.

54. A 75-year-old male with mild dementia, atrial fibrillation, osteoarthritis, and depression presents after sustaining a fall in his home 1 week ago. His son states, "He is a little banged up but otherwise fine." Your evaluation should include all of the following EXCEPT:

A) Asking about potential neglect and abuse.
B) CT scan of the brain.
C) Medication review.
D) Neurologic examination.
E) Observation of the patient ambulating.

See p. 702.

55. A 75-year-old female fell and injured her hip. She did not fracture it but has significant pain. She has a remote history of peptic ulcer disease. She takes lisinopril for hypertension and phenytoin for a seizure disorder. Which pain medication will be safest for her to take?

A) Aspirin.
B) Meperidine.
C) Oxycodone.
D) Piroxicam.
E) Propoxyphene.

See p. 712.

56. You are considering treating a 65-year-old male with supplemental testosterone because of low serum testosterone levels associated with fatigue, muscle weakness, and mild depression. After initiating testosterone, it is most important to check which of the following?

A) Creatinine.
B) Hemoglobin.
C) Potassium.
D) Sodium.

See p. 571.

57. The most appropriate next step for a 60-year-old male with a PSA level 12.5 ng/mL is:

A) One month of a fluoroquinolone followed by repeat rectal exam.
B) Referral for prostate biopsy.
C) Repeat PSA in 6–12 months.
D) Transrectal ultrasound of the prostate.

See p. 572.

58. A 30-year-old male presents with difficulty obtaining an erection sufficient for penetration. He has GERD and takes cimetidine. He reports a good relationship with his wife and denies depression. He does not smoke and rarely drinks alcohol. The most appropriate intervention now is:

A) To order a testosterone level.
B) To perform cardiac stress testing.
C) To refer him to a urologist.
D) To replace cimetidine with omeprazole.
E) To send him to a psychologist.

See p. 576.

59. Sudden cardiac death in adolescent athletes is MOST OFTEN due to:

A) Hypertrophic cardiomyopathy.
B) Long QT syndrome.
C) Myocardial infarction.
D) Tetralogy of Fallot.

See p. 484.

60. A 17-year-old female runner with secondary amenorrhea should be further evaluated with all of the following EXCEPT:

A) Assessing calcium intake.
B) MRI of the pituitary.
C) Screening for eating disorders.
D) Urine β-hCG.

See pp. 482–483.

61. Gynecomastia in an adolescent male occurs as a response to which of the following mechanisms?

A) Excessive DHEA.
B) Excessive estrogen compared to testosterone.

C) Excessive growth hormone.

D) Excessive progesterone compared to testosterone.

E) Rapidly developing obesity.

See p. 564.

62. Treatment for a patient in diabetic ketoacidosis includes all of the following EXCEPT:

A) Aggressive volume replacement.

B) Frequent glucose monitoring.

C) Insulin.

D) Potassium.

E) Sodium bicarbonate.

See p. 351.

63. A 33-year-old male with depression had been taking paroxetine 60 mg daily for a year for depression. Because of sexual problems, he decided to try another medication, and his doctor prescribed bupropion. He stopped the paroxetine one day and started bupropion the next. He comes in 5 days later feeling dizzy, nauseated, and fatigued. He complains of myalgias and insomnia. These symptoms are most likely caused by:

A) Adverse effects of bupropion.

B) Hyperthyroidism.

C) Major depression.

D) Serotonin syndrome.

E) SSRI discontinuation syndrome.

See p. 778.

64. A FREQUENT side effect of metformin is:

A) Constipation.

B) Hypoglycemia.

C) Lactic acidosis.

D) Renal failure.

E) Weight loss.

See p. 355.

65. A 40-year-old male presents with generalized weakness for 1 month. He has lost some weight, approximately 10 pounds. He briefly lost consciousness yesterday while getting out of bed. He denies depression, drug, or alcohol use, and any significant medical history. He is hypotensive but not tachycardic. He has orthostatic hypotension

as well. Lab tests reveal mild anemia, low sodium, elevated potassium, and normal TSH, BUN, creatinine, and glucose. To confirm your presumptive diagnosis you order:

A) 24-hour urine catecholamines.

B) Free T4 and T3.

C) Plasma metanephrines.

D) Serum cortisol and ACTH.

E) Serum testosterone.

See p. 348.

66. A 29-year-old female day-care teacher presents with a severely pruritic rash that started at her wrists and has progressed to the web spaces of her fingers, under her arms, around her waist, and around her nipples. On exam, she has multiple excoriations and few small, erythematous papules. The MOST APPROPRIATE next step is:

A) Biopsy of normal-appearing skin.

B) Biopsy of one of the papules.

C) Empiric treatment with topical clotrimazole.

D) Empiric treatment with topical lindane 1%.

E) Empiric treatment with topical permethrin 5%.

See p. 308.

67. You find a new and suspicious skin lesion in a patient who has had a liver transplant for hepatitis C. You plan to perform a biopsy. If the skin lesion turns out to be malignant, it will most likely be:

A) Basal cell carcinoma.

B) Distant metastasis from liver cancer.

C) Melanoma.

D) Squamous cell carcinoma.

See p. 585.

68. A patient presents with thickened, yellowish, dystrophic toenails. What is the most appropriate next step?

A) Recommend that the patient return for toenail removal.

B) Send nail scrapings for KOH stain and/or fungal culture.

C) Start treatment with a topical antifungal.

D) Start treatment with an oral antifungal.

See p. 586.

69. The major Jones criteria for rheumatic fever include all of the following EXCEPT:

A) Carditis.
B) Fever.
C) Polyarthritis.
D) Subcutaneous nodules.
E) Sydenham chorea.

See p. 373.

70. A 62-year-old female presents to the ED with a sudden hole in her right visual field developing today. She also has a right temporal headache present for the last 2 weeks, shoulder and neck pain for a month, and weight loss of 5 pounds. She is slightly hypertensive and has a prominent tender vessel at the right side of her head. Her CBC is normal but the ESR is 85 mm/hour. What is the most appropriate course of action?

A) Administer IV methylprednisolone and admit for further evaluation.
B) Admit for cardiac monitoring and rule out myocardial infarction.
C) Discharge to home with oral antibiotics.
D) Discharge to home with referral to an ophthalmologist in the next week.
E) Perform a CT scan of the brain and discharge to home if normal.

See p. 376.

71. A 60-year-old female with diabetic nephropathy is hospitalized with chest pain and a cardiac catheterization is planned. Which one of the following is the best option to reduce her risk of contrast-induced nephropathy?

A) Administer ketorolac and IV saline.
B) Administer mannitol and IV saline.
C) Administer N-acetylcysteine and IV saline.
D) Administer sodium bicarbonate and IV saline.

See p. 181.

72. A 58-year-old male with hypertension, diabetes, heart failure, and chronic kidney disease (stage 4, GFR ~25 mL/min/1.73 m²) presents for follow-up. His current medications are insulin, aspirin, metoprolol, and lisinopril. His blood pressure is 142/86 and he has significant dependent edema. His labs reveal a serum potassium of

5.3 meq/L. To achieve his blood pressure to goal (<130/80) while avoiding adverse events, the best initial step is:

A) Discontinue lisinopril.
B) Furosemide 20 mg PO QAM.
C) Hydrochlorothiazide 12.5 mg PO QAM.
D) Increase lisinopril.
E) Losartan 25 mg PO daily.

See p. 209.

73. Which of the following is most likely to cause hypokalemia?

A) Excessive use of "lite" salt.
B) Hypoaldosteronism.
C) Hypomagnesemia.
D) Overdose of propranolol.
E) Renal tubular acidosis type 4.

See pp. 196–197.

74. The fractional excretion of sodium (FENa) is useful for determining:

A) If the patient has true hyponatremia.
B) Whether the patient has oliguric or anuric renal failure.
C) Whether the renal failure is due to acute tubular necrosis or another cause.
D) Whether the renal failure is due to intrinsic renal disease or a prerenal cause.
E) Why the patient has hyponatremia.

See p. 203.

75. All of the following are consistent with a diagnosis of SIADH (syndrome of inappropriate antidiuretic hormone secretion) EXCEPT:

A) High urine osmolality.
B) Low plasma osmolality.
C) Low urine sodium.
D) Normal adrenal function.
E) Normal thyroid function.

See pp. 203–204.

76. A 21-year-old male is brought in the ED by his girlfriend after he overdosed on aspirin. He took "a bottle, maybe 100 pills or so," but he denies other ingestions. He complains only of nausea. He becomes more somnolent during the

evaluation. He is slightly tachycardic and febrile with a normal blood pressure. His blood gas shows: pH 7.38, PaCO$_2$ 23 mm Hg, PaO$_2$ 98 mm Hg HCO$_3$ 15meq/L. His creatinine, CBC, and electrolytes are normal, except for low potassium. What is the best description of this patient's blood gas?

A) Metabolic acidosis and metabolic alkalosis.
B) Metabolic acidosis and respiratory alkalosis.
C) Metabolic alkalosis and respiratory acidosis.
D) Normal blood gas (no acidosis or alkalosis).

See p. 163.

77. An otherwise healthy 70-year-old female is admitted and started on ceftriaxone and azithromycin for pneumonia. On hospital day 3, her serum creatinine is found to have tripled from admission. She is mildly nauseated and has an erythematous, macular rash on her trunk and arms. Her CBC shows that her white cell count has declined from admission, but she now has a prominent eosinophilia. Urinalysis shows 1 + protein, and urine sediment shows white cell casts and eosinophils. The most appropriate next step is:

A) Add metronidazole to her antibiotic regimen.
B) Bolus with IV 0.9% saline.
C) Consult a nephrologist for possible renal biopsy.
D) Discontinue ceftriaxone and consider an alternative antibiotic.
E) Start furosemide to improve urine output.

See p. 215.

78. You perform joint aspiration on a patient with a painful, swollen knee. Microscopic exam of the fluid shows rhomboid-shaped, positively birefringent crystals. Which one of the following is the most likely to alleviate the patient's symptoms?

A) Acetaminophen daily.
B) Allopurinol daily.
C) Ceftriaxone IM.
D) Corticosteroid injection into the knee.

See p. 381.

79. A 23-year-old male with HIV stopped taking all of his medications 3 months ago because of cost. He was feeling fine until 3 weeks ago when

he developed a cough. He now has daily fevers (T~101°F), a nonproductive cough, dyspnea on exertion, fatigue, chills, and tightness in his chest with inspiration. His exam is notable for fever, diaphoresis, bilateral crackles with inspiration, and mild tachypnea. Chest x-ray shows diffuse bilateral interstitial infiltrates. Which of the following is the most likely causative agent for this pulmonary infection?

A) Adenovirus.
B) Cryptococcus neoformans.
C) Mycobacterium tuberculosis.
D) *Pneumocystis jiroveci* (PCP).
E) Toxoplasma gondii.

See p. 323.

80. Each of the following patients is found to have asymptomatic bacteruria. Which one should be treated with a course of antibiotics?

A) An 88-year-old female nursing home resident.
B) A 20-year-old pregnant patient.
C) A 75-year-old male with an indwelling Foley catheter for BPH.
D) All of the above.

See p. 300.

81. Which of the following will cause a low SAAG ascites?

A) Nephrotic syndrome.
B) Portal hypertension.
C) Bud-Chiari syndrome.
D) Cirrhosis.

See p. 277.

82. Which of the following is not useful in the treatment of hepatic encephalopathy?

A) Lactulose.
B) Polyethylene glycol (Go-lytely).
C) Oral neomycin.
D) Enemas for acute encephalopathy.

See p. 279.

83. Which of the following is NOT useful in the treatment of alcoholic liver disease with portal hypertension?

A) Pentoxifylline (Trental).
B) Nadolol.
C) Isosorbide dinitrate.
D) Cilostazol (Pletal).

See p. 277.

84. Which of the following is generally true in alcohol- or toxin-related liver disease?

A) AST is >2 times than ALT.
B) ALT is >2 times than AST.
C) ALT and AST are both elevated to the same degree.
D) The GGT is specific for liver disease and higher than either the ALT or AST.

See p. 283.

85. The most common cause of pancreatitis in the United States is:

A) Alcohol.
B) Cholelithiasis.
C) Thiazide diuretics.
D) Viruses.

See p. 285.

86. Which of the following is true about the treatment of pancreatitis?

A) Antibiotics should be used in most cases of pancreatitis.
B) Enteral feedings with the feeding tube in the jejunum is the preferred method of nutrition.
C) Pseudocysts must be drained for pancreatitis to resolve.
D) The Ransom criteria can be used at the time of admission to accurately predict mortality.

See p. 286.

87. Which of the following does NOT promote gastric emptying in gastric paresis?

A) Erythromycin.
B) Metoclopramide.
C) Azithromycin.
D) Cisapride.

See pp. 288–289.

88. Appropriate antibiotic treatment of diverticulitis includes all of the following EXCEPT:

A) Ciprofloxacin + metronidazole.
B) Amoxicillin clavulanate.
C) Trimethoprim/Sulfamethoxazole + metronidazole.
D) Clindamycin + metronidazole.

See p. 291.

89. All of the following are causes of nonalcoholic fatty liver disease EXCEPT:

A) Statin use.
B) Hypothyroidism.
C) Diabetes.
D) Obesity.

See p. 282.

90. The most common cause of the development of drug resistance in HIV is:

A) Failure to include zidovudine in the treatment regimen.
B) Failure to initiate treatment until the patient has a known AIDS-defining illness.
C) Poor compliance with medications.
D) Failure to include a protease inhibitor in the treatment regimen.

See p. 319.

91. At what CD4 + level should one initiate prophylactic treatment for *Pneumocystis jiroveci* (previously *Pneumocystis carinii*)?

A) CD4 + ≤50.
B) CD4 + ≤75.
C) CD4 + ≤100.
D) CD4 + ≤200.

See p. 326.

92. Which of the following statements regarding Pap smear screening in an HIV + woman is true?

A) No modification is needed in the Pap smear regimen.
B) If the CD4 + count is normal and the patient has 2 normal Pap smears at 1-year intervals, you can go back to routine screening.
C) If the patient has a CD4 + count of <200, screening should be done Q 6 months regardless of whether or not the patient has had negative Pap smears.
D) Pap smears can be suspended in HIV positive patients because they will likely die from HIV before they die from cervical cancer.

See p. 329.

93. Which of the following statements best reflects the current thinking about treating influenza?

A) Rimantadine and amantadine are most effective against influenza B.

B) Treatment with oseltamivir (Tamiflu) is highly effective thus negating the need for influenza vaccine.

C) Oseltamivir must be started within 48 hours of symptom onset to be of benefit.

D) There is no resistance of influenza A to oseltamivir.

See p. 295.

94. The most common bacterial organism causing meningitis in adults is:

A) Pneumococcus.

B) Meningococcus.

C) Haemophilus.

D) Listeria.

See p. 299.

95. The recommended empirical antibiotic treatment for meningitis in an adult is:

A) Ceftriaxone.

B) Ceftriaxone + vancomycin.

C) Ceftriaxone + ciprofloxacin.

D) Ceftriaxone + TMP/SMX.

See p. 299.

96. Which of the following patients needs isoniazid treatment?

A) A patient with no risk factors who has a PPD reaction of 5 mm.

B) A patient with recent exposure to TB and a PPD reaction of 5 mm.

C) A health-care worker with a PPD reaction of 5 mm.

D) A health-care worker with a PPD reaction of 10 mm and a positive chest radiograph.

See p. 303.

97. All of the following can be used for malaria prophylaxis EXCEPT:

A) Doxycycline.

B) Mefloquine.

C) Azithromycin.

D) Atovaquone/proguanil (Malarone).

See p. 313.

98. Which of the following drugs is LEAST LIKELY to slow proteinuria?

A) Enalapril.

B) Losartan.

C) Verapamil.

D) Nifedipine.

See pp. 85–86.

99. Which of the following profiles are you likely to see in a patient with a prerenal cause of elevated creatinine?

A) Urine sodium <20, fractional excretion of sodium <1%.

B) Urine sodium <20, fractional excretion of sodium >2%.

C) Urine sodium >40, fractional excretion of sodium <1%.

D) Urine sodium >40, fractional excretion of sodium >2%.

See p. 200.

100. Aldosterone resistance (such as occurs with diabetic nephropathy) *or* hypoaldosteronism will present with which of the following?

A) Hypokalemia.

B) Hyperkalemia.

C) Hyperphosphatemia.

D) Hypophosphatemia.

See p. 182.

101. Which of the following regimens is NOT recommended for treatment of a simple cystitis?

A) Amoxicillin 500 mg PO TID for 3 days.

B) Levoflxacin 250 mg PO daily for 3 days.

C) Nitrofurantoin 100 mg PO TID for 7 days.

D) TMP/SMX 1 PO TID for 3 days.

See p. 32.

102. Which of the following statements is true regarding the diagnosis of urolithiasis?

A) >90% of patients will have blood in their urine at the time of diagnosis.
B) Urolithiasis may be difficult to differentiate from aortic dissection at the initial time of presentation.
C) Hematuria will reliably differentiate urolithiasis from aortic dissection.
D) A negative FAST ultrasound scan is considered the standard and if negative rules out urolithiasis.

See p. 189.

103. The definition of nephrotic syndrome requires all of the following EXCEPT:

A) Hypoalbuminemia.
B) Urine albumin excretion >3 grams per day.
C) Edema.
D) Renal biopsy.

See p. 195.

104. Based on current U.S. guidelines, which of the following patients should have a carotid endarterectomy?

A) 60-year-old female with a unilateral symptomatic 70% carotid plaque.
B) 60-year-old male or female with an asymptomatic 69% carotid plaque.
C) Patient of either gender with bilateral 50% carotid plaque, symptomatic or asymptomatic.
D) None of the above meets current qualification criterion.

See p. 608.

105. If cost were NOT an issue, which of the following drugs/drug combinations would be the ideal regimen for the secondary prevention of stroke?

A) Aspirin + clopidogrel (Plavix).
B) Aspirin + dipyridamole.
C) Aspirin alone.
D) Clopidogrel alone.

See p. 607.

106. Which of the following drugs is NOT associated with rebound headaches?

A) Acetaminophen.
B) DHE.
C) Nortriptyline.
D) Sumatriptan.

See pp. 616–617.

107. Which one of the following agents is most effective for controlling the pain of peripheral neuropathy?

A) Tricyclic antidepressant.
B) Gabapentin or other newer antiepileptic drug (eg, Topamax).
C) Oxycodone or other narcotic.
D) Carbamazepine or other traditional antiepileptic.

See p. 613.

108. Which one of the following entities presents with reflexes preserved?

A) Guillain-Barré.
B) Amyotrophic lateral sclerosis.
C) Charcot-Marie-Tooth disease.
D) Diabetic neuropathy.

See p. 622.

109. The risk of having a second seizure after a first febrile seizure is:

A) 2%–5%; the same as the rest of the population.
B) 6%–10%; slightly higher than the general population.
C) 11%–15%; significantly higher than the general population.
D) Unknown.

See p. 637.

110. You determine that a 77-year-old female has Parkinson disease that is interfering with her daily life. The best drug or drug combination to alleviate her symptoms and improve her function is:

A) A COMT inhibitor (eg, Entacapone).
B) A dopamine agonist (eg, Requip).
C) Levodopa/carbidopa (eg, Sinemet).
D) Apomorphine.

See p. 628.

111. Skinnier, politically correct Santas are in vogue this year. Your patient is in a tizzy: he has played Santa for years without the need for pillows. He wants to keep up his tradition as St. Nick. What can you tell him about weight-reduction surgery?

A) "Sorry, even though you may lose weight, it will not help your overall health."

B) "You must have a BMI >40 kg/m² before qualifying for bariatric surgery regardless of other underlying conditions."

C) "You must have a BMI of >35 kg/m² and significant reversible disease to qualify for bariatric surgery."

D) "The reindeer union says it won't work if Santa's weight is <300 pounds—they need to keep 8 reindeer working the sleigh at all times."

See p. 810.

112. Which of the following patients has an indication for cataract surgery?

A) Vision 20/100 bilaterally in a patient who has no visual complaints or functional impairment.

B) Vision 20/20 OD and 10/100 OS in a patient who can see well enough to do everything she desires.

C) Vision 20/30 OD and 20/30 OS in a patient who is bothered by her inability to quilt.

D) Vision unknown in a patient who can carry out all ADLs to her own satisfaction.

See p. 660.

113. All of the following intraocular muscles are innervated by cranial nerve III EXCEPT:

A) Inferior oblique.
B) Inferior rectus.
C) Lateral rectus.
D) Medial rectus.
E) Superior rectus.

See p. 662.

114. The presence of an RAPD (relative afferent pupillary defect) is indicative of:

A) Cataracts.
B) Large retinal detachment.
C) Bleed into the anterior chamber.
D) Severe refractive error.

See pp. 640–641.

115. A 70-year-old male patient presents with complaint of severe unilateral visual loss. He has no other symptoms. Here is an image of his fundus. His diagnosis is:

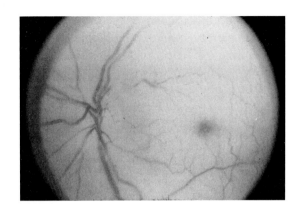

A) Acute glaucoma.
B) Acute venous disruption.
C) Acute arterial occlusion.
D) Diabetic retinopathy.

See pp. 657–658.

116. You are seeing a 57-year-old-male in your practice who has complaint of bitemporal headache. He checked the Web and decided that he has giant cell (temporal) arteritis. The only thing is that his ESR is only 30 mm/hour. The CRP is not much more edifying. You appropriately respond to him:

A) "You may still have temporal arteritis because 15% or more will have normal ESR and CRP."

B) "You seem to be displaying drug-seeking behavior because you came in to the ER with the same complaint 1 month ago."

C) "You may still have temporal arteritis, but we need to perform a temporal bone biopsy."

D) "You may still have temporal arteritis, but we will need to submit your head to the state lab for formal testing. You don't mind, do you?"

See p. 374.

117. A diagnosis of rheumatoid arthritis can be made after symptoms have been present for at least:

A) 15 minutes.
B) 2 weeks.
C) 6 weeks.
D) 3 months.

See p. 369.

118. You make a diagnosis of rheumatoid (RA) arthritis based on laboratory and clinical criteria. The best time to begin DMARDs (disease modifying antirheumatic drugs) is:

A) At the time of diagnosis.
B) After failure of 2 NSAIDs.
C) After the failure of prednisone.
D) When complications of rheumatoid arthritis occur.

See p. 370.

119. What is the general course of rheumatoid arthritis during pregnancy?

A) Worsening during pregnancy.
B) Worsening during pregnancy but only if methotrexate is used.
C) RA may remit during pregnancy and methotrexate is relatively contraindicated.
D) Morning sickness is worse in those with RA.

See pp. 371–372.

120. Which one of these drugs for gout is relatively contraindicated in those with renal insufficiency?

A) Allopurinol.
B) Probenecid.
C) Prednisone.
D) Colchicine.

See p. 382.

121. With regard to therapy for giant cell arteritis, which of the following statements best describes the appropriate relationship of aspirin, prednisone, and giant cell arteritis?

A) ASA (81 mg/day) can be used as adjunctive therapy for those on prednisone.
B) ASA (325 mg/day) can be used as adjunctive therapy for those on prednisone.
C) High-dose ASA (650 mg/day) can be used in those who do not tolerate prednisone.
D) ASA has no role in the treatment of giant cell arteritis.

See p. 376.

122. Which of the following screening tests is recommended universally for all children in the United States?

A) Eye exam at 24 months.
B) Hearing testing at 1 or 2 days.
C) Hemoglobin at 12 months.
D) Lead level at 12 months.

See p. 441.

123. A 12-month-old female presents to the ED after 24 hours of vomiting, diarrhea, and fever. She is lethargic, tachycardic, and hypotensive with poor skin turgor. What is the most appropriate initial method of providing her fluids?

A) Half-normal saline, 20 mL/kg bolus.
B) Half-normal saline with 5% dextrose, 10 mL/kg bolus.
C) Normal saline, 100 mL/kg bolus.
D) Normal saline, 20 mL/kg bolus.

See p. 39.

124. The best first-line drug treatment for osteoarthritis pain is:

A) Acetaminophen.
B) Celecoxib (Celebrex).
C) Ibuprofen.
D) Naproxen.

See p. 377.

125. The best initial pharmacologic therapy for fibromyalgia pain is:

A) Duloxetine.
B) Ibuprofen.
C) Nortriptyline.
D) Tramadol.

See p. 390.

126. Which of the following should NOT go into the calculus of which antibiotic to use for a patient with community-acquired pneumonia?

A) Appearance of infiltrate on chest x-ray (lobar versus atypical).
B) Comorbid medical conditions.
C) Likelihood of resistant organisms (based on recent antibiotic use, day-care exposure, etc).
D) Patient age.

See p. 157.

127. The use of Depo-Provera should be limited to 2 years because of the risk of:

A) Osteoporosis.
B) Breast cancer.
C) Ovarian cancer.
D) Prolonged or permeant amenorrhea.

See p. 697.

128. Bleeding in a nonpregnant, amenorrheic patient in response to a progesterone challenge (eg, medroxyprogsterone given for 10 days and then stopped) indicates that the patient has sufficient endogenous:

A) FSH.
B) LH.
C) Progesterone.
D) Estrogen.

See p. 361.

129. You get the following results on a vaginal wet prep: pH 5.0 and a positive "whiff" test. The rest of the results got lost. With the information available, the most likely diagnosis is:

A) Vulvovaginal candidiasis.
B) Bacterial vaginosis.
C) Vaginal trichomoniasis.
D) Physiologic vaginal discharge.

See p. 543.

130. When is screening for group B streptococcus in the pregnant female recommended?

A) 30–32 weeks' gestation.
B) 32–34 weeks' gestation.
C) 35–37 weeks' gestation.
D) Intrapartum only.

See pp. 492–493.

131. This fetal tracing shown on page 904, is:

A) Reassuring.
B) Worrisome.
C) An indication for immediate C-section.
D) An indication for the addition of Pitocin.

See pp. 495–496.

132. You are called to see a partner's patient who is G3P2 at 32 weeks' gestation and is having regular contractions. After monitoring and an exam, you suspect that she is in labor. The MOST IMPORTANT step, and the first step to take now, is:

A) Administration of corticosteroids to hasten fetal lung maturation.
B) Administration a tocolytic such as terbutaline.
C) Insertion of a cervical cerclage to delay delivery.
D) Antibiotic therapy (ampicillin) from now until delivery.

See p. 506.

133. At spontaneous rupture of membranes during an otherwise normal labor, you note meconium-stained amniotic fluid. An hour later, this G3P2 female at 41 weeks' gestation delivers a vigorous female infant. The most appropriate intervention now is:

A) Routine neonatal resuscitation with stimulation and warming.
B) Bulb suction of the oropharynx and nasopharynx on the perineum.
C) Tracheal suctioning under direct supervision.
D) Endotracheal intubation and ventilation.

See p. 435.

134. Each of the following infants is undergoing neonatal resuscitation. Which one should receive chest compressions?

A) An infant with a 1-minute Apgar of 3 and a heart rate of 100 bpm.
B) A cyanotic infant receiving blow-by oxygen with a heart rate of 80 bpm.
C) A cyanotic infant receiving positive pressure ventilation with a heart rate of 50 bpm.
D) A cyanotic infant with a heart rate of 60 who is about to be started on positive pressure ventilation.

See p. 437.

135. A 15-month-old male is brought to the clinic by his parents. Like everyone else at his home, he has had some rhinorrhea and diarrhea in the last week. However, 4 hours ago the patient developed episodes of inconsolable crying accompanied by lying in the fetal position for 15–20 minutes at a time. At first his parents were

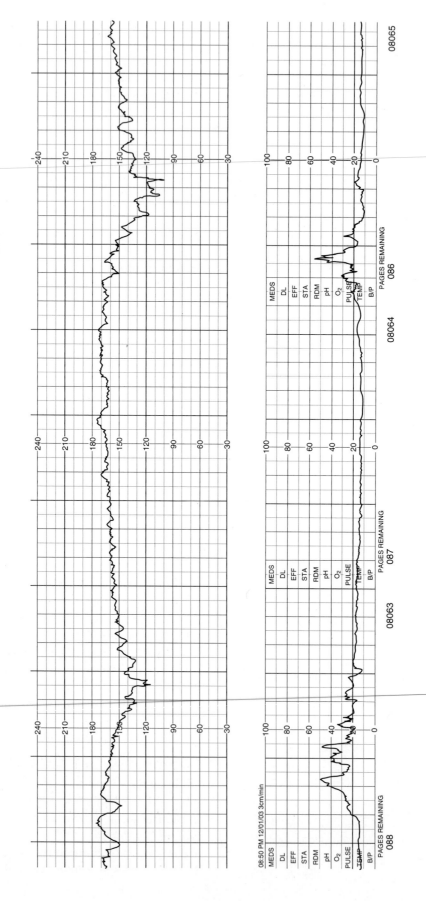

puzzled but not too worried, but these episodes have occurred 6–7 times now and he has become more lethargic. Finally, he had a bloody bowel movement, so they decided to bring him in to the office. On exam, he is afebrile, lethargic but arousable, and well-hydrated. His abdomen appears benign. What is your leading diagnosis?

A) Cholecystitis.
B) Gastroenteritis.
C) Intussusception.
D) Volvulus.

See p. 448.

136. Which of the following lesions is considered premalignant on colonoscopy?

A) Sessile polyp.
B) Hyperplastic polyp.
C) Tubular adenoma.
D) Pedunculated polyp.

See p. 262.

137. Which of these drugs is indicated for control of an acute flare of Crohn disease?

A) Any 5-ASA moiety.
B) Oral prednisone.
C) Sulfasalazine.
D) Thalidomide.

See p. 265.

138. HPV vaccine is indicated for all of the following EXCEPT:

A) 24-year-old female with cervical dysplasia.
B) 9-year-old female who has never been sexually active.
C) 18-year-old female with known HPV.
D) Immunosuppressed 15-year-old female who is HIV positive.

See p. 489.

139. Sensitivity is best defined as

A) True positives/(true positives + false negatives).
B) True positives.
C) True positives/(true positives + true negatives).
D) True positives/(true positives + false positives).

See p. 863.

140. Which of the following foods does NOT contain gluten?

A) Oats.
B) Rye.
C) Rice.
D) Sticky rice.

See p. 269.

141. Which of the following is recommended for treating *Giardia*?

A) Metronidazole.
B) Vancomycin.
C) Ciprofloxacin.
D) Azithromycin.

See p. 543.

142. A patient comes to the ED after sustaining a needle stick. She is a nurse who had just finished drawing blood for culture on a patient with AIDS, and somehow she stuck herself through her glove. She bled a little. She washed the area copiously. What is the most appropriate next step?

A) Prescribe zidovudine and lamivudine for 4 weeks.
B) Prescribe zidovudine for 2 weeks.
C) Reassure the patient as her risk of contracting HIV is negligible.
D) Test her for HIV and treat based on the results.

See p. 330.

143. A 19-year-old college student presents to the ED with complaints of fever, headache, myalgias, and confusion. She has had a splenectomy but is otherwise healthy. The exam is notable for somnolence, fever, and nuchal rigidity. Because of her inability to follow directions, the neurologic exam is difficult to complete, but it appears to be nonfocal. There are several other seriously ill patients in the ED to triage. Which of the following interventions should not wait an hour and must be done now?

A) Administer ceftriaxone, vancomycin, dexamethasone.
B) Consult a neurosurgeon.
C) Perform lumbar puncture.
D) Obtain blood cultures.
E) Order CT of the brain.

See p. 299.

144. The patient is enrolled in hospice, and 3 months later you are called by the nursing home because of an acute condition change. When you see the patient, he is unresponsive, with labored breathing and mottled feet. All of the following can be signs of impending death EXCEPT:

A) Cheyne-Stokes breathing.
B) Fever.
C) Cyanosis and mottling.
D) Increased urine output.
E) Talking to someone who is already dead.

See p. 858.

145. As you start a patient on fluoxetine for depression, you counsel him about the adverse effects of this class of medications. All of the following are common adverse effects of SSRIs EXCEPT:

A) Anxiety.
B) Diarrhea.
C) Headaches.
D) Hypersexuality.
E) Insomnia.

See p. 778.

146. During a visit for a physical exam, you note that this 33-year-old female has checked "depression" on her health screening questionnaire. You ask her more about this and find that she has felt that her mood has been depressed for ≥15 years. She generally feels fatigued and has low self-esteem, but she denies suicidal ideation and feelings of guilt and worthlessness. What diagnosis best characterizes her symptoms?

A) Avoidant personality disorder.
B) Borderline personality disorder.
C) Dysthymia.
D) Major depressive disorder.

See p. 767.

147. Which of the following symptoms would LEAST likely result from a panic attack and therefore would prompt further investigation in a patient with known panic disorder?

A) Chest pain.
B) Dyspnea.
C) Palpitations.
D) Syncope.

See p. 772.

148. A 23-year-old male presents with symptoms suggestive of panic attacks, an underlying anxiety disorder, and possibly panic disorder. You refer him for counseling services and recommend starting a medication. Which of the following drugs is the LEAST effective treatment for panic disorder?

A) Bupropion.
B) Nortriptyline.
C) Sertraline.
D) Venlafaxine.

See p. 773.

149. Which case is typically cited as a legal precedent for withdrawing a medical intervention that results in death from the underlying disease?

A) Cruzan.
B) Tarasoff.
C) M'Naghten.
D) Quinlan.

See p. 839.

150. You are watching a really bad grade B movie. Who do you think will win?

A) Mothra.
B) King Ghidora.
C) Biollante.
D) Godzilla.
E) Mechagodzilla.

Never bet against Godzilla

Answers

1. *Answer: A.*
2. *Answer: B.*
3. *Answer: B.*
4. *Answer: A.*
5. *Answer: A.*
6. *Answer: C.*
7. *Answer: D.*
8. *Answer: B.*
9. *Answer: D.*
10. *Answer: C.*
11. *Answer: B.*
12. *Answer: D.*
13. *Answer: A.*
14. *Answer: B.*
15. *Answer: B.*
16. *Answer: C.*
17. *Answer: D.*
18. *Answer: C.*
19. *Answer: C.*
20. *Answer: A.*
21. *Answer: B.*
22. *Answer: D.*
23. *Answer: B.*
24. *Answer: C.*
25. *Answer: D.*
26. *Answer: C.*
27. *Answer: D.*
28. *Answer: C.*
29. *Answer: B.*
30. *Answer: D.*
31. *Answer: B.*
32. *Answer: D.*
33. *Answer: C.*
34. *Answer: D.*
35. *Answer: B.*
36. *Answer: B.*
37. *Answer: A.*
38. *Answer: D.*
39. *Answer: B.*
40. *Answer: D.*
41. *Answer: B.*
42. *Answer: B.*
43. *Answer: D.*
44. *Answer: D.*
45. *Answer: C.*
46. *Answer: E.*
47. *Answer: D.*
48. *Answer: C.*
49. *Answer: E.*
50. *Answer: C.*
51. *Answer: B.*
52. *Answer: A.*
53. *Answer: C.*
54. *Answer: B.*
55. *Answer: C.*
56. *Answer: B.*
57. *Answer: B.*
58. *Answer: D.*
59. *Answer: A.*
60. *Answer: B.*
61. *Answer: B.*
62. *Answer: E.*
63. *Answer: E.*
64. *Answer: E.*
65. *Answer: D.*
66. *Answer: E.*
67. *Answer: D.*
68. *Answer: B.*
69. *Answer: B.*
70. *Answer: A.*
71. *Answer: D.*
72. *Answer: B.*
73. *Answer: C.*
74. *Answer: D.*
75. *Answer: C.*
76. *Answer: B.*
77. *Answer: D.*
78. *Answer: D.*
79. *Answer: D.*
80. *Answer: B.*
81. *Answer: A.*
82. *Answer: B.*
83. *Answer: D.*
84. *Answer: A.*
85. *Answer: B.*
86. *Answer: B.*
87. *Answer: C.*
88. *Answer: D.*
89. *Answer: A.*
90. *Answer: C.*
91. *Answer: D.*
92. *Answer: C.*
93. *Answer: C.*
94. *Answer: A.*
95. *Answer: B.*
96. *Answer: B.*
97. *Answer: C.*
98. *Answer: D.*
99. *Answer: A.*
100. *Answer: B.*
101. *Answer: A.*
102. *Answer: B.*
103. *Answer: D.*
104. *Answer: A.*
105. *Answer: B.*
106. *Answer: C.*
107. *Answer: A.*
108. *Answer: B.*
109. *Answer: A.*
110. *Answer: C.*
111. *Answer: B.*
112. *Answer: C.*
113. *Answer: C.*
114. *Answer: B.*
115. *Answer: C.*
116. *Answer: A.*
117. *Answer: C.*
118. *Answer: A.*
119. *Answer: C.*
120. *Answer: B.*
121. *Answer: A.*
122. *Answer: B.*
123. *Answer: D.*
124. *Answer: A.*
125. *Answer: C.*
126. *Answer: A.*
127. *Answer: A.*
128. *Answer: D.*
129. *Answer: B.*
130. *Answer: C.*
131. *Answer: B.*
132. *Answer: A.*
133. *Answer: A.*
134. *Answer: C.*
135. *Answer: C.*
136. *Answer: C.*
137. *Answer: B.*
138. *Answer: B.*
139. *Answer: A.*
140. *Answer: C.*
141. *Answer: A.*
142. *Answer: A.*
143. *Answer: A.*
144. *Answer: D.*
145. *Answer: D.*
146. *Answer: C.*
147. *Answer: D.*
148. *Answer: A.*
149. *Answer: D.*
150. *Answer: D.*

Index

Page numbers followed by *f* or *t* indicate figures or tables, respectively.